Aulton's Pharmaceutics

The Design and Manufacture of Medicines

Edited by

Michael E. Aulton BPharm PhD FAAPS FRPharmS

THIRD EDITION

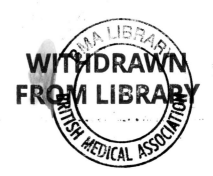
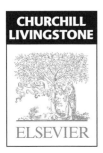

CHURCHILL LIVINGSTONE

ELSEVIER

EDINBURGH   LONDON   NEW YORK   OXFORD   PHILADELPHIA   ST LOUIS   SYDNEY   TORONTO   2007

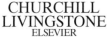

CHURCHILL
LIVINGSTONE
ELSEVIER

An imprint of Elsevier Limited

© Harcourt Publishers Limited 2001
© 2007, Elsevier Limited. All rights reserved.

The right of Michael E. Aulton to be identified as editor of this work has been asserted by him in accordance with the Copyright, Designs and Patents Act 1988

No part of this publication may be reproduced, stored in a retrieval system, or transmitted in any form or by any means, electronic, mechanical, photocopying, recording or otherwise, without the prior permission of the Publishers. Permissions may be sought directly from Elsevier's Health Sciences Rights Department, 1600 John F. Kennedy Boulevard, Suite 1800, Philadelphia, PA 19103-2899, USA: phone: (+1) 215 239 3804; fax: (+1) 215 239 3805; e-mail: healthpermissions@elsevier.com. You may also complete your request on-line via the Elsevier homepage (www.elsevier.com), by selecting 'Support and Contact' and then 'Copyright and Permission'.

First edition 1988
Second edition 2002
Third edition 2007

ISBN-13: 9780443101083

International Edition ISBN-13: 9780443101076

British Library Cataloguing in Publication Data
A catalogue record for this book is available from the British Library

Library of Congress Cataloging in Publication Data
A catalog record for this book is available from the Library of Congress

Note
Knowledge and best practice in this field are constantly changing. As new research and experience broaden our knowledge, changes in practice, treatment and drug therapy may become necessary or appropriate. Readers are advised to check the most current information provided (i) on procedures featured or (ii) by the manufacturer of each product to be administered, to verify the recommended dose or formula, the method and duration of administration, and contraindications. It is the responsibility of the practitioner, relying on their own experience and knowledge of the patient, to make diagnoses, to determine dosages and the best treatment for each individual patient, and to take all appropriate safety precautions. To the fullest extent of the law, neither the Publisher nor the Editor assumes any liability for any injury and/or damage to persons or property arising out or related to any use of the material contained in this book.

The Publisher

ELSEVIER your source for books, journals and multimedia in the health sciences
www.elsevierhealth.com

Working together to grow
libraries in developing countries

www.elsevier.com | www.bookaid.org | www.sabre.org

ELSEVIER   BOOK AID International   Sabre Foundation

Printed in Hungary

The Publisher's policy is to use **paper manufactured from sustainable forests**

Preface

This is the third edition of *Pharmaceutics;* the first edition was published in 1988 and the second in 2002. The pedigree of the book is actually much older than that. It was originally known as *Tutorial Pharmacy* and edited by John Cooper and Colin Gunn and later by Sidney Carter.

The philosophy of this third edition remains unchanged, i.e. it is designed and written intentionally for newcomers to the design of dosage forms – other expert texts can take you into much more detail in each of the subject areas considered here once you have mastered these basics. The subject matter of the book remains in essence the same but the detail has been changed significantly because pharmaceutics has changed. Since the last edition there have been changes in the way dosage forms are designed and drugs are delivered. These developments are reflected in this new edition.

The structure and the content of this edition have changed to reflect modern thinking and current university curricula throughout the world. More importantly, every chapter has received attention and has been updated appropriately. Some of the basic science remains virtually unchanged – and will always remain so – but other areas, particularly biopharmaceutics, some areas of drug delivery and our understanding of the significance of the solid state, have changed enormously in recent years. The current and future use of biotechnology products has also been reflected in this new edition.

Several completely new chapters have been included to widen the comprehensive nature of this text. Two new chapters discuss the principles and practice of sterilization as they pertain to the design and manufacture of dosage forms. A chapter has been included on the important area of wound dressings. The section on product stability and the stability testing of medicinal products has been completely rewritten and expanded to include more of the relevant chemistry. All of these are written by experts who are new authors to the book.

The involvement of a wide range of authors continues in this edition, each an accepted expert in the field on which they have written and, just as importantly, each has experience and ability in imparting that information to undergraduate pharmacy and pharmaceutical science students and those practitioners in the pharmaceutical and associated industries that are new to the subject. Many authors from the previous edition remain as they are still world leaders in their field. Other chapters have been written by a new generation of experts. The new authorship reflects modern knowledge and thinking in pharmaceutics.

I wish you well in your studies if you are an undergraduate or with your career if you are working in industry or the hospital service. I sincerely hope that this book helps you with your understanding of pharmaceutics – the design and manufacture of medicines.

M.E.A.   Leicester

Acknowledgements

The Editor wishes to take this opportunity to thank the following who have assisted with the preparation of this text.

The contributors – for the work, time and quality that they have put into their texts, always under pressure from numerous other commitments, and also from me. Modern life has few spare moments and so the time that they spent in contributing so knowledgeably and professionally to this text is warmly appreciated.

The many secretaries and artists – who assisted the authors in the preparation of their work.

My wife Christine – for typing and other secretarial assistance, and help in a million other ways which enabled me to spend time on this edition of the book.

Ellen Green and Janice Urquhart of Elsevier – for their special expertise and assistance in the commissioning and preparation of this third edition. Ellen has recently retired from Elsevier so I wish her every happiness for the future.

The many academic and industrial pharmaceutical scientists – who helped during the design of the contents and organization of this edition to ensure that it corresponds as closely as possible with modern practice and with the curricula of current pharmacy and pharmaceutical science courses internationally.

Those publishing companies – who have given their permission to reproduce material in this edition.

Mike Aulton

Contributors

Göran Alderborn MSci PhD
Professor in Pharmaceutical Technology, Department of Pharmacy, Uppsala University, Uppsala, Sweden

Marianne Ashford BSc PhD MRPharmS
Project Manager, Pharmaceutical & Analytical Research & Development Department, AstraZeneca, Macclesfield, UK

David Attwood BPharm PhD DSc CChem FRSC
Professor of Pharmacy, School of Pharmacy and Pharmaceutical Sciences, University of Manchester, Manchester, UK

Michael E. Aulton BPharm PhD FAAPS FRPharmS
Emeritus Professor, School of Pharmacy, De Montfort University, Leicester, UK, and Scientific Advisor, Molecular Profiles, Nottingham, UK

Andrew R. Barnes PhD MRPharmS CChem FRSC
Quality Assurance Manager, UHB Medicines, University Hospital Birmingham, Birmingham, UK

Brian W. Barry BSc PhD DSc FRPharmS CChem FRSC
Emeritus Professor, School of Pharmacy, Bradford University, Bradford, UK

Michael R. Billany BSc MRPharmS
Principal Lecturer in Formulation Science, Leicester School of Pharmacy, De Montfort University, Leicester, UK

Graham Buckton BPharm PhD DSc FRPharmS FRSC
Professor of Pharmaceutics, School of Pharmacy, University of London, London, UK

John H. Collett PhD DSc FRPharmS
Professor of Pharmaceutics, University of Manchester, Manchester, UK

Daan J. A. Crommelin PhD
Scientific Director, Dutch Top Institute Pharma, Leiden and Utrecht Institute for Pharmaceutical Sciences, UIPS, Utrecht University, The Netherlands

Gillian M. Eccleston BSc PhD CChem FRCS FRPharmS
Professor of Pharmaceutics, Department of Pharmaceutical Science, University of Strathclyde, Glasgow, UK

John T. Fell BSc PhD
Honorary Reader, School of Pharmacy and Pharmaceutical Sciences, University of Manchester, Manchester, UK

Josephine Ferdinando PhD
Senior Vice President, Global Pharmaceutical Sciences Shire R&D, Basingstoke, UK

Geoffrey W. Hanlon BSc PhD MRPharmS
Professor of Pharmaceutical Microbiology, School of Pharmacy and Biomolecular Sciences, University of Brighton, UK

Norman A. Hodges BPharm MRPharmS PhD
Principal Lecturer in Pharmaceutical Microbiology, School of Pharmacy and Biomolecular Sciences, University of Brighton, Brighton, UK

Keith G. Hutchison BSc(Pharm) PhD
Vice President, Research and Development, Capsugel Division of Pfizer, Bornem, Belgium

Brian E. Jones BPharm MPharm FRPharmS
Scientific Advisor, Qualicaps Europe SA, Alcobendas (Madrid), Spain, and Honorary Lecturer, Department of Drug Delivery, Welsh School of Pharmacy, Cardiff University, Cardiff, UK

Jean-Yves Maillard BSc PhD
Senior Lecturer in Pharmaceutical Microbiology, Welsh School of Pharmacy, Cardiff University, Cardiff, UK

Christopher Marriott PhD DSc FRPharmS CChem FRSC
Emeritus Professor of Pharmaceutics, Department of Pharmacy, King's College, London, UK

Albert Mekking BSc MSc
Manager, Clinical Production, OctoPlus BV, Leiden, The Netherlands

R. Christian Moreton BPharm MSc PhD MRPharmS MInstPkg(Dip)
Vice President, Pharmaceutical Sciences, Idenix Pharmaceuticals, Cambridge, MA, USA

Stuart C. Porter PhD BPharm MRPharmS
President, PPT Pharma Services, Hatfield, Pennsylvania, USA

W. John Pugh BPharm PhD MRPharmS
Lecturer in Physical Pharmacy, Welsh School of
Pharmacy, Cardiff University, Cardiff, UK

John N. Staniforth BSc PhD
Honorary Visiting Professor, Department of Pharmacy
and Pharmacology, University of Bath, Bath, UK

Malcolm P. Summers BSc(Pharm) PhD CChem MRSC
MRPharmS
Director, European Regulatory Affairs, Kendle
International, Ely, UK

Kevin M. G. Taylor BPharm PhD MRPharmS
Professor of Clinical Pharmaceutics, School of
Pharmacy, University of London and University College
London Hospitals, London, UK

Peter M. Taylor BSc PhD
Principal Lecturer in Pharmaceutics, Leicester School
of Pharmacy, De Montfort University, Leicester, UK

Josef J. Tukker PhD
Manager, Pharmedia, Houten and Pharmacy Manager,
GE Healthcare
The Netherlands

Andrew M. Twitchell BSc(Pharm) PhD MRPharmS
Compounding Manager, Nova Laboratories,
Leicester, UK

Susannah E. Walsh BSc PhD MBA
Senior Lecturer in Microbiology, Leicester School of
Pharmacy, De Montfort University, Leicester, UK

Ewoud van Winden PhD
Director, Regulon SA, Athens, Greece

James I. Wells
BSc(Pharm) MSc PhD MRPharmS MInstPkg
Pharmaceutical Consultant

Peter York
BSc(Pharm) DSc PhD FRPharmS CChem FRSC
Professor of Physical Pharmaceutics, Institute of
Pharmaceutical Innovation, University of Bradford,
Bradford, UK

Contents

ix

CONTENTS

x

What is 'pharmaceutics'?

One of the earliest impressions that many new pharmacy and pharmaceutical science students have of their chosen subject is the large number of long and sometimes unusual-sounding names that are used to describe the various subject areas within pharmacy and the pharmaceutical sciences. The aim of this section is to explain to the reader what is meant by just one of them – *pharmaceutics*. I will describe how the term has been interpreted for the purpose of this book and how pharmaceutics fits into the overall scheme of pharmaceutical science and the process of designing a new medicine. I will also lead the reader through the organization of this book and explain the reasons why an understanding of the material contained in its chapters is important in the design of modern drug delivery systems.

The word 'pharmaceutics' is used in pharmacy and pharmaceutical science to encompass many subject areas that are all associated with the steps to which a drug is subjected towards the end of its development, i.e. it is the stages that follow the discovery or synthesis or the drug, its isolation and purification, and testing for advantageous pharmacological effects and absence of serious toxicological problems. Put at its simplest – *pharmaceutics converts a drug into a medicine*.

Just a comment here about the word 'drug'. This is the pharmacologically active ingredient in a medicine. 'Drug' is the correct word but because it is often confused by the general public with the common term for a substance of misuse, alternatives are used increasingly, such as 'medicinal agent', 'active ingredient' or 'active pharmaceutical ingredient (API)'. I still use the simpler, and still correct, word 'drug' here. To me, phrases like 'active ingredient' suggest that the other ingredients of a dosage form have no activity or function. This book will teach you loud and clear that this is not the case.

Pharmaceutics, and therefore this book, is concerned with the scientific and technological aspects of the design and manufacture of dosage forms. Arguably, it is the most diverse of all the subject areas in pharmaceutical science and encompasses:

- an understanding of the basic physical chemistry necessary for the efficient design of dosage forms (physical pharmaceutics)
- an understanding of relevant body systems and how drugs arrive there following administration (biopharmaceutics)
- the design and formulation of medicines (dosage form design)
- the manufacture of these medicines on both a small (compounding) and large (pharmaceutical technology) scale and
- the avoidance and elimination of microorganisms in medicines (pharmaceutical microbiology).

Medicines are drug delivery systems. That is, they are means of administering drugs to the body in a safe, efficient, reproducible and convenient manner. The introductory chapter to the book discusses the overall considerations that must be made so that the conversion of drug to medicine can take place. It emphasizes the fact that medicines are very rarely drugs alone but require additives to make them into dosage forms and this in turn introduces the concept of formulation. The chapter explains that there are three major considerations in the design of dosage forms:

1. the physicochemical properties of the drug itself
2. biopharmaceutical considerations, such as how the administration route of a dosage form affects the rate and extent of drug absorption into the body, and
3. therapeutic considerations of the disease state to be treated, which in turn decide the most suitable type of dosage form, possible routes of administration and the most suitable duration of action and dose frequency for the drug in question.

This first chapter provides an excellent introduction to the subject matter of this book and clearly justifies the need for the formulation scientist and pharmacist to understand the science contained in this text. New readers are encouraged to read this chapter first, thoroughly and carefully, so that they can grasp the basics of the subject before delving into the more detailed information that follows.

The book is then divided into various Parts that group the chapters into related subject areas. Part 1 collects some of the more important physicochemical knowledge required to design and prepare dosage forms. The chapters have been designed to give the reader an insight into those scientific and physicochemical principles that are important to the formulation scientist. They are not intended as a substitute for a thorough understanding of physical chemistry and many specific, more detailed, texts are available with this information.

For many reasons, which are discussed in the book, the vast majority of dosage forms are administered orally in the form of solid products such as tablets and capsules. This means that one of the most important stages in drug administration is the dissolution of solid particles to form a solution in the gastrointestinal tract. The formulation scientist thus needs knowledge of both liquid and solid materials, in particular the properties of drugs in solution and the factors influencing their dissolution from solid particles. Once solutions are formed, the formulation scientist must understand the properties of these solutions. The reader will see later in the book how drug release from the dosage form and absorption of the drug by the body are strongly dependent on the properties of the drug in solution, such as degree of dissociation and speed of diffusion of the drug molecules. Knowledge of the flow properties of liquids is useful in solving certain problems relating to the manufacture and performance of solutions and semi-solids as dosage forms in their own right.

The properties of interfaces are described next. These are important to an understanding of adsorption onto solid surfaces as involved in the dissolution of solid particles and the study of disperse systems such as colloids, suspensions and emulsions. The scientific background to the systems mentioned is also discussed.

Part 2 collects together those aspects of pharmaceutics associated with powdered materials. By far the majority of drugs are solid (mainly crystalline) powders and, unfortunately, most of these have numerous adverse characteristics that must be overcome during the design of medicines to enable their satisfactory manufacture and subsequent performance in dosage forms.

The book therefore explains the concept of the solid state and how the internal and surface properties of solids are important and need to be characterized. This is followed by an explanation of the more macroscopic properties of powders that influence their performance during the design and manufacture of dosage forms – particle size and its measurement, size reduction and size separation of powders from those of other sizes. There follows an explanation of the many problems associated with the mixing and flow of powders. In high-speed tablet and capsule production, for example, powders must contain a satisfactory mix of all the ingredients in order to achieve uniformity of dosage in each dosage form, and fast and uniform powder flow in high-speed tableting and encapsulation machines. For convenience, the mixing of liquids and semi-solids is also discussed here as the basic theory is the same.

Another extremely important area that must be understood before a satisfactory dosage form can be designed and manufactured is the microbiological aspects of medicines development and production. It is necessary to eliminate microorganisms from the product both before and during manufacture. Microbiology is a very wide-ranging subject. This book concentrates only on those aspects of microbiology that are directly relevant to the design, production and distribution of dosage forms. This mainly involves avoiding (asepsis) and eliminating (sterilization) their presence (contamination) in medicines, and preventing the growth of any microorganism which might enter the product during storage and use of the medicine (preservation). Techniques for testing that these intentions have been achieved are also described. The principles and practice of sterilization are discussed also. The relevant parts of pharmaceutical microbiology and sterilization are considered in Part 3.

It is not possible to begin to design a satisfactory dosage form without an understanding of how drugs are absorbed into the body, the various routes that can be used for this purpose and the fate of the drugs once they enter the body and reach their site(s) of action.

The terms 'bioavailability' and 'biopharmaceutics' are defined and explained in Part 4. The factors influencing the bioavailability of a drug and methods of its assessment are described. This is followed by a consideration of the manner in which the frequency of drug administration and the rate at which it is released affect its concentration in the blood plasma at any given time. This book concentrates on the preparation, administration, release and absorption of drugs but stops short at the cellular level and leaves to other texts the detail of how drugs enter individual cells, how they act, how they are metabolized and eliminated.

Having gathered this understanding of the basics of pharmaceutics, the formulation scientist should now be equipped to begin a consideration of the design and manufacture of the most suitable dosage forms for the drug in question.

The first stage of this process is known as preformulation. This, as the name implies, is a consideration of the steps that need to be performed before formulation proper can begin. Preformulation involves a full understanding of the physicochemical properties of drug molecules and excipients and how they interact in dosage forms. An early grasp of this knowledge is of great use to the formulation scientist as the data gathered will strongly influence the design of the future dosage form. Results of tests carried out at this stage of development can give a much clearer indication of the possible (and indeed impossible) dosage forms for a new drug candidate.

The chapters collected together in Part 5 cover the formulation of, the rate and extent of drug release from, advantages and disadvantages of, and large-scale manufacture of the many dosage forms. Dosage forms suitable for the administration of drugs through almost every possible body orifice and external surface are discussed, as well as a consideration of novel and future drug delivery systems that will be necessary for tomorrow's biotechnology products.

The pack and any possible interactions between it and the drug or medicine it contains are so vitally linked that the pack must not be considered as an afterthought. Packaging considerations should be uppermost in the minds of the formulators as soon as they receive the drug powder on which to work. The technology of packaging and filling of products is also discussed.

At this point we consider further the possible routes of microbiological contamination of medicines and the ways in which this can be prevented or minimized and how the presence of preservatives in the medicine can minimize its consequences.

Before finalizing on the formulation and packaging of the dosage form there must be a clear understanding of the stability of drug(s) and other additives in the formulation with respect to the reasons why and the rates at which they degrade. There must be an awareness of the means of inhibiting decomposition and increasing the shelf life of a product. These points are discussed.

The book ends at the 'hard end' of manufacturing, and includes a discussion of the design of manufacturing facilities, manufacturing construction materials and the use of steam (it is still used!).

At this point the pharmaceutical technologist passes the product on to another aspect of pharmacy – the interface with the patient, i.e. dispensing and pharmacy practice. These disciplines are dealt with in the companion volume *Pharmaceutical Practice*, 3rd edition (2003), eds A J Winfield and R M E Richards (Elsevier/Churchill Livingstone).

Design of dosage forms

P. York

PRINCIPLES OF DOSAGE FORM DESIGN

Drugs are rarely administered as pure chemical substances alone and are almost always given as formulated preparations or medicines. These can vary from relatively simple solutions to complex drug delivery systems through the use of appropriate additives or excipients in the formulations. The excipients provide varied and specialized pharmaceutical functions. It is the formulation additives that, amongst other things, solubilize, suspend, thicken, preserve, emulsify, modify dissolution, improve the compactability and flavour drug substances to form various medicines or dosage forms.

The principal objective of dosage form design is to achieve a predictable therapeutic response to a drug included in a formulation which is capable of large-scale manufacture with reproducible product quality. To ensure product quality, numerous features are required: chemical and physical stability, with suitable preservation against microbial contamination if appropriate, uniformity of dose of drug, acceptability to users, including both prescriber and patient, as well as suitable packaging and labelling. Ideally, dosage forms should also be independent of patient-to-patient variation, although in practice, this feature remains difficult to achieve. However, recent developments which rely on the specific metabolic activity of individual patients or implants that respond, for example, to externally applied sound or magnetic fields to trigger a drug delivery function are beginning to accommodate this requirement.

Consideration should be given to differences in bioavailability between apparently similar formulations and possible causative reasons. In recent years, increasing attention has therefore been directed towards eliminating variation in bioavailability characteristics, particularly for medicinal products containing an equivalent dose of a drug substance, as it is recognized that formulation factors can influence their therapeutic performance. To optimize the bioavailability of drug substances, it is often necessary to carefully select the most appropriate chemical form of the drug. For example, such selection should address solubility requirements, drug particle size and physical form and consider appropriate additives and manufacturing aids coupled to selecting the most appropriate administration route(s) and dosage form(s). Additionally, suitable manufacturing processes and packaging are required.

There are numerous dosage forms into which a drug substance can be incorporated for the convenient and efficacious treatment of a disease. Dosage forms can be designed for administration by alternative delivery routes to maximize therapeutic response. Preparations can be taken orally or injected, as well as being applied to the skin or inhaled, and Table 1.1 lists the range of dosage forms which can be used to deliver drugs by the various administration routes. However, it is necessary to relate the drug substance to the clinical indication being treated before the correct combination of drug and dosage form can be made since each disease or illness often requires a specific type of drug therapy. In addition, factors governing choice of administration route and the specific requirements of that route which affect drug absorption need to be taken into account when designing dosage forms.

Many drugs are formulated into several dosage forms of varying strengths, each having selected pharmaceutical characteristics which are suitable for a specific application. One such drug is the glucocorticoid prednisolone used in the suppression of inflammatory and allergic disorders. Through the use of different chemical forms and formulation additives, a range of effective antiinflammatory preparations is available, including tablet, enteric-coated tablet, injections, eye drops and enema. The extremely low aqueous solubility of the base prednisolone and acetate salt makes these forms useful in tablet and slowly absorbed intramuscular suspension injection forms, whilst the soluble sodium phosphate salt enables a soluble tablet form and solutions for eye and ear drops, enema and intravenous injection to be prepared. The analgesic paracetamol is also available in a range of dosage forms and strengths to meet the specific needs of the user, including tablets, dispersible tablets, paediatric soluble tablets, paediatric oral solution, sugar-free oral solution, oral suspension, double-strength oral suspension and suppositories.

In addition, whilst many new drugs based on low molecular weight organic compounds continue to be discovered and transformed into medicinal products, the development of drugs from biotechnology is ever increasing. Such active compounds are macromolecular and of relatively large molecular weight, and these include materials such as peptides, proteins and viral components. These drug substances present different challenges in their formulation and processing into medicines due to their alternative biological, chemical and structural properties. Nevertheless, the underlying principles of dosage form design remain applicable. At present, these therapeutic agents are principally formulated into parenteral and respiratory dosage forms. Delivery of these biotechnologically based drug substances via these routes of administration imposes additional constraints upon the selection of appropriate formulation excipients.

It is therefore apparent that before a drug substance can be successfully formulated into a dosage form, many factors must be considered. These can be broadly grouped into three categories:

1. biopharmaceutical considerations, including factors affecting the absorption of the drug substance from different administration routes
2. drug factors, such as the physical and chemical properties of the drug substance
3. therapeutic considerations, including consideration of the clinical indication to be treated and patient factors.

Table 1.1 Dosage forms available for different administration routes

Administration route	Dosage forms
Oral	Solutions, syrups, suspensions, emulsions, gels, powders, granules, capsules, tablets
Rectal	Suppositories, ointments, creams, powders, solutions
Topical	Ointments, creams, pastes, lotions, gels, solutions, topical aerosols, transdermal patches
Parenteral	Injections (solution, suspension, emulsion forms), implants, irrigation and dialysis solutions
Respiratory	Aerosols (solution, suspension, emulsion, powder forms), inhalations, sprays, gases
Nasal	Solutions, inhalations
Eye	Solutions, ointments, creams
Ear	Solutions, suspensions, ointments, creams

High-quality and efficacious medicines will be formulated and prepared only when all these factors are considered and related to each other. This is the underlying principle of dosage form design.

BIOPHARMACEUTICAL ASPECTS OF DOSAGE FORM DESIGN

Biopharmaceutics can be regarded as the study of the relationship between the physical, chemical and biological sciences applied to drugs, dosage forms and drug action. Clearly, understanding the principles of this subject is important in dosage form design, particularly with regard to drug absorption, as well as drug distribution, metabolism and excretion. In general, a drug substance must be in solution form before it can be absorbed via absorbing membranes and epithelia of the skin, gastrointestinal tract and lungs into body fluids. Drugs are absorbed in two general ways: by passive diffusion and by specialized transport mechanisms. In passive diffusion, which is thought to control the absorption of must drugs, the process is driven by the concentration gradient existing across the cellular barrier, with drug molecules passing from regions of high to low concentration. Lipid solubility and degree of ionization of the drug at the absorbing site influence the rate of diffusion. Several specialized transport mechanisms are postulated, including active and facilitated transport. Once absorbed, the drug can exert a therapeutic effect either locally or at a site of action remote from the site of administration. In the latter case, the drug has to be transported in body fluids (as shown in Fig. 1.1).

When the dosage form is designed to deliver drugs via the buccal, respiratory, rectal, intramuscular or subcutaneous routes, the drug passes directly into the circulation blood from absorbing tissues, whilst the intravenous route provides the most direct route of all. When delivered by the oral route, onset of drug action will be delayed because of required transit time in the gastrointestinal tract, the absorption process and hepatoenteric blood circulation features. The physical form of the oral dosage form will also influence absorption rate and onset of action, with solutions acting faster than suspensions, which in turn generally act faster than capsules and

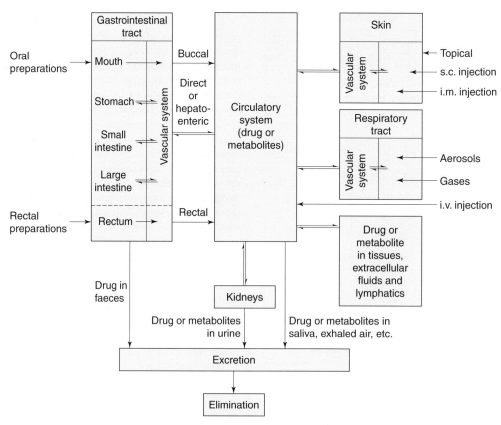

Fig. 1.1 Pathways a drug may take following the administration of a dosage form by different routes.

tablets. Dosage forms can thus be listed in order of time of onset of therapeutic effect (see Table 1.2). However, all drugs irrespective of their delivery route remain foreign substances to the human body and distribution, metabolic and elimination processes commence immediately following drug absorption until eliminated from the body via the urine, faeces, saliva, skin or lungs in unchanged or metabolized form.

Routes of drug administration

The absorption pattern of drugs varies considerably between individual drug substances as well as between the different administration routes. Dosage forms are designed to provide the drug in a suitable form for absorption from each selected route of administration. The following discussion considers briefly the routes of drug administration and whilst dosage forms are mentioned, this is intended only as an introduction since they will be dealt with in greater detail later in this book.

Oral route

The oral route is the most frequently used route for drug administration. Oral dosage forms are intended usually for systemic effects resulting from drug absorption through the various epithelia and mucosa of the gastrointestinal tract. A few drugs, however, are intended to dissolve in the mouth for rapid absorption or for local effect in the tract due to poor absorption by this route or low aqueous solubility. Compared with other routes, the oral route is the simplest, most convenient and safest means of drug administration. However, disadvantages include relatively slow onset of action, possibilities of irregular absorption and destruction of certain drugs by the enzymes and secretions of the gastrointestinal tract. For example, insulin-containing preparations are inactivated by the action of stomach fluids.

Whilst drug absorption from the gastrointestinal tract follows the general principles described later in this book, several specific features should be emphasized. Changes in drug solubility can result from reactions with other materials present in the gastrointestinal tract, as for example the interference of absorption of tetracyclines through the formation of insoluble complexes with calcium, which can be available from foodstuffs or formulation additives. Gastric emptying time is an important factor for effective drug absorption from the intestine. Slow gastric emptying can be detrimental to drugs inactivated by the gastric juices and can delay absorption of drugs more effectively absorbed from the intestine. In addition, since environmental pH can influence the ionization and lipid solubility of drugs, the pH change occurring along the gastrointestinal tract, from a pH of about 1 in the stomach to approximately 7 or 8 in the large intestine, is important to both degree and site of drug absorption. Since membranes are more permeable to unionized rather than ionized forms and since most drugs are weak acids or bases, it can be shown that weak acids, being largely unionized, are well absorbed from the stomach. In the small intestine (pH about 6.5), with its extremely large absorbing surface, both weak acids and weak bases are well absorbed.

The most popular oral dosage forms are tablets, capsules, suspensions, solutions and emulsions. Tablets are prepared by compaction and contain drugs and formulation additives which are included for specific functions, such as disintegrants which promote tablet break-up into granules and powder particles in the gastrointestinal tract, facilitating drug dissolution and absorption. Tablets are often coated, either to provide a protective barrier to environmental factors for drug stability purposes or to mask unpleasant drug taste, as well as to protect drugs from the acid conditions of the stomach (enteric coating). Increasing use is being made of modified-release tablet products such as fast-dissolving systems and controlled, delayed or sustained-release formulations. Benefits of controlled-release tablet formulations, achieved for example by the use of polymeric-based tablet cores or coating membranes, include reduced frequency of drug-related side-effects and maintaining steady drug-plasma levels for extended periods, important when medications are delivered for chronic conditions or where constant levels are required to achieve optimal efficacy, as in treating angina and hypertension.

Capsules are solid dosage forms containing drug and, usually, appropriate filler(s), enclosed in a hard or soft

Table 1.2 Variation in time of onset of action for different dosage forms	
Time of onset of action	**Dosage forms**
Seconds	i.v. injections
Minutes	i.m. and s.c. injections, buccal tablets, aerosols, gases
Minutes to hours	Short-term depot injections, solutions, suspensions, powders, granules, capsules, tablets, modified-release tablets
Several hours	Enteric-coated formulations
Days to weeks	Depot injections, implants
Varies	Topical preparations

shell composed of gelatin. As with tablets, uniformity of dose can be readily achieved and various sizes, shapes and colours of shell are commercially available. The gelatin shell readily ruptures and dissolves following oral administration and in most cases drugs are released from capsules faster than from tablets. Recently, renewed interest has been shown in filling semi-solid and microemulsion formulations into hard gelatin capsules to provide rapidly dispersing dosage forms for poorly soluble drugs.

Suspensions, which contain finely divided drugs suspended in a suitable vehicle, are a useful means of administering large amounts of drugs that would be inconvenient if taken in tablet or capsule form. They are also useful for patients who experience difficulty in swallowing tablets and capsules and for paediatric use. Whilst dissolution of drugs is required prior to absorption, fine particles with a large surface area are presented to dissolving fluids which facilitate drug dissolution in the gastrointestinal tract, absorption and thereby the onset of drug action. Not all oral suspensions, however, are formulated for systemic effects and several are designed for local effects in the gastrointestinal tract. On the other hand, solutions, including formulations such as syrups and linctuses, are absorbed more rapidly than solid dosage forms or suspensions since drug dissolution is not required.

Rectal route

Drugs given rectally in solution, suppository or emulsion form are generally administered for local rather than systemic effects. Suppositories are solid forms intended for introduction into body cavities (usually rectal but also vaginal and urethral) where they melt, releasing the drug, and the choice of suppository base or drug carrier can greatly influence the degree and rate of drug release. This route of drug administration is also indicated for drugs inactivated by the gastrointestinal fluids when given orally or when the oral route is precluded, as for example when a patient is vomiting or unconscious. Drugs administered rectally enter the systemic circulation without passing through the liver, an advantage for drugs significantly inactivated by the liver following oral route absorption. Disadvantageously, the rectal route is inconvenient and drug absorption is often irregular and difficult to predict.

Parenteral route

A drug administered parenterally is one injected via a hollow needle into the body at various sites and to varying depths. The three main parenteral routes are subcutaneous (s.c.), intramuscular (i.m.) and intravenous (i.v.).

Other routes such as intracardiac and intrathecal are used less frequently. The parenteral route is preferred when rapid absorption is essential, as in emergency situations or when patients are unconscious or unable to accept oral medication, and in cases when drugs are destroyed, inactivated or poorly absorbed following oral administration. Absorption after parenteral drug delivery is rapid and, in general, blood levels attained are more predictable than those achieved by oral dosage forms.

Injectable preparations are usually sterile solutions or suspensions of drugs in water or other suitable physiologically acceptable vehicles. As referred to previously, drugs in solution are rapidly absorbed and thus injection suspensions are slower acting than solution injections. In addition, since body fluids are aqueous, by using suspended drugs in oily vehicles, a preparation exhibiting slower absorption characteristics can be formulated to give a depot preparation, providing a reservoir of drug which is slowly released into the systemic circulation. Such preparations are administered by intramuscular injection deep into skeletal muscles (e.g. several penicillin-containing injections). Alternatively, depot preparations can be achieved by subcutaneous implants or pellets, which are compacted or moulded discs of drug placed in loose subcutaneous tissue under the outer layers of the skin. Such systems include solid microspheres, polymeric biodegradable polymeric microspheres (e.g. polylactide co-glycollic acid homo- and copolymers) containing proteins or peptides (e.g. human growth hormone and leuprolide). More generally, subcutaneous injections are aqueous solutions or suspensions which allow the drug to be placed in the immediate vicinity of blood capillaries. The drug then diffuses into the capillaries. Inclusion of vasoconstrictors or vasodilators in subcutaneous injections will clearly influence blood flow through the capillaries, thereby modifying the capacity for absorption. This principle is often used in the administration of local anaesthetics with the vasoconstrictor adrenaline, which delays drug absorption. Conversely, improved drug absorption can result when vasodilators are included. Intravenous administration involves injection of sterile aqueous solutions directly into a vein at an appropriate rate. Volumes delivered can range from a few millilitres, as in emergency treatment or for hypnotics, up to litre quantities, as in replacement fluid treatment or nutrient feeding.

Given the generally negative patient acceptance of this important route of drug delivery, primarily associated with pain and inconvenience, recent developments have focused on 'needle-free' injection systems and devices which propel drug in aqueous solution or powder form at high velocity directly through the external layers of the skin.

Topical route

Drugs are applied topically, that is to the skin, mainly for local action. Whilst this route can also be used for systemic drug delivery, percutaneous absorption is often poor and erratic, although several transdermal patches delivering drug for systemic distribution (e.g. glyceryl trinitrate patches for the prophylaxis and treatment of angina) are available. Drugs applied to the skin for local effect include antiseptics, antifungals, antiinflammatory agents, as well as skin emollients for protective effects.

Pharmaceutical topical formulations – ointments, creams and pastes – are composed of drug in a suitable semi-solid base which is either hydrophobic or hydrophilic in character. The bases play an important role in determining the drug release character from the formulation. Ointments are hydrophobic, oleaginous-based dosage forms whereas creams are semi-solid emulsions. Pastes contain more solids than ointments and thus are stiffer in consistency. For topical application in liquid form other than solution, lotions, suspensions of solids in aqueous solution or emulsions are used. Recently, interest in transdermal electrotransport systems has grown. Here, a low electrical potential maintained across the skin can improve drug transport.

Application of drugs to other topical surfaces such as the eye, ear and nose is common and ointments, creams, suspensions and solutions are utilized. Ophthalmic preparations are required, amongst other features, to be sterile. Nasal dosage forms include solutions or suspensions delivered by drops or fine aerosol from a spray. Ear formulations in general are viscous to prolong contact with affected areas.

Respiratory route

The lungs provide an excellent surface for absorption when the drug is delivered in gaseous, aerosol mist or ultrafine solid particle form. For drug particles presented as an aerosol or solid form, particle size largely determines the extent to which they penetrate the alveolar region, the zone of rapid absorption. Drug particles that are in the region 0.5–1 μm diameter reach the alveolar sacs. Particles smaller than this range are either exhaled or, if larger, deposited upon larger bronchial airways. This delivery route is particularly useful for the direct treatment of asthmatic problems, using both powder aerosols (e.g. sodium cromoglycate) and metered aerosols containing the drug in liquefied inert propellant (e.g. salbutamol sulphate aerosol). Importantly, this delivery route is being increasingly recognised as a useful means of administering the therapeutic agents emerging from biotechnology requiring systemic distribution and targeted delivery, such as peptides and proteins.

DRUG FACTORS IN DOSAGE FORM DESIGN

Each type of dosage form requires careful study of the physical and chemical properties of drug substances to achieve a stable, efficacious product. These properties, such as dissolution, crystal size and polymorphic form, solid-state stability and drug–additive interaction, can have profound effects on the physiological availability and physical and chemical stability of the drug. By combining such information and knowledge with those from pharmacological and biochemical studies, the most suitable drug form and additives can be selected for the formulation of chosen dosage forms.

Whilst comprehensive property evaluation will not be required for all types of formulations, those properties which are recognized as important in dosage form design and processing are listed in Table 1.3. Also listed in Table 1.3 are the stresses to which the formulation might be exposed during processing and manipulation into dosage forms, as well as the procedures involved. Variations in physicochemical properties, occurring for example between batches of the same material or resulting from alternative treatment procedures, can modify formulation requirements as well as processing and dosage form performance. For instance, the fine milling of poorly soluble drug substances can modify their wetting and dissolution characteristics, important properties during granulation and product performance respectively. Careful evaluation of these properties and understanding of the effects of these stresses upon these parameters are therefore important in dosage form design and processing as well as product performance.

Particle size and surface area

Particle size reduction results in an increase in the specific surface (i.e. surface area per unit weight) of powders. Drug dissolution rate, absorption rate, dosage form content uniformity and stability are all dependent to varying degrees on particle size, size distribution and interactions of solid surfaces. In many cases, for both drugs and additives, particle size reduction is required to achieve the desired physiochemical characteristics.

It is now generally recognized that poorly aqueous soluble drugs showing a dissolution rate-limiting step in the absorption process will be more readily bioavailable when administered in a finely subdivided form with larger surface than as a coarse material. Examples include griseofulvin, tolbutamide, indomethacin, spironolactone and nifedipine. The fine material, often in micrometre or submicrometre (nanometre) form with

Table 1.3 Properties of drug substances important in dosage form design and potential stresses occurring during processes, with range of manufacturing procedures

Properties	Processing stresses	Manufacturing procedures
Particle size, surface area	Pressure	Precipitation
Particle surface chemistry	Mechanical	Filtration
Solubility	Radiation	Emulsification
Dissolution	Exposure to liquids	Milling
Partition coefficient	Exposure to gases and liquid vapours	Mixing
Ionization constant	Temperature	Drying
Crystal properties, polymorphism		Granulation
Stability		Compaction
Organoleptic		Autoclaving
Molecular weight		Crystallization
		Handling
		Storage
		Transport

large specific surface, dissolves at faster rates which can lead to improved drug absorption by passive diffusion. On the other hand, with formulated nitrofurantoin preparations an optimal particle size of 150 μm reduced gastrointestinal distress whilst still permitting sufficient urinary excretion of this urinary antibacterial agent.

Rates of drug dissolution can be adversely affected, however, by unsuitable choice of formulation additives, even though solids of appropriate particle size are used. Tableting lubricant powders, for example, can impart hydrophobicity to a formulation and inhibit drug dissolution. Fine powders can also increase air adsorption or static charge, leading to wetting or agglomeration problems. Micronizing drug powders can lead to changes in crystallinity and particle surface energy which cause reduced chemical stability. Drug particle size also influences content uniformity in solid dosage forms, particularly for low-dose formulations. It is important in such cases to have as many particles as possible per dose to minimize potency variation between dosage units. Other dosage forms are also affected by particle size, including suspensions (for controlling flow properties and particle interactions), inhalation aerosols (for optimal penetration of drug particles to absorbing mucosa) and topical formulations (for freedom from grittiness).

Solubility

All drugs, regardless of their administration route, must exhibit at least limited aqueous solubility for therapeutic efficiency. Thus relatively insoluble compounds can exhibit erratic or incomplete absorption, and it might be appropriate to use more soluble salt or other chemical derivatives. Alternatively, micronizing, complexation or solid dispersion techniques might be employed. Solubility, and especially degree of saturation in the vehicle, can also be important in the absorption of drugs already in solution in liquid dosage forms since precipitation in the gastrointestinal tract can occur, modifying bioavailability.

Solubilities of acidic or basic compounds are pH dependent and can be altered by forming salts, with different salts exhibiting different equilibrium solubilities. However, the solubility of a salt of a strong acid is less affected by changes in pH than the solubility of a salt of a weak acid. In the latter case, when pH is lower, the salt hydrolyses to an extent dependent of pH and pK_a, resulting in decreased solubility. Reduced solubility can also occur for slightly soluble salts of drugs through the common ion effect. If one of the ions involved is added as a different, more soluble salt, the solubility product can be exceeded and a portion of the drug precipitates.

Dissolution

As mentioned above, for a drug to be absorbed it must first be dissolved in the fluid at the site of absorption. For example, an orally administered drug in tablet form is not absorbed until drug particles are dissolved or solubilized by the fluids at some point along the gastrointestinal tract, depending on the pH-solubility profile of the drug substance. Dissolution describes the process by which the drug particles dissolve.

During dissolution, the drug molecules in the surface layer dissolve, leading to a saturated solution around the particles to form the diffusion layer. Dissolved drug molecules then pass throughout the dissolving fluid to contact absorbing mucosa and are absorbed. Replenishment of diffusing drug molecules in the diffusion layer is achieved by further drug dissolution and the absorption process continues. If dissolution is fast or the drug remains in solution form, the rate of absorption is primarily dependent upon its ability to traverse the absorbing membrane. If, however, drug dissolution is slow due to its physicochemical properties or formulation factors, then dissolution may be the rate-limiting step in absorption and influence drug bioavailability. The dissolution of a drug is described in a simplified manner by the Noyes–Whitney equation:

$$\frac{dm}{dt} = kA(C_S - C) \qquad (1.1)$$

where $\frac{dm}{dt}$ is the dissolution rate, k is the dissolution rate constant, A is the surface area of dissolving solid, C_S is the drug's solubility and C is the concentration of drug in the dissolution medium at time t. The equation reveals that dissolution rate can be raised by increasing the surface area (reducing particle size) of the drug, by increasing the solubility of the drug in the diffusing layer and by increasing k which incorporates the drug diffusion coefficient and diffusion layer thickness. During the early phases of dissolution, $C_S > C$ and if the surface area, A, and experimental conditions are kept constant then k can be determined for compacts containing drug alone. The constant k is termed the intrinsic dissolution rate constant and is a characteristic of each solid drug compound in a given solvent under fixed hydrodynamic conditions.

Drugs with k values below 0.1 mg^{-1} cm^{-2} usually exhibit dissolution rate-limiting absorption. Particulate dissolution can also be examined where an effort is made to control A, and formulation effects can be studied.

Dissolution rate data, when combined with solubility, partition coefficient and pK_a results, provide an insight into the potential in vivo absorption characteristics of a drug. However, in vitro tests only have significance when they are related to in vivo results. Once such a relationship has been established, in vitro dissolution tests can be used as a predictor of in vivo behaviour. The importance of dissolution testing has been widely recognized by official compendia, as well as drug registration authorities, with the inclusion of dissolution specifications using standardized testing procedures for a range of preparations.

Partition coefficient and pK_a

As pointed out earlier, for relatively insoluble compounds the dissolution rate is often the rate-determining step in the overall absorption process. Alternatively, for soluble compounds the rate of permeation across biological membranes is the rate-determining step. Whilst dissolution rate can be changed by modifying the physicochemical properties of the drug and/or altering the formulation composition, the permeation rate is dependent upon the size, relative aqueous and lipid solubility and ionic charge of drug molecules, factors which can be altered through molecular modifications. The absorbing membrane acts as a lipophilic barrier to the passage of drugs which is related to the lipophilic nature of the drug molecule. The partition coefficient, for example between oil and water, is a measure of lipophilic character.

The majority of small molecular weight drugs are weak acids or bases and, depending on the pH, exist in an ionized or unionized form. Membranes of absorbing mucosa are more permeable to unionized forms of drugs than to ionized species because of the greater lipid solubility of the unionized forms and the highly charged nature of the cell membrane which results in the binding or repelling of the ionized drug, thereby decreasing penetration.

The dominating factors that therefore influence the absorption of weak acids and bases are the pH at the site of absorption and the lipid solubility of the unionized species. These factors, together with the Henderson–Hasselbalch equations for calculating the proportions of ionized and unionized species at a particular pH, constitute the pH-partition theory for drug absorption. However, these factors do not describe completely the process of absorption since certain compounds with low partition coefficients and/or which are highly ionized over the entire physiological pH range show good bioavailability and therefore other factors are clearly involved.

Crystal properties: polymorphism

Practically all drug substances are handled in powder form at some stage during manufacture into dosage forms. However, for those substances composed of, or containing, powders or compacted powders in the finished product, the crystal properties and solid-state form of the drug must be carefully considered. It is well recognized that drug substances can be amorphous (i.e. without regular molecular lattice arrangements), crystalline, anhydrous, at various degrees of hydration or solvated with other entrapped solvent molecules, as well as varying in crystal hardness, shape and size. In addition, many drug stances can exist in more than one form with different molecular packing arrangements in the crystal lattice. This property is termed polymorphism and different polymorphs may be prepared by manipulation of conditions of particle formation during crystallization such as solvent, temperature and rate of cooling. It is known that only one form of a pure drug substance is stable at a given temperature and pressure, with the other forms, termed metastable, converting at different rates to the stable crystalline form. The different polymorphs vary in physical properties such as dissolution and solid-state stability, as well as processing behaviour in terms of powder flow and compaction during tableting in some cases.

These different crystalline forms can be of considerable importance in relation to ease or difficulty of formulation and as regards stability and biological activity. As might be expected, higher dissolution rates are obtained for metastable polymorphic forms; for example, the metastable form of chlortetracyline hydrochloride exhibits improved rate and extent of bioavailability. In some cases, amorphous forms are more active than crystalline forms.

The polypeptide hormone insulin, widely used in the regulation of carbohydrate, fat and protein metabolism, also demonstrates how differing degrees of activity can result from the use of different crystalline forms of the same agent. In the presence of acetate buffer, zinc combines with insulin to form an extremely insoluble complex of the proteinaceous hormone. This complex is an amorphous precipitate or crystalline product depending on environmental pH. The amorphous form, containing particles of no uniform shape and smaller than 2 μm, is absorbed following i.m. or s.c. injection and has a short duration of action, whilst the crystalline product, consisting of 10–40 μm sized rhombohedral crystals, is more slowly absorbed and has a longer duration of action. Insulin preparations which are intermediate in duration of action are prepared by taking physical mixtures of these two products.

Polymorphic transitions can also occur during milling, granulating, drying and compacting operations (e.g. tran-sitions during milling for digoxin and spironolactone). Granulation can result in solvate formation or, during drying, a solvated or hydrated molecule may be lost to form an anhydrous material. Consequently, the formulator must be aware of these potential transformations which can result in undesirable modified product performance, even though routine chemical analyses may not reveal any changes. Reversion from metastable forms, if used, to the stable form may also occur during the lifetime of the product. In suspensions, this may be accompanied by changes in the consistency of the preparation which affects its shelf life and stability. Such changes can often be prevented by additives, such as hydrocolloids and surface-active agents.

Stability

The chemical aspects of formulation generally centre on the chemical stability of the drug and its compatibility with the other formulation ingredients. In addition, it should be emphasized that the packaging of the dosage form is an important factor contributing to product stability and must be an integral part of stability testing programmes. It has been mentioned previously that one of the principles of dosage form design is to ensure that the chemical integrity of drug substances is maintained during the usable life of the product. At the same time, chemical changes involving additives and any physical modifications to the product must be carefully monitored to optimize formulation stability.

In general, drug substances decompose as a result of the effects of heat, oxygen, light and moisture. For example, esters such as aspirin and procaine are susceptible to solvolytic breakdown, whilst oxidative decomposition occurs for substances such as ascorbic acid. Drugs can be classified according to their sensitivity to breakdown:

1. stable in all conditions (e.g. kaolin)
2. stable if handled correctly (e.g. aspirin)
3. only moderately stable even with special handling (e.g. vitamins)
4. very unstable (e.g. certain antibiotics in solution form).

Whilst the mechanisms of solid-state degradation are complex and often difficult to analyse, a full understanding is not a prerequisite in the design of a suitable formulation containing solids. For example, in cases where drug substances are sensitive to hydrolysis, steps such as minimum exposure to moisture during preparation, low moisture content specifications in the final product and moisture-resistant packaging can be used. For oxygen-sensitive drugs, antioxidants can be included in the formulation and, as with light-sensitive materials, suitable packaging can reduce or eliminate the problem. For drugs administered in liquid form, the stability in solution as well as the effects of pH over the physiological range of 1–8 should be understood. Buffers may be required to control the pH of the preparation to improve stability; where liquid dosage forms are sensitive to microbial attack, preservatives are required.

In these formulations, and indeed in all dosage forms incorporating additives, it is also important to ensure that the components, which may include additional drug substances as in multivitamin preparations, do not produce chemical interactions themselves. Interactions between drug(s) and added excipients such as antioxidants, preservatives, suspending agents, colorants, tablet lubricants and packaging materials do occur and must be checked for during formulation. Over recent years data from thermal analysis techniques, particularly microcalorimetry and differential scanning calorimetry (DSC), when critically examined, have been found useful in rapid screening for possible drug–additive and drug–drug interactions. For example, using DSC it has been demonstrated that the widely used tableting lubricant magnesium stearate interacts with aspirin and should be avoided in formulations containing this drug.

Organoleptic properties

Modern medicines require that pharmaceutical dosage forms are acceptable to the patient. Unfortunately, many drug substances in use today are unpalatable and unattractive in their natural state and dosage forms containing such drugs, particularly oral preparations, may require the addition of approved flavours and/or colours.

The use of flavours applies primarily to liquid dosage forms intended for oral administration. Available as concentrated extracts, solutions, adsorbed onto powders or microencapsulated, flavours are usually composed of mixtures of natural and synthetic materials. The taste buds of the tongue respond quickly to bitter, sweet, salt or acid elements of a flavour. In addition, unpleasant taste can be overcome by using water-insoluble derivatives of drugs which have little or no taste. An example is the use of amitriptyline pamoate, although other factors, such as bioavailability, must remain unchanged. If an insoluble derivative is unavailable or cannot be used, a flavour or perfume can be used. However, unpleasant drugs in capsules or prepared as coated particles or tablets may be easily swallowed, avoiding the taste buds.

Selection of flavour depends upon several factors but particularly on the taste of the drug substance. Certain flavours are more effective at masking various taste elements; for example, citrus flavours are frequently used to combat sour or acid-tasting drugs. Solubility and stability of the flavour in the vehicle are also important. In addition, the age of the intended patient should also be considered, since children for example prefer sweet tastes, as well as the psychological links between colours and flavours (e.g. yellow colour is associated with lemon flavour). Sweetening agents may also be required to mask bitter tastes. Sucrose continues to be used but alternatives, such as sodium saccharin which is 200–700 times sweeter depending on concentration, are available. Sorbitol is recommended for diabetic preparations.

Colours are employed to standardize or improve an existing drug colour, to mask a colour change or complement a flavour. Whilst colours are obtained both from natural sources (e.g. carotenoids) or synthesized (e.g. amaranth), the majority used are synthetically produced. Dyes may be aqueous (e.g. amaranth) or oil soluble (e.g. Sudan IV) or insoluble in both (e.g. aluminium lakes). Lakes, which are generally calcium or aluminium complexes of water-soluble dyes, are particularly useful in tablets and tablet coatings because of greater stability to light than corresponding dyes, which also vary in their stability to pH and reducing agents. However, in recent years, the inclusion of colours in formulations has become extremely complex because of the banning of many traditionally used colours in many countries.

Other drug properties

At the same time as ensuring that dosage forms are chemically and physically stable and are therapeutically efficacious, it is also relevant to establish that the selected formulation is capable of efficient and, in most cases, large-scale manufacture. In addition to those properties previously discussed such as particle size and crystal form, other characteristics such as hygroscopicity, flowability and compactability are particularly valuable when preparing solid dosage forms where the drugs constitute a large percentage of the formulation. Hygroscopic drugs can require low moisture manufacturing environments and need to avoid water during preparation. Poorly flowing formulations may require the addition of flow agents (e.g. fumed silica). Studies of the compactability of drug substances are frequently undertaken using instrumented tablet machines in formulation laboratories to examine the tableting potential of the material in order to foresee any potential problems during compaction, such as lamination or sticking, which may require modification to the formulation or processing conditions.

THERAPEUTIC CONSIDERATIONS IN DOSAGE FORM DESIGN

The nature of the clinical indication, disease or illness against which the drug is intended is an important factor when selecting the range of dosage forms to be prepared.

Factors such as the need for systemic or local therapy, duration of action required, and whether the drug will be used in emergency situations, need to be considered. In the vast majority of cases a single drug substance is prepared into a number of dosage forms to satisfy both the particular preferences of the patient or physician and the specific needs of a certain clinical situation. For example, many asthmatic patients use inhalation aerosols, from which the drug is rapidly absorbed into the systematic circulation following deep inhalation for rapid emergency relief, and oral products for chronic therapy.

Patients requiring urgent relief from angina pectoris, a coronary circulatory problem, place tablets of nitroglycerin sublingually for rapid drug absorption directly into the blood capillaries there. Thus, whilst systemic effects are generally obtained following oral and parenteral drug administration, other routes can be employed as the drug and situation demand. Local effects are generally restricted to dosage forms applied directly such as those applied to the skin, ear, eye, throat and lungs. Some drugs may be well absorbed by one route and not another and must therefore be considered individually.

The age of the patient also plays a role in defining the types of dosage forms made available. Infants generally prefer liquid dosage forms, usually solutions and mixtures, given orally. Also, by having liquid preparations, the amount of drug administered can be readily adjusted by dilution to give the required dose for the particular patient, taking weight, age and patient's condition into account. Children can have difficulty in swallowing solid dosage forms and for this reason many oral preparations are prepared as pleasantly flavoured syrups or mixtures. Adults generally prefer solid dosage forms, primarily because of their convenience. However, alternative liquid preparations are usually available for those unable to take tablets and capsules.

Interest has grown in the design of drug-containing formulations which deliver drugs to specific 'targets' in the body, for example the use of liposomes and nanoparticles, as well as providing drugs over longer periods of time at controlled rates. Alternative technologies for preparing particles with required properties – crystal engineering – provide new opportunities. Supercritical fluid processing using carbon dioxide as a solvent or anti-solvent is one such method, allowing fine tuning of crystal properties and particle design and fabrication.

Undoubtedly, these new technologies and others, as well as sophisticated formulations, will be required to deal with the advent of gene therapy and the need to deliver such labile macromolecules to specific targets and cells in the body. Interest is also likely to be directed to individual patient requirements such as age, weight and physiological and metabolic factors, features which can influence drug absorption and bioavailability.

SUMMARY

This chapter has demonstrated that the formulation of drugs into dosage forms requires the interpretation and application of a wide range of information from several study areas. Whilst the physical and chemical properties of drugs and additives need to be understood, the factors influencing drug absorption and the requirements of the disease to be treated also have to be taken into account when identifying potential delivery routes. The formulation and associated preparation of dosage forms demand the highest standards with careful examination, analysis and evaluation of wide-ranging information by pharmaceutical scientists to achieve the objective of creating high-quality, safe and efficacious dosage forms.

BIBLIOGRAPHY

Amidon, G.L., Lennernas, H., Shah, V.P., Crison, J.R. (1995) A theoretical basis for a biopharmaceutical drug classification: the correlation of in vitro drug product dissolution and bioavailability. *Pharmaceutical Research*, **12**, 413-420.

British Pharmacopoeial Commission (2005) *British Pharmacopoeia*. Stationery Office, London.

Byrn, S.R., Pfeiffer, R.R., Stowell, J.G. (1999) *Solid State Chemistry of Drugs*, 2nd edn. SSCI, West Lafayette.

Florence, A.T., Attwood, D. (2006) *Physicochemical Principles of Pharmacy*, 4th edn. Pharmaceutical Press, Royal Pharmaceutical Society of Great Britain, London.

Hillary, A.M., Lloyd, A.W., Swarbrick, J. (2001) *Drug Delivery and Targeting*. Taylor and Francis, London.

Martindale, W. (2003) *The extra pharmacopoeia*, 34th edn. Pharmaceutical Press, Royal Pharmaceutical Society of Great Britain, London.

Shekunov, B.Yu, York, P. (2000) Crystallisation processes in pharmaceutical technology and drug delivery design. *Journal of Crystal Growth*, **211**, 122-136.

PART 1

SCIENTIFIC PRINCIPLES OF DOSAGE FORM DESIGN

Dissolution and solubility

M. E. Aulton

INTRODUCTION

Solutions are encountered frequently in pharmaceutical development, either as dosage form in their own right or as a clinical trials material. Equally importantly, almost all drugs function in solution in the body.

This chapter discusses the principles underlying the formation of solutions from solute and solvent and the factors that affect the rate and extent of the dissolution process. It will discuss this process particularly in the context of a solid dissolving in a liquid as this is the situation most likely to be encountered during the formation of a drug solution, either during manufacturing or during drug delivery.

Further properties of solutions are discussed in the subsequent chapters in Part 1 of this book. Because of the number of principles and properties that need to be considered, the contents of each of these chapters should only be regarded as introductions to the various topics. The student is encouraged, therefore, to refer to the bibliography cited at the end of each chapter in order to augment the present contents. The textbook written by Florence & Attwood (2006) is recommended particularly. It uses a large number of pharmaceutical examples to aid understanding of physicochemical principles.

DEFINITION OF TERMS

This chapter will begin by clarifying some of the key terms relevant to solutions.

Solution, solubility and dissolution

A *solution* may be defined as a mixture of two or more components that form a single phase that is homogeneous down to the molecular level. The component that determines the phase of the solution is termed the *solvent*; it usually (but not necessarily) constitutes the largest proportion of the system. The other component(s) are termed *solute(s)* and these are dispersed as molecules or ions throughout the solvent, i.e. they are said to be *dissolved* in the solvent.

The transfer of molecules or ions from a solid state into solution is known as *dissolution*. Fundamentally this process is controlled by the relative affinity between the molecules of the solid substance and those of the solvent. The *extent* to which the dissolution proceeds under a given set of experimental conditions is referred to as the *solubility* of the solute in the solvent. The solubility of a substance is the *amount* of it that passes into solution when *equilibrium* is established between the solute in solution and the excess (undissolved) substance. The solution that is obtained under these conditions is said to be *saturated*. A solution with a concentration less than that at equilibrium is said to be *subsaturated*. Solutions with a concentration greater than equilibrium can be obtained. These are known as *supersaturated* solutions

Since the above definitions are general ones, they may be applied to all types of solution involving any of the three states of matter (gas, liquid, solid) dissolved in any of the three states of matter, i.e. solid-in-liquid, liquid-in-solid, solid-in-vapour, vapour-in-liquid, etc. However, when the two components forming a solution are either both gases or both liquids then it is more usual to talk in terms of *miscibility* rather than solubility. Otherwise all principles are the same.

One point to emphasize at this stage is that the rate of solution (dissolution rate) and amount which can be dissolved (solubility) are not the same and are not necessarily related. In practice, high drug solubility is usually associated with a high dissolution rate, but there are exceptions; an example is the commonly used film coating material hydroxypropyl methylcelluose (HPMC) which is very water soluble yet takes many hours to hydrate and dissolve.

PROCESS OF DISSOLUTION

Dissolution mechanisms

The majority of drugs and excipients are crystalline solids. Liquid, semi-solid and amorphous drugs and excipients do exist but these are in the minority. For now, we will restrict our discussion to dissolution of crystalline solids into liquid solvents. Also, to simplify the discussion, it will be assumed that the drug is molecular in nature. The same discussion applies to ionic drugs. Again, to avoid undue repetition in the explanations that follow, it can be assumed that most solid crystalline materials, whether drugs or excipients, will dissolve in a similar manner.

The dissolution of a solid in a liquid may be regarded as being composed of two consecutive stages.

1. First is an *interfacial reaction* that results in the liberation of solute molecules from the solid phase to the liquid phase. This involves a phase change so that molecules of solid become molecules of solute in the solvent in which the crystal is dissolving.
2. After this, the solute molecules must migrate through the boundary layers surrounding the crystal to the bulk of solution.

These stages, and the associated solution concentration changes, are illustrated in Figure 2.1.

These two stages of dissolution are now discussed in turn.

Interfacial reaction

Leaving surface Dissolution involves the replacement of crystal molecules by solvent molecules. This is illustrated in Figure 2.2.

The process of the removal of drug molecules from a solid, and their replacement by solvent molecules, is determined by the relative affinity of the various molecules involved. The solvent/solute forces of attraction must overcome the cohesive forces of attraction between the molecules of the solid.

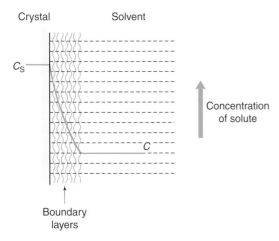

Fig. 2.1 Diagram of boundary layers and concentration change surrounding a dissolving particle.

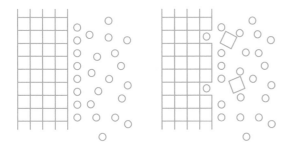

Fig. 2.2 Schematic representation of the replacement of crystal molecules with solvent molecules during dissolution.

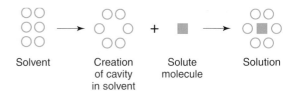

Fig. 2.3 The theory of cavity creation in the mechanism of dissolution.

Moving into liquid On leaving the solid surface, the drug molecule must become incorporated in the liquid phase, i.e. within the solvent. Liquids are thought to contain a small amount of so-called 'free volume' in the form of 'holes' that, at a given instant, are not occupied by the solvent molecules themselves (this is discussed further in Chapter 3). Individual solute molecules are thought to occupy these 'holes', as is shown in Figure 2.3.

The process of dissolution may be considered, therefore, to involve the relocation of solute molecules from an environment where they are surrounded by other identical molecules, with which they form intermolecular attractions, into a cavity in a liquid where it is surrounded by non-identical molecules, with which it may interact to a different degree.

Diffusion through the boundary layer

This step involves transport of the drug molecules away from the solid/liquid interface into the bulk of the liquid phase under the influence of diffusion or convection. Boundary layers are static or slow-moving layers of liquid that surround all solid surfaces that are surrounded by liquid (discussed further in Chapter 4). Mass transfer takes place more slowly (usually by diffusion; Chapter 3) through these static or slow-moving layers that inhibit the movement of solute molecules from the surface of the solid to the bulk of the solution. The solution in contact with the solid will be saturated (because it is in direct contact with undissolved solid). During diffusion, the concentration of the solution in the boundary layers changes from being saturated (C_s) at the crystal surface to being equal to that of the bulk of the solution (C) at its outermost limit, as shown in Figure 2.1.

Energy/work changes during dissolution

In order for the process of dissolution to occur spontaneously at a constant pressure, the accompanying change in free energy or Gibbs free energy (ΔG) must be negative. The free energy (G) is a measure of the energy available to the system to perform work. Its value decreases during a spontaneously occurring process until an equilibrium position is reached when no more energy can be made available, i.e. $\Delta G = 0$ at equilibrium.

In most cases heat is absorbed when dissolution occurs and the process is usually defined as an *endothermic* one. In some systems, where marked affinity between solute and solvent occurs, the overall enthalpy change becomes negative so that heat is evolved and the process is an *exothermic* one.

DISSOLUTION RATES OF SOLIDS IN LIQUIDS

Like any reaction that involves consecutive stages, the overall rate of dissolution will be dependent on whichever of these steps is the slowest (the *rate-determining* or *rate-limiting step*). In dissolution the interfacial step (as above) is virtually instantaneous and so the rate of dissolution will most frequently be determined by the rate of the slower step (b above) of diffusion of dissolved solute through the static boundary layer of liquid that exists at a solid/liquid interface. On the rare occasions when the release of the molecule from the solid into solution is slow and the transport across the boundary layer to the bulk solution is faster, dissolution is said to be *interfacially controlled*.

The rate of diffusion will obey Fick's Law of Diffusion. Fick's Law states that the rate of change in concentration of dissolved material with time is directly proportional to the concentration difference between the two sides of the diffusion layer, i.e.

$$\frac{dC}{dt} \propto \Delta C \tag{2.1}$$

or

$$\frac{dC}{dt} = k\Delta C \tag{2.2}$$

where C is the concentration of solute in solution at any point and at time t, and the constant k is the rate constant (s^{-1}).

In the present context ΔC is the difference in concentration of solution at the solid surface (C_1) and the bulk of the solution (C_2). At equilibrium, the solution in contact with the solid (C_1) will be saturated (concentration = C_S) as discussed above. Thus $\Delta C = C_1 - C_2 = C_S - C$.

If C_2 is less than saturated, the molecules will move from the solid to the bulk (as during dissolution). If the concentration of the bulk (C_2) is greater than this, the solution is referred to as supersaturated and movement of solid molecules will be in the direction of bulk to surface (as occurs during crystallization).

An equation known as the Noyes–Whitney (1897) equation was developed to define the dissolution from a single spherical particle. This equation has found great usefulness in the estimation or prediction of the dissolution of pharmaceutical particles. The rate of mass transfer of solute molecules or ions through a static diffusion layer (dm/dt) is directly proportional to the area available for molecular or ionic migration (A), the concentration difference (ΔC) across the boundary layer and is inversely proportional to the thickness of the boundary layer (h).

This relationship is shown in Eqn 2.3 and in a slightly modified form in Eqn 2.4.

$$\frac{dm}{dt} = \frac{k_1 A \Delta C}{h} \tag{2.3}$$

$$\frac{dm}{dt} = \frac{k_1 A (C_S - C)}{h} \tag{2.4}$$

The constant k_1 is known as the *diffusion coefficient*, usually given the symbol D, and has the units of m^2/s.

If the volume of the solvent is large, or solute is removed from the bulk of the dissolution medium by some process at a faster rate than it passes into solution, then C remains close to zero and the term $(C_S - C)$ in Eqn 2.4 may be approximated to C_S. In practice, if the volume of the dissolution medium is so large that C is not allowed to exceed 10% of the value of C_S, then the same approximation may be made. In either of these circumstances dissolution is said to occur under 'sink' conditions and Eqn 2.4 may be simplified to:

$$\frac{dm}{dt} = \frac{DAC_S}{h} \tag{2.5}$$

Sink conditions may arise in vivo when a drug is absorbed into the body from its solution in the gastrointestinal fluids at a faster rate than it dissolves in those fluids from a solid dosage form such as a tablet. The phrase is illustrative of the solute 'disappearing down a sink'!

If solute is allowed to accumulate in the dissolution medium to such an extent that the above approximation is no longer valid, i.e. when $C > C_S/10$, then 'non-sink' conditions are said to be in operation. When C builds up to such an extent that it equals C_S, i.e. the dissolution medium is saturated with solute, it is clear from Eqn 2.4 that the overall dissolution rate will be zero.

Factors affecting the rate of dissolution

These factors may be derived from a consideration of the terms that appear in the Noyes–Whitney equation (Eqn 2.4) and knowledge of the factors that in turn affect these terms. Most of the effects of these factors are included in the summary given in Table 2.1.

The various factors that affect the in vitro rate of diffusion-controlled dissolution of solids into liquids can be predicted by examination of the Noyes–Whitney equation (Eqn 2.3). Clearly, increases in those factors on the top of the right-hand side of the Noyes–Whitney equation will increase the rate of diffusion (and therefore dissolution) and increases in factors at the bottom of the equation will result in their decrease. The opposite situation obviously applies regarding reduction in these parameters. Each of these is discussed briefly below.

Surface area of undissolved solid (A)

Size of solid particles   The surface area of isodiametric particles is inversely proportional to their particle size. Much practical evidence exists to show that, in general, milling or other means of particle size reduction will increase the rate of dissolution of sparingly soluble drugs. An added complication is that particle size will

Table 2.1 Factors affecting in vitro dissolution rates of solids in liquids	
Term in Noyes–Whitney equation	Affected by
A, surface area of undissolved solid	Size of solid particles Dispersibility of powdered solid in dissolution medium Porosity of solid particles
C_S solubility of solid in dissolution medium	Temperature Nature of dissolution medium Molecular structure of solute Crystalline form of solid Presence of other compounds
C, concentration of solute in solution at time t	Volume of dissolution medium Any process that removes dissolved solute from the dissolution medium
k, dissolution rate constant	Thickness of boundary layer Diffusion coefficient of solute in the dissolution medium

change during dissolution process, because large particles will become smaller and small particles will eventually disappear. This effect is shown in Figure 2.4.

Compacted masses of solid may also disintegrate into smaller particles, thus increasing the surface area available for dissolution as the disintegration process progresses. (This effect is shown in Figure 31.7 and explained further in the associated discussion.)

Dispersibility of powdered solid in dissolution medium   If particles tend to form coherent masses in the dissolution medium then the surface area available for dissolution is reduced. This effect may be overcome by the addition of a wetting agent to improve the dispersion into primary powder particles.

Porosity of solid particles   Pores in some materials, particularly granulated ones, may be large enough to allow access of the dissolution medium and outward diffusion of dissolved solute molecules.

Solubility of solid in dissolution medium (C_S)

Temperature   Dissolution may be an exothermic or an endothermic process and so temperature changes will influence the energy balance and thus the energy available to promote dissolution.

Nature of dissolution medium   Factors such as solubility parameters, cosolvents and pH will affect the rate of dissolution. These are referred to in the text.

Molecular structure of solute   Factors such as the use of salts of either weakly acidic or weakly basic drugs, or esterification of neutral compounds, can influence solubility and dissolution rate.

Crystalline form of solid   The presence of polymorphs, hydrates, solvates or the amorphous form of the drug all can have an influence on dissolution rate.

Presence of other compounds   The common ion effect, complex formation and the presence of solubilizing agents can affect the rate of dissolution.

Concentration of solute in solution at time t (C)

Volume of dissolution medium   If volume of the dissolution medium is small, C can approach C_S. If it is large then C may be negligible with respect to C_S and thus 'sink' conditions will operate. This can be controlled in vitro but must be taken into account in vivo as the volume of the stomach contents can vary greatly (hence the common instruction 'To be taken with a glass of water'). Also, the volume of the fluid in the rectum and vagina can be small (see Chapter 40) and so this consideration can be important in drug delivery from suppositories and pessaries.

Any process that removes dissolved solute from the dissolution medium   For example, adsorption on to an insoluble adsorbent, partition into a second liquid that is immiscible with the dissolution medium, removal of solute by dialysis or by continuous replacement of solution by fresh dissolution medium.

Dissolution rate constant (k)

Thickness of boundary layer   Affected by degree of agitation, which depends, in turn, on speed of stirring or shaking, shape, size and position of stirrer, volume of dissolution medium, shape and size of container, viscosity of dissolution medium.

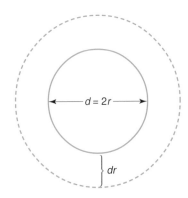

Fig. 2.4   The reduction in surface area and volume during the dissolution of a spherical particle.

Diffusion coefficient of solute in the dissolution medium The diffusion coefficient of solute in the dissolution medium is affected by the viscosity of dissolution medium, and the molecular characteristics and size of diffusing molecules.

It should be borne in mind that pharmaceutical scientists are often concerned with the rate of dissolution of a drug from a formulated product such as a tablet or a capsule, as well as with the dissolution rates of pure solids. In practice, the rate of dissolution can have either zero-order, first-order, second-order or cube-root kinetics. These are discussed later in the book when relevant to particular dosage forms. Later chapters in this book can also be consulted for information on the influence of formulation factors on the rates of release of drugs into solution from various dosage forms.

Intrinsic dissolution rate

Since the rate of dissolution is dependent on so many factors, it is advantageous to have a measure of the rate of dissolution which is independent of some of these – rate of agitation and area of solute available in particular. In the latter case, this will change greatly in a conventional tablet formulation as the tablet breaks up into granules and then into primary powder particles as it comes in contact with water.

A useful parameter is the *intrinsic dissolution rate* (IDR). IDR is the rate of mass transfer per area of dissolving surface and typically has the units of mg cm^{-2} min^{-1}. IDR should be independent of boundary layer thickness and volume of solvent (i.e. it is assumed that sink conditions have been achieved). Thus:

$$IDR = k_1 C_S \qquad (2.6)$$

Thus IDR measures the intrinsic properties of the drug only as a function of the dissolution media, e.g. its pH, ionic strength, presence of counter ions, etc., and is independent of many other factors.

Techniques for measuring IDR are discussed briefly below and in Chapter 24.

Measurement of dissolution rates

Many methods have been described in the literature, particularly in relation to the determination of the rate of release of drugs into solution from tablet and capsule formulations, because such release may have an important effect on the therapeutic efficiency of these dosage forms (Chapters 21, 31, 34 and 35). Attempts have been made to classify the methods for determining dissolution rates. These classifications are based mainly on whether or not the mixing processes that take place in the various

methods occur by natural convection, arising from density gradients produced in the dissolution medium, or by forced convection brought about by stirring or shaking the system. The following brief descriptions are given as examples of the more commonly used methods that are illustrated in Figure 2.5. Chapter 31 in particular gives a more detailed description of apparatus used for the dissolution testing of solid dosage forms.

Flask-stirrer method

In this method a round-bottomed flask is used. The use of a round-bottomed container helps to avoid the problems that may arise from the formation of 'mounds' of particles in different positions on the flat bottom of a normal laboratory beaker.

Rotating basket method

This method is described in most pharmacopoeias for the determination of the dissolution rates of drugs from tablets and capsules. Details of the apparatus and methods of operation are given in these official compendia.

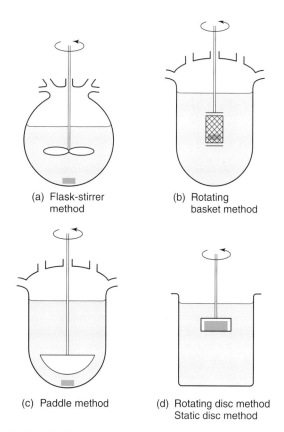

(a) Flask-stirrer method

(b) Rotating basket method

(c) Paddle method

(d) Rotating disc method Static disc method

Fig. 2.5 Methods of measuring dissolution rates.

Basically, these methods involve placing the tablet or capsule inside a stainless steel wire basket, which is rotated at a fixed speed whilst immersed in the dissolution medium that is contained in a wide-mouthed cylindrical vessel. The bottom of this vessel is either flat or spherical. Samples of the dissolution medium are removed at specified times, filtered and assayed.

Paddle method

This is another official method. The dissolution vessel described in the rotating basket method, i.e. a cylindrical vessel with a spherical bottom, is also used in this method. Agitation is provided by a rotating paddle and the dosage form is allowed to sink to the bottom of the dissolution vessel before agitation is commenced.

Rotating and static disc methods

In these methods the compound to be assessed for rate of dissolution is compressed into a non-disintegrating disc. This is mounted in a holder so that only one face of the disc is exposed to the dissolution medium. The holder and disc are immersed in the dissolution medium and either held in a fixed position in the static disc method or rotated at a given speed in the rotating disc method. Samples of dissolution medium are removed after known times, filtered and assayed. Further information on this methodology can be found in Chapter 24.

In this method it is assumed that the surface area, from which dissolution can occur, remains constant. Under these conditions the amount of substance dissolved per unit time and unit surface area can be determined. This is the *intrinsic dissolution rate* and should be distinguished from the measurements obtained from the previously described methods. In the non-disc methods the surface area of the drug that is available for dissolution changes considerably during the course of the determination because the dosage form usually disintegrates into many smaller particles and the size of these particles then decreases as dissolution proceeds. Since these changes are not usually monitored, the dissolution rate is measured in terms of the total amount of drug dissolved per unit time.

It should be appreciated from a consideration of the comments made earlier relating to factors affecting dissolution rate that not only will different dissolution rate methods yield different results but also changes in the experimental variables in a given method are likely to lead to changes in the results. This latter point is particularly important since dissolution rate tests are usually performed in a comparative manner to determine, for example, the difference between two polymorphic forms of the same compound or between the rates of release of a drug from two formulations. Thus, standardization of the experimental methodology is essential if such comparisons are to be meaningful and useful.

Finally, it should also be realized that, although the majority of dissolution testing is concerned with pure drugs or with conventional tablet or capsule formulations, knowledge of the rates of drug release from other types of dosage form is also important. Reference should be made therefore to later chapters in this book for information on the dissolution methods applied to specific dosage forms.

SOLUBILITY

The solution produced when equilibrium is established between undissolved and dissolved solute in a dissolution process is termed a *saturated solution*. The amount of substance that passes into solution in order to establish this equilibrium at constant temperature and so produce a saturated solution is known as the *solubility* of the substance. It is possible to obtain supersaturated solutions but these are unstable and precipitation of the excess solute tends to occur readily.

Methods of expressing solubility and concentration

Solubilities may be expressed by any of the variety of concentration terms explained below. In general, solubility is expressed in terms of the maximum mass or volume of solute that will dissolve in a given mass or volume of solvent at a particular temperature and at equilibrium.

Expressions of concentration

Quantity per quantity

Concentrations are often expressed simply as the weight or volume of solute that is contained in a given weight or volume of the solution. The majority of solutions encountered in pharmaceutical practice consist of solids dissolved in liquids. Consequently, concentration is expressed most commonly by the weight of solute contained in a given volume of solution. Although the SI unit is kg m^{-3} the terms that are used in practice are based on more convenient or appropriate weights and volumes. For example, in the case of a solution with a concentration of 1 kg m^{-3} the strength may be denoted by any one of the following concentration terms, depending on the circumstances:

1 g L^{-1}, 0. 1 g per 100 mL, 1 mg mL^{-1}, 5 mg in 5 mL or 1 μg μL^{-1}.

Percentage

Pharmaceutical scientists have a preference for quoting concentrations in percentages. The concentration of a solution of a solid in a liquid is given by:

$$\frac{\text{concentration}}{\text{in \% w/v}} = \frac{\text{weight of solute}}{\text{volume of solution}} \times 100 \quad (2.7)$$

Equivalent percentages based on weight and volume ratios (% v/w, % v/v and % w/w expressions) can also be used for solutions of liquids in liquids and solutions of gases in liquids.

It should be realized that if concentration is expressed in terms of weight of solute in a given *volume* of solution then changes in volume caused by temperature fluctuations will alter the concentration.

Parts

Pharmacopoeias give information on the approximate solubilities of official substances in terms of the number of 'parts' of solute dissolved in a stated number of 'parts' of solution. Use of this method to describe the strength of a solution of a solid in a liquid suggests that a certain number of parts by weight (g) of solid are contained in a given number of parts by volume (mL) of solution. In the case of solutions of liquids in liquids, parts by volume of solute in parts by volume of solution are intended whereas with solutions of gases in liquids, parts by weight of gas in parts by weight of solution are inferred. The use of 'parts' in scientific work, or indeed in practice, is not recommended as there is the chance for some degree of ambiguity.

Molarity

This is the number of moles of solute contained in 1 dm^3 (or, more commonly in pharmaceutical science, 1 litre) of solution. Thus, solutions of equal molarity contain the same number of solute molecules in a given volume of solution. The unit of molarity is mol L^{-1} (equivalent to 10^3 mol m^{-3} if converted to the strict SI unit).

Molality

This is the number of moles of solute divided by the mass of the solvent, i.e. its SI unit is mol kg^{-1}. Although it is less likely to be encountered in pharmaceutical science than the other terms, it does offer a more precise description of concentration because it is unaffected by temperature.

Mole fraction

This is often used in theoretical considerations and is defined as the number of moles of solute divided by the total number of moles of solute and solvent, i.e.:

$$\text{mole fraction of solute}\,(x_1) = \frac{n_1}{n_1 + n_2} \quad (2.8)$$

where n_1 and n_2 are the numbers of moles of solute and solvent, respectively.

Milliequivalents and normal solutions

The concentrations of solutes in body fluids and in solutions used as replacements for these fluids are usually expressed in terms of the number of millimoles (1 millimole = one-thousandth of a mole) in a litre of solution. In the case of electrolytes, however, these concentrations may still be expressed in terms of milliequivalents per litre. A milliequivalent (mEq) of an ion is, in fact, one-thousandth of the gram equivalent of the ion, which is, in turn, the ionic weight expressed in grams divided by the valency of the ion. Alternatively:

$$1\,\text{mEq} = \frac{\text{ionic weight in mg}}{\text{valency}} \quad (2.9)$$

Knowledge of the concept of chemical equivalents is also required in order to understand the use of 'normality' as a means of expressing the concentration of solutions. A normal solution, i.e. one with a concentration of 1 N, is one that contains the equivalent weight of the solute, expressed in grams, in 1 litre of solution. It was expected that this term would have disappeared following the introduction of SI units but it is still encountered in some volumetric assay procedures.

Qualitative descriptions of solubility

Pharmacopoeias also express approximate solubilities that correspond to descriptive terms such as 'freely soluble' and 'sparingly soluble'. The interrelationship between such terms and approximate solubilities is shown in Table 2.2.

Prediction of solubility

Probably the most sought after information about solutions in formulation problems is 'what is the best solvent for a given solute?'. Theoretical prediction of precise solubilities is an involved and occasionally unsuccessful operation but, from knowledge of the structure and properties of solute and solvent, you can make an educated guess. This guess is best expressed in subjective terms, such as 'very soluble' or 'sparingly soluble', as described

Table 2.2 Descriptive solubilities

Description	Approximate weight of solvent (g) necessary to dissolve 1 g of solute
Very soluble	< 1
Freely soluble	Between 1 and 10
Soluble	Between 10 and 30
Sparingly soluble	Between 30 and 100
Slightly soluble	Between 100 and 1000
Very slightly soluble	Between 1000 and 10 000
Practically insoluble	> 10 000

above. Often (particularly in pre- or early formulation) this is all the information that the formulator requires. A more precise value can be obtained later in the development process.

Speculation on what is likely to be a good solvent is usually based on the 'like dissolves like' principle. That is, a solute dissolves best in a solvent with similar chemical properties. The concept traditionally follows two rules.

1. Polar solutes dissolve in polar solvents.
2. Non-polar solutes dissolve in non-polar solvents.

Chemical groups that confer polarity to their parent molecules are known as *polar groups*. In the context of solubility, a *polar molecule* has a high dipole moment.

To rationalize the above rules, you can consider the forces of attraction between solute and solvent molecules. The following explains the basic physicochemical properties of solutions that lead to such observations.

Physicochemical prediction of solubility

Similar types of intermolecular force may contribute to solute–solvent, solute–solute and solvent–solvent interactions. The attractive forces exerted between polar molecules are much stronger, however, than those that exist between polar and non-polar molecules or between non-polar molecules themselves. Consequently, a polar solute will dissolve to a greater extent in a polar solvent, where the strength of the solute/solvent interaction will be comparable to that between solute molecules, than in a non-polar solvent, where the solute/solvent interaction will be relatively weak. In addition, the forces of attraction between the molecules of a polar solvent will be too great to facilitate the separation of these molecules by the insertion of a non-polar solute between them, because the solute–solvent forces will again be relatively weak. Thus, solvents for non-polar solutes tend to be restricted to non-polar liquids.

The above considerations thus follow the very general 'like dissolves like' principle, i.e. a polar substance will dissolve in a polar solvent and a non-polar substance will dissolve in a non-polar solvent. Such generalizations should be treated with caution, because the intermolecular forces involved in the process of dissolution are influenced by factors that are not obvious from a consideration of the overall polarity of a molecule. For example, the possibility of intermolecular hydrogen bond formation between solute and solvent may be more significant than polarity.

Solubility parameters Attempts have been made to define a parameter that indicates the ability of a liquid to act as a solvent. The most satisfactory approach, introduced by Hildebrand & Scott (1962), is based on the concept that the solvent power of a liquid is influenced by its intermolecular cohesive forces and that the strength of these forces can be expressed in terms of a *solubility parameter*. The initial parameters, which are concerned with the behaviour of non-polar, non-interacting liquids, are referred to as *Hildebrand solubility parameters*. Whilst these provide good quantitative predictions of the behaviour of a small number of hydrocarbons, they only provide a broad qualitative description of the behaviours of most liquids, because of the influence of factors such as hydrogen bond formation and ionization. The concept has been extended, however, by the introduction of *partial solubility parameters*, e.g. Hansen parameters and interaction parameters. These have improved the quantitative treatment of systems in which polar effects and interactions occur.

Solubility parameters, in conjunction with the electrostatic properties of liquids, e.g. dielectric constant and dipole moment, have often been linked by empirical or semi-empirical relationships either to these parameters or to solvent properties. Studies on solubility parameters are reported in the pharmaceutical literature. The use of dielectric constants as indicators of solvent power has also received attention but deviations from the behaviour predicted by such methods may occur in practice.

Mixtures of liquids are often used as solvents. If the two liquids have similar chemical structures, e.g. benzene and toluene, then neither tends to associate in the presence of the other and the solvent properties of a 50:50 mixture would be the mean of those of each pure liquid. If the liquids have dissimilar structures, e.g. water and propanol, then the molecules of one of them tend to associate with each other and so form regions of high concentration within the mixture. The solvent properties of this type of system are not so simply related to its composition as in the previous case. Studies have included the prediction of the solubilities of various compounds in ethanol/water mixtures and of phenobarbitone and hydrocortisone in ethanol/propylene glycol/water mixtures.

Solubility of solids in liquids

Solutions of solids in liquids are the most common type of solution encountered in pharmaceutical practice. A pharmaceutical scientist should therefore be aware of the general method of determining the solubility of a solid in a liquid and the various precautions that should be taken during such determinations.

Determination of the solubility of a solid in a liquid

The following points should be observed in all solubility determinations.

- The solvent and solute must be as pure as possible. The presence of small amounts of many impurities may either increase or decrease the measured solubility. This is a particular problem with early preformulation samples which are often impure and here special care must be taken (discussed further in Chapter 24).
- A saturated solution must be obtained before any solution is removed for analysis and then all undissolved material removed prior to analysis.
- The method of separating a sample of saturated solution from undissolved solute must be satisfactory.
- The method of analysing the solution must be sufficiently accurate and reliable.
- Temperature must be adequately controlled.

A saturated solution is obtained either by stirring excess powdered solute with solvent for several hours at the required temperature, until equilibrium has been attained, or by warming the solvent with an excess of the solute and allowing the mixture to cool to the required temperature. It is essential that some undissolved solid should be present at the completion of the cooling stage in order to ensure that the solution is saturated and not supersaturated.

A sample of the saturated solution is obtained for analysis by separating out undissolved solid from the solution. Filtration is usually used, but precautions should be taken to ensure that:

- it is carried out at the temperature of the solubility determination in order to prevent any change in the equilibrium between dissolved and undissolved solute
- loss of any volatile component does not occur
- adsorption of sample material onto surfaces within the filter is minimized

Membrane filters that can be used in conjunction with conventional syringes fitted with suitable in-line adapters have proved to be successful.

The amount of solute contained in the sample of saturated solution may be determined by a variety of methods, e.g. gravimetric analysis, UV spectrophotometry and chromatographic methods (particularly HPLC). The selection of an appropriate method is affected by the nature of the solute and the solvent and by the concentration of the solution.

Factors affecting the solubility of solids in liquids

Knowledge of these factors, together with their practical applications, as discussed below, is an important aspect of a pharmaceutical scientist's expertise. Additional information, which shows how some of these factors may be used to improve the solubilities and bioavailabilities of drugs, is given in Chapters 25 and 21, respectively.

Temperature The dissolution process is usually an endothermic one, i.e. heat is normally absorbed when dissolution occurs. In this type of system a rise in temperature will lead to an increase in the solubility of a solid with a positive heat of solution. Conversely, in the case of the less commonly occurring systems that exhibit exothermic dissolution, then an increase in temperature will result in a decrease in solubility.

Plots of solubility versus temperature, referred to as *solubility curves*, are often used to describe the effect of temperature on a given system. Some examples are shown in Figure 2.6. Most of the curves are continuous ones. However, abrupt changes in slope may be observed with some systems if a change in the nature of the dissolving solid occurs at a specific transition temperature. For example, sodium sulfate exists as the decahydrate $Na_2SO_4.10H_2O$ up to 32.5°C and its dissolution in water

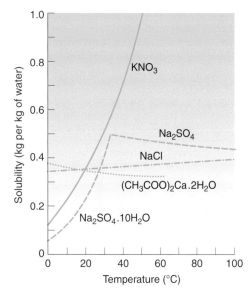

Fig. 2.6 Solubility curves for various substances in water.

is an endothermic process. Its solubility therefore increases with rise in temperature until 32.5°C is reached. Above this temperature the solid is converted into the anhydrous form (Na_2SO_4) and the dissolution of this compound is exothermic. The solubility therefore exhibits a change from a positive to a negative slope as the temperature exceeds the transition value.

Molecular structure of solute It should be appreciated from the previous comments in this chapter on the prediction of solubility that the natures of the solute and solvent will be of paramount importance in determining the solubility of a solid in a liquid. It should also be realized that even a small change in the molecular structure of a compound can have a marked effect on its solubility in a given liquid. For example, the introduction of a hydrophilic hydroxyl group can produce a large improvement in water solubility as evidenced by the more than 100-fold difference in the solubility of phenol compared with benzene.

In addition, the conversion of a weak acid to its sodium salt leads to a much greater degree of ionic dissociation of the compound when it dissolves in water. The overall interaction between solute and solvent is increased markedly and the solubility consequently rises. A specific example of this effect is provided by a comparison of the aqueous solubilities of salicylic acid and its sodium salt, which are 1 in 550 and 1 in 1, respectively.

The reduction in aqueous solubility of a parent drug by its esterification may also be cited as an example of the effects of changes in the chemical structure of the solute. Such a reduction in solubility may provide a suitable method for:

- masking the taste of a parent drug. For example, chloramphenicol palmitate has been used in paediatric suspensions rather than the more soluble and very bitter chloramphenicol base
- protecting the parent drug from excessive degradation in the gut, e.g. erythromycin propionate is less soluble and consequently less readily degraded than erythromycin
- increasing the ease of absorption of drugs from the gastrointestinal tract, e.g. erythromycin propionate is also more readily absorbed than erythromycin.

Nature of solvent: cosolvents The importance of the nature of the solvent has already been discussed in terms of the statement 'like dissolves like' and in relation to solubility parameters. In addition, the point has been made that mixtures of solvents may be employed. Such mixtures are often used in pharmaceutical practice in order to obtain aqueous-based systems that contain solutes in excess of their solubilities in pure water. This is achieved by using cosolvents such as ethanol or propylene glycol, which are miscible with water and which act as better solvents for the solute in question.

For example, the aqueous solubility of metronidazole is about 100 mg in 10 mL. The solubility of this drug can be increased exponentially by the incorporation of one or more water-miscible cosolvents so that a solution containing 500 mg in 10 mL (and thus suitable for parenteral administration in the treatment of anaerobic infection) can be obtained.

Crystal characteristics: polymorphism and solvation When the conditions under which crystallization is allowed to occur are varied then some substances produce crystals in which the constituent molecules are aligned in different ways with respect to one another in the lattice structure. These different crystalline forms of the same substance, which are known as *polymorphs*, consequently possess different lattice energies and this difference is reflected by changes in other properties. For example, the polymorphic form with the lowest free energy will be the most stable and possess the highest melting point. Other less stable (or metastable) forms will tend to transform into the most stable one at rates that depend on the energy differences between the metastable and stable forms.

Many drugs exhibit polymorphism, e.g. steroids, barbiturates and sulfonamides. Polymorphs are explained more fully in Chapter 8, which also includes an explanation of why polymorphs appear to have different solubilities. Examples of the importance of polymorphism with respect to the bioavailabilities of drugs are given in Chapter 21.

The effect of polymorphism on solubility is particularly important from a pharmaceutical point of view, because it provides a means of increasing the solubility of a crystalline material, and hence its rate of dissolution, by using a metastable polymorph.

Although the more soluble polymorphs are metastable and will convert to the stable form, the rate of such conversion is often slow enough for the metastable form to be regarded as being sufficiently stable from a pharmaceutical point of view. The degree of conversion should obviously be monitored during storage of the drug product to ensure that its efficacy is not altered significantly. There are products on the market containing a more soluble, but less stable, polymorph of the drug. But the chosen polymorph is 'stable enough' to survive the approved storage conditions and shelf life.

Conversion to the less soluble and most stable polymorph may contribute to the growth of crystals in suspension formulations. Examples of the importance of polymorphism with respect to the occurrence of crystal growth in suspensions are given in Chapter 27.

The absence of crystalline structure that is usually associated with an *amorphous* powder (discussed in Chapter 8) may also lead to an increase in the solubility of a drug when compared with that of its crystalline form.

In addition to the effect of polymorphism, the lattice structures of crystalline materials may be altered by the incorporation of molecules of the solvent from which crystallization occurred. The resultant solids are called *solvates* and the phenomenon is referred to correctly as *solvation* and sometimes incorrectly and confusingly as *pseudopolymorphism*. The alteration in crystal structure that accompanies solvation will affect the internal energetics of the solid so that the solubilities of solvated and unsolvated crystals will differ.

If water is the solvating molecule, i.e. a *hydrate* is formed, then the interaction between the substance and water that occurs in the crystal phase reduces the amount of energy liberated when the solid hydrate dissolves in water. Consequently, hydrated crystals tend to exhibit a lower aqueous solubility than their unhydrated forms. This decrease in solubility can lead to precipitation from solutions of drugs.

In contrast, the aqueous solubilities of other, i.e. non-aqueous, solvates are often greater than those of the unsolvated forms. Examples of the effects of solvation and the attendant changes in solubilities of drugs on their bioavailabilities are given in Chapter 21.

Particle size of the solid The changes in interfacial free energy that accompany the dissolution of particles of varying sizes cause the solubility of a substance to increase with decreasing particle size, as indicated by Eqn 2.10.

$$\log \frac{S}{S_0} = \frac{2\gamma M}{2.303RT\rho r} \qquad (2.10)$$

where S is the solubility of small particles of radius r, S_o is the normal solubility (i.e. of a solid consisting of fairly large particles), γ is the interfacial energy, M is the molecular weight of the solid, ρ is the density of the bulk solid, R is the gas constant and T is the thermodynamic temperature.

The increase in solubility with decrease in particle size ceases when the particles have a very small radius (less than about 1 μm), and any further decrease in size causes a decrease in solubility. It has been postulated that this change arises from the presence of an electrical charge on the particles and that the effect of this charge becomes more important as the particle size decreases. Such solubility changes are rarely a problem in conventional dosage forms and drug delivery but could be significant with nanotechnology products.

pH If the pH of a solution of either a weakly acidic drug or a salt of such a drug is reduced then the proportion of unionized acid molecules in the solution increases. Precipitation may occur, therefore, because the solubility of the unionized species is less than that of the ionized form. Conversely, in the case of solutions of weakly basic drugs or their salts, precipitation is favoured by an increase in pH. Such precipitation is an example of one type of chemical incompatibility that may be encountered in the formulation of liquid medicines.

This relationship between pH and solubility of ionized solutes is extremely important with respect to the ionization of weakly acidic and basic drugs as they pass through the gastrointestinal tract and can experience pH changes between about 1 and 8. This will affect the degree of ionization of the drug molecule which in turn influences their solubility and their ability to be absorbed. This aspect is discussed elsewhere in this book in some detail and the reader is referred in particular to Chapters 3 and 21.

The relationship between pH, the solubility and pK_a of weakly acidic or weakly basic drugs is given a modification of the Henderson–Hasselbalch equation. To avoid repetition here, the reader is referred to the relevant section of Chapter 3.

Common ion effect The equilibrium in a saturated solution of a sparingly soluble salt in contact with undissolved solid may be represented by:

$$\underset{\text{(solid)}}{AB} \Leftrightarrow \underset{\text{(ions)}}{A^+ + B^-} \qquad (2.11)$$

From the Law of Mass Action, the equilibrium constant K for this reversible reaction is given by Eqn 2.12:

$$K = \frac{[A^+][B^-]}{[AB]} \qquad (2.12)$$

where the square brackets signify concentrations of the respective components. Since the concentration of a solid may be regarded as being constant then:

$$K'_S = [A^+][B^-] \qquad (2.13)$$

where K'_S is a constant, which is known as the *solubility product* of compound AB.

If each molecule of the salt contains more than one ion of each type, e.g. $A_x^+ B_y^-$, then in the definition of the solubility product, the concentration of each ion is expressed to the appropriate power, i.e.:

$$K'_S = [A^+]^x [B^-]^y$$

These equations for the solubility product are only applicable to solutions of sparingly soluble salts.

If K'_S is exceeded by the product of the concentration of the ions, i.e. $[A^+][B^-]$ (or $[A^+]^x[B^-]^y$ if appropriate) then the equilibrium shown above, Eqn 2.11, moves towards the left in order to restore the equilibrium, and solid AB is precipitated. The product $[A^+][B^-]$ will be increased by the addition of more A^+ ions produced by the dissociation of another compound, e.g. $AX \rightarrow A^+ + X^-$, where A^+ is the common ion. Solid AB will be precipitated and the solubility of this compound is therefore decreased. This is known as the *common ion effect*. The addition of common B^- ions would have the same effect.

The precipitating effect of common ions is, in fact, less than that predicted from Eqn 2.13. The reason for this is explained in the following section.

Effect of indifferent electrolytes on the solubility product   The solubility of a sparingly soluble electrolyte may be increased by the addition of a second electrolyte that does not possess ions common to the first, i.e. an different electrolyte.

The definition of the solubility product of a sparingly soluble electrolyte in terms of the concentration of ions produced at equilibrium, as indicated by Eqn 2.13, is only an approximation from the more exact thermodynamic relationship expressed by Eqn 2.14:

$$K'_S = a_{A^+} \, a_{B^-} \qquad (2.14)$$

where K'_S is the solubility product of compound AB and a_{A^+} and a_{B^-} are known as the activities of the respective ions. The activity of a particular ion may be regarded as its 'effective concentration'. In general, this has a lower value than the actual concentration, because some ions produced by dissociation of the electrolyte are strongly associated with oppositely charged ions and do not contribute so effectively as completely unallocated ions to the properties of the system. At infinite dilution, the wide separation of ions prevents any interionic association, and the molar concentration (c_{A^+}) and activity (a_{A^+}) of a given ion (A^+) are then equal, i.e.:

$$a_A = c_{A^+} \ or \ \frac{a_{A^+}}{c_{A^+}} = 1 \qquad (2.15)$$

As the concentration increases, the effects of interionic association are no longer negligible, and the ratio of activity to molar concentration becomes less than unity, i.e.:

$$f_{A^+} = \frac{a_{A^+}}{c_{A^+}} \qquad (2.16)$$

or

$$a_{A^+} = c_{A^+} \cdot f_{A^+} \qquad (2.17)$$

where f_{A^+} is known as the activity coefficient of A^+. If concentrations and activity coefficients are used instead of activities in Eqn 2. 14 then:

$$K_S = (c_{A^+} \cdot c_{B^-}) \, (f_{A^+} \cdot f_{B^-}) \qquad (2.18)$$

The product of the concentrations, i.e. ($c_{A^+} \cdot c_{B^-}$), will be a constant (K'_S) as shown by Eqn 2.13, and ($f_{A^+} \cdot f_{B^-}$) may be equated to $f_{A^+B^-}$, where $f_{A^+B^-}$ is the mean activity coefficient of the salt AB, i.e.:

$$K_S = K'_S f_{A^+B^-} \qquad (2.19)$$

Since $f_{A^+B^-}$ varies with the overall concentration of ions present in solution (the ionic strength), and since K_S is a constant, it follows that K'_S must also vary with the ionic strength of the solution in an inverse manner to the variation of $f_{A^+B^-}$. Thus, in a system containing a sparingly soluble electrolyte without a common ion, the ionic

strength will have an appreciable value and the mean activity coefficient $f_{A^+B^-}$ will be less than one.

From Eqn 2.19 it will be seen that K'_S will, therefore, be greater than K_S. In fact, the concentration solubility product K'_S will become larger and larger as the ionic strength of the solution increases. The solubility of AB will therefore increase as the concentration of added electrolyte increases.

This argument also accounts for the fact that if no allowance is made for the variation in activity with ionic strength of the medium, the precipitating effect of common ions is less than that predicted from the Law of Mass Action.

Effect of non-electrolytes on the solubility of electrolytes   The solubility of electrolytes depends on the dissociation of dissolved molecules into ions. The case of this dissociation is affected by the dielectric constant of the solvent, which is a measure of the polar nature of the solvent. Liquids with a high dielectric constant (e.g. water) are able to reduce the attractive forces that operate between oppositely charged ions produced by dissociation of an electrolyte.

If a water-soluble non-electrolyte, such as alcohol, is added to an aqueous solution of a sparingly soluble electrolyte, the solubility of the latter is decreased because the alcohol lowers the dielectric constant of the solvent and ionic dissociation of the electrolyte becomes more difficult.

Effect of electrolytes on the solubility of non-electrolytes   Non-electrolytes do not dissociate into ions in aqueous solution, and in dilute solution the dissolved species therefore consists of single molecules. Their solubility in water depends on the formation of weak intermolecular bonds (hydrogen bonds) between their molecules and those of water. The presence of a very soluble electrolyte, the ions of which have a marked affinity for water, will reduce the solubility of a non-electrolyte by competing for the aqueous solvent and breaking the intermolecular bonds between the non-electrolyte and water. This effect is important in the precipitation of proteins.

Complex formation   The apparent solubility of a solute in a particular liquid may be increased or decreased by the addition of a third substance which forms an intermolecular complex with the solute. The solubility of the complex will determine the apparent change in the solubility of the original solute. Use is made of formation of a complex as an aid to solubility in the preparation of solution of mercuric iodide (HgI_2). The latter is not very soluble in water but it is soluble in aqueous solutions of potassium iodide because of the formation of a water-soluble complex, $K_2(HgI_4)$.

Solubilizing agents   These agents are capable of forming large aggregates or micelles in solution when their concentrations exceed certain values. In aqueous solution the centre of these aggregates resembles a separate organic phase and organic solutes may be taken up by the aggregates, thus producing an apparent increase in their solubilities in water. This phenomenon is known as *solubilization*. A similar phenomenon occurs in organic solvents containing dissolved solubilizing agents because the centre of the aggregates in these systems constitutes a more polar region than the bulk of the organic solvent. If polar solutes are taken up into these regions their apparent solubilities in the organic solvents are increased.

Solubility of gases in liquids

The amount of gas that will dissolve in a liquid is determined by the natures of the two components and by temperature and pressure.

Provided that no reaction occurs between the gas and liquid then the effect of pressure is indicated by Henry's Law which states that at constant temperature, the solubility of a gas in a liquid is directly proportional to the pressure of the gas above the liquid. The law may be expressed by Eqn 2.20:

$$w = kp \qquad (2.20)$$

where w is the mass of gas dissolved by unit volume of solvent at an equilibrium pressure p and k is a proportionality constant. Although Henry's Law is most applicable at high temperatures and low pressures, when solubility is low, it provides a satisfactory description of the behaviour of most systems at normal temperatures and reasonable pressures, unless solubility is very high or reaction occurs. Eqn 2.20 also applies to the solubility of each gas in a solution of several gases in the same liquid provided that p represents the partial pressure of a particular gas.

The solubility of most gases in liquids decreases as the temperature rises. This provides a means of removing dissolved gases. For example, water for injections free from either carbon dioxide or air may be prepared by boiling water with minimum exposure to air and prevention of access of air during cooling. The presence of electrolytes may also decrease the solubility of a gas in water by a 'salting out' process, which is caused by the marked attraction exerted between electrolyte and water.

Solubility of liquids in liquids

The components of an ideal solution are miscible in all proportions. Such complete miscibility is also observed in some real binary systems, e.g. ethanol and water, under normal conditions. However, if one of the components tends to self-associate because the attractions between its own molecules are greater than those between its molecules and those of the other component, i.e. if a positive deviation from Raoult's Law occurs, the miscibility of the components may be reduced. The extent of the reduction depends on the strength of the self-association and, therefore, on the degree of deviation from Raoult's Law (Raoult's Law is discussed more fully in Chapter 3). Thus, partial miscibility may be observed in some systems whereas virtual immiscibility may be exhibited when the self-association is very strong and the positive deviation from Raoult's Law is large.

In those cases where partial miscibility occurs under normal conditions then the degree of miscibility is usually dependent on the temperature. This dependency is indicated by the *phase rule*, introduced by J. Willard Gibbs, which is expressed quantitatively by Eqn 2.21:

$$F = C - P + 2 \qquad (2.21)$$

where P and C are the numbers of phases and components in the system, respectively, and F is the number of degrees of freedom, i.e. the number of variable conditions such as temperature, pressure and composition, that must be stated in order to define completely the state of the system at equilibrium.

The overall effect of temperature variation on the degree of miscibility in these systems is usually described by means of phase diagrams, which are graphs of temperature versus composition at constant pressure. For convenience of discussion of their phase diagrams, the partially miscible systems may be divided into the following types:

Systems showing an increase in miscibility with rise in temperature

A positive deviation from Raoult's Law arises from a difference in the cohesive forces that exist between the molecules of each component in a liquid mixture. This difference becomes more marked as the temperature decreases and the positive deviation may then result in a decrease in miscibility sufficient to cause the separation of the mixture into two phases. Each phase consists of a saturated solution of one component in the other liquid. Such mutually saturated solutions are known as *conjugate solutions*.

The equilibria that occur in mixtures of partially miscible liquids may be followed either by shaking the two liquids together at constant temperature and analysing samples from each phase after equilibrium has been attained, or by observing the temperature at which known proportions of the two liquids, contained in sealed glass ampoules, become miscible, as shown by the disappearance of turbidity.

Systems showing a decrease in miscibility with rise in temperature

A few mixtures, which probably involve compound formation, exhibit a lower critical solution temperature

(CST), e.g. triethylamine plus water and paraldehyde plus water. The formation of a compound produces a negative deviation from Raoult's Law, and miscibility therefore increases as the temperature falls, as shown in Figure 2.7.

Systems showing upper and lower critical solution temperatures

The decrease in miscibility with increase in temperature in systems having a lower CST is not indefinite. Above a certain temperature, positive deviations from Raoult's Law become important and miscibility starts to increase again with further rise in temperature. This behaviour produces a closed-phase diagram as shown in Figure 2.8. This behaviour is shown by the nicotine–water system.

In some mixtures where an upper and lower CST are expected, these points are not, in fact, observed since a phase change by one of the components occurs before the relevant CST is reached. For example, the ether–water system should exhibit a lower CST, but water freezes before the temperature is reached.

Effects of added substances on critical solution temperatures

It has already been stated that a CST is an invariant point at constant pressure. However, these temperatures are very sensitive to impurities or added substances. The effects of additives are summarized by Table 2.3.

Blending

The increase in miscibility of two liquids caused by the addition of a third substance is referred to as *blending*.

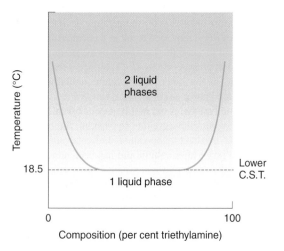

Fig. 2.7 Temperature–composition diagram for the triethylamine–water system exhibiting a decrease in miscibility with rise in temperature.

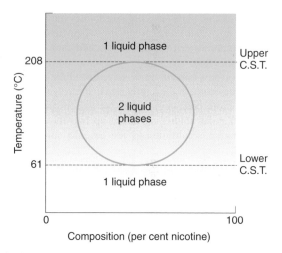

Fig. 2.8 Temperature–composition diagram for the nicotine–water system exhibiting upper and lower critical solution temperatures.

The use of propylene glycol as a blending agent, which improves the miscibility of volatile oils and water, can be explained in terms of a ternary-phase diagram. This diagram is a triangular plot which indicates the effects of changes in the relative proportions of the three components at constant temperature and pressure and it presents a good example of the interpretation and use of such phase diagrams.

Distribution of solutes between immiscible liquids

Partition coefficients

When a substance which is soluble in both components of a mixture of immiscible liquids is dissolved in such a mixture, when equilibrium is attained at constant temperature, it is found that the solute is distributed between the two liquids in such a way that the ratio of the activities of the substance in each liquid is a constant. This is known as the Nernst Distribution Law, expressed by Eqn 2.22:

$$\frac{a_A}{a_B} = \text{constant} \tag{2.22}$$

where a_A and a_B are the activities of the solute in solvents A and B, respectively. When the solutions are dilute or when the solute behaves ideally, the activities may be replaced by concentrations (C_A and C_B):

$$\frac{C_A}{C_B} = K \tag{2.23}$$

The constant K is known as the *distribution coefficient* or *partition coefficient*. In the case of sparingly soluble substances, K is approximately equal to the ratio of the solubilities (S_A and S_B) of the solute in each liquid. Thus:

Table 2.3   The effects of additives on critical solution temperature (CST)

Type of CST	Solubility of additive in each component	Effect on CST	Effect on miscibility
Upper	Approx. equally soluble in both components	Lowered	Increased
Upper	Readily soluble in one component but not in other	Raised	Decreased
Lower	Approx. equally soluble in both components	Raised	Increased
Lower	Readily soluble in one component but not in other	Lowered	Decreased

$$\frac{S_A}{S_B} = K \qquad (2.24)$$

In most other systems, however, deviation from ideal behaviour invalidates Eqn 2.24. For example, if the solute exists as monomers in solvent A and as dimers in solvent B, the distribution coefficient is given by Eqn 2.25, in which the square root of the concentration of the dimeric form is used:

$$K = \frac{C_A}{\sqrt{C_B}} \qquad (2.25)$$

If the dissociation into ions occurs in the aqueous layer, B, of a mixture of immiscible liquids, then the degree of dissociation (α) should be taken into account, as indicated by Eqn 2.26:

$$K = \frac{C_A}{C_B(1 - \alpha)} \qquad (2.26)$$

The solvents in which the concentrations of the solute are expressed should be indicated when partition coefficients are quoted. For example, a partition coefficient of 2 for a solute distributed between oil and water may also be expressed as a partition coefficient between water and oil of 0.5. This can be represented as $K^{oil}_{water} = 2$ and $K^{water}_{oil} = 0.5$. The abbreviation K^o_w is often used for the former and this notation has become the most commonly used.

Solubility of solids in solids

If two solids are either melted together and then cooled or dissolved in a suitable solvent that is then removed by evaporation, the solid that is redeposited from the melt or the solution will either be a one-phase solid solution or a two-phase eutectic mixture.

In a solid solution, as in other types of solution, the molecules of one component (the solute) are dispersed molecularly throughout the other component (the solvent). Complete miscibility of two solid components is only achieved if:

- the molecular size of the solute is similar to that of the solvent so that a molecule of the former can be substituted for one of the latter in its crystal lattice structure, or

- the solute molecules are much smaller than the solvent molecules so that the former can be accommodated in the spaces of the solvent lattice structure.

These two types of solvent mechanism are referred to as *substitution* and *interstitial* effects, respectively. Since these criteria are only satisfied in relatively few systems then it is more common to observe *partial miscibility* of solids. Thus, dilute solutions of solids in solids may be encountered in systems of pharmaceutical interest; for example, when the solvent is a polymeric material with large spaces between its intertwined molecules that can accommodate solute molecules.

Unlike a solution, a *simple eutectic* consists of an intimate mixture of the two microcrystalline components in a fixed composition. However, both solid solutions and eutectics provide a means of dispersing a relatively water-insoluble drug in a very fine form, i.e. as molecules or microcrystalline particles, respectively, throughout a water-soluble solid. When the latter carrier solid is dissolved away, the molecules or small crystals of insoluble drug may dissolve more rapidly than a conventional powder because the contact area between drug and water is increased. The rate of dissolution and, consequently, the bioavailabilities of poorly soluble drugs may be improved, therefore, by the use of solid solutions or eutectics.

SUMMARY

This chapter has shown that dissolution must be considered as a change in phase of a molecule or ion. Most often this is from solid to liquid. Simple diffusional mechanisms and equations usually define this rate and extent of this process. The concept of solubility in a pharmaceutical context has also been discussed. The chapter that follows will describe the properties of the solution thus produced.

REFERENCES

Florence, A.T., Attwood, D. (2006) *Physicochemical Principles of Pharmacy*, 4th edn. Pharmaceutical Press Ltd, London.

Hildebrand, J.H., Scott, R.L. (1962) *Regular Solutions*. Prentice-Hall, New Jersey.

Noyes, A.A., Whitney, W.R. (1897) The rate of solution of solid substances in their own solutions. *Journal of the American Chemical Society*, **19**, 930.

BIBLIOGRAPHY

Barton, A.F.M. (1983) *Handbook of Solubility Parameters and other Cohesion Parameters*. CRC Press, Boca Raton, Florida.

Beerbower, A., Wu, P.L., Martin, A. (1984) Expanded solubility parameter approach. I. Naphthalene and benzoic acid in individual solvents. *Journal of Pharmaceutical Science*, **73,** 179-188.

British Pharmacopoeia (latest edition). Stationery Office, London.

Carstensen, J.T. (1972) *Theory of Pharmaceutical Systems, Vol. 1. General Principles*. Academic Press, London.

Eyring, H., Henderson, D., Jost, W. (1971) *Physical Chemistry: An Advanced Treatise, Volume VIIIA Liquid State*. Academic Press, London.

Haleblian, J., McCrone, W. (1969) Pharmaceutical applications of polymorphism. *Journal of Pharmaceutical Science*, **58**, 911-929.

Hildebrand, J.H., Prausnitz, J.M., Scott, R.L. (1970) *Regular and Related Solutions: The Solubility of Gases, Liquids and Solids*. Van Nostrand Reinhold, New York.

Leeson, L., Cartsensen, J. T. (1974) *Dissolution Technology*. IPT Academy of Pharmaceutical Science, Washington DC.

Martin, A., Wu, P.L., Beerbower, A. (1984) Expanded solubility parameter approach. II. p-Hydroxybenzoic acid and methyl p-hydroxybenzoate in individual solvents. *Journal of Pharmaceutical Science*, **73**, 188-194.

Price, N.C., Dwek, R.A. (1979) *Principles and Problems in Physical Chemistry for Biochemists*, 2nd edn. Clarendon Press, Oxford.

Rowe, R.C., Sheskey, P.J., Owen, S.C. (2006) *Handbook of Pharmaceutical Excipients,* 5th edn. The Pharmaceutical Press, London.

Rowlinson, J.S., Swinton, F.L. (1982) *Liquids and Liquid Mixtures*, 3rd edn. Butterworth Scientific, London.

Swarbrick, J. (1970) Drug dissolution and bioavailability. In: Swarbrick, J. (ed.) *Current Concepts in the Pharmaceutical Sciences: Biopharmaceutics*. Lea and Febiger, Philadelphia.

United States Pharmacopeia and National Formulary (latest edition). United States Pharmacopeial Convention, Rockville, Maryland, USA.

Wallwork, S.C., Grant, D.J.W. (1977) *Physical Chemistry for Students of Pharmacy and Biology*, 3rd edn. Longman, London.

Williams, V.R., Mattice, W.L., Williams, H. (1978) *Basic Physical Chemistry for the Life Sciences*, 3rd edn. W. H. Freeman, San Francisco.

3

Properties of solutions

M. E. Aulton

CHAPTER CONTENTS

INTRODUCTION

The aim of this chapter is to provide information on certain properties of solutions that relate to their applications in pharmaceutical science. This chapter deals mainly with the physicochemical properties of solutions that are important with respect to pharmaceutical systems. These aspects are covered in sufficient detail to introduce the pharmaceutical scientist to these properties to allow an understanding of their importance in dosage form design and drug delivery. Much is published elsewhere in far greater detail and any reader requiring this additional information can trace some of this by referring to the bibliography at the end of the chapter.

TYPES OF SOLUTION

Solutions may be classified based on the physical states (i.e. gas, liquid or solid) of the solute(s) and solvent. Although a variety of different types can exist, solutions of pharmaceutical interest virtually all possess liquid solvents. In addition, the solutes are predominantly solid substances. Consequently, most of the information in this chapter is relevant to solutions of solids in liquids.

Vapour pressures of solids, liquids and solutions

An understanding of many of the properties of solutions requires an appreciation of the concept of an ideal solution and its use as a reference system, to which the behaviours of real (non-ideal) solutions can be compared. This concept is itself based on a consideration of vapour pressure. The present section serves as an introduction to the later discussions on ideal and non-ideal solutions.

The kinetic theory of matter indicates that the thermal motion of molecules of a substance in its gaseous state is more than adequate to overcome the attractive forces that exist between the molecules. Thus, the molecules will undergo a completely random movement within the confines of the container. The situation is reversed, however, when the temperature is lowered sufficiently so that a *condensed phase* is formed. Here the thermal motions of the molecules are now insufficient to overcome completely the intermolecular attractive forces and some degree of order in the relative arrangement of molecules occurs. This condensed state may be either liquid or solid.

If the intermolecular forces are so strong that a high degree of order, the structure of which is hardly influenced by thermal motions, is brought about then the substance is usually in the solid state.

In the liquid condensed state, the relative influences of thermal motion and intermolecular attractive forces are intermediate between those in the gaseous and solid states. Thus, the effects of interactions between the permanent and induced dipoles, i.e. the so-called van der Waals forces of attraction, lead to some degree of coherence between the molecules of liquids. Consequently, liquids occupy a definite volume with a surface, unlike gases, and whilst there is evidence of structure within liquids, such structure is much less apparent than in solids.

Although both solids and liquids are condensed systems with cohering molecules, some of the surface molecules in these systems will occasionally acquire sufficient energy to overcome the attractive forces exerted by adjacent molecules. The molecules can therefore escape from the surface to form a vapour phase. If temperature is maintained constant, equilibrium will be established eventually between the vapour phase and the condensed phase. The pressure exerted by the vapour at this equilibrium is referred to as the *vapour pressure* of the substance.

All condensed systems have the inherent ability to give rise to a vapour pressure. However, the vapour pressures exerted by solids are usually much lower than those exerted by liquids, because the intermolecular forces in solids are stronger than those in liquids. Thus, the escaping tendency for surface molecules is higher in liquids. Consequently, surface loss of vapour from liquids by the process of evaporation is more common than surface loss of vapour from solids by sublimation.

In the case of a liquid solvent containing a dissolved solute, molecules of both solvent and solute may show a tendency to escape from the surface and so contribute to the vapour pressure. The relative tendencies to escape will depend on the relative numbers of the different molecules in the surface of the solution, and on the relative strengths of the attractive forces between adjacent solvent molecules on the one hand and between solute and solvent molecules on the other hand. Because the intermolecular forces between solid solutes and liquid solvents tend to be relatively strong, such solute molecules do not generally

escape from the surface of a solution nor contribute to the vapour pressure. In other words, the solute is generally non-volatile and the vapour pressure arises solely from the dynamic equilibrium that is set up between the rates of evaporation and condensation of solvent molecules contained in the solution. In a mixture of miscible liquids, i.e. a liquid in liquid solution, the molecules of both components are likely to evaporate and contribute to the overall vapour pressure exerted by the solution.

Ideal solutions: Raoult's Law

The concept of an ideal solution has been introduced in order to provide a model system that can be used as a standard, to which real or non-ideal solutions can be compared. In the model, it is assumed that the strengths of all intermolecular forces are identical. Thus solvent/solvent, solute/solvent and solute/solute interactions are the same and are equal to the strength of the intermolecular interactions in either the pure solvent or pure solute. Because of this equality, the relative tendencies of solute and solvent molecules to escape from the surface of the solution will be determined only by their relative numbers in the surface.

Since a solution is homogeneous by definition then the relative number of these surface molecules will be the same as the relative number in the whole of the solution. The latter can be expressed conveniently by the mole fractions of the components because, for a binary solution (one with two components), $x_1 + x_2 = 1$, where x_1 and x_2 are the mole fractions of the solute and solvent, respectively.

The total vapour pressure (P) exerted by a binary solution is given by Eqn 3.1:

$$P = p_1 + p_2 \qquad (3.1)$$

where p_1 and p_2 are the partial vapour pressures exerted above the solution by the solute and solvent, respectively. Raoult's Law states that the partial vapour pressure (p) exerted by a volatile component in a solution at a given temperature is equal to the vapour pressure of the pure component at the same temperature (p°) multiplied by its mole fraction in the solution (x), i.e.:

$$p = p^\circ x \qquad (3.2)$$

Thus from Eqns 3.1 and 3.2:

$$P = p_1 + p_2 = p_1^\circ x_1 + p_2^\circ x_2 \qquad (3.3)$$

where p_1° and p_2° are the vapour pressures exerted by pure solute and pure solvent, respectively. If the total vapour pressure of the solution is described by Eqn 3.3, then Raoult's Law is obeyed by the system.

One of the consequences of the preceding comments is that an ideal solution may be defined as one that obeys

Raoult's Law. In addition, ideal behaviour should be expected to be exhibited only by real systems composed of chemically similar components, because it is only in such systems that the condition of equal intermolecular forces between components (as assumed in the ideal model) is likely to be satisfied. Consequently, Raoult's Law is obeyed over an appreciable concentration range by relatively few systems in reality.

Mixtures of benzene + toluene, n-hexane + n-heptane, ethyl bromide + ethyl iodide and binary mixtures of fluorinated hydrocarbons are systems that exhibit ideal behaviour. Note the chemical similarity of the two components of the mix in each example.

Real or non-ideal solutions

The majority of real solutions do not exhibit ideal behaviour because solute–solute, solute–solvent and solvent–solvent forces of interaction are unequal. These inequalities alter the effective concentration of each component so that it cannot be represented by a normal expression of concentration, such as the mole fraction term x that is used in Eqns 3.2 and 3.3. Consequently, deviations from Raoult's Law are often exhibited by real solutions and the previous equations are not obeyed in such cases. These equations can be modified, however, by substituting each concentration term (x) by a measure of the effective concentration; this is provided by the so-called *activity* (or *thermodynamic activity*), a. Thus, Eqn 3.2 is converted into Eqn 3.4:

$$p = p^{\circ}a \qquad (3.4)$$

and the resulting equation is applicable to all systems whether they are ideal or non-ideal. It should be noted that if a solution exhibits ideal behaviour then a equals x, whereas a will not equal x if deviations from such behaviour are apparent. The ratio of activity divided by the mole fraction is termed the *activity coefficient* (f) and it provides a measure of the deviation from ideality. Thus when $a = x$, $f = 1$.

If the attractive forces between solute and solvent molecules are weaker than those exerted between the solute molecules themselves or between the solvent molecules themselves then the components will have little affinity for each other. The escaping tendency of the surface molecules in such a system is increased when compared with an ideal solution. In other words, p_1, p_2 and therefore P are greater than expected from Raoult's Law and the thermodynamic activities of the components are greater than their mole fractions, i.e. $a_1 > x_1$ and $a_2 > x_2$. This type of system is said to show a *positive deviation* from Raoult's Law and the extent of the deviation increases as the miscibility of the components decreases. For example, a mixture of alcohol and benzene shows a smaller

deviation than the less miscible mixture of water + diethyl ether whilst the virtually immiscible mixture of benzene + water exhibits a very large positive deviation.

Conversely, if the solute and solvent molecules have a strong mutual affinity (that sometimes may result in the formation of a complex or compound) then a negative deviation from Raoult's Law occurs. Thus, p_1, p_2 and thus P are lower than expected and $a_1 < x_1$ and $a_2 < x_2$. Examples of systems that show this type of behaviour include chloroform + acetone, pyridine + acetic acid and water + nitric acid.

Although most systems are non-ideal and deviate either positively or negatively from Raoult's Law, such deviations are small when a solution is dilute. This is because the effect that a small amount of solute has on interactions between solvent molecules is minimal. Thus, dilute solutions tend to exhibit ideal behaviour and the activities of their components approximate to their mole fractions, i.e. a_1 approximately equals x_1 and a_2 approximately equals x_2. Conversely, large deviations may be observed when the concentration of a solution is high.

Knowledge of the consequences of such marked deviations is particularly important in relation to the distillation of liquid mixtures. For example, the complete separation of the components of a mixture by fractional distillation may not be achievable if large positive or negative deviations from Raoult's Law give rise to the formation of so-called azeotropic mixtures with minimum and maximum boiling points, respectively.

IONIZATION OF SOLUTES

Many solutes dissociate into ions if the dielectric constant of the solvent is high enough to cause sufficient separation of the attractive forces between the oppositely charged ions. Such solutes are termed *electrolytes* and their ionization (or dissociation) has several consequences that are often important in pharmaceutical practice. Some of these consequences are indicated below.

Hydrogen ion concentration and pH

The dissociation of water can be represented by Eqn 3.5:

$$H_2O \leftrightarrow H^+ + OH^- \qquad (3.5)$$

It should be realized that this is a simplified representation because the hydrogen and hydroxyl ions do not exist in a free state but combine with undissociated water molecules to yield more complex ions such as H_3O^+ and $H_7O_4^-$.

In pure water the concentrations of H^+ and OH^- ions are equal and at 25°C both have the values of 1×10^{-7} mol L^{-1}. The Lowry–Brönsted theory of acids and bases defines an acid as a substance which donates a proton (or hydrogen ion) so it follows that the addition of an acidic solute to water will result in a hydrogen ion concentration that exceeds the pure water value. Conversely, the addition of a base, which is defined as a substance that accepts protons, will decrease the concentration of hydrogen ions in solution. The hydrogen ion concentration range decreases from 1 mol L^{-1} for a strong acid down to 1×10^{-14} mol L^{-1} for a strong base.

In order to avoid the frequent use of inconvenient numbers that arise from this very wide range, the concept of pH has been introduced as a more convenient measure of hydrogen ion concentration. pH is defined as the negative logarithm of the hydrogen ion concentration [H$^+$] as shown by Eqn 3.6:

$$pH = -\log_{10}[H^+] \tag{3.6}$$

so that the pH of a neutral solution like pure water is 7. This is because, as mentioned above, the concentration of H$^+$ ions (and thus OH$^-$ ions) in pure water is 1×10^{-7} mol L^{-1}. The pHs of acidic solutions will be less than 7 and the pH of alkaline solutions will be greater than 7.

pH has several important implications in pharmaceutical practice. It has an effect on:

- the degree of ionization of drugs that are weak acids or bases
- the solubilities of drugs that are weak acids or bases
- the ease of absorption of drugs from the gastrointestinal tract into the blood. For example, many (about 75%) drugs are weak bases or their salts. These drugs dissolve more rapidly in the low pH of the acidic stomach. However, there will be little or no absorption of the drug there as it will be too ionized. Drug absorption normally will have to wait until the more alkaline intestine where the ionization of the dissolved base is reduced
- the stabilities of many drugs
- body tissues (both extremes of pH are injurious).

These implications have great consequence during peroral drug delivery as the pH experienced by the drug could range from pH 1 to 8 at it passes down the gastrointestinal tract. The interrelationship between degree of ionization, solubility and pH is discussed below in this chapter. The biopharmaceutical consequences are discussed in Chapter 21.

Dissociation (or ionization) constants; pK_a and pK_b

Many drugs are either weak acids or weak bases. In solutions of these drugs, equilibria exist between undissociated molecules and their ions. In a solution of a weakly acidic drug HA, the equilibrium may be represented by Eqn 3.7:

$$HA \leftrightarrow H^+ + A^- \tag{3.7}$$

Similarly, the protonation of a weakly basic drug B can be represented by Eqn 3.8:

$$B + H^+ \leftrightarrow BH^+ \tag{3.8}$$

In solutions of most salts of strong acids or strong bases in water, such equilibria are shifted strongly to one side of the equation because these compounds are virtually completely ionized. In the case of aqueous solutions of weaker acids and bases, the degree of ionization is much more variable and indeed, as will be seen, controllable.

The *ionization constant* (or *dissociation constant*) K_a of a partially ionized weakly acid species can be obtained by applying the Law of Mass Action to yield Eqn 3.9 in which [I^+] and [I^-] represent the concentrations of the dissociated ionized species and [U] is the concentration of the unionized species.

$$K_a = \frac{[I^+][I^-]}{[U]} \tag{3.9}$$

For the case of a weak acid this can be written (from Eqn 3.7) as:

$$K_a = \frac{[H^+][A^-]}{[HA]} \tag{3.10}$$

Taking logarithms of both sides of Eqn 3.10 yields:

$$\log_{10} K_a = \log_{10}[H^+] + \log_{10}[A^-] - \log_{10}[HA] \tag{3.11}$$

The signs in this equation may be reversed to give Eqn 3.12:

$$-\log_{10} K_a = -\log_{10}[H^+] - \log_{10}[A^-] + \log_{10}[HA] \tag{3.12}$$

The symbol pK_a is used to represent the negative logarithm of the acid dissociation constant K_a in an analogous way that pH is used to represent the negative logarithm of the hydrogen ion concentration (as Eqn 3.6). Therefore:

$$pK_a = -\log_{10} K_a \tag{3.13}$$

Now Eqn 3.12 may therefore be rewritten as Eqn 3.14:

$$pK_a = pH + \log_{10}[HA] - \log_{10}[A^-] \tag{3.14}$$

or

$$pK_a = pH + \log_{10}\frac{[HA]}{[A^-]} \tag{3.15}$$

or even:

$$pH = pK_a + \log_{10}\frac{[A^-]}{[HA]} \tag{3.16}$$

Eqns 3.15 and 3.16 are known as the Henderson–Hasselbalch equations for a weak acid.

Ionization constants of both acidic and basic drugs are usually expressed in terms of pK_a. The equivalent acid dissociation constant (K_a) for the protonation of a weak base is given (from Eqn 3.8) by Eqn 3.17. Note the equation appears to be inverted, but it is written in terms of K_a rather than K_b (the base dissociation constant):

$$K_a = \frac{[H^+][B]}{[BH^+]} \quad (3.17)$$

Taking negative logarithms yields Eqn 3.18:

$$-\log_{10} K_a = -\log_{10}[H^+] - \log_{10}[B] + \log_{10}[BH^+] \quad (3.18)$$

or

$$pK_a = pH + \log_{10}\frac{[BH^+]}{[B]} \quad (3.19)$$

or

$$pH = pK_a + \log_{10}\frac{[B]}{[BH^+]} \quad (3.20)$$

Eqns 3.19 and 3.20 are known as the Henderson–Hasselbalch equations for a weak base.

Link between pH, pK$_a$, degree of ionization and solubility of weakly acidic or basic drugs

There is a direct link for most polar ionic compounds between the degree of ionization and aqueous solubility. As has been shown above, in turn, the degree of ionization is controlled by the pK$_a$ of the molecule and the pH of its surrounding environment. This interrelationship is shown diagrammatically in Figure 3.1.

Taking the weak acid line first, it can be seen that at high pH the drug is fully ionized and at its maximum solubility. Under low pH conditions the opposite is true. The shape of the curve is defined by the Henderson–Hasselbalch equation for weak acids (Eqn 3.15) that shows the link between pH, pK$_a$ and degree of ionization

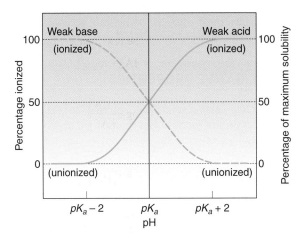

Fig. 3.1 Change in degree of ionization and relative solubility of weakly acidic and weakly basic drugs as a function of pH.

for a weakly acidic drug. It can also be seen from Figure 3.1 that when the pH is equal to the pK$_a$ of the drug, that drug is 50% ionized. This is also predicted from the Henderson–Hasselbalch equation.

Refer again to Eqn 3.16 as this will show that when $[A^-] = [HA]$, log $([A^-]/[HA])$ will equal log 1 (i.e. zero) and thus pH = pK$_a$. Put another way, when the pH of the surrounding solution equals the pK$_a$, then the concentration of the ionized species $[A^-]$ will equal the concentration of the unionized species $[HA]$, i.e. the drug is 50% ionized. The Henderson–Hasselbalch equations also show that a drug is almost completely ionized or non-ionized (as appropriate) when two pH units away from its pK$_a$.

Examination of the equivalent line for a weak base will indicate that it is probably not a coincidence that most drugs for peroral delivery are weak bases. A weak base will be ionized and at its most soluble in the acidic stomach and non-ionized and therefore more easily absorbed in the more alkaline small intestine. The choice of the pK$_a$ for a drug is thus of paramount importance in peroral drug delivery.

Use of the Henderson–Hasselbalch equations to calculate degree of ionization of weakly acidic or basic drugs

Various analytical techniques, e.g. spectrophotometric and potentiometric methods, may be used to determine ionization constants but the temperature at which the determination is performed should be specified because the values of the constants vary with temperature.

The degree of ionization of a drug in a solution can be calculated from rearranged Henderson–Hasselbalch equations for weak acids and bases (Eqns 3.15 and 3.19, respectively) if the pK$_a$ value of the drug and the pH of the solution are known. The resulting equations for weak acids and weak bases are Eqns 3.21 and 3.22, respectively:

$$\log_{10}\frac{[HA]}{[A^-]} = pK_a - pH \quad (3.21)$$

$$\log_{10}\frac{[BH^+]}{[B]} = pK_a - pH \quad (3.22)$$

Such calculations are particularly useful in determining the degree of ionization of drugs in various parts of the gastrointestinal tract and in the plasma. The following examples are therefore related to this type of situation.

Calculation examples:
1. The pK$_a$ value of aspirin, which is a weak acid, is about 3.5. If the pH of the gastric contents is 2.0 then from Eqn 3.21:

$$\log_{10}\frac{[HA]}{[A^-]} = pK_a - pH = 3.5 - 2.0 = 1.5$$

so that the ratio of the concentration of unionized acetylsalicyclic acid to acetylsalicylate anion is given by:

$$[HA]:[A^-] = \text{antilog } 1.5 = 31.62:1$$

2. The pH of plasma is 7.4 so that the ratio of unionized:ionized aspirin in this medium is given by:

$$\log_{10}\frac{[HA]}{[A^-]} = pK_a - pH = 3.5 - 7.4 = -3.9$$

and

$$[HA]:[A^-] = \text{antilog} -3.9 = 1.259 \times 10^{-4}:1$$

3. The pK_a of the weakly *acidic* drug sulphapyridine is about 8.0 and if the pH of the intestinal contents is 5.0 then the ratio of unionized:ionized drug is given by:

$$\log_{10}\frac{[HA]}{[A^-]} = pK_a - pH = 8.0 - 5.0 = 3.0$$

and

$$[HA]:[A^-] = \text{antilog } 3.0 = 10^3:1$$

4. The pK_a of the *basic* drug amidopyrine is 5.0. In the stomach the ratio of ionized:unionized drug is calculated from Eqn 3.22 as follows:

$$\log\frac{[BH^+]}{[B]} = pK_a - pH = 5.0 - 2.0 = 3.0$$

and

$$[BH^+]:[B] = \text{antilog } 3.0 = 10^3:1$$

while in the intestine the ratio is given by:

$$\log\frac{[BH^+]}{[B]} = pK_a - pH = 5.0 - 5.0 = 0$$

and

$$[BH^+]:[B] = \text{antilog } 0 = 1:1$$

Buffer solutions and buffer capacity

Buffer solutions will maintain a constant pH even when small amounts of acid or alkali are added to the solution. Buffers usually contain mixtures of a weak acid and one of its salts, although mixtures of a weak base and one of its salts may be used. The latter suffer from the disadvantage that arises from the volatility of many bases.

The action of a buffer solution can be appreciated by considering, as an example, a simple system such as a solution of a mixture of acetic acid and sodium acetate in water. The acetic acid, being a weak acid, will be confined virtually to its undissociated form because its ionization will be suppressed by the presence of common acetate ions produced by complete dissociation of the sodium salt. The pH of this solution can be described by Eqn 3.23, which is Eqn 3.16 in which $[A^-]$ is the con-centration of acetate ions and [HA] is the concentration of acetic acid in the buffer solution:

$$pH = pK_a + \log\frac{[A^-]}{[HA]} \qquad (3.23)$$

It can be seen from Eqn 3.23 that the pH will remain constant as long as the logarithm of the ratio [acetate]/[acetic acid] does not change. When a small amount of an acid is added to the solution it will convert some of the salt into acetic acid but if the concentrations of both acetate ion and acetic acid are reasonably large then the effect of the change will be negligible and the pH will remain constant. Similarly, the addition of a small amount of base will convert some of the acetic acid into its salt form but the pH will be virtually unaltered if the overall changes in concentrations of the two species are relatively small.

If large amounts of acid or base are added to a buffer then changes in the ratio of ionized to unionized species become appreciable and the pH will then alter. The ability of a buffer to withstand the effects of acids and bases is an important property from a practical point of view. This ability is expressed in terms of *buffer capacity* (β). This can be defined as being equal to the amount of strong acid or strong base, expressed as moles of H^+ or OH^- ion, required to change the pH of 1 litre of the buffer by 1 pH unit. From the remarks above, it should be clear that buffer capacity increases as the concentrations of the buffer components increase. In addition, the capacity is also affected by the ratio of the concentrations of weak acid and its salt, maximum capacity (β_{max}) being obtained when the ratio of acid to salt = 1, i.e. pH equals the pK_a of the acid.

The components of various buffer systems and the concentrations required to produce different pHs are listed in several reference books, such as the pharmacopoeias. When selecting a suitable buffer, the pK_a value of the acid should be close to the required pH and the compatibility of its components with other ingredients in the system should be considered. The toxicity of buffer components must also be taken into account if the solution is to be used for medicinal purposes.

COLLIGATIVE PROPERTIES

When a non-volatile solute is dissolved in a solvent, certain properties of the resultant solution are largely independent of the nature of the solute and are determined by the concentration of solute particles. These properties are known as *colligative properties*. In the case of a non-electrolyte the solute particles will be molecules but if the solute is an electrolyte then its degree of dissociation will determine whether the particles will be ions only or a mixture of ions and undissociated molecules.

The most important colligative property from a pharmaceutical point of view is referred to as *osmotic pressure*.

However, since all colligative properties are related to each other by virtue of their common dependency on the concentration of the solute molecules, the remaining colligative properties (which include lowering of vapour pressure of the solvent, elevation of its boiling point and depression of its freezing point) are of pharmaceutical interest. These other observations offer alternative means to osmotic pressure measurements as methods of comparing the colligative properties of different solutions.

Osmotic pressure

The osmotic pressure of a solution is the external pressure that must be applied to the solution in order to prevent it being diluted by the entry of solvent via a process that is known as *osmosis*. This process refers to the spontaneous diffusion of solvent from a solution of low solute concentration (or a pure solvent) into a more concentrated one through a semi-permeable membrane. Such a membrane separates the two solutions and is permeable only to solvent molecules.

Since the process occurs spontaneously at constant temperature and pressure, the laws of thermodynamics indicate that it will be accompanied by a decrease in the *free energy* (G) of the system. This free energy may be regarded as the energy available for the performance of useful work. When an equilibrium position is attained then there is no remaining difference between the energies of the states that are in equilibrium. The rate of increase in free energy of a solution caused by an increase in the number of moles of one component is termed the *partial molar free energy* ($\bar{G}$) or *chemical potential* (μ) of that component. For example, the chemical potential of the solvent in a binary solution is given by Eqn 3.24. The subscripts outside the bracket on the left-hand side indicate that temperature, pressure and amount of component 1 (the solute in this case) remain constant:

$$\left(\frac{\partial G}{\partial n_2}\right)_{T, P, n_1} = \bar{G}_2 = \mu_2 \qquad (3.24)$$

Since (by definition) only solvent molecules can pass through the semi-permeable membrane, the driving force for osmosis arises from the inequality of the chemical potentials of the solvent on opposing sides of the membrane. Thus the direction of osmotic flow is from the dilute solution (or pure solvent), where the chemical potential of the solvent is highest because of the higher concentration of solvent molecules, into the concentrated solution, where the concentration and, consequently, the chemical potential of the solvent are reduced by the presence of more solute. The chemical potential of the solvent in the more concentrated solution can be increased by forcing its molecules closer together under the

influence of an externally applied pressure. Osmosis can be prevented, therefore, by such means, hence the definition of osmotic pressure.

The relationship between osmotic pressure (π) and concentration of a non-electrolyte is given for dilute solutions, which may be assumed to exhibit ideal behaviour, by the van't Hoff equation (Eqn 3.25):

$$\pi V = n_2 RT \qquad (3.25)$$

where V is the volume of solution, n_2 is the number of moles of solute, T is the absolute temperature and R is the gas constant. This equation, which is similar to the ideal gas equation, was derived empirically but it does correspond to a theoretically derived equation if approximations based on low solute concentrations are taken into account.

If the solute is an electrolyte, Eqn 3.25 must be modified to allow for the effect of ionic dissociation, because this will increase the number of particles in the solution. This modification is achieved by insertion of the van't Hoff correction factor (i) to give:

$$\pi V = in_2 RT \qquad (3.26)$$

$$\text{where i} = \frac{\text{observed colligative property}}{\begin{array}{c}\text{colligative property expected if}\\\text{dissociation did not occur}\end{array}}$$

Osmolality and osmolarity

The amount of osmotically active particles in a solution is sometimes expressed in terms of osmoles or milliosmoles. These osmotically active particles may be either molecules or ions. *Osmoles* refers to the number of particles dissolved in a solution, regardless of charge. For substances that maintain their molecular structure when they dissolve (e.g. glucose), osmolarity and the molarity are essentially the same. For substances that dissociate when they dissolve, the osmolarity is the number of free particles times the molarity. Thus a 1 molar solution of pure NaCl solution would be 2 osmolar (1 for Na^+, and 1 for Cl^-).

The concentration of a solution may therefore be expressed in terms of its *osmolarity* or its *osmolality*. Osmolarity is the number of osmoles per litre of solution and osmolality is the number of osmoles per kilogram of solvent.

Isoosmotic solutions

If two solutions are separated by a perfect semi-permeable membrane, i.e. a membrane which is permeable only to solvent molecules, and no net movement of solvent occurs across the membrane then the solutions are said to be *isoosmotic* and will have equal osmotic pressures.

Isotonic solutions

Biological membranes do not always function as perfect semi-permeable membranes and some solute molecules in addition to water are able to pass through them. If two isoosmotic solutions remain in osmotic equilibrium when separated by a biological membrane, they may be described as being *isotonic* with respect to that particular membrane.

Adjustment of isotonicity is particularly important for formulations intended for parenteral routes of administration. Excessively hypotonic or hypertonic solutions can cause biological damage.

DIFFUSION IN SOLUTION

The components of a solution, by definition, form a homogeneous single phase. This homogeneity arises from the process of diffusion, which occurs spontaneously and is consequently accompanied by a decrease in the free energy (*G*) of the system. *Diffusion* may be defined as the spontaneous transference of a component from a region in the system which has a high chemical potential into a region where its chemical potential is lower. Although such a gradient in chemical potential provides the driving force for diffusion, the laws that describe this phenomenon are usually expressed, more conveniently, in terms of concentration gradients. An example is Fick's First Law which is discussed in Chapter 2.

The most common explanation of the mechanism of diffusion in solution is based on the lattice theory of the structure of liquids. Lattice theories postulate that liquids have crystalline or quasicrystalline structures. The concept of a crystal type of lattice is only intended to provide a convenient starting point and should not be interpreted as a suggestion that liquids possess rigid structures. The theories also postulate that a reasonable proportion of the volume occupied by the liquid is, at any moment, empty, i.e. there are 'holes' in the liquid lattice network, which constitute the so-called *free volume* of the liquid.

Diffusion can therefore be regarded as the process by which solute molecules move from hole to hole within a liquid lattice. In order to achieve such movement, a solute molecule must acquire sufficient kinetic energy at the right time so that it can break away from any bonds that tend to anchor it in one hole and then jump into an adjacent hole. If the average distance of each jump is δ cm and the frequency with which the jumps occur is $\phi\,s^{-1}$ then the *diffusion coefficient* (*D*) is given by:

$$D = \frac{\delta^2 \phi}{6} \ cm^2 s^{-1} \qquad (3.27)$$

The diffusion coefficient is assumed to have a constant value for a particular system at a given temperature. This assumption is only strictly true at infinite dilution and the value of *D* may therefore exhibit some concentration dependency. In a given solvent the value of *D* decreases as the size of the diffusing solute molecule increases. In water, for example, *D* is of the order of 2×10^{-5} cm^2 s^{-1} for solutes with molecular weights of approximately 50 Da and it decreases to about 1×10^{-6} cm^2 s^{-1} when the molecular weight increases to a few thousand Da.

The value of δ for any given solute is reasonably constant. Differences in the diffusion coefficient of a substance in solution in various solvents arise mainly from changes in jump frequency (ϕ), which is determined, in turn, by the free volume or looseness of packing in the solvent.

When the size of the solute molecules is not appreciably larger than that of the solvent molecules then it has been shown that the diffusion coefficient of the former is related to its molecular weight (*M*) by the relationship:

$$DM^{1/2} = constant \qquad (3.28)$$

When the solute is much greater in size than the solvent, diffusion arises largely from transport of solvent molecules in the opposite direction and the relationship becomes:

$$DM^{1/3} = constant \qquad (3.29)$$

This latter equation forms the basis of the Stokes–Einstein equation (Eqn 3.30) for the diffusion of spherical particles that are larger than surrounding liquid molecules. Since the mass (*m*) of a spherical particle is proportional to the cube of its radius (*r*), i.e. $r \propto m^{1/3}$, it follows from Eqn 3.29 that $Dm^{1/3}$ and consequently *D* and *r* are constants for such a system. The Stokes–Einstein equation is usually written in the form:

$$D = \frac{kT}{6\pi r \eta} \qquad (3.30)$$

where *k* is the Boltzmann constant, *T* is the absolute temperature and η is the viscosity of the liquid. The appearance of a viscosity term in this type of equation is not unexpected because the reciprocal of viscosity, which is known as the *fluidity* of a liquid, is proportional to the free volume in a liquid. Thus, jump frequency (ϕ) and diffusion coefficient (*D*) will increase as the viscosity of a liquid decreases or as the number of 'holes' in its structure increases.

The experimental determination of diffusion coefficients of solutes in liquid solvents is not easy because the effects of other factors that may influence the movement of solute in the system, e.g. temperature and density gradients, mechanical agitation and vibration, must be eliminated.

SUMMARY

This chapter has outlined the key fundamental issues relating to the properties of solutions. The issues discussed are of relevance both to dosage forms, which themselves comprise solutions, and to the fate of the drug molecule once in solution following administration.

BIBLIOGRAPHY

Chang, R. (1981) *Physical Chemistry with Applications to Biological Systems*, 2nd edn. Macmillan, Basingstoke.

Florence, A.T., Attwood, D. (2006) *Physicochemical Principles of Pharmacy*, 4th edn. Pharmaceutical Press, London.

Martin, A. (1993) *Physical Pharmacy*, 4th edn. Lea and Febiger, Philadelphia.

4

Rheology

C. Marriott

VISCOSITY, RHEOLOGY AND THE FLOW OF FLUIDS

The *viscosity* of a fluid may be described simply as its resistance to flow or movement. Thus water, which is easier to stir than syrup, is said to have the lower viscosity. The reciprocal is *fluidity*. *Rheology* (a term invented by Bingham and formally adopted in 1929) may be defined as the study of the flow and deformation properties of matter.

Historically the importance of rheology in pharmacy was merely as a means of characterizing and classifying fluids and semi-solids. For example, in the *British Pharmacopoeia* a viscosity standard has for many years been used to control substances such as liquid paraffin. However, the increased reliance on the dissolution testing of dosage forms and the use of polymers has given added importance to a knowledge of flow properties. Furthermore, advances in the methods of evaluation of the viscoelastic properties of semi-solids and biological materials have produced useful correlations with bioavailability and function.

A proper understanding of the rheological properties of pharmaceutical materials is essential to the preparation, development, evaluation and performance of pharmaceutical dosage forms. This chapter describes rheological behaviour and techniques of measurement and will form a basis for the applied studies described in later chapters.

NEWTONIAN FLUIDS

Viscosity coefficients for Newtonian fluids

Dynamic viscosity

The definition of viscosity was put on a quantitative basis by Newton, who was the first to realize that the rate of flow (γ) was directly related to the applied stress (σ): the constant of proportionality is the *coefficient of dynamic viscosity* (η), more usually referred to simply as the viscosity. Simple fluids which obey this relationship are referred to as *Newtonian* fluids and those which do not are known as *non-Newtonian*.

The phenomenon of viscosity is best understood by a consideration of a hypothetical cube of fluid made up of infinitely thin layers (laminae) which are able to slide over one another like playing cards in a pack or deck (Fig. 4.1a). When a tangential force is applied to the uppermost layer, it is assumed that each subsequent layer will move at progressively decreasing velocity and that the bottom layer will be stationary (Fig. 4.1b). A velocity gradient will therefore exist and this will be equal to the velocity of the upper layer in m s^{-1} divided by the height of the cube in metres. The resultant gradient, which is effectively the rate of flow but is usually referred to as the rate of shear, γ, will have units of reciprocal seconds (s^{-1}). The applied stress, known as the shear stress, σ, is derived by dividing the applied force by the area of the upper layer and will have units of N m^{-2}.

As Newton's Law can be expressed as:

$$\sigma = \eta\gamma \qquad (4.1)$$

then

$$\eta = \frac{\sigma}{\gamma} \qquad (4.2)$$

and η will have units of N m^{-2}s. Thus by reference to Eqn 4.1, it can be seen that a Newtonian fluid of viscosity 1 N m^{-2}s would produce a velocity of 1 m s^{-1} for a cube of 1 m dimension with an applied force of 1 N. Because the name for the derived unit of force per unit area in the SI system is the pascal (Pa), then viscosity should be referred to in Pa s. It is common to

centipoise (cP), which is one-hundredth of a Poise (1 dyn cm^{-2}s). These are the units of viscosity in the now redundant cgs system of units that, although no longer official and not recommended, are still relatively commonly used.

The values of the viscosity of water and some examples of other fluids of pharmaceutical interest are given in Table 4.1.

Kinematic viscosity

The dynamic viscosity is not the only coefficient that can be used to characterize a fluid. The *kinematic viscosity* (v) is also used and may be defined as the dynamic viscosity divided by the density of the fluid (ρ):

$$v = \frac{\eta}{\rho} \qquad (4.3)$$

and the SI units will be m^2 s^{-1} or, more usefully, mm^2 s^{-1}. The cgs unit was the Stoke (10^{-4} m^2 s^{-1}) and the centistoke (cS) might still be found in the literature.

Table 4.1 Viscosities of some fluids of pharmaceutical interest

Fluid	Dynamic viscosity at 20°C (mPa s)
Chloroform	0.58
Water	1.002
Ethanol	1.20
Glyceryl trinitrate	36.0
Olive oil	84.0
Castor oil	986.0
Glycerol	1490.0

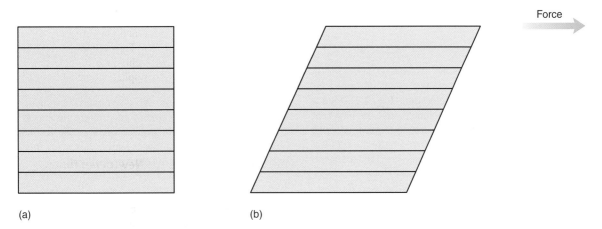

Force

(a)　　　　　　　　　(b)

Fig. 4.1 Representation of the effect of shearing a 'block' of fluid.

Relative and specific viscosities

The *viscosity ratio* or *relative viscosity* (η_r) of a solution is the ratio of the viscosity of a solution to the viscosity of its solvent (η_o):

$$\eta_r = \frac{\eta}{\eta_o} \qquad (4.4)$$

and the *specific viscosity* (η_{sp}) is given by:

$$\eta_{sp} = \eta_r - 1 \qquad (4.5)$$

In these calculations the solvent can be of any nature, although in pharmaceutical products it is often water.

$$\eta = \eta_o (1 + 2.5\phi) \qquad (4.6)$$

where ϕ is the volume fraction of the colloidal phase (the volume of the dispersed phase divided by the total volume of the dispersion). The Einstein equation may be rewritten as:

$$\frac{\eta}{\eta_o} = 1 + 2.5\,\phi \qquad (4.7)$$

when from Eqn 4.4 it can be seen that the left-hand side of Eqn 4.7 is equal to the relative viscosity. It can also be rewritten as:

$$\frac{\eta}{\eta_o} - 1 = \frac{\eta - \eta_o}{\eta_o} = 2.5\phi \qquad (4.8)$$

when the left-hand side equals the specific viscosity. Eqn 4.8 can be rearranged to produce:

$$\frac{\eta_{sp}}{\phi} = 2.5 \qquad (4.9)$$

and as the volume fraction will be directly related to concentration C, Eqn 4.9 can be rewritten as:

$$\frac{\eta_{sp}}{C} = k \qquad (4.10)$$

When the dispersed phase is a high molecular mass polymer then a colloidal solution will result and, provided moderate concentrations are used, Eqn 4.10 can be expressed as a power series:

$$\frac{\eta_{sp}}{C} = k_1 + k_2 C + k_3 C^2 \qquad (4.11)$$

Intrinsic viscosity

If η_{sp}/C, the *viscosity number* or *reduced viscosity*, is determined at a range of polymer concentrations and plotted as a function of concentration (Fig. 4.2), then a linear relationship should be obtained, and the intercept produced on extrapolation of the line to the ordinate will yield the constant k_1 which is referred to as the *limiting viscosity number* or the *intrinsic viscosity*, [η], when the units of concentration are in g dL^{-1}.

The limiting viscosity number may be used to determine the approximate molecular mass (M) of polymers using the Mark–Houwink equation:

$$[\eta] = KM^\alpha \qquad (4.12)$$

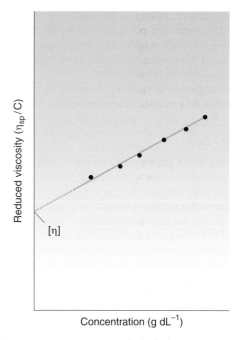

Fig. 4.2 Plot of concentration (g dL^{-1}) against reduced viscosity (η_{sp}/C), which by extrapolation gives the limiting viscosity number or intrinsic viscosity ([η]).

where K and α are constants that must be obtained at a given temperature for the specific polymer–solvent system. However, once these constants are known then viscosity determinations provide a quick and precise method of molecular mass determination of pharmaceutical polymers such as dextrans, which are used as plasma extenders. Also the values of the two constants provide an indication of the shape of the molecule in solution: spherical molecules yield values of $\alpha = 0$, whereas extended rods have values greater than 1.0. A randomly coiled molecule will yield an intermediate value (≈ 0.5).

The specific viscosity may be used in the following equation to determine the volume of a molecule in solution:

$$\eta_{sp} = 2.5C\frac{NV}{M} \qquad (4.13)$$

where C is concentration, N is Avogadro's number, V is the hydrodynamic volume of each molecule and M is the molecular mass. However, it does suffer from the obvious disadvantage that the assumption is made that all polymeric molecules form spheres in solution.

Huggins' constant

Finally, the constant k_2 in Eqn 4.11 is referred to as Huggins' constant and is equal to the slope of the plot shown in Figure 4.2. Its value gives an indication of the interaction between the polymer and the solvent, such that a positive slope is produced for a polymer that interacts weakly with the solvent, and the slope becomes less positive as the interaction increases. A change in the value of Huggins' constant can be used to evaluate the interaction of drug molecules in solution with polymers.

Boundary layers

From Figure 4.1 it can be seen that the rate of flow of a fluid over an even surface will be dependent upon the distance from the surface. The velocity, which will be almost zero at the surface, increases with increasing distance from the surface until the bulk of the fluid is reached and the velocity becomes constant. The region over which differences in velocity are observed is referred to as the *boundary layer*. The boundary layer arises because of the intermolecular forces between the liquid molecules and those of the surface resulting in reduction of movement of the layer adjacent to the wall to zero. Its depth is dependent upon the viscosity of the fluid and the rate of flow in the bulk fluid. High viscosity and a low flow rate would result in a thick boundary layer, which will become thinner as either the viscosity falls or the flow rate is increased. The boundary layer represents an important barrier to heat and mass transfer.

In the case of a capillary tube then the two boundary layers meet at the centre of the tube, such that the velocity distribution is parabolic (Fig. 4.3). With an increase in either the diameter of the tube or the fluid velocity, the proximity of the two boundary layers is reduced and the velocity profile becomes flattened at the centre (Fig. 4.3).

Laminar, transitional and turbulent flow

The conditions under which a fluid flows through a pipe, for example, can markedly affect the character of the flow. The type of flow that occurs can be best understood

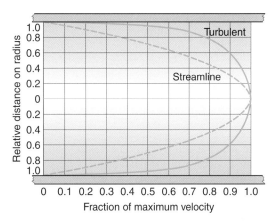

Fig. 4.3 Velocity distributions across a circular cross-section pipe.

by reference to experiments conducted by Reynolds in 1883. The apparatus used (Fig. 4.4) consisted of a straight glass tube through which the fluid flowed under the influence of a force provided by a constant head of water. At the centre of the inlet of the tube, a fine stream of dye was introduced. At low flow rates the dye formed a coherent thread which remained undisturbed in the centre of the tube and grew very little in thickness along the length. This type of flow is described as *streamlined flow* or *laminar flow*, and the liquid is considered to flow as a series of concentric cylinders in a manner analogous to an extending telescope.

If the speed of the fluid is increased a critical velocity is reached at which the thread begins to waver and then to break up, although no mixing occurs. This is known as *transitional flow*. When the velocity is increased to high values the dye instantaneously mixes with the fluid in the tube, as all order is lost and irregular motions are imposed on the overall movement of the fluid. Such flow is described as *turbulent flow*. In this type of flow the movement of molecules is

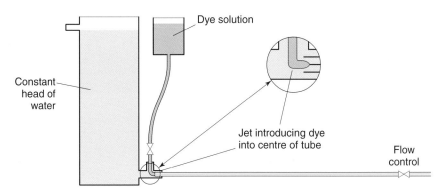

Fig. 4.4 Reynolds' apparatus.

totally haphazard, although the average movement will be in the direction of flow.

Reynolds' experiments indicated that the flow conditions were affected by four factors, namely the diameter of the pipe and the viscosity, density and velocity of the fluid. Furthermore, it was shown that these factors could be combined to give the following equation:

$$Re = \frac{\rho u d}{\eta} \qquad (4.14)$$

where ρ is the density, u is the velocity and η is the dynamic viscosity of the fluid, and d is the diameter of the circular cross-section pipe. Re is known as Reynolds' number and, provided compatible units are used, it will be dimensionless.

Values of Reynolds' number in a circular cross-section pipe have been determined that can be associated with a particular type of flow. If it is below 2000 then streamline flow will occur, but if it is above 4000 then flow will be turbulent. In between these two values the nature of the flow will depend upon the surface over which the fluid is flowing. For example, if the surface is smooth then streamline flow may not be disturbed and may exist at values of Reynolds' number above 2000. However, if the surface is rough or the channel tortuous then flow may well be turbulent at values below 4000, and even as low as 2000. Consequently, although it is tempting to state that values of Reynolds' number between 2000 and 4000 are indicative of transitional flow, such a statement would only be correct for a specific set of conditions. This also explains why it is difficult to demonstrate transitional flow practically.

Nevertheless, Reynolds' number is still an important parameter and can be used to predict the type of flow that will occur in a particular situation. The importance of knowing the type of flow lies in the fact that with streamline flow, there is no component at right angles to the direction of flow, so that fluid cannot move across the tube. This component is strong for turbulent flow and interchange across the tube is rapid. Thus in the latter case, for example, mass will be rapidly transported, whereas in streamline flow the fluid layers will act as a barrier to such transfer, which can only occur by molecular diffusion.

Determination of the flow properties of simple fluids

A wide range of instruments exist that can be used to determine the flow properties of Newtonian fluids. However, only some of these are capable of providing data that can be used to calculate viscosities in fundamental units. The design of many instruments precludes the calculation of absolute viscosities as they are capable of providing data only in terms of empirical units.

This chapter will not describe all the types of instrument used to measure viscosity and consequently the section is limited to simple instruments specified in the *European Pharmacopoeia* (Ph Eur) or the *British Pharmacopoeia* (BP).

Capillary viscometers

A capillary viscometer can be used to determine viscosity provided that the fluid is Newtonian and the flow is streamlined. The rate of flow of the fluid through the capillary is measured under the influence of gravity or an externally applied pressure.

Ostwald U-tube viscometer Such instruments are described in pharmacopoeias and are the subject of a specification of the International Standards Organization (ISO). A range of capillary bores is available and an appropriate one should be selected so that a flow time of approximately 200 seconds is obtained; the wider-bore viscometers are thus for use with fluids of higher viscosity. For fluids where there is a viscosity specification in the BP, the size of instrument that must be used in the determination of their viscosity is stated.

The instrument is shown in Figure 4.5 and flow through the capillary occurs under the influence of gravity. The maximum shear rate, γ_m is given by:

$$\gamma_m = \frac{\rho g r_c}{2\eta} \qquad (4.15)$$

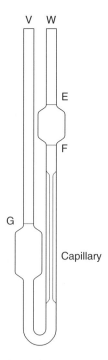

Fig. 4.5 A U-tube viscometer.

where ρ is the density of the fluid, g the acceleration due to gravity, r_c the radius of the capillary and η the absolute viscosity. Consequently, for a fluid of viscosity 1 mPa s, the maximum shear rate is approximately 2×10^3 s^{-1} if the capillary has a diameter of 0.64 mm, but it will be of the order of 10^2 s^{-1} for a fluid with a viscosity of 1490 mPa s if the capillary has a diameter of 2.74 mm.

The liquid is introduced into the viscometer up to mark G through arm V using a pipette long enough to prevent wetting the sides of the tube. The viscometer is then clamped vertically in a constant-temperature water bath and allowed to reach the required temperature. The level of the liquid is adjusted and is then blown or sucked into tube W until the meniscus is just above mark E. The time for the meniscus to fall between marks E and F is recorded. Determinations should be repeated until three readings all within 0.5 seconds are obtained. Care should be taken not to introduce air bubbles and that the capillary does not become partially occluded with small particles.

Suspended-level viscometer This instrument is a modification of the U-tube viscometer which avoids the need to fill the instrument with a precise volume of fluid. It also addresses the fact that the pressure head in the U-tube viscometer is continually changing as the two menisci approach one another. This is also described in the BP and the Ph Eur and is shown in Figure 4.6.

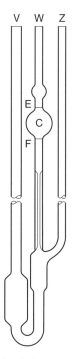

Fig. 4.6 A suspended-level viscometer.

A volume of liquid which will at least fill bulb C is introduced via tube V. The only upper limit on the volume used is that it should not block the ventilating tube Z. The viscometer is clamped vertically in a constant-temperature water bath and allowed to attain the required temperature. Tube Z is closed and fluid is drawn into bulb C by the application of suction through tube W until the meniscus is just above the mark E. Tube W is then closed and tube Z opened so that liquid can be drawn away from the bottom of the capillary. Tube W is then opened and the time the fluid takes to fall between marks E and F is recorded. If at any time during the determination the end of the ventilating tube Z becomes blocked by the liquid, the experiment must be repeated. The same criteria for reproducibility of timings described with the U-tube viscometer must be applied.

Because the volume of fluid introduced into the instrument can vary between the limits described above, this means that measurements can be made at a range of temperatures without the need to adjust the volume.

Calculation of viscosity from capillary viscometers

Poiseuille's Law states that for a liquid flowing through a capillary tube:

$$\eta = \frac{\pi r^4 t P}{8 L V} \qquad (4.16)$$

where r is the radius of the capillary, t is the time of flow, P is the pressure difference across the ends of the tube, L is the length of the capillary and V is the volume of liquid. As the radius and length of the capillary as well as the volume flowing are constants for a given viscometer, then:

$$\eta = K t P \qquad (4.17)$$

where K is equal to $\dfrac{\pi r^4}{8 L V}$

The pressure difference, P, depends upon the density, ρ, of the liquid, the acceleration due to gravity, g, and the difference in heights of the two menisci in the two arms of the viscometer. Because the value of g and the level of the liquids are constant, these can be included in a constant and Eqn 4.17 can be written for the viscosities of an unknown and a standard liquid:

$$\eta_1 = K' t_1 r_1 \qquad (4.18)$$

$$\eta_2 = K' t_2 r_2 \qquad (4.19)$$

Thus, when the flow times for two liquids are compared using the same viscometer, division of Eqn 4.18 by Eqn 4.19 gives:

$$\frac{\eta_1}{\eta_2} = \frac{K' t_1 \rho_1}{K' t_2 \rho_2} \qquad (4.20)$$

and reference to Eqn 4.4 shows that Eqn 4.20 will yield the viscosity ratio.

However, as Eqn 4.3 indicates that the kinematic viscosity is equal to the dynamic viscosity divided by the density, then Eqn 4.20 may be rewritten as:

$$\frac{v_1}{v_2} = \frac{t_1}{t_2} \tag{4.21}$$

For a given viscometer a standard fluid such as water can be used for the purposes of calibration. Then, Eqn 4.21 may be rewritten as:

$$v = ct \tag{4.22}$$

where c is the viscometer constant.

This is the equation that appears in the BP and explains the continued use of the kinematic viscosity as it means that liquids of known viscosity but of differing density from the test fluid can be used as the standard. A series of oils of given viscosity are available commercially and are recommended for the calibration of viscometers if water cannot be used.

Falling-sphere viscometer

This viscometer is based upon Stokes' Law (Chapter 6). When a body falls through a viscous medium, it experiences a resistance or viscous drag which opposes the downward motion. Consequently, if a body falls through a liquid under the influence of gravity, an initial acceleration period is followed by motion at a uniform terminal velocity when the gravitational force is balanced by the viscous drag. Eqn 4.23 will then apply to this terminal velocity when a sphere of density ρ_s and diameter d falls through a liquid of viscosity η and density ρ_l. The terminal velocity is u and g is the acceleration due to gravity:

$$3\pi\eta du = \frac{\pi}{6} d^3 g (\rho_s - \rho_l) \tag{4.23}$$

The viscous drag is given by the left-hand side of equation, whereas the right-hand side represents the force responsible for the downward motion of the sphere under the influence of gravity. Eqn 4.23 may be used to calculate viscosity by rearrangement to give:

$$\eta = \frac{d^2 g (\rho_s - \rho_l)}{18u} \tag{4.24}$$

Eqn 4.3 gives the relationship between η and the kinematic viscosity, such that Eqn 4.24 may be rewritten as:

$$v = \frac{d^2 g (\rho_s - \rho_l)}{18u\rho_l} \tag{4.25}$$

In the derivation of these equations it is assumed that the sphere falls through a fluid of infinite dimensions. However, for practical purposes the fluid must be contained in a vessel of finite dimensions. Therefore it is necessary to include a correction factor to allow for the end and wall effects. The correction normally used is due to Faxen and may be given as:

$$F = 1 - 2.104\frac{d}{D} + 2.09\frac{d^3}{D^3} - 0.95\frac{d^5}{D^5} \tag{4.26}$$

where D is the diameter of the measuring tube and d is the diameter of the sphere. The last term in Eqn 4.26 accounts for the end effect and may be ignored as long as only the middle third of the depth is used for measuring the velocity of the sphere. In fact, the middle half of the tube can be used if D is at least 10 times d, and the second and third terms, which account for the wall effects, can be replaced by 2.1 d/D.

The apparatus used to determine u is shown in Figure 4.7. The liquid is placed in the fall tube which is clamped vertically in a constant-temperature bath. Sufficient time must be allowed for temperature equilibration to occur and for air bubbles to rise to the surface. A steel sphere which has been cleaned and brought to the temperature of the experiment is introduced into the fall tube through a narrow guide tube. The passage of the sphere is monitored by a method that avoids parallax, and the time it takes to fall between the etched marks A and B is recorded. It is usual to take the average of three readings, of which all are within 0.5%, as the fall time, t, to calculate the viscosity. If the same sphere and fall tube are used then Eqn 4.25 reduces to:

$$v = Kt\left(\frac{\rho_s}{\rho_l} - 1\right) \tag{4.27}$$

where K is a constant that may be determined by the use of a liquid of known kinematic viscosity.

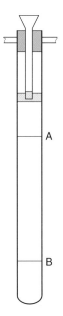

Fig. 4.7 A falling-sphere viscometer.

The BP specifies the use of a falling-sphere viscometer complying with the relevant British Standard. This type of viscometer is really only of use with Newtonian fluids. A variation has involved measuring the time taken for a sphere to roll through the fluid contained in an inclined tube. This instrument can only be used after calibration with standard fluids as fundamental derivation of viscosity is impossible.

NON-NEWTONIAN FLUIDS

The characteristics described in the previous sections apply only to fluids that obey Newton's Law (Eqn 4.1) and which are consequently referred to as Newtonian. However, most pharmaceutical fluids do not follow this law as the viscosity of many fluids varies with the rate of shear. The reason for these deviations is that the fluids concerned are not simple fluids such as water and syrup, but may be disperse or colloidal systems, including emulsions, suspensions and gels. These materials are known as non-Newtonian and with the increasing use of sophisticated polymer-based delivery systems, more examples of such behaviour are found in pharmaceutical science.

Types of non-Newtonian behaviour

More than one type of deviation from Newton's law can be recognized, and it is the type of deviation that occurs that can be used to classify the particular material.

If a Newtonian fluid is subjected to an increasing rate of shear, γ, and the corresponding shear stress, σ, recorded then a plot of γ against σ will produce the linear relationship shown in Figure 4.8a. Such a plot is usually referred to as a flow curve or rheogram. The slope of this plot will give the viscosity of the fluid and its reciprocal the fluidity. Eqn 4.1 implies that this line will pass through the origin.

Plastic (or Bingham) flow

Figure 4.8b indicates an example of *plastic flow* or *Bingham flow*, when the rheogram does not pass through the origin but intersects with the shear stress axis at a point usually referred to as the yield value, σ_y. This implies that a plastic material does not flow until such a value of shear stress has been exceeded, and at lower stresses the substance behaves as a solid (elastic) material. Plastic materials are often referred to as Bingham bodies in honour of the worker who carried out many of

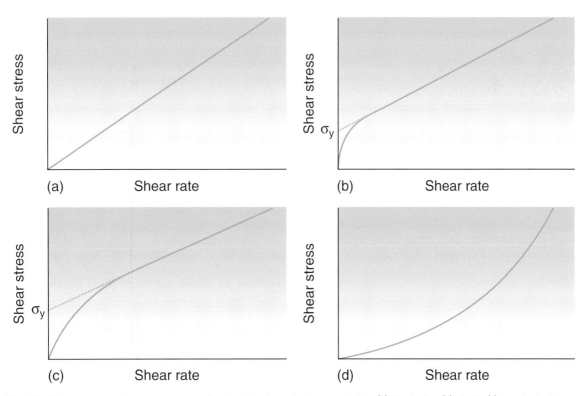

Fig. 4.8 Flow curves or rheograms representing the behaviour of various materials. (a) Newtonian, (b) plastic, (c) pseudoplastic and (d) dilatant.

the original studies with such materials. The equation he derived may be given as:

$$\sigma = \sigma_y + \eta_p \gamma \qquad (4.28)$$

where η_p is the plastic viscosity and σ_y the Bingham yield stress or value (Fig. 4.8b). The equation implies that the rheogram is a straight line intersecting the shear stress axis at the yield value σ_y. In practice, flow occurs at a lower shear stress than σ_y and the flow curve gradually approaches the extrapolation of the linear portion of the line shown in Figure 4.8b. This extrapolation will also give the Bingham or apparent yield value; the slope is the plastic viscosity.

Plastic flow is exhibited by concentrated suspensions, particularly if the continuous phase is of high viscosity or if the particles are flocculated.

Pseudoplastic flow

The rheogram shown in Figure 4.8c arises at the origin and, as no yield value exists, the material will flow as soon as a shear stress is applied; the slope of the curve gradually decreases with increasing rate of shear. The viscosity is derived from the slope and therefore decreases as the shear rate is increased. Materials exhibiting this behaviour are said to be pseudoplastic, and no single value of viscosity can be considered as characteristic. The viscosity can only be calculated from the slope of a tangent drawn to the curve at a specific point. Such viscosities are known as *apparent viscosities* and are only of any use if quoted in conjunction with the shear rate at which the determination was made, as it would need several apparent viscosities to characterize a pseudoplastic material and, indeed, the most satisfactory representation is by means of the entire flow curve. However, it is frequently noted that at higher shear stresses the flow curve tends towards linearity, indicating that a minimum viscosity has been attained. When this is the case, such a viscosity can be a useful means of classification.

There is no completely satisfactory quantitative explanation of pseudoplastic flow; probably the most widely used is the Power Law, which is given as:

$$\sigma^n = \eta'\gamma \qquad (4.29)$$

where η' is a viscosity coefficient and the exponent n an index of pseudoplasticity. When $n = 1$, then η' becomes the dynamic viscosity (η) and Eqn 4.29 the same as Eqn 4.1, but as a material becomes more pseudoplastic then the value of n will fall. In order to obtain the values of the constants in Eqn 4.29, log σ must be plotted against log γ, from which the slope will produce n and the intercept η'. The equation may only apply over a limited range (approximately one decade) of shear rates, and so it may not be applicable for all pharmaceutical materials and other models may have to be considered in order to fit the data. For example, the model known as Herschel–Bulkley can be given as:

$$\sigma = \sigma_y + K\gamma^n - 1 \qquad (4.30)$$

where K is a viscosity coefficient. This can be of use for flow curves that are curvilinear and which intersect with the stress axis.

The materials that exhibit this type of flow include aqueous dispersions of natural and chemically modified hydrocolloids, such as tragacanth, methylcellulose and carmellose, and synthetic polymers such as polyvinylpyrrolidone and polyacrylic acid. The presence of long, high molecular weight molecules in solution results in entanglement together with the association of immobilized solvent. Under the influence of shear, the molecules tend to become disentangled and align themselves in the direction of flow. They thus offer less resistance to flow and this, together with the release of some of the entrapped water, accounts for the lower viscosity. At any particular shear rate, an equilibrium will be established between the shearing force and the re-entanglement brought about by Brownian motion.

Dilatant flow

The opposite type of flow to pseudoplasticity is depicted by the curve in Figure 4.8d, in that the viscosity increases with increase in shear rate. As such materials increase in volume during shearing, they are referred to as *dilatant* and exhibit shear thickening. An equation similar to that for pseudoplastic flow (Eqn 4.29) may be used to describe dilatant behaviour, but the value of the exponent n will be greater than 1 and will increase as dilatancy increases.

This type of behaviour is less common than plastic or pseudoplastic flow but may be exhibited by dispersions containing a high concentration ($\approx 50\%$) of small, deflocculated particles. Under conditions of zero shear, the particles are closely packed and the interparticulate voids are at a minimum (Fig. 4.9), which the vehicle is sufficient to fill. Consequently, at low shear rates such as those created during pouring, such fluids can adequately lubricate the relative movement of the particles. As the shear rate is increased the particles become displaced from their uniform distribution and the clumps that are produced result in the creation of larger voids, into which the vehicle drains, so that the resistance to flow is increased and viscosity rises. The effect is progressive with increase in shear rate until eventually the material may appear paste-like as flow ceases. Fortunately, the effect is reversible and removal of the shear stress results in the re-establishment of the fluid nature.

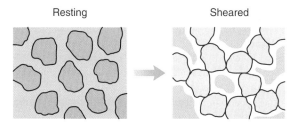

Fig. 4.9 Representation of the cause of dilatant behaviour.

Dilatancy can be a problem during the processing of dispersions and the granulation of tablet masses when high-speed mills and blenders are employed. If the material being processed becomes dilatant in nature then the resultant solidification could overload and damage the motor. Changing the batch or supplier of the material used could lead to processing problems that can only be avoided by rheological evaluation of the dispersions prior to their introduction in the production process.

Time-dependent behaviour

In the description of the different types of non-Newtonian behaviour it was implied that although the viscosity of a fluid might vary with shear rate, it was independent of the length of time that the shear rate was applied, and also that replicate determinations at the same shear rate would always produce the same viscosity. This must be considered as the ideal situation, as most non-Newtonian materials are colloidal in nature and the flowing elements, whether they are particles or macromolecules, may not adapt immediately to the new shearing conditions.

Therefore, when such a material is subjected to a particular shear rate, the shear stress and consequently the viscosity will decrease with time. Furthermore, once the shear stress has been removed, even if the structure that has been broken down is reversible, it may not return to its original structure (rheological ground state) instantly. The common feature of all these materials is that if they are subjected to a gradually increasing shear rate, followed immediately by a shear rate decreasing to zero, then the down curve will be displaced with regard to the up curve and the rheogram will exhibit a hysteresis loop (Fig. 4.10). In the case of plastic and pseudoplastic materials, the down curve will be displaced to the right of the up curve (Fig. 4.10), whereas for dilatant substances the reverse will be true (Fig. 4.11). The presence of the hysteresis loop indicates that a breakdown in structure has occurred, and the area within the loop may be used as an index of the degree of breakdown.

The term used to describe such behaviour is *thixotropy*, which means 'to change by touch'. Although

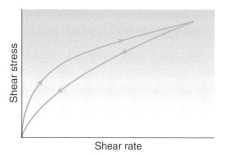

Fig. 4.10 Rheogram produced by a thixotropic pseudoplastic material.

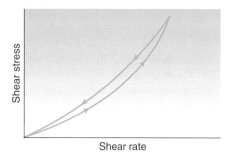

Fig. 4.11 Rheogram produced by a thixotropic dilatant material.

strictly the term should only be applied to an isothermal sol-gel transformation, it has become common to describe as thixotropic any material that exhibits a reversible time-dependent decrease in apparent viscosity. Thixotropic systems are usually composed of asymmetric particles or macromolecules that are capable of interacting by numerous secondary bonds to produce a loose three-dimensional structure, so that the material is gel-like when unsheared. The energy imparted during shearing disrupts these bonds, so that the flowing elements become aligned and the viscosity falls, as a gel-sol transformation has occurred. When the shear stress is eventually removed the structure will tend to reform, although the process is not immediate and will increase with time as the molecules return to the original state under the influence of Brownian motion. Furthermore, the time taken for recovery, which can vary from minutes to days depending upon the system, will be directly related to the length of time the material was subjected to the shear stress, as this will affect the degree of breakdown.

In some cases the structure that has been destroyed is never recovered, no matter how long the system is left unsheared. Repeat determinations of the flow curve will then produce only the down curve which was obtained in the experiment that resulted in the destruction. It is suggested that such behaviour be referred to as 'shear destruction' rather than thixotropy which, as will be appreciated from the above, is a misnomer in this case.

An example of such behaviour is the gels produced by high molecular weight polysaccharides, which are stabilized by large numbers of secondary bonds. Such systems undergo extensive reorganization during shearing such that the three-dimensional structure is reduced to a two-dimensional one; the gel-like nature of the original is then never recovered.

The occurrence of such complex behaviour creates problems in the quantification of the viscosity of these materials because not only will the apparent viscosity change with shear rate, but there will also be two viscosities that can be calculated for any given shear rate (i.e. from the up curve and the down curve). It is usual to attempt to calculate one viscosity for the up curve and another for the down curve. This must of course assume that each of the curves achieves linearity over some of its length, otherwise a defined shear rate must be used; only the former situation is truly satisfactory. Each of the lines used to derive the viscosity may be extrapolated to the shear stress axis to give an associated yield value. However, only the one derived from the up curve has any significance, as that derived from the down curve will relate to the broken-down system.

Consequently, the most useful index of thixotropy can be obtained by integration of the area contained within the loop. This will not, of course, take into account the shape of the up and down curves, and consequently two materials may produce loops of similar area but with completely different shapes, representing totally different flow behaviours. In order to prevent confusion, it is best to adopt a method whereby an estimate of area is accompanied by yield value(s). This is particularly important when complex up curves exhibiting bulges are obtained, although it is now acknowledged that when these have been reported in the literature, they might well have been a consequence of the design of the instrument, rather than providing information on the three-dimensional structure of the material. The evidence for this is based on the flow curves produced using more modern instruments, which do not exhibit the same, if any, bulges.

Determination of the flow properties of non-Newtonian fluids

With such a wide range of rheological behaviours it is extremely important to carry out measurements that will produce meaningful results. It is crucial therefore not to use a determination of viscosity at one shear rate (such as would be acceptable for a Newtonian fluid), as it could lead to completely erroneous comparative results. Figure 4.12 shows rheograms that are an example of the four different types of flow behaviour, all of which intersect at point A, which is equivalent to a shear rate of 100 s^{-1}. Therefore, if a measurement was made at this one shear rate, all four materials would be shown to have the same viscosity although they each exhibit different properties and behaviours. Single-point determinations are probably an extreme example but are used to emphasize the importance of properly designed experiments.

Rotational viscometers

These instruments rely on the viscous drag exerted on a body when it is rotated in the fluid to determine its viscosity. The major advantage of such instruments is that wide ranges of shear rate can be achieved, and usually a programme of shear rates can be produced automatically. Thus, the flow curve of a material may be obtained directly. A number of commercial instruments are available but all share a common feature in that various measuring geometries can be used; often these have been concentric cylinder (or couette) and cone-plate, although parallel-plate geometry is sometimes preferred.

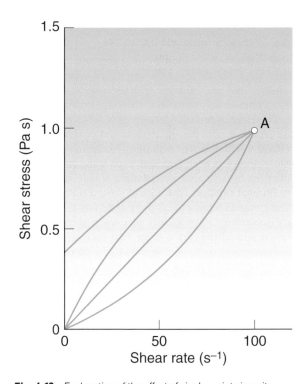

Fig. 4.12 Explanation of the effect of single-point viscosity determination and the resultant errors.

Concentric cylinder In this geometry there are two coaxial cylinders of different diameters, the outer forming the cup containing the fluid in which the inner cylinder or bob is positioned centrally (Fig. 4.13). In older types of instrument the outer cylinder is rotated and the viscous drag exerted by the fluid is transmitted to the inner cylinder as a torque, so that it rotates against a transducer or a fine torsion wire. The stress on this inner cylinder is indicated by the angular deflection, θ, once equilibrium (i.e. steady flow) has been attained. The torque, T, can then be calculated from:

$$C\theta = T \qquad (4.31)$$

where C is the torsional constant of the wire. The viscosity is then given by:

$$\eta = \frac{\left(\dfrac{1}{r_1^2} - \dfrac{1}{r_2^2}\right)T}{4\pi h\omega} \qquad (4.32)$$

where r_1 and r_2 are the radii of the inner and outer cylinders respectively, h is the height of the inner cylinder, and ω is the angular velocity of the outer cylinder.

A rheometer of this type is described in the BP, although any instrument that has equivalent accuracy and precision may be used.

Cone-plate The geometry of a cone-plate viscometer is composed of a flat circular plate with a wide-angle cone placed centrally above it (Fig. 4.14). The tip of the cone just touches the plate and the sample is loaded into the included gap. When the plate is rotated the cone will be caused to rotate against a torsion wire in the same way as

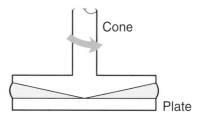

Fig. 4.14 Cone-plate geometry.

the inner cylinder described above. Provided the gap angle is small (of the order of 1°), the viscosity will be given by:

$$\eta = \frac{3\omega T}{2\pi r^3 \alpha} \qquad (4.33)$$

where ω is the angular velocity of the plate, T is the torque, r is the radius of the cone and α is the angle between the cone and the plate.

Rotational viscometers in use Whether cone-plate or concentric cylinder geometry is used, instruments, particularly the more modern examples, have been modified to make measurements both easier and more accurate. The common modification is to make one part of the geometry, usually the plate or the outer cylinder, stationary and to rotate the other member at a constant speed. A torque sensor can then measure the developed shear stress. An alternative is to rotate the upper member under a constant stress when the developed shear rate is measured.

Such controlled stress instruments consist of a specially designed induction motor which generates a torque that is independent of the degree or rate of rotation. Torque is not measured directly. It is defined by the way the power is fed to the motor, which is connected to the measuring geometry through a rigid drive chain so that no motion is lost in the deflection of a torque sensor. It is then necessary only to detect the movement of the drive system and its associated measuring geometry by, for example, an optical encoder, in order to obtain the shear rate or strain. Both designs have been the subject of considerable sophistication, including the use of microcomputers for programming and data analysis. Also, having one part of the geometry stationary means that it can be circulated with water or other fluid at a temperature appropriate to the measurement.

Concentric cylinder viscometers are very useful for Newtonian and non-Newtonian fluids provided the latter are not too solid-like in nature. Wide ranges of shear rate can be achieved by varying the diameters of the cylinders. However, this geometry does suffer from disadvantages. The major one is that the shear rate across the gap is not constant, and this is especially the case when the gap is large. Also, the end effects can be significant, as Eqn 4.32 only takes into account the surfaces of the walls of the cylinders and not the ends. These end effects are

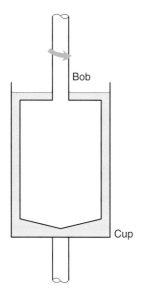

Fig. 4.13 Concentric cylinder geometry.

usually accounted for by calibration of the instrument with a fluid of known viscosity.

Frictional heating can be a problem at high shear rates, and so temperature control is essential with such instruments. Filling and cleaning are often difficult when the gap is small, but if it is large then the volume of sample required may be prohibitive.

Viscoelasticity

In the experiments described for rotational viscometers, two observations are often made with pharmaceutical materials.

1. With cone-plate geometry, the sample appears to 'roll up' at high shear rates and is ejected from the gap.
2. With concentric cylinder geometry, the sample will climb up the spindle of the rotating inner cylinder (Weissenberg effect).

The reason for both these phenomena is the same; that is, the liquids are not exhibiting purely viscous behaviour but are viscoelastic. Such materials display solid and liquid properties simultaneously, and the factor that governs the actual behaviour is time. A whole spectrum of viscoelastic behaviour exists, from materials that are predominantly liquid to those that are predominantly solid. Under a constant stress, all these materials will dissipate some of the energy in viscous flow and store the remainder, which will be recovered when the stress is removed. The type of response can be seen in Figure 4.15a, where a small, constant stress has been applied to a 2% gelatin gel and the resultant change in shape (strain) is measured.

In the region A–B an initial elastic jump is observed, followed by a curved region B–C when the material is attempting to flow as a viscous fluid but is being retarded by its solid characteristics. At longer times equilibrium is established, such that for a system like this, which is ostensibly liquid, viscous flow will eventually predominate and the curve will become linear (C–D). If the concentration of gelatin in the gel had been increased to 30% then the resultant material would be more solid-like and no flow would be observed at longer times, and the curve would level out as shown in Figure 4.15b. In the case of the liquid system, when the stress is removed only the stored energy will be recovered, and this is exhibited by an initial elastic recoil (D–E, Fig. 4.15a) equivalent to the region A–B and a retarded response E–F equivalent to B–C. There will be a displacement from the starting position (F–G) and this will be related to the amount of energy lost in viscous flow. For the higher-concentration gel all the energy will be recovered, so that only the regions D–E and E–F are observed.

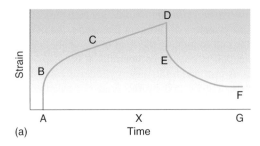

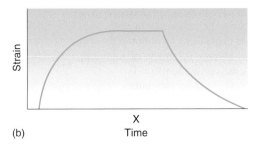

Fig. 4.15 Creep (or compliance) curves for (a) an uncrosslinked system and (b) a crosslinked system.

This significance of time can be observed from the point X on the time axis. Although both systems are viscoelastic, and, indeed, are produced by different concentrations of the same biopolymer, in Figure 4.15a the sample is flowing like a high-viscosity fluid, whereas in Figure 4.15b it is behaving like a solid.

Creep testing

Both the experimental curves shown in Figure 4.15 are examples of a phenomenon known as creep. If the measured strain is divided by the stress – which, it should be remembered, is constant – then a compliance will be produced. As compliance is the reciprocal of elasticity, it will have the units $m^2 N^{-1}$ or Pa^{-1}. The resultant curve, which will have the same shape as the original strain curve, then becomes known as a creep compliance curve. If the applied stress is below a certain limit (known as the linear viscoelastic limit) it will be directly related to the strain and the creep compliance curve will have the same shape and magnitude regardless of the stress used to obtain it. This curve therefore represents a fundamental property of the system, and derived parameters are characteristic and independent of the experimental method. For example, although it is common to use either cone-plate or concentric cylinders with viscoelastic pharmaceuticals, almost any measuring geometry can be used provided the shape of the sample can be defined.

It is common to analyse the creep compliance curve in terms of a mechanical model, an example of which is shown in Figure 4.16. This figure also indicates the regions on the curve shown in Figure 4.15a to which the components of the model relate. Thus, the instantaneous jump can be described by a perfectly elastic spring and the region of viscous flow by a piston fitted into a cylinder containing an ideal Newtonian fluid (this arrangement is referred to as a dashpot). In order to describe the behaviour in the intermediate region, it is necessary to combine both these elements in parallel, such that the movement of the spring is retarded by the piston; this combination is known as a Voigt unit. It is implied that the elements of the model do not move until the preceding one has become fully extended. Although it is not feasible to associate the elements of the model with the molecular arrangement of the material, it is possible to ascribe viscosities to the fluids in the cylinders and elasticities (or compliances) to the springs.

Thus, a viscosity can be calculated for the single dashpot (Fig. 4.16) from the reciprocal of the slope of the linear part of the creep compliance curve. This viscosity will be several orders of magnitude greater than that obtained by the conventional rotational techniques. It may be considered to be that of the rheological ground state (η_0) as the creep test is non-destructive and should produce the same viscosity however many times it is repeated on the same sample. This is in direct contrast to continuous

shear measurements, which destroy the structure being measured and with which it is seldom possible to obtain the same result on subsequent experiments on the same sample. The compliance (J_0) of the spring can be measured directly from the height of region A–B (Fig. 4.15a) and the reciprocal of this value will yield the elasticity, E_0. It is often the case that this value, together with η_0, provides an adequate characterization of the material.

However, the remaining portion of the curve can be used to derive the viscosity and elasticity of the elements of the Voigt unit. The ratio of the viscosity to the elasticity is known as the retardation time, τ, and is a measure of the time taken for the unit to deform to 1/e of its total deformation. Consequently, more rigid materials will have longer retardation times and the more complex the material, the greater number of Voigt units that are necessary to describe the creep curve.

It is also possible to use a mathematical expression to describe the creep compliance curve:

$$J(t) = J_0 - \sum_{i=1}^{n} J_i(1 - e^{t/\tau_i}) + t/\eta_0 \qquad (4.34)$$

where $J(t)$ is the compliance at time t, and J_i and τ_i are the compliance and retardation time, respectively, of the 'ith' Voigt unit. Both the model and the mathematical approach interpret the curve in terms of a line spectrum. It is also possible to produce a continuous spectrum in terms of the distribution of retardation times.

What is essentially the reverse of the creep compliance test is the stress relaxation test, where the sample is subjected to a predetermined strain and the stress required to maintain that strain is measured as a function of time. In this instance, a spring and dashpot in series (Maxwell unit) can be used to describe the behaviour. Initially the spring will extend instantaneously, and will then contract more slowly as the piston flows in the dashpot. Eventually the spring will be completely relaxed but the dashpot will be displaced, and in this case the ratio of viscosity to elasticity is referred to as the relaxation time.

Dynamic testing

Both creep and relaxation experiments are considered to be static tests. Viscoelastic materials can also be evaluated by means of dynamic experiments, whereby the sample is exposed to a forced sinusoidal oscillation and the transmitted stress measured. Once again, if the linear viscoelastic limit is not exceeded then the stress will also vary sinusoidally (Fig. 4.17). However, because of the nature of the material, energy will be lost so that the amplitude of the stress wave will be less than that of the strain wave and it will also lag behind the strain wave. If the amplitude ratio and the phase lag can be measured,

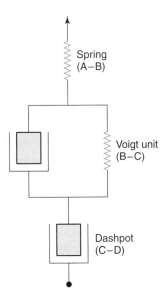

Fig. 4.16 Mechanical model representation of a creep compliance curve.

Spring (A–B)

Voigt unit (B–C)

Dashpot (C–D)

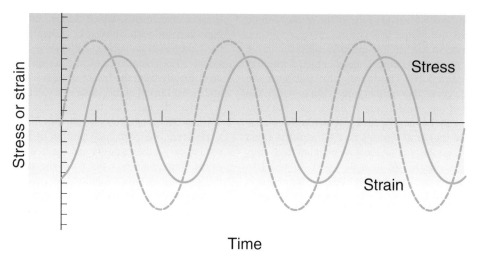

Fig. 4.17 Sine waves showing the stress wave lagging behind the strain wave during dynamic testing.

then the elasticity, referred to as the storage modulus, G', is given by:

$$G' = \left(\frac{\sigma}{\gamma}\right)\cos\delta \qquad (4.35)$$

where σ is the stress, γ is the strain and δ is the phase lag. A further modulus, G'', known as the loss modulus, is given by:

$$G'' = \left(\frac{\sigma}{\gamma}\right)\sin\delta \qquad (4.36)$$

This can be related to viscosity, η', by:

$$\eta' = \frac{G''}{\omega} \qquad (4.37)$$

where ω is the frequency of oscillation in rad (s^{-1}). From Eqns 4.35 and 4.36 it can be seen that:

$$\frac{G''}{G'} = \tan\delta \qquad (4.38)$$

and $\tan\delta$ is known as the loss tangent. Thus, a perfectly elastic material would produce a phase lag of 0°, whereas for a perfect fluid it would be 90°.

Finally, the concepts of liquid-like and solid-like behaviour can be explained by the dimensionless Deborah number (De), which finds expression as:

$$De = \frac{\tau}{T} \qquad (4.39)$$

where τ is a characteristic time of the material and T is a characteristic time of the deformation process. For a perfectly elastic material, τ will be infinite, whereas for a Newtonian fluid it will be zero. High Deborah numbers can be produced either by high values of τ or by small values of T. The latter will occur in situations where high rates of strain are experienced, for example slapping water with the hand. Also, even solid materials would be predicted to flow if a high enough stress was applied for a sufficiently long time.

Suspensions

Many pharmaceutical products, particularly those for children, are presented as suspensions and their rheological properties are important. In general these properties must be adjusted so that:

- the product is easily administered (e.g. easily poured from a bottle or forced through a syringe needle)
- sedimentation is either prevented or retarded; if it does occur, redispersion is easy
- the product has an elegant appearance.

The rheological properties of suspensions are markedly affected by the degree of flocculation (see Chapter 6). The reason for this is that the amount of free continuous phase is reduced, as it becomes entrapped in the diffuse floccules. Consequently, the apparent viscosity of a flocculated suspension is normally higher than that of a suspension, which is in all ways similar with the exception that it is deflocculated. In addition, when a disperse system is highly flocculated then the possibility of interaction between floccules occurs and structured systems result. If the forces bonding floccules together are capable of withstanding weak stresses then a yield value will result. Below this value, the suspension will behave like a solid. Once the yield value has been exceeded the amount of structural breakdown increases with increased shear stress. Therefore, flocculated suspensions will exhibit plastic or, more usually, pseudoplastic behaviour. Obviously, if the breakdown and reformation of the bonds between floccules are time dependent then thixotropic behaviour will also be observed.

The formation of structures does not occur in deflocculated suspensions and so their rheological behaviour is determined by that of the continuous phase together with the effect of distortion of the flow lines around the particles; in this situation the Einstein equation (Eqn 4.6) may apply. As the suspension becomes more concentrated and the particles come into contact, then dilatancy will occur.

Deflocculated particles in Newtonian vehicles

When such systems sediment, a compact sediment or cake is produced which is difficult to redisperse. The rate of sedimentation can be reduced by increasing the viscosity of the continuous medium, which will remain Newtonian. However, there is a limit to which this viscosity can be increased because difficulty will be experienced, for example, in pouring the suspension from a bottle. Furthermore, if sedimentation does occur, then subsequent redispersion may be even more difficult.

Deflocculated particles in non-Newtonian vehicles

Only pseudoplastic or plastic dispersion media can be used in the formulation of suspensions and both will retard the sedimentation of small particles, as their apparent viscosities will be high under the small stresses associated with sedimentation. Also, as the medium will undergo structural breakdown under the higher stresses involved in shaking and pouring, both these processes are facilitated.

The hydrocolloids used as suspending agents, such as acacia, tragacanth, methylcellulose, gelatin and sodium carboxymethylcellulose, all impart non-Newtonian properties, normally pseudoplasticity, to the suspensions. Thixotropy can occur and this is particularly the case with the mineral clays, such as bentonite (which must only be used in suspensions for external use). The three-dimensional gel network traps the deflocculated particles at rest and their sedimentation is retarded and may be completely prevented. The gel network is destroyed during shaking so that administration is facilitated. It is desirable that the gel network is reformed quickly so that dispersion of the particles is maintained.

Flocculated particles in Newtonian vehicles

Such particles will still sediment but because the aggregates are diffuse, a large volume sediment is produced and, as such, is easier to disperse. These systems are seldom improved by an increase in the viscosity of the continuous phase as this will only influence the rate of sedimentation. The major problem is one of pharmaceutical inelegance, in that the sediment does not fill the whole of the fluid volume. Methods of improving such products are given in Chapter 27.

Flocculated particles in non-Newtonian vehicles

These systems combine the advantages of both methods. Furthermore, variations in the properties of the raw materials to be suspended are unlikely to influence the performance of a product made on production scale. Consequently, less difference will be observed between batches made by the same method and plant.

Emulsions

Because nearly all but the most dilute of medicinal emulsions exhibit non-Newtonian behaviour, their rheological characteristics have a marked effect on their usefulness. The fluid emulsions are usually pseudoplastic and those approaching a semi-solid nature behave plastically and exhibit marked yield values. The semi-solid creams are usually viscoelastic. A considerable variety of pharmaceutical products can be formulated by altering the concentration of the disperse phase and the nature and concentration of the emulsifying agent. The latter can be used to confer viscoelastic properties on a topical cream merely by varying the ratio of surface-active agent to long-chain alcohol. Further aspects of pharmaceutical emulsions and topical creams are discussed in Chapters 27 and 38, respectively.

EFFECT OF RHEOLOGICAL PROPERTIES ON BIOAVAILABILITY

The presence of the diffusion coefficient which is inversely related to viscosity in the constant k_1 of the Noyes–Whitney equation (Chapter 2, Eqns 2.3 and 2.4) means that the rate of dissolution of a drug particle will be decreased as the viscosity of the dissolution medium is increased. This will apply to both in vitro and in vivo situations, and usually the medium into which the drug is dissolving will exhibit Newtonian behaviour. However, in the stomach the presence of the high molecular weight glycoproteins from mucus in acid solution will only be Newtonian up to a concentration of about 2%, beyond which it will exhibit non-Newtonian behaviour. In addition, the use of hydrocolloids will contribute to this effect and it has been shown that their inclusion in formulations can affect bioavailability. However, both increases and decreases in bioavailability have been reported, and it is not clear whether the effect is simply due to the modification of rheological properties or whether there has been an effect on gastrointestinal transit.

Attempts to predict this decrease in absorption have been made by the inclusion of natural or synthetic polymers in the dissolution medium used for in vitro studies. Some studies have shown that it is not the bulk viscosity of the dissolution medium that is of importance, but rather the 'effective viscosity'. Also, it is by no means certain that these polymers will behave in the same manner as the macromolecules that will be encountered in the gastrointestinal tract. Furthermore, it is impossible to carry out a dissolution test in an environment that relates to conditions in the region of the gut wall.

This viscosity effect will also operate at other drug delivery sites. For example, the absorption of drugs by the skin and from injection sites will be decreased by an increase in the viscosity of the vehicle. Indeed, in the case of injections, the creation of a depot with a highly viscoelastic nature should result in prolonged delivery of the drug.

A proper understanding of rheological behaviour, both in the formulation and, if possible, at the absorption site, is essential in any evaluation of bioavailability.

BIBLIOGRAPHY

Barnes, H.A., Hutton, J.F., Walters, K. (1989) *An Introduction to Rheology*. Elsevier Science, Amsterdam.

Barry, B.W. (1974) Rheology of pharmaceutical and cosmetic semisolids. In: Bean H.S., Beckett, A.W., Carless, J.E. (eds) *Advances in Pharmaceutical Sciences*, Vol 4. Academic Press, London.

Ferry, J.D. (1980) *Viscoelastic Properties of Polymers*. John Wiley, New York.

Lapasin, R., Pricl, S. (1999) *Rheology of Industrial Polysaccharides: Theory and Applications*. Aspen Publishers, Gaithersburg.

Ross-Murphy, S.B. (1994) Rheological methods. In: Ross-Murphy, S.B. (ed.) *Physical Techniques for the Study of Food Biopolymers*. Blackie Academic and Professional, Glasgow.

Schnaare, R., Block, L., Rohan, L. (2005) Rheology. In: Hendrickson, R. (ed.) *Remington's The Science and Practice of Pharmacy*, 21st edn. Lippincott, Williams and Wilkins, Philadelphia.

Surface and interfacial phenomena

J. T. Fell

INTRODUCTION

The boundary between two phases is generally described as an *interface*. When one of the phases is a gas or a vapour and the other a liquid or solid, the term *surface* is frequently used. Matter at interfaces usually has different characteristics from that in the bulk of the media and as a consequence, the study of interfaces has developed into a separate branch of chemistry – surface chemistry. In pharmaceutical sciences interfacial phenomena play an important role in the processing of a wide variety of formulations. The subsequent behaviour of these formulations in vivo is often governed by an interfacial process.

Interfaces are categorized according to the phases they separate, as follows: liquid/liquid (L/L), liquid/vapour (L/V), solid/vapour (S/V) and solid/liquid (S/L). It is often convenient to consider each interface separately.

SURFACE TENSION AND SURFACE FREE ENERGY

Consider the case of a single component liquid. The molecules in the liquid are subject to attractive forces from adjacent molecules. Figure 5.1 shows the attractive forces experienced by a molecule at the surface of the liquid. In the bulk of the liquid the molecules are subjected to equal attraction in all directions. At the surface, however, the net attractive force is towards the bulk of the liquid. This net inward attraction reduces the number of molecules in the surface and increases the intermolecular distance. It is this that gives the surface different characteristics from the bulk and gives rise to surface tension and surface free energy.

A useful approach to understanding these terms is to examine Figure 5.2. This shows parallel wires, joined at the top, on which there is a freely moving slider of length l and mass m_1. If a film of soap solution is formed between the upper wire and the slider, the film will

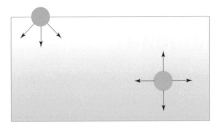

Fig. 5.1 Attractive forces at the surface and in the bulk of a material.

rapidly contract owing to the surface tension forces (as the system attempts to minimize its free energy). The slider can be held in the original position by attaching a weight to it, m_2, and this will give a measure of the surface tension. The same weight will hold the film in equilibrium even if it is expanded or contracted. This is because the surface is not stretched or contracted as such but remains the same, with molecules entering or leaving the bulk to compensate for the change in area.

The surface tension is therefore independent of the area of the film, but depends on the chemical nature of the interfaces and their length. In the example in Figure 5.2 there are two interfaces, on the front and the back of the film; the total length of the film/air interface is $2l$. The surface tension is the force acting parallel to the surface at right angles to a line of 1 m length anywhere in the surface. Its units are typically mN m^{-1}. In the above example the surface tension (γ) is the force acting perpendicular to the surface, divided by the length of the surface, and is:

$$\gamma = \frac{(m_1 + m_2)g}{2l} = \frac{F}{2l} \tag{5.1}$$

where g is the acceleration due to gravity.

As explained earlier, if the film shown in Figure 5.2 is expanded, no force is required. Work is done, however, because the area is increased. If the slider is moved a

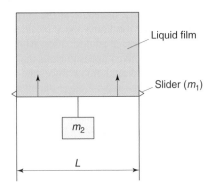

Fig. 5.2 Liquid film attached to a freely moving slider.

distance, x, the increase in total surface area is $2lx$ as there are two surfaces, the front and back of the film. The work done is Fx. The surface free energy is defined as the work required to increase the surface area by 1 m^2. Typical units are mJ m^{-2}. The work done per unit area in expanding the film is:

$$\frac{Fx}{2lx} = \frac{F}{2l} = \gamma \tag{5.2}$$

The surface tension and the surface free energy are thus dimensionally equivalent (J = N m) and numerically equal.

The above concepts were derived from a consideration of a liquid/vapour system. Identical arguments can be used for liquid/liquid systems, the terminology being changed to *interfacial free energy* and *interfacial tension*. In principle, the above argument also applies to solids, although it is easier to visualize the existence of the surface free energy of solids in terms of the unbalanced forces projecting from the interface, rather than the net inward attraction exerted on the molecules residing at the interface.

In this chapter, the symbol γ will be used to denote both surface and interfacial tension. When it is necessary to distinguish between different surface or interfacial tensions, subscripts will be used. For example, $\gamma_{L/L}$ is the interfacial tension between two liquids and $\gamma_{L/V}$ is the surface tension between a liquid and its vapour. For more specific cases, γ_A will represent the surface tension of a liquid A and $\gamma_{A/B}$ the interfacial tension between liquids A and B.

Liquid/vapour systems

Curved surfaces

A pressure difference exists across curved surfaces to balance the influence of surface tension. Knowledge of this is important in some methods used in the determination of surface tension.

Consider a bubble of vapour in a liquid. In the absence of any external forces, the bubble will be spherical in shape and will remain the same size because the surface tension forces are balanced by an internal excess pressure. This excess pressure is given by:

$$\Delta p = \frac{2\gamma}{r} \tag{5.3}$$

where Δp is the excess pressure and r is the radius of the bubble. For non-spherical surfaces which can be described by two radii of curvature, the equation becomes:

$$\Delta p = \gamma \left(\frac{1}{r_1} + \frac{1}{r_2} \right) \tag{5.4}$$

This is known as the Laplace equation; γ is always positive. For p to be positive, r must be positive, which means that the pressure is always greater on the concave side.

These equations (5.3 and 5.4) apply to any curved liquid interface, e.g. the system described above, a liquid film around a bubble in air or the meniscus of a bulk liquid.

Influence of temperature

For the majority of liquids an increase in temperature leads to a decrease in surface tension. The exceptions are some molten metals. This decrease in surface tension with increasing temperature is approximately linear. As the temperature approaches the critical temperature for a liquid (i.e. the temperature when the liquid structure is lost), the intermolecular cohesion forces approach zero and the surface tension becomes very small.

Liquid/liquid systems

The interfacial tension between two immiscible liquids arises as a result of an imbalance of forces, in an identical manner to the surface tension between a liquid and its vapour. Interfacial tensions generally lie between the surface tensions of the two liquids under consideration. Table 5.1 lists the surface tensions of several liquids and their interfacial tensions against water.

Spreading

If a small quantity of an immiscible liquid is placed on a clean surface of a second liquid, it may spread to cover the surface with a film or remain as a drop or lens (Fig. 5.3). Which of the two applies depends on how the system achieves a state of minimum free energy. The ability of one liquid to spread over another can be assessed in terms of the spreading coefficient (S). A positive or zero value of S is required for spreading to occur.

$$S = \gamma_A - (\gamma_B + \gamma_{A/B}) \qquad (5.5)$$

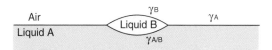

Fig. 5.3 Spreading of one liquid on another.

An alternative approach is to examine spreading in terms of the *work of cohesion* and *work of adhesion*. The work of cohesion applies to a single liquid and is the work required to pull apart a column of liquid of unit cross-sectional area and create two liquid/air interfaces.

$$W_{A/A} = 2\gamma_A \qquad (5.6)$$

The work of adhesion is the work required to separate a unit cross-sectional area of a liquid/liquid interface between two different liquids (A and B) to form two different liquid/air interfaces. This is given by the Dupre equation:

$$W_{A/B} = \gamma_A + \gamma_B - \gamma_{A/B} \qquad (5.7)$$

Hence, by substitution into Eqn 5.5:

$$S = W_{A/B} - W_{A/A} \qquad (5.8)$$

Therefore, spreading occurs when the liquid placed on, for example, a water surface adheres to the water more strongly than it coheres to itself.

In practice, when two immiscible liquids are placed in contact, the bulk liquids will eventually become mutually saturated. This will change the values of the various surface and interfacial tensions. Hence, there is an initial spreading coefficient which is an immediate value, and a final spreading coefficient after mutual saturation has taken place. For benzene or hexanol on water, the initial spreading coefficients are positive. When mutual saturation has occurred the values of the surface and interfacial tensions are reduced, so that the final spreading coefficients are negative. Hence benzene or hexanol spreads immediately on water and then the spreading stops, leaving a monomolecular layer of benzene or hexanol, with the remainder of the liquid in the form of flat lenses.

Measurement of surface and interfacial tension

There are several methods available for the measurement of surface and interfacial tension. Four will be described here. Further details and descriptions of other methods can be obtained by consulting the bibliography.

Wilhelmy plate methods

The apparatus consists of a thin mica, glass or platinum plate attached to a suitable balance (Fig. 5.4). When used

Table 5.1 The surface tensions of some common liquids and their interfacial tensions against water at 20°C (mN m⁻¹)

Liquid	Surface tension	Interfacial tension against water
Water	72	–
n-Octanol	27	8.5
Carbon tetrachloride	27	45
Chloroform	27	33
Olive oil	36	33
n-Hexane	18	51

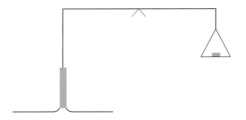

Fig. 5.4   Wilhelmy plate method.

as a detachment method, the plate is immersed in the liquid, and the liquid container is gradually lowered. The reading on the balance immediately prior to detachment is noted. The detachment force is equal to the surface tension multiplied by the perimeter of the surface detached:

$$(W_L - W)g = 2(L + T)\gamma \tag{5.9}$$

where W_L is the reading on the balance prior to detachment, W is the weight of the plate in air and L and T are the length and thickness of the plate, respectively. Immersion of the plate into the lower of two liquids in a container and subsequent detachment will give the interfacial tension.

Alternatively, the plate can be used in a static mode, where the change in force required to keep the plate at a constant depth is measured. This is useful for assessing changes in surface tension with time.

The method requires the contact angle that the liquid makes with the plate to be zero. This can be achieved by scrupulous cleaning and by roughening the surface of the plate. In addition, it must be ensured that the edge of the plate lies in a horizontal plane.

Ring method (du Nuoy tensiometer)

This method measures the force required to detach a platinum ring from a surface or an interface. Figure 5.5 shows the set-up for an interface. Again, the detachment

force is equal to the surface tension multiplied by the perimeter of liquid detached, hence:

$$F = 2\pi(R_1 + R_2)\gamma \tag{5.10}$$

where F is the detachment force and R_1 and R_2 are the inner and outer radii of the ring. Again, a zero contact angle of the liquid on the ring must be assured or the equation will not hold. This can be achieved by careful cleaning and flaming of the platinum loop or by the use of a silicone-treated ring for oils. The ring must also lie horizontally in the surface.

As the shape of the liquid supported by the ring during detachment is complex and hence the surface tension forces do not act vertically, the above simple equation is imprecise and correction factors must be applied for accurate determinations.

Drop weight and drop volume methods

If the volume or weight of a drop as it is detached from a tip of known radius is determined, the surface or interfacial tension can be calculated from:

$$\gamma = \frac{\phi mg}{2\pi r} = \frac{\phi V\rho g}{2\pi r} \tag{5.11}$$

where m is the mass of the drop, V is the volume of the drop, ρ is the density of the liquid, r is the radius of the tip, g is the acceleration due to gravity and ϕ is a correction factor. A typical apparatus is shown in Figure 5.6. The method is easily adapted for both surface and interfacial tensions and is therefore popular. The correction factor is required as not all the drop leaves the tip on detachment. The correction factors are shown in Figure 5.7 and depend on the radius of the tip and the

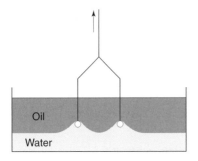

Fig. 5.5   Du Nuoy tensiometer being used to measure interfacial tension.

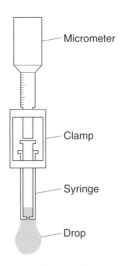

Fig. 5.6   Drop volume or drop weight method.

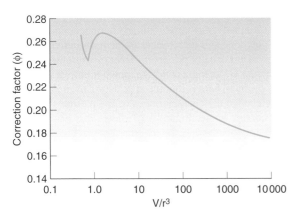

Fig. 5.7 Correction factors for the drop volume or drop weight method.

drop volume. It is important that the tip is completely wetted by the liquid, and that the drop does not 'climb' up the outside of the tube. The drop should also be formed slowly, especially in the stage immediately preceding detachment.

Capillary rise method

Although this method is little used in pharmaceutical research, it is considered to be the most accurate way of measuring surface tension and has been used to establish values for many liquids. As the surface of the liquid is undisturbed during the measurement, time effects can be followed.

If a capillary tube is placed in a liquid, provided the angle of contact that the liquid makes with the capillary tube is less than 90°, the liquid will rise in the tube to a certain height. Figure 5.8 shows a diagrammatic representation of this.

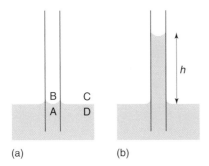

(a) (b)

Fig. 5.8 Stages in the rise of a liquid up a capillary tube.

If the tube is small in diameter, the meniscus can be considered to be hemispherical and the radius of curvature will be:

$$r_t = r_m \cos\theta \qquad (5.12)$$

where r_t is the radius of the capillary tube, r_m is the radius of curvature of the meniscus and θ is the contact angle. Hence, from the Laplace equation (Eqn 5.3) for this system:

$$\Delta p = \frac{2\gamma \cos\theta}{r_t} \qquad (5.13)$$

which is the pressure difference between atmospheric and that immediately below the meniscus. Referring to Figure 5.8, the pressure at point B is atmospheric, whereas that at point A is less by an amount given by Eqn 5.4. At point C the pressure is atmospheric, as it also is at point D, as the liquid here is effectively flat, i.e. the radius of curvature of the meniscus is large. The pressure difference between D and A causes the liquid to rise in the capillary tube until the difference is balanced by the hydrostatic pressure of the column of liquid. At this equilibrium point:

$$\frac{2\gamma \cos\theta}{r_t} = h\left(\rho_L - \rho_V\right)g \qquad (5.14)$$

where $\rho_L - \rho_V$ is the density difference between the liquid and its vapour, g is the acceleration due to gravity and h is the height of the liquid in the capillary tube.

As contact angles are difficult to reproduce, experiments are always run at $\theta = 0$ ($\cos\theta = 1$), achieved by careful cleaning. Hence the equation reduces to:

$$\gamma = \frac{r_t h\left(\rho_L - \rho_V\right)}{2} g \qquad (5.15)$$

The capillaries used must be circular in cross-section and of uniform bore. As with all methods of measuring surface and interfacial tension, cleanliness at all stages of the experiment is vital and adequate temperature control must be ensured.

Solid/vapour and solid/liquid systems

Liquid surfaces and interfaces are open to direct, simple experimental procedures for determining surface and interfacial tensions. Methods for determining similar parameters for solids are indirect and difficult. The system of most interest pharmaceutically is the behaviour of a liquid in contact with a solid.

Contact angle

If a drop of liquid is placed on a flat, smooth, horizontal solid surface, it may spread completely but is more likely to form a drop. This drop will exhibit a definite angle against the solid, known as the *contact angle* (Fig. 5.9). By equating the horizontal component of the various interfacial tensions, the following equation (Young's equation) is derived:

$$\gamma_{S/V} = \gamma_{S/L} + \gamma_{L/V}\cos\theta \qquad (5.16)$$

The work of adhesion between the solid and the liquid is given by the appropriate form of the Dupre equation (Eqn 5.7):

$$W_{S/L} = \gamma_{S/V} + \gamma_{L/V} - \gamma_{S/L} \qquad (5.17)$$

Combining this with Eqn 5.16 gives the following:

$$W_{S/L} = \gamma_{L/V}(1 + \cos\theta) \qquad (5.18)$$

This means that the work of adhesion between the solid and the liquid can be determined in terms of measurable quantities.

In a similar manner to liquids, a spreading coefficient (*S*) for a liquid on a solid may be defined as:

$$S = \gamma_{L/V}(\cos\theta - 1) \qquad (5.19)$$

which will give a measure of how well a liquid will spread on a solid. If a liquid is penetrating into a capillary, for example the pores in a powder bed or a tablet, the value of interest is the adhesion tension (AT), given by:

$$AT = \gamma_{L/V}\cos\theta \qquad (5.20)$$

As $\gamma_{L/V}$ is always positive, the spontaneity of these processes will be controlled by $\cos\theta$. For example, for penetration into capillaries under no extra applied pressure, the adhesion tension must be positive, hence $\cos\theta$ must be positive, i.e. the contact angle, θ, must be less than 90°.

The determination of contact angles for materials that are available as flat, smooth, solid surfaces is relatively straightforward. A drop of liquid is placed on the surface and the angle it makes with the surface can be measured directly by magnifying the drop in some way. Unfortunately, most materials of pharmaceutical interest are powders, and direct measurement on individual particles is not usually possible. Direct measurement can be achieved by compressing the powder into a compact. The problem here is that the application of high pressure may change the characteristics of the particles and alter the contact angle. Figure 5.10 shows this has occurred with amylobarbitone, the measured contact angle changing as the pressure is increased. The *h-ε* method also uses a compact, but prepared at a lower pressure and saturated with the test liquid. A liquid drop is then formed on the surface of this saturated compact and the maximum height of this drop is related to the contact angle.

Another method that uses a compact is dynamic contact angle analysis. Here the powder is compressed into a thin rectangular plate and the method used is the same as the Wilhelmy plate method for measuring surface tension. The liquid forms a contact angle with the plate, as shown in Figure 5.11. The contact angle is given by:

$$\cos\theta = \frac{F}{\gamma^2(L + T)} \qquad (5.21)$$

Compare this to the determination of surface tension by the Wilhelmy plate.

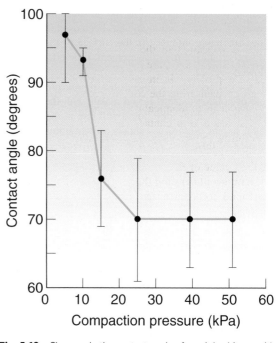

Fig. 5.10 Changes in the contact angle of amylobarbitone with the pressure used to form the compact (from Buckton et al (1996) *Powder Technology*, 46: 201-208, with permission from Elsevier Science).

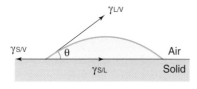

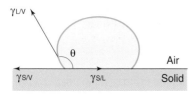

Fig. 5.9 Contact angles of liquids on solids.

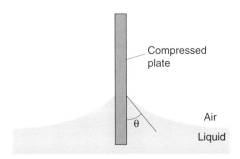

Fig. 5.11 Measurement of contact angles using dynamic contact angle analysis.

Table 5.2 The contact angles of some pharmaceutical solids against their saturated aqueous solutions

Material	Contact angle (°)
Acetylsalicylic acid	74
Amylobarbitone	102
Diazepam	83
Lactose	30
Magnesium stearate	121
Paracetamol	59
Digoxin	49
Ampicillin	35
Indomethacin	90
Sulfanilamide	64

To measure the contact angle of a powder without compaction, the Washburn method can be used. Here, a powder bed is formed in a tube fitted with a sintered glass filter at the base. The base of the tube is immersed in liquid and the liquid will penetrate into the capillaries between the powder particles, as shown earlier in Figure 5.8. The rate of penetration is measured and if the capillaries in the powder bed are regarded as being a bundle of capillary tubes, the rate of penetration is given by:

$$\frac{L^2}{t} = \gamma \frac{\cos\theta\, r}{2\eta} \qquad (5.22)$$

where L is the length penetrated in time t, r is the radius of the capillaries, η is the liquid viscosity and γ and θ are the surface tension and the contact angle of the liquid, respectively.

L^2/t is measured in the experiment and the liquid characteristics η and γ are known or can be easily measured; the problem is in determining r. This can be solved by measuring the rate of penetration, L^2/t, into the powder in an identical state of packing, using a liquid that has a zero contact angle against the powder. Substituting this into Eqn 5.22 gives a value for r which can then be used in the equation to determine the required value of θ.

Examples illustrating the range of contact angle values found for pharmaceutical powders are given in Table 5.2.

Pharmaceutical applications

Many pharmaceutical processes involve interactions at the interfaces described. The preparation of emulsions and suspensions, described in Chapters 6 and 27, involves interactions at the liquid/liquid and liquid/solid interfaces, respectively. Interactions between a liquid and a solid are particularly common. Granulation, prior to tableting, involves the mixing of a powder with a liquid binder and the success of the process will, in part, depend on the spreading of the liquid over the solid.

A rational approach to the selection of a granulating agent, based on the measurement of spreading coefficients and other surface properties, has been described by Rowe (1989). Similarly, film coating requires the spread of liquid over a tablet surface. The successful dissolution of a tablet or capsule necessitates penetration of the liquid into the pores of the dosage form. In all these examples, the contact angle and the surface tension of the liquid are important. Surface-active agents are commonly employed in formulation as they reduce the contact angle and hence aid in the wetting of a solid by reducing $\gamma_{L/V}$, and also absorbing at the solid/liquid interface and reducing $\gamma_{S/V}$.

ADSORPTION

Liquid/vapour and liquid/liquid systems

Surface-active agents

Many molecules have structures that contain two separate regions: a hydrophilic (water-liking) region, which confers on the compound a solubility in water, and a hydrophobic (water-hating) region, which renders the material soluble in hydrocarbon solvents. Because of this dual structure, it is energetically favourable for these materials, when dissolved, to adsorb at interfaces, orientating themselves in such a manner that the regions are associated with the appropriate solvent or air. Such materials are termed *surface-active agents* (or *surfactants*). Details of their structures and properties are given in Chapters 6 and 27.

Pure liquid surfaces have a tendency to contract as a result of surface tension forces. The packing of the surface with surface-active molecules favours expansion of the surface. The surface-active molecules reduce the surface tension of the liquid by an amount equal to the expanding (or surface) pressure. Surfactants will lower surface tension to different degrees. An approximation, Traube's Rule, states that for a particular homologous series of surfactants in dilute solution, the concentration necessary to produce an equal lowering of surface tension decreases by a factor of three for each additional –CH$_2$– group. The formation of the adsorbed surface layer will not be instantaneous, but will be governed by the diffusion of the surfactant to the interface. The time taken to reach equilibrium will depend on factors such as molecular size, shape and the presence of impurities. For immiscible liquids, the reduction in interfacial tension may be such that emulsification takes place readily. Detailed aspects of this are dealt with in Chapter 6.

In certain cases a 'negative adsorption' may occur, i.e. the solute molecules migrate away from the surface. In these cases, examples of which are solutions of sugars and electrolytes, small increases in surface tension are observed.

Surface excess concentration

The extent of the distribution of a solute between an interface and the bulk phase is generally expressed in terms of a *surface excess, n*. This is the amount of a material present at the interface in excess of that which would have been there if the bulk phase extended to the interface without a change in composition.

The *surface excess concentration, Γ*, is *n/A* where *A* is the area of the interface.

The adsorption of material at any interface is given by the Gibbs adsorption equation. Its general form is:

$$d\gamma = - \Sigma\Gamma_i du_i \qquad (5.23)$$

where $d\gamma$ is the change in interfacial tension, Γ_i is the surface excess concentration of the *i*th component and u_i is the chemical potential of the *i*th component.

In the specific case of a solute partitioning between the surface and the bulk of a liquid, the equation becomes:

$$\Gamma = \frac{C}{RT}\frac{d\gamma_{L/V}}{dC} \qquad (5.24)$$

where *C* is the overall solute concentration, *R* is the gas constant, *T* is the absolute temperature and $d\gamma_{L/V}/dC$ is the change of surface tension with concentration. The above is applicable to dilute solutions. For concentrated solutions, activities must be substituted for concentration. Equation 5.24 has been verified experimentally by direct measurement of surface concentrations after removal of the surface layer with a microtome blade. The equation enables calculation of the surface excess from surface tension data.

As the concentration of a surface-active agent in aqueous solution is increased, the surface layer will eventually become saturated. Figure 5.12 shows a typical plot of surface tension against concentration. When the surface layer is saturated, further increases in concentration can no longer change the surface tension and the surfactant molecules form micelles (small aggregates of molecules) as an alternative means of 'protecting' the hydrophobic regions. Details of these are given in Chapter 6.

The discontinuity of the plot in Figure 5.12 is called the *critical micelle concentration*. Immediately before this, the surfactant molecules are closely packed at the surface and this gives a method of determining the surface area occupied by each molecule, *A*, from:

$$A = \frac{1}{N_A \Gamma} \qquad (5.25)$$

where N_A is the Avogadro constant and *Γ* is the surface excess concentration calculated from the slope of the plot $d\gamma_{L/V}/d \log C$ immediately before the critical micelle concentration (remembering that *Γ* is a concentration expressed in terms of surface area).

Because of their structures, many drugs are surface active in nature and this activity may play a part in their pharmacological effects. Examples are some antihistamines, the phenothiazine tranquillizers and antidepressants.

Monomolecular films (monolayers)

Certain insoluble materials can, when dissolved in a suitable volatile solvent, be made to spread on the surface of water to form a film one molecule thick. This may be

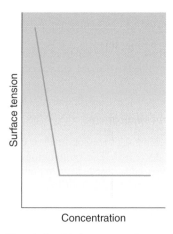

Fig. 5.12 The relationship between surface tension and concentration for a typical surfactant.

regarded as an extreme case of adsorption, as all the molecules are at the surface. Surface excess concentrations can be calculated directly from knowledge of the amount of material and the surface area. The monolayer will reduce the surface tension of the water by an amount equal to the surface pressure. The surface pressure, which is the expanding pressure due to the monolayer opposing the contracting tension of the water, can be measured directly by enclosing the film between moveable barriers.

$$\pi = \gamma_o - \gamma_m \qquad (5.26)$$

where π is the surface pressure, γ_o is the surface tension of the 'clean' liquid and γ_m the surface tension of the liquid covered with a monolayer.

Monolayers exist in different physical states which are in some ways analogous to the three states of matter: solid, liquid and gas. Pharmaceutically, monolayers have been used to study polymers which are used for film coating and packaging, and as models for cell membranes.

Solid/vapour systems

Although adsorption in solid/liquid systems is of more interest pharmaceutically, the interpretation of results is often achieved using equations developed for solid/vapour systems. This system will therefore be described first.

If a gas or vapour is brought into contact with a solid, some of it will become attached to the surface. This reduces the imbalance of attractive forces and hence the surface free energy. Adsorption here must be distinguished from absorption, where penetration into the solid may take place. In some cases it may be impossible to distinguish between the two. Here the general term *sorption* is used. Adsorption may be by relatively weak non-specific forces (van der Waals forces), this being termed *physical adsorption*.

Alternatively, the adsorption may be by stronger specific valence forces – *chemisorption*. Physical absorption is rapid and reversible, and multilayer adsorption is possible. Chemisorption is specific, may require an activation energy, and therefore be slow and not readily reversible. Only monomolecular chemisorbed layers are possible.

Adsorption studies using gases or vapour generally involve the determination of the amount of gas or vapour adsorbed, x, by a given mass, m, of the adsorbent at constant temperature. Determinations are carried out at different equilibrium pressures, p (the pressure attained after adsorption has taken place), to yield an adsorption isotherm. When vapours are used the results are generally expressed in terms of a *relative vapour pressure, p/p_o*, where p_o is the saturated vapour pressure. Prior to the studies the solid adsorbent must have any adsorbed material removed by placing it under vacuum or heating.

The isotherms obtained can generally be classified into five types, shown in Figure 5.13. Type I isotherms exhibit a rapid rise in adsorption up to a limiting value. They are referred to as Langmuir-type isotherms and are due to the adsorption being restricted to a monolayer. Hence adsorption of the chemisorption type will give this type of curve. Type II isotherms represent multilayer physical adsorption on non-porous materials. Types III and V occur when the adsorption in the first layer is weak, and are rare. Type IV is considered to be due to condensation of vapour in fine capillaries within a porous solid. There have been many attempts to develop equations to fit the experimentally observed isotherm. Among the most widely used expressions are the following:

Langmuir adsorption isotherm

The equation was derived by assuming that only monolayer coverage was possible, and so it is only

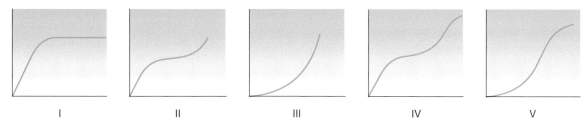

Fig. 5.13 Classification of isotherms for the adsorption of vapours by solids. Ordinates x/m, abscissae p/p_o.

applicable to type I isotherms. The equation is usefully written as:

$$\frac{pm}{x} = \frac{1}{b}p + \frac{1}{ab} \qquad (5.27)$$

where p, m and x are as defined previously and b and a are constants, b being the amount of gas required to produce a monolayer over the whole surface of the absorbent. Hence plotting pm/x against p should give a straight line with a slope $1/b$ and intercept $1/ab$.

Freundlich adsorption isotherm

This is given as:

$$\frac{x}{m} = kp^{1/n} \qquad (5.28)$$

where n and k are constants for a particular system. Plots of log x/m against log p should therefore give straight lines. The equation does not predict a limiting value as does the Langmuir equation.

Brunauer, Emmett and Teller (BET) equation

This equation takes into account multilayer adsorption and so describes type II isotherms. It is usually written in the form:

$$\frac{p}{V(p_o - p)} = \frac{1}{V_m c} + \frac{c - 1}{V_m c} \times \frac{p}{p_o} \qquad (5.29)$$

where p_o is the saturation vapour pressure, V is the equilibrium volume of gas adsorbed per unit mass of adsorbent, V_m is the volume of gas required to cover unit mass of adsorbent with monolayer, and c is a constant. The equation reduces to the Langmuir equation if adsorption is restricted to monolayer formation.

One direct practical application of the adsorption of gases of pharmaceutical interest is the determination of the surface area of powders. If the isotherm is determined and the point of monolayer formation identified, knowledge of the surface area of the adsorbing species will give a value for the surface area of the powder.

Solid/liquid systems

The adsorption of most interest is that of a solute, in solution, on to a solid. The equations most widely used to interpret the data are those of Langmuir and Freundlich. The pressure terms are replaced by concentration terms; hence the Langmuir equation becomes:

$$\frac{x}{m} = \frac{abC}{1 + bC} \qquad (5.30)$$

where x is the amount of solute adsorbed by a weight, m, of adsorbent, C is the concentration of the solution at equilibrium, and b and a are constants.

Adsorption from solution

Several factors will affect the extent of adsorption from solution. These include the following.

Solute concentration   An increase in the concentration of the solute will result in an increase in the amount of absorption that occurs at equilibrium until a limiting value is reached. It should be noted that for most cases of adsorption from solution, the relative amount of solute removed is greater in dilute solutions.

Temperature   Adsorption is generally exothermic, and hence an increase in temperature leads to a decrease in adsorption.

pH   The influence of pH is usually through a change in the ionization of the solute and the influence will depend on which species is more strongly adsorbed.

Surface area of adsorbent   An increased surface area, achieved by a reduction in particle size or the use of a porous material, will increase the extent of adsorption.

Pharmaceutical applications of adsorption from solution

The phenomenon of adsorption from solution finds practical application of pharmaceutical interest in chromatographic techniques and in the removal of unwanted materials. In addition, adsorption may give rise to certain formulation problems.

Successive adsorption and desorption forms the basis for both TLC and HPLC chromatographic analysis (Chapter 24). Materials such as activated charcoal can be given in cases of orally taken poisons to adsorb the toxic materials. In addition, adsorbents may be used in haemodialysis to remove the products of dialysis from the dialysing solution, allowing the solution to be recycled.

Adsorption may cause problems in formulation where drugs or other materials such as preservatives are adsorbed by containers, thereby reducing the effective concentration. In addition, certain additives, such as the parabens, may be adsorbed on to the solid material present in a suspension, leading to a loss in antimicrobial activity (Allwood 1982). Glyceryl trinitrate is a volatile liquid given in the form of tablets. The vapour may be sorbed by the container, leading to further volatilization and loss of potency. The adsorption of insulin on to intravenous administration sets has been reported, as has the sorption of phenylmercuric acetate, used as a preservative in eye drops, on to polyethylene containers (Aspinall et al 1980).

Adsorption may be put to a positive use in the enhancement of the dissolution rate of hydrophobic drugs by adsorption of surface-active agents onto the surface of the drug particles.

REFERENCES

Allwood, M.C. (1982) The adsorption of esters of *p*-hydroxybenzoic acid by magnesium trisilicate. *International Journal of Pharmaceutics,* **11**, 101-107.

Aspinall, J.D., Duffy, T.D., Saunders, M.B., Taylor, C.G. (1980) The effect of low density polyethylene containers on some hospital manufactured eye-drop formulations: sorption of phenyl mercuric acetate. *Journal of Clinical and Hospital Pharmacy,* **5**, 21-30.

Rowe, R.C. (1989) Binder-substrate interactions in granulation: a theoretical approach based on surface free energy and polarity. *International Journal of Pharmaceutics,* **52**, 149-154.

BIBLIOGRAPHY

Adamson, A.W. (1980) *Physical Chemistry of Surfaces*, 4th edn. John Wiley, New York.

Florence, A.T., Attwood, D. (2006) *Physicochemical Principles of Pharmacy*, 4th edn. Pharmaceutical Press, London.

Shaw, D.J. (1992) *Introduction to Colloid and Surface Chemistry*, 4th edn. Butterworths, London.

CHAPTER CONTENTS

INTRODUCTION

A disperse system consists essentially of one component, the *disperse phase*, dispersed as particles or droplets throughout another component, the *continuous phase*. By definition, those dispersions in which the size of the dispersed particles is within the range 10^{-9} m (1 nm) to about 10^{-6} m (1 μm) are termed colloidal. However, the upper size limit is often extended to include emulsions and suspensions which are very polydisperse systems in which the droplet size frequently exceeds 1 μm, but which show many of the properties of colloidal systems.

Some examples of colloidal systems of pharmaceutical interest are shown in Table 6.1. Many natural systems such as suspensions of microorganisms, blood and isolated cells in culture are also colloidal dispersions.

This chapter will examine the properties of both coarse dispersions, such as emulsions, suspensions and aerosols, and also fine dispersions, such as micellar systems, which fall within the defined size range of true colloidal dispersions.

Colloids can be broadly classified as those that are *lyophobic* (solvent-hating) and those that are *lyophilic* (solvent-liking). The terms *hydrophobic* and *hydrophilic* are used when the solvent is water. Surfactant molecules

Table 6.1   Types of disperse systems

Dispersed phase	Dispersion medium	Name	Examples
Liquid	Gas	Liquid aerosol	Fogs, mists, aerosols
Solid	Gas	Solid aerosol	Smoke, powder aerosols
Gas	Liquid	Foam	Foam on surfactant solutions
Liquid	Liquid	Emulsion	Milk, pharmaceutical emulsions
Solid	Liquid	Sol, suspension	Silver iodide sol, aluminium hydroxide suspension
Gas	Solid	Solid foam	Expanded polystyrene
Liquid	Solid	Solid emulsion	Liquids dispersed in soft paraffin, opals, pearls
Solid	Solid	Solid suspension	Pigmented plastics, colloidal gold in glass, ruby glass

tend to associate in water into aggregates called micelles and these constitute hydrophilic colloidal dispersions. Proteins and gums also form lyophilic colloidal systems because of a similar affinity between the dispersed particles and the continuous phase. On the other hand, dispersions of oil droplets in water or water droplets in oil are examples of lyophobic dispersions.

It is because of the subdivision of matter in colloidal systems that they have special properties. A common feature of these systems is a large surface-to-volume ratio of the dispersed particles. As a consequence, there is a tendency for the particles to associate in order to reduce their surface area. Emulsion droplets, for example, eventually coalesce to form a macrophase, so attaining a minimum surface area and hence an equilibrium state. This chapter will examine how the stability of colloidal dispersions can be understood by a consideration of the forces acting between the dispersed particles. Approaches to the formulation of emulsions, suspensions and aerosols will be described and the instability of these coarse dispersions will be discussed using a theory of colloid stability. The association of surface-active agents into micelles and the applications of these colloidal dispersions in the solubilization of poorly water-soluble drugs will also be considered.

COLLOIDS

Preparation and purification of colloidal systems

Lyophilic colloids

The affinity of lyophilic colloids for the dispersion medium leads to the spontaneous formation of colloidal dispersions. For example, acacia, tragacanth, methylcellulose and certain other cellulose derivatives readily disperse in water. This simple method of dispersion is a general one for the formation of lyophilic colloids.

Lyophobic colloids

The preparative methods for lyophobic colloids may be divided into those methods that involve the breakdown of larger particles into particles of colloidal dimensions (dispersion methods) and those in which the colloidal particles are formed by aggregation of smaller particles such as molecules (condensation methods).

Dispersion methods   The breakdown of coarse material may be carried out by the use of a colloid mill or ultrasonics.

Colloid mills   These mills cause the dispersion of coarse material by shearing in a narrow gap between a static cone (the stator) and a rapidly rotating cone (the rotor).

Ultrasonic treatment   The passage of ultrasonic waves through a dispersion medium produces alternating regions of cavitation and compression in the medium. The cavities collapse with great force and cause the breakdown of coarse particles dispersed in the liquid.

With both these methods the particles will tend to reunite unless a stabilizing agent such as a surface-active agent is added.

Condensation methods   These involve the rapid production of supersaturated solutions of the colloidal material under conditions in which it is deposited in the dispersion medium as colloidal particles and not as a precipitate. The supersaturation is often obtained by means of a chemical reaction that results in the formation of the colloidal material. For example, colloidal silver iodide may be obtained by reacting together dilute solutions of silver nitrate and potassium iodide; colloidal sulphur is produced from sodium thiosulfate and hydrochloric acid solutions; and ferric chloride boiled with excess of water produces colloidal hydrated ferric oxide.

A change of solvent may also cause the production of colloidal particles by condensation methods. If a saturated solution of sulphur in acetone is poured slowly into hot water, the acetone vaporizes, leaving a colloidal dispersion of sulphur. A similar dispersion may be obtained when a solution of a resin, such as benzoin in alcohol, is poured into water.

Dialysis

Colloidal particles are not retained by conventional filter papers but are too large to diffuse through the pores of membranes such as those made from regenerated cellulose products, e.g. collodion (cellulose nitrate evaporated from a solution in alcohol and ether) and cellophane. The smaller particles in solution are able to pass through these membranes. Use is made of this difference in diffusibility to separate micromolecular impurities from colloidal dispersions. The process is known as dialysis. The process of dialysis may be hastened by stirring so as to maintain a high concentration gradient of diffusible molecules across the membrane and by renewing the outer liquid from time to time.

Ultrafiltration   By applying pressure (or suction), the solvent and small particles may be forced across a membrane whilst the larger colloidal particles are retained. The process is referred to as ultrafiltration. It is possible to prepare membrane filters with known pore size and use of these allows the particle size of a colloid to be determined. However, particle size and pore size cannot be properly correlated because the membrane permeability is affected by factors such as electrical repulsion, when both the membrane and particle carry the same charge, and particle adsorption which can lead to blocking of the pores.

Electrodialysis   An electric potential may be used to increase the rate of movement of ionic impurities through a dialysing membrane and so provide a more rapid means of purification. The concentration of charged colloidal particles at one side and at the base of the membrane is termed electrodecantation.

Pharmaceutical applications of dialysis   Dialysis is the basis of a method, haemodialysis, whereby small molecular weight impurities from the body are removed by passage through a membrane. Other applications involving dialysis include the use of membranes for filtration, and as models for the diffusion of drugs through natural membranes.

Properties of colloids

Size and shape of colloidal particles

Size distribution   Within the size range of colloidal dimensions specified above, there is often a wide distribution of sizes of the dispersed colloidal particles. The molecular weight or particle size is therefore an average value the magnitude of which is dependent on the experimental technique used in its measurement. When determined by the measurement of colligative properties such as osmotic pressure, a number average value, M_n, is obtained which, in a mixture containing n_1, n_2, n_3 ... moles of particle of mass M_1, M_2, M_3 ... respectively, is defined by:

$$M_n = \frac{n_1 M_1 + n_2 M_2 + n_3 M_3 + \cdots}{n_1 + n_2 + n_3 + \cdots} = \frac{\Sigma n_i M_i}{\Sigma n_i} \quad (6.1)$$

In the light-scattering method for the measurement of particle size, larger particles produce greater scattering and the weight rather than the number of particles is important, giving a weight average value, M_w, defined by:

$$M_w = \frac{m_1 M_1 + m_2 M_2 + m_3 M_3 + \cdots}{m_1 + m_2 + m_3 + \cdots} = \frac{\Sigma n_i M_i^2}{\Sigma n_i M_i} \quad (6.2)$$

In Eqn 6.2, m_1, m_2, and m_3 ... are the masses of each species, and m_i is obtained by multiplying the mass of each species by the number of particles of that species; that is, $m_i = n_i M_i$. A consequence is that $M_w > M_n$, and only when the system is monodisperse will the two averages be identical. The ratio M_w/M_n expresses the degree of polydispersity of the system.

Shape   Many colloidal systems, including emulsions, liquid aerosols and most dilute micellar solutions, contain spherical particles. Small deviations from sphericity are often treated using ellipsoidal models. Ellipsoids of revolution are characterized by their axial ratio, which is the ratio of the half-axis a to the radius of revolution b (see Fig. 6.1). Where this ratio is greater than unity, the ellipsoid is said to be a prolate (rugby ball-shaped) ellipsoid, and when less than unity an oblate (discus-shaped) ellipsoid.

High molecular weight polymers and naturally occurring macromolecules often form random coils in aqueous solution. Clay suspensions are examples of systems containing plate-like particles.

Kinetic properties

In this section several properties of colloidal systems, which relate to the motion of particles with respect to the dispersion medium, will be considered. Thermal motion manifests itself in the form of Brownian motion, diffusion and osmosis. Gravity (or a centrifugal field) leads to sedimentation. Viscous flow is the result of an externally

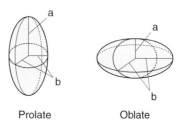

Fig. 6.1   Model representation of ellipsoids of revolution.

applied force. Measurement of these properties enables molecular weights or particle size to be determined.

Brownian motion   Colloidal particles are subject to random collisions with the molecules of the dispersion medium with the result that each particle pursues an irregular and complicated zigzag path. If the particles (up to about 2 μm diameter) are observed under a microscope or the light scattered by colloidal particles is viewed using an ultramicroscope, an erratic motion is seen. This movement is referred to as Brownian motion after Robert Brown who first reported his observation of this phenomenon with pollen grains suspended in water in 1827.

Diffusion   As a result of Brownian motion, colloidal particles spontaneously diffuse from a region of higher concentration to one of lower concentration. The rate of diffusion is expressed by Fick's First Law:

$$\frac{dm}{dt} = - DA \frac{dC}{dx} \qquad (6.3)$$

where dm is the mass of substance diffusing in time dt across an area A under the influence of a concentration gradient dC/dx (the minus sign denotes that diffusion takes place in the direction of decreasing concentration). D is the diffusion coefficient and has the dimensions of area per unit time. The diffusion coefficient of a dispersed material is related to the frictional coefficient, f, of the particles by Einstein's Law of Diffusion:

$$Df = k_B T \qquad (6.4)$$

where k_B is the Boltzmann constant and T temperature.

Therefore, as the frictional coefficient is given by the Stokes equation:

$$f = 6\pi\eta a \qquad (6.5)$$

where η is the viscosity of the medium and a the radius of the particle (assuming sphericity), then:

$$D = k_B T/6\pi\eta a = RT/6\pi\eta a N_A \qquad (6.6)$$

N_A is the Avogadro constant, R is the universal gas constant and $k_B = R/N_A$. The diffusion coefficient may be obtained by an experiment measuring the change in concentration, via refractive index gradients, when the solvent is carefully layered over the solution to form a sharp boundary and diffusion is allowed to proceed. A more commonly used method is that of dynamic light scattering which is based on the frequency shift of laser light as it is scattered by a moving particle, the so-called Doppler shift. The diffusion coefficient can be used to obtain the molecular weight of an approximately spherical particle, such as egg albumin and haemoglobin, by using Eqn 6.6 in the form:

$$D = \frac{RT}{6\pi\eta N_A} \sqrt[3]{\frac{4\pi N_A}{3M\bar{v}}} \qquad (6.7)$$

where M is the molecular weight and $\bar{v}$ is the partial specific volume of the colloidal material $\bar{v}$.

Sedimentation   Consider a spherical particle of radius a and density σ falling in a liquid of density ρ and viscosity η. The velocity v of sedimentation is given by Stokes' Law:

$$v = 2a^2 g(\sigma - \rho)/9\eta \qquad (6.8)$$

where g is acceleration due to gravity.

If the particles are only subjected to the force of gravity then, due to Brownian motion, the lower size limit of particles obeying Eqn 6.8 is about 0.5 μm. A stronger force than gravity is therefore needed for colloidal particles to sediment and use is made of a high-speed centrifuge, usually termed an ultracentrifuge, which can produce a force of about $10^6 g$. In a centrifuge, g is replaced by $\omega^2 x$, where ω is the angular velocity and x the distance of the particle from the centre of rotation, and Eqn 6.8 becomes:

$$v = \frac{2a^2 g (\sigma - \rho) \omega^2 x}{9\eta} \qquad (6.9)$$

The ultracentrifuge is used in two distinct ways in investigating colloidal material. In the *sedimentation velocity* method, a high centrifugal field is applied, up to about $4 \times 10^5 g$, and the movement of the particles, monitored by changes in concentration, is measured at specified time intervals. In the *sedimentation equilibrium* method, the colloidal material is subjected to a much lower centrifugal field until sedimentation and diffusion tendencies balance one another, and an equilibrium distribution of particles throughout the sample is attained.

Sedimentation velocity The velocity dx/dt of a particle in a unit centrifugal force can be expressed in terms of the Svedberg coefficient s:

$$s = (dx/dt)/\omega^2 x \qquad (6.10)$$

Under the influence of the centrifugal force, particles pass from position x_1 at time t_1 to position x_2 at time t_2. The differences in concentration with time can be measured using changes in refractive index and the application of the schlieren optical arrangement whereby photographs can be taken showing these concentrations as peaks. Integration of Eqn 6.10 using the above limits gives:

$$s = \frac{\ln x_2 / x_1}{\omega^2 (t_2 - t_1)} \qquad (6.11)$$

By suitable manipulation of Eqns 6.9, 6.10 and 6.11, an expression giving molecular weight M can be obtained:

$$M = \frac{RTs}{D(1 - \bar{v}\rho)} = \frac{RT \ln x_2 / x_1}{D(1 - \bar{v}\rho)(t_2 - t_1)\omega^2} \qquad (6.12)$$

where $\bar{v}$ is the partial specific volume of the particle.

Sedimentation equilibrium Equilibrium is established when sedimentation and diffusional forces balance.

Combination of sedimentation and diffusion equations is made in the analysis giving:

$$M = \frac{2RT \ln C_2/C_1}{\omega^2 (1 - \bar{v}\rho)(x_2^2 - x_1^2)}$$

(6.13)

where C_1 and C_2 are the sedimentation equilibrium concentrations at distances x_1 and x_2 from the axis of rotation. A disadvantage of the sedimentation equilibrium method is the length of time required to attain equilibrium, often as long as several days. A modification of the method in which measurements are made in the early stages of the approach to equilibrium significantly reduces the overall measurement time.

Osmotic pressure The determination of molecular weights of dissolved substances from colligative properties such as the depression of freezing point or the elevation of boiling point is a standard procedure. However, of the available methods, only osmotic pressure has a practical value in the study of colloidal particles because of the magnitude of the changes in the properties. For example, the depression of freezing point of a 1% w/v solution of a macromolecule of molecular weight 70 000 Da is only 0.0026 K, far too small to be measured with sufficient accuracy by conventional methods and also very sensitive to the presence of low molecular weight impurities. In contrast, the osmotic pressure of this solution at 20°C would be 350 N m^{-2} or about 35 mm of water. Not only does the osmotic pressure provide an effect that is measurable, but also the effect of any low molecular weight material, which can pass through the membrane, is virtually eliminated.

However, the usefulness of osmotic pressure measurement is limited to a molecular weight range of about 10^4–10^6 Da; below 10^4 Da the membrane may be permeable to the molecules under consideration and above 10^6 Da the osmotic pressure will be too small to permit accurate measurement.

If a solution and solvent are separated by a semi-permeable membrane, the tendency to equalize chemical potentials (and hence concentrations) on either side of the membrane results in a net diffusion of solvent across the membrane. The pressure necessary to balance this osmotic flow is termed the *osmotic pressure*.

For a colloidal solution the osmotic pressure, Π, can be described by:

$$\Pi/C = RT/M + BC$$

(6.14)

where C is the concentration of the solution, M the molecular weight of the solute and B a constant depending on the degree of interaction between the solvent and solute molecules.

Thus a plot of Π/C versus C is linear with the value of the intercept at $C \to 0$ giving RT/M enabling the molecular weight of the colloid to be calculated. The molecu-

lar weight obtained from osmotic pressure measurements is a number average value.

A potential source of error in the determination of molecular weight from osmotic pressure measurements arises from the *Donnan membrane effect*. The diffusion of small ions through a membrane will be affected by the presence of a charged macromolecule that is unable to penetrate the membrane because of its size. At equilibrium the distribution of the diffusible ions is unequal, being greater on the side of the membrane containing the non-diffusible ions. Consequently, unless precautions are taken to correct for this effect or eliminate it, the results of osmotic pressure measurements on charged colloidal particles such as proteins will be invalid.

Viscosity Viscosity is an expression of the resistance to flow of a system under an applied stress. An equation of flow applicable to colloidal dispersions of spherical particles was developed by Einstein (Chapter 4):

$$\eta = \eta_o (1 + 2.5\phi)$$

(6.15)

where η_o is the viscosity of the dispersion medium and η the viscosity of the dispersion when the volume fraction of colloidal particles present is ϕ.

A number of viscosity coefficients may be defined with respect to Eqn 6.15. These include *relative viscosity*:

$$\eta_{rel} = \eta/\eta_o = 1 + 2.5\phi$$

(6.16)

and *specific viscosity*:

$$\eta_{sp} = \eta/\eta_o - 1 = (\eta - \eta_o)/\eta_o = 2.5\phi$$

$$\text{or } \eta_{sp}/\phi = 2.5$$

(6.17)

Since volume fraction is directly related to concentration, Eqn 6.17 may be written as:

$$\eta_{sp}/C = k$$

(6.18)

where C is the concentration expressed as grams of colloidal particles per 100 mL of total dispersion and k is a constant. If η is determined for a number of concentrations of macromolecular material in solution and η_{sp}/C is plotted versus C then the intercept obtained on extrapolation of the linear plot to infinite dilution is known as the *intrinsic viscosity* $[\eta]$.

This constant may be used to calculate the molecular weight of the macromolecular material by making use of the Mark–Houwink equation:

$$[\eta] = KM^\alpha$$

(6.19)

where K and α are constants characteristic of the particular polymer-solvent system. These constants are obtained initially by determining $[\eta]$ for a polymer fraction whose molecular weight has been determined by another method such as sedimentation, osmotic pressure or light scattering. The molecular weight of the unknown polymer fraction may then be calculated. This method is suitable for use with polymers like the dextrans used as blood plasma substitutes.

Optical properties

Light scattering When a beam of light is passed through a colloidal sol, some of the light may be absorbed (when light of certain wavelengths is selectively absorbed, a colour is produced), some is scattered and the remainder transmitted undisturbed through the sample. Due to the light scattered, the sol appears turbid; this is known as the *Tyndall effect*. The turbidity of a sol is given by the expression:

$$I = I_o \exp^{-\tau l} \qquad (6.20)$$

where I_o is the intensity of the incident beam, I that of the transmitted light beam, l the length of the sample and τ the turbidity.

Light-scattering measurements are of great value for estimating particle size, shape and interactions, particularly of dissolved macromolecular materials, as the turbidity depends on the size (molecular weight) of the colloidal material involved. Measurements are simple in principle but experimentally difficult because of the need to keep the sample free from dust, the particles of which would scatter light strongly and introduce large errors.

As most colloids show very low turbidities, instead of measuring the transmitted light (which may differ only marginally from the incident beam), it is more convenient and accurate to measure the scattered light, at an angle (usually 90°) relative to the incident beam. The turbidity can then be calculated from the intensity of the scattered light, provided the dimensions of the particle are small compared to the wavelength of the incident light, by the expression:

$$\tau = \frac{16\pi}{3} R_{90} \qquad (6.21)$$

R_{90} is known as the Rayleigh ratio after Lord Rayleigh who laid the foundations of the light-scattering theory in 1871. The light-scattering theory was modified for use in the determination of the molecular weight of colloidal particles by Debye in 1947 who derived the following relationship between turbidity and molecular weight:

$$HC/\tau = 1/M + 2BC \qquad (6.22)$$

C is the concentration of the solute and B an interaction constant allowing for non-ideality. H is an optical constant for a particular system depending on the refractive index change with concentration and the wavelength of light used. A plot of HC/τ against concentration results in a straight line of slope $2B$. The intercept on the HC/τ axis is $1/M$, allowing the molecular weight to be calculated. The molecular weight derived by the light-scattering technique is a weight average value.

Light-scattering measurements are particularly suitable for finding the size of the micelles of surface-active agents and for the study of proteins and natural and synthetic polymers.

For spherical particles, the upper limit of the Debye equation is a particle diameter of approximately one-twentieth of the wavelength λ of the incident light; that is, about 20–25 nm. The light-scattering theory becomes more complex when one or more dimensions exceed $\lambda/20$ because the particles can no longer be considered as point sources of scattered light. By measuring the light scattering from such particles as a function of both the scattering angle θ and the concentration C, and extrapolating the data to zero angle and zero concentration, it is possible to obtain information on not only the molecular weight but also the particle shape.

Because the intensity of the scattered light is inversely proportional to the fourth power of the wavelength of the light used, blue light ($\lambda \approx 450$ nm) is scattered much more than red light ($\lambda \approx 650$ nm). With incident white light, a scattering material will therefore tend to be blue when viewed at right angles to the incident beam, which is why the sky appears to be blue, the scattering arising from dust particles in the atmosphere.

Ultramicroscopy Colloidal particles are too small to be seen with an optical microscope. Light scattering is employed in the ultramicroscope first developed by Zsigmondy, in which a cell containing the colloid is viewed against a dark background at right angles to an intense beam of incident light. The particles, which exhibit Brownian motion, appear as spots of light against the dark background. The ultramicroscope is used in the technique of microelectrophoresis for measuring particle charge.

Electron microscopy The electron microscope, capable of giving actual pictures of the particles, is used to observe the size, shape and structure of colloidal particles. The success of the electron microscope is due to its high resolving power, defined in terms of d, the smallest distance by which two objects are separated yet remain distinguishable. The smaller the wavelength of the radiation used, the smaller is d and the greater the resolving power. An optical microscope, using visible light as its radiation source, gives a d of about 0.2 μm. The radiation source of the electron microscope is a beam of high-energy electrons having wavelengths in the region of 0.01 nm; d is thus about 0.5 nm. The electron beams are focused using electromagnets and the whole system is under a high vacuum of about 10^{-3}–10^{-5} Pa to give the electrons a free path.

With wavelengths of the order indicated, the image cannot be viewed directly, so use is made of a fluorescent screen.

A major disadvantage of the electron microscope for viewing colloidal particles is that normally only dried samples can be examined. Consequently, it usually gives no information on solvation or configuration in solution and, moreover, the particles may be affected by sample preparation. A recent development which overcomes these problems is environmental scanning electron microscopy (ESEM) which allows the observation of material in the wet state.

Electrical properties

Electrical properties of interfaces Most surfaces acquire a surface electric charge when brought into contact with an aqueous medium, the principal charging mechanisms being as follows.

Ion dissolution Ionic substances can acquire a surface charge by virtue of unequal dissolution of the oppositely charged ions of which they are composed. For example, the particles of silver iodide in a solution with excess $[I^-]$ will carry a negative charge, but the charge will be positive if excess $[Ag^+]$ is present. Since the concentrations of Ag^+ and I^- determine the electric potential at the particle surface, they are termed potential determining ions. In a similar way, H^+ and OH^- are potential-determining ions for metal oxides and hydroxides of, for example, magnesium and aluminium hydroxides.

Ionization Here the charge is controlled by the ionization of surface groupings; examples include the model system of polystyrene latex which frequently has carboxylic acid groupings at the surface which ionize to give negatively charged particles. In a similar way, acidic drugs such as ibuprofen and nalidixic acid also acquire a negative charge.

Amino acids and proteins acquire their charge mainly through the ionization of carboxyl and amino groups to give $-COO^-$ and NH_3^+ ions. The ionization of these groups and so the net molecular charge depends on the pH of the system. At a pH below the pK_a of the COO^- group the protein will be positively charged because of the protonation of this group, $-COO^- \rightarrow COOH$, and the ionization of the amino group, $-NH_2 \rightarrow -NH_3^+$, which has a much higher pK_a. Whereas at higher pH, where the amino group is no longer ionized, the net charge on the molecule is now negative because of the ionization of the carboxyl group. At a certain definite pH, specific for each individual protein, the total number of positive charges will equal the total number of negative charges and the net charge will be zero. This pH is termed the isoelectric point of the protein and the

protein exists as its zwitterion. This may be represented as follows:

$$R — NH_2 — COO^- \qquad \text{Alkaline solution}$$
$$\downarrow\uparrow$$
$$R — NH_3^+ —COO^- \qquad \text{Isoelectric point (zwitterion)}$$
$$\downarrow\uparrow$$
$$R — NH_3^+ —COOH \qquad \text{Acidic solution}$$

A protein is least soluble (the colloidal sol is least stable) at its isoelectric point and is readily desolvated by very water-soluble salts such as ammonium sulfate. Thus insulin may be precipitated from aqueous alcohol at pH 5.2.

Erythrocytes and bacteria usually acquire their charge by ionization of surface chemical groups such as sialic acid.

Ion adsorption A net surface charge can be acquired by the unequal adsorption of oppositely charged ions. Surfaces in water are more often negatively charged than positively charged, because cations are generally more hydrated than anions. Consequently, the former have the greater tendency to reside in the bulk aqueous medium whereas the smaller, less hydrated and more polarizing anions have the greater tendency to reside at the particle surface. Surface-active agents are strongly adsorbed and have a pronounced influence on the surface charge, imparting either a positive or negative charge depending on their ionic character.

The electrical double layer Consider a solid charged surface in contact with an aqueous solution containing positive and negative ions. The surface charge influences the distribution of ions in the aqueous medium; ions of opposite charge to that of the surface, termed counter-ions, are attracted towards the surface, ions of like charge, termed co-ions, are repelled away from the surface. However, the distribution of the ions will also be affected by thermal agitation which will tend to redisperse the ions in solution. The result is the formation of an electrical double layer made up of the charged surface and a neutralizing excess of counter-ions over co-ions (the system must be electrically neutral) distributed in a diffuse manner in the aqueous medium.

The theory of the electric double layer deals with this distribution of ions and hence with the magnitude of the electric potentials which occur in the locality of the charged surface. For a fuller explanation of what is a rather complicated mathematical approach, the reader is referred to a textbook of colloid science (e.g. Shaw 1992). A somewhat simplified picture of what pertains from the theories of Gouy, Chapman and Stern follows.

The double layer is divided into two parts (see Fig. 6.2a): the inner, which may include adsorbed ions, and the diffuse part where ions are distributed as influenced by electrical forces and random thermal motion.

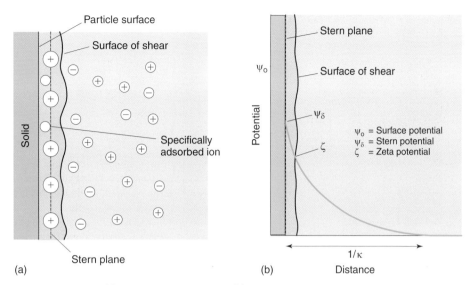

Fig. 6.2 The electric double layer. (a) Schematic representation. (b) Changes in potential with distance from particle surface.

The two parts of the double layer are separated by a plane, the Stern plane, at about a hydrated ion radius from the surface; thus counter-ions may be held at the surface by electrostatic attraction and the centre of these hydrated ions forms the Stern plane.

The potential changes linearly from ψ_o (the surface potential) to ψ_δ (the Stern potential) in the Stern layer and decays exponentially from ψ_δ to zero in the diffuse double layer (Fig. 6.2b). A plane of shear is also indicated in Figure 6.2. In addition to ions in the Stern layer, a certain amount of solvent will be bound to the ions and the charged surface. This solvating layer is held to the surface, and the edge of the layer, termed the surface or plane of shear, represents the boundary of relative movement between the solid (and attached material) and the liquid. The potential at the plane of shear is termed the zeta, ζ, or electrokinetic, potential and its magnitude may be measured using microelectrophoresis or any other of the electrokinetic phenomena. The thickness of the solvating layer is ill defined and the zeta potential therefore represents a potential at an unknown distance from the particle surface; its value, however, is usually taken as being slightly less than that of the Stern potential.

In the discussion above it was stated that the Stern plane existed at a hydrated ion radius from the particle surface; the hydrated ions are electrostatically attracted to the particle surface. It is possible for ions/molecules to be more strongly adsorbed at the surface, termed *specific adsorption*, than by simple electrostatic attraction. In fact, the specifically adsorbed ion/molecule may be uncharged as is the case with non-ionic surface-active agents. Surface-active ions specifically adsorb by the hydrophobic effect and can have a significant effect on the Stern potential, causing ψ_o and ψ_δ to have opposite signs, as in Figure 6.3a, or for ψ_δ to have the same sign as ψ_o but be greater in magnitude, as in Figure 6.3b.

Figure 6.2b shows an exponential decay of the potential to zero with distance from the Stern plane. The distance over which this occurs is $1/\kappa$, referred to as the Debye–Hückel length parameter or the thickness of the electrical double layer. The parameter κ is dependent on the electrolyte concentration of the aqueous media. Increasing the electrolyte concentration increases the value of κ and consequently decreases the value of $1/\kappa$; that is, it compresses the double layer. As ψ_δ stays constant this means that the zeta potential will be lowered.

As indicated earlier, the effect of specifically adsorbed ions may be to lower the Stern potential and hence the zeta potential without compressing the double layer. Thus the zeta potential may be reduced by additives to the aqueous system in either (or both) of two different ways.

Electrokinetic phenomena This is the general description applied to the phenomena that arise when attempts are made to shear off the mobile part of the electrical double layer from a charged surface. There are four such phenomena: namely, electrophoresis, sedimentation potential, streaming potential and electroosmosis. All of these electrokinetic phenomena may be used to measure the zeta potential but electrophoresis is the easiest to use and has the greatest pharmaceutical application.

Electrophoresis The movement of a charged particle (plus attached ions) relative to a stationary liquid under the influence of an applied electric field is termed electrophoresis. When the movement of the particles is observed with a microscope, or the movement of light spots scattered by particles too small to be observed with

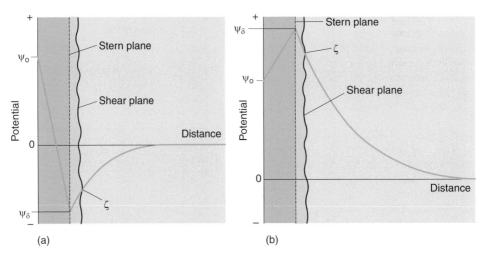

Fig. 6.3 Changes in potential with distance from solid surface. (a) Reversal of charge sign of Stern potential ψ_δ, due to adsorption of surface-active or polyvalent counter-ion. (b) Increase in magnitude of Stern potential ψ_δ, due to adsorption of surface-active co-ions.

the microscope is observed using an ultramicroscope, this constitutes microelectrophoresis.

A microscope equipped with an eyepiece graticule is used and the speed of movement of the particle under the influence of a known electric field is measured. This is the electrophoretic velocity, v, and the electrophoretic mobility, u, is given by:

$$u = v/E \qquad (6.23)$$

where v is measured in m s^{-1}, and E, the applied field strength in V m^{-1}, so that u has the dimensions of m^2 s^{-1} V^{-1}. Typically a stable lyophobic colloidal particle may have an electrophoretic mobility of 4×10^{-8} m^2 s^{-1} V^{-1}. The equation used for converting the electrophoretic mobility, u, into the zeta potential depends on the value of κa (κ is the Debye–Hückel reciprocal length parameter described previously and a the particle radius). For values of $\kappa a > 100$ (as is the case for particles of radius 1 μm dispersed in 10^{-3} mol dm^{-3} sodium chloride solution) the Smoluchowski equation can be used:

$$u = \varepsilon \zeta / \eta \qquad (6.24)$$

where ε is the permittivity and η the viscosity of the liquid used. For particles in water at 25°C, $\zeta = 12.85 \times 10^{-5}$ u volts and, for the mobility given above, a zeta potential of 0.0514 volts or 51.4 millivolts is obtained. For values of $\kappa a < 100$, a more complex relationship which is a function of κa and the zeta potential is used.

The technique of microelectrophoresis finds application in the measurement of zeta potentials, of model systems (like polystyrene latex dispersions) to test colloid stability theory, of coarse dispersions (like suspensions and emulsions) to assess their stability, and in identification of charge groups and other surface characteristics of water-insoluble drugs and cells such as blood and bacteria.

Other electrokinetic phenomena The other electrokinetic phenomena are as follows. *Sedimentation potential,* the reverse of electrophoresis, is the electric field created when particles sediment; *streaming potential,* the electric field created when liquid is made to flow along a stationary charged surface, e.g. a glass tube or a packed powder bed; *and electroosmosis,* the opposite of streaming potential, the movement of liquid relative to a stationary charged surface, e.g. a glass tube, by an applied electric field.

Physical stability of colloidal systems

In colloidal dispersions, frequent encounters between the particles occur due to Brownian movement. Whether these collisions result in permanent contact of the particles (coagulation), which leads eventually to the destruction of the colloidal system as the large aggregates formed sediment out, or temporary contact (flocculation) or whether the particles rebound and remain freely dispersed (a stable colloidal system) depends on the forces of interaction between the particles.

These forces can be divided into three groups: electrical forces of repulsion, forces of attraction and forces arising from solvation. An understanding of the first two explains the stability of lyophobic systems, and all three forces must be considered in a discussion of the stability of lyophilic dispersions. Before considering the interaction of these forces, it is necessary to define the terms *aggregation,* *coagulation* and *flocculation* as used in colloid science.

Aggregation is a general term signifying the collection of particles into groups. Coagulation signifies that the particles are closely aggregated and difficult to redisperse – a primary minimum phenomenon of the DLVO theory of colloid stability (see next section). In flocculation, the aggregates have an open structure in which the particles remain a small distance apart from one another. This may be a secondary minimum phenomenon (see the DLVO theory) or a consequence of bridging by a polymer or polyelectrolyte, as explained later in this chapter.

As a preliminary to discussion on the stability of colloidal dispersions, a comparison of the general properties of lyophobic and lyophilic sols is given in Table 6.2.

Stability of lyophobic systems *DLVO theory* In considering the interaction between two colloidal particles, Derjaguin and Landau and, independently, Verwey and Overbeek in the 1940s produced a quantitative approach to the stability of hydrophobic sols. In what has come to be known as the *DLVO theory of colloid stability*, they assumed that the only interactions involved are electrical repulsion, V_R, and van der Waals

attraction, V_A, and that these parameters are additive. Therefore the total potential energy of interaction V_T (expressed schematically in the curve shown in Fig. 6.4) is given by:

$$V_T = V_A + V_R \qquad (6.25)$$

Repulsive forces between particles Repulsion between particles arises due to the osmotic effect produced by the increase in the number of charged species on overlap of the diffuse parts of the electrical double layer. No simple equations can be given for repulsive interactions; however, it can be shown that the repulsive energy that exists between two spheres of equal but small surface potential is given by:

$$V_R = 2\pi\varepsilon a \psi_o^2 \exp[-\kappa H] \qquad (6.26)$$

where ε is the permittivity of the polar liquid, a the radius of the spherical particle of surface potential ψ_o, κ is the Debye–Hückel reciprocal length parameter and H the

Table 6.2 Comparison of properties of lyophobic and lyophilic sols

Property	Lyophobic	Lyophilic
Effect of electrolytes	Very sensitive to added electrolyte, leading to aggregation in an irreversible manner. Depends on: (a) type and valency of counter ion of electrolyte, e.g. with a negatively charged sol, $La^{3+} > Ba^{2+} > Na^+$ (b) Concentration of electrolyte. At a particular concentration sol passes from disperse to aggregated state. For the electrolyte types in (a) the concentrations are about 10^{-4}, 10^{-3}, 10^{-1} mol dm^{-3} respectively. These generalizations, (a) and (b), form what is known as the Schulze–Hardy rule	Dispersions are stable generally in the presence of electrolytes. May be salted out by high concentrations of very soluble electrolytes. Effect is due to desolvation of the lyophilic molecules and depends on the tendency of the electrolyte ions to become hydrated. Proteins more sensitive to electrolytes at their isoelectric points. Lyophilic colloids when salted out may appear as amorphous droplets known as a coacervate
Stability	Controlled by charge on particles	Controlled by charge and solvation of particles
Formation of dispersion	Dispersions usually of metals, inorganic crystals, etc., with a high interfacial surface-free energy due to large increase in surface area on formation. A positive ΔG of formation, dispersion will never form spontaneously and is thermodynamically unstable. Particles of sol remain dispersed due to electrical repulsion	Generally proteins, macromolecules, etc., which disperse spontaneously in a solvent. Interfacial free energy is low. There is a large increase in entropy when rigidly held chains of a polymer in the dry state unfold in solution. The free energy of formation is negative, a stable thermodynamic system
Viscosity	Sols of low viscosity, particles unsolvated and usually symmetrical	Usually high. At sufficiently high concentration of disperse phase a gel may be formed. Particles solvated and usually asymmetric

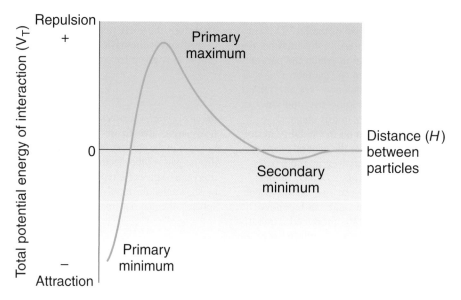

Fig. 6.4 Schematic curve of total potential energy of interaction, V_T, versus distance of separation, H, for two particles. $V_T = V_R + V_A$.

distance between particles. An estimation of the surface potential can be obtained from zeta potential measurements. As can be seen, the repulsion energy is an exponential function of the distance between the particles and has a range of the order of the thickness of the double layer.

Attractive forces between particles The energy of attraction, V_A, arises from van der Waals universal forces of attraction, the so-called dispersion forces, the major contribution to which are the electromagnetic attractions described by London in 1930. For an assembly of molecules, dispersion forces are additive, summation leading to long-range attraction between colloidal particles. As a result of the work of de Boer and Hamaker in 1936, it can be shown that the attractive interaction between spheres of the same radius, a, can be approximated to:

$$V_A = -Aa/12H \qquad (6.27)$$

where A is the Hamaker constant for the particular material derived from London dispersion forces. Eqn 6.27 shows that the energy of attraction varies as the inverse of the distance between particles.

Total potential energy of interaction Consideration of the curve of total potential energy of interaction V_T versus distance between particles, H (Fig. 6.4), shows that attraction predominates at small distances, hence the very deep primary minimum. The attraction at large interparticle distances, that produces the secondary minimum, arises because the fall-off in repulsive energy with distance is more rapid than that of attractive energy. At intermediate distances, double layer repulsion may pre-

dominate, giving a primary maximum in the curve. If this maximum is large compared with the thermal energy k_BT of the particles, the colloidal system should be stable, i.e. the particles should stay dispersed. Otherwise, the interacting particles will reach the energy depth of the primary minimum and irreversible aggregation, i.e. coagulation, occurs. If the secondary minimum is smaller than k_BT the particles will not aggregate but will always repel one another but if it is significantly larger than k_BT a loose assemblage of particles will form which can be easily redispersed by shaking, i.e. flocculation occurs.

The depth of the secondary minimum depends on particle size, and particles may need to be of radius 1 μm or greater before the attractive force is sufficiently great for flocculation to occur.

The height of the primary maximum energy barrier to coagulation depends upon the magnitude of V_R, which is dependent on ψ_o and hence the zeta potential. In addition, it depends on electrolyte concentration via κ, the Debye–Hückel reciprocal length parameter. Addition of electrolyte compresses the double layer and reduces the zeta potential; this has the effect of lowering the primary maximum and deepening the secondary minimum (Fig. 6.5). This latter means that there will be an increased tendency for particles to flocculate in the secondary minimum and this is the principle of the *controlled flocculation* approach to pharmaceutical suspension formulation described later. The primary maximum may also be lowered (and the secondary minimum deepened) by adding substances, such as ionic surface-active agents, which are specifically adsorbed within the Stern layer. Here ψ_δ is

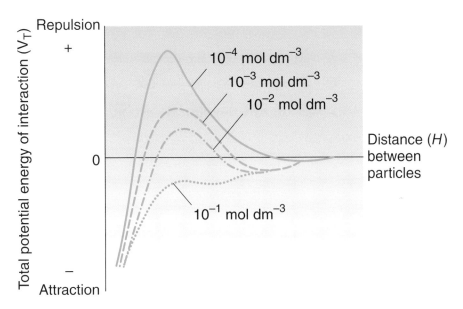

Fig. 6.5 Schematic curves of total potential energy of interaction, V_T, versus distance of separation, H, showing the effect of adding electrolyte at constant surface potential.

reduced and hence the zeta potential; the double layer is usually not compressed.

Stability of lyophilic systems Solutions of macromolecules, lyophilic colloidal sols, are stabilized by a combination of electrical double layer interaction and solvation and both of these stabilizing factors must be sufficiently weakened before attraction predominates and the colloidal particles coagulate. For example, gelatin has a sufficiently strong affinity for water to be soluble even at its isoelectric pH where there is no double layer interaction.

Hydrophilic colloids are unaffected by the small amounts of added electrolyte which cause hydrophobic sols to coagulate; however, when the concentration of electrolyte is high, particularly with an electrolyte whose ions become strongly hydrated, the colloidal material loses its water of solvation to these ions and coagulates, i.e. a 'salting out' effect occurs.

Variation in the degree of solvation of different hydrophilic colloids affects the concentration of soluble electrolyte required to produce their coagulation and precipitation. The components of a mixture of hydrophilic colloids can therefore be separated by a process of fractional precipitation, which involves the 'salting out' of the various components at different concentrations of electrolyte. This technique is used in the purification of antitoxins.

Lyophilic colloids can be considered to become lyophobic by the addition of solvents such as acetone and alcohol. The particles become desolvated and are then very sensitive to precipitation by added electrolyte.

Coacervation and microencapsulation Coacervation is the separation of a colloid-rich layer from a lyophilic sol on addition of another substance. This layer, which is present in the form of an amorphous liquid, constitutes the coacervate. Simple coacervation may be brought about by a 'salting out' effect on addition of electrolyte or addition of a non-solvent. Complex coacervation occurs when two oppositely charged lyophilic colloids are mixed, e.g. gelatin and acacia. Gelatin at a pH below its isoelectric point is positively charged, acacia above about pH 3 is negatively charged; a combination of solutions at about pH 4 results in coacervation. Any large ions of opposite charge, for example cationic surface-active agents (positively charged) and dyes used for colouring aqueous mixtures (negatively charged), may react in a similar way.

If the coacervate is formed in a stirred suspension of an insoluble solid, the macromolecular material will surround the solid particles. The coated particles can be separated and dried and this technique forms the basis of one method of microencapsulation. A number of drugs including aspirin have been coated in this manner. The coating protects the drug from chemical attack and microcapsules may be given orally to prolong the action of the medicament.

Effect of addition of macromolecular material to lyophobic colloidal sols When added in small amounts, many polyelectrolyte and polymer molecules (lyophilic colloids) can adsorb simultaneously on to two particles and are long enough to bridge across the energy barrier between the particles. This can even occur with neutral polymers when the lyophobic particles have a high zeta potential (and would thus be considered a stable sol). A structured floc results (Fig. 6.6a).

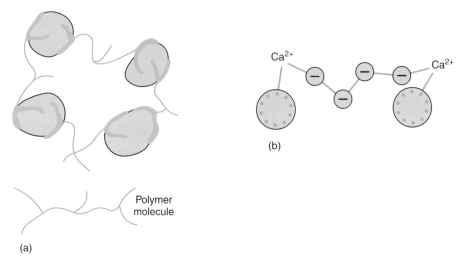

Fig. 6.6 Diagram of flocs formed by (a) polymer bridging and (b) polyelectrolyte bridging in the presence of divalent ions of opposite charge.

With polyelectrolytes, where the particles and polyelectrolyte have the same sign, flocculation can often occur when divalent and trivalent ions are added to the system (Fig. 6.6b). These complete the 'bridge' and only very low concentrations of these ions are needed. Use is made of this property of small quantities of polyelectrolytes and polymers in removing colloidal material, resulting from sewage, in water purification.

On the other hand, if larger amounts of polymer are added, sufficient to cover the surface of the particles, then a lyophobic sol may be stabilized to coagulation by added electrolyte – the so-called steric stabilization or protective colloid effect.

Steric stabilization (protective colloid action) It has long been known that non-ionic polymeric material such as gums, non-ionic surface-active agents and methylcellulose adsorbed at the particle surface can stabilize a lyophobic sol to coagulation even in the absence of a significant zeta potential. The approach of two particles with adsorbed polymer layers results in a steric interaction when the layers overlap, leading to repulsion. In general, the particles do not approach each other closer than about twice the thickness of the adsorbed layer and hence passage into the primary minimum is inhibited. An additional term has thus to be included in the potential energy of interaction for what is called steric stabilization, V_S:

$$V_T = V_A + V_R + V_S \qquad (6.28)$$

The effect of V_S on the potential energy against distance between particles curve is seen in Figure 6.7, showing that repulsion is generally seen at all shorter distances provided that the adsorbed polymeric material does not move from the particle surface.

Steric repulsion can be explained by reference to the free energy changes that take place when two polymer-covered particles interact. Free energy ΔG, enthalpy ΔH and entropy ΔS changes are related according to:

$$\Delta G = \Delta H - T\Delta S \qquad (6.29)$$

The Second Law of Thermodynamics implies that a positive value of ΔG is necessary for dispersion stability, a negative value indicating that the particles have aggregated.

A positive value of ΔG can arise in a number of ways, for example when ΔH and ΔS are both negative and $T\Delta S$ $>\Delta H$. Here the effect of the entropy change opposes aggregation and outweighs the enthalpy term; this is termed *entropic stabilization*. Interpenetration and compression of the polymer chains decrease the entropy as these chains become more ordered. Such a process is not spontaneous: 'work' must be expended to interpenetrate and compress any polymer chains existing between the colloidal particles and this work is a reflection of the repulsive potential energy. The enthalpy of mixing of these polymer chains will also be negative. Stabilization by these effects occurs in non-aqueous dispersions.

Again, a positive ΔG occurs if both ΔH and ΔS are positive and $T\Delta S$ $>\Delta H$. Here enthalpy aids stabilization, entropy aids aggregation. Consequently, this effect is termed *enthalpic stabilization* and is common with aqueous dispersions, particularly where the stabilizing polymer has polyoxyethylene chains. Such chains are hydrated in aqueous solution due to H-bonding between water molecules and the 'ether oxygens' of the ethylene oxide groups. The water molecules have thus become more structured and lost degrees of freedom. When interpenetration and

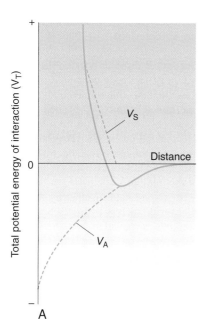

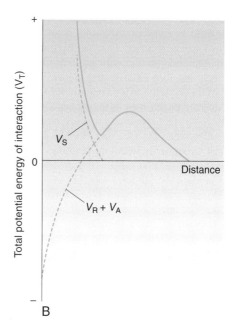

Fig. 6.7 Schematic curves of the total potential energy of interaction versus distance for two particles, showing the effect of the steric stabilization term V_S (a) in the absence of electrostatic repulsion, the solid line representing $V_T = V_A + V_S$; (b) in the presence of electrostatic repulsion, the solid line representing $V_T = V_R + V_A + V_S$.

compression of ethylene oxide chains occur, there is an increased probability of contact between ethylene oxide groups, resulting in some of the bound water molecules being released (see Fig. 6.8). The released water molecules have greater degrees of freedom than those in the bound state. For this to occur, they must be supplied with energy,

obtained from heat absorption, i.e. there is a positive enthalpy change. Although there is a decrease in entropy in the interaction zone, as with entropic stabilization, this is overridden by the increase in the configurational entropy of the released water molecules.

GELS

The majority of gels are formed by aggregation of colloidal sol particles, the solid or semi-solid system so formed being interpenetrated by a liquid. The particles link together to form an interlaced network, thus imparting rigidity to the structure; the continuous phase is held within the meshes. Often only a small percentage of disperse phase is required to impart rigidity; for example, 1% of agar in water produces a firm gel. A gel rich in liquid may be called a jelly; if the liquid is removed and only the gel framework remains, this is termed a xerogel. Sheet gelatin, acacia tears and tragacanth flakes are all xerogels.

Types of gel

Gelation of lyophobic sols

Gels may be flocculated lyophobic sols where the gel can be looked upon as a continuous floccule (Fig. 6.9a). Examples are aluminium hydroxide and magnesium hydroxide gels.

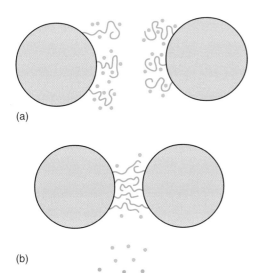

Fig. 6.8 Enthalpic stabilization. (a) Particles with stabilizing polyoxyethylene chains and H-bonded water molecules. (b) Stabilizing chains overlap, water molecules released $\rightarrow + \Delta H$.

Clays such as bentonite, aluminium magnesium silicate (Veegum) and to some extent kaolin form gels by flocculation in a special manner. They are hydrated aluminium (aluminium/magnesium) silicates whose crystal structure is such that they exist as flat plates. The flat part or 'face' of the particle carries a negative charge due to O^- atoms and the edge of the plate carries a positive charge due to Al^{3+}/ Mg^{2+} atoms. As a result of electrostatic attraction between the face and edge of different particles, a gel structure is built up, forming what is usually known as a 'card house floc' (Fig. 6.9b).

The forces holding the particles together in this type of gel are relatively weak – van der Waals forces in the secondary minimum flocculation of aluminium hydroxide, electrostatic attraction in the case of the clays; because of this these gels show the phenomenon of *thixotropy*, a non-chemical isothermal gel-sol-gel transformation. If a thixotropic gel is sheared (for example, by simple shaking) these weak bonds are broken and a lyophobic sol is formed. On standing, the particles collide, flocculation occurs and the gel is reformed. Flocculation in gels is the reason for their anomalous rheological properties (see Chapter 4). This phenomenon of thixotropy is employed in the formulation of pharmaceutical suspensions, e.g. bentonite in calamine lotion, and in the paint industry.

Gelation of lyophilic sols

Gels formed by lyophilic sols can be divided into two groups depending on the nature of the bonds between the chains of the network. Gels of *type I* are irreversible systems with a three-dimensional network formed by covalent bonds between the macromolecules. Typical examples of this type of gel are the swollen networks that have been formed by the polymerization of monomers of water-soluble polymers in the presence of a cross-linking agent. For example, poly (2-hydroxyethylmethacrylate) [poly(HEMA)], crosslinked with ethylene glycol dimethacrylate [EGDMA], forms a three-dimensional structure (Fig. 6.10), that swells in water but cannot dissolve because the crosslinks are stable. Such polymers have been used in the fabrication of expanding implants that imbide body fluids and swell to a predetermined volume. Implanted in the dehydrated state, these polymers swell to fill a body cavity or give form to surrounding tissues. They also find use in the fabrication of implants for the prolonged release of drugs, such as antibiotics, into the immediate environment of the implant.

Type II gels are held together by much weaker intermolecular bonds such as hydrogen bonds. These gels are heat reversible, a transition from the sol to gel occurring on either heating or cooling. Poly(vinyl alcohol) solutions, for example, gel on cooling below a certain temperature referred to as the gel point. Because of their gelling properties, poly(vinyl alcohol)s are used as jellies for application of drugs to the skin. On application, the gel dries rapidly, leaving a plastic film with the drug in intimate contact with the skin. Concentrated aqueous solutions of high molecular weight poly(oxyethylene)-poly(oxypropylene)-poly(oxyethylene) block copolymers, commercially available as Pluronic™ or Synperonic™ surfactants, form gels on heating. These compounds are amphiphilic and many form micelles with a hydrophobic core comprising the poly(oxypropylene) blocks, surrounded by a shell of the hydrophilic poly(oxyethylene) chains. Unusually, water is a poorer solvent for these compounds at higher temperatures and consequently warming a solution with a concentration above the critical micelle concentration leads to the formation of more micelles. If the solution is sufficiently

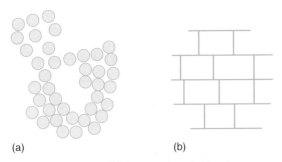

(a)   (b)

Fig. 6.9 Gel structure. (a) Flocculated lyophobic sol, e.g. aluminium hydroxide. (b) 'Card house' floc of clays, e.g. bentonite.

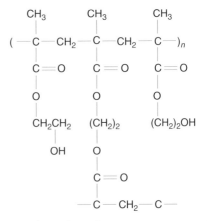

Fig. 6.10 Poly (HEMA): poly (2-hydroxyethyl methacrylate) crosslinked with ethylene glycol dimethacrylate (EGDMA).

concentrated gelation may occur as the micelles pack so closely as to prevent their movement (see Fig. 6.11). Gelation is a reversible process, the gels returning to the sol state on cooling.

SURFACE-ACTIVE AGENTS

Certain compounds, because of their chemical structure, have a tendency to accumulate at the boundary between two phases. Such compounds are termed amphiphiles, surface-active agents or surfactants. The adsorption at the various interfaces between solids, liquids and gases results in changes in the nature of the interface which are of considerable importance in pharmacy. Thus, the lowering of the interfacial tension between oil and water phases facilitates emulsion formation, the adsorption of surfactants on insoluble particles enables these particles to be dispersed in the form of a suspension, their adsorption on solid surfaces enables these surfaces to be more readily wetted, and the incorporation of insoluble compounds within micelles of the surfactant can lead to the production of clear solutions.

Surface-active compounds are characterized by having two distinct regions in their chemical structure, termed hydrophilic (water-liking) and hydrophobic (water-hating) regions. The existence of two such regions in a molecule is referred to as amphipathy and the molecules are consequently often referred to as amphipathic molecules. The hydrophobic portions are usually saturated or unsaturated hydrocarbon chains or, less commonly, heterocyclic or aromatic ring systems. The hydrophilic regions can be anionic, cationic or nonionic. Surfactants are generally classified according to the nature of the hydrophilic group. Typical examples are given in Table 6.3.

A wide variety of drugs has also been reported to be surface active, this surface activity being a consequence of the amphipathic nature of the drugs. The hydrophobic portions of the drug molecules are usually more complex than those of typical surface-active agents, being composed of aromatic or heterocyclic ring systems. Examples include tranquillizers such as chlorpromazine which are based on the large tricyclic phenothiazine ring system; the antidepressant drugs such as imipramine which also possess tricyclic ring systems; and the antihistamines such as diphenhydramine which are based on a diphenylmethane group. Further examples of surface-active drugs are given in Attwood & Florence (1983).

Surface activity

The dual structure of amphipathic molecules is the unique feature that is responsible for the surface activity of these compounds. It is a consequence of their adsorption at the solution–air interface, the means by which the hydrophobic region of the molecule 'escapes' from the hostile aqueous environment by protruding into the vapour phase above. Similarly, adsorption at the interface between non-aqueous solutions occurs in such a way that the hydrophobic group is in solution in the non-aqueous phase, leaving the hydrophilic group in contact with the aqueous solution.

The molecules at the surface of a liquid are not completely surrounded by other like molecules as they are in the bulk of the liquid. As a result there is a net inward force of attraction exerted on a molecule at the surface from the molecules in the bulk solution, which results in a tendency for the surface to contract. The contraction of the surface is spontaneous; that is, it is accompanied by a decrease in free energy. The contracted surface thus represents a minimum free energy state and any attempt to expand the surface must involve an increase in the free energy. The surface tension is a measure of the contracting power of the surface. Surface-active molecules in aqueous solution orientate themselves at the surface in such a way as to remove the hydrophobic group from the aqueous phase and hence achieve a minimum free energy state. As a result, some of the water molecules at the surface are replaced by non-polar groups. The attractive forces between these groups and the water molecules, or between the groups themselves, are less than those existing between water molecules. The contracting power of the surface is thus reduced and so therefore is the surface tension.

A similar imbalance of attractive forces exists at the interface between two immiscible liquids. The value of the interfacial tension is generally between those of the surface tensions of the two liquids involved except where

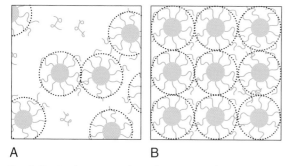

Fig. 6.11 Poly(oxyethylene)–poly(oxypropylene)–poly(oxyethylene) block copolymers. (a) Micelle formation. (b) Formation of a cubic gel phase by packing of micelles.

A   B

Table 6.3 Classification of surface-active agents

Anionic

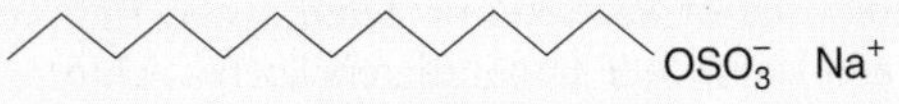

Alkyl sulfate

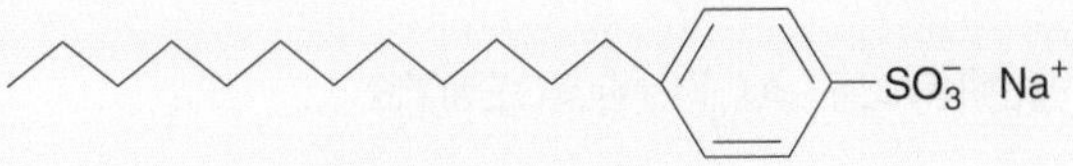

Alkylbenzene sulfonate

Cationic

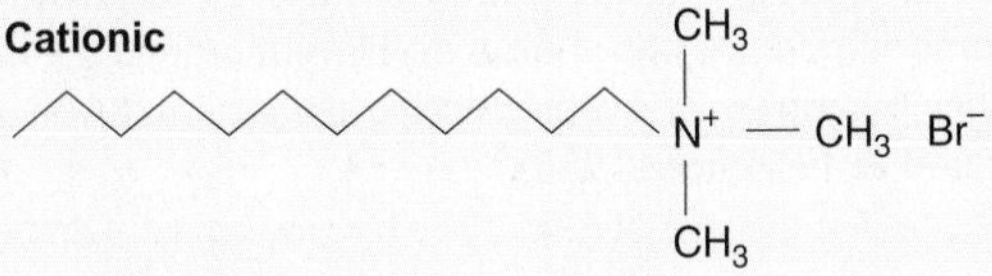

Alkyltrimethylammonium bromide

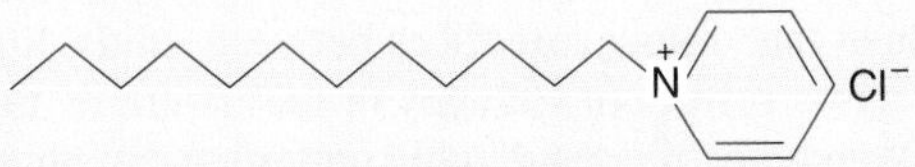

Alkylpyridinium chloride

Zwitterionic

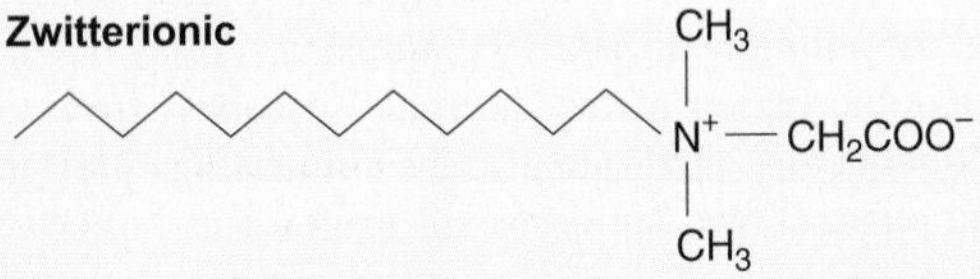

Alkyl betaine

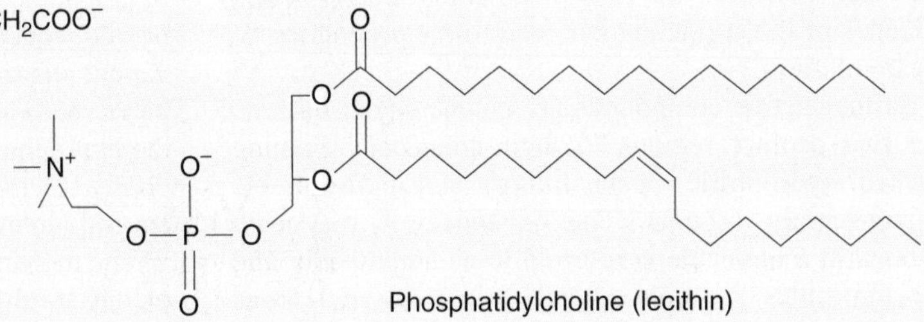

Phosphatidylcholine (lecithin)

Nonionic

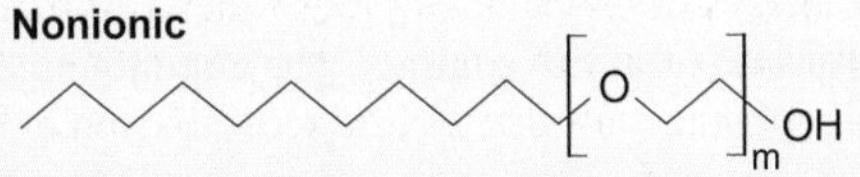

Alcohol ethoxylate

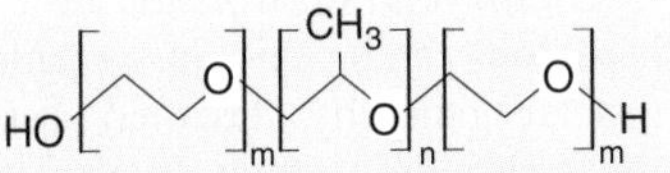

Polyoxyethylene-polyoxypropylene-polyoxyethylene block copolymer

there is interaction between them. Intrusion of surface-active molecules at the interface between two immiscible liquids leads to a reduction of interfacial tension, in some cases to such a low level that spontaneous emulsification of the two liquids occurs.

Micelle formation

The surface tension of a surfactant solution decreases progressively with increase of concentration as more surfactant molecules enter the surface or interfacial layer. However, at a certain concentration this layer becomes saturated and an alternative means of shielding the hydrophobic group of the surfactant from the aqueous environment occurs through the formation of aggregates (usually spherical) of colloidal dimensions, called *micelles*. The hydrophobic chains form the core of the micelle and are shielded from the aqueous environment by the surrounding shell composed of the hydrophilic groups that serve to maintain solubility in water.

The concentration at which micelles first form in solution is termed the *critical micelle concentration* or CMC. This onset of micelle formation can be detected by a variety of experimental techniques. A change of slope occurs when physical properties such as surface tension, conductivity, osmotic pressure, solubility and light-scattering intensity are plotted as a function of concentration (see Fig. 6.12) and such techniques can be used to measure the CMC. The CMC decreases with increase of the length of the hydrophobic chain. With non-ionic surfactants, which are typically composed of a hydrocarbon chain and an oxyethylene chain (see Table 6.3), an increase of the hydrophilic oxyethylene chain length causes an increase of the CMC. Addition of electrolytes to ionic surfactants decreases the CMC and increases the micellar size. The effect is simply explained in terms of a reduction in the magnitude of the forces of repulsion between the charged head groups in the micelle, allowing the micelles to grow and also reducing the work required for their formation.

The primary reason for micelle formation is the attainment of a state of minimum free energy. The free energy change, ΔG, of a system is dependent on changes in both the entropy, S, and enthalpy, H, which are related by the expression $\Delta G = \Delta H - T\Delta S$. For a micellar system at normal temperatures, the entropy term is by far the most important in determining the free energy changes ($T\Delta S$ constitutes approximately 90–95% of the ΔG value). The explanation most generally accepted for the entropy change is concerned with the structure of water. Water possesses a relatively high degree of structure due to hydrogen bonding between adjacent molecules. If an ionic or strongly polar solute is added to water, it will disrupt this structure but the solute molecules can form hydrogen bonds with the water molecules that more than compensate for the disruption or distortion of the bonds existing in pure water. Ionic and polar materials thus tend to be easily soluble in water. No such compensation occurs with non-polar groups and their solution in water is accordingly resisted, the water molecules forming extra structured clusters around the non-polar region. This increase in structure of the water molecules around the hydrophobic groups leads to a large negative entropy change. To counteract this, and achieve a state of minimum free energy, the hydrophobic groups tend to withdraw from the aqueous phase, either by orientating themselves at the interface with the hydrocarbon chain away from the aqueous phase or by self-association into micelles.

This tendency for hydrophobic materials to be removed from water, due to the strong attraction of water molecules for each other and not for the hydrophobic solute, has been termed *hydrophobic bonding*. However, because there is, in fact, no actual bonding between the hydrophobic groups the phenomenon is best described as the hydrophobic effect. When the non-polar groups approach each other until they are in contact, there will be a decrease in the total number of water molecules in contact with the non-polar groups. The formation of the hydrophobic bond in this way is thus equivalent to the partial removal of hydrocarbon from an aqueous environment and a consequent loss of the ice-like structuring which always surrounds the hydrophobic molecules. The increase in entropy and decrease in free energy which accompany the loss of structuring make the formation of the hydrophobic bond an energetically favourable process. An alternative explanation of the free energy decrease emphasizes the increase in internal freedom of the hydrocarbon chains which occurs when these chains are transferred from the aqueous environment, where their motion is restrained by the hydrogen-bonded water molecules, to the interior of the micelle. It has been suggested that the increased mobility of the hydrocarbon chains, and of course their mutual attraction, constitute the principal hydrophobic factor in micellization.

It should be emphasized that micelles are in dynamic equilibrium with monomer molecules in solution, continuously breaking down and reforming. It is this factor that distinguishes micelles from other colloidal particles and the

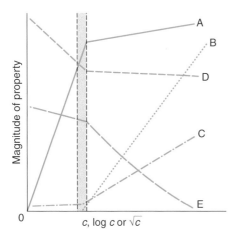

Fig. 6.12 Solution properties of an ionic surfactant as a function of concentration, *c*. (A) Osmotic pressure (against *c*); (B) solubility of a water-insoluble solubilisate (against *c*); (C) intensity of light scattered by the solution (against *c*); (D) surface tension (against log *c*); (E) molar conductivity (against $\sqrt{c}$).

reason why they are called *association colloids*. The concentration of surfactant monomers in equilibrium with the micelles stays approximately constant at the CMC value when the solution concentration is increased above the CMC, i.e. the added surfactant all goes to form micelles.

A typical micelle is a spherical or near-spherical structure composed of some 50–100 surfactant molecules. The radius of the micelle will be slightly less than that of the extended hydrocarbon chain (approximately 2.5 nm) with the interior core of the micelle having the properties of a liquid hydrocarbon. For ionic micelles, about 70–80% of the counter-ions will be attracted close to the micelle, thus reducing the overall charge. The compact layer around the core of an ionic micelle which contains the head groups and the bound counter-ions is called the *Stern layer* (see Fig. 6.13a). The outer surface of the Stern layer is the shear surface of the micelle. The core and the Stern layer together constitute what is termed the 'kinetic micelle'. Surrounding the Stern layer is a diffuse layer called the *Gouy–Chapman electrical double layer* that contains the remaining counter-ions required to neutralize the charge on the kinetic micelle. The thickness of the double layer is dependent on the ionic strength of the solution and is greatly compressed in the presence of electrolyte. Non-ionic micelles have a hydrophobic core surrounded by a shell of oxyethylene chains which is often termed the *palisade layer* (Fig. 6.13b). As well as the water molecules that are hydrogen bonded to the oxyethylene chains, this layer is also capable of mechanically entrapping a considerable number of water molecules. Micelles of non-ionic surfactants tend, as a consequence, to be highly hydrated. The outer surface of the palisade layer forms the shear surface; that is, the hydrating molecules form part of the kinetic micelle.

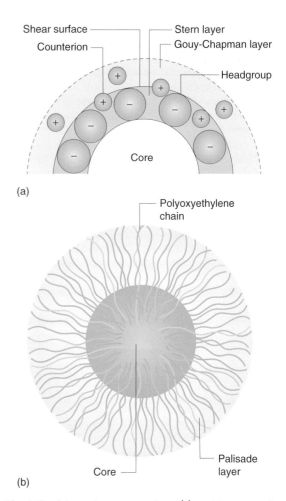

(a)

(b)

Fig. 6.13 Schematic representation of (a) partial cross-section on an anionic micelle and (b) a non-ionic micelle.

Solubilization

As mentioned previously, the interior core of a micelle can be considered as having the properties of a liquid hydrocarbon and is thus capable of dissolving materials that are soluble in such liquids. This process, whereby water-insoluble or partly soluble substances are brought into aqueous solution by incorporation into micelles, is termed *solubilization*. The site of solubilization within the micelle is closely related to the chemical nature of the solubilisate. It is generally accepted that non-polar solubilisates (aliphatic hydrocarbons, for example) are dissolved in the hydrocarbon core (Fig. 6.14a). Water-insoluble compounds containing polar groups are orientated with the polar group at the surface of the ionic micelle amongst the micellar charged head groups, and the hydrophobic group buried inside the hydrocarbon core of the micelle (Fig. 6.14b). Slightly polar solubilisates without a distinct amphiphilic structure partition between the micelle

surface and core (Fig. 6.14c). Solubilization in non-ionic polyoxyethylated surfactants can also occur in the polyoxyethylene shell (palisade layer) which surrounds the core (Fig. 6.14d); thus *p*-hydroxy benzoic acid is entirely within this region hydrogen bonded to the ethylene oxide groups, whilst esters such as the parabens are located at the shell core junction.

The maximum amount of solubilisate that can be incorporated into a given system at a fixed concentration is termed the *maximum additive concentration* (MAC). The simplest method of determining the MAC is to prepare a series of vials containing surfactant solution of known concentration. Increasing concentrations of solubilisate are added and the vials are then sealed and agitated until equilibrium conditions are established. The maximum concentration of solubilisate forming a clear solution can be determined by visual

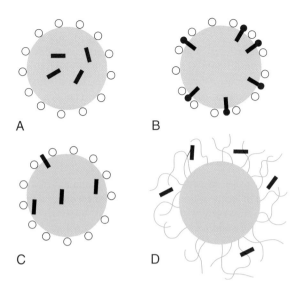

Fig. 6.14 Schematic representation of sites of solubilization in ionic and non-ionic micelles. (a) Non-polar solubilisate; (b) amphipathic solubilisate; (c) slightly polar solubilisate; (d) polar solubilisate in polyoxyethylene shell of a non-ionic micelle.

inspection or from turbidity measurements on the solutions. Solubility data are expressed as a solubility versus concentration curve or as phase diagrams. The latter are preferable since a three-component phase diagram completely describes the effect of varying all three components of the system: namely, the solubilisate, the solubilizer and the solvent.

Pharmaceutical applications of solubilization

A wide range of insoluble drugs has been formulated using the principle of solubilization, some of which will be considered here.

Phenolic compounds such as cresol, chlorocresol, chloroxylenol and thymol are frequently solubilized with soap to form clear solutions which are widely used for disinfection. Pharmacopoeial solutions of chloroxylenol, for example, contain 5% v/v chloroxylenol with terpineol in an alcoholic soap solution.

Non-ionic surfactants can be used to solubilize iodine; such iodine-surfactant systems (referred to as iodophors) are more stable than iodine–iodide systems. They are preferable in instrument sterilization since corrosion problems are reduced. Loss of iodine by sublimation from iodophor solutions is significantly less than from simple iodine solutions. There is also evidence of an ability of the iodophor solution to penetrate hair follicles of the skin, so enhancing the activity.

The low solubility of steroids in water presents a problem in their formulation for ophthalmic use. Because

such formulations are required to be optically clear, it is not possible to use oily solutions or suspensions and there are many examples of the use of non-ionic surfactants as a means of producing clear solutions which are stable to sterilization. In most formulations, solubilization has been effected using polysorbates or polyoxyethylene sorbitan esters of fatty acids.

The polysorbate non-ionics have also been employed in the preparation of aqueous injections of the water-insoluble vitamins A, D, E and K.

Whilst solubilization is an excellent means of producing an aqueous solution of a water-insoluble drug, it should be realized that it may well have effects on the drug's activity and absorption characteristics. As a generalization, it may be said that low concentrations of surface-active agents increase absorption, possibly due to enhanced contact of the drug with the absorbing membrane, whilst concentrations above the CMC either produce no additional effect or cause decreased absorption. In the latter case the drug may be held within the micelles so that the concentration available for absorption is reduced. For a survey of this topic, the review by Attwood & Florence (1983) can be consulted.

Solubilization and drug stability

Solubilization has been shown to have a modifying effect on the rate of hydrolysis of drugs. Non-polar compounds solubilized deep in the hydrocarbon core of a micelle are likely to be better protected against attack by hydrolysing species than more polar compounds located closer to the micellar surface. For example, the alkaline hydrolysis of benzocaine and homatropine in the presence of several non-ionic surfactants is retarded, the less polar benzocaine showing a greater increase in stability compared to homatropine because of its deeper penetration into the micelle. An important factor in considering the breakdown of a drug located close to the micellar surface is the ionic nature of the surface-active agent. For base-catalysed hydrolysis anionic micelles should give an enhanced protection due to repulsion of the attacking OH^- group. For cationic micelles there should be the converse effect. Whilst this pattern has been found, enhanced protection by cationic micelles also occurs, suggesting that in these cases the positively charged polar head groups hold the OH^- groups and thus block their penetration into the micelle.

Protection from oxidative degradation has also been found with solubilized systems.

As indicated earlier, drugs may be surface active. Such drugs form micelles and this self-association has been found in some cases to increase the drug's stability. Thus micellar solutions of penicillin G have been reported to be 2.5 times as stable as monomeric solutions under conditions of constant pH and ionic strength.

Detergency

Detergency is a complex process whereby surfactants are used for the removal of foreign matter from solid surfaces, be it removal of dirt from clothes or cleansing of body surfaces. The process includes many of the actions characteristic of specific surfactants. Thus the surfactant must have good wetting characteristics so that the detergent can come into intimate contact with the surface to be cleaned. The detergent must have the ability to remove the dirt into the bulk of the liquid; the dirt/water and solid/water interfacial tensions are lowered and thus the work of adhesion between the dirt and solid is reduced, so that the dirt particle may be easily detached. Once removed, the surfactant can be adsorbed at the particle surface, creating charge and hydration barriers which prevent deposition. If the dirt is oily it may be emulsified or solubilized.

COARSE DISPERSE SYSTEMS

Suspensions

A pharmaceutical suspension is a coarse dispersion in which insoluble particles, generally greater than 1 μm in diameter, are dispersed in a liquid medium, usually aqueous.

An aqueous suspension is a useful formulation system for administering an insoluble or poorly soluble drug. The large surface area of dispersed drug ensures a high availability for dissolution and hence absorption. Aqueous suspensions may also be used for parenteral and ophthalmic use and provide a suitable form for the application of dermatological materials to the skin. Suspensions are used similarly in veterinary practice and a closely allied field is that of pest control. Pesticides are frequently presented as suspensions for use as fungicides, insecticides, ascaricides and herbicides.

An acceptable suspension possesses certain desirable qualities among which are the following: the suspended material should not settle too rapidly; the particles which do settle to the bottom of the container must not form a hard mass but should be readily dispersed into a uniform mixture when the container is shaken; and the suspension must not be too viscous to pour freely from the orifice of the bottle or to flow through a syringe needle.

Physical stability of a pharmaceutical suspension may be defined as the condition in which the particles do not aggregate and in which they remain uniformly distributed throughout the dispersion. Since this ideal situation is seldom realized, it is appropriate to add that if the particles do settle they should be easily resuspended by a moderate amount of agitation.

The major difference between a pharmaceutical suspension and a colloidal dispersion is one of size of dispersed particles, with the relatively large particles of a suspension liable to sedimentation due to gravitational forces. Apart from this, suspensions show most of the properties of colloidal systems. The reader is referred to Chapter 27 for an account of the formulation of suspensions.

Controlled flocculation

A suspension in which all the particles remain discrete would, in terms of the DLVO theory, be considered to be stable. However, with pharmaceutical suspensions, in which the solid particles are very much coarser, such a system would sediment because of the size of the particles. The electrical repulsive forces between the particles allow the particles to slip past one another to form a close packed arrangement at the bottom of the container, with the small particles filling the voids between the larger ones. The supernatant liquid may remain cloudy after sedimentation due to the presence of colloidal particles that will remain dispersed. Those particles lowermost in the sediment are gradually pressed together by the weight of the ones above. The repulsive barrier is thus overcome, allowing the particles to pack closely together. Physical bonding leading to 'cake' or 'clay' formation may then occur due to the formation of bridges between the particles resulting from crystal growth and hydration effects, forces greater than agitation usually being required to disperse the sediment. Coagulation in the primary minimum, resulting from a reduction in the zeta potential to a point where attractive forces predominate, thus produces coarse compact masses with a 'curdled' appearance, which may not be readily dispersed.

On the other hand, particles flocculated in the secondary minimum form a loosely bonded structure, called a *flocculate* or *floc*. A suspension consisting of particles in this state is said to be flocculated. Although sedimentation of flocculated suspensions is fairly rapid, a loosely packed, high-volume sediment is obtained in which the flocs retain their structure and the particles are easily resuspended. The supernatant liquid is clear because the colloidal particles are trapped within the flocs and sediment with them. Secondary minimum flocculation is therefore a desirable state for a pharmaceutical suspension.

Particles greater than 1 μm radius should, unless highly charged, show a sufficiently deep secondary minimum for flocculation to occur because the attractive force between particles, V_A, depends on particle size. Other contributing factors to secondary minimum flocculation are shape (asymmetric particles, especially those that are elongated, being more satisfactory than spherical ones) and concentration. The rate of flocculation depends on the number of particles present, so that the greater the number of particles, the more collisions there will be and flocculation is more likely to occur. However, it may be necessary, as with highly charged particles, to control the depth of the secondary minimum to induce a satisfactory flocculation state. This can be achieved by addition of electrolytes or ionic surface-active agents which reduce the zeta potential and hence V_R, resulting in the displacement of the whole of the DLVO plot to give a satisfactory secondary minimum, as indicated in Figure 6.5. The production of a satisfactory secondary minimum leading to floc formation in this manner is termed *controlled flocculation*.

A convenient parameter for assessing a suspension is the sedimentation volume ratio, F, which is defined as the ratio of the final settled volume V_u to the original volume V_o:

$$F = V_u/V_o \qquad (6.30)$$

The ratio F gives a measure of the aggregated-deflocculated state of a suspension and may usefully be plotted, together with the measured zeta potential, against concentration of additive, enabling an assessment of the state of the dispersion to be made in terms of the DLVO theory. The appearance of the supernatant liquid should be noted and the redispersibility of the suspensions evaluated.

It should be pointed out that in using the controlled flocculation approach to suspension formulation, it is important to work at a constant, or narrow, pH range because the magnitude of the charge on the drug particle can vary greatly with pH.

Other additives such as flavouring agents may also affect particle charge.

Steric stabilization of suspensions

As described earlier in this chapter, colloidal particles may be stabilized against coagulation in the absence of a charge on the particles by the use of non-ionic polymeric material – the concept of steric stabilization or protective colloid action. This concept may be applied to pharmaceutical suspensions where naturally occurring gums such as tragacanth and synthetic materials like non-ionic surfactants and cellulose polymers may be used to produce satisfactory suspensions. These materials may increase the viscosity of the aqueous vehicle and thus slow the rate of sedimentation of the particles but they will also form adsorbed layers around the particles so that the approach of their surfaces and aggregation to the coagulated state is hindered.

Repulsive forces arise as the adsorbed layers interpenetrate and, as explained above, these have an enthalpic component due to release of water of solvation from the polymer chains and an entropic component due to movement restriction. As a result, the particles will not usually approach one another closer than twice the thickness of the adsorbed layer.

However, as indicated above in the discussion on controlled flocculation, from a pharmaceutical point of view an easily dispersed aggregated system is desirable. To produce this state, a balance between attractive and repulsive forces is required. This is not achieved by all polymeric materials, and the equivalent of deflocculated and caked systems may be produced. The balance of forces appears to depend on both the thickness and the concentration of the polymer in the adsorbed layer. These parameters determine the Hamaker constant and hence the attractive force, which must be large enough to cause aggregation of the particles comparable to flocculation. The steric repulsive force, which depends on the concentration and degree of solvation of the polymer chains, must be of sufficient magnitude to prevent close approach of the uncoated particles, but low enough so that the attractive force is dominant, leading to aggregation at about twice the adsorbed layer thickness. It has been found, for example, that adsorbed layers of certain polyoxyethylene-polyoxypropylene block copolymers will product satisfactory flocculated systems, whilst many nonyl phenyl ethoxylates will not. With both types of surfactant, the molecular moieties producing steric repulsion are hydrated ethylene oxide chains, but the concentration of these in the adsorbed layers varies, giving the results indicated above.

Wetting problems

One of the problems encountered in dispersing solid materials in water is that the powder may not be readily wetted (see Chapter 5). This may be due to entrapped air or to the fact that the solid surface is hydrophobic. The wettability of a powder may be described in terms of the contact angle, θ, which the powder makes with the surface of the liquid. This is described by:

$$\gamma_{S/V} = \gamma_{S/L} + \gamma_{L/V} \cos\theta$$

or

$$\cos\theta = \frac{\gamma_{S/V} - \gamma_{S/L}}{\gamma_{L/V}} \qquad (6.31)$$

where $\gamma_{S/V}$, $\gamma_{S/L}$ and $\gamma_{L/V}$ are the respective interfacial tensions.

For a liquid to completely wet a powder, there should be a decrease in the surface free energy as a result of the immersion process. Once the particle is submerged in the liquid, the process of spreading wetting becomes important. In most cases where water is involved, the reduction of contact angle may only be achieved by reducing the magnitude of $\gamma_{L/V}$ and $\gamma_{S/L}$ by the use of a wetting agent. The wetting agents are surfactants that not only reduce $\gamma_{L/V}$ but also adsorb on to the surface of the powder, thus reducing $\gamma_{S/V}$. Both of these effects reduce the contact angle and improve the dispersibility of the powder.

Problems may arise because of the build-up of an adhering layer of suspension particles on the walls of the container just above the liquid line that occurs as the walls are repeatedly wetted by the suspension. This layer subsequently dries to form a hard, thick crust. Surfactants reduce this adsorption by coating both the glass and particle surfaces such that they repel, reducing adsorption.

Rheological properties of suspensions

Flocculated suspensions tend to exhibit plastic or pseudoplastic flow, depending on concentration, while concentrated deflocculated dispersions tend to be dilatant. This means that the apparent viscosity of flocculated suspensions is relatively high when the applied shearing stress is low, but it decreases as the applied stress increases and the attractive forces producing the flocculation are overcome. Conversely, the apparent viscosity of a concentrated deflocculated suspension is low at low shearing stress, but increases as the applied stress increases. This effect is due to the electrical repulsion that occurs when the charged particles are forced close together (see the DLVO plot of potential energy of interaction between particles; Fig. 6.4), causing the particles to rebound, creating voids into which the liquid flows, leaving other parts of the dispersion dry. In addition to the rheological problems associated with particle charge, the sedimentation behaviour is also of course influenced by the rheological properties of the liquid continuous phase.

Emulsions

An emulsion is a system consisting of two immiscible liquid phases, one of which is dispersed throughout the other in the form of fine droplets. A third component, the emulsifying agent, is necessary to stabilize the emulsion.

The phase that is present as fine droplets is called the disperse phase and the phase in which the droplets are suspended is the continuous phase. Most emulsions will have droplets with diameters of 0.1–100 µm and are inherently unstable systems; smaller globules exhibit colloidal behaviour and have the stability of a hydrophobic colloidal dispersion.

Pharmaceutical emulsions usually consist of water and an oil. Two main types of emulsion can exist, oil-in-water (o/w) and water-in-oil (w/o), depending upon whether the continuous phase is aqueous or oily. More complicated emulsion systems may exist; for example, an oil droplet enclosing a water droplet may be suspended in water to form a water-in-oil-in-water emulsion (w/o/w). Such systems, and their o/w/o counterparts, are termed *multiple emulsions* and are of interest as delayed-action drug delivery vehicles. Traditionally, emulsions have been used to render oily substances such as castor oil in a more palatable form. It is possible to formulate together oil-soluble and water-soluble medicaments in emulsions, and drugs may be more easily absorbed owing to the finely divided condition of emulsified substances.

A large number of bases used for topical preparations are emulsions, water miscible being o/w type and greasy bases w/o. The administration of oils and fats by intravenous infusion, as part of a total parenteral nutrition programme, has been made possible by the use of suitable non-toxic emulsifying agents like lecithin. Here, the control of particle size of emulsion droplets is of paramount importance in the prevention of formation of emboli.

Microemulsions

Unlike the coarse emulsions described above, microemulsions are homogeneous, transparent systems that are thermodynamically stable. Moreover, they form spontaneously when the components are mixed in the appropriate ratios. They can be dispersions of oil in water or water in oil but the droplet size is very much smaller, 5–140 nm, than in coarse emulsions. They are essentially swollen micellar systems, but obviously the distinction between a micelle containing solubilized oil and an oil droplet surrounded by an interfacial layer largely composed of surfactant is difficult to assess.

An essential requirement for their formation and stability is the attainment of a very low interfacial tension. It is generally not possible to achieve the required lowering of interfacial tension with a single surfactant and it is necessary to include a second amphiphile, usually a medium chain length alcohol, in the formulation. The second amphiphile is referred to as the *cosurfactant*.

Although microemulsions have many advantages over coarse emulsions, particularly their transparency and stability, they require much larger amounts of surfactant for their formulation which restricts the choice of acceptable components.

Theory of emulsion stabilization

Interfacial films When two immiscible liquids, e.g. liquid paraffin and water, are shaken together a temporary emulsion will be formed. The subdivision of one of the phases into small globules results in a large increase in surface area and hence interfacial free energy of the system. The system is thus thermodynamically unstable which results, in the first place, in the dispersed phase being in the form of spherical droplets (the shape of minimum surface area for a given volume) and, secondly, in coalescence of these droplets, causing phase separation, the state of minimum surface free energy.

The adsorption of a surface-active agent at the globule interface will lower the o/w interfacial tension, the process of emulsification will be made easier and the stability may be enhanced. However, if a surface-active agent such as sodium dodecyl sulfate is used, the emulsion, on standing for a short while, will still separate out into its constituent phases. On the other hand, substances like acacia, which are only slightly surface active, produce stable emulsions. Acacia forms a strong viscous interfacial film around the globules and it is thought that the characteristics of the interfacial film are most important in considering the stability of emulsions.

Pioneering work on emulsion stability by Schulman & Cockbain in 1940 showed that a mixture of an oil-soluble alcohol such as cholesterol and a surface-active agent such as sodium cetyl (hexadecyl) sulfate was able to form a stable complex condensed film at the oil/water interface. This film was of high viscosity, sufficiently flexible to permit distortion of the droplets, resisted rupture and gave an interfacial tension lower than that produced by either component alone. The emulsion produced was stable, the charge arising from the sodium cetyl sulfate contributing to the stability as described for lyophobic colloidal dispersions. For complex formation at the interface, the correct 'shape' of molecule is necessary. Thus Schulman & Cockbain found that sodium cetyl sulfate stabilized an emulsion of liquid paraffin when elaidyl alcohol (the *trans* isomer) was the oil-soluble component but not when the *cis* isomer, oleyl alcohol, was used.

In practice, the oil-soluble and water-soluble components are dissolved in the appropriate phases and on mixing the two phases, the complex is formed at the interface. Alternatively, an emulsifying wax may be used consisting of a blend of the two components. The wax is dispersed in the oil phase and the aqueous phase added at the same temperature. Examples of such mixtures are given in Table 6.4.

This principle is also applied with the non-ionic emulsifying agents. For example, mixtures of sorbitan monooleate and polyoxyethylene sorbitan esters (e.g. polysorbate 80) have good emulsifying properties.

Table 6.4 Emulsifying waxes

Product	Oil-soluble component	Water-soluble component
Emulsifying wax (anionic)	Cetostearyl alcohol	Sodium lauryl (dodecyl) sulphate
Cetrimide emulsifying wax (cationic)	Cetostearyl alcohol	Cetrimide (hexadecyl trimethyl ammonium bromide)
Cetomacrogol emulsifying wax (non-ionic)	Cetostearyl alcohol	Cetomacrogol (polyoxyethylene monohexadecyl ether)

Non-ionic surfactants are widely used in the production of stable emulsions and have the advantage over ionic surfactants of being less toxic and less sensitive to electrolytes and pH variation. These emulsifying agents are not charged and there is no electrical repulsive force contributing to stability. It is likely, however, that these substances, and the cetomacrogol emulsifying wax included in Table 6.4, sterically stabilize the emulsions as discussed under suspensions.

Hydrophilic colloids as emulsion stabilizers A number of hydrophilic colloids are used as emulsifying agents in pharmaceutical science. These include proteins (gelatin, casein) and polysaccharides (acacia, cellulose derivatives and alginates). These materials, which generally exhibit little surface activity, adsorb at the oil/water interface and form multilayers. Such multilayers have viscoelastic properties, resist rupture and presumably form mechanical barriers to coalescence. However, some of these substances have chemical groups which ionize, e.g. acacia consists of salts of arabic acid, proteins contain both amino and carboxylic acid groupings, thus providing electrostatic repulsion as an additional barrier to coalescence. Most cellulose derivatives are not charged. However, there is evidence from studies on solid suspensions that these substances sterically stabilize and it would appear probable that there will be a similar effect with emulsions.

Solid particles in emulsion stabilization Emulsions may be stabilized by finely divided solid particles if they are preferentially wetted by one phase and possess sufficient adhesion for one another so that they form a film around the dispersed droplets.

Solid particles will remain at the interface as long as a stable contact angle, θ, is formed by the liquid/liquid interface and the solid surface. The particles must also be of sufficiently low mass for gravitational forces not to affect the equilibrium. If the solid is preferentially wetted by one of the phases, then more particles can be accommodated at the interface if the interface is convex towards that phase. In other words, the liquid whose contact angle (measured through the liquid) is less than 90° will form the continuous phase (see Fig. 6.15). Aluminium and magnesium hydroxides and clays such as bentonite are preferentially wetted by water and thus stabilize o/w emulsions, e.g. liquid paraffin and magnesium hydroxide emulsion. Carbon black and talc are more readily wetted by oils and stabilize w/o emulsions.

Emulsion type

When an oil, water and an emulsifying agent are shaken together, what decides whether an o/w or w/o emulsion will be produced? A number of simultaneous processes have to be considered, for example, droplet formation, aggregation and coalescence of droplets, and interfacial film formation. On shaking together oil and water, both phases initially form droplets. The phase that persists in droplet form for the longer time should become the disperse phase and it should be surrounded by the continuous phase formed from the more rapidly coalescing droplets. The phase volumes and interfacial tensions will determine the relative number of droplets produced and hence the probability of collision, i.e. the greater the number of droplets, the higher the chance of collision, so that the phase present in greater amount should finally become the continuous phase. However, emulsions containing well over 50% of disperse phase are common.

A more important consideration is the interfacial film produced by the adsorption of emulsifier at the o/w interface. Such films significantly alter the rates of coalescence by acting as physical and chemical barriers to coalescence. As indicated in the previous section, the barrier at the surface of an oil droplet may arise because of electrically charged groups producing repulsion between approaching droplets, or because of the steric repulsion, enthalpic in origin, from hydrated polymer chains. The greater the number of charged molecules present, or the greater the number of hydrated polymer chains at the interface, the greater will be the tendency to reduce oil droplet coalescence. On the other hand, the interfacial barrier for approaching water droplets arises primarily because of the non-polar or hydrocarbon portion of the interfacial film. The longer the hydrocarbon chain length and the greater the number of molecules present per unit area of film, the greater is the tendency for water droplets to be prevented from coalescing. Thus it may be said generally that it is the dominance of the polar or non-polar characteristics of the emulsifying agent which plays a major part in the type of emulsion produced.

It would appear, then, that the type of emulsion formed, depending as it does on the polar/non-polar characteristics of the emulsifying agent, is a function of the relative solubility of the emulsifying agent, the phase in which it is more soluble being the continuous phase. This is a statement of what is termed the Bancroft rule, an empirical observation made in 1913.

The foregoing helps to explain why charged surface-active agents such as sodium and potassium oleates which are highly ionized and possess strong polar groups favour o/w emulsions, whereas calcium and magnesium soaps which are little dissociated tend to produce w/o emulsions. Similarly, non-ionic sorbitan esters favour w/o emulsions whilst o/w emulsions are produced by the more hydrophilic polyoxyethylene sorbitan esters.

By reason of the stabilizing mechanism involved, polar groups are far better barriers to coalescence than their non-polar counterparts. It is thus possible to see why o/w emulsions can be made with greater than 50% disperse phase and w/o emulsions are limited in this respect and invert (change type) if the amount of water present is significant.

Hydrophile–lipophile balance The fact that a more hydrophilic interfacial barrier favours o/w emulsions whilst a more non-polar barrier favours w/o emulsions is employed in the hydrophile–lipophile balance (HLB) system for assessing surfactants and emulsifying agents, which was introduced by Griffin in 1949. Here an HLB number is assigned to an emulsifying agent that is characteristic of its relative polarity. Although originally conceived for non-ionic emulsifying agents with polyoxyethylene hydrophilic groups, it has since been applied with varying success to other surfactant groups, both ionic and non-ionic.

By means of this number system, an HLB range of optimum efficiency for each class of surfactant is established, as seen in Figure 6.16. This approach is empirical but it does allow comparison between different chemical types of emulsifying agent.

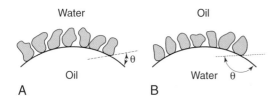

Fig. 6.15 Emulsion stabilization using solid particles. (a) Preferential wetting of solid by water, leading to an o/w emulsion. (b) Preferential wetting of solid by oil, leading to a w/o emulsion.

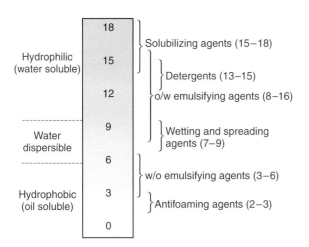

Fig. 6.16 HLB scale showing classification of surfactant function.

There are several formulae for calculating HLB values of non-ionic surfactants. We can estimate values for polysorbates (tweens) and sorbitan esters (spans) from:

$$HLB = (E + P)/5 \qquad (6.32)$$

where E is the percentage by weight of oxyethylene chains and P is the percentage by weight of polyhydric alcohol groups (glycerol or sorbitol) in the molecule. If the surfactant contains only polyoxyethylene as the hydrophilic group then we can use a simpler form of the equation:

$$HLB = E/5 \qquad (6.33)$$

Alternatively, we can calculate HLB values directly from the chemical formula using empirically determined group numbers. The formula is then:

$$HLB = 7 + \Sigma(\text{hydrophilic group numbers})$$
$$- \Sigma(\text{lipophilic group numbers}) \qquad (6.34)$$

Group numbers of some commonly occurring groups are given in Table 6.5. Finally, the HLB of polyhydric alcohol fatty acid esters such as glyceryl monostearate may be obtained from the saponification value, S, of the ester and the acid number, A, of the fatty acid using:

$$HLB = 20\,[1 - S/A] \qquad (6.35)$$

In addition, it has been suggested that certain emulsifying agents of a given HLB value appear to work best with a particular oil phase and this has given rise to the concept of a *required HLB value* for any oil or combination of oils. However, this does not necessarily mean that every surfactant having the required HLB value will produce a good emulsion; specific surfactants may interact with the oil, with another component of the emulsion or even with each other.

For reasons mentioned earlier, mixtures of surface-active agents give more stable emulsions than when used singly. The HLB of a mixture of surfactants, consisting of fraction x of A and $(1 - x)$ of B, is assumed to be an algebraic mean of the two HLB numbers:

$$HLB_{mixt} = x\,HLB_A + (1-x)\,HLB_B \qquad (6.36)$$

It has been found that, at the optimum HLB for a particular emulsion, the mean particle size of the emulsion is at a minimum and this factor contributes to the stability of the emulsion system. The use of HLB values in the formulation of emulsions is discussed in Chapter 27.

Phase viscosity The emulsification process and the type of emulsion formed are influenced to some extent by the viscosity of the two phases. Viscosity can be expected to affect interfacial film formation because the migration of molecules of emulsifying agent to the oil/water interface is diffusion controlled. Droplet movement prior to coalescence is also affected by the viscosity of the medium in which the droplets are dispersed.

Table 6.5 Group contributions to HLB values	
Group	**Contribution**
SO_4Na	+38.7
COOK	+21.1
COONa	+19.1
SO_3Na	+11.0
N (tertiary amine)	+9.4
Ester (sorbitan ring)	+6.8
Ester (free)	+2.4
COOH	+2.1
OH (free)	+1.9
-O-(ether)	+1.3
OH (sorbitan)	+0.5
CH, CH_2 etc	0
OCH_2CH_2	+0.33
$OCH(CH_3)CH_2$	−0.15
(alkyl)	−0.475
CF_2, CF_3	−0.870

Stability of emulsions

A stable emulsion may be defined as a system in which the globules retain their initial character and remain uniformly distributed throughout the continuous phase. The function of the emulsifying agent is to form an interfacial film around the dispersed droplets; the physical nature of this barrier controls whether or not the droplets will coalesce as they approach one another. If the film is electrically charged then repulsive forces will contribute to stability.

Separation of an emulsion into its constituent phases is termed *cracking* or *breaking*. It follows that any agent that will destroy the interfacial film will crack the emulsion. Some of the factors that cause an emulsion to crack are:

- the addition of a chemical that is incompatible with the emulsifying agent, thus destroying its emulsifying ability. Examples include surface-active agents of opposite ionic charge, e.g. the addition of cetrimide (cationic) to an emulsion stabilized with sodium oleate (anionic); addition of large ions of opposite charge, e.g. neomycin sulfate (cationic) to aqueous cream (anionic); addition of electrolytes such as calcium and magnesium salts to an emulsion stabilized with anionic surface-active agents
- bacterial growth – protein materials and non-ionic surface-active agents are excellent media for bacterial growth
- temperature change – protein emulsifying agents may be denatured and the solubility characteristics of non-ionic emulsifying agents change with a rise in temperature; heating above 70°C destroys most emulsions. Freezing will also crack an emulsion; this may be because the ice formed disrupts the interfacial film around the droplets.

Other ways in which an emulsion may show instability are as follows.

Flocculation   Even though a satisfactory interfacial film is present around the oil droplets, secondary minimum flocculation, as described earlier in this chapter under the discussion on the DLVO theory of colloid stability, is likely to occur with most pharmaceutical emulsions. The globules do not coalesce and may be redispersed by shaking. However, due to the closeness of approach of droplets in the floccule, if any weaknesses in the interfacial films occur then coalescence may follow. Flocculation should not be confused with creaming (see below). The former is due to the interaction of attractive and repulsive forces and the latter due to density differences in the two phases. Both may occur.

Phase inversion   As indicated under the section on emulsion type, phase volume ratio is a contributory factor to the type of emulsion formed. Although it was stated there that stable emulsions containing more than 50% of disperse phase are common, attempts to incorporate excessive amounts of disperse phase may cause cracking of the emulsion or phase inversion (conversion of an o/w emulsion to w/o or vice versa). It can be shown that uniform spheres arranged in the closest packing will occupy 74.02% of the total volume irrespective of their size. Thus Ostwald suggested that an emulsion which resembles such an arrangement of spheres would have a maximum disperse phase concentration of the same order. Although it is possible to obtain more concentrated emulsions than this, because of the non-uniformity of size of the globules and the possibility of deformation of shape of the globules, there is a tendency for emulsions containing more than about 70% disperse phase to crack or invert.

Further, any additive that alters the HLB of an emulsifying agent may alter the emulsion type; thus addition of a magnesium salt to an emulsion stabilized with sodium oleate will cause the emulsion to crack or invert.

The addition of an electrolyte to anionic and cationic surfactants may suppress their ionization due to the common ion effect and thus a w/o emulsion may result even though normally an o/w emulsion would be produced. For example, pharmacopoeial White Liniment is formed from turpentine oil, ammonium oleate, ammonium chloride and water. With ammonium oleate as emulsifying agent, an o/w emulsion would be expected but the suppression of ionization of the ammonium oleate by the ammonium chloride (the common ion effect), and a relatively large volume of turpentine oil, produce a w/o emulsion.

Emulsions stabilized with non-ionic emulsifying agents such as the polysorbates may invert on heating. This is due to the breaking of the H-bonds responsible for the hydrophilic characteristics of the polysorbate; its HLB value is thus altered and the emulsion inverts.

Creaming   Many emulsions cream on standing. The disperse phase, according to its density relative to that of the continuous phase, rises to the top or sinks to the bottom of the emulsion, forming a layer of more concentrated emulsion. The commonest example is milk, an o/w emulsion, with cream rising to the top of the emulsion.

As mentioned earlier, flocculation may occur as well as creaming but not necessarily so. Droplets of the creamed layer do not coalesce, as may be found by gentle shaking which redistributes the droplets throughout the continuous phase. Although not so serious an instability factor as cracking, creaming is undesirable from a pharmaceutical point of view because a creamed emulsion is inelegant in appearance, provides the possibility of inaccurate dosage and increases the likelihood of coalescence since the globules are close together in the cream.

Those factors which influence the rate of creaming are similar to those involved in the sedimentation rate of suspension particles and are indicated by Stokes' Law as follows:

$$v = \frac{2a^2 g (\sigma - \rho)}{9\eta} \qquad (6.37)$$

where v is the velocity of creaming, a the globule radius, σ and ρ the densities of disperse phase and dispersion medium respectively, and η the viscosity of the dispersion medium. A consideration of this equation shows that the rate of creaming will be decreased by:

- a reduction in the globule size
- a decrease in the density difference between the two phases, and
- an increase in the viscosity of the continuous phase.

A decrease of creaming rate may therefore be achieved by homogenizing the emulsion to reduce the globule size and increasing the viscosity of the continuous phase η by the use of thickening agents such as tragacanth or methylcellulose. It is seldom possible to satisfactorily adjust the densities of the two phases.

Assessment of emulsion stability Approximate assessments of the relative stabilities of a series of emulsions may be obtained from estimations of the degree of separation of the disperse phase as a distinct layer, or from the degree of creaming. Whilst separation of the emulsion into two layers, i.e. cracking, indicates gross instability, a stable emulsion may cream, creaming being simply due to density differences and easily reversed by shaking. Some coalescence may, however, take place due to the close proximity of the globules in the cream; similar problems occur with flocculation.

However, instability in an emulsion results from any process which causes a progressive increase in particle size and a broadening of the particle size distribution, so that eventually the dispersed particles become so large that they separate out as free liquid. Accordingly, a more precise method for assessing emulsion stability is to follow the globule size distribution with time. An emulsion approaching the unstable state is characterized by the appearance of large globules as a result of the coalescence of others.

Foams

A foam is a coarse dispersion of a gas in a liquid which is present as thin films or lamellae of colloidal dimensions between the gas bubbles.

Foams find application in pharmacy as aqueous and non-aqueous spray preparations for topical, rectal and vaginal medication and for burn dressings. Equally important, however, is the destruction of foams and the use of antifoaming agents. These are of importance in manufacturing processes, preventing foam in, for example, liquid preparations. In addition, foam inhibitors like the silicones are used in the treatment of flatulence, for the elimination of gas, air or foam from the gastrointestinal tract prior to radiography and for the relief of abdominal distension and dyspepsia.

Due to their high interfacial area (and surface free energy), all foams are unstable in the thermodynamic sense. Their stability depends on two major factors: the tendency for the liquid films to drain and become thinner, and their tendency to rupture due to random disturbances such as vibration, heat and diffusion of gas from small bubbles to large bubbles. Gas diffuses from the small bubbles to the large because the pressure in the former is greater. This is a phenomenon of curved interfaces, the pressure difference Δp being a function of the interfacial tension, γ, and the radius, r, of the droplet according to $\Delta p = 2\gamma/r$.

Pure liquids do not foam. Transient or unstable foams are obtained with solutes such as short chain acids and alcohols which are mildly surface active. However, persistent foams are formed by solutions of surfactants. The film in such foams consists of two monolayers of adsorbed surface-active molecules separated by an aqueous core. The surfactants stabilize the film by means of electrical double layer repulsion or steric stabilization as described for colloidal dispersions.

Foams are often troublesome and knowledge of the action of substances that cause their destruction is useful. There are two types of antifoaming agent:

- *foam breakers* such as ether and *n*-octanol. These substances are highly surface active and are thought to act by lowering the surface tension over small regions of the liquid film. These regions are rapidly pulled out by surrounding regions of higher tension, small areas of film are therefore thinned out and left without the properties to resist rupture
- *foam inhibitors,* such as polyamides and silicones. It is thought that these are adsorbed at the air/water interface in preference to the foaming agent, but they do not have the requisite ability to form a stable foam. They have a low interfacial tension in the pure state and may be effective by virtue of rapid adsorption.

Aerosols

Aerosols are colloidal dispersions of liquids or solids in gases. In general, mists and fogs possess liquid disperse phases whilst smoke is a dispersion of solid particles in gases. However, no sharp distinction can be made between the two kinds because liquid is often associated with the solid particles. A mist consists of fine droplets of liquid that may or may not contain dissolved or suspended material. If the concentration of droplets becomes high it may be called a *fog*.

While all the disperse systems mentioned above are less stable than colloids that have a liquid as dispersion medium, they have many properties in common with the latter and can be investigated in the same way. Particle size is usually within the colloidal range but if larger than 1 μm, the life of an aerosol is short because the particles settle out too quickly.

Preparation of aerosols

In common with other colloidal dispersions, aerosols may be prepared by either dispersion or condensation methods. The latter involve the initial production of supersaturated vapour of the material that is to be dispersed. This may be achieved by supercooling the vapour. The supersaturation eventually leads to the formation of nuclei, which grow into particles of colloidal dimensions. The preparation of aerosols by dispersion methods is of greater interest in pharmacy and may be achieved by the use of pressurized containers with, for example, liquefied gases such as propellants. If a solution or suspension of active ingredients is contained in the liquid propellant or in a mixture of this liquid and an additional solvent, then when the valve on the container is opened the vapour pressure of the propellant forces the mixture out of the container. The large expansion of the propellant at room temperature and atmospheric pressure produces a dispersion of the active ingredients in air. Although the particles in such dispersions are often larger than those in colloidal systems, these dispersions are still generally referred to as aerosols.

Application of aerosols in pharmacy

The use of aerosols as a dosage form is particularly important in the administration of drugs via the respiratory system. In addition to local effects, systemic effects may be obtained if the drug is absorbed into the blood stream from the lungs. Topical preparations (Chapter 38) are also well suited for presentation as aerosols. Therapeutic aerosols for inhalation are discussed in more detail in Chapter 36.

REFERENCES

Attwood, D., Florence, A. T. (1983) *Surfactant Systems: Their Chemistry, Pharmacy and Biology*. Chapman and Hall, London.
Shaw, D. J. (1992) *Introduction to Colloid and Surface Chemistry*, 4th edn. Butterworth-Heinemann, Oxford.

BIBLIOGRAPHY

Florence, A. T., Attwood, D. (2006) *Physicochemical Principles of Pharmacy*, 4th edn. Pharmaceutical Press, London.
Rosen, M. J. (1989) *Surfactants and Interfacial Phenomena*, 2nd edn. John Wiley, New York.

Kinetics of product stability

W. J. Pugh

INTRODUCTION

Kinetics is the study of the rate at which processes occur. The changes may be chemical (decomposition of a drug, radiochemical decay) or physical (transfer across a boundary such as the intestinal lining or skin). Kinetic studies are useful in providing information that:

- gives an insight into the mechanisms of the changes involved and
- allows prediction of the degree of change that will occur after a given time has elapsed.

In general, the theories and laws of chemical kinetics are well founded and provide a sound basis for the application of such studies to pharmaceutical problems that involve chemical reactions, e.g. the decomposition of medical compounds.

This chapter is concerned with chemical reactions. It is not the intention of this chapter to discuss in detail the chemistry of instability and methods of prolonging the effective life of a medicine. These are discussed in Chapter 44 and preformulation considerations are discussed in Chapter 24.

HOMOGENEOUS AND HETEROGENEOUS REACTIONS

Homogeneous reactions occur in a single phase, i.e. true solutions or gases, and proceed uniformly throughout the whole of the system. *Heterogeneous reactions* involve more than one phase and are often confined to the phase boundary, their rates being dependent on the supply of fresh reactants to this boundary. Examples are decomposition of drugs in suspensions and enzyme-catalysed reactions.

MOLECULARITY

Molecularity is the number of molecules involved in forming the product. This follows from the balanced (stoichiometrical) equation describing the reaction. For example, in the following two-step reaction:

$N_2O_5 \rightarrow 2NO_2 + \frac{1}{2}O_2$ is a slow, unimolecular reaction

and

$\frac{1}{2}O_2 + \frac{1}{2}O_2 \rightarrow O_2$ is a fast, bimolecular reaction.

ORDER

This is the number of concentration terms that determine the rate. In a unimolecular process a molecule will react if it has sufficiently high energy. The number of high-energy molecules depends on how many molecules are present, i.e. on their concentration in solution (or pressure in a gas). In a bimolecular process, two molecules must collide to react and the likelihood of collision depends on the concentrations of each species. The Law of Mass Action states that the rate depends on the product of concentrations of the reactants.

Thus in the first step of the example reaction:

$$N_2O_5 = 2NO_2 + \frac{1}{2}O_2$$

the rate of reaction $= k_1[N_2O_5]$. Here k_1 is the rate constant. The square brackets here, and throughout this chapter, mean 'concentration of' the entity within the brackets. In this case there is only one concentration term and the reaction is known as *first order*.

In the second step:

$$\frac{1}{2}O_2 + \frac{1}{2}O_2 = O_2$$

the rate of reaction $= k_2[\frac{1}{2}O_2][\frac{1}{2}O_2] = k_2[\frac{1}{2}O_2]^2$, where k_2 is the reaction rate constant. Thus there are two concentration terms and the reaction is known as *second order*.

Each of these is discussed in more detail below.

First-order processes

The rate is determined by one concentration term. These are by far the most important processes in pharmaceutical science. Many drug decompositions during storage and the passage of drugs from one body compartment to another, e.g. lumen of the intestine into blood, follow first-order kinetics. The rate of reaction is most simply defined as the concentration change divided by the corresponding time change.

$$\frac{dc}{dt} = -kc \qquad (7.1)$$

The negative sign is used because concentration falls as time increases. This makes the rate constant, k, positive.

The differential equation above describes infinitely small changes. For real changes these small changes are summed (integrated) usually from the start of the process (time $= 0$, concentration $= c_o$) to the concentration, c, remaining at any other time, t, as follows.

$$\int_c^{c_o} \frac{dc}{c} = -k \int_t^o dt \qquad (7.2)$$

$$[\ln c]_c^{c_o} = -k[t]_t^o \qquad (7.3)$$

$$\ln c_o - \ln c = -k\{(0)\}(t) \qquad (7.4)$$

$$\ln c = \ln c_o - kt \qquad (7.5)$$

$$(y) \qquad a \quad + b(x)$$

Thus a plot of $\ln c$ against t is a straight line with intercept c_0 and gradient $-k$.

The units of k are given by rearranging Eqn 7.1, i.e.:

$$\frac{dc}{cdt} = -k \qquad (7.6)$$

Thus the rate constant has the dimensions of time^{-1} and typical units of s^{-1}.

Note that because k contains no concentration term, it is not necessary to convert experimental data to concentration values in order to estimate it. Any convenient property of the system which is directly proportional to concentration can be used, such as UV absorbance, conductivity, pressure and radioactivity. For example, absorbance (A) is related to concentration, c, by Beer's Law, i.e. $c = \alpha A$, where α is a proportionality constant. Substitution into Eqn 7.5 gives:

$$\ln \alpha A = \ln \alpha A_o - kt \qquad (7.7)$$

hence

$$\ln A = \ln A_o - kt \qquad (7.8)$$

Thus, although the intercept of the graph will alter, the gradient remains the same.

Example 7.1

Consider the following example. A tritiated cardiac stimulant is administered by i.v. injection. Blood samples have the following radioactivity counts per second (cps).

t (min)	0	30	60	90	120	150
cps	59.7	24.3	9.87	4.01	1.63	0.67
ln (cps)	4.09	3.19	2.29	1.39	0.49	−0.41

From Figure 7.1, it can be seen that the rate constant for absorption from the blood is 0.03 min^{-1}.

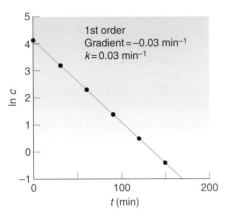

Fig. 7.1 First order.

Pseudo first-order processes

Consider the hydrolysis of ethyl acetate:

$$CH_3COOEt + H_2O \rightarrow CH_3COOH + EtOH$$

Strictly the reaction is second order and the rate of reaction is expressed as:

$$\text{Rate} = k\,[CH_3COOEt]\,[H_2O]$$

However, in a dilute aqueous solution of ethyl acetate, $[H_2O]$ is very large compared to $[CH_3COOEt]$ and hardly alters during the course of the reaction. $[H_2O]$ can be taken as a constant and incorporated into the second-order rate constant, now k', where $k' = k[H_2O]$:

$$\text{Rate} = k'\,[CH_3COOEt]$$

Thus the reaction is, in effect, first order with a rate constant k'. This applies to many drug decompositions by hydrolysis in aqueous solution.

Second-order processes

The rate depends on the product of two concentration terms. In the simplest case they refer to the same species. For example:

$$2HI \rightarrow H_2 + I_2$$

Here the reaction is not simply a matter of a HI molecule falling apart, but relies on the collision of two HI molecules. The rate of reaction for this example is given from the Law of Mass Action by:

$$\text{Rate} = k\,[HI]\,[HI] = k\,[HI]^2$$

For a second-order process:

$$\frac{dc}{dt} = -kc^2 \tag{7.9}$$

$$\int_c^{c_0} c^{-2}\,dc = -k \int_t^o dt \tag{7.10}$$

$$[-c^{-1}]_c^{c_0} = -k\,[t]_t^o \tag{7.11}$$

$$\frac{1}{c} = \frac{1}{c_0} + kt \tag{7.12}$$
$$(y) \quad a + b(x)$$

Thus the gradient of a plot of $1/c$ against t gives the rate constant, k.

Units of k from Eqn 7.9 are:

$$\frac{dc}{c^2dt} = -k \tag{7.13}$$

i.e. conc^{-1} time^{-1} and typical units are L mole^{-1} s^{-1} or similar.

Example 7.2

Consider the following decomposition data.

t (days)	0	30	60	90	120	150
c (mmole L^{-1})	100	2.17	1.10	0.74	0.56	0.44

From Figure 7.2, it can be seen that the rate constant is 0.015 L mmole^{-1} day^{-1}.

If the reaction is between two different species, A and B, it is unlikely that their starting concentrations will be equal. Let their initial concentrations be a_0 and b_0 (where $a_0 > b_0$), falling to a and b at time t. Since equal numbers of molecules of A and B are lost in the decomposition, the rate can be defined as da/dt (or db/dt). Thus:

$$da/dt = -kab \tag{7.14}$$

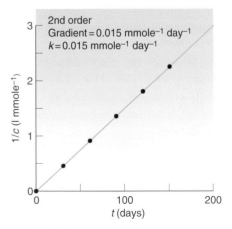

Fig. 7.2 Second order.

Integration by partial fractions gives:

$$\ln(a/b) = \ln(a_o/b_o) + k(a_o - b_o)t \qquad (7.15)$$
$$(y) \quad = \quad a \quad + \quad b(x)$$

Thus a plot of $\ln(a/b)$ against t is a straight line with gradient $k(a_o - b_o)$.

Zero-order processes

In a zero-order reaction the rate of process (decomposition, dissolution, drug release) is *independent* of the concentration of the reactants, i.e. the rate is constant. A constant rate of drug release from a dosage form is highly desirable. Zero-order kinetics often apply to processes occurring at phase boundaries, where the concentration at the surface remains constant either because reaction sites are saturated (enzyme kinetics, drug receptor interaction) or it is replenished constantly by diffusion of fresh material from within the bulk of one phase. This diffusion criterion applies to hydrolysis of drugs in suspensions and delivery from controlled-release dosage forms such as transdermal patches.

$$\frac{dc}{dt} = -k \qquad (7.16)$$

$$\int_c^{c_o} cdc = -k \int_t^o dt \qquad (7.17)$$

$$[c]_c^{c_o} = -k[t]_t^o \qquad (7.18)$$

$$c_o - c = -k\{(0) - (t)\} \qquad (7.19)$$

$$c = c_o - kt \qquad (7.20)$$

$$(y) \quad a + b(x)$$

Thus, a plot of c against t is a straight line with gradient k. Units of k from Eqn 7.16 are concentration^{-1} time^{-1} with typical units of mole L^{-1} s^{-1} or similar.

Example 7.3

The concentration of steroid remaining in a transdermal patch is as follows:

t (h)	0	30	60	90	120	150
Amount (µg)	20	16.4	12.8	9.2	5.6	2

Note: strictly speaking, 'amount' is not the same as 'concentration' but in this case concentration can be considered to be µg patch^{-1}.

From Figure 7.3, it can be seen that the rate constant is 0.12 µg h^{-1}(patch^{-1}).

Half-Life $t_{1/2}$

This is the time taken for the concentration (of, say, a drug in solution or in the body) to reduce by a half.

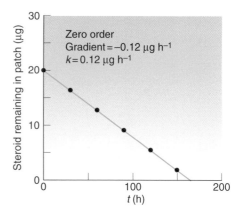

Fig. 7.3 Zero order.

Rearrangement of the integrated equations for t (Eqns 7.5, 7.14 and 7.20) gives the relationships in the first line below and substituting $c = c_o/2$ at $t_{1/2}$ gives those in the second line.

	Zero order	First order	Second order
$t =$	$(c - c_o)/k$	$\ln(c_o/c)/k$	$(1/c - 1/c_o)/k$
$t_{1/2}$	$c_o/2k$	$0.693/k$	$1/c_o k$

Note that for first-order reactions, the half-life, $t_{1/2}$, is independent of concentration.

Summary of Parameters

Table 7.1 summarizes the parameters for zero-order, first-order and second-order processes.

DETERMINATION OF ORDER AND RATE CONSTANT FROM EXPERIMENTAL DATA

This can be achieved in two ways:
- substituting the data into the integrated equations and observing which plot is a straight line
- finding $t_{1/2}$ values at different stages of the reaction and noting if and how they vary with 'starting' concentration.

Example 7.4

The following data apply to decomposition of a drug.

t (h)	0	10	20	30	40	50	60
c(mg L^{-1})	10	6.2	3.6	2.2	1.3	0.8	0.6
$\ln c$	2.30	1.83	1.28	0.79	0.26	−0.22	−0.51
$1/c$	0.10	0.161	0.278	0.455	0.769	1.250	1.667

Table 7.1 Summary of parameters

	Zero order	First order	Second order ($a = b$)
Linear equation	$c = c_0 - kt$	$\ln c = \ln c_0 - kt$	$1/c = 1/c_0 + kt$
Intercept	c_0	$\ln c_0$	$1/c_0$
Gradient	$-k$	$-k$	k
Units of k	conc time^{-1}	time^{-1}	conc^{-1} time^{-1}
e.g.	mole L^{-1} s^{-1}	s^{-1}	L mole^{-1} s^{-1}
Half-life ($t_{1/2}$)	$c_0/2k$	$0.693/k$	$1/c_0 k$

Data plotting method

The data are plotted in Figure 7.4. The plot of c against t (Fig. 7.4a) is obviously not linear so the reaction is not zero order. A plot of $1/c$ against time (Fig. 7.4b) is also not linear so reaction is not second order.

However, a plot of $\ln c$ against t (Fig. 7.4c) is linear so the reaction is first order. From the graph, the gradient

(i.e. $-k$) = -0.048 h^{-1} and the first-order rate constant = 0.048 h^{-1}.

Half-life method

This involves the selection of a set of convenient 'initial' concentrations and then determining the times taken to fall to half these values.

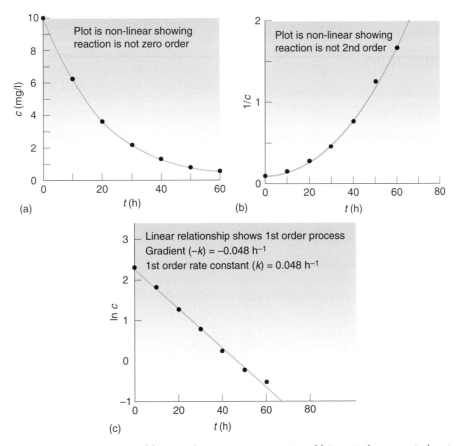

Fig. 7.4 (a) Plot of concentration against time. (b) Plot of 1/concentration against time. (c) Plot of ln (concentration) against time.

Example 7.5

The 'c_0' values are obtained by interpolation of the concentration versus time plot of the data in Example 7.4.

'c_0'	10	8	6	4	2
t at 'c_0'	0	5	11	18	32
t at 'c_0'/2	12	18	24	32	45
$t_{1/2}$	12	13	13	14	13

Within experimental error $t_{1/2}$ seems independent of 'c_0', suggesting that the reaction is first order. To confirm this it is necessary to check whether $t_{1/2}$ values correspond to zero or second-order kinetics.

If the reaction was zero order, then $c_0/2t_{1/2}$ would be a constant value (k). Similarly for a second-order reaction, $k = 1/c_0t_{1/2}$ would be constant. Calculating these gives:

'c_0'	10	8	6	4	2
'c_0'/2$t_{1/2}$	0.42	0.31	0.23	0.14	0.08
1/'c_0'$t_{1/2}$	0.008	0.009	0.013	0.018	0.038

Thus, neither set of values is constant, confirming that the reaction is neither zero or second order.

The first-order rate constant is found from the mean $t_{1/2}$ value of 13 h, i.e. $k = 0.693/t_{1/2} = 0.053$ h^{-1}.

COMPLEX REACTIONS

The theories so far have assumed that a single reaction pathway is involved and that the product does not, in turn, affect the kinetics. Neither of these assumptions may be true and the *overall* order, being the result of several reactions, may not be zero, first or second order but have a fractional value.

There are three basic types of complex behaviour.

Parallel (side) reactions

Here reactants A form a mixture of products:

$$B \xleftarrow{k_1} A \xrightarrow{k_2} C$$

Usually only one of the products is desirable, the others are byproducts.

$$(\text{Yield of B/Yield of C}) = k_1/k_2 \qquad (7.21)$$

Series (consecutive) reactions

$$A \xrightarrow{k_1} B \xrightarrow{k_2} C$$

If $k_1 \gg k_2$ then a build-up of B occurs. The second (slower) step is then the 'rate-determining' step of the

reaction, and the overall order is approximately that of the rate-determining step. Thus the reaction:

$$2N_2O_5 \rightarrow 4NO_2 + O_2$$

is composed of two consecutive reactions as discussed previously:

$$N_2O_5 \rightarrow 2NO_2 + \tfrac{1}{2}O_2 \qquad (\text{slow – first order})$$

$$\tfrac{1}{2}O_2 + \tfrac{1}{2}O_2 \rightarrow O_2 \qquad (\text{fast – second order})$$

The overall reaction is first order, defined by the slower first step.

Reversible reactions

Here the product can re-form into the reactants:

$$A \underset{k_{-1}}{\overset{k_1}{\rightleftharpoons}} B + C$$

Here there are two reactions occurring simultaneously:

- first-order decomposition of A, with a rate constant of k_1
- second-order formation of A from B and C. The rate constant of the reverse reaction is often written as k_{-1}, i.e. with subscript −1. This can cause confusion. The negative sign merely implies that it refers to the reverse of a reaction numbered 1 (A → B + C). It does NOT mean that if k_1 is 0.5 h^{-1} then the rate constant for the reverse reaction is −0.5 h^{-1}.

Michaelis–Menten equation

These three basic reaction types can be combined in different ways. One important combination describes processes that occur at interfaces. These appear repeatedly in the life sciences, e.g. enzyme–substrate, transmitter–receptor and drug–receptor binding. The kinetics are described by the Michaelis–Menten equation. This assumes that the enzyme, E, and substrate, S, form an unstable complex, ES, which can either re-form S or a new product, P.

$$E + S \underset{k_2}{\overset{k_1}{\rightleftharpoons}} ES \xrightarrow{k_3} P + E \qquad (7.21)$$

The overall reaction rate is the rate at which P is formed. This is first order depending on [ES], i.e. the concentration of ES. Thus dP/d$t = k_3[ES]$ (note that there is no negative sign because P increases as t increases).

Unfortunately we normally have no way of measuring [ES]. However, the rate at which [ES] changes is the rate at which it forms from E and S, ($k_1[E][S]$), minus the rates at which it decomposes to reform E and S, ($k_2[ES]$), or to form P, ($k_3[ES]$). Thus:

$$\frac{d[ES]}{dt} = k_1[E][S] - k_2[ES] - k_3[ES] \qquad (7.22)$$

$$\frac{d[ES]}{dt} = k_1[E][S] - (k_2 + k_3)[ES] \qquad (7.23)$$

In practice $[ES]$ is small as the complex decomposes rapidly. Changes in $[ES]$ soon become negligible compared to other concentration changes in the system. Then $[ES]$ is almost a constant, i.e. $d[ES]/dt$ = zero, and the system is said to be at a 'steady state'.

Thus at the steady state:

$$\frac{d[ES]}{dt} = \text{zero} = k_1[E][S] - (k_2 + k_3)[ES] \qquad (7.24)$$

and rearrangement gives:

$$[ES] = \frac{k_1[E][S]}{(k_2 + k_3)} \qquad (7.25)$$

Writing $(k_2 + k_3)/k_1$ as K gives:

$$[ES] = \frac{[E][S]}{K} \text{ or} \qquad (7.26)$$

$$[ES] = \frac{[E]}{K/[S]} \qquad (7.27)$$

To proceed further, we need to know $[ES]$, i.e. the concentration of the unstable intermediate. In practice we only know the total concentration of enzyme that we put into the mixture, $[E_0]$. Since this now exists in free and complexed forms then:

$$[E_0] = [E] + [ES] \qquad (7.28)$$

Substituting $[E] = [E_0] - [ES]$ in Eqn 7.27 and then writing $J = K/[S]$ gives:

$$[ES] = \frac{[E_0] - [ES]}{K/[S]} = \frac{[E_0]}{J} - \frac{[ES]}{J} \qquad (7.29)$$

$$[ES] + \frac{[ES]}{J} = \frac{[E_0]}{J} \qquad (7.30)$$

$$[ES]\left(1 + \frac{1}{J}\right) = \frac{[E_0]}{J} \qquad (7.31)$$

$$[ES]\left(\frac{J+1}{J}\right) = \frac{[E_0]}{J} \qquad (7.32)$$

$$[ES] = \frac{[E_0]}{(J+1)} = \frac{[E_0]}{((K/[S]) + 1)} \qquad (7.33)$$

The overall rate of reaction, V, is given by the Michaelis–Menten equation:

$$V = \frac{dP}{dt} = k_3[ES] \qquad (7.34)$$

$$V = \frac{k_3[E_0]}{\frac{K}{[S]} + 1} \qquad (7.35)$$

Thus the rate, V, is not constant but declines from its initial value, V_0, as $[S]$ falls, i.e. as the substrate is used up. V_0 is found from the initial gradient of the plot of $[P]$ against t (Fig. 7.5).

If these V_0 values are found for a range of substrate concentrations, $[S]$, and the enzyme concentration $[E_0]$ is maintained constant, the familiar plateau curve results (Fig. 7.6). The plateau shape arises from the mathematical properties of the Michaelis–Menten equation.

$$V_0 = \frac{k_3[E_0]}{K}[S] \qquad (7.36)$$

$$V_0 = k_3[E_0] \qquad (7.37)$$

k_3 and $[E_0]$ are constants so this process is zero order. $k_3[E_0]$ is the maximum rate, V_{max}, for a given enzyme concentration.

Viewed simply, the enzyme reactive sites are saturated by substrate molecules. This plateau curve is very common and often signifies a process occurring at a saturatable interphase, a heterogeneous process.

Equation 7.35 is often inverted to give a linear relationship between $1/V_0$ and $1/[S]$.

$$\frac{1}{V_0} = \frac{1}{k_3 E_0} + \frac{K}{k_3 E_0}\left(\frac{1}{[S]}\right) \qquad (7.38)$$

$$\frac{1}{V_0} = \frac{1}{V_{max}} + \frac{K}{V_{max}}\left(\frac{1}{[S]}\right) \qquad (7.39)$$

V_{max}, K and k_3 are found from the gradient and intercept of this Lineweaver–Burke plot (Fig. 7.7). Workers in the field of enzyme inhibition or drug–receptor interaction often estimate K from the intercept on the abscissa (x-axis) of the plot. This is the value of $1/[S]$ where $1/V_0$ = zero. Substitution into Eqn 7.11 gives:

$$1/[S] = -1/K \qquad (7.40)$$

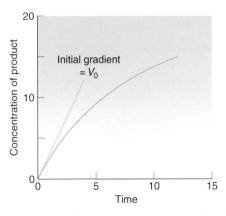

Fig. 7.5 Estimation of initial velocity of enzyme-catalysed reaction.

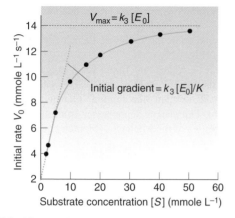

Fig. 7.6 Michaelis–Menten plot for enzyme-catalysed reaction.

Thus from Figure 7.7, it can be seen that $V_{max} = 15.1$ mmole $L^{-1}s^{-1}$ and $K = 5.7$. The way in which these parameters are altered by inhibitors enables us to say whether the inhibition is reversible/irreversible and competitive/noncompetitive. See York (1992) for further details.

EFFECT OF TEMPERATURE ON REACTION RATE

Generally, increasing temperature increases rate of reaction, and an often quoted rough guide is that a 10°C rise doubles the rate constant. Better descriptions are given by the Arrhenius theory and the more rigorous transition state theory (see, for example, Martin 1993).

Arrhenius theory

This can be developed from simple basic ideas and leads to an equation that is formally identical with the transition state theory.

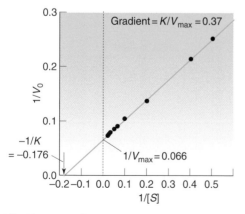

Fig. 7.7 Lineweaver–Burke plot of data in Figure 7.6.

Consider the simple bimolecular reaction:

$$2HI \rightarrow H_2 + I_2$$

The original proposition was that if two molecules collided they would react. The collision number, Z, can be calculated from the kinetic theory of gases, and it was found that the number of molecules reacting per second, μ, was much smaller than Z. The theory was modified to propose that the colliding molecules must have sufficient energy to form an unstable intermediate, which breaks down to form the product.

The fraction of molecules with at least this activation energy, E, was calculated by Boltzmann as $e^{-E/RT}$ so that:

$$\mu = Ze^{-E/RT} \tag{7.41}$$

This equation adequately describes simple reactions like the decomposition of HI, but for even slightly more complex reactions such as:

$$N(CH_3)_3 + CH_3I = N(CH_3)_4I$$

μ is thousands of times smaller than $Ze^{-E/RT}$. This is because the nitrogen atom is shielded by a mass of C and H atoms, so that only very few collisions occur between the nitrogen and the carbon of the approaching CH_3I. Thus an orientation factor, P, often with a very small value, must also be included.

$$\mu = PZe^{-E/RT} \tag{7.42}$$

The rate constant k is proportional to μ. So, writing k as $\alpha\mu$ gives:

$$k = \alpha PZe^{-E/RT} \tag{7.43}$$

Over a small temperature range the change in Z with T is negligible compared to that in the $e^{-E/RT}$ term, so that αPZ is a constant, A. A is called the 'frequency factor' since it is related to the frequency of correctly aligned collisions.

$$k = Ae^{-E/RT} \tag{7.44}$$

This is the Arrhenius equation, which may also be written as:

$$\ln k = \ln A - \frac{E}{R}\left(\frac{1}{T}\right) \tag{7.45}$$

$$(y) \quad a \quad + \quad b(x)$$

or in $\log_{10}$ form:

$$\log k = \log A - \frac{E}{2.303R}\left(\frac{1}{T}\right) \tag{7.46}$$

so that a plot of $\ln k$ (or $\log k$) against $(1/T)$ is a straight line, enabling calculation of E and A from the gradient and intercept. (Remember that T must be in K, not °C.) The same equation holds for zero- and first-order reactions. Here the molecule will react if it has energy $\geq E$.

The collision and orientation factors are inapplicable and A is now the proportionality constant α. However, it is still termed the frequency factor.

Example 7.6

From the following data, estimate the rate constant at 25°C.

Temp (°C)	k (day^{-1})	T (K)	$1/T$	$\ln k$
70	0.0196	343	2.92×10^{-3}	−3.93
60	0.0082	333	3.00×10^{-3}	−4.80
50	0.0028	323	3.10×10^{-3}	−5.88
40	0.0011	313	3.20×10^{-3}	−6.81
25		298	3.36×10^{-3}	

A plot of $\ln k$ against $1/T$ is a good straight line (Fig. 7.8).

Reading $\ln k$ off the graph at $1/T = 3.36 \times 10^{-3}$ (corresponding to 25°C) is −8.5, giving $k_{25} = 2.03 \times 10^{-4}$ day^{-1}.

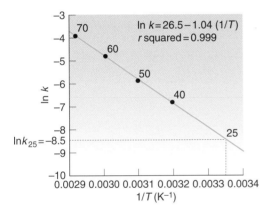

Fig. 7.8 Variation of $\ln k$ with $1/T$ (Arrhenius plot).

Regression analysis (see, for example, Bolton 1984) gives the equation for the best straight line as $\ln k = 26.4 − 10408\ 1/T$; correlation coefficient, r, of 0.999. Hence $k_{25} = 1.98 \times 10^{-4}$ day^{-1}.

The 95% confidence interval is $(1.35–2.95) \times 10^{-4}$ day^{-1}, showing that even good-quality experimental data yield disappointingly imprecise results on extrapolation.

The decomposition is first order and so obeys the equation:

$$\ln c = \ln c_0 - kt \qquad (7.47)$$

At the shelf life $t_{10\%}$, $c = 0.9c_0$, thus:

$$t_{10\%} = \frac{\ln(c_0/0.9c_0)}{k} = \frac{\ln 1.11}{1.98 \times 10^{-4}}$$

Thus, $t_{10\%} = 527$ days (95% confidence interval = 354–773 days).

REFERENCES

Bolton, S. (1984) *Pharmaceutical Statistics*. Marcel Dekker, New York.

Martin, A. (1993) *Physical Pharmacy*, 4th edn. Lea and Febiger. Philadelphia.

York, J.L. (1992) Enzymes: classification, kinetics and control. In: Devlin, T.M. (ed.) *Textbook of Biochemistry*, 3rd edn. John Wiley, New York.

BIBLIOGRAPHY

Rogers, A.R. (1963) An accelerated storage test with programmed temperature rise. *Journal of Pharmacy and Pharmacology*, **15**, 101T-105T.

Saunders, L., Fleming, R. (1971) *Mathematics and Statistics for Use in the Biological and Pharmaceutical Sciences,* 2nd edn. Pharmaceutical Press, London.

PART 2

PARTICLE SCIENCE AND POWDER TECHNOLOGY

8

Solid-state properties

G. Buckton

SOLID STATE

The three states of matter are solid, liquid and gas (or vapour). In a sealed container, vapours will diffuse to occupy the total space, liquids will flow to fill part of the container completely, whereas solids will retain their original shape unless a compressive force is applied to them. From this simple consideration it becomes clear that solids are unique because their physical form (the packing of the molecules and the size and shape of the particles) can have an influence on the way the material will behave. At normal room temperature and pressure, the majority of drugs and excipients exist as solids, thus the study of solid-state properties is of enormous pharmaceutical importance.

Solid particles are made up of molecules that are held in close proximity to each other by intermolecular forces. The strength of interaction between two molecules is due to the individual atoms within the molecular structure. For example, hydrogen bonds occur due to an electrostatic attraction involving one hydrogen atom and one electronegative atom, such as oxygen. For molecules which cannot hydrogen bond, attraction is due to van der Waals forces. The term 'van der Waals forces' is generally taken to include dipole-dipole (Keesom), dipole-induced dipole (Debye) and induced dipole-induced dipole (London) forces. Here a dipole is where the molecule has a small imbalance of charge from one end to the other, making it behave like a small bar magnet. When the molecules pack together to form a solid, these dipoles align and give attraction between the positive pole of one and the negative pole on the next. Induced dipoles are where the free molecule does not have an imbalance of charge, but an imbalance is caused by bringing a second molecule into close proximity with the first.

CRYSTALLIZATION

Materials in the solid state can be crystalline or amorphous (or a combination of both). Crystalline materials are those in which the molecules are packed in a defined order, and this same order repeats over and over again throughout the particle. In Figure 8.1a, an ordered packing of a molecule is shown; here the shape of the molecule is represented with a 'hockey stick' style image, which is representing a planar structure with a functional group pointing up at the end. This isn't a real molecule – it has been drawn to provide an easy representation of a possible crystal packing arrangement. A characteristic property of a crystal is that it has a melting point. The melting point is the temperature at which the crystal lattice breaks down, due to the molecules having gained sufficient energy from the heating process to overcome the attractive forces that hold the crystal together. It follows that crystals with weak forces holding the molecules together (such as paraffins, which only have van der Waals interactions) have low melting points, whereas crystals with strong lattices (i.e. those held together with strong attractive forces, such as extensive hydrogen bonding) have high melting points.

Crystals are produced by inducing a change from the liquid to the solid state. There are two options: one is to cool a molten sample to below the melting point. Pharmaceutical examples of crystallizing through cooling include the formation of suppositories, creams and semi-solid matrix oral dosage forms. The other method of crystallization is to have a solution of the material and to change the system so that the solid is formed. At a given temperature and pressure, any *solute* (where the solute is the material that has been dissolved and the liquid is the *solvent*) has a certain maximum amount that can be dissolved in any liquid (called a *saturated solu-*

tion). If crystals are to be formed from a solution, it is necessary to have more solute present than can be dissolved, which is known as a supersaturated solution. As crystals form from a supersaturated solution, the systems will progress until there are solid particles in equilibrium with a saturated solution. In order to make a solid precipitate out of solution one can:

- remove the liquid by evaporation, thus making the concentration of solute rise in the remaining solvent (this is the way sea salt is prepared)
- cool the solution, as most materials become less soluble as the temperature is decreased
- add another liquid which will mix with the solution, but in which the solute has a low solubility. This second liquid is often called an *antisolvent*.

Many drugs are crystallized by adding water as an antisolvent to a solution of the drug in an organic liquid. For example, if a drug is almost insoluble in water but freely soluble in ethanol, the drug could be crystallized by adding water to a near-saturated solution of the drug in ethanol.

The processes by which a crystal forms are called nucleation and growth. Nucleation is the formation of a small mass onto which a crystal can grow. Growth is the addition of more solute molecules onto the nucleation site. In order to achieve nucleation and growth, it is necessary to have a supersaturated solution. As mentioned above, a *supersaturated solution* is one where the amount of solute dissolved in the liquid is greater than the true solubility. Supersaturated solutions are not thermodynamically stable, so in these circumstances the system will adjust in order to move back to the true solubility, and to do this, the excess solute will precipitate. However, in some circumstances the process of nucleation can be slow. Most students will at some stage have had a supersaturated solution which has not crystallized but on simply scratching the side of the beaker with a glass rod, crystallization was induced. The scratching action produces a small amount of rough surface that acts as a nucleation site and causes the supersaturated solute to precipitate rapidly.

POLYMORPHISM

If the crystallization conditions are changed in any way, it is possible that the molecules may start to form crystals with a different packing pattern to that which occurred when the original conditions were used. The change in conditions could be a different solvent, a change in the stirring or different impurities being present. In Figure 8.1b, an alternative packing arrangement is shown to that

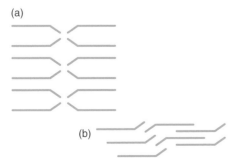

(a)

(b)

Fig. 8.1 A representation of two polymorphic forms of a crystal consisting of a molecule represented by a 'hockey stick' shape.

which occurred for the same molecule in Figure 8.1a. As both the packing arrangements in Figure 8.1 are repeating ordered systems, they are both crystals; these would be called *polymorphic forms*.

By looking at the packing arrangements in Figure 8.1, it can be seen that the molecules in (a) are more spaced out than those in (b), which means that the two crystal forms would have different densities (i.e. the same mass of material would be housed in different volumes). It looks as though it would be easier to physically pull a molecule off structure (a) than (b), as the molecules in (b) are more interwoven into the structure. If this were the case then (a) would have a lower melting point than (b), and (a) may dissolve more easily. Also if an attempt were made to mill the two crystals, it looks like (a) would break easily, as there are natural break lines (either vertically or horizontally), whereas (b) does not seem to have an obvious weak line to allow easy breakage. This could mean that the milling and compaction (tableting) properties of the two forms will differ. In summary, a change in the packing arrangement of the same molecule, giving two different crystal forms, could result in significant changes in the properties of the solid.

Many organic molecules, including drugs and excipients, exhibit polymorphism. Often this is of a form called *monotropic polymorphism*, which means that only one polymorphic form is stable and any other polymorph that is formed will eventually convert to the stable form. However, some materials exhibit *enantropic polymorphism*, which means that under different conditions (temperature and pressure) the material can reversibly transform between alternative stable forms; this type of behaviour will not be considered further here. Considering monotropic polymorphism, the true stable form has the highest melting point and all other forms are described as metastable. This means that the other forms exist for a period of time, and thus appear stable, but given a chance they will convert to the true stable form. Different metastable forms can exist for very short times or many months before they convert to the stable form, depending upon the conditions under which they are stored.

In general there will be a correlation between the melting point of the different polymorphs and the rate of dissolution, because the one with the lowest melting point will most easily give up molecules to dissolve, whereas the most stable form (highest melting point) will not give up molecules to the solvent.

High melting point = strong lattice = hard to remove a molecule = low dissolution rate (and vice versa).

It is relatively easy to understand that changes in polymorphic form can cause changes in the rate at which a drug will dissolve. However, it is less easy to understand why this can lead to a change in the apparent solubility.

Nonetheless, it is true that when a metastable polymorphic form is dissolved, it can give a greater amount of material in solution than the saturated solubility. In other words, metastable forms can dissolve to give supersaturated solutions. These supersaturated solutions will eventually return to the equilibrium solubility, due to the stable crystal form precipitating from solution, but that process may not be instantaneous. In fact, the supersaturated solution can often exist long enough to cause an increase in bioavailability of a poorly soluble drug. In Figure 8.2 the solubility of two different polymorphs of sulphamethoxydiazine is shown. It can be seen that Form III has a higher solubility than Form II and that this lasts throughout the 90-minute experiment. However, if crystals of Form II are added to the solution of Form III then the solubility reverts rapidly to that of Form II, because the excess solute in the supersaturated solution will have seed crystals of Form II on which to precipitate.

Polymorphism and bioavailability

Many drugs are hydrophobic and have very limited solubility in water. For drugs of this type, the rate at which they dissolve (slow dissolution rate), due to their limited aqueous solubility, can result in only a small percentage

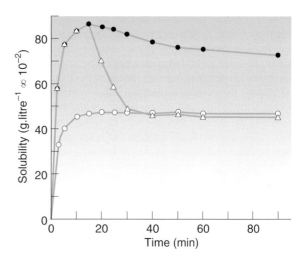

Fig. 8.2 The solubility time relationship for sulpha-methoxydiazine. **Open circles**: solubility of polymorphic Form III, which rises to the drug's equilibrium solubility and plateaux. **Filled circles**: solubility of polymorphic form II, which dissolves to twice the extent of Form III and then shows a gradual decline with time, as the stable form crystallizes from solution. **Triangles**: the effect of adding crystals of Form III to the solution of Form II at the peak of solubility. It can be seen that the amount dissolved falls rapidly from the supersaturated level to the true equilibrium solubility because the added crystals of Form II act as nucleation sites. (Reproduced from Ebian et al 1973, with permission.)

of the administered drug actually being available to the patient (low bioavailability). A classic example of the importance of polymorphism in bioavailability is that of chloramphenicol palmitate suspensions. In Figure 8.3 the blood serum level is plotted as a function of time after dosing. It can be seen that the stable α-polymorph produces low serum levels, whereas the metastable β-polymorph yields much higher serum levels when the same dose is administered.

For drugs that are freely soluble in water the bioavailability is not likely to be limited by the dissolution, so it would be surprising for polymorphism to influence bioavailability in this way. However, for drugs with low aqueous solubility, the polymorphic form must be well controlled in order to ensure that the bioavailability is the same each time the product is made, and throughout the shelf life of the product. It would be risky to deliberately make a product using anything other than the stable form of a drug, as other polymorphic forms could convert to the stable form during the shelf life of the product, which could result in a reduction in bioavailability and thus therapeutic effect of certain products.

In conclusion, the stable polymorphic form will have the slowest dissolution rate, so there may be occasions when it would be desirable to speed the dissolution by using a metastable form. However, the risk associated with using the metastable form is that it will convert back to the stable form during the product life, and give a consequent change in properties.

As polymorphism can have such serious consequences for bioavailability of drugs with low aqueous solubility, it is essential that manufacturers check for the existence of polymorphism and ensure that they use the same appropriate polymorphic form every time they make a product. New drugs are therefore screened to see how many polymorphs (and solvates and hydrates – see below) exist, and then to identify which one is the most stable. The screening process requires a lot of work in crystallizing from different solvent systems, with variations in method and conditions, in order to try to cause different polymorphs to form. The products are then checked with spectroscopy (e.g. Raman) and X-ray diffraction to see if they have different internal packing. Sadly, there are examples of products being taken to market with what is believed to be the stable form, only for the stable form to be produced at a later stage. In these circumstances, the stable form may have been inhibited from being formed by a certain impurity, which may have been lost due to an alteration in the method of chemical synthesis of the drug, so the stable form suddenly is produced. Having then seen the stable form, if the drug is poorly soluble it would be probable that the bioavailability would reduce. Also, having made the stable form, it is often then very hard to stabilize the metastable form again. This can result in products having to be recalled from the market and reformulated and retested clinically. The fact that major pharmaceutical companies, all of whom take the study of physical form very seriously, have seen the stable form arrive after product launch shows that it is difficult to be sure that you are working with the most stable form of the drug.

As was mentioned above, many properties other than rate of solution can change when a material is in a different polymorphic form. For example, paracetamol is a high-dose drug with poor compression properties, which can make it difficult to form into tablets. This is because there is an upper limit on the size of tablet that can be swallowed easily, so for high-dose drugs the amount of compressible excipient that can be added is modest. Consequently, researchers have tried to use different polymorphic forms of paracetamol to find one that is more compressible.

HYDRATES AND SOLVATES

It is possible for materials to crystallize and in so doing to trap molecules of the solvent within the lattice. If the solvent used is water, the material will be described as a *hydrate*. This entrapment is often in an exact molar ratio with the crystallizing material; for example, a monohydrate will have one molecule of water for each molecule of the crystallizing material. It is possible to have many different levels of hydrate; for example, some drugs can exist as a monohydrate, dihydrate and trihydrate (respectively one, two and three molecules

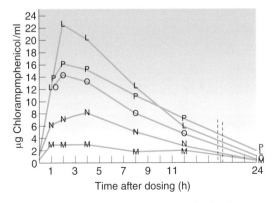

Fig. 8.3 Comparison of mean blood serum levels after administration of chloramphenicol palmitate suspensions using varying ratios of the stable (α) and the metastable (β) polymorphs. M = 100% α polymorph, N = 25:75 β:α,O = 50:50 β:α, P = 75:25 β:α, L = 100% β-polymorph. (Reproduced from Aguiar et al 1976, with permission.)

of water to each molecule of drug). Morris (1999) notes that about 11% (over 16 000 compounds) of all structures recorded on the Cambridge Structural Database exist as hydrates. Of the classes of hydrate materials that were similar to drugs, about 50% were monohydrates (one water molecule for each one of host), over 20% were dihydrates (2 water molecules: 1 host), 8% were trihydrates (3 water molecules:1 host) and 8% were hemihydrates (1 water molecule:2 host); other hydrate levels (up to 10 water:1 host) became progressively less common.

If solvents other than water are present in a crystal lattice, the material is called a *solvate*. For example, if ethanol is present it would be an ethanolate. In general, it is undesirable to use solvates for pharmaceuticals as the presence of retained organic vapours would be regarded as an unnecessary impurity in the product. If the organic vapour were toxic in any way it would obviously be inappropriate for pharmaceuticals. For this reason discussion will be limited to hydrates.

Hydrates often have very different properties from the anhydrous form, in the same way as two different polymorphs have different properties from each other. For this reason, the difference between hydrates and anhydrous forms is described as pseudopolymorphism. With polymorphism, the stable form will have the highest melting point and the slowest dissolution rate (see above). However, with hydrates it is possible for the hydrate form to have either a faster or slower dissolution rate than the anhydrous form. The most usual situation is for the anhydrous form to have a faster dissolution rate than the hydrate; an example of this is shown in Figure 8.4 for theophylline. In this situation, water could hydrogen bond between two drug molecules and tie the lattice together; this would give a much stronger, more stable lattice and thus a slower dissolution rate. It can be seen from Figure 8.4 that the anhydrous theophylline rises to a high concentration in solution and then falls again until the amount dissolved is the same as that recorded for the hydrate. The reason for this is that the hydrate has come to the true equilibrium solubility, whereas the anhydrous form had initially formed a supersaturated solution (as has been described for metastable polymorphic forms above).

Although anhydrous forms are usually more rapidly soluble than the hydrate, there are examples of the opposite being true. In such circumstances one could think of water as a wedge pushing two molecules apart and preventing the optimum interaction between the molecules in the lattice. Here water would be weakening the lattice and would result in a more rapid dissolution rate. An example of the hydrate form speeding up dissolution is shown in Figure 8.5 for erythromycin.

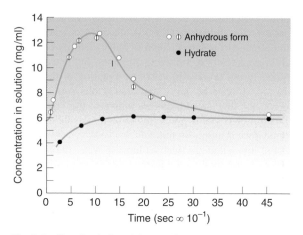

Fig. 8.4 The dissolution of theophylline monohydrate rising to an equilibrium solubility, compared with that for theophylline anhydrous which forms a supersaturated solution with a peak over twice that of the dissolving hydrate, before crystallizing to form the true equilibrium solubility. (Reproduced from Shefter & Higuchi 1963, with permission.)

AMORPHOUS STATE

When a material is in the solid state but the molecules are not packed in a repeating long-range ordered fashion, it is said to be amorphous. Amorphous solids have very different properties from the crystal form of the same material. For example, crystals have a melting point (the break-up of

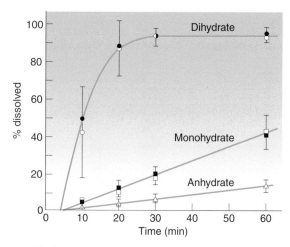

Fig. 8.5 The dissolution behaviour for erythromycin as the anhydrate, monohydrate and dihydrate, showing a progressively faster dissolution rate as the level of hydrate is increased. (Reproduced from Allen et al 1978, with permission.)

the crystal lattice), whereas the amorphous form does not (as it does not have a crystal lattice to break!).

Polymeric materials (or other large molecular weight species) have molecules that are so large and flexible that it is not possible for them to align perfectly to form crystals. For these materials it will be usual to have ordered regions within the structure surrounded by disorder, so they are described as semi-crystalline. For materials such as these, it will not be possible to produce a completely crystalline sample; however, the degree of crystallinity can vary depending upon processing conditions. This can affect the properties of the material and thus how they function in pharmaceutical products.

For low molecular weight materials, the amorphous form may be produced if the solidification process was too fast for the molecules to have a chance to align in the correct way to form a crystal (this could happen when a solution is spray dried). Alternatively, a crystal may be formed but then may be broken. This could happen if a crystal were exposed to energy, such as milling. A simple analogy is that a crystal is like a brick wall, which has ordered long-range packing. If the wall is hit hard, perhaps during demolition, the bricks will separate (Fig. 8.6). Unlike the brick wall, however, a disrupted crystal will be unstable and will revert back to the crystal form. This conversion may be rapid or very slow and, as with polymorphism, its pharmaceutical significance will depend on how long the partially amorphous form survives.

Amorphous forms have a characteristic temperature at which there is a major change in properties. This is called the glass transition temperature (Tg). If the sample is stored below the Tg, the amorphous form will be brittle, described as being in the glassy state. If the sample is above its Tg, it becomes rubbery. The Tg, although not well understood, is a point at which the molecules in the glass exhibit a major change in mobility. The lack of mobility when the sample is glassy allows the amorphous form to exist for a longer time, whereas when Tg is below the storage temperature, the increased molecular mobility allows rapid conversion to the crystalline form.

The glass transition temperature of an amorphous material can be lowered by adding a small molecule, called a plasticizer, that fits between the glassy molecules, giving them greater mobility. Water has a good plasticizing effect on many materials, so the glass transition temperature will usually reduce when in the presence of water vapour.

Most amorphous materials are able to absorb large quantities of water vapour. Absorption is a process whereby one molecule passes into the bulk of another material and should not be confused with adsorption, which is where something concentrates at the surface of another material. In Figure 8.6, the way in which water can access amorphous regions is shown. Figure 8.7 shows the amount of water that is adsorbed to a crystalline material (Fig. 8.7a) in comparison with that absorbed into an amorphous form of the same material (Fig. 8.7b). It can be seen that the amount absorbed is many times greater than that adsorbed. This large difference in water content at any selected relative humidity is important in many materials. For example, it is possible that certain drugs can degrade by hydrolysis when amorphous but remain stable when crystalline. The extent of hydrolysis of an antibiotic which had been processed to yield different levels of crystalline:amorphous forms is shown in Table 8.1; the extent of degradation is greater when the amorphous content is increased.

In Figure 8.7 it can be seen that the amorphous form absorbs a very large amount of water until 50% RH, after which there is a weight loss. The reason for the loss is that the sample has crystallized. Crystallization occurs because the absorbed water has plasticized the sample to such an extent that the Tg has dropped below room temperature and allowed sufficient molecular mobility that the molecules are able to align and crystallize. The water is lost during this process as absorption can only occur in the amorphous form, so it cannot endure into the crystalline state. However, some water is retained in this example (Fig. 8.7a, b), because lactose is able to form a monohydrate. The amount of water required to form a monohydrate with lactose is 5% w/w (calculated from the molecular weight of lactose and water), which is much less than the 11% that was present in the amorphous form (Fig. 8.7b).

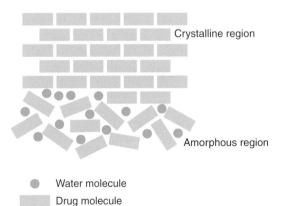

Crystalline region

Amorphous region

● Water molecule

▭ Drug molecule

Fig. 8.6 The disruption of a crystal (represented as a brick wall) giving the possibility for water vapour absorption in the amorphous region.

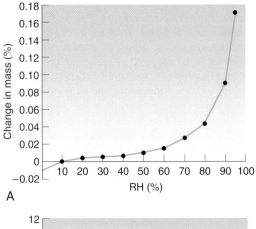

A

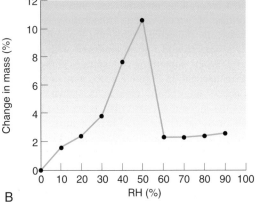

B

Fig. 8.7 (a) A water sorption isotherm for crystalline lactose monohydrate; the quantity of water adsorbed to the crystal surface is small. (b) A water sorption isotherm for amorphous lactose, showing a rise to ca 11% water content due to absorption, followed by water loss as the sample crystallizes and the absorbed water is expelled.

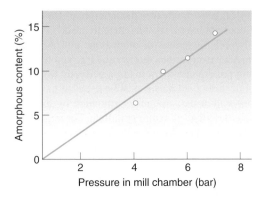

Fig. 8.8 The amorphous content induced in crystalline lactose as a consequence of milling in an air jet mill at different air pressures. (Redrawn from Briggner et al 1994, with permission.)

treated in a simple ball mill, and extensively amorphous when micronized. Although the example in Figure 8.9 is an extreme behaviour, it is not unusual for highly processed materials to become partially amorphous. Although milling does not necessarily make all materials partially amorphous, the chance of seeing disruption to the crystalline lattice will increase with the amount of energy used in the milling.

The fact that processing can make crystalline materials partially amorphous means that it is possible that very complex materials can be formed that contain different metastable states. For example, in Figure 8.3 the plasma levels of two polymorphs of chloramphenicol palmitate

Table 8.1 The chemical stability of cephalothin sodium related to the amorphous content of the sample (data derived from Pikal et al 1978)

Sample	% amorphous	% stable drug after storage at 31% RH 50°C
Crystalline	0	100
Freeze dried	12	100
Freeze dried	46	85
Spray dried	53	44

In Figure 8.8 the amorphous content of lactose is seen to increase in proportion to the length of time it was left in an air jet mill (micronizer). In Figure 8.9 it can be seen that a drug substance became partially amorphous when

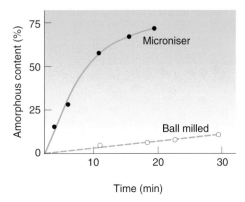

Fig. 8.9 The amorphous content of a model drug substance following milling in a ball mill and a micronizer. (Redrawn from Ahmed et al 1996, with permission.)

were shown; if the β-polymorph were milled it is possible that it may also become partially amorphous, which could make the plasma level even higher than when the crystalline form were used. However, milling the β-polymorph could also provide the necessary energy to convert it to the stable α-polymorph, which would reduce the effective plasma level. Equally, milling could disrupt the α-polymorph giving a partially amorphous form that may have a higher bioavailability than the crystal. In other words, the effect of processing on the physical form can be very complicated, and often unpredictable. It is possible to produce a physical form that is partially amorphous and partially crystalline. The crystalline component could then be stable or metastable. Inevitably, with time (for low molecular weight species) the sample will revert to only contain the stable crystalline form, with no amorphous content and none of the metastable polymorph(s), but as this does not necessarily happen instantly, the physical form and its complexity are of great importance.

CRYSTAL HABIT

All the discussion above has related to the internal packing of molecules. It has been shown that they may have no long-range order (amorphous) or different repeating packing arrangements (polymorphic crystals) or have solvent included (solvates and hydrates). Each of these changes in internal packing of a solid will give rise to changes in properties. However, it is also possible to change the external shape of a crystal. The external shape is called the crystal habit and this is a consequence of the rate at which different faces grow. Changes in internal packing usually (but not always) give an easily distinguishable change in habit. However, for the same crystal packing, it is possible to change the external appearance by changes in the crystallization conditions.

With any crystalline material, the largest face is always the slowest growing. The reason for this is shown in Figure 8.10, where it can be seen that if drug is deposited on two faces of the hexagonal crystal habit, then the first consequence is that the face where drug is deposited actually becomes a smaller part of the crystal, whereas the other faces get larger. Eventually, the fastest growing faces will no longer exist (Fig. 8.10). The growth on different faces will depend on the relative affinities of the solute for the solvent and the growing faces of the crystal. Every molecule is made up of different functional groups – some are relatively polar (such as carboxylic acid groups) whereas others are non-polar (such as a methyl group). Depending on the packing geometry of the molecules into the lattice, some crystal faces may have

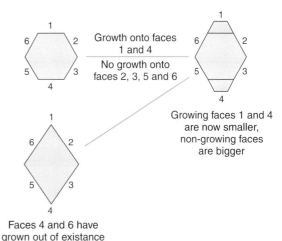

Fig. 8.10 Demonstration of how growth onto faces 1 and 4 of a hexagonal crystal form result in the formation of a diamond.

more exposed polar groups and others may be relatively non-polar. If the crystal were growing from an aqueous solution, drug would deposit on the faces that make the crystal more polar (i.e. the non-polar faces would grow, making the more polar faces dominate). If, however, the same crystal form were growing from a non-polar solvent, then the opposite would be true.

Obviously the external shape can alter the properties of drugs and excipients. For example, the dissolution rate of a drug can change if the surface area to volume ratio is altered. An extreme difference would be between a long needle and a sphere (Fig. 8.11). A sphere of 20 μm radius has approximately the same volume (mass) as a needle of $335 \times 10 \times 10$ μm; however, the surface area of the needle is 2.7 times greater than that of the sphere. As dissolution rate is directly proportional to surface area, the needle would dissolve much faster than the sphere. Crystals do not grow to make spheres, although through milling, crystals can develop rounded geometries, the closest to a sphere would be a cube, which would still

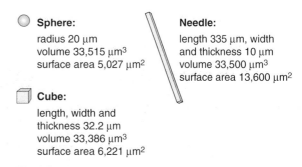

Sphere:
radius 20 μm
volume 33,515 μm³
surface area 5,027 μm²

Cube:
length, width and thickness 32.2 μm
volume 33,386 μm³
surface area 6,221 μm²

Needle:
length 335 μm, width and thickness 10 μm
volume 33,500 μm³
surface area 13,600 μm²

Fig. 8.11 The relative surface areas of a sphere, cube and needle that have similar volumes of material.

have under half the surface area of the needle shown in Figure 8.11.

As well as changes in dissolution rate, different crystal habits can cause changes in powder flow (which is important as, for example, the die of a tableting machine is filled by volume and requires good powder flow in order to guarantee content uniformity of the product) and sedimentation and caking of suspensions.

It is technically possible to engineer changes in crystal habit, by deliberately manipulating the rate of growth of different faces of the crystal. This is done by intentionally adding a small amount of impurity to the solution. The impurity must preferentially interact with one face of the growing crystal, and in so doing it will stop growth on that face, so the remaining face(s) grow more rapidly. The impurity would either be a very similar molecule to that of the crystallizing material, so that part of the molecule is included in the lattice but the remainder of the molecule blocks further layers from attaching, or it may be a surfactant that adsorbs to one growing face.

SURFACE NATURE OF PARTICLES

Dry powder inhalers

Dry powder inhalers often have a micronized drug, which has to be small enough to be inhaled, mixed with a larger carrier particle which is often lactose. The carrier particle is there to make the powder suitable for handling and dosing, as micronized particles have poor flow properties. The shape and surface properties of the drug and/or carrier particles can be critical parameters in controlling the dose of drug that is delivered. It may be necessary to adjust the surface roughness of carrier particles. Figure 8.12a is a cartoon of a rough carrier particle; this would hold the micronized drug too strongly, essentially trapped within the rough regions of the carrier, so the inhaled dose would be very low. In Figure 8.12b, a smooth particle of the same drug is seen. Here the drug will easily be displaced from the carrier during inhalation but it may not stay mixed with the carrier during filling of the inhaler and dosing. In Figure 8.12c, a rough carrier particle has first been mixed with micronized carrier and then with micronized drug. Using this approach, the drug is free to detach, as the micronized carrier is trapped in all the crevices on the carrier surface.

The hypothesis relating to the use of fine carrier particles to enhance the delivery of micronized drug from large carrier particles is not proved beyond doubt. It remains possible that interactions between the fine carrier and fine drug may be the reason for the enhanced delivery.

It should of course be noted that the cartoons in Figure 8.12 simplify the real situation greatly. In Figure 8.13 a

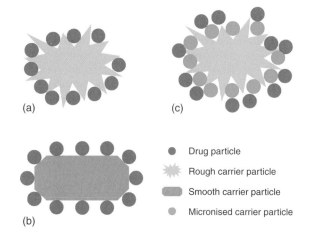

Fig. 8.12 A hypothesis that surface roughness may relate to dry release from carrier particles in dry powder inhalers. (a) Micronized drug trapped in the rough regions of the carrier particle giving low inhaled dose. (b) Micronized drug can be readily removed from a smooth carrier particle. (c) Micronized drug may be removed readily (thus high inhaled dose) if the carrier is first treated with micronized carrier particles, in order to fill the rough voids.

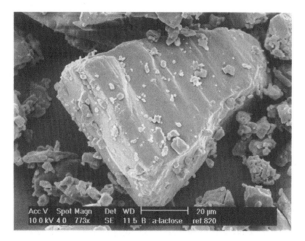

Fig. 8.13 An electron micrograph showing a large lactose carrier particle with added fine lactose, some of which is seen to be at rough spots on the large carrier, but also there is a lot of non-adsorbed fine lactose content. This shows that Figure 8.12 is an enormous simplification of the real system.

real lactose particle is shown along with added micronized particles. It can be seen that the large lactose particle (lactose particles are often described as 'tomahawk' shaped) has rough ridges on its surface and there are some very fine particles aligned to some extent in the rough areas. It is also clear that many fine particles are not on the surface of the lactose and that some fine particles are on smooth regions of the lactose.

For products such as these it is becomingly increasingly important to first measure the surface nature of samples and then to control the form in order to achieve the desired delivery of drug. The surface shape of the carrier is an important consideration for the design of this type of product. A further concern is the surface energy as this can influence the way in which the drug and carrier are attached to each other.

Surface energy

Molecules at the surface of a material have a net inward force exerted on them from the molecules in the bulk; this is the basis of surface energy. Surface energy is important as every interaction (except the mixing of two gasses) starts by an initial contact between two surfaces. If this surface interaction is favoured then the process will probably proceed, whereas if it is not favoured then the process will be limited. A good example of the role of surface energy is the wetting of a powder by a liquid; here the powder cannot dissolve until the liquid makes good contact with it. A practical example is instant coffee, where some brands are hard to wet and dissolve whereas others dissolve easily. Changes in the wetting of powders can affect the processes of wet granulation, suspension formation, film coating and drug dissolution.

The measurement and understanding of surface energy are relatively simple for pure liquids, because there is a single value of surface energy (= surface tension). However, for solids and especially powders, the situation is far more complex. Even on the same crystal form, it would be expected that every crystal face, edge and defect could experience different forces pulling from the bulk and thus could have a different surface energy. From the discussion above, it would be reasonable to assume that different physical forms of the same drug could have quite different surface energies. Thus for the same drug, it is possible that changes in habit and/or polymorphic form and/or the presence of a solvate or hydrate would change the surface energy. For amorphous forms, the molecules at the surface have greater freedom to move and reorientate than do molecules in crystal surfaces, so the amorphous form could have changes in surface energy with time (and with physical state in relation to T_g).

The conventional way of determining the surface energy of a solid is to place a drop of liquid onto the solid surface and measure the contact angle. The contact angle is defined as the angle between the solid surface and the tangent drawn at the three-phase interface, measured through the liquid. Examples of contact angles are shown in Chapter 5. Perfect wetting of a solid by a liquid will result in a contact angle of 0°. Contact angles are the result of a balance of three interfacial forces: γ_{LV} being the liquid surface tension, γ_{LS} between the liquid and the solid, and γ_{SV} between the solid and the vapour. The relative magnitude of these forces will determine whether the drop of liquid spreads on the solid or not, and consequently, by use of the contact angle (θ), it is possible to calculate the solid surface energy if the surface tension of the liquid is known:

$$\gamma_{SV} = \gamma_{SL} + \gamma_{LV} \cos \theta \text{ (Young's equation)} \quad (8.1)$$

For smooth solid surfaces, contact angles are an ideal way of assessing surface energy. However, powders present problems as it is not possible to place a drop of liquid on the surface. Consequently a compromise will always be required when measuring a contact angle for powdered systems. An example of such a compromise would be to make a compact of the powder in order to produce a smooth flat surface. However, the disadvantage of this is that the process of compaction may well change the surface energy of the powder.

A preferred option by which to assess the surface energy of powders would be vapour sorption.

Vapour sorption

When a powder is exposed to a vapour, or gas, the interaction will take one of the following forms:

- adsorption of the vapour to the powder surface (adsorption is described in Chapter 5)
- absorption into the bulk
- deliquescence
- hydrate/solvate formation.

Absorption into the bulk can occur if the sample is amorphous, whereas the interaction will be limited to adsorption if the powder is crystalline. The extent and energetics of interaction between vapours and powder surfaces allow the surface energy to be calculated. The other processes listed are deliquescence, which is where the powder dissolves in the vapour, and hydrate formation which has been discussed above.

It is possible therefore to use adsorption and/or absorption behaviour as a method by which the powder surface energy can be determined. There are three basic approaches to this: gravimetric (measuring weight change), calorimetric (measuring heat change) and chromatographic (measuring retention to a solid using analysis such as flame ionization of the eluted carrier from a column). Each of these techniques has found application in studies of batch-to-batch variability of materials. An example of a critical case could be that a certain drug shows extensive variability in respirable dose from a dry powder inhaler. Assuming that the size distribution was acceptable in all cases, it would be necessary to understand why some batches yielded unacceptable doses. These vapour sorption techniques could then be used to assess the surface energy and then define values that would be acceptable in order to get good drug dosing, and equally to define batches of drug that will give unacceptable products.

Gravimetric methods use sensitive microbalances as a means of determining the extent of vapour sorption to a powder surface. The calorimetric approaches measure the enthalpy change associated with vapour/powder interaction, which gives clear information on the nature of the powder surface. By use of the principles of gas chromatography it is possible to pack the powder, for which the surface energy is required, into a column and then to inject different vapours into the column with a carrier gas. Obviously, the time taken for the vapour to come out of the other end of the column is a measure of how favourable was the interaction between the powder and the vapour. It is then possible to calculate the surface energy of the powder from the retention time of different vapours in the column. Gas chromatography is normally used with a column of known properties with unknown vapours. However, in this experiment the unknown is the solid column and the materials with known properties are the injected vapours. For this reason this technique is called inverse phase gas chromatography.

REFERENCES

Aguiar, A.J., Krc, J. Jr., Kinkel, A.W., Sanyn, J.C. (1967) *Journal of Pharmaceutical Sciences,* **56**, 847-853.

Ahmed, H., Buckton, G., Rawlins, D.A. (1996) *International Journal of Pharmaceutics,* **130**, 195-201.

Allen, P.V., Rahn, P.D., Sarapu, A.C., Vanderwielen, A.J. (1978) *Journal of Pharmaceutical Sciences,* **67**, 1087-1093.

Briggner, L-E., Buckton, G., Bystrom, K., Darcy, P. (1994) *International Journal of Pharmaceutics,* **105**, 125-135.

Ebian, A.R., Moustafa, M.A., Khalil, S.A., Motawi, M.M. (1973) *Journal of Pharmacy and Pharmacology,* **25**, 13-20.

Morris, K.R. (1999) Structural aspects of hydrates and solvates. In: Brittain, H.G. (ed.) *Polymorphism in Pharmaceutical Solids.* Marcel Dekker, New York.

Pikal, M.J., Lukes, A.L., Lang, J.E., Gaines, K. (1978) *Journal of Pharmaceutical Sciences,* **67**, 767-773.

Shefter, E., Higuchi, T. (1963) *Journal of Pharmaceutical Sciences,* **52**, 781-791.

BIBLIOGRAPHY

Brittain, H.G. (ed.) (1999) *Polymorphism in Pharmaceutical Solids.* Marcel Dekker, New York.

Buckton, G. (1995) *Interfacial Phenomena in Drug Delivery and Targeting.* Harwood Academic Press, Amsterdam.

Florence, A.T., Attwood, D. (2006) *Physicochemical Principles of Pharmacy,* 4th edn. Pharmaceutical Press, London.

Mersmann, A. (ed.) (1994) *Crystallization Technology Handbook.* Marcel Dekker, New York.

Particle size analysis

J. N. Staniforth, M. E. Aulton

PARTICLE SIZE AND THE LIFETIME OF A DRUG

The dimensions of particulate solids are important in achieving optimum production of efficacious medicines. Figure 9.1 shows an outline of the lifetime of a drug. During stages 1 and 2, when a drug is synthesized and formulated, the particle size of drug and other powders is determined and this influences the subsequent physical performance of the medicine and the pharmacological performance of the drug.

Particle size influences the production of formulated medicines as solid dosage forms (stage 3, Fig. 9.1). Both tablets and capsules are produced using equipment that controls the mass of drug and other particles by volumetric filling. Therefore, any interference with the uniformity of fill volumes may alter the mass of drug incorporated into the tablet or capsule and hence reduce the content uniformity of the medicine. Powders with different particle sizes have different flow and packing properties, which alter the volumes of powder during each encapsulation or tablet compression event. In order to avoid such problems, the particle sizes of drug and other powder may be defined during formulation so that problems during production are avoided.

Following administration of the medicine (stage 4, Fig. 9.1), the dosage form should release the drug into solution at the optimum rate. This depends on several factors, one of which will be the particle size of drug as predicted from the following theoretical considerations. Noyes and Whitney first showed that the rate of solution of a solid was related to the law of diffusion, and proposed that the following equations could be used to predict the rate of solution of a wide variety of solutes.

$$\frac{dm}{dt} = c(C_S - C) \qquad (9.1)$$

$$c = \frac{1}{t} \log_e \frac{C_S}{C_S - C} \qquad (9.2)$$

where C is the concentration of solute in solution at time, t, C_S is the solubility of solute and c is a constant which can be determined from a knowledge of solute solubility. The constant c was more precisely defined by Danckwerts, who showed that the mean rate of solution per unit area under turbulent conditions was given by:

$$\frac{dm}{dt} = D\sigma(C_S - C) \qquad (9.3)$$

where D is a diffusion coefficient and σ is the rate of production of fresh surface. $D\sigma$ can be interpreted as a liquid film mass transfer coefficient, which will tend to vary inversely with particle size as a reduction in size generally increases the specific surface area of particles. Thus particles having small dimensions will tend to increase the rate of solution. For example, the drug griseofulvin has a low solubility by oral administration but is rapidly distributed following absorption; the solubility of griseofulvin can be greatly enhanced by particle size reduction, so that blood levels equivalent to, or better than, those obtained with crystalline griseofulvin can be produced using a microcrystalline form of the drug. A reduction of particle size to improve rate of solution and hence bioavailability is not always beneficial. For example, small particle-size nitrofurantoin has an increased rate of solution which produces toxic side-effects because of its more rapid absorption.

It is clear from the lifetime of a drug outlined above that knowledge and control of particle size are of importance for both the production of medicines containing particulate solids and the efficacy of the medicine following administration.

PARTICLE SIZE

Dimensions

When determining the size of a relatively large solid, it would be unusual to measure fewer than three dimensions, but if the same solid were broken up and the fragments milled, the resulting fine particles would be irregular, with different numbers of faces, and it would be difficult or impractical to determine more than one or two dimensions. For this reason a solid particle is often considered to approximate to a sphere which can then be characterized by determining the diameter of that sphere. Because measurement is then based on a hypothetical sphere, which represents only an approximation to the true size and shape of the particle, the dimension is referred to as the *equivalent diameter* of the particle.

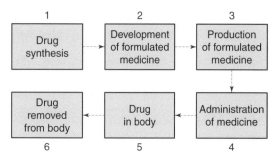

Fig. 9.1 Schematic representation of the lifetime of a drug.

Equivalent diameters

It is possible to generate more than one sphere which is equivalent to a given irregular particle shape. Figure 9.2 shows the two-dimensional projection of a particle with two different diameters constructed about it.

The *projected area diameter* is based on a circle of equivalent area to that of the projected image of a solid particle; the *perimeter diameter* is based on a circle having the same perimeter as the particle. Unless the particles are unsymmetrical in three dimensions then these two diameters will be independent of particle orientation.

This is not true for *Feret's* and *Martin's diameters* (Fig. 9.3), the values of which are dependent on both the orientation and the shape of the particles. These are statistical diameters which are averaged over many different orientations to produce a mean value for each particle diameter. Feret's diameter is determined from the mean distance between two parallel tangents to the projected outline of the particle. Martin's diameter is the mean chord length of the projected particle perimeter, which can be considered as the boundary separating equal particle areas (A and B in Fig. 9.3).

It is also possible to determine the equivalent particle size of powder particles based on other factors such as volume, surface, sieve aperture, sedimentation characteristics, etc. Some of the more commonly used equivalent diameters are defined in Table 9.1; there are others. In general, the method used to determine particle size dictates the type of equivalent diameter that is measured. This is explained under each particle size analysis method described later in this chapter. Interconversion of the various equivalent particle sizes may be carried out and this can be done automatically as part of the size analysis.

Particle size distribution

A particle population which consists of spheres or equivalent spheres of the same diameter is said to be *monosized* and its characteristics can be described by a single diameter or equivalent diameter.

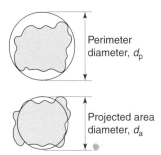

Fig. 9.2 Different equivalent diameters constructed around the same particle.

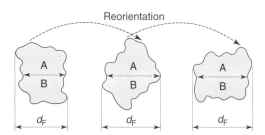

Fig. 9.3 Influence of particle orientation on statistical diameters. The change in Feret's diameter is shown by the distances, d_F; Martin's diameter d_M corresponds to the dotted lines in the mid part of each image.

However, it is unusual for particles to be completely monosized and such a sample will rarely, if ever, be seen in a pharmaceutical system. Most powders contain particles with a range of different equivalent diameters. In order to be able to define a size distribution or compare the characteristics of two or more powders consisting of particles with many different diameters, the size distribution can be broken down into different size ranges, which can be presented in the form of a histogram plotted from data such as those in Table 9.2.

Such a histogram presents an interpretation of the particle size distribution and enables the percentage of particles having a given equivalent diameter to be determined. A histogram allows different particle size distributions to be compared. For example, the histogram in Figure 9.4a is a representation of particles that are *normally distributed* symmetrically about a central value. The peak frequency value, known as the *mode*, separates the *normal curve* into two identical halves, because the size distribution is fully symmetrical. The data in Table 9.2 are normally distributed.

Not all particle populations are characterized by symmetrical, or normal, size distributions and the frequency distributions of such populations exhibit skewness. The size distribution shown in Figure 9.4b contains a larger proportion of fine particles than the powder. A frequency curve such as this with an elongated tail towards higher size ranges is *positively skewed*; the reverse case exhibits *negative skewness*. These skewed distributions can sometimes be normalized by replotting the equivalent particle diameters using a logarithmic scale, and are thus usually referred to as *log normal distributions*.

In some size distributions more than one mode occurs: Figure 9.4c shows bimodal frequency distribution for a powder which has been subjected to milling. Some of the coarser particles from the unmilled population remain unbroken and produce a mode towards the highest particle size, whereas the fractured (size reduced) particles have a new mode which appears lower down the size range.

Table 9.1   Equivalent diameters of irregular particles

Equivalent diameter	Symbol	Definition	Equation
Drag diameter (or frictional drag diameter)	d_d	Diameter of a sphere having the same resistance to motion in a fluid as the particle in a fluid of the same density (ρ_f) and same viscosity (η), and moving at the same velocity (v) (d_d approximates to d_s when the particle Reynolds number (Re_p) is small and particle motion is streamlined, i.e. $Re_p < 0.2$)	$F_D = C_D A \rho f \dfrac{v^2}{2}$ where $C_D A = f(d_d)$ (i.e. $F_D = 3\pi d_d \eta v$)
Feret's diameter	d_F	The mean value of the distance between pairs of parallel tangents to the projected outline of the particle. This can be considered as the boundary separating equal particle areas (see text and Fig. 9.3)	None
Free-falling diameter	d_f	Diameter of a sphere having the same density and same free-falling speed as the particle in a fluid of the same density and viscosity	None
Martin's diameter	d_M	The mean chord length of the projected outline of the particle (see text and Fig. 9.3)	None
Projected area diameter	d_a	Diameter of a circle having the same area (A) as the projected area of the particle resting in a stable position (see text and Fig. 9.2)	$A = \dfrac{\pi}{4} d_a^2$
Perimeter diameter	d_p	Diameter of a circle having the same perimeter as the projected outline of the particle (see text and Fig. 9.2)	None
Sieve diameter	d_A	The width of the minimum square aperture through which the particle will pass (see text and Fig. 9.7)	None
Stokes diameter	d_{St}	The free-falling diameter (d_f, see above) of a particle in the laminar flow region ($Re_p < 0.2$)	Under these conditions $d_{St}^2 = \dfrac{d_v^3}{d_d}$
Surface diameter	d_s	Diameter of a sphere having the same external surface area (S) as the particle	$S = \pi d_s^2$
Surface volume diameter	d_{sv}	Diameter of a sphere having the same external surface area to volume ratio as the particle	$d_{sv} = \dfrac{d_v^3}{d_s^2}$
Volume diameter	d_v	Diameter of a sphere having the same volume (V) as the particle	$V = \dfrac{\pi}{6} d_v^3$

An alternative to the histogram representation of particle size distribution is obtained by sequentially adding the percent frequency values, as shown in Table 9.2, to produce a cumulative percent frequency distribution. If the addition sequence begins with the coarsest particles, the values obtained will be *cumulative percent frequency undersize* (or more commonly *cumulative percent undersize*); the reverse case produces a *cumulative percent oversize*.

It is possible to compare two or more particle populations using the cumulative distribution representation. Figure 9.5 shows two cumulative percent frequency distributions. For example, the size distribution in Figure

Table 9.2 Frequency and cumulative frequency distribution data for a nominal particle size analysis procedure

Range of equivalent diameters of particles measured (known as the *size fraction*) (μm)	Mean diameter of each size fraction (μm)	Number of particles in each size fraction (frequency)	Percent particles in each size fraction (% frequency)	Number of particles in the sample smaller than the mean diameter of each size fraction	Cumulative percent frequency smaller than the mean diameter of each size fraction (cum. % undersize)	Number of particles in the sample larger than the mean diameter of each size fraction	Cumulative percent frequency larger than the mean diameter of each size fraction (cum. % oversize)
<9.9	–	0	0.0	0	0	2200	100.0
10–29.9	20	100	4.5	50	2.3	2150	97.7
30–49.9	40	200	9.1	200	9.1	2000	90.9
50–69.9	60	400	18.2	500	22.7	1700	77.3
70–89.9	80	800	36.4	1100	50.0	1100	50.0
90–109.9	100	400	18.2	1700	77.3	500	22.7
110–129.9	120	200	9.1	2000	90.9	200	9.1
130–149.9	140	100	4.5	2150	97.9	50	2.3
150>		0	0.0	2200	100.0	0	0.0

9.5a shows that this powder has a larger range or spread of equivalent diameters than the powder represented in Figure 9.5b. The particle diameter corresponds to the point that separates the cumulative frequency curve into two equal halves, above and below which 50% of the particles lie (point *a* in Fig. 9.5a). Just as the median divides a symmetrical cumulative size distribution curve into two equal halves, so the lower and upper quartile points at 25% and 75% divide the upper and lower ranges of a symmetrical curve into equal parts (points *b* and *c*, respectively, in Fig. 9.5a).

Statistical methods to summarize size distribution data

Although it is possible to describe particle size distributions qualitatively, it is always more satisfactory to compare particle size data quantitatively. This is made possible by summarizing the distributions using statistical methods.

In order to quantify the degree of skewness of a particle population, the *interquartile coefficient of skewness (IQCS)* can be determined as follows:

$$IQCS = \frac{(c - a) - (a - b)}{(c - a) + (a - b)} \quad (9.4)$$

where *a* is the median diameter and *b* and *c* are the lower and upper quartile points (see Fig. 9.5).

The IQCS can take any value between −1 and +1. If the IQCS is zero then the size distribution is practically symmetrical between the quartile points. To ensure unambiguity in interpreting values for IQCS, a large number of size intervals is required.

To quantify the degree of symmetry of a particle size distribution, a property known as *kurtosis* can be determined. The symmetry of a distribution is based on a

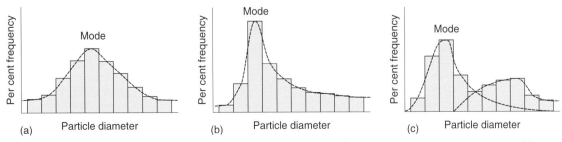

Fig. 9.4 Frequency distribution curves corresponding to (a) a normal distribution, (b) a positively skewed distribution and (c) a bimodal distribution.

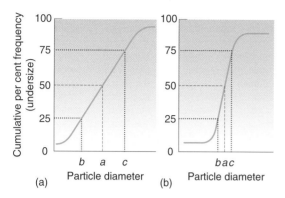

Fig. 9.5 Cumulative frequency distribution curves. Point *a* corresponds to the median diameter; *b* is the lower quartile point and *c* is the upper quartile point.

comparison of the height or thickness of the tails and the 'sharpness' of the peaks with those of a normal distribution. 'Thick'-tailed 'sharp' peaked curves are described as *leptokurtic*, whereas 'thin'-tailed 'blunt' peaked curves are *platykurtic* and the normal distribution is *mesokurtic*.

The coefficient of kurtosis, *k* (Eqn. 9.5), has a value of 0 for a normal curve, a negative value for curves showing platykurtosis and positive values for leptokurtic size distributions:

$$k = \frac{N\Sigma(d-x)^4}{(\Sigma(d-x)^2)^2} - 3 \qquad (9.5)$$

where *d* is any particle diameter, *x* is mean particle diameter and *N* is number of particles. Again, a large number of data points is required to provide an accurate analysis.

Mean particle sizes

As explained above, it is impossible for any single number to fully describe the size distribution of particles in a real pharmaceutical powder sample. However, mainly to simplify matters for our own convenience, pharmaceutical scientists have a desire to describe a power in a single number representing the mean size of the sample. The mean of the particle population, the median (Fig. 9.5) and the mode (Fig. 9.4) are all measures of central tendency. They provide a single value near the middle of the size distribution that attempts to represent a central particle diameter. Whereas the mode and median diameters can be obtained for an incomplete particle size distribution, the mean diameter can only be determined when the size distribution is complete and the upper and lower size limits are known. It is possible to define the 'mean' particle size in several ways.

Arithmetic means

Arithmetic means are achieved by summating a particular parameter for all the individual particles in a sample and dividing the value achieved by the total number of particles. Means can be related to the diameter, surface, volume or mass of a particle. In the equation below, *x* is the mean particle size and the subscripts *L*, *S*, *V* and *M* indicate mean size based on length (diameter), surface area, volume and mass, respectively. ΣdL is the sum of the diameters of all the particles, etc., and ΣdN is the total number of particles in the sample.

$$x_L = \frac{\Sigma dL}{\Sigma dN} \qquad (9.6)$$

$$x_S = \sqrt{\frac{\Sigma dS}{\Sigma dN}} \qquad (9.7)$$

$$x_V = \sqrt[3]{\frac{\Sigma dV}{\Sigma dN}} \qquad (9.8)$$

$$x_W = \frac{\Sigma dM}{\Sigma dN} \qquad (9.9)$$

Such means are strictly referred to a *number mean* or *number average* particle sizes as they are based on the number of particles. Equivalent sets of equations exist based on, for example, the mass of individual particles, giving *mass mean* or *mass average* particle size. In this case the two types of mean will differ as numerous small particles contribute little to the mass. Consequently number average particle sizes are smaller than the equivalent mass average ones.

Geometric means

As explained above, not all powder samples show an arithmetic distribution of particle sizes; some (particularly after milling) follow a log-normal distribution. In a log-normal distribution the frequency, *f*, of the occurrence of any given particle of equivalent diameter *d* is given by:

$$f = \frac{\Sigma N}{2\pi \ln \sigma_g} \cdot \exp\left[-\frac{(\ln d - \ln x_{gN})^2}{2\ln^2\sigma_g}\right] \qquad (9.10)$$

where x_{gN} is the number geometric mean diameter and σ_g is the geometric standard deviation.

Interconversion of mean sizes

For powders exhibiting a log-normal distribution of particle size, a series of relationships, sometimes known as the Hatch–Choate equations, links the different mean diameters of a size distribution. There are numerous combinations of these and the reader is referred to Allen (1997) for further details if required.

Influence of particle shape

The techniques discussed above for representing particle size distribution are all based on the assumption that particles could be adequately represented by an equivalent circle or sphere. In many pharmaceutically relevant cases, particles deviate markedly from circularity and sphericity, and the use of a single equivalent diameter measurement may be inappropriate. For example, a powder consisting of monosized fibrous particles would appear to have a wider size distribution according to statistical diameter measurements. However, the use of an equivalent diameter based on projected area would also be misleading. Under such circumstances it may be desirable to return to the concept of characterizing a particle using more than one dimension. Thus, the breadth of the fibre could be obtained using a projected circle inscribed within the fibre (d_i) and the fibre length could be measured using a projected circle circumscribed around the fibre d_c (Fig. 9.6).

The ratio of inscribed circle to circumscribed circle diameters can also be used as a simple shape factor to provide information about the circularity of a particle. The ratio d_i/d_c will be 1 for a circle and diminish as the particle becomes more acicular.

Such comparisons of equivalent diameters determined by different methods offer considerable scope for both particle size and particle shape analysis. For example, measurement of particle size to obtain a projected area diameter, d_a, and an equivalent volume diameter, d_b, provides information concerning the surface:volume ratio or bulkiness of a group of particles, which can also be useful in interpreting particle size data.

PARTICLE SIZE ANALYSIS METHODS

In order to obtain equivalent diameters with which to interpret the particle size of a powder, it is necessary to carry out a size analysis using one or more different methods. Particle size analysis methods can be divided into different categories based on several different criteria: size range of analysis; wet or dry methods; manual or automatic methods; speed of analysis. Particle size instrumentation is developing quickly but a summary of the principles of these different methods is presented below based on the salient features of each technique.

Sieve methods

Equivalent diameter

Sieve diameter, d_A, as defined in Table 9.1 and shown diagrammatically in Figure 9.7 for different-shaped particles.

Range of analysis

The International Standards Organization (ISO) sets a lowest sieve diameter of 45 μm and, as powders are usually defined as having a maximum diameter of 1000 μm, this could be considered to be the upper limit. In practice, sieves can be obtained for size analysis over a range from 5 to 125 000 μm. These ranges are indicated diagrammatically in Figure 9.8.

Sample preparation and analysis conditions

Sieve analysis is usually carried out using dry powders, although for powders in liquid suspension or which agglomerate during dry sieving, a process of wet sieving can be used.

Principles of measurement

Sieve analysis utilizes a woven, punched or electroformed mesh, often in brass or stainless steel, with

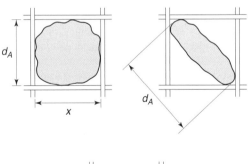

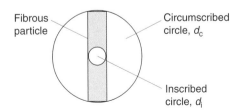

Fig. 9.6 A simple shape factor is shown which can be used to quantify circularity. The ratio of two different diameters (d_i/d_c) is unity for a circle and falls for acicular particles.

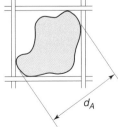

Fig. 9.7 Sieve diameter d_A is the size of the size aperture for various shaped particles x.

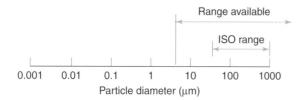

Fig. 9.8 Range of analysis for sieves.

known aperture diameters which form a physical barrier to particles. Most sieve analyses utilize a series, stack or 'nest' of sieves, which has the smallest mesh above a collector tray followed by meshes that become progressively coarser towards the top of the stack of sieves. A sieve stack usually comprises 6–8 sieves with an apperture progression based on a $\sqrt{2}$ or $2\sqrt{2}$ change in diameter between adjacent sieves. Powder is loaded on to the coarsest sieve at the top of the assembled stack and the nest is subjected to mechanical vibration. After a suitable time the particles are considered to be retained on the sieve mesh with an aperture corresponding to the sieve diameter. Sieving is rarely complete as some particles can take a long time to orientate themselves over the sieve apertures and pass through. Thus sieving times should not be arbitrary and it is recommended that sieving be continued until less than 0.2% of material passes a given sieve aperture in any 5-minute interval.

Alternative techniques

Another form of sieve analysis, called *air-jet sieving*, uses individual sieves rather than a complete nest of sieves. Starting with the finest-aperture sieve and progressively removing the undersize particle fraction by sequentially increasing the apertures of each sieve, particles are encouraged to pass through each aperture under the influence of a partial vacuum applied below the sieve mesh. A reverse air jet circulates beneath the sieve

mesh, blowing oversize particles away from the mesh to prevent blocking. Air-jet sieving is often more efficient and reproducible than using mechanically vibrated sieve analysis, although with finer particles agglomeration can become a problem.

Automatic methods

Sieve analysis is still largely a non-automated process, although an automated wet sieving technique has been described.

Microscope methods

Equivalent diameters

Projected area diameter, d_a; perimeter diameter, d_p; Feret's diameter, d_F and Martin's diameter, d_M (all defined in Table 9.1).

Range of analysis

This is shown diagrammatically in Figure 9.9.

Sample preparation and analysis conditions

Specimens prepared for light microscopy must be adequately dispersed on a microscope slide to avoid analysis of agglomerated particles. Specimens for scanning electron microscopy are prepared by fixing to aluminium stubs before sputter coating with a film of gold a few nanometres in thickness. Specimens for transmission electron microscopy are often set in resin, sectioned by microtome and supported on a metal grid before metallic coating.

Principles of measurement

Size analysis by light microscopy is carried out on the two-dimensional images of particles which are generally assumed to be randomly oriented in three dimensions. In many cases this assumption is valid, although for den-

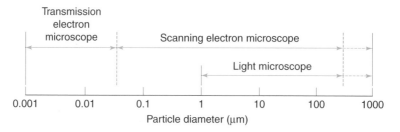

Fig. 9.9 Range of analysis for microscopy.

drites, fibres or flakes it is very improbable that the particles will orient with their minimum dimensions in the plane of measurement. Under such conditions, size analysis is carried out accepting that they are viewed in their most stable orientation. This will lead to an overestimation of size, as the largest dimensions of the particle will be observed as the smallest dimension will most often orientate vertically.

The two-dimensional images are analysed according to the desired equivalent diameter. Using a conventional light microscope, particle size analysis can be carried out using a projection screen with screen distances related to particle dimensions by a previously derived calibration factor using a graticule. A graticule can also be used which has a series of opaque and transparent circles of different diameters, usually in a $\sqrt{2}$ progression. Particles are compared with the two sets of circles and are sized according to the circle that corresponds most closely to the equivalent particle diameter being measured. The field of view is divided into segments to facilitate measurement of different numbers of particles.

Alternative techniques

Alternatives to light microscopy include scanning electron microscopy (SEM) and transmission electron microscopy (TEM). Scanning electron microscopy is particularly appropriate when a three-dimensional particle image is required; in addition, the very much greater depth of field of an SEM compared to a light microscope may also be beneficial. Both SEM and TEM analysis allow the lower particle sizing limit to be greatly extended over that possible with a light microscope.

Automatic methods

Semi-automatic methods of microscope analysis use some form of precalibrated variable distance to split particles into different size ranges. One technique, called a particle comparator, utilizes a variable-diameter light spot projected on to a photomicrograph or electron photomicrograph of a particle under analysis. The variable iris controlling the light spot diameter is linked electronically to a series of counter memories, each corresponding to a different size range (Fig. 9.10). Alteration of the iris diameter causes the particle count to be directed into the appropriate counter memory following activation of a switch by the operator.

A second technique uses a double-prism arrangement mounted in place of the light microscope eyepiece. The image from the prisms is usually displayed on a video monitor. The double-prism arrangement allows light to pass through to the monitor unaltered, where the usual single particle image is produced. When the prisms are

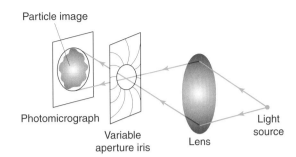

Fig. 9.10 Particle comparator.

sheared against one another, a double image of each particle is produced and the separation of the split images corresponds to the degree of shear between the prisms (Fig. 9.11). Particle size analysis can be carried out by shearing the prisms until the two images of a single particle make touching contact. The prism-shearing mechanism is linked to a precalibrated micrometer scale from which the equivalent diameter can be read directly. Alternatively, a complete size distribution can be obtained more quickly by subjecting the prisms to a sequentially increased and decreased shear distance between two preset levels corresponding to a known size range. All particles whose images separate and overlap sequentially under a given shear range are considered to fall in this size range, and are counted by operating a switch which activates the appropriate counter memory. Particles whose images do not overlap in either shear sequence are undersize and particles whose images do

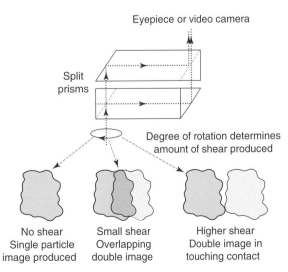

Fig. 9.11 Image-shearing eyepiece.

not separate in either shear mode are oversize and will be counted in a higher size range.

Fully automatic size analysis has the advantage of being more objective and very much faster, and also enables a much wider variety of size and shape parameters to be processed. Automatic microscopy is usually associated with microprocessor-controlled manipulation of an analogue signal derived from some form of video monitor used to image particles directly from a light microscope or from photomicrographs of particles. Alternatively, the signal from an electron microscope can in some cases be processed directly without an intermediate digital imaging system. Automatic microscopy allows both image analysis and image processing to be carried out.

Electrical stream sensing zone method (Coulter counter)

Equivalent diameter

Volume diameter, d_v (Table 9.1).

Range of analysis

This is shown in Figure 9.12.

Sample preparation and analysis conditions

Powder samples are dispersed in an electrolyte to form a very dilute suspension, which is usually subjected to ultrasonic agitation for a period to break up any particle agglomerates. A dispersant may also be added to aid particle deagglomeration.

Principles of measurement

The particle suspension is drawn through an aperture (Fig. 9.13) accurately drilled through a sapphire crystal set into the wall of a hollow glass tube. Electrodes, situated on either side of the aperture and surrounded by an electrolyte solution, monitor the change in electrical signal that occurs when a particle momentarily occupies the orifice and displaces its own volume of

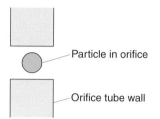

Fig. 9.13 Particle passing through the measuring aperture of an electrical stream sensing zone apparatus.

electrolyte. The volume of suspension drawn through the orifice is determined by the suction potential created by a mercury thread rebalancing in a convoluted U-tube (Fig. 9.14). The volume of electrolyte fluid which is displaced in the orifice by the presence of a particle causes a change in electrical resistance between the electrodes that is proportional to the volume of the particle. The change in resistance is converted into a voltage pulse which is amplified and processed electronically. Pulses falling within precalibrated limits or thresholds are used to split the particle size distribution into many different size ranges. In order to carry out size analysis over a wide diameter range, it will be necessary to change the orifice diameter used, to prevent coarser particles blocking a small-diameter orifice. Conversely, finer particles in a large-diameter orifice will cause too small a relative change in volume to be accurately quantified.

Alternative techniques

Since the electrical stream sensing zone method principle was first described there have been some modifications to the basic method such as use of alternative orifice designs and hydrodynamic focusing, but in general the particle detection technique remains the same.

Another type of stream sensing analyser utilizes the attenuation of a light beam by particles drawn through the sensing zone. Some instruments of this type use the change in reflectance, whereas others use the change in transmittance of light. It is also possible to use ultrasonic waves generated and monitored by a piezoelectric crystal at the base of a flow-through tube containing particles in fluid suspension.

Laser light-scattering methods

Equivalent diameters

Projected area diameter, d_a, and, following computation, volume diameter, d_v (both defined in Table 9.1).

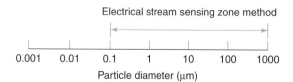

Fig. 9.12 Range of analysis for electrical stream sensing zone method.

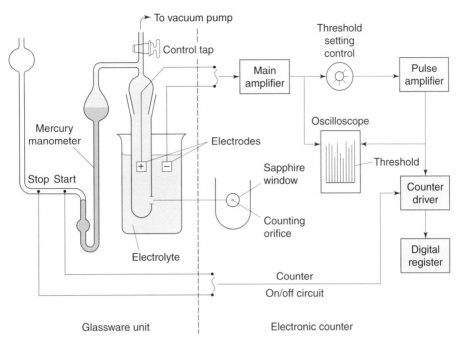

Fig. 9.14 Diagram of electrical stream sensing zone apparatus.

Range of analysis

This is shown in Figure 9.15.

Sample preparation and analysis conditions

Depending on the type of measurement to be carried out and the instrument used, particles can be presented either in liquid or in air suspension.

Principles of measurement

Both the large-particle and small-particle analysers are based on the interaction of laser light with particles.

    Fraunhofer diffraction For particles that are much larger than the wavelength of light, any interaction with particles causes light to be scattered in a forward direc-

tion with only a small change in angle. This phenomenon is known as Fraunhofer diffraction and produces light intensity patterns that occur at regular angular intervals and are proportional to the particle diameter producing the scatter (Fig. 9.16). The composite diffraction pattern produced by different diameter particles may be considered to be the sum of all the individual patterns produced by each particle in the size distribution.

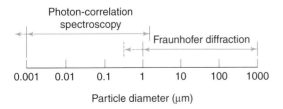

Fig. 9.15 Range of analysis for laser light–scattering methods.

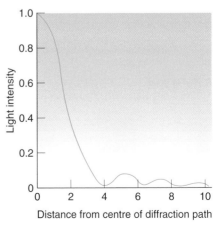

Fig. 9.16 Diffraction pattern intensity distribution.

Light emitted by a helium-neon laser is incident on the sample of particles and diffraction occurs. In some cases the scattered light is focused by a lens directly on to a photodetector, which converts the signals into an equivalent area diameter. In other cases the scattered light is directed by a lens on to a rotating filter, which is used to convert equivalent area diameters into volume diameters which are quantified by final focusing on to a photodetector using a second lens. The light flux signals occurring on the photodetector are converted into electrical current, which is digitized and processed into size distribution data using a microprocessor (Fig. 9.17).

Small particle sizes can be analysed based on light diffraction or by photon correlation spectroscopy.

In the former case Fraunhofer diffraction theory is still useful for the particle fraction that is significantly larger than the wavelength of laser light. As particles approach the dimension of the wavelength of the light, some light is still scattered in the forward direction, according to Mie scatter theory, but there is also some side scatter at different wavelengths and polarizations. Use of the Mie theory requires knowledge of the refractive index of the sample material for calculation of particle size distributions.

Photon-correlation spectroscopy In the case of photon-correlation spectroscopy (PCS) the principle of Brownian motion is used to measure particle size. Brownian motion is the random movement of a small particle or macromolecule caused by collisions with the smaller molecules of the suspending fluid. It is independent of external variations, except viscosity of the suspending fluid and its temperature, and as it randomizes particle orientations, any effects of particle shape are minimized. Brownian motion is independent of the suspending medium and although increasing the viscosity

does slow down the motion, the amplitude of the movements is unaltered. Because the suspended small particles are always in a state of motion, they undergo diffusion. Diffusion is governed by the mean free path of a molecule or particle, which is the average distance of travel before diversion by collision with another molecule. PCS analyses the constantly changing patterns of laser light scattered or diffracted by particles in Brownian motion and monitors the rate of change of scattered light during diffusion.

Particle movement during Brownian diffusion, D, is a three-dimensional random walk where the mean distance travelled, $\bar{x}$, does not increase linearly with time, t, but according to the following relationship:

$$X^- = \sqrt{Dt} \tag{9.11}$$

A basic property of molecular kinetics is that each particle or macromolecule has the same average thermal or kinetic energy, E, regardless of mass, size or shape:

$$E = kT \tag{9.12}$$

where k is Boltzmann's constant and T is absolute temperature (Kelvin).

Thus at $T = 0$ K, molecules possess zero kinetic energy and therefore do not move. E can also be equated with the driving force, F, of particle motion:

$$F = \frac{E}{X} \tag{9.13}$$

At equilibrium:

$$F = F_d \tag{9.14}$$

where F_d is the drag force resisting particle motion. According to Stokes' theory, discussed below:

$$F_D = 3\pi d_h . \eta . v_{st} \tag{9.15}$$

where d_h is the hydrodynamic diameter, v_{st} the Stokes velocity of the particle and η the fluid viscosity, i.e.:

$$E = F\bar{x} = 3\pi d_h . \eta . v_{st} \tag{9.16}$$

but

$$\bar{x}^2 = Dt \tag{9.17}$$

and

$$v_{st} = \bar{x}/t \tag{9.18}$$

substituting,

$$E = 3\pi d_h . \eta . D \tag{9.19}$$

since

$$E = kt, \tag{9.20}$$

$$D = \frac{kT \times 10^7}{3\pi \eta d_n} \tag{9.21}$$

or

$$D = \frac{1.38 \times 10^{-12} T}{3\pi \eta d} \, \text{m}^2 \text{s}^{-1} \tag{9.22}$$

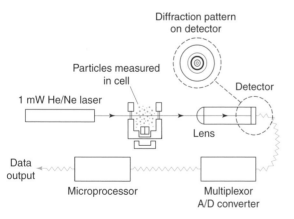

Fig. 9.17 Schematic diagram of laser diffraction pattern particle sizer.

Equation 9.22 is known as the Stokes–Einstein equation and is the basis for calculation of particle diameters using photon-correlation spectroscopy.

Alternative techniques

There is a wide variety of different instruments based on laser Doppler anemometry or velocimetry, and diffraction measurements. The instruments vary according to their ability to characterize different particle size ranges, produce complete size distributions, measure both solid and liquid particles, and determine molecular weights, diffusion coefficients, zeta potential or electrophoretic mobility.

Automatic methods

Most of the instruments based on laser light scattering produce a full particle size analysis automatically. The data are often presented in graphical and tabular form but in some instruments only a mean diameter is produced.

Sedimentation methods

Equivalent diameters

d_d, (frictional) drag diameter and d_{St}, Stokes diameter (Table 9.1).

Range of analysis

This is represented in Figure 9.18.

Sample preparation and analysis conditions

Particle size distributions can be determined by examining the powder as it sediments out. In cases where the powder is not uniformly dispersed in a fluid, it can be introduced as a thin layer on the surface of the liquid. If the powder is hydrophobic it may be necessary to add a dispersing agent to aid wetting. In cases where the powder is soluble in water, it will be necessary to use non-aqueous liquids or carry out the analysis in a gas.

Principles of measurement

Techniques of size analysis by sedimentation can be divided into two main categories according to the method of measurement used. One type is based on measurement of particles in a retention zone; a second type uses a non-retention measurement zone.

An example of a non-retention zone measurement method is known as the pipette method. In this method, known volumes of suspension are drawn off and the concentration differences are measured with respect to time.

One of the most popular of the pipette methods was that developed by Andreasen and Lundberg and commonly called the Andreasen pipette (Fig. 9.19). The Andreasen fixed-position pipette consists of a 200 mm tall graduated cylinder which can hold about 500 mL of suspension fluid. A pipette is located centrally in the cylinder and is held in position by a ground-glass stopper so that its tip coincides with the zero level. A three-way tap allows fluid to be drawn into a 10 mL reservoir, which can then be emptied into a beaker or centrifuge tube. The amount of powder can be determined by weight following drying or centrifuging; alternatively, chemical analysis of the particles can be carried out.

The largest size present in each sample is then calculated from Stokes' equation. Stokes' Law is an expression of the drag factor in a fluid and is linked to the flow conditions characterized by a Reynolds number. Drag is one of three forces acting on a particle sedimenting in a gravitational field. A drag force, F_d, acts upwards, as

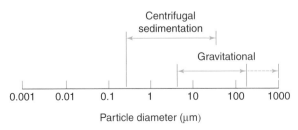

Fig. 9.18 Range of analysis for sedimentation methods.

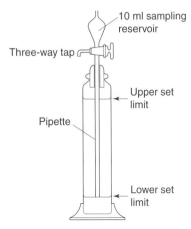

Fig. 9.19 Diagram of Andreasen pipette.

does a buoyancy force, F_b; a third force is gravity, F_g, which acts as the driving force of sedimentation. At the constant terminal velocity, which is rapidly achieved by sedimenting particles, the drag force becomes synonymous with particle motion. Thus for a sphere of diameter d and density ρ_s, falling in a fluid of density ρ_f, the equation of motion is:

$$F_d = \frac{\pi}{6}(\rho_s - \rho_f)F_g \cdot d^3 \qquad (9.23)$$

According to Stokes (Eqn. 9.15):

$$F_D = 3\pi \, d_h.\eta.v_{st}$$

where v_{St} is the Stokes terminal velocity, i.e. sedimentation rate. That is:

$$v_{st} = \frac{(\rho_s - \rho_f)F_g d^2}{18\eta} \qquad (9.24)$$

as $v_{St} = h/t$ where h is sedimentation height or distance and t is sedimentation time. By rearrangement, Stokes' equation is obtained:

$$d_{st} = \sqrt{\frac{18\eta h}{(\rho_s - \rho_f)F_g t}} \qquad (9.25)$$

Stokes' equation for determining particle diameters is based on the following assumptions:

- near-spherical particles
- motion equivalent to that in a fluid of infinite length
- terminal velocity conditions
- low settling velocity so that inertia is negligible
- large particle size relative to fluid molecular size, so that diffusion is negligible
- no particle aggregation
- laminar flow conditions, characterized by particle Reynolds numbers ($Re_p = \rho u d_{particle}/\eta$) of less than approximately 0.2.

The second type of sedimentation size analysis, using retention zone methods, also uses Stokes' Law to quantify particle size. One of the most common retention zone methods uses a sedimentation balance. In this method the amount of sedimented particles falling on to a balance pan suspended in the fluid is recorded. The continual increase in weight of sediment is recorded with respect to time.

Alternative techniques

One of the limitations of gravitational sedimentation is that below a diameter of approximately 5 μm, particle settling becomes prolonged and is subject to interference from convection, diffusion and Brownian motion. These effects can be minimized by increasing the driving force of sedimentation by replacing gravitational

forces with a larger centrifugal force. Once again, sedimentation can be monitored by retention or non-retention methods, although the Stokes equation requires modification because particles are subjected to different forces according to their distance from the axis of rotation. To minimize the effect of distance on the sedimenting force, a two-layer fluid system can be used. A small quantity of concentrated suspension is introduced on to the surface of a bulk sedimentation liquid known as spin fluid. Using this technique of disc centrifugation, all particles of the same size are in the same position in the centrifugal field and hence move with the same velocity.

Automatic methods

In general, gravity sedimentation methods tend to be less automated than those using centrifugal forces. However, an adaptation of a retention zone gravity sedimentation method is known as a Micromerograph and measures sedimentation of particles in a gas rather than a fluid. The advantages of this method are that sizing is carried out relatively rapidly and the analysis is virtually automatic.

SELECTION OF A PARTICLE SIZE ANALYSIS METHOD

The selection of a particle size analysis method may be constrained by the instruments already available in a laboratory but wherever possible, the limitations on the choice of method should be governed by the properties of the powder particles and the type of size information required. For example, size analysis over a very wide range of particle diameters may preclude the use of a gravity sedimentation method; alternatively, size analysis of aerosol particles would probably not be carried out using an electric sensing zone method. As a general guide, it is often most appropriate to determine the particle size distribution of a powder in an environment that most closely resembles the conditions in which the powder will be processed or handled. There are many different factors influencing the selection of an analysis method: these are summarized in Table 9.3 and may be used together with information from a preliminary microscopic analysis and any other known physical properties of the powder, such as solubility, density, cohesivity, in addition to analysis requirements such as speed of measurement, particle size data processing or the physical separation of different particle size powders for subsequent processing.

Table 9.3 Summary of particle size analysis instrument characteristics

Analysis method		Sample measurement environment				Other functions	Rapid analysis	Size data printout available	Approximate size range (mm)				Initial cost	
		Gas	Aqueous liquid	Non-aqueous liquid	Replica				0.001-10	1-10	10-100	100-1000	High	Low
Sieve		✓	✓	✓							✓	✓		✓
Light	Manual	✓	✓	✓						✓	✓	✓		✓
	Semi-automatic	✓	✓	✓						✓	✓	✓		✓
	Automatic	✓	✓	✓		✓	✓	✓		✓	✓	✓	✓	
Electron		✓	✓	✓	✓				✓	✓	✓	✓	✓	
Electrical stream sensing zone			✓	✓					✓	✓	✓	✓	✓	
Laser light scattering	Diffraction	✓	✓	✓		✓	✓	✓		✓	✓	✓	✓	
	Droppler anemometry	✓	✓	✓		✓	—	✓	✓	✓	✓	✓	✓	
Sedimentation	Gravitational	✓	✓	✓			×	×	✓	✓	✓			✓
	Centrifugal		✓	✓			×	×	✓	✓			✓	

REFERENCE

Allen, T. (1997) *Particle Size Measurement*, vols 1 and 2, 5th edn. Chapman and Hall, London.

BIBLIOGRAPHY

Ahuja, S., Scypinski, S. (eds) (2001) *Handbook of Modern Pharmaceutical Analysis*. Elsevier, Edinburgh.

Barnett, M.I., Nystrom, C. (1982) Coulter counters and microscopes for the measurement of particles in the sieve range. *Pharmaceutical Technology*, **6**, 49-50.

Gotoh, K., Masuda, H., Higashitan, K. (1997) *Powder Technology Handbook*, 2nd edn. Marcel Dekker, New York.

Kay, B.H. (1981) *Direct Characterization of Fine Particles*. John Wiley, New York.

Lieberman, H., Lachman, L., Schwartz, J.B. (1990) *Pharmaceutical Dosage Forms: Tablets*, vol 2, 2nd edn. Marcel Dekker, New York.

Manual on Test Sieving Methods (1985) (ASTM Special Technical Publication). American Society for Testing and Materials Standards, Pennsylvania.

Niazi, S.K. (ed.) (2004) *Handbook of Pharmaceutical Manufacturing Formulations, vol 2: Uncompressed Solid Products, Part V. Powder Flow Properties*. CRC Press, Boca Raton, Florida.

Rhodes, M. (ed.) (1990) *Principles of Powder Technology*. John Wiley, Chichester.

Swarbrick, J., Boylan, J.C. (2002) *Encyclopedia of Pharmaceutical Technology*. Marcel Dekker, New York.

10

Particle size reduction

J. N. Staniforth, M. E. Aulton

INTRODUCTION

The significance of particle size has been discussed in Chapter 9 and some of the reasons for carrying out a size reduction operation have already been noted. In addition, the function of size reduction (also called comminution) may be to aid efficient processing of solid particles by facilitating powder mixing or the production of suspensions. There are also some special functions of size reduction, such as exposing cells in plant tissue prior to extraction of the active principles or reducing the bulk volume of a material to improve transportation efficiency.

INFLUENCE OF MATERIAL PROPERTIES ON SIZE REDUCTION

Crack propagation and toughness

Size reduction or comminution is carried out by a process of crack propagation, whereby localized stresses produce strains in the particles which are large enough to cause bond rupture and thus propagate the crack. In general, cracks are propagated through regions of a material that possess the most flaws or discontinuities, and are related to the strain energy in specific regions according to Griffith's theory of crack propagation. The stress in a material is concentrated at the tip of a crack and the stress multiplier can be calculated from an equation developed by Inglis:

$$\sigma_K = 1 + 2\left(\frac{L}{2r}\right) \qquad (10.1)$$

where σ_K is the multiplier of the mean stress in a material around a crack, L is the length of the crack and r is the radius of curvature of the cracks tip. For a simple geometric figure such as a circular discontinuity $L = 2r$ and the stress multiplier σ_K will have a value of 3.

In the case of a thin disc-shaped crack, shown in cross-section in Figure 10.1, the crack is considered to have occurred at molecular level between atomic surfaces

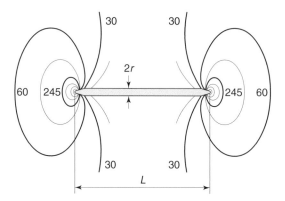

Fig. 10.1 Stress concentrations at the edges of a disc-shaped crack; *r* is the radius of curvature of the crack tip; *L* is the crack length.

separated by a distance of 2×10^{-10} m for a crack 3 μm long, which gives a stress multiplier of approximately 245. The stress concentration diminishes towards the mean stress according to the distance from the crack tip (Fig. 10.1). Once a crack is initiated, the crack tip propagates at a velocity approaching 40% of the speed of sound in the solid. This crack propagation is so rapid that excess energy from strain relaxation is dissipated through the material and concentrates at other discontinuities, where new cracks are propagated. Thus a cascade effect occurs and almost instantaneous brittle fracture occurs.

Not all materials exhibit this type of brittle behaviour and some can resist fracture at much larger stresses. This occurs because these tougher materials can undergo plastic flow, which allows strain energy relaxation without crack propagation. When plastic flow occurs, atoms or molecules slip over one another and this process of deformation requires energy. Brittle materials can also exhibit plastic flow and Irwin and Orowan suggested a modification of Griffiths' crack theory to take this into account. The new relationship has a fracture stress, σ, which varies inversely with the square root of crack length, L:

$$\sigma = \frac{Ep}{\sqrt{L}} \qquad (10.2)$$

where *Ep* is the energy required to form unit area of double surface.

It can therefore be seen that the ease of comminution depends on the brittleness or plasticity of the material because of their relationship with crack initiation and crack propagation.

Surface hardness

In addition to the toughness of the material described above, size reduction may also be influenced by surface hardness. The hardness of a material can be described by

its position in a scale devised by a German mineralogist called Mohs. Mohs' scale is a table of minerals; at the top of the table is diamond, with Mohs hardness >7, and this has a surface that is so hard that it can scratch anything below it. At the bottom of the table is talc, with Mohs hardness <3, and this is soft enough to be scratched by anything above it.

A more quantitative measurement of surface hardness was devised by Brinell. This involves placing a hard spherical indenter (e.g. hardened steel or sapphire) in contact with the test surface and applying a known constant load to the sphere. The indenter will penetrate into the surface and when the sphere is removed, the permanent deformation of the sample is measured. From this the hardness of the material can be calculated. A similar Vickers hardness test employs a square-pyramidal diamond as the indenter tip. Such determinations of hardness may prove useful as a guide to the ease with which size reduction can be carried out. In general, harder materials are more difficult to comminute and can lead to abrasive wear of metal mill parts, which can then result in product contamination. Conversely, materials with a large elastic component, such as rubber, are extremely soft yet difficult to size reduce.

Materials such as rubber which are soft under ambient conditions, waxy substances such as stearic acid which soften when heated, and 'sticky' materials such as gums are capable of absorbing large amounts of energy through elastic and plastic deformation without crack initiation and propagation. This type of material, which resists comminution at ambient or elevated temperatures, can be more easily size reduced by lowering the temperature below the glass transition point of the material. When this is carried out the material undergoes a transition from plastic to brittle behaviour and crack propagation is facilitated.

Other factors that influence the process of size reduction include the moisture content of the feed material. In general, a material with a moisture content below 5% is suitable for dry grinding and one with greater than 50% requires wet grinding to be carried out.

Energy requirements of size reduction process

Only a very small amount of the energy put into a comminution operation actually effects size reduction. This has been estimated to be as little as 2% of the total energy consumption, the remainder being lost in many ways, including:

- elastic deformation of particles
- plastic deformation of particles without fracture
- deformation to initiate cracks that cause fracture
- deformation of metal machine parts

- interparticulate friction
- particle–machine wall friction
- heat
- sound
- vibration

A number of hypotheses and theories have been proposed in an attempt to relate energy input to the degree of size reduction produced.

Rittinger's hypothesis is usually interpreted according to the energy, E, used in a size reduction process, which is proportional to the new surface area produced, S_n, or:

$$E = \kappa_R (S_n - S_i) \qquad (10.3)$$

where S_i is the initial surface area and κ_R is Rittinger's constant of energy per unit area.

Kick's theory states that the energy used in deforming or fracturing a set of particles of equivalent shape is proportional to the ratio of the change in size, or:

$$E = \kappa_K \log \frac{d_i}{d_n} \qquad (10.4)$$

where κ_K is Kick's constant of energy per unit mass, d_i is the initial particle diameter and d_n the new particle diameter.

Bond's theory states that the energy used in crack propagation is proportional to the new crack length produced, which is often related to the change in particle dimensions according to the following equation:

$$E = 2\kappa_B \left(\frac{1}{d_n} - \frac{1}{d_i} \right) \qquad (10.5)$$

Here κ_B is known as Bond's work index and represents the variation in material properties and size reduction methods with dimensions of energy per unit mass.

Walker proposed a generalized differential form of the energy–size relationship that can be shown to link the theories of Rittinger and Kick, and in some cases that of Bond:

$$\partial E = -\kappa_W \frac{\partial d}{d^n} \qquad (10.6)$$

where K_W is Walker's constant and d is a size function that can be characterized by an integrated mean size or by a weight function, n is an exponent. When $n = 1$ for particles defined by a weight function, integration of Walker's equation corresponds to a Kick-type theory, when $n = 2$ a Rittinger-type solution results and when $n = 1.5$ Bond's theory is given.

When designing a milling process for a given particle, the most appropriate energy relationship will be required in order to calculate energy consumptions. It has been considered that the most appropriate values for n are 1 for coarse particles >1 μm where Kick-type behaviour occurs, and 2 for Rittinger-type milling of particles <1 μm. The third value of $n = 1.5$ is the average of these two extremes and indicates a possible solution where neither Kick's nor Rittinger's theory is appropriate.

Other workers have found that n cannot be assumed to be constant, but varies according to a particle size function, so that:

$$n = f(d) \qquad (10.7)$$

or

$$E = -\kappa \frac{d}{d^{f(d)}} \qquad (10.8)$$

As the particle size increases, $f(d)$ tends to 1, and as the size reduces, $f(d)$ tends to 2.

INFLUENCE OF SIZE REDUCTION ON SIZE DISTRIBUTION

In Chapter 9, several different size distributions were discussed and these were based on either a normal or a log-normal distribution of particle sizes. During a size reduction process the particles of feed material will be broken down and particles in different size ranges undergo different amounts of breakage. This uneven milling leads to a change in the size distribution, which is superimposed on the general movement of the normal or log-normal curve towards smaller particle diameters. Changes in size distributions that occur as milling proceeds have been demonstrated experimentally and this showed that an initial normal particle size distribution was transformed through a size-reduced bimodal population into a much finer powder with a positively skewed, leptokurtic particle population (Fig. 10.2) as milling continued. The initial, approximately normal, size distribution was transformed into a size-reduced bimodal

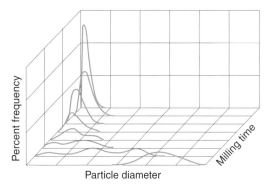

Fig. 10.2 Changes in particle size distributions with increased milling time.

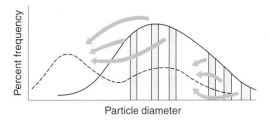

Fig. 10.3 Transformation of approximate normal particle size distribution into finer bimodal population following milling.

population through differences in the fracture behaviour of coarse and fine particles (Fig. 10.3). If milling is continued a unimodal population reappears, as the energy input is not great enough to cause further fracture of the finest particle fraction (Fig 10.4).

The lower particle size limit of a milling operation is dependent on the energy input and on material properties. With particle diameters below approximately 5 µm, interactive cohesive forces between the particles generally predominate over comminution stresses as the comminution forces are distributed over increasing surface areas. This eventually results in particle agglomeration as opposed to particle fracture and size reduction ceases. In some cases particle agglomeration occurs to such a degree that subsequent milling actually causes size enlargement.

SIZE REDUCTION METHODS

There are many different types of size reduction techniques and the apparatus available for pharmaceutical powders continues to develop. This chapter illustrates the principles associated with current techniques that are classified according to the milling process employed to subdivide the powder particles. Examples of each type are given below. The approximate size reduction range achievable with each technique is illustrated, although it should be remembered that the extent of size reduction is always related to milling time.

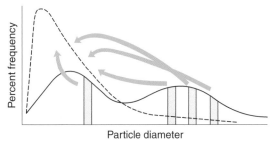

Fig. 10.4 Transformation of a fine bimodal particle population into a finer unimodal distribution following prolonged milling.

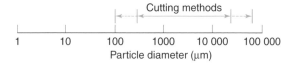

Fig. 10.5 Size reduction range for cutting methods.

Cutting methods

Size reduction range

This is indicated in Figure 10.5.

Principles of operation

A cutter mill (Fig. 10.6) consists of a series of knives attached to a horizontal rotor which act against a series of stationary knives attached to the mill casing. During milling, size reduction occurs by fracture of particles between the two sets of knives, which have a clearance of a few millimetres. A screen is fitted in the base of the mill casing and acts to retain material in the mill until a sufficient degree of size reduction has been effected.

The high shear rates present in cutter mills are useful in producing a coarse degree of size reduction of dried granulations prior to tableting.

Compression methods

Size reduction range

These are indicated in Figure 10.7.

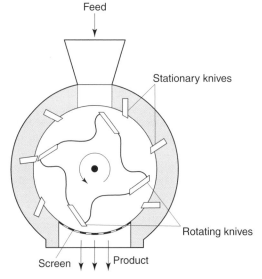

Fig. 10.6 Cutter mill.

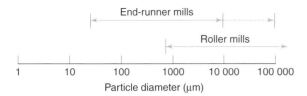

Fig. 10.7 Size reduction range for compression methods.

Principles of operation

Size reduction by compression can be carried out on a small laboratory scale using a mortar and pestle. End-runner and edge-runner mills are mechanized forms of mortar and pestle-type compression comminution. Such techniques are now rarely used in pharmaceutical production.

Alternative techniques

Another form of compression mill uses two cylindrical rolls mounted horizontally and rotated about their long axes. In roller mills, one of the rolls is driven directly while the second is rotated by friction as material is drawn through the gap between the rolls. This form of roller mill should not be confused with the type used for milling ointments, where both rollers are driven but at different speeds, so that size reduction occurs by attrition (see below).

Impact methods

Size reduction range

These are shown in Figure 10.8.

Principles of operation

Size reduction by impact is carried out using a hammer mill (Fig. 10.9). Hammer mills consist of a series of four or more hammers, hinged on a central shaft which is enclosed within a rigid metal case. During milling the hammers swing out radially from the rotating central shaft. The angular velocity of the hammers produces strain rates up to 80 s^{-1}, which are so high that most particles undergo brittle fracture. As size reduction continues, the inertia of

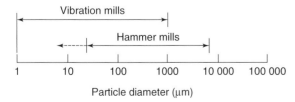

Fig. 10.8 Size reduction range for impact methods.

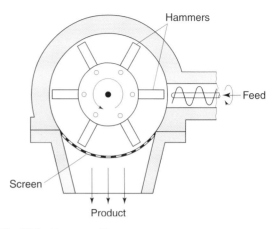

Fig. 10.9 Hammer mill.

particles hitting the hammers reduces markedly and subsequent fracture is less probable, so that hammer mills tend to produce powders with narrow size distributions. Particles are retained within the mill by a screen that allows only adequately comminuted particles to pass through. Particles passing through a given mesh can be much finer than the mesh apertures, as particles are carried around the mill by the hammers and approach the mesh tangentially. For this reason, square, rectangular or herringbone slots are often used. According to the purpose of the operation, the hammers may be square-faced, tapered to a cutting edge or have a stepped form.

Alternative techniques

An alternative to hammer milling which produces size reduction is vibration milling (Fig. 10.10). Vibration mills are filled to approximately 80% total volume with porcelain or steel balls. During milling the whole body of the mill is vibrated and size reduction occurs by repeated

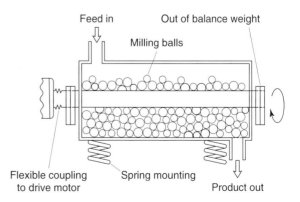

Fig. 10.10 Vibration mill.

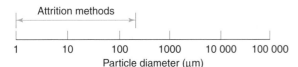

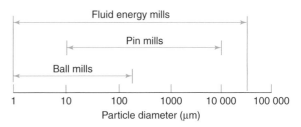

Fig. 10.11 Size reduction range for attrition methods.

Fig. 10.12 Size reduction range for combined impact and attrition methods.

impaction. Comminuted particles fall through a screen at the base of the mill. The efficiency of vibratory milling is greater than that for conventional ball milling described below.

Attrition methods

Size reduction range

This is indicated in Figure 10.11.

Principles of operation

Roller mills use the principle of attrition to produce size reduction of solids in suspensions, pastes or ointments. Two or three porcelain or metal rolls are mounted horizontally with an adjustable gap, which can be as small as 20 μm. The rollers rotate at different speeds so that the material is sheared as it passes through the gap and is transferred from the slower to the faster roll, from which it is removed by means of a scraper.

Combined impact and attrition methods

Size reduction range

This is indicated in Figure 10.12.

Principles of operation

A ball mill is an example of a comminution method which produces size reduction by both impact and attri-

tion of particles. Ball mills consist of a hollow cylinder mounted such that it can be rotated on its horizontal longitudinal axis (Fig. 10.12). The cylinder contains balls that occupy 30–50% of the total volume, ball size being dependent on feed and mill size. Mills usually contain balls with many different diameters owing to self-attrition, and this helps to improve the product as the large balls tend to break down the coarse feed materials and the smaller balls help to form the fine product by reducing void spaces between balls.

The amount of material in a mill is of considerable importance: too much feed produces a cushioning effect and too little causes loss of efficiency and abrasive wear of the mill parts.

The factor of greatest importance in the operation of the ball mill is the speed of rotation. At low angular velocities (Fig. 10.13a) the balls move with the drum until the force due to gravity exceeds the frictional force of the bed on the drum, and the balls then slide back en masse to the base of the drum. This sequence is repeated, producing very little relative movement of balls so that size reduction is minimal. At high angular velocities (Fig. 10.13b), the balls are thrown out on to the mill wall by centrifugal force and no size reduction occurs. At about two-thirds of the critical angular velocity where centrifuging occurs (Fig. 10.13c), a cascading action is produced. Balls are lifted on the rising side of the drum

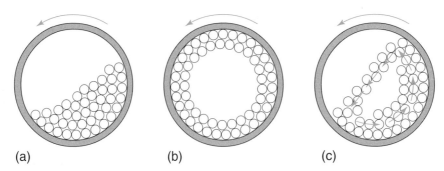

(a)   (b)   (c)

Fig. 10.13 Ball mill in operation, showing correct cascade action.

until their dynamic angle of repose is exceeded. At this point they fall or roll back to the base of the drum in a cascade across the diameter of the mill. By this means, the maximum size reduction occurs by impact of the particles with the balls and by attrition. The optimum rate of rotation is dependent on mill diameter but is usually of the order of 0.5 revolutions per second.

Alternative techniques

Fluid energy milling is another form of size reduction method that acts by particle impaction and attrition. A typical form of fluid energy or jet mill is shown in Figure 10.14. This type of mill or 'micronizer' consists of a hollow toroid which has a diameter of 20–200 mm. A fluid, usually air, is injected as a high-pressure jet through nozzles at the bottom of the loop. The high velocity of the air gives rise to zones of turbulence into which solid particles are fed. The high kinetic energy of the air causes the particles to impact *with other particles* with sufficient momentum for fracture to occur. Turbulence ensures that the level of particle–particle collisions is high enough to produce substantial size reduction by impact and some attrition.

A particle size classifier is incorporated in the system so that particles are retained in the toroid until suffi-

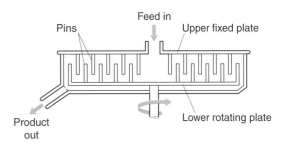

Fig. 10.15   Pin mill.

ciently fine and are then entrained in the air stream that exhausts from the mill.

Other types of fluid energy mill replace the turbulent zone technique with horizontally opposed air jets through which the feed material is forced. Alternatively, a single air jet is used to feed particles directly on to a target plate, where impaction causes fracture.

In addition to ball mills and fluid energy mills, there are other methods of comminution that act by producing particle impact and attrition. These include *pin mills*, in which two discs with closely spaced pins rotate against one another at high speeds (Fig. 10.15). Particle size reduction occurs by impaction with the pins and by attrition between pins as the particles travel outwards under the influence of centrifugal force.

SELECTION OF PARTICLE SIZE REDUCTION METHOD

Different mills can produce differing endproduct from the same starting material. For example, particle shape may vary according to whether size reduction occurs as a result of impact or attrition. In addition, the proportion of fines in the product may vary, so that other properties of the powder will be altered.

The subsequent usage of a powder usually controls the degree of size reduction but in some cases the precise particle size required is not critical. In these circumstances the important factor is that, in general, the cost of size reduction increases as particle size decreases, so that it is economically undesirable to mill particles to a finer degree than necessary. Once the particle size required has been established, the selection of mills capable of producing that size may be modified from knowledge of the particle properties, such as hardness, toughness, etc. The influences of various process and material variables on selection of a size reduction method are summarized in Table 10.1.

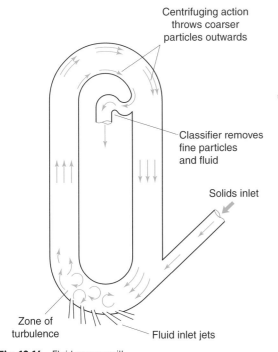

Fig. 10.14   Fluid energy mill.

Table 10.1 Selection of size reduction mills according to particle properties and product size required

Mohs' 'hardness'	Tough	Sticky	Abrasive	Friable
(a) Fine powder product (< 50 μm)				
1–3 (soft)	Ball, vibration (under liquid nitrogen)	Ball, vibration		Ball, vibration, pin, fluid energy
3–5 (intermediate)	Ball, vibration			Ball, vibration, fluid energy
5–10 (hard)	Ball, vibration, fluid energy		Ball, vibration, fluid energy	
(b) Coarse powder product (50–1000 μm)				
1–3 (soft)	Ball, vibration, roller, pin, hammer, cutter (all under liquid nitrogen)	Ball, pin		Ball, roller, pin, hammer, vibration
3–5 (intermediate)	Ball, roller, pin, hammer, vibration, cutter			Ball, roller, pin, vibration, hammer
5–10 (hard)	Ball, vibration		Ball vibration, roller	
(c) Very coarse product (> 1000 μm)				
1–3 (soft)	Cutter, edge runner	Roller, edge runner, hammer		Roller, edge runner, hammer
3–5 (intermediate)	Edge runner, roller, hammer			Roller, hammer
5–10 (hard)	Roller		Roller	

BIBLIOGRAPHY

Austin, L.G., Brame, K. (1983) A comparison of the bond method for sizing wet tumbling ball mills with a size-mass balance simulation model. *Powder Technology*, **34**, 261-274.

Gotoh, K., Masuda, H., Higashitan, K. (1997) *Powder Technology Handbook*, 2nd edn. Marcel Dekker, New York.

Lachman, L., Lieberman, H.A., Kanig, J.L. (latest edition) *Theory and Practice of Industrial Pharmacy*. Lea and Febiger, Philadelphia.

Lieberman, H., Lachman, L., Schwartz, J.B. (1990)*Pharmaceutical Dosage Forms: Tablets*, vol 2, 2nd edn. Marcel Dekker, New York.

Mecham, W.J., Jardine, L.J., Reedy, G.T., Steindler, M.J. (1983) General statistical description of the fracture particulates formed by mechanical impacts of brittle materials. *Industrial and Engineering Chemistry Fundamentals*, **22**, 384-391.

Niazi, S.K. (ed.) (2004) *Handbook of Pharmaceutical Manufacturing Formulations*: vol 2 *Uncompressed Solid Products, Part V. Powder Flow Properties*. CRC Press, Boca Raton, Florida.

Paramanathan, B.K., Bridgwater, J. (1983) Attrition of solids, Pts I & II. *Chemical Engineering Science*, **38**, 197-224.

Rhodes, M. (ed.) (1990) *Principles of Powder Technology*. John Wiley, New York.

Swarbrick, J., Boylan, J.C. (2002) *Encyclopedia of Pharmaceutical Technology*. Marcel Dekker, New York.

Voller, V.R. (1983) A note on energy-size reduction relationships in comminution. *Powder Technology*, **36**, 281-286.

Wheeler, D.A. (1982) Size reduction. *Processing*, **Dec**, 55-58.

11

Particle size separation

J. N. Staniforth, M. E. Aulton

INTRODUCTION

Objectives of size separation

The significance of particle size and the principles involved in differentiating a powder into fractions of known particle size and in reducing particle dimensions have been considered in Chapters 9 and 10. In this chapter the methods by which size separation can be achieved will be discussed, together with the standards that are applied to powders for pharmaceutical purposes.

Solid separation is a process by which powder particles are removed from gases or liquids, and has two main aims:

1. to recover valuable products or byproducts
2. to prevent environmental pollution.

Although size separation uses many similar techniques to those used in solid separation it has a different aim, which is to classify powders into separate particle size ranges or 'cuts', and is therefore linked to particle size analysis. However, an important difference exists between size separation and size analysis: following size separation, powder in a given particle size range is available for separate handling or subsequent processing. This means that whereas a particle size analysis method such as microscopy would be of no use as a size separation method, the principle of sieving could be used for both purposes.

Size separation efficiency

The efficiency with which a powder can be separated into different particle size ranges is related to the particle and fluid properties and the separation method used. Separation efficiency is determined as a function of the effectiveness of a given process in separating particles into oversize and undersize fractions.

In a continuous size separation process, the production of oversize and undersize powder streams from a single feed stream can be represented by the following equation:

$$f_F = f_o + f_u \qquad (11.1)$$

where f_F, f_o and f_u are functions of the mass flow rates of the feed material, oversize product and undersize product streams, respectively. If the separation process is 100% efficient then all oversize material will end up in the oversize product stream and all undersize material will end up in the undersize product stream. Invariably, industrial separation processes produce an incomplete size separation, so that some undersize material is retained in the oversize stream and some oversize material may find its way into the undersize stream.

Considering the oversize material, a given powder feed stream will contain a certain proportion of true oversize material, δ_F; the oversize product stream will contain a fraction, δ_o, of true oversize particles, and the undersize stream will contain a fraction, δ_u, of true oversize material (Fig. 11.1).

The efficiency of the separation of oversize material can be determined by considering the relationship between mass flow rates of feed and product streams and the fractional contributions of true size grade in the streams. For example, the efficiency E_o of a size separation process for oversize material in the oversize stream is given by:

$$E_o = \frac{f_o \delta_o}{f_F \delta_F} \qquad (11.2)$$

and the separation efficiency for undersize material in the undersize stream is given by:

$$E_u = \frac{f_u (1 - \delta_o)}{f_F (1 - \delta_F)} \qquad (11.3)$$

The total efficiency, E_t, for the whole size separation process is given by:

$$E_t = E_u \cdot E_o \qquad (11.4)$$

Separation efficiency determination can be applied to each stage of a complete size classification and is often referred to as *grade efficiency*. In some cases knowledge of grade efficiency is insufficient, for example where a precise particle size cut is required. A *sharpness index* can be used to quantify the sharpness of cut-off in a given size range. A sharpness index, S, can be determined in several different ways, for example by taking the percentage values from a grade efficiency curve at the 25% and 75% levels (L_{25} and L_{75}, respectively):

$$S_{25/75} = \frac{L_{25}}{L_{75}} \qquad (11.5)$$

or at other percentile points, such as the 10% and 90% levels:

$$S_{10/90} = \frac{L_{10}}{L_{90}} \qquad (11.6)$$

SIZE SEPARATION METHODS

Some of the major types of size separation equipment are discussed briefly below. These have been chosen to illustrate the basic principles of size separation. The actual equipment in use in pharmaceutical processing continues to develop yet remains based on the principles illustrated.

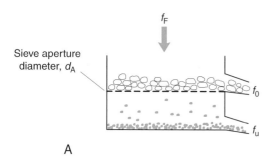

A

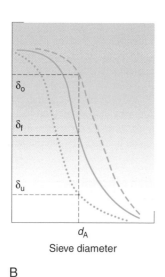

B

Fig. 11.1 Size separation efficiency determination. (a) Separation operation. (b) Size distributions of feed, oversize and undersize material to obtain values for d_o, d_f and d_u.

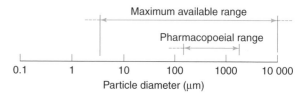

Fig. 11.2 Separation range for sieving.

Size separation by sieving

Separation ranges

These are shown in Figure 11.2.

Principles of operation

The principles of sieving in order to achieve particle size analysis are described in Chapter 9. There may be some differences in the methods used to achieve size separation rather than size analysis. The wire mesh used for the construction of size analysis test sieves should be of uniform circular cross-section, and the sieve mesh should possess adequate strength to avoid distortion and should also be resistant to chemical action with any of the material to be sifted. Commonly used materials for the construction of test sieve meshes for size analysis are brass and bronze, but it is probably more common and more suitable to use stainless steel meshes in process sieves used for size separation.

The use of sieving in size separation usually requires processing of larger volumes of powder than are commonly found in size analysis operations. For this reason, the sieves used for size separation are often larger in area than those used for size analysis.

There are several techniques for encouraging particles to separate into their appropriate size fractions efficiently. In dry sieving processes these are based on mechanical disturbances of the powder bed and include the following.

Agitation methods Size separation is achieved by electrically induced oscillation, mechanically induced vibration of the sieve meshes or by gyration in which sieves are fitted to a flexible mounting which is connected to an out-of-balance flywheel. In the latter case, the eccentric rotation of the flywheel imparts a rotary movement of small amplitude and high intensity to the sieve and causes the particles to spin, thereby continuously changing their orientation and increasing their potential to pass through a given sieve aperture. The output from gyratory sieves is often considerably greater than that obtained using oscillation or vibration methods.

Agitation methods can be made continuous by inclination of the sieve and the use of separate outlets for the undersize and oversize powder streams.

Brushing methods A brush is used to reorientate particles on the surface of a sieve and prevent apertures becoming blocked. A single brush can be rotated about the midpoint of a circular sieve or, for large-scale processing, a horizontal cylindrical sieve is employed with a spiral brush rotating about its longitudinal axis.

Centrifugal methods In this type of equipment, particles are thrown outwards on to a vertical cylindrical sieve under the action of a high-speed rotor inside the cylinder. The current of air created by the rotor move-

ment also assists in sieving, especially where very fine powders are being processed.

Wet sieving can also be used to effect size separation and is generally more efficient than dry sieving methods.

Standards for powders based on sieving

Standards for powders used pharmaceutically are provided in pharmacopoeias, which indicate that 'the degree of coarseness or fineness of a powder is differentiated and expressed by reference to the nominal mesh aperture size of the sieves used'. Grades of powder are specified and defined in most pharmacopoeias. An example is shown in Table 11.1.

It should be noted that the term 'sieve number' has been used as a method of quantifying particle size in pharmacopoeias and is still favoured in some parts of the world. However, various monographs use the term differently and in order to avoid confusion it is strongly recommended to always refer to particle sizes according to the appropriate equivalent diameters expressed in millimetres, micrometres or nanometres, as appropriate.

Size separation by fluid classification

Sedimentation methods

Separation ranges

These are shown in Figure 11.3.

Principles of operation

The principles of liquid classification using sedimentation methods are described in Chapter 9. Size separation

---

Table 11.1 Example of powder grades specified in pharmacopoeias

Description of grade of powder	Coarsest sieve diameter (μm)	Sieve diameter through which no more than 40% of powder must pass (μm)
Coarse	1700	355
Moderately coarse	710	250
Moderately fine	355	180
Fine	180	–
Very fine	125	–

Some pharmacopoeias define another size fraction, known as *ultrafine powder*, in which the maximum diameter of at least 90% of the particles must be no greater than 5 μm and none of the particles should have diameters greater than 50 μm.

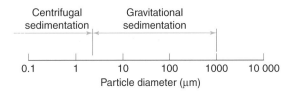

Fig. 11.3 Separation range for sedimentation techniques.

by sedimentation utilizes the differences in settling velocities of particles with different diameters, and these can be related according to Stokes' equations, see Eqns 9.11 and 9.21.

One of the simplest forms of sedimentation classification uses a chamber containing a suspension of solid particles in a liquid, which is usually water. After predetermined times, particles less than a given diameter can be recovered using a pipette placed a fixed distance below the surface of the liquid. Size fractions can be collected continuously using a pump mechanism in place of a pipette.

Alternatively, a single separation can be carried out simply by removing the upper layer of suspension fluid after the desired time. Disadvantages of these simple methods are that they are batch processes and discrete particle fractions cannot be collected, as samples contain every particle diameter up to the limiting diameter and not specific size ranges.

Alternative techniques

An alternative technique is to use a continuous settling chamber so that particles in suspension enter a shallow container, as shown in Figure 11.4. The particle Reynolds' number of the system ($Pud_{particle}/\eta$) is below approximately 0.2 to ensure that streamline sedimentation occurs.

Particles entering at the top of the chamber are acted upon by a driving force which can be divided into two components: a horizontal component of particle velocity which is equal to the suspension fluid velocity, and a vertical component which corresponds to Stokes' settling velocity and is different for each particle size. These two components are constant for each particle, so that the settling path will be given by a curve whose slope depends on particle diameter. The coarsest particles will have the steepest settling paths and will sediment closest to the inlet, whereas the finest particles with low Stokes velocity component will have the shallowest settling paths and will sediment furthest from the fluid suspension feed stream (see Fig. 11.4). Particles separated into the different hopper-type discharge points can be removed continuously.

Very fine particles will not sediment efficiently under the influence of gravity due to Brownian diffusion. In order to increase the driving force of sedimentation, centrifugal methods can be used to separate particles of different sizes in the submicrometre range.

Simple cylindrical centrifuges can be used to remove single size cuts from a fluid stream but where separation is required over a wider number of size ranges, multiple-chamber centrifuges can be used. In this type of centrifuge there are a number of spinning cylinders of

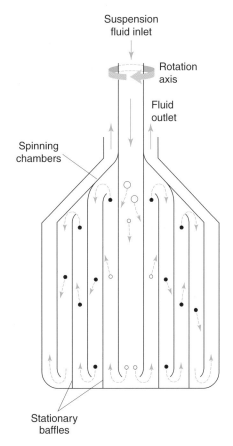

Fig. 11.5 Multiple-chamber separation centrifuge.

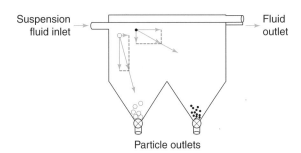

Fig. 11.4 Continuous settling chamber showing vectors of particle movement for different sizes.

different diameters set inside a closed chamber (Fig. 11.5). Fine particles in liquid suspension are fed in through the top of the inner or central cylinder. As in continuous-flow gravity sedimentation, the particles are acted on by two component forces, one due to fluid flow and, in this case, one due to centrifugal force. The coarsest particles will have the shallowest trajectories and will be carried to the walls of the inner cylinder (Fig. 11.6); all other particles remain entrained in the liquid and flow out at the base of the cylinder and via a baffle or weir into the top of the next cylinder out, where the centrifugal force is higher. This sequence continues so that only the finest particles reach the outermost spinning cylinder.

Another type of sedimentation method is based on separation from particles dispersed in air and is known as *mechanical air classification*.

Elutriation methods

Separation ranges

These are shown in Figure 11.7.

Principles of operation

In sedimentation methods the fluid is stationary and the separation of particles of various sizes depends solely on particle velocity. Therefore, the division of particles into size fractions depends on the *time* of sedimentation.

Elutriation is a technique in which the fluid flows in an opposite direction to the sedimentation movement, so that in gravitational elutriators particles move vertically downwards while the fluid travels vertically upwards. If the upward velocity of the fluid is less than the settling velocity of the particle, sedimentation occurs and the particle moves downwards against the flow of fluid.

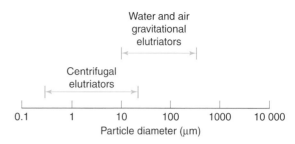

Fig. 11.7 Separation ranges for elutriation methods.

Conversely, if the settling velocity of the particle is less than the upward fluid velocity, the particle moves upwards with the fluid flow. Therefore, in the case of elutriation, particles are divided into different size fractions depending on the *velocity* of the fluid.

Elutriation and sedimentation are compared in Figure 11.8, where the arrows are vectors; that is, they show the direction and magnitude of particle movement. This figure indicates that if particles are suspended in a fluid moving up a column, there will be a clear cut into two fractions of particle size. In practice this does not occur, as there is a distribution of velocities across the tube in which a fluid is flowing – the highest velocity is found in the centre of the tube and the lowest velocity at the tube walls. Therefore, the size of particles that will be separated depends on their position in the tube: the largest particles in the centre, the smallest towards the outside. In practice, particles can be seen to rise with the fluid and then to move outwards to the tube wall, where the velocity is lower and they start to fall. A separation into two size fraction occurs but the size cut will not be clearly defined. Assessing the sharpness of size cuts is discussed in more detail above.

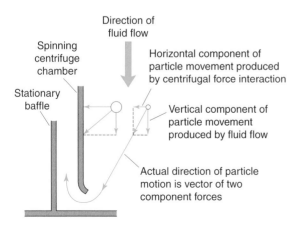

Fig. 11.6 Influence of particle size on particle movement in multiple-chamber centrifuge.

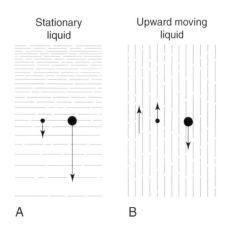

Fig. 11.8 Comparison of (a) sedimentation and (b) elutriation.

Separation of powders into several size fractions can be effected by using a number of elutriators connected in series. The suspension is fed into the bottom of the narrowest column, overflowing from the top into the bottom of the next widest column and so on (Fig. 11.9). Because the mass flow remains the same, as the column diameter increases the fluid velocity decreases and therefore particles of decreasing size will be separated.

Alternative techniques

Air may be used as the counterflow fluid in place of water for elutriation of soluble particles into different size ranges. There are several types of air elutriator, which differ according to the airflow patterns used. An example of an upward airflow elutriator is shown in Figure 11.10. Particles are held on a supporting mesh through which air is drawn. Classification occurs within a very short distance of the mesh and any particles remaining entrained in the air stream are accelerated to a collecting chamber by passage through a conical section of tube. Further separation of any fine particles still entrained in the air flow may be carried out subsequently using different air velocities.

It may be required to separate finer particles than can be achieved using gravitational elutriation, and in these cases counterflow centrifugal methods can be used. Particles in air suspension are fed into a rotating hollow torus at high speed, tangential to the outer wall. Coarse particles move outwards to the walls against the inwardly spiralling air flow, which leaves the elutriator in the centre. The desired particle size fraction can be

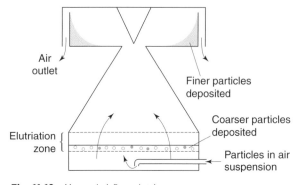

Fig. 11.10   Upward airflow elutriator.

separated by selecting the appropriate airflow rate and rotor speed.

Cyclone methods

Separation range

This is shown in Figure 11.11.

Principles of operation

Cyclone separation can take the form of a centrifugal elutriation process, similar to the one described above, or a centrifugal sedimentation process in which particles sediment out of a helical gas or liquid stream.

Probably the most common type of cyclone used to separate particles from fluid streams is the reverse-flow cyclone (Fig. 11.12). In this system, particles in air or liquid suspension are often introduced tangentially into the cylindrical upper section of the cyclone, where the relatively high fluid velocity produces a vortex that throws solid particles out on to the walls of the cyclone. The particles are forced down the conical section of the cyclone under the influence of the fluid flow – gravity interactions are a relatively insignificant mechanism in this process. At the tip of the conical section the vortex of fluid is above the critical velocity at which it can escape through the narrow outlet and forms an inner vortex which travels back up the cyclone and out through a central outlet or vortex finder. Coarser particles

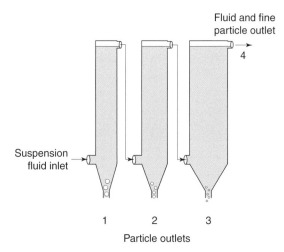

Fig. 11.9   Multistage elutriator. Particle outlets 1–4 collect fractions of decreasing particle size.

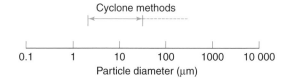

Fig. 11.11   Separation ranges for cyclone methods.

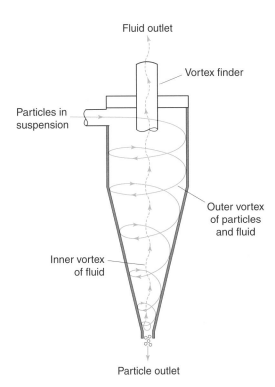

Fig. 11.12 Reverse-flow cyclone separation.

separate from the fluid stream and fall out of the cyclone through the dust outlet, whereas finer particles remain entrained in the fluid stream and leave the cyclone through the vortex finder. In some cases, the outer vortex is allowed to enter a collector connected to the base of the cyclone, but the coarser particles still appear to separate from the fluid stream and remain in the collector. A series of cyclones having different flow rates or differ-ent dimensions could be used to separate a powder into different particle size ranges.

SELECTION OF A SIZE SEPARATION PROCESS

Selection of a specific size separation may be limited by pharmacopoeial requirements but for general cases, the most efficient method should be selected based on particle properties. Of these, size is particularly important as each separation method is most efficient over a particular size range, as indicated in the foregoing text.

Particles that have just undergone size reduction will already be in suspension in a fluid, whether air or water, and can be separated quickly by elutriation or cyclone separation methods, so that oversize material can be returned to the mill.

Alternatively, many powders used pharmaceutically are soluble in water and size separation may have to be restricted to air classification methods.

BIBLIOGRAPHY

Allen, T. (1997) *Particle Size Measurement*, vols 1 and 2, 5th edn. Chapman and Hall, London.
Gotoh, K., Masuda, H., Higashitan, K. (1997) *Powder Technology Handbook*, 2nd edn. Marcel Dekker, New York.
Manual on Test Sieving Methods (1985) ASTM Special Technical Publication. American Society for Testing and Materials Standards, Pennsylvania.
Rhodes, M. (ed.) (1990) *Principles of Powder Technology*. John Wiley, Chichester.
Schweitzer, P.A. (ed.) (1997) *Handbook of Separation Techniques for Chemical Engineers*. McGraw-Hill Professional, New York.
Svarovsky, L. (1981) Solid gas separation. In: Williams, J.C., Allen, T. (eds) *Handbook of Powder Technology*, vol. 3. Elsevier, Amsterdam.

12

Mixing

A. M. Twitchell

MIXING PRINCIPLES

Importance of mixing

There are very few pharmaceutical products that contain only one component. In the vast majority of cases, several ingredients are needed to ensure that the required dosage form functions as required. If, for example, a pharmaceutical company wishes to produce a tablet dosage form containing a drug which is active at a dose of 1 mg, other components (e.g. a diluent, binder, disintegrant and lubricant) will be needed both to enable the product to be manufactured and for it to be handled by the patient.

Whenever a product contains more than one component, a mixing or blending stage will be required in the manufacturing process. This may be to ensure an even distribution of the active component(s), an even appearance or that the dosage form releases the drug at the correct site and at the desired rate. The unit operation of mixing is therefore involved at some stage in the production of practically every pharmaceutical preparation. This is illustrated below by the list of products which invariably utilize mixing processes of some kind.

- Tablets, capsules, sachets and dry powder inhalers – mixtures of solid particles
- Linctuses – mixtures of miscible liquids
- Emulsions and creams – mixtures of immiscible liquids
- Pastes and suspensions – dispersions of solid particles

This chapter considers the objectives of the mixing operation, how mixing occurs, and the ways in which a satisfactory mix can be produced and maintained.

Definition and objectives of mixing

Mixing may be defined as a unit operation that aims to treat two or more components, initially in an unmixed or partially mixed state, so that each unit (particle, molecule, etc.) of the components lies as nearly as possible in contact with a unit of each of the other components.

If this is achieved, it produces a theoretical 'ideal' situation, i.e. a *perfect mix*. As will be shown, however, this situation is not normally practicable, is actually unnecessary and, indeed, is sometimes undesirable.

How closely it is attempted to approach the 'ideal' situation depends on the product being manufactured and the objective of the mixing operation. For example, when mixing a small amount of a potent drug in a powder mix, the degree of mixing must be of a high order to ensure a consistent dose. Similarly, when dispersing two immisci-

ble liquids or dispersing a solid in a liquid, a well-mixed product is required to ensure product quality/stability. In the case of mixing lubricants with granules during tablet production, however, there is a danger of 'overmixing' and the subsequent production of a weak tablet with an increased disintegration time (discussed in Chapter 31).

Types of mixtures

Mixtures may be categorized into three types that differ fundamentally in their behaviour.

Positive mixtures

Positive mixtures are formed from materials such as gases or miscible liquids which mix *spontaneously* and *irreversibly* by diffusion and tend to approach a perfect mix. There is no input of energy required with positive mixtures if the time available for mixing is unlimited, although input of energy will shorten the time required to obtain the desired degree of mixing. In general, materials which mix by positive mixing do not present any problems during product manufacture.

Negative mixtures

With negative mixtures, the components will tend to separate out. If this occurs quickly, then energy must be continuously input to keep the components adequately dispersed, e.g. with a suspension formulation where there is a dispersion of solids in a liquid of low viscosity. With other negative mixtures, the components tend to separate very slowly, e.g. emulsions, creams and viscous suspensions. Negative mixtures are generally more difficult to form and to maintain and require a higher degree of mixing efficiency than do positive mixtures.

Neutral mixtures

Neutral mixtures are said to be static in behaviour, i.e. the components have no tendency to mix spontaneously or segregate spontaneously once work has been input to mix them. Examples of this type of mixture include mixed powders, pastes and ointments.

It should be noted that in an ointment the type of mixture could change during processing. For example, if the viscosity of the base increases, the mixture may change from a negative to a neutral mixture. Similarly, if the particle size, degree of wetting or liquid surface tension changes the mixture type may also change.

Neutral mixes are capable of demixing, but this requires energy input (discussed in more detail in the Powder Segregation section later in this chapter).

The mixing process

To discuss the principles of the mixing process, a situation will be considered where there are equal quantities of two powdered components of the same size, shape and density that are required to be mixed, the only difference between them being their colour. This situation will not, of course, occur practically but it will serve to simplify the discussion of the mixing process and allow some important considerations to be illustrated with the help of statistical analysis.

If the components are represented by coloured cubes, then a two-dimensional representation of the initial unmixed or completely segregated state can be shown as in Figure 12.1a.

From the definition of mixing, the ideal situation or *perfect mix* in this case would be produced when each particle lies adjacent to a particle of the other component (i.e. each particle lies as closely as possible in contact with a particle of the other component). This is shown in Figure 12.1b where it can be seen that the components are as evenly distributed as possible. If this mix was viewed in three dimensions then behind and in front of each coloured particle would be a white particle and vice versa.

Powder mixing, however, is a 'chance' process and while the situation shown in Figure 12.1b could arise, the odds against it are so great that for practical purposes it can be considered impossible. For example, if there are only 200 particles present, the chance of a perfect mix occurring is approximately 1 in 10^{60} and is similar to the chance of the situation in Figure 12.1a occurring after prolonged mixing. In practice, the best type of mix likely to be obtained will have the components under consideration distributed as indicated in Figure 12.1c. This is referred to as a *random mix* which can be defined as a mix where the *probability* of selecting a particular type of particle is the *same* at all positions in the mix and is equal to the *proportion* of such particles in the total mix.

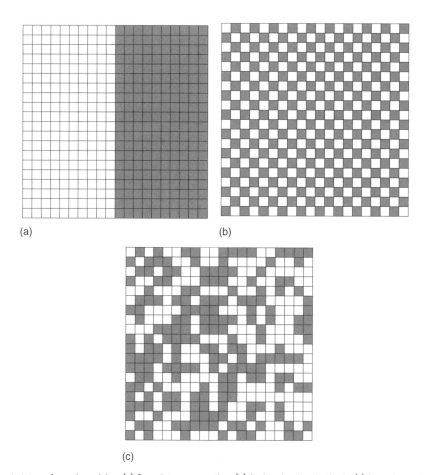

(a)   (b)

(c)

Fig. 12.1   Different states of powder mixing. (a) Complete segregation. (b) An ideal or 'perfect' mix. (c) A random mix.

If any two adjacent particles are selected from the random mix shown:

- the chance of picking two coloured particles = 1 in 4 (25%)
- the chance of picking two white particles = 1 in 4 (25%)
- and the chance of picking one of each = 2 in 4 (50%).

If any two particles are selected from the perfect mix shown in Figure 12.1b, there will always be one coloured and one white particle.

Thus if the samples taken from a random mix contain only two particles, then in 25% of cases the sample will contain no white particles and in 25% it will contain no coloured particles. It may help in this and subsequent discussions to imagine one of the coloured particles as being the active drug and the other the inert excipient.

It can be seen that, in practice, the components will not be perfectly evenly distributed, i.e. there will not be full mixing. But if an overall view is taken, the components can be described as being mixed since in the total sample the amount of each component is approximately similar (48.8% coloured and 51.2% white). If, however, Figure 12.1c is considered as 16 different blocks of 25 particles, then it can be seen that the number of coloured particles in the blocks varies from six to 19 (24% to 76% of the total number of particles in each block). Careful examination of Figure 12.1c shows that as the number of particles in the sample increases then the closer will be the proportion of each component to that which would occur with a perfect mix. This is a very important consideration in powder mixing and is discussed in more detail in the following sections.

Scale of scrutiny

Often a mixing process produces a large 'bulk' of mixture that is subsequently subdivided into individual dose units (e.g. a tablet, capsule or 5 mL spoonful) and it is important that each dosage unit contains the correct amount/concentration of active component(s). It is the weight/volume of the *dosage unit* which dictates how closely the mix must be examined/analysed to ensure it contains the correct dose/concentration. This weight/volume is known as the *scale of scrutiny* and is the amount of material within which the quality of mixing is important. For example, if the unit weight of a tablet is 200 mg then a 200 mg sample from the mix needs to be 'scrutinized' and analysed to see if mixing is adequate. The scale of scrutiny therefore = 200 mg.

The number of *particles* in the scale of scrutiny will depend on the sample weight, particle size and particle density, and will increase as the sample weight increases

and the particle size and density decrease. This number should be sufficient to ensure an acceptably small deviation from the required dose in the dosage forms.

Another important factor to consider when carrying out a mixing process is the proportion of the active component in the dosage form/scale of scrutiny. This is illustrated in Figure 12.2 and in Table 12.1, the latter also demonstrating the importance of the number of particles in the scale of scrutiny.

Figure 12.2 shows a random mix containing only 10% coloured particles. If the blocks of 25 particles are examined it can be seen that the number of coloured particles varies from 0 to 8 or 0% to 32%. Thus, the number of coloured particles as a percentage of the theoretical content varies from 0% to 320%. This is considerably greater than the range of 48 to 152% when the proportion of coloured particles was 0.5 or 50% (Fig. 12.1c).

Table 12.1 shows how the content of a minor active constituent (present in a proportion of one part in a thousand, i.e. 0.1%) typically varies with the number of particles in the scale of scrutiny when sampling a random mix. In the example shown, when there are 1000 particles in the scale of scrutiny, three samples contain no active constituent and two have twice the amount that should be present. With 10 000 particles in the scale of scrutiny, the deviation is reduced but samples may still deviate from the theoretical content of 10 particles by ±50%. Even with 100 000 particles, deviation from theoretical content may be ±15% which is unacceptable for a pharmaceutical mixture. The difficulty in mixing potent substances can be appreciated if it is realized that there may only be approximately 75 000 particles of diameter 150 μm in a tablet weighing 200 mg.

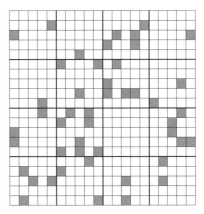

Fig. 12.2 Particle distribution in a representative random mix containing 10% active ingredient.

Table 12.1 Number of particles of a minor active constituent present in samples taken from a 1:1000 random powder mix with different numbers of particles in the scale of scrutiny

Sample number	Number of particles in scale of scrutiny		
	1000	10 000	100 000
1	1	7	108
2	0	10	91
3	1	15	116
4	2	8	105
5	0	13	84
6	1	10	93
7	1	6	113
8	2	5	92
9	0	12	104
10	1	13	90

The figures in the table are the numbers of particles of the minor constituent in the samples.

The information in Figures 12.1 and 12.2 and Table 12.1 leads to two important conclusions:

1. the lower the proportion of active component present in the mixture, the more difficult it is to achieve an acceptably low deviation in active content
2. the more particles there are present in a unit dose/scale of scrutiny, the lower the likely deviation in content.

One way of reducing the deviation, therefore, would be to increase the number of particles in the scale of scrutiny by decreasing the particle size. This may, however, lead to particle aggregation due to the increased cohesion and adhesion that occurs with smaller particles, which in turn may reduce the ease of mixing.

It should be noted that with liquid solutions, even very small samples are likely to contain many million 'particles'. Deviation in content is therefore likely to be very small with miscible liquids even if they are randomly mixed. Diffusion effects in miscible liquids arising from the existence of concentration gradients in an unmixed system mean that they tend to approach a perfect mix.

Mathematical treatment of the mixing process

It should be appreciated that there will always be some variation in composition of samples taken from a random mix. The aim during formulation and processing is to minimize this variation to acceptable levels by selecting an appropriate scale of scrutiny, particle size and mixing pro-

cedure (the latter involving the correct choice of mixer, rotation speed, etc.). The following section uses a simplified statistical approach to illustrate some of the factors that influence dose variation within a batch of a dosage form and demonstrates the difficulties encountered with drugs that are active in low doses (potent drugs).

Consider the situation where samples are taken from a random mix in which the particles are all of the same size, shape and density. The variation in the proportion of a component in samples taken from the random mix can be calculated from Eqn 12.1:

$$SD = \sqrt{\frac{p(1-p)}{n}} \qquad (12.1)$$

where SD is the standard deviation in the proportion of the component in the samples (content sample deviation), p is the proportion of the component in the total mix and n is the total number of particles in the sample.

Equation 12.1 shows that as the number of particles present in the sample increases, the standard deviation of the content decreases (i.e. there is less variation in sample content), as illustrated previously by the data in Figure 12.2 and Table 12.1. The situation with respect to the effect of the proportion of the active component in the sample is not as clear from Equation 12.1. As p is decreased, the value of content standard deviation decreases, and this may lead to the incorrect conclusion that it is beneficial to have a low proportion of the active component. A more useful parameter to determine is the percentage coefficient of variation (% CV), which indicates the average deviation as a percentage of the mean amount of active component in the samples. Thus, % CV = (content standard deviation/mean content) × 100. The value of % CV will increase as p decreases, as illustrated below.

Consider the situation where $n = 100\,000$ and $p = 0.5$. Using Equation 12.1, it can be calculated that the SD = 1.58×10^{-3} and % CV = $(1.58 \times 10^{-3}/0.5) \times 100 = 0.32\%$. Thus on average, the content will deviate from mean content by 0.32% which is an acceptably low value for a pharmaceutical product.

If, however, p is reduced to 0.001 and n remains at 100 000 there is a reduction in SD to 9.99×10^{-5} but the % CV = $(9.99 \times 10^{-5}/0.001) \times 100 = 10\%$. Thus in this latter case, the content will deviate from theoretical content on average by 10% which would be unacceptable for a pharmaceutical product.

It might be considered that the variation in content could be reduced by increasing the sample size (increasing the scale of scrutiny), as this would increase the number of particles in each sample. The dose of a drug will, however, be fixed and any increase in the sample size will cause a reduction in the proportion of the active component in the mix. The consequence of increasing the sample size depends on the initial proportion of the active component. If p is relatively high initially, increasing the sample size causes the %CV in content to increase. If p is small, increasing the sample size has little effect. Inserting appropriate values into Equation 12.1 can substantiate this.

In a true random mix the content of samples taken from the mix will follow a normal distribution. With a normal distribution, 68.3% of samples will be within ±1 SD of the overall proportion of the component (p), 95.5% will be within ±2 SD of p and 99.7% of samples will be within ±3 SD of p. For example, if $p = 0.5$ and the standard deviation in content = 0.02, then for 99.7% of samples the proportion of the component will be between 0.44 and 0.56. In other words, if 1000 samples were analysed, 997 samples would contain between 44% and 56% of drug (mean = 50%).

A typical specification for a pharmaceutical product is that the active component should not deviate by more than ±5% of the mean or specified content, i.e. the acceptable deviation = $p \times (5/100)$ or $p \times 0.05$. NB: this is not the same as a standard deviation of 5%.

If a product contains an active component which makes up half of the weight of the dosage form ($p = 0.5$) and it is required that 99.7% of samples contain within ±5% of p, then the number of particles required in the product can be estimated as described below.

As 99.7% of samples will be within ±3 SD and ±5% of p then Equation 12.2 can be used to calculate the standard deviation required:

$$3 \times SD = p \times (\% \text{ acceptable deviation}/100) \quad (12.2)$$

In this case, $3 \times SD = 0.5 \times 0.05$

so
$$\frac{0.5 \times 0.05}{3} = \sqrt{\frac{p(1-p)}{n}}$$

$$6.94 \times 10^{-5} = 0.5(1-0.5)/n$$

and therefore $n = 3600$.

The above calculation indicates that 3600 particles are required in each sample or dosage form in order to be 99.7% sure that the content is within ±5% of the theoretical amount.

If, however, the product contains a potent drug where $p = 1 \times 10^{-3}$, the number of particles needed to meet the same criteria can be estimated to be 3.6×10^6.

Estimation of the particle size required when formulating a dosage form

Using the preceding information, it is possible to estimate the particle size required so that a formulation may meet a desired specification. For example, imagine it is necessary to produce a tablet weighing 50 mg which contains 50 μg of a potent steroid, and that the product spec-

ification requires 99.7% of tablets to contain between 47.5 μg and 52.5 μg of the steroid. If the mean particle density of the components is 1.5 g/cm³ (1500 kg/m³), what particle size should the steroid and excipients be?

As there is 50 μg of the steroid in a 50 mg tablet, the proportion of active component (p) = 1×10^{-3}. The specification allows the content to vary by ±2.5 μg, and so the % deviation allowed = $(2.5/50) \times 100 = 5\%$. Under these circumstances, the calculations described in the previous section show that, providing a random mix is achieved, the number of particles required in the tablet = 3.6×10^6. The 50 mg tablet must therefore contain at least 3.6×10^6 particles and each particle must weigh less than $50/3.6 \times 10^6$ mg = 1.39×10^{-5} mg = 1.39×10^{-11} kg. Since the density of a particle = particle mass/particle volume, the volume of each particle must be less than $1.39 \times 10^{-11}/1500$ m³ = 9.27×10^{-15} m³.

The volume of a particle (assuming it is spherical) = $4\pi r^3/3$ and so:

r^3 must be $<9.27 \times 10^{-15} \times 3/4\pi$ m³, i.e.
$r^3 < 2.21 \times 10^{-15}$ m³ and therefore
$r < 1.30 \times 10^{-5}$ m (and therefore d $<26 \mu$m).

This calculation indicates that in order to meet the product specification, the particle size of the components needs to be of the order of 26 μm. There would therefore be practical difficulties in making this product, as particles of this size tend to become very cohesive, flow poorly (see Chapter 13) and are difficult to mix.

In order to appreciate the effect of changing the scale of scrutiny, it is suggested that the reader calculates in a similar manner what particle size would be required if the tablet weight were increased to 250 mg. It should be remembered that the tablet weight or scale of scrutiny will affect both the number of particles present and the proportion of active component.

In summary, the above calculations illustrate the difficulty in mixing potent (low-dose) substances and the importance of both the number of particles in the scale of scrutiny and proportion of the active component.

Evaluation of the degree of mixing

Manufacturers require some means of monitoring a mixing process for a variety of reasons. These could be to:

- indicate the degree/extent of mixing
- follow a mixing process
- indicate when sufficient mixing has occurred
- assess the efficiency of a mixer
- determine the mixing time required for a particular process.

Many evaluation methods involve the generation of a *mixing index* that compares the content standard deviation of samples taken from a mix under investigation (S_{ACT}) with the content standard deviation of samples from a fully random mix (S_R). Comparison with a random mix is made since this is theoretically likely to be the best mix that is practically achievable. The simplest form of a mixing index (M) can be calculated as:

$$M = \frac{S_R}{S_{ACT}} \qquad (12.3)$$

At the start of the mixing process the value of S_{ACT} will be high and that for M will be low. As mixing proceeds, S_{ACT} will tend to decrease as the mix approaches a random mix (see Fig. 12.3). If the mix becomes random, $S_{ACT} = S_R$ and $M = 1$. There is typically an exponential decrease in S_{ACT} as the mixing time or number of mixer rotations increases although the shape of the curve will depend on the powder properties and mixer design and utilization. Other more complicated equations for calculating the mixing index have been used but they all tend to rely on similar principles to those described.

In order to evaluate a mixing process in this way, there are two basic requirements. First, a sufficient number of samples which are representative of the mix as a whole must be removed and analysed. A minimum of 10 samples is usually taken, these being removed from different depths into the mixer and from the middle and sides. Samples are often taken with a 'sampling thief' which is a device which can be inserted into the mix and samples withdrawn with minimum disruption to the powder bed. Garcia et al (1995) and Venables & Wells (2001) have discussed some of the problems associated with removing representative samples and analysing powder blends. Second, a suitable analytical technique must be available so that the value of S_{ACT} is a true reflection of the variation in content in the samples and not due to variation arising from the method of analysis.

When mixing formulations where the proportion of active component is high, it is possible to achieve an acceptably low variation in content without obtaining a random mix. Thus it may be possible to stop the mixing process before a random mix is achieved and therefore reduce manufacturing costs. Equation 12.2 can be used to generate an estimated acceptable standard deviation value (S_E) that will allow the product to meet its specification. For example, if the proportion of active component present in the formulation is 0.5 and the acceptable variation from mean content is ±5% for 99.7% of samples, then:

$$S_E = \frac{0.5 \times (5/100)}{3} = 8.3 \times 10^{-3}$$

Therefore, if when the mix is analysed the content standard deviation in the proportion of the active component is $<8.3 \times 10^{-3}$ (%CV <1.67), the product should meet the specification. This approach is illustrated in Figure 12.4.

MECHANISMS OF MIXING AND DEMIXING

Powders

In order that powders may be mixed, the powder particles need to move relative to each other. There are three main mechanisms by which powder mixing occurs, namely *convection*, *shear* and *diffusion*.

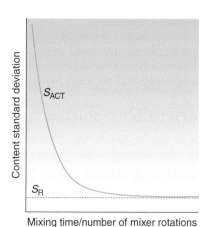

Fig. 12.3 The reduction in content standard deviation as a random mix is approached. S_{ACT} represents the content standard deviation of samples taken from the mix and S_R the standard deviation expected from a random mix.

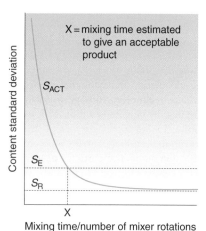

Fig. 12.4 The reduction in mixing time possible if a random mix is not required. S_{ACT} represents the content standard deviation of samples taken from the mix, S_E the estimated acceptable standard deviation and S_R the standard deviation expected from a random mix.

Convective mixing arises when there is the transfer of relatively large groups of particles from one part of the powder bed to another, e.g. as might occur when a mixer blade or paddle moves through the mix. This type of mixing contributes mainly to the macroscopic mixing of powder mixtures and tends to produce a large degree of mixing fairly quickly (as evidenced by a rapid drop in S_{ACT}). Mixing does not, however, occur *within* the group of particles moving together as a unit and thus in order to achieve a random mix, an extended mixing time is required.

Shear mixing occurs when a 'layer' of material moves/flows over another 'layer'. This might be due to the removal of a mass by convective mixing creating an unstable shear/slip plane which causes the powder bed to collapse. It may also occur in high-shear mixers or tumbling mixers where the action of the mixer induces velocity gradients within the powder bed and hence 'shearing' of one layer over another.

In order to achieve a true random mix, movement of individual particles is required. This occurs with *diffusive mixing*. When a powder bed is forced to move or flow, it will 'dilate', i.e. the volume occupied by the bed will increase. This arises because the powder particles will become less tightly packed and there is an increase in the air spaces or voids between them. Under these circumstances there is the potential for the powder particles to fall, under gravitational forces, through the void spaces created. Mixing of individual particles in this way is referred to as diffusive mixing. Diffusive mixing has the potential to produce a random mix but generally results in a low speed of mixing.

All three mixing mechanisms are likely to occur in a mixing operation. Which mechanism predominates and the extent to which each occurs will depend on the mixer type, mixing process conditions (mixer load, speed, etc.) and the flowability of the components of the powder.

Liquids

The three main mechanisms by which liquids are mixed are *bulk transport*, *turbulent mixing* and *molecular diffusion*.

Bulk transport is analogous to the convective mixing of powders and involves the movement of a relatively large amount of material from one position in the mix to another, e.g. due to a mixer paddle. It too tends to produce a large degree of mixing fairly quickly, but leaves the liquid within the moving material unmixed.

Turbulent mixing arises from the haphazard movement of molecules when forced to move in a turbulent manner. The constant changes in speed and direction of movement mean that induced turbulence is a highly effective mechanism for mixing. Within a turbulent fluid there are,

however, small groups of molecules moving together as a unit, referred to as eddies. These eddies tend to reduce in size and eventually break up, being replaced by new eddies. Turbulent mixing alone may therefore leave small unmixed areas within the eddies and in areas near the container surface which will exhibit streamlined flow (see Chapter 4).

Mixing of individual molecules in these regions will occur by the third mechanism, which is *molecular diffusion* (analogous to diffusive mixing in powders). This will occur with miscible fluids wherever a concentration gradient exists and will eventually produce a well-mixed product, although considerable time may be required if this is the only mixing mechanism. In most mixers all three mechanisms will occur, bulk transport and turbulence arising from the movement of a stirrer or mixer paddle set at a suitable speed.

Powder segregation (demixing)

Segregation is the opposite effect to mixing, i.e. components tend to separate out. This is very important in the preparation of pharmaceutical products because if it occurs, an already formed random mix may change to a non-random mix, or a random mix may never be achieved. Care must be taken to avoid segregation occurring during handling after powders have been satisfactorily mixed, e.g. during transfer to filling machines or in the hopper of a tablet/capsule/sachet filling machine. Segregation will cause an increase in content variation in samples taken from the mix and may cause a batch to fail a uniformity of content test. If segregation of granules occurs in a hopper of a filling machine, an unacceptable variation in weight may result.

Segregation arises because powder mixes encountered in practice are not composed of monosized spherical particles but contain particles that differ in size, shape and density. These variations in particle properties mean that they will tend to behave differently when forced to move and hence tend to separate. Particles exhibiting similar properties tend to congregate together, giving regions in the powder bed which have a higher concentration of a particular component. Segregation is more likely to occur, or may occur to a greater extent, if the powder bed is subjected to vibration and when the particles have greater flowability.

Particle size effects

A difference in the particle sizes of components of a formulation is the main cause of segregation in powder mixes in practice. Smaller particles tend to fall through the voids between larger particles and thus move to the bottom of the mass. This is known as *percolation segregation*. It may occur in static powder beds if the percolating particles are so small that they can fall into the void spaces between larger particles, but occurs to a greater extent as the bed 'dilates' on being disturbed. Domestically, percolation segregation is often observed in cereal packets or jars of coffee where the smaller 'particles' congregate towards the bottom of the container.

Percolation can occur whenever a powder bed containing particles of different size is disturbed in such a way that particle rearrangement occurs, e.g. during vibration, stirring or pouring.

During mixing, larger particles will tend to have greater kinetic energy imparted to them (owing to their larger mass) and therefore move greater distances than smaller particles before they come to rest. This may result in separation of particles of different size; an effect referred to as *trajectory segregation*. This effect, along with percolation segregation, accounts for the occurrence of the larger particles at the edge of a powder heap when it is poured from a container.

During mixing, or when a material is discharged from a container, very small particles ('dust') in a mix may tend to be 'blown' upwards by turbulent air currents as the mass tumbles, and remain suspended in the air during mixing. When the mixer is stopped or material discharge is complete, these particles will sediment and subsequently form a layer on top of the coarser particles. This is called *elutriation segregation* and is also referred to as *dusting out* or *fluidization segregation*.

Particle density effects

If components are of different density, the more dense particles will have a tendency to move downwards even if their particle sizes are similar. Trajectory segregation may also occur with particles of the same size but different densities due to their difference in mass. The effect of density on percolation segregation may be potentiated if the denser particles are also smaller. Alternatively, size and density effects may cancel each other out if the larger particles are denser. Often materials used in pharmaceutical formulations have similar densities and density effects are not generally too important. An exception to this is in fluidized beds, where density differences are often more serious than particle size differences.

Particle shape effects

Spherical particles exhibit the greatest flowability and therefore are more easily mixed, but they also segregate more easily than non-spherical particles. Irregular or needle-shaped particles may become interlocked, decreasing

the tendency to segregate once mixing has occurred. Non-spherical particles will also have a greater surface area to weight ratio (specific surface area), which will tend to decrease segregation by increasing any cohesive effects (greater contact surface area) but will increase the likelihood of 'dusting out'.

It should be remembered that the particle size distribution and particle shape may change during processing (due to attrition, aggregation, etc.) and therefore the tendency to segregate may also change.

Non-segregating mixes will improve with continued increases in mixing time, as shown in Figure 12.3. This may not, however, occur for segregating mixes, where there is often an optimum mixing time. This arises since the factors causing segregation generally require a longer time to take effect than the time needed to produce a reasonable degree of mixing. During the initial stages of the process, the rate of mixing is greater than the rate of demixing. After a period of time, however, the rate of demixing may predominate until eventually an equilibrium situation will be reached where the two effects are balanced. This is illustrated in Figure 12.5 which demonstrates that, if factors exist which may cause segregation, then a random mix will not be achieved and there may both an optimum mixing time and a time range over which an acceptable mix can be produced.

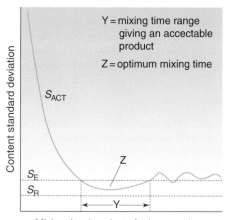

Fig. 12.5 Possible effect of extended mixing time on the content standard deviation of samples taken from a mix prone to segregation. S_{ACT} represents the content standard deviation of samples taken from the mix, S_E the estimated acceptable standard deviation and S_R the standard deviation expected from a random mix.

Approaches to minimize segregation

If segregation is a problem with a formulation there are a number of approaches that may be attempted to rectify the situation. These include the following:

- Selection of particular size fractions (e.g. by sieving to remove fines or lumps) to achieve drug and excipients of the same narrow particle size range.
- Milling of components (size reduction) to either reduce the particle size range (this may need to be followed by a sieving stage to remove fines) or to ensure all particles are below approximately 30 μm at which size segregation does not tend to cause serious problems (but may give rise to aggregation).
- Controlled crystallization during production of the drug/excipients to give components of a particular crystal shape or size range.
- Selection of excipients which have a density similar to the active component(s); there is usually a range of excipients which will produce a product of the required properties.
- Granulation of the powder mix (size enlargement) so that large numbers of different particles are evenly distributed in each segregating 'unit'/granule (see Fig. 29.1).
- Reduce the extent to which the powder mass is subjected to vibration or movement after mixing (e.g. avoid the use of pneumatic transfer systems).
- Use filling machine hoppers designed so that powder residence time is minimized.
- Use equipment where several operations can be carried out without transferring the mix, e.g. a fluidized-bed drier or high-speed mixer/granulator for mixing and granulating.
- Production of an 'ordered' mix. This technique is also referred to as *adhesive* or *interactive* mixing and is described in more detail below.

Ordered mixing

It would be expected that a mix composed of very small and much larger particles would segregate because of the size differences. Sometimes, however, if one powder is sufficiently small (micronized) it may become adsorbed onto 'active sites' on the surface of a larger 'carrier' particle. Here it will exhibit a greater resistance to being dislodged. This has the effect of minimizing segregation while maintaining good flow properties. It was first noticed by Travers & White (1971) during the mixing of micronized sodium bicarbonate with sucrose crystals when the mixture was found to exhibit minimal segregation. The phenomenon is referred to as ordered mixing, as the particles are not independent of each other and there is a degree of order to the mix. If a carrier particle is removed then some of the adsorbed smaller particles will automatically be removed with it. Ordered mixing has also been used in the production of dry antibiotic formulations to which water is added before use to form a liquid or syrup product. In these cases the antibiotic in fine powder form is blended with, and adsorbed onto the surface of, larger sucrose or sorbitol particles (Nikolakakis & Newton 1989).

Ordered mixing probably occurs to a certain extent in every pharmaceutical powder mix due to interactions and cohesive/adhesive forces between constituents. It is most likely to occur when smaller particles exist, as these have a high specific surface area and thus the attractive forces holding the particles to the adsorption site are more likely to be greater than the gravitational forces trying to separate the components.

Pharmaceutical mixes are therefore likely to be partly ordered and partly random, the extent of each depending on the component properties. With an ordered mix, it may be possible to achieve a degree of mixing which is superior to that of a random mix which may be beneficial for potent drugs.

Ordered mixing has been shown to be important in direct-compression tablet formulations (Chapter 31) in preventing segregation of drug from direct compression bases.

Dry powder inhaler formulations also utilize ordered mixing to deliver drugs to the lungs (Chapter 36). In this case the drug needs to be in a micronized form in order to reach its site of action. By adsorbing the drug onto larger carrier particles (usually lactose), it is possible to manufacture a product which will provide an even dosage on each inhalation.

Segregation in ordered mixes

Although ordered mixes can reduce or prevent segregation, it may still occur if:

- *the carrier particles vary in size* – different-sized particles will have different surface area to weight ratios and will contain different amounts of adsorbed material per unit mass. If the different-sized carrier particles separate (e.g. by percolation segregation), drug-rich areas where the smaller carrier particles congregate may result. This is referred to as *ordered unit segregation*
- *there is competition for the active sites on the carrier particle* – if another component competes for sites on the carrier it may displace the original adsorbed material which may then segregate due to its small size. This is known as *displacement segregation* and has been shown to occur under certain circumstances with the addition of the lubricant magnesium stearate to tablet formulations
- *there are insufficient carrier particles* – each carrier particle can only accommodate a certain amount of

adsorbed material on its surface. If there is any excess small-sized material that is not adsorbed on to the carrier particles, this may quickly separate. This is referred to as *saturation segregation* and may limit the proportion of the active component that can be used in the formulation.

With an ordered mix, particles may be dislodged if the mix is subjected to excessive vibration. The extent to which this occurs depends on the forces of attraction between the components and therefore on how tightly the adsorbed particles are attached to the surface. The orientation of the particles is also important, particles protruding out from the surface being more likely to be dislodged than those lying parallel to the surface.

MIXING OF POWDERS

Practical considerations

When mixing formulations in which there is a relatively low proportion of active ingredient(s), a more even distribution may be obtained by sequentially building up the amount of material in the mixer. This may be achieved by initially mixing the active component(s) with an approximately equal volume of diluent(s). Further amounts of diluents, equal to the amount of material in the mixer, can then be added and mixed, the process being continued until all material has been added. It may be more appropriate to preblend the active component with a diluent in a smaller mixer prior to transferring it to the main mixer in cases where the amount of active ingredient is very low.

Care must be taken to ensure that the volume of powder in mixer is appropriate, as both over- and underfilling may significantly reduce mixing efficiency. In the case of overfilling, for example, sufficient bed dilation may not take place for diffusive mixing to occur to the required extent or the material may not be able to flow in a way that enables shear mixing to occur satisfactorily. Similarly, underfilling may mean the powder bed does not move in the required manner in the mixer or that an increased number of mixing operations may be needed for a batch of material.

The mixer used should produce the mixing mechanisms appropriate for the formulation. For example, diffusive mixing is generally preferable if potent drugs are to be mixed, and high shear is needed to break up aggregates of cohered material and ensure mixing at a particulate level. The impact or attrition forces generated if too-high shear forces are used may, however, damage fragile material and thus produce fines. The mixer design should be such that it is dust tight, can be easily cleaned and the product can be fully discharged. These features

reduce the risk of cross-contamination between batches and protect the operator from the product.

In order to determine the appropriate mixing time, the process should be checked by removing and analysing representative samples after different mixing intervals. This may also indicate if segregation is occurring within the mixer and whether problems occur if the mixing time is extended.

When particles rub past each other as they move within the mixer, static charges will be produced. These tend to result in 'clumping' and a reduction in diffusive mixing and cause material to adhere to machine or container surfaces. To avoid this, mixers should be suitably earthed to dissipate the static charge and the process should be carried out at a relative humidity greater (although not excessively) than approximately 40%.

Powder-mixing equipment

Tumbling mixers/blenders

Tumbling mixers are commonly used for mixing/blending of granules or free-flowing powders. There are many different designs of tumbling mixer, e.g. double-cone, twin-shell, cube, Y-cone and drum mixers, some of which are shown diagrammatically in Figure 12.6. It is now common to use *intermediate bulk containers* (IBCs)

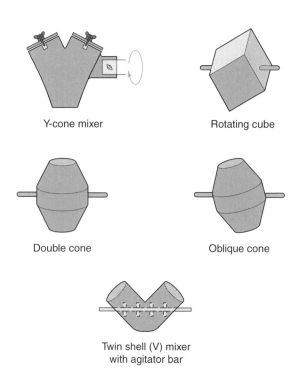

Y-cone mixer   Rotating cube

Double cone   Oblique cone

Twin shell (V) mixer
with agitator bar

Fig. 12.6 Different designs of tumbling mixers.

as both the mixer bowl and to feed the hopper of a tablet or as the capsule machine or as the hopper itself. The shape of an IBC used for this purpose is illustrated in Figure 12.7.

Mixing containers are generally mounted so that they can be rotated about an axis. When operated at the correct speed, the tumbling action indicated in Figure 12.8 is achieved. Shear mixing will occur as a velocity gradient is produced, the top layer moving with the greatest velocity and the velocity decreasing as the distance from the surface increases. When the bed tumbles it dilates, allowing particles to move downwards under gravitational force, and so diffusive mixing occurs. Too high a rotation speed will cause the material to be held on the mixer walls by centrifugal force and too low a speed will generate insufficient bed expansion and little shear mixing. Addition of 'prongs', baffles or rotating bars will also cause convective mixing (e.g. the V-mixer with agitator bar in Fig. 12.6).

Tumbling mixers are available to mix from approximately 50 g, e.g. for laboratory-scale development work, to over 100 kg at a production scale. The material typically occupies about a half to two-thirds of the mixer volume. The rate at which the product is mixed will depend on the mixer design and rotation speed since they influence the movement of the material in the mixer.

Tumbling mixers are good for free-flowing powders/granules but poor for cohesive/poorly flowing powders because the shear forces generated are usually insufficient to break up any aggregates. Care also needs to be taken if there are significant differences in particle

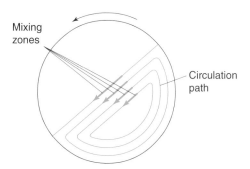

Fig. 12.8 Movement of the powder bed in a tumbling mixer.

size present since segregation is likely to occur. A common use of tumbling mixers is in the blending of lubricants, glidants or external disintegrants with granules prior to tableting.

Tumbling mixers can also be used to produce ordered mixes, although the process is often slow because of the cohesiveness of the adsorbing particles.

The Turbula shaker-mixer (WAB, Switzerland) is a more sophisticated form of tumbling mixer which utilizes inversional motion in addition to the rotational and translational motion of traditional tumbling mixers. This leads to more efficient mixing and makes it less likely that material of different size and density will segregate.

High-speed mixer-granulators

In pharmaceutical product manufacture it is often preferable to use one piece of equipment to carry out more than one function. An example of this is the use of a mixer-granulator (one design of which is shown diagrammatically in Fig. 12.9). As the name suggests, it can both mix and granulate a product, thus removing the need to transfer the product between pieces of equipment and thereby reducing the opportunity for segregation to occur. The centrally mounted impeller blade at the bottom of mixer rotates at high speed, throwing the material towards the mixer bowl wall by centrifugal force. The

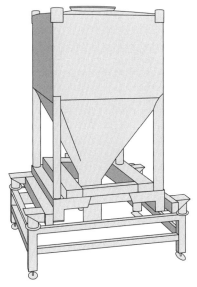

Fig. 12.7 Typical intermediate bulk container.

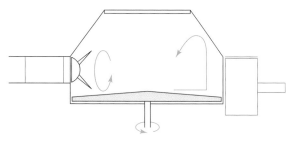

Fig. 12.9 Diagrammatic representation of a high-speed mixer-granulator.

material is then forced upwards before dropping back down towards the centre of the mixer. The particulate movement within the bowl tends to mix the components quickly owing to high shear forces (arising from the high velocity) and the expansion in bed volume which allows diffusive mixing. Once mixed, granulating agent can be added and granules formed in situ using a slower impeller speed and the action of the side-mounted chopper blade. Further details of granule production using this method can be found in Chapter 29.

Because of the high-speed movement within a mixer-granulator, care needs to be taken if the material being mixed fractures easily. This, and the problems associated with overmixing of lubricants, means that this type of mixer is not normally used for blending lubricants.

Fluidized-bed mixers

The main use of fluidized-bed equipment is in the drying of granules (Chapter 30) or the coating of multiparticulates (Chapter 33). Fluidized-bed equipment can, however, be used to mix powders prior to granulation in the same bowl. This is discussed in Chapter 29.

Agitator mixers

This type of mixer depends on the motion of a blade or paddle through the product, and hence the main mixing mechanism is convection. Examples include the ribbon mixer, the planetary mixer and the Nautamixer.

In the *ribbon mixer* (Fig. 12.10), mixing is achieved by the rotation of helical blades in a hemispherical trough. 'Dead spots' are difficult to eliminate in this type of mixer and the shearing action caused by the movement of the blades may be insufficient to break up drug aggregates. The mixer does, however, mix poorly flowing material and is less likely to cause segregation than a tumbling mixer.

A drawing of an industrial *planetary mixer* is shown in Figure 12.11. Similar designs are used for both powder and semi-solid mixing. The mixing bowl is shown in the lowered position for filling and emptying. The bowl is raised up to the mixing blade for the mixing process. The mixing blade is set off centre and is carried on a rotating arm. It therefore travels round the circumference

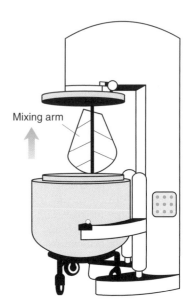

Fig. 12.11 Planetary mixer for powders and semi-solids.

of the mixing bowl while simultaneously rotating around its own axis (Fig. 12.12). This is therefore a double rotation similar to that of a spinning planet around the sun – hence the name – and is designed so that the blade covers all the volume of the mixer.

The *Nautamixer* (Fig. 12.13) consists of a conical vessel fitted at the base with a rotating screw which is fastened to the end of a rotating arm at the upper end. The screw conveys the material to near the top where it cascades back into the mass. The mixer thus combines convective mixing (as the material is raised by the helical

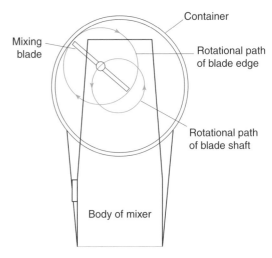

Fig. 12.12 Planetary mixer – top view, showing path of paddle.

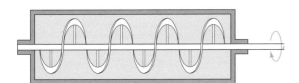

Fig. 12.10 Ribbon agitator powder mixer.

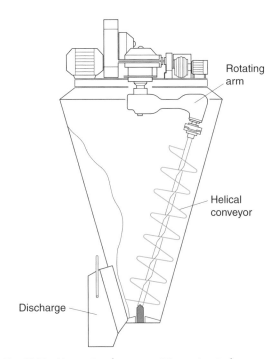

Rotating arm

Helical conveyor

Discharge

Fig. 12.13   Nautamixer (courtesy of Nautamixer Ltd).

conveyor) and shear and diffusive mixing (as the material cascades downwards). In general, agitator mixers are more difficult to clean than other mixer types.

Scale-up of powder mixing

The extent of mixing achieved at a small laboratory scale during development work may not necessarily be mirrored when the same formulation is mixed at a full production scale, even if the same mixer design is used for both. Often, mixing efficiency and the extent of mixing are improved on scale-up owing to increased shear forces. This is likely to be beneficial in most cases, although when blending lubricants, care is needed to avoid overlubrication which may, for example, lead to soft tablets and delayed disintegration and dissolution.

Problems associated with a deficiency of some of the components of a formulation, which have been encountered at a production scale but not in development work, have been traced to adsorption of a minor constituent (e.g. a drug or colorant) onto the mixer wall or mixing blade.

Drug particle characteristics may also change when the drug is manufactured on a large scale. This in turn may affect the movement of the particles in the mixer or the interaction with other components and hence the tendency to mix and segregate.

The optimum mixing time and conditions should therefore be established and validated at a production scale so that the appropriate degree of mixing is obtained without segregation, overlubrication or damage to component particles. Minimum and maximum mixing times which give a satisfactory product should be determined if appropriate so that the 'robustness' of the mixing process is established.

MIXING OF MISCIBLE LIQUIDS AND SUSPENSIONS

Mobile liquids with a low viscosity are easily mixed with each other. Similarly, solid particles are readily suspended in mobile liquids though the particles are likely to settle rapidly when mixing is discontinued. Viscous liquids are more difficult to stir and mix but they reduce the sedimentation rate of suspended particles (discussed further in Chapter 27).

Mixers for miscible liquids and suspensions

Propeller mixers

A common arrangement for medium-scale fluid mixing is a propeller-type stirrer which is often used clamped to the edge of a vessel. A propeller has angled blades, which cause the circulation of the fluid in both an axial and radial direction. An off-centre mounting discourages the formation of a vortex, which may form when the stirrer is mounted centrally. A vortex forms when the centrifugal force imparted to the liquid by the propeller blades causes it to back up round the sides of the vessel and form a depression around the shaft. As the speed of rotation is increased, air may be sucked into the fluid due to the formation of a vortex; this can cause frothing and possible oxidation (Fig. 12.14a). Another method of suppressing a vortex is to fit vertical baffles into the vessel. These divert the rotating fluid from its circular path into the centre of the vessel where the vortex would otherwise form (Fig. 12.14b).

The ratio of the diameter of a propeller stirrer to the diameter of the vessel is commonly 1:10 to 1:20 and it typically operates at speeds of 1–20 rev/s. The propeller stirrer depends for its action on a satisfactory axial and radial flow pattern which will not occur if the fluid is too viscous. There must be a fast flow of fluid towards the propeller which can only occur if the fluid is mobile.

Turbine mixers

A turbine mixer may be used for more viscous fluids and a typical construction is given in Figure 12.15.

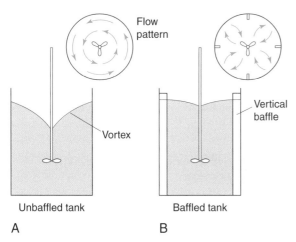

Fig. 12.14 Propeller mixer with (a) unbaffled tank and (b) baffled tank.

The impeller has four flat blades surrounded by perforated inner and outer diffuser rings. The rotating impeller draws the liquid into the mixer 'head' and forces the liquid through the perforations with considerable radial velocity sufficient to overcome the viscous drag of the bulk of the fluid. One drawback is the absence of an axial component but a different head

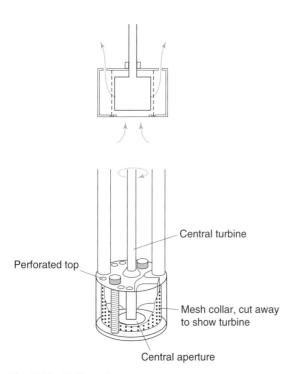

Fig. 12.15 Turbine mixer.

with the perforations pointing upwards can be fitted if this is desired. As the liquid is forced through the small orifices of the diffuser rings at high velocity, large shear forces are produced. When mixing immiscible liquids, if the orifices are sufficiently small and velocity sufficiently high, the shear forces produced enable the generation of droplets of the dispersed phase which are small enough to produce stable dispersions (water-in-oil or oil-in-water). Turbine mixers of this type are therefore often fitted to vessels used for the large-scale production of emulsions and creams (described in Chapter 46).

Turbine-type mixes will not cope with liquids of very high viscosity since the material will not be drawn into the mixer head. These liquids are best treated as semi-solids and handled in the same equipment as used for such materials.

In-line mixers

As an alternative to mixing fluids in batches in vessels, mobile miscible components may be fed through an 'in-line' mixer designed to create turbulence in a flowing fluid stream. In this case, a continuous mixing process is possible.

MIXING OF SEMI-SOLIDS

The problems that arise during the mixing of semi-solids (ointments and pastes) stem from the fact that, unlike liquids, semi-solids will not flow easily. Material that finds its way to a 'dead spot' will remain there. For this reason, suitable mixers must have rotating elements with narrow clearances between themselves and the mixing vessel wall and they must produce a high degree of shear mixing since diffusion and convective mixing cannot occur.

Mixers for semi-solids

Planetary mixers

This type of mixer is commonly found in the domestic kitchen (e.g. Kenwood type mixers) and larger machines which operate on the same principle are used in the pharmaceutical industry (shown in Fig. 12.11).

When used for the mixing of semi-solids, they are designed so that there is only a small clearance between the vessel and the paddle in order to ensure sufficient shear. However, 'scraping down' of the bowl is usually necessary several times during a run to mix the contents well since some materials are forced to the top of the bowl.

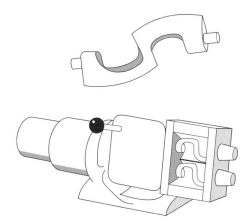

Fig. 12.16 Sigma blade mixer.

Sigma blade mixers

This robust mixer will deal with stiff pastes and ointments and depends for its action on the close intermeshing of the two blades which resemble the Greek letter Σ in shape – hence the name. The clearance between the blades and the mixing trough is kept small by the design shown in Figure 12.16.

It is very difficult, using primary mixers, to completely disperse powder particles in a semi-solid base so that they are invisible to the eye. The mix is usually subjected to the further action of a roller mill or colloid mill so as to 'rub out' these particles by the intense shear generated by rollers or cones set with a very small clearance between them.

REFERENCES

Garcia, T.P., Elsheimer, B., Tarczynski, F. (1995) Examination of components of variance for a production scale, low dose powder blend and resulting tablets. *Drug Development and Industrial Pharmacy*, **21**(18), 2035-2045.

Nikolakakis, N., Newton, M. (1989) Solid state adsorption of antibiotics onto sorbitol. *Journal of Pharmacy and Pharmacology*, **41**, 145.

Travers, D. N., White, R. C. (1971) The mixing of micronized sodium bicarbonate with sucrose crystals. *Journal of Pharmacy and Pharmacology*, **23**(12), 260S–261S.

Venables, H.J., Wells, J.I. (2001) Powder mixing. *Drug Development and Industrial Pharmacy*, **27**(7), 599.

BIBLIOGRAPHY

Harnby, N., Nienow, A.W., Edwards, M.F. (1997) *Mixing in the Process Industries*. Butterworth-Heinemann, Oxford.

Kaye, B.H. (1997) *Powder Mixing*. Chapman and Hall, London.

Miyanam, I.K. (1991) Mixing. In: Linoya, K., Gotoh, K., Higashitani, K. (eds) *Powder Technology Handbook*. Marcel Dekker, New York.

Rothman, H. (1981) High speed mixing in the pharmaceutical industry. *Manufacturing Chemist and Aerosol News*, **52**(4), 47-49.

Rumpf, H. (1990) *Particle Technology*. Chapman and Hall, London.

Staniforth, J.N. (1982) Advances in powder mixing and segregation in relation to pharmaceutical processing. *International Journal of Pharmaceutical Technology and Product Manufacture*, **3**(Suppl), 1-12.

Williams, J.C. (1990) Mixing and segregation of powders. In: Rhodes, M.J. (ed.) *Principles of Powder Technology*. John Wiley, Chichester.

13

Powder flow

J. N. Staniforth, M. E. Aulton

INTRODUCTION

Powders are generally considered to be composed of solid particles of the same or different chemical compositions having equivalent diameters less than 1000 μm. However, the term 'powder' will also be used here to describe groups of particles formed into granules which may have overall dimensions greater than 1000 μm.

The largest pharmaceutical use of powders is to produce tablets and capsules. Together with mixing and compaction properties, the flowability of a powder is of critical importance in the production of pharmaceutical dosage forms. Some of the reasons for producing free-flowing pharmaceutical powders include:

- uniform feed from bulk storage containers or hoppers into the feed mechanisms of tableting or capsule-filling equipment, allowing uniform particle packing and a constant volume-to-mass ratio which maintains tablet weight uniformity
- reproducible filling of tablet dies and capsule dosators, which improves weight uniformity and allows tablets to be produced with more consistent physicomechanical properties
- uneven powder flow can result in excess entrapped air within powders, which in some high-speed tableting conditions may promote capping or lamination
- uneven powder flow can result from excess fine particles in a powder, which increase particle–die-wall friction, causing lubrication problems, and increase dust contamination risks during powder transfer.

There are many industrial processes that require powders to be moved from one location to another and this is achieved by many different methods, such as gravity feeding, mechanically assisted feeding, pneumatic transfer, fluidization in gases and liquids and hydraulic transfer. In each of these examples powders are required to flow and, as with other operations described earlier, the efficiency with which they do so is dependent on both process design and particle properties.

PARTICLE PROPERTIES

Adhesion and cohesion

The presence of molecular forces produces a tendency for solid particles to stick to themselves and to other surfaces. Adhesion and cohesion can be considered as two parts of the same phenomenon: cohesion occurs between like surfaces, such as component particles of a bulk solid, whereas adhesion occurs between two unlike surfaces, for example between a particle and a hopper wall.

Cohesive forces acting between particles in a powder bed are composed mainly from short-range non-specific van der Waals forces which increase as particle size decreases and vary with changes in relative humidity. Other attractive forces contributing to interparticulate cohesion may be produced by surface tensional forces between adsorbed liquid layers at the particle surfaces and electrostatic forces arising from contact or frictional charging, which may have short half-lives but increase cohesion through improving interparticulate contacts and hence increasing the quantity of van der Waals interactions. Cohesion provides a useful method of characterizing the drag or frictional forces acting within a powder bed to prevent powder flow.

Measurement of adhesive/cohesive properties

Adhesive/cohesive forces acting between a single pair of particles or a particle and substrate surface can be accurately determined using a specially adapted ultracentrifuge to apply very high forces strong enough to separate the two surfaces. However, it is more usual when studying powder flow to characterize adhesion/cohesion in a bed of powder.

Shear strength   Cohesion can be defined as the stress (force per unit area) necessary to shear a powder bed under conditions of zero normal load. Using this criterion, the shear strength of a powder can be determined

from the resistance to flow caused by cohesion or friction and can be measured using a shear cell.

The shear cell (Fig. 13.1) is a relatively simple piece of apparatus which is designed to measure shear stress, τ, at different values of normal stress, σ. There are several types of shear cell, such as the Jenike and the Portishead, which use different methods of applying the stresses and measuring the shear strengths. In order to carry out a shear strength determination, powder is packed into the two halves of the cell and a normal stress is applied to the lid of the assembled cell. A shearing stress across the two halves of the cell is applied and the shear stress is determined by dividing the shear force by the cross-sectional area of the powder bed. The measured shear stress will increase as the normal stress is increased.

In order to calculate the cohesion in a powder bed using the shear cell method, the shear stress is extrapolated back to zero normal stress, as the shear stress at zero normal stress is, by definition, equal to the cohesion of the powder. For a non-cohesive powder, the extrapolated shear stress will pass through the origin, equivalent to zero shear stress.

Tensile strength   The tensile strength of a powder bed is a characteristic of the internal friction or cohesion of the particles. In tensile strength determinations, the powder bed is caused to fail in tension by splitting, rather than failing in shear by sliding, as is the case with shear strength determinations. The powder is packed into a split plate, one half of which is fixed and the other half free to move (Fig. 13.2). The table is then tilted towards the vertical until the angle is reached at which the powder cohesion is overcome and the mobile half-plate breaks away from the static half-plate. The tensile strength, σ_t, of the powder can then be determined from Eqn 13.1:

$$\sigma_t = \frac{Mg \sin \theta}{A} \qquad (13.1)$$

where M is the mass of the mobile half-plate + powder, θ the angle of the tilted table to the horizontal at the point of failure and A is the cross-sectional area of the powder bed.

The tensile strength values of different powders have been found to correlate reasonably well with another measurement of powder cohesion – angle of repose.

Angle of repose   An object, such as a particle, will begin to slide when the angle of inclination is large

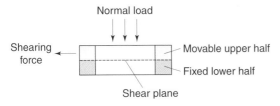

Fig. 13.1   Diagrammatic representation of Jenike shear cell.

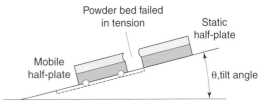

Fig. 13.2   Measurement of tensile strength of a powder bed using tilting table method.

enough to overcome frictional forces. Conversely, an object in motion will stop sliding when the angle of inclination is below that required to overcome adhesion/cohesion. This balance of forces causes a powder poured from a container on to a horizontal surface to form a heap. Initially the particles stack until the approach angle for subsequent particles joining the stack is large enough to overcome friction. They then slip and roll over each other until the gravitational forces balance the interparticulate forces. The sides of the heap formed in this way make an angle with the horizontal which is called the angle of repose and is a characteristic of the internal friction or cohesion of the particles.

The value of the angle of repose will be high if the powder is cohesive and low if the powder is non-cohesive. If the powder is very cohesive, the heap may be characterized by more than one angle of repose. Initially the interparticulate cohesion causes a very steep cone to form but, on the addition of further powder, this tall stack may suddenly collapse, causing air to be entrained between particles and partially fluidizing the bed, thus making it more mobile. The resulting heap has two angles of repose: a large angle remaining from the initial heap and a shallower angle formed by the powder flooding from the initial heap (Fig. 13.3).

In order to overcome this problem, it has been suggested that determinations of angles of repose be carried out using different concentrations of very cohesive powders and non-cohesive powders. The angles of repose are plotted against mixture concentration and extrapolated to 100% cohesive powder content so as to obtain the appropriate angle of repose (Fig. 13.4).

Particle properties and bulk flow

In the discussion concerning adhesion/cohesion it is clear that an equilibrium exists between forces responsible for

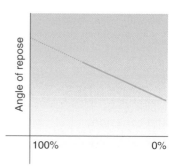

Fig. 13.4 Determination of angle of repose for very cohesive powders.

promoting powder flow and those preventing powder flow, i.e. at equilibrium:

$$\Sigma f(\text{driving forces}) = \Sigma f(\text{drag forces}) \qquad (13.2)$$

that is:

Σf(gravitational force, particle mass, angle of inclination of powder bed, static head of powder, mechanical force ...) = Σf(adhesive forces, cohesive forces, other surface forces, mechanical interlocking...) (13.3)

Some of these forces are modified or controlled by external factors related to particle properties, such as size, shape and density.

Particle size effects

Because cohesion and adhesion are phenomena that occur at surfaces, particle size will influence the flowability of a powder. In general, fine particles with very high surface-to-mass ratios are more cohesive than coarser particles which are influenced more by gravitational forces. Particles larger than 250 μm are usually relatively free flowing but as the size falls below 100 μm, powders become cohesive and flow problems are likely to occur. Powders having a particle size less than 10 μm are usually extremely cohesive and resist flow under gravity, except possibly as large agglomerates.

Particle shape

Powders with similar particle sizes but dissimilar shapes can have markedly different flow properties owing to differences in interparticulate contact areas. For example, a group of spheres has minimum interparticulate contact and generally optimal flow properties, whereas a group of particle flakes or dendritic particles has a very high surface-to-volume ratio and poorer flow properties.

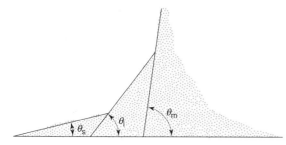

Fig. 13.3 Cohesive powder poured in a heap and showing different angles of repose: θ_m maximum angle formed by cohesive particles θ_s shallowest angle formed by collapse of cohesive particle heap, resulting in flooding. In some cases a third angle, θ_i is identifiable as an intermediate slope produced by cohesive particles stacking on flooded powder.

Particle density (true density)

Because powders normally flow under the influence of gravity, dense particles are generally less cohesive than less dense particles of the same size and shape.

Packing geometry

A set of particles can be filled into a volume of space to produce a powder bed which is in static equilibrium owing to the interaction of gravitational and adhesive/cohesive forces. By slight vibration of the bed, particles can be mobilized so that if the vibration is stopped, the bed is once more in static equilibrium but occupies a different spatial volume than before. The change in bulk volume has been produced by rearrangement of the packing geometry of the particles. In general, such geometric rearrangements result in a transition from loosely packed particles to more tightly packed ones, so that the equilibrium balance moves from left to right in Eqn 13.2 and cohesion increases. This also means that more tightly packed powders require a higher driving force to produce powder flow than more loosely packed particles of the same powder.

Characterization of packing geometry by porosity and bulk density

A set of monosized spherical particles can be arranged in many different geometric configurations. At one extreme, when the spheres form a cubic arrangement, the particles are most loosely packed and have a porosity of 48% (Fig. 13.5a). At the other extreme, when the spheres form a rhombohedral arrangement, they are most densely packed and have a porosity of only 26% (Fig. 13.5b). The porosity used to characterize packing geometry is linked to the bulk density of the powder. Bulk density, ρ_B, is a characteristic of a powder rather than individual particles and is given by the mass, M, of powder occupying a known volume, V, according to the relationship:

$$\rho_B = \frac{M}{V} \, kgm^{-3} \qquad (13.4)$$

The bulk density of a powder is always less than the true density of its component particles because the powder contains interparticulate pores or voids. This statement reveals that whereas a powder can only possess a single true density, it can have many different bulk densities, depending on the way in which the particles are packed and the bed porosity. However, a high bulk density value does not necessarily imply a close-packed low-porosity bed, as bulk density is directly proportional to true density.

bulk density α true density

i.e. bulk density = k true density   (13.5)

or:

$$k = \frac{\text{bulk density}}{\text{true density}} \qquad (13.6)$$

The constant of proportionality, k, is known as the *packing fraction* or *fractional solids content*. For example, the packing fraction for dense, randomly packed spheres is approximately 0.65, whereas the packing fraction for a set of dense, randomly packed discs is 0.83. Also:

$$1 - k = e \qquad (13.7)$$

where e is the *fractional voidage* of the powder bed, which is usually expressed as a percentage and termed the bed porosity. Another way of expressing fractional voidage is to use the ratio of particle volume V_P to bulk powder volume V_B, i.e.:

$$e = \frac{1 - V_P}{V_B} \qquad (13.8)$$

A simple ratio of void volume V_v to particle volume V_P represents the voids ratio:

$$\frac{V_v}{V_p} = \frac{e}{(1 - e)} \qquad (13.9)$$

which provides information about the stability of the powder mass.

For powders having comparable true densities, an increase in bulk density causes a decrease in porosity. This increases the number of interparticulate contacts and contact areas and causes an increase in cohesion. In very coarse particles this may still be insufficient to overcome the gravitational influence on particles. Conversely, a decrease in bulk density may be associated with a reduction in particle size and produce a loose-packed powder bed which, although porous, is unlikely to flow because of the inherent cohesiveness of the fine particles.

The use of porosity as a means of characterizing packing geometrics can sometimes be misleading. For example, monosize cubic crystals could be considered to be

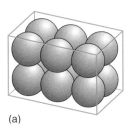
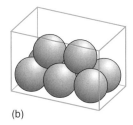

(a)   (b)

Fig. 13.5 Different geometric packings of spherical particles. (a) Cubic packing. (b) Rhombohedral packing.

loosely packed with a porosity of 20%, as the closest packed cubic arrangement would have a porosity close to 0%. By comparison, a system of spheronized crystals of the same size with a porosity of 30% could be considered to be more closely packed, as the closest packed spherical arrangement has a porosity of 26%. In this example the powder with the higher porosity is relatively more closely packed than that with the lower porosity.

In powders where the particle shape or cohesiveness promotes arch or bridge formation, two equilibrium states could have similar porosities but widely different packing geometries. In such conditions, interparticulate pore size distributions can be useful for comparing packing geometry.

For example, Figure 13.6a shows a group of particles in which arching has occurred and Figure 13.6b shows a similar group of particles in which arch formation is absent. The total porosity of the two systems can be seen to be similar but the pore size distributions (Fig. 13.7) reveal that the powder in which arch formation has occurred is generally more tightly packed than that in which arching is absent.

Factors affecting packing geometry

Particle size and size distribution Void spaces between coarse particles may become filled with finer particles in a powder with a wide size range, resulting in a more closely packed cohesive powder.

Particle shape and texture These influence the minimum porosity of the powder bed. Arches or bridges within the powder bed will be formed more readily through the interlocking of non-isometric, highly textured particles. This tendency for irregular-shaped particles to produce open structures supported by small or large powder arches causes them to have a larger difference in porosity between loose packing and tight packing geometries than more regularly shaped particles.

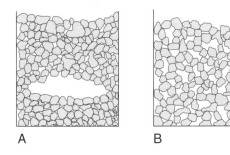

A　　　　　　　**B**

Fig. 13.6 Two equidimensional powders having the same porosity but different packing geometries.

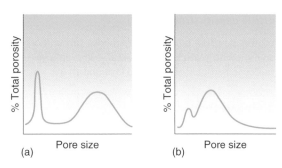

(a)　　　Pore size　　　(b)　　　Pore size

Fig. 13.7 (a) Interparticulate pore size distribution corresponding to close–packed bed containing a powder arch. (b) Interparticulate pore size distribution corresponding to loosely packed bed.

Surface properties The presence of electrostatic forces can add to interparticulate attractions and promote closer particle packing, resulting in increased cohesion.

Handling and processing conditions The way in which a powder has been handled prior to flow or packing influences the type of packing geometry.

PROCESS CONDITIONS: HOPPER DESIGN

Flow through an orifice

There are many examples of this type of flow to be found in the manufacture of pharmaceutical solid dosage forms, for example when granules or powders flow through the opening in a hopper or bin used to feed powder to tableting machines, capsule-filling machines or sachet-filling machines. Because of the importance of such flow in producing unit doses containing the same or very similar powder masses, and the importance of flow behaviour in other industries, the behaviour of particles being fed through orifices has been extensively studied.

A hopper or bin can be modelled as a tall cylindrical container having a closed orifice in the base and initially full of a free-flowing powder which has a horizontal upper surface (Fig. 13.8a). When the orifice at the base of the container is opened, flow patterns develop as the powder discharges (Fig. 13.8a–f).

The observed sequence is as follows:

1. On opening the orifice, there is no instantaneous movement at the surface but particles just above the orifice fall freely through it (Fig. 13.8b).
2. A depression forms at the upper surface and spreads outwards to the sides of the hopper (Fig. 13.8c, d).

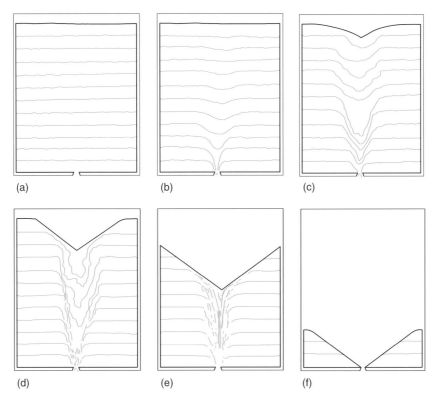

Fig. 13.8 Development of flow through an orifice. The horizontal lines are formed by indicator particles to show the course of the discharge.

3. Provided that the container is tall and not too narrow, the flow pattern illustrated in Figure13.8e and shown schematically in Figure 13.9 is rapidly established. Particles in zone A move rapidly over the slower moving particles in zone B, whereas those in zone E remain stationary. The particles in zone A feed into zone C, where they move quickly downwards and out through the orifice. The more slowly moving particles in zone B do not enter zone C.

4. Both powder streams in zones B and C converge to a 'tongue' just above the orifice, where the movement is most rapid and the particle packing is least dense. In a zone just above the orifice, the particles are in free flight.

Important practical consequences of this flow pattern are that if a square-bottomed hopper or bin is repeatedly refilled and partially emptied, the particles in a zone towards the base and sides of the container (Fig. 13.8f) will not be discharged and may degrade. Alternatively, this static zone may provide a segregation potential for previously homogeneous powders.

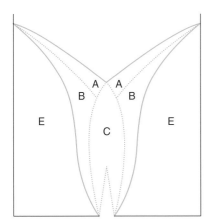

Fig. 13.9 Fully developed flow of a free-flowing powder through an orifice.

Factors affecting flow rates through orifices

The flow patterns described above, together with powder flow rates through orifices, are dependent on many different factors, some of which are particle related and some process related. Particle-related effects, notably particle size, are discussed above. Process-related effects include the following.

Orifice diameter Flow rate is directly proportional to $D_o{}^A$. The rate of powder flow through an orifice is proportional to a function of orifice diameter, D_o. A is a constant with a value of approximately 2.6. Provided that the height of the powder bed, called the head of powder, remains considerably greater than the orifice diameter, flow rate is virtually independent of powder head. This situation is unlike that relating to liquid flow through an orifice, where the flow rate falls off continuously as the head diminishes. The constant rate of flow for powders is a useful property as it means that if a bulk powder is filled into dies, sachets, capsules or other enclosures, they will receive equal weights if filled for equal times.

Hopper width At different positions within a powder bed, the consolidating stresses and shear or tensile strengths are different (Fig. 13.10b). If the bed strength at a given point in the hopper is great enough to resist the driving forces promoting flow, then a stable arch will be formed. At all other points in the powder, the bed strength will not be high enough to support an arch against the stresses within it, and flow will occur. The stresses acting on a stable arch are proportional to the width of the container and vary with diameter, as exemplified in Figure 13.10a, b. The relationship between the stress on the arch and the arch strength, resulting in part from consolidating pressures at different points in the hopper (Fig. 13.10c), shows that with the exception of a region close to the hopper outlet and another at the point where the cylindrical section meets the conical section of the hopper, powder arches are weaker than the stresses on them. This suggests that powder flow will occur in all other regions (Fig. 13.10d) and allows the hopper design to be adjusted so that the minimum hopper widths are always large enough to produce arch stresses greater than

arch strengths, and thereby ensure continuous, uniform powder flow.

Head size Figure 13.10b shows the way in which pressure within the powder changes with powder head size (powder depth). The pressure below the upper free surface increases to a constant governed by frictional factors. The pressure again falls off towards the hopper outlet and drops below atmospheric at the orifice, causing air to be drawn up into the region close to the base so as to equalize this negative pressure and allow flow to continue.

Hopper wall angle It was noted above, in the description of flow through an orifice, that a flat-bottomed bin retains a certain volume of powder in the form of a drained cone centred on the orifice. In order to prevent this behaviour and to ensure that all the powder is discharged from a hopper, the walls are frequently angled inwards as the outlet is approached. The wall angle that is required to ensure that powder empties freely is determined by the particle–wall adhesion component of friction within powders, and is characterized by a wall-friction angle, ϕ. Powders with very low wall-friction angles will empty freely, even from hoppers with very shallow slopes, whereas powders with very high wall-friction angles will empty poorly even from steep-walled hoppers. In between these two extremes, powder discharge characteristics will be determined by the relationship between wall friction and hopper angle, as shown in Figure 13.11.

Mass flow and funnel flow

Powder that discharges freely from a hopper is said to undergo mass flow when particles that enter the hopper first leave it first. This first-in-first-out sequence holds throughout the bed, so that powder can be considered to leave in near-horizontal bands which move down the hopper en masse (Fig. 13.12a).

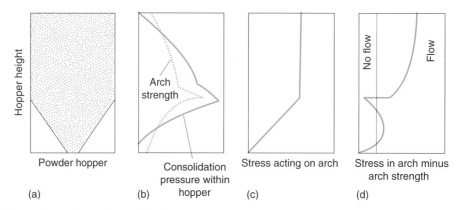

Fig. 13.10 Influence of stress interactions within a hopper on powder flow.

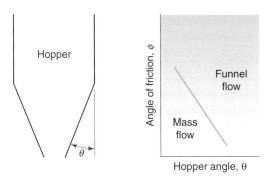

Fig. 13.11 Influence of hopper wall angle and particle–wall friction on powder flow.

Powders that do not discharge freely, due to either high adhesion/cohesion or hopper angles that are too shallow, may undergo funnel flow (Fig. 13.12b). Particles which are loaded into the hopper last are among the first to leave, forming a 'pipe', 'rat-hole' or 'funnel', extending from the upper free powder surface to the hopper outlet and producing uneven erratic flow. Another problem associated with funnel flow may occur when the rat-hole collapses. This produces a sudden rapid discharge of powder which can entrain relatively large volumes of air, causing the particles to partially fluidize and flood out of the hopper. This 'flooding' or 'flushing' may be succeeded by periods when the bed is quiescent and flow is slow or interrupted.

In general, most powders will discharge by mass flow from hoppers with θ angles of about 20°, and by funnel flow from hoppers with angles of approximately 50°.

Mass flow rate

Throughout this section it has been shown that specific particle properties and individual design criteria influence powder flow. However, in a given practical situation powder flowability is the resultant of the relative influ-

ences of all these factors. An equation has been derived which relates some particulate properties, such as bulk density, ρ_B, and angle of repose, α, and hopper design criteria such as orifice diameter, D_o, and a discharge coefficient, C, to mass flow rate of powder, M:

$$M = \pi/4 \; C\rho_B \; [(g \; D_o^5)/2 \tan \alpha]^{1/2} \qquad (13.10)$$

where g is the acceleration due to gravity.

CHARACTERIZATION OF POWDER FLOW

When examining the flow properties of a powder, it is useful to be able to quantify the type of behaviour in terms of speed and (possibly more importantly) uniformity of flow. Many different methods are available, either directly, using dynamic or kinetic methods, or indirectly, generally by measurements carried out on static beds. A wide range of equipment is available to cater for the wide range of powder types and particle sizes encountered in pharmaceutical applications. The apparatus and techniques described below are illustrative of the principles on which most equipment is based.

Indirect methods

Angle of repose

Angles of repose have been used as indirect methods of quantifying powder flowability, because of their relationship with interparticulate cohesion. There are many different methods of determining angles of repose and some of these are shown in Table 13.1. The different methods may produce different values for the same powder, although these may be self-consistent. It is also possible that different angles of repose could be obtained for the same powder, owing to differences in the way the samples were handled prior to measurement. For these reasons, angles of repose tend to be variable and are not always representative of flow under specific conditions.

As a general guide, powders with angles of repose greater than 50° have unsatisfactory flow properties, whereas minimum angles close to 25° correspond to very good flow properties.

Bulk density measurements

The bulk density of a powder is dependent on particle packing and changes as the powder consolidates. A consolidated powder is likely to have a greater arch strength than a less consolidated one and may therefore be more resistant to powder flow. The ease with which a powder consolidates can be used as an indirect method of quantifying powder flow.

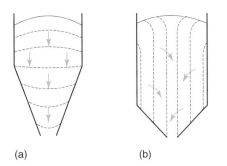

(a)   (b)

Fig. 13.12 (a) Mass flow hopper. (b) Funnel flow hopper.

Table 13.1 Methods of measuring angle of repose

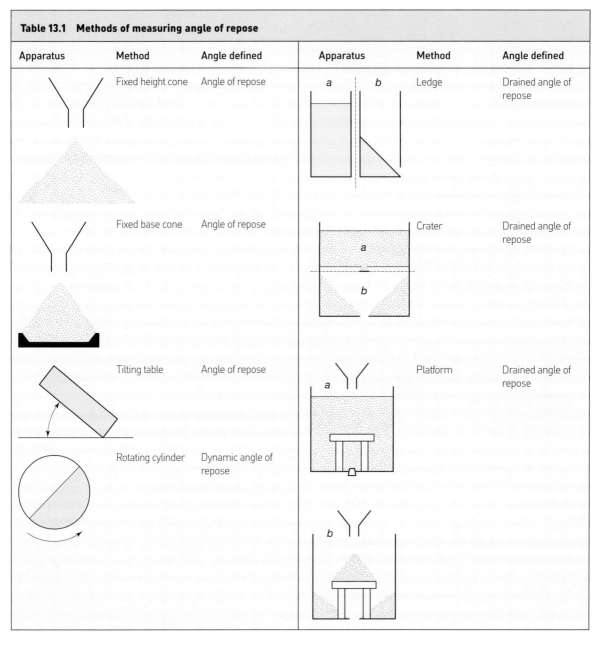

Apparatus	Method	Angle defined	Apparatus	Method	Angle defined
	Fixed height cone	Angle of repose		Ledge	Drained angle of repose
	Fixed base cone	Angle of repose		Crater	Drained angle of repose
	Tilting table	Angle of repose		Platform	Drained angle of repose
	Rotating cylinder	Dynamic angle of repose			

Figure 13.13 shows a mechanical tapping device or jolting volumeter which can be used to follow the change in packing volume that occurs when void space diminishes and consolidation occurs. The powder contained in the measuring cylinder is mechanically tapped by means of a constant velocity rotating cam and increases from an initial bulk density P_{Bmin} (also known as fluff or poured bulk density) to a final bulk density P_{Bmax} (also known as equilibrium, tapped or consoli-dated bulk density) when it has attained its most stable, i.e. unchanging, arrangement.

Hausner found that the ratio P_{Bmin}/P_{Bmax} was related to interparticulate friction and, as such, could be used to predict powder flow properties. He showed that powders with low interparticulate friction, such as coarse spheres, had ratios of approximately 1.2 whereas more cohesive, less free-flowing powders such as flakes have Hausner ratios greater than 1.6.

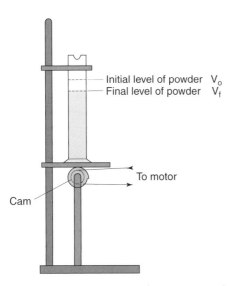

Initial level of powder V_0
Final level of powder V_f

To motor

Cam

Fig. 13.13 Mechanical tapping device (jolting volumeter).

Another indirect method of measuring powder flow from bulk densities was developed by *Carr*. The percentage compressibility of a powder (Carr's Index) is a direct measure of the potential powder arch or bridge strength and stability and is calculated according to Eqn 13.11:

$$\% \text{ compressibility} = \frac{\rho_{B\,\text{max}} - \rho_{B\,\text{min}}}{\rho_{B\,\text{max}}} \times 100 \quad (13.11)$$

Table 13.2 shows the generalized relationship between descriptions of powder flow and percent compressibility, according to Carr.

Table 13.2 Relationship between powder flowability and % compressibility

% Compressibility range	Flow description
5–15	Excellent (free-flowing granules)
12–16	Good (free-flowing powdered granules)
18–21	Fair (powdered granules)
23–28	Poor (very fluid powders)
28–35	Poor (fluid cohesive powders)
35–38	Very poor (fluid cohesive powders)
>40	Extremely poor (cohesive powders

Critical orifice diameter

In order to carry out measurements of critical orifice diameter, powder is filled into a shallow tray to a uniform depth with near-uniform packing. The base of the tray is perforated with a graduated series of holes, which are blocked either by resting the tray on a plane surface or by the presence of a simple shutter. The critical orifice diameter is the size of the smallest hole through which powder discharges when the tray is lifted or the shutter removed. Sometimes repetition of the experiment produces different critical orifice diameters, and in these cases maximum and minimum values are sometimes quoted.

Critical orifice diameter is a direct measure of powder cohesion and arch strength since:

$$\tan \alpha = \frac{r}{x} \quad (13.12)$$

where r is the particle radius and x is the orifice radius, and:

$$\tan \theta_F = \frac{\tan \phi}{1 - \tan \phi \frac{r}{x} - \frac{r^2}{x^2}} \quad (13.13)$$

where θ_F is the angle of form, which is the obtuse angle between the contracting powder dome and the horizontal, and tan ϕ is a coefficient of friction.

An alternative critical orifice method for determining powder flowability uses a cylinder with a series of interchangeable base plate discs having different diameter orifices. Using this system, flowability indices related to orifice diameters have been used as a method of specifying materials for use in filling given capsule sizes or producing particular tablet sizes at a specified rate.

Direct methods

Hopper flow rate

The simplest method of determining powder flowability directly is to measure the rate at which powder discharges from a hopper. A simple shutter is placed over the hopper outlet and the hopper is filled with powder. The shutter is then removed and the time taken for the powder to discharge completely is recorded. By dividing the discharged powder mass by this time, a flow rate is obtained which can be used for quantitative comparison of different powders.

Hopper or discharge tube outlets should be selected to provide a good model for a particular flow application. For example, if a powder discharges well from a hopper into a tablet machine feed frame but does not flow reproducibly into the tablet die, then it is likely that more useful information will be generated by selecting experimental conditions to model those occurring in flow from the feeder to the die rather than those in flow from the hopper to the feeder.

Recording flowmeter

A recording flowmeter is essentially similar to the method described above except that powder is allowed to discharge from a hopper or container onto a balance. The digital signal from the balance records the increase in powder mass with time. Recording flowmeters allow mass flow rates to be determined and also provide a means of quantifying uniformity of flow.

IMPROVEMENT OF POWDER FLOWABILITY

Alteration of particle size and size distribution

Because coarse particles are generally less cohesive than fine particles and an optimum size for free flow exists, there is a distinct disadvantage in using a finer grade of powder than is necessary.

The size distribution can also be altered to improve flowability by removing a proportion of the fine particle fraction or by increasing the proportion of coarser particles, such as occurs through granulation.

Alteration of particle shape or texture

In general, for a given particle size, more spherical particles have better flow properties than more irregular particles. The process of spray-drying can be used to produce near-spherical excipients, for example spray-dried lactose. Under certain circumstances, drug particles that are normally acicular can be made more spherical by spray drying or by temperature-cycling crystallization.

The surface texture of particles may also influence powder flowability, as particles with very rough surfaces will be more cohesive and have a greater tendency to interlock than smooth-surfaced particles. The shape and texture of particles can also be altered by control of production methods, such as crystallization conditions.

Alteration of surface forces

Reduction of electrostatic charges can improve powder flowability and this can be achieved by altering process conditions to reduce frictional contacts. For example, where powder is poured down chutes or conveyed along pipes pneumatically, the speed and length of transportation should be minimized. Electrostatic charges in pow-

der containers can be prevented or discharged by efficient earth connections.

The moisture content of particles is also of importance to powder flowability, as adsorbed surface moisture films tend to increase bulk density and reduce porosity. In cases where moisture content is excessive, powders should be dried and, if hygroscopic, stored and processed under low-humidity conditions.

Formulation additives: flow activators

Flow activators are commonly referred to pharmaceutically as 'glidants', although some also have lubricant or antiadherent properties. Flow activators improve the flowability of powders by reducing adhesion and cohesion.

A flow activator with an exceptionally high specific surface area is colloidal silicon dioxide, which may act by reducing the bulk density of tightly packed powders. Colloidal silicon dioxide also improves flowability of formulations, even those containing other glidants, although in some cases it can cause flooding.

Where powder flowability is impaired through increased moisture content, a small proportion of very fine magnesium oxide may be used as a flow activator. Used in this way, magnesium oxide appears to disrupt the continuous film of adsorbed water surrounding the moist particles.

The use of silicone-treated powder, such as silicone-coated talc or sodium bicarbonate, may also be beneficial in improving the flowability of moist or hygroscopic powder.

Alteration of process conditions

Use of vibration-assisted hoppers

In cases where the powder arch strength within a bin or hopper is greater than the stresses in it due to gravitational effects, powder flow will be interrupted or prevented. If the hopper cannot be redesigned to provide adequate downward stresses and if the physical properties of the particles cannot be adjusted or the formulation altered, then extreme measures are required. One method of encouraging powder flow where arching or bridging has occurred within a hopper is to add to the stresses due to gravitational interactions by vibrating the hopper mechanically. Both the amplitude and the frequency of vibration can be altered to produce the desired effect, and may vary from a single cycle or shock, produced by a compressed-air device or hammer, to higher frequencies produced, for example, by out-of-balance electric motors mounted on a hopper frame.

Use of force feeders

The flow of powders that discharge irregularly or flood out of hoppers can be improved by fitting vibrating baffles, known as live-bottom feeders, at the base of the conical section within a hopper.

The outflowing stream from a hopper can be encouraged to move towards its required location using a slightly sloping moving belt or, in the case of some tableting machines, the use of mechanical force feeders. Force feeders are usually made up of a single or two counter-rotating paddles at the base of the hopper just above the die table in place of a feed frame. The paddles presumably act by preventing powder arching over dies and thereby improve die filling, especially at high turret speeds.

SUMMARY

In most pharmaceutical technology operations, it is difficult to alter one process without adversely influencing another. In the case of alterations made in order to improve powder flow, relative particle motion will be promoted and can lead to demixing or segregation. In extreme cases, improving powder flow to improve weight uniformity may reduce content uniformity through increased segregation.

BIBLIOGRAPHY

Gotoh, K., Masuda, H., Higashitan, K. (1997) *Powder Technology Handbook*, 2nd edn. Marcel Dekker, New York.

Lieberman, H. (1996) *Pharmaceutical Dosage Forms: Disperse Systems*, vol 2, 2nd edn. Marcel Dekker, New York.

Lieberman, H. (1998) *Pharmaceutical Dosage Forms: Disperse Systems*, vol 3, 2nd edn. Marcel Dekker, New York.

Lieberman, H., Lachman, L., Schwartz, J.B. (1990) *Pharmaceutical Dosage Forms: Tablets*, vol 2, 2nd edn. Marcel Dekker, New York.

McNaughton, K. (ed.) (1981) *Solids Handling*. McGraw-Hill, New York.

Rhodes, M. (1990) *Principles of Powder Technology*. John Wiley, Chichester.

Sadek, H.M., Olsen, J.L., Smith, H.L., Onay, S. (1982) A systematic approach to glidant selection. *Pharmaceutical Technology*, **6**(Feb.), 42-44, 46, 50, 52, 54, 56, 59-60, 62.

Niazi, S.K. (ed.) (2004) *Handbook of Pharmaceutical Manufacturing Formulations: volume 2 Uncompressed Solid Products, Part V. Powder Flow Properties*. CRC Press, Boca Raton, Florida.

Shahinpoor, M. (ed.) (1983) *Advances in the Mechanics and the Flow of Granular Materials*, vols 1 and 2. Gulf Publishing, Houston.

Singley, M.E., Chaplin, R.V. (1982) Flow of particulate materials. *Transactions of the American Society of Agricultural Engineers*, **25**, 1360-1373.

Swarbrick, J., Boylan, J.C. (2002) *Encyclopedia of Pharmaceutical Technology*. Marcel Dekker, New York.

Taubmann, H.J. (1982) The influence of flow activators on the flow behaviour of powders. *Aufbereitungs-Technik*, **23**, 423-428.

PART 3

PHARMACEUTICAL MICROBIOLOGY AND STERILIZATION

14

Fundamentals of microbiology

G. W. Hanlon

INTRODUCTION

Microorganisms are ubiquitous in nature and are vital components in the cycle of life. The majority are free-living organisms growing on dead or decaying matter whose prime function is the turnover of organic materials in the environment. Pharmaceutical microbiology, however, is concerned with the relatively small group of biological agents that cause human disease, spoil prepared medicines or can be used to produce compounds of medical interest.

In order to understand microorganisms more fully, living organisms of similar characteristics have been grouped together into taxonomic units. The most fundamental division is between prokaryotic and eukaryotic cells, which differ in a number of respects (Table 14.1) but particularly in the arrangement of their nuclear material. Eukaryotic cells contain chromosomes, which are separate from the cytoplasm and contained within a limiting nuclear membrane, i.e. they possess a true nucleus. Prokaryotic cells do not possess a true nucleus and their nuclear material is free within the cytoplasm, although it may be aggregated into discrete areas called nuclear bodies. Prokaryotic organisms make up the lower forms of life and include Eubacteria and Archaeobacteria. Eukaryotic cell types embrace all the higher forms of life, of which only the fungi will be dealt with in this chapter.

One characteristic shared by all microorganisms is the fact that they are small; however, it is a philosophical argument whether all infectious agents can be regarded as living. Some are little more than simple chemical entities incapable of any free-living existence. Viroids, for example, are small circular, single-stranded RNA molecules not complexed with protein. One particularly well-studied viroid has only 359 nucleotides (one-10th the size of the smallest known virus) and yet causes a disease in potatoes. Prions are small, self-replicating proteins devoid of any nucleic acid. The prion associated with Creutzfeld–Jakob disease in humans, scrapie in sheep and bovine spongiform encephalitis in cattle has only 250 amino acids and is highly resistant to inactivation by normal sterilization procedures.

Viruses are more complex than viroids or prions, possessing both protein and nucleic acid. Despite being among the most dangerous infectious agents known, they are still not regarded as living. Table 14.2 shows the major groups of viruses infecting humans.

VIRUSES

Viruses are obligate intracellular parasites with no intrinsic metabolic activity, being devoid of ribosomes and energy-producing enzyme systems. They are thus incapable of leading an independent existence and cannot be cultivated on cell-free media, no matter how nutritious. The size of human viruses ranges from the largest poxviruses, measuring about 300 nm, to the picornaviruses, such as the poliovirus which is approximately 20 nm. When one considers that a bacterial coccus measures 1000 nm in diameter, it can be appreciated that only the very largest virus particles may be seen under the light microscope, and electron microscopy is required for visualizing the majority. It will also be apparent that few of these viruses are large enough to be retained on the (0.2 μm) membrane filters used to sterilize thermolabile liquids.

Viruses consist of a core of nucleic acid (either DNA as in vaccinia virus or RNA as in poliovirus) surrounded by a protein shell or capsid. Most DNA viruses have linear, double-stranded DNA but in the case of the parvovirus it is single stranded. The majority of RNA-containing viruses contain one molecule of single-stranded RNA, although in reoviruses it is double stranded. The protein capsid comprises 50–90% of the weight of the virus and, as nucleic acid can only synthesize approximately 10% its own weight of protein, the capsid must be made up of a number of identical protein molecules. These individual protein units are called capsomeres and are not in themselves symmetrical but are arranged around the nucleic acid core in characteristic symmetrical patterns. Additionally, many of the larger viruses possess a lipoprotein envelope surrounding the

Table 14.1 Differences between prokaryotic and eukaryotic organisms		
Structure	Prokaryotes	Eukaryotes
Cell wall structure	Usually contains peptidoglycan	Peptidoglycan absent
Nuclear membrane	Absent	Present. Possess a true nucleus
Nucleolus	Absent	Present
Number of chromosome	One	More than one
Mitochondria	Absent	Present
Mesosomes	Present	Absent
Ribosomes	70S	80S

Table 14.2   The major groups of viruses that infect humans

Family	Capsid	Nucleic acid	Envelope	Example
Adenoviridae	Icosahedral	dsDNA	No	Human adenovirus
Arenaviridae	Helical	ssRNA	Yes	Lassa fever virus
Flaviviridae	Icosahedral	ssRNA	Yes	Yellow fever virus
				Hepatitis C virus
Hepadnaviridae	Icosahedral	dsDNA	No	Hepatitis B virus
Herpesviridae	Icosahedral	dsDNA	Yes	Herpes simplex virus
				Cytomegalovirus
				Varicella zoster virus
Orthomyxoviridae	Helical	ssRNA	Yes	Influenza virus
Papoviridae	Icosahedral	dsDNA	No	Papillomavirus
Paramyxoviridae	Helical	ssRNA	Yes	Respiratory syncytial virus
				Measles virus
				Mumps virus
Picornaviridae	Icosahedral	ssRNA	No	Rhinovirus
				Poliovirus
				Coxsackie virus
Poxviridae	Complex	dsDNA	Yes	Molluscum contagiosum
				Vaccinia virus
				Variola virus
Reoviridae	Icosahedral	dsRNA	No	Rotavirus
				Colorado tick fever virus
Retroviridae	Icosahedral	ssRNA	Yes	HIV
Rhabdoviridae	Helical	ssRNA	Yes	Rabies virus
Togaviridae	Icosahedral	ssRNA	Yes	Rubella virus

capsid arising from the membranes within the host cell. In many instances the membranes are virus modified to produce projections outwards from the envelope, such as haemagglutinins or neuraminidase. The enveloped viruses are often called ether sensitive, as ether and other organic solvents may dissolve the membrane.

The arrangement of the capsomeres can be of a number of types.

- Helical – the classic example is tobacco mosaic virus (TMV), which resembles a hollow tube with capsomeres arranged in a helix around the central nucleic acid core. Other examples include mumps and influenza virus.
- Icosahedral – these often resemble spheres on cursory examination but when studied more closely, they are seen to be made up of icosahedra that have 20 triangular faces, each containing an identical number of capsomeres. Examples include the poliovirus and adenovirus.
- Complex – the poxviruses and bacterial viruses (bacteriophages) make up a group whose members have a geometry that is individual and complex.

Reproduction of viruses

Because viruses have no intrinsic metabolic capability, they require the functioning of the host cell machinery in order to manufacture and assemble new virus particles. It is this intimate association between the virus and its host that makes the treatment of viral infections so complex. Any chemotherapeutic approach which damages the virus will almost inevitably cause injury to the host cells and hence lead to side-effects. An understanding of the life cycle of the virus is vital in determining suitable target sites for antiviral chemotherapy. The replication of viruses within host cells can be broken down into a number of stages.

Adsorption to host cell

The first step in the infection process involves virus adsorption on to the host cell. This usually occurs via an interaction between protein or glycoprotein moieties on the virus surface with specific receptors on the host cell outer membrane. Different cells possess receptors for different viruses. For example, the AIDS virus (HIV) possesses two proteins involved in adsorption to

T lymphocytes and these are known as gp41 and gp120. The viral protein gp120 binds to a receptor called CD4 on the T lymphocyte membrane and gp41 binds to a second receptor called fusin or CXCR4. Both attachments are necessary for infection and lead to conformational changes in the HIV envelope proteins, resulting in membrane fusion.

Penetration

Enveloped viruses fuse the viral membrane with the host cell membrane and release the nucleocapsid directly into the cytoplasm. Naked virions generally penetrate the cell by phagocytosis. Bacteriophages are viruses which specifically attack bacteria and these inject their DNA into the host cell while the rest of the virus remains on the outside.

Uncoating

In this stage the capsid is removed as a result of attack by cellular proteases and this releases the nucleic acid into the cytoplasm. These first three stages are similar for both DNA and RNA viruses.

Nucleic acid and protein synthesis

The detailed mechanisms by which DNA- and RNA-containing viruses replicate inside the cell are outside the scope of this chapter and the reader is referred to the bibliography for further information. After nucleic acid replication, early viral proteins are produced, the function of which is to switch off host cell metabolic activity and direct the activities of the cell towards the synthesis of proteins necessary for the assembly of new virus particles.

Assembly of new virions

Again, there are differences in the detail of how the viruses are assembled within the host cell but construction of new virions occurs at this stage and up to 100 new virus particles may be produced per cell.

Release of virus progeny

The newly formed virus particles may be liberated from the cell as a burst, in which case the host cell ruptures and dies. Infection with influenza virus results in a lytic response. Alternatively, the virions may be released gradually from the cell by budding of the host cell plasma membrane. These are often called 'persistent' infection; an example is hepatitis B.

Latent infections

In some instances a virus may enter a cell but not go through the replicative cycle outlined above and the host cell may be unharmed. The genome of the virus is conserved and may become integrated into the host cell genome where it may be replicated along with the host DNA during cell division. At some later stage the latent virus may become reactivated and progress through a lytic phase, causing cell damage/death and the release of new virions. Examples of this type of infection are those which occur with the herpes simplex viruses associated with cold sores, genital herpes and also chickenpox where the dormant virus may reactivate to give shingles later in life.

Oncogenic viruses

Oncogenic viruses have the capacity to transform the host cell into a cancer cell. In some cases this may lead to relatively harmless, benign growths, such as warts caused by papovavirus, but in other cases more severe, malignant tumours may arise. Cellular transformation may result from viral activation or mutation of normal host genes, called protooncogenes, or the insertion of viral oncogenes.

Bacteriophages

Bacteriophages (phages) are viruses that attack bacteria but not animal cells. It is generally accepted that the interaction between phage and bacterium is highly specific, and there is probably at least one phage for each species of bacterium. In many cases the infection of a bacterial cell by a phage results in lysis of the bacterium; such phages are termed virulent. Some phages, however, can infect a bacterium without causing lysis. In this case the phage DNA becomes incorporated within the bacterial genome. The phage DNA can then be replicated along with the bacterial cell DNA; this is then termed a prophage. Bacterial cells carrying a prophage are called lysogenic and phages capable of inducing lysogeny are called temperate. Occasionally some of the prophage genes may be expressed and this will confer on the bacterial cell the ability to produce new proteins. The ability to produce additional proteins as a result of prophage DNA is termed lysogenic conversion.

The discovery of bacteriophages in the early 20th century is attributed to two workers, Frederick Twort and Felix d'Herelle. In 1896 Ernest Hankin had made an observation that the waters of the Ganges River possessed antibacterial properties which may have led to a reduction in cases of dysentery and cholera in the areas surrounding the river. Twort and d'Herelle independently came to the conclusion that this effect must be due to a virus. Twort did not carry on with his research but d'Herelle quickly established the potential of bacteriophages in antibacterial therapy 10 years before the advent of antibiotics. It was the discovery of penicillin by Alexander Fleming in 1928 that led to the demise of bacteriophage therapy but interest is now increasing again due to the emergence of antibiotic-resistant strains of bacteria.

ARCHAEOBACTERIA

Archaeobacteria are a fascinating group of prokaryotic microorganisms that are frequently found living in hostile environments. They differ in a number of respects from Eubacteria, particularly in the composition of their cell walls. They comprise methane producers, sulfate reducers, halophiles and extreme thermophiles. However, they are of little significance from a pharmaceutical or clinical standpoint and so will not be considered further.

EUBACTERIA

Eubacteria constitute the major group of prokaryotic cells that have pharmaceutical and clinical significance. They cover a diverse range of microorganisms, from the primitive parasitic rickettsias that share some of the characteristics of viruses, through the more typical free-living bacteria to the branching, filamentous actinomycetes, which at first sight resemble fungi rather than bacteria.

Atypical bacteria

Rickettsiae

The family Rickettsiaceae includes three clinically important genera, *Rickettsia, Coxiella* and *Bartonella*. Although these are prokaryotic cells, they differ from most other bacteria both in their structure and in the fact that the majority of species lead an obligate intracellular existence. This means that, with a few exceptions, they cannot be grown on cell-free media, although unlike many viruses they do possess some independent enzymes. They have a pleomorphic appearance, ranging from coccoid through to rod-shaped cells; multiplication is by binary fission. Their cell wall composition bears similarities to that of Gram-negative bacteria and in general they stain this way. The genus *Rickettsia* has a number of species that give rise to human diseases, in particular epidemic typhus (*R. prowazekii*), murine typhus (*R. typhi*) and spotted fevers (various species).

These are characterized by transmission via insect vectors, particularly mites, ticks, fleas and lice.

The mode of transmission by these vectors varies depending upon the insect concerned. In the case of lice and fleas, the microorganisms multiply within the insect and get into the faeces. These insects then colonize humans and transmit the microorganism when the faeces or the insect itself is crushed onto the skin. No bite is necessary and the faeces may also be inhaled. Mites and ticks pick up the microorganism when they take a blood meal from an infected animal. They then pass on the infection to humans when they accidentally bite us.

Coxiella burnetii is the only species in the genus *Coxiella* and this gives rise to a disease called Q fever. Although the source of the disease is infected animals, usually no insect vector is involved and the most common route of transmission is by inhalation of infected dust. *Bartonella quintana* is the causative agent of trench fever which, as the name suggests, occurs typically under conditions of war and deprivation. Each of the infections described here can be treated with doxycycline, although the duration of therapy may vary depending upon the nature of the disease and its severity.

Chlamydiae

These are obligate intracellular parasitic bacteria that possess some independent enzymes but lack the ability to generate ATP. Two cellular forms are identified: a small (0.3 μm) highly infectious elementary body which, after infection, enlarges to give rise to the replicative form called the initial or reticulate body (0.8–1.2 μm). These divide by binary fission within membrane-bound vesicles in the cytoplasm of infected cells. Insect vectors are not required for the transmission of infection. Chlamydiae lack peptidoglycan in their cell walls and have weak Gram-negative characteristics.

Chlamydia trachomatis is the most important member of the group, being responsible for the disease trachoma, characterized by inflammation of the eyelids, which can lead to scarring of the cornea. This is the most common cause of infectious blindness worldwide. It is estimated that 400 million people are infected, with at least 6 million totally blind. The same species is also recognized as one of the major causes of sexually transmitted disease. *C. psittaci* and *C. pneumoniae* are responsible for respiratory tract infections. Chlamydial infections are responsive to treatment by tetracyclines, either topical or systemic as appropriate.

Mycoplasmas

The mycoplasmas are a group of very small (0.3–0.8 μm) prokaryotic microorganisms that are capable of growing on cell-free media but which lack cell walls. The cells are surrounded by a double-layered plasma membrane that contains substantial amounts of phospholipids and sterols. This structure has no rigidity owing to the absence of peptidoglycan, and so the cells are susceptible to osmotic lysis. The lack of peptidoglycan is also the reason for these bacteria being resistant to the effects of cell wall-acting antibiotics such as the penicillins, and also the enzyme lysozyme. Members of this group are pleomorphic, varying in shape from coccoid to filamentous. Most are facultative anaerobes capable of growth at 35°C, and on solid media produce colonies with a characteristic 'fried egg' appearance. They contain a number of genera, of which the most important from a clinical point of view are *Mycoplasma* and *Ureaplasma*. *M. pneumoniae* is a major cause of respiratory tract infections in children and young adults, whereas *U. urealyticum* has been implicated in non-specific genital infections. Despite being resistant to the β-lactam antibiotics, these infections can be effectively treated using either tetracyclines or erythromycin.

Actinomycetes

Many of the macroscopic features of the actinomycetes are those that are more commonly found among the filamentous fungi but they are indeed prokaryotic cells. They are a diverse group of Gram-positive bacteria morphologically distinguishable from other bacteria because they have a tendency to produce branching filaments and reproductive spores. *Nocardia* contain a number of species that have been shown to be pathogenic to humans, but they occur principally in tropical climates. Reproduction in this genus is by fragmentation of the hyphal strands into individual cells, each of which can form a new mycelium. The genus *Streptomyces* contains no human pathogens but most species are saprophytic bacteria found in the soil. They are aerobic microorganisms producing a non-fragmenting, branching mycelium that may bear spores. The reason for their pharmaceutical importance is their ability to produce a wide range of therapeutically useful antibiotics, including streptomycin, chloramphenicol, oxytetracycline, erythromycin and neomycin.

Typical bacteria

Shape, size and aggregation

Bacteria occur in a variety of shapes and sizes, determined not only by the nature of the organisms themselves but also by the way in which they are grown (Fig. 14.1). In general, bacterial dimensions lie in the range 0.75–5 μm. The most common shapes are the sphere (coccus) and the rod (bacillus).

Genus		Approximate dimensions (μm)
Staphylococcus Irregular clusters of spherical cells. Resemble bunch of grapes. Non-motile	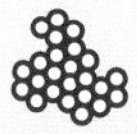	0.5–1.5
Streptococcus Spherical or ovoid cells occurring in pairs or in chains. Non-motile	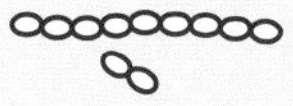	<2.0
Neisseria Small Gram-negative cocci. Occur in pairs with adjacent sides flattened. Non-motile	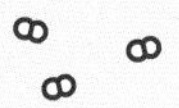	0.6–1.0
Lactobacillus Shape variable between long and slender to short coccobacillus. Non-motile, chain formation common	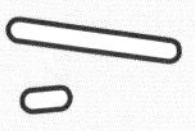	0.5–0.8 × 2–9
Escherichia Short rods, motile by peritrichous flagella	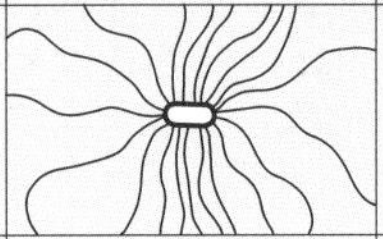	1.1–1.5 × 2–6
Bacillus Large endospore-forming rods. Motile by lateral flagella (not shown). Gram-positive	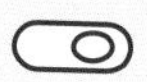	0.3–2.2 × 1.2–7.0
Vibrio Short curved or straight rods. Sometimes 'S' shaped. Motile by single polar flagella	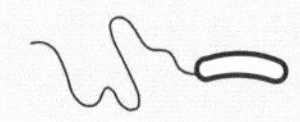	0.5 × 1.5–3.0
Spirochaeta Thin, flexible, helically coiled cells. Motile, possess axial fibrils (not shown)	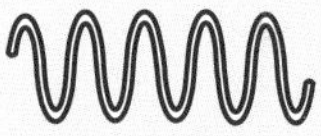	0.2–0.75 × 5–500
Spirillum Long, slender cells in rigid spirals. Number of turns varies. Motile bipolar flagellation	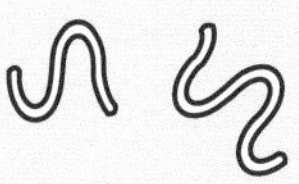	0.2–1.7 × 0.5–60
Streptomyces Slender, non-septate branching filaments. Form reproductive spores. Non-motile	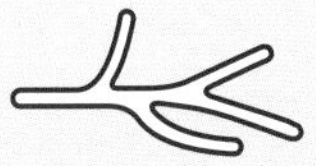	0.5–2.0 (diameter)

Fig. 14.1 Morphology of different bacterial genera.

Some bacteria grow in the form of rods with a distinct curvature, e.g. vibrios are rod-shaped cells with a single curve resembling a comma, whereas a spirillum possesses a partial rigid spiral; spirochaetes are longer and thinner, exhibit a number of turns and are also more flexible. Rod-shaped cells occasionally grow in the form of chains but this is dependent upon growth conditions rather than being a characteristic of the species.

Cocci, however, show considerable variation in aggregation, which is characteristic of the species. The plane of cell division and the strength of adhesion of the cells determine the extent to which they aggregate after division. Cocci growing in pairs are called diplococci, those in four are tetrads and groups of eight are sarcina. If a chain of cells is produced resembling a string of beads this is termed a streptococcus, whereas an irregular cluster similar in appearance to a bunch of grapes is called a staphylococcus. In many cases this is sufficiently characteristic to give rise to the name of the bacterial genus, e.g. *Staphylococcus aureus*, *Streptococcus pneumoniae*.

Anatomy

Figure 14.2 is a diagrammatic representation of a typical bacterial cell. The various components are described below.

Capsule Many bacteria produce extracellular polysaccharides, which may take the form of either a discrete capsule firmly adhered to the cell or a more diffuse layer of slime. Not all bacteria produce a capsule and even those that can will only do so under certain circumstances. Many encapsulated pathogens, when first isolated, give rise to colonies on agar which are smooth (S) but subculturing leads to the formation of rough colonies (R). This S to R transition is due to loss in capsule production. Reinoculation of the R cells into an animal results in the resumption of capsule formation, indicating that the capacity has not been lost irrevocably.

The function of the capsule is generally regarded as protective, as encapsulated cells are more resistant to disinfectants, desiccation and phagocytic attack. In some organisms, however, it serves as an adhesive mechanism; for example, *Streptococcus mutans* is an inhabitant of the mouth that metabolizes sucrose to produce a polysaccharide capsule enabling the cell to adhere firmly to the teeth. This is the initial step in the formation of dental plaque, which is a complex array of microorganisms and organic matrix that adheres to the teeth and ultimately leads to decay. The substitution of sucrose by glucose prevents capsule formation and hence eliminates plaque.

A similar picture emerges with *Staph. epidermidis*. This bacterium forms part of the normal microflora of the skin and until recently was thought of as non-pathogenic. With the increased usage of indwelling medical devices, coagulase-negative staphylococci, in particular *Staph. epidermidis*, have emerged as the major cause of device-related infections. The normal microbial flora have developed the ability to produce extracellular polysaccharide, which enables the cells to form resistant biofilms attached to the devices. These biofilms are very difficult to eradicate and have profound resistance to antibiotics and disinfectants. It is now apparent that the dominant mode of growth for aquatic bacteria is not planktonic (free swimming) but sessile, i.e. attached to surfaces and covered with protective extracellular polysaccharide or glycocalyx.

Cell wall Bacteria can be divided into two broad groups by the use of the Gram-staining procedure (see later in this chapter for details), which reflects differences in cell wall structure. The classification is based upon the ability of the cells to retain the dye methyl violet after washing with a decolourizing agent such as absolute alcohol. Gram-positive cells retain the stain whereas Gram-negative cells do not. As a *very rough* guide, the majority of small rod-shaped cells are Gram negative. Most large rods, such as the Bacillaceae, lactobacilli and actinomycetes, are Gram positive. Similarly, most cocci are Gram positive, although there are notable exceptions, such as the Neisseriaceae.

Bacteria are unique in that they possess peptidoglycan in their cell walls. This is a complex molecule with repeating units of *N*-acetylmuramic acid and *N*-acetylglucosamine (Fig. 14.3). This extremely long molecule is wound around the cell and crosslinked by polypeptide bridges to form a structure of great rigidity. The degree and nature of crosslinking vary between bacterial species. Crosslinking imparts to the cell its characteristic shape and has principally a protective function. Peptidoglycan (also called murein or mucopeptide) is the site of action of a number of antibiotics, such as penicillin, bacitracin, vancomycin and cycloserine. The enzyme lysozyme is also capable of hydrolysing the β–1–4 linkages between *N*-acetylmuramic acid and *N*-acetylglucosamine.

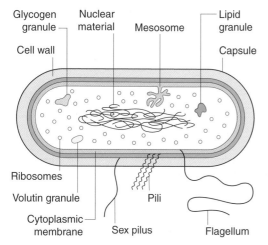

Glycogen granule Nuclear material Mesosome Lipid granule

Cell wall Capsule

Ribosomes

Volutin granule Pili

Cytoplasmic membrane Sex pilus Flagellum

Fig. 14.2 Diagrammatic representation of a typical bacterial cell.

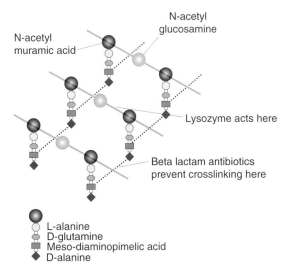

N-acetyl muramic acid

N-acetyl glucosamine

Lysozyme acts here

Beta lactam antibiotics prevent crosslinking here

● L-alanine
○ D-glutamine
■ Meso-diaminopimelic acid
◆ D-alanine

Fig. 14.3   Peptidoglycan.

Figure 14.4 shows simplified diagrams of a Gram-positive and a Gram-negative cell wall. The Gram-positive cell wall is much simpler in layout, containing peptidoglycan interspersed with teichoic acid polymers. These latter are highly antigenic but do not provide structural support. Functions attributed to teichoic acids include the regulation of enzyme activity in cell wall synthesis, sequestration of essential cations, cellular adhesion and mediation of the inflammatory response in disease. In general, proteins are not found in Gram-positive cell walls. Gram-negative cell walls are more complex, comprising a much thinner layer of peptidoglycan surrounded by an outer bilayered membrane. This outer membrane acts as a diffusional barrier and is the

main reason why many Gram-negative cells are much less susceptible to antimicrobial agents than are Gram-positive cells.

The lipopolysaccharide component of the outer membrane can be shed from the wall upon cell death. It is a highly heat-resistant molecule known as endotoxin, which has a number of toxic effects on the human body, including fever, shock and even death. For this reason it is important that solutions for injection or infusion are not just sterile but are also free from endotoxins.

Cytoplasmic membrane   The cytoplasmic membranes of most bacteria are very similar and are composed of protein, lipids, phospholipids and a small amount of carbohydrate. The components are arranged into a bilayer structure with a hydrophobic interior and a hydrophilic exterior. The cytoplasmic membrane has a variety of functions.

- It serves as an osmotic barrier.
- It is selectively permeable and is the site of carrier-mediated transport.
- It is the site of ATP generation and cytochrome activity.
- It is the site of cell wall synthesis.
- It provides a site for chromosome attachment.

The cytoplasmic membrane has very little tensile strength and the internal hydrostatic pressure of up to 20 bar forces it firmly against the inside of the cell wall. Treatment of bacterial cells with lysozyme may remove the cell wall and, as long as the conditions are isotonic, the resulting cell will survive. These cells are called protoplasts and, as the cytoplasmic membrane is now the limiting structure, the cell assumes a spherical shape. Protoplasts of Gram-negative bacteria are difficult to obtain because the layer of lipopolysaccharide protects the peptidoglycan from attack. In these cases mixtures of EDTA and lysozyme are used and the resulting cells, which still retain fragments of cell envelope, are termed spheroplasts.

Nuclear material   The genetic information necessary for the functioning of the cell is contained within a single circular molecule of double-stranded DNA. When unfolded, this would be about 1000 times as long as the cell itself and so exists within the cytoplasm in a considerably compacted state. It is condensed into discrete areas called chromatin bodies that are not surrounded by a nuclear membrane. Rapidly dividing cells may contain more than one area of nuclear material but these are copies of the same chromosome, not different chromosomes, and arise because DNA replication proceeds ahead of cell division.

In addition to the main chromosome, cells may contain extra pieces of circular double-stranded DNA which are called plasmids. These can encode a variety of products

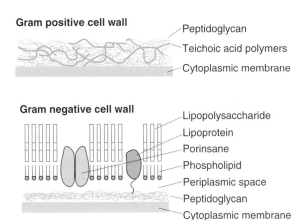

Gram positive cell wall

Peptidoglycan
Teichoic acid polymers
Cytoplasmic membrane

Gram negative cell wall

Lipopolysaccharide
Lipoprotein
Porinsane
Phospholipid
Periplasmic space
Peptidoglycan
Cytoplasmic membrane

Fig. 14.4   Structural components of bacterial cell walls.

which are not necessary for the normal functioning of the cell but confer some sort of selective advantage. For example, the plasmids may contain genes conferring antibiotic resistance or the ability to synthesize toxins or virulence factors. Plasmids replicate autonomously (i.e. independent of the main chromosome) and in some cases are able to be transferred from one cell to another (maybe of a different species).

Mesosomes These are irregular invaginations of the cytoplasmic membrane which are quite prominent in Gram-positive bacteria but less so in Gram-negative bacteria. It has been proposed that they have a variety of functions, including cross-wall synthesis during cell division and furnishing an attachment site for nuclear material, facilitating the separation of segregating chromosomes during cell division. They have also been implicated in enzyme secretions and may act as a site for cell respiration. However, it has also been suggested that they are simply artefacts which arise as a result of preparation for electron microscopy.

Ribosomes The cytoplasm of bacteria is densely populated with ribosomes, which are complexes of RNA and protein in discrete particles 20 nm in diameter. They are the sites of protein synthesis within the cell and the numbers present reflect the degree of metabolic activity of the cell. They are frequently found organized in clusters called polyribosomes or polysomes. Prokaryotic ribosomes have a sedimentation coefficient of 70S, compared to 80S ribosomes of eukaryotic cells. This distinction aids the selective toxicity of a number of antibiotics. The 70S ribosome is made up of RNA and protein and can dissociate into one 30S and one 50S subunit.

Inclusion granules Certain bacteria tend to accumulate reserves of materials after active growth has ceased, and these become incorporated within the cytoplasm in the form of granules. The most common are glycogen granules, volutin granules (containing polymetaphosphate) and lipid granules (containing poly β-hydroxybutyric acid). Other granules, such as sulphur and iron, may also be found in the more primitive bacteria.

Flagella A flagellum is made up of protein called flagellin and it operates by forming a rigid helix that turns rapidly like a propeller. This can propel a motile cell up to 200 times its own length in 1 second. Under the microscope bacteria can be seen to exhibit two kinds of motion: swimming and tumbling. When tumbling, the cell stays in one position and spins on its own axis but when swimming, it moves in a straight line. Movement towards or away from a chemical stimulus is referred to as chemotaxis. The flagellum arises from the cytoplasmic membrane and is composed of a basal body, hook and filament. The number and arrangement of flagella depend upon the organism and vary from a single flagellum (monotrichous) to a complete covering (peritrichous).

Pili and fimbriae These terms are often used interchangeably but in reality these structures are functionally distinct from each other. Fimbriae are smaller than flagella and are not involved in motility. They are found all over the surface of certain bacteria (mainly Gram-negative cells) and are believed to be associated with adhesiveness and pathogenicity. They are also antigenic. Pili (of which there are different types) are larger and of a different structure to fimbriae and are involved in the transfer of genetic information from one cell to another. This is of major importance in the transfer of drug resistance between cell populations.

Endospores Under conditions of specific nutrient deprivation some genera of bacteria, in particular *Bacillus* and *Clostridium*, undergo a differentiation process at the end of logarithmic growth and change from an actively metabolizing vegetative form to a resting spore form. The process of sporulation is not a reproductive mechanism, as found in certain actinomycetes and filamentous fungi, but serves to enable the organism to survive periods of hardship. A single vegetative cell differentiates into a single spore. Subsequent encounter with favourable conditions results in germination of the spore and the resumption of vegetative activities.

Endospores are very much more resistant to heat, disinfectants, desiccation and radiation than are vegetative cells, making them difficult to eradicate from foods and pharmaceutical products. Heating at 80°C for 10 minutes would kill most vegetative bacteria, whereas some spores will resist boiling for several hours. The sterilization procedures now routinely used for pharmaceutical products are thus designed specifically with reference to the destruction of the bacterial spore.

The mechanism of this extreme heat resistance was a perplexing issue for many years. At one time it was thought to be due to the presence of a unique spore component, dipicolinic acid (DPA). This compound is found only in bacterial spores where it is associated in a complex with calcium ions. The isolation of heat-resistant DPA-less mutants, however, led to the demise of this theory. Spores do not have a water content appreciably different from that of vegetative cells, but the distribution within the different compartments is unequal and this is thought to generate the heat resistance. The central core of the spore houses the genetic information necessary for growth after germination and this becomes dehydrated by expansion of the cortex against the rigid outer protein coats. Water is thus squeezed out of the central core. Osmotic pressure differences also help to maintain this water imbalance. Endospores are also highly unusual because of their ability to remain dormant and ametabolic for prolonged periods of time. Bacterial spores have been isolated from lake sediments where they were deposited 1000 years previously and there have even been claims of spores revived from geological specimens up to 40 million years old.

The sequence of events involved in sporulation is illustrated in Figure 14.5. It is a continuous process, although for convenience it may be divided into six stages. The complete process takes about 8 hours, although this may vary depending on the species and the conditions used. Occurring simultaneously with the morphological changes is a number of biochemical events that have been shown to be associated with specific stages and occur in an exact sequence. One important biochemical event is the production of antibiotics. Peptides possessing antimicrobial activity have been isolated from the majority of *Bacillus* species and many of these have found pharmaceutical applications. Examples of antibiotics include bacitracin, polymyxin and gramicidin. Similarly, the proteases produced by *Bacillus* species during sporulation are used extensively in a wide variety of industries.

Microscopy and staining of bacteria

Bacterial cells contain about 80% water by weight and this results in a very low refractility, i.e. they are transparent when viewed under ordinary transmitted light. Consequently, in order to visualize bacteria under the microscope, the cells must be killed and stained with some compound that scatters the light or, if live preparations are required, special adaptations must be made to the microscope. Such adaptations are found in phase-

contrast, dark-ground and differential-interference contrast microscopy.

The microscopic examination of fixed and stained preparations is a routine procedure in most laboratories but it must be appreciated that not only are the cells dead, but they may also have been altered morphologically by the often quite drastic staining process. The majority of stains used routinely are basic dyes, i.e. the chromophore has a positive charge and this readily combines with the abundant negative charges present both in the cytoplasm in the form of nucleic acids and on the cell surface. These dyes remain firmly adhered even after washing with water. This type of staining is called simple staining and all bacteria and other biological material are stained the same colour. Differential staining is a much more useful process as different organisms or even different parts of the same cell can be stained distinctive colours.

To prepare a film ready for staining, the glass microscope slide must be carefully cleaned to remove all traces of grease and dust. If the culture of bacteria is in liquid form then a loopful of suspension is transferred directly to the slide. Bacteria from solid surfaces require suspension with a small drop of water on the slide to give a faintly turbid film. A common fault with inexperienced workers is to make the film too thick. The films must then be allowed to dry in air. When thoroughly dry the film is fixed by passing the back of the slide through a small Bunsen flame until the area is just too hot to touch on the palm of the hand. The bacteria are killed by this procedure and also stuck on to the slide. Fixing also makes the

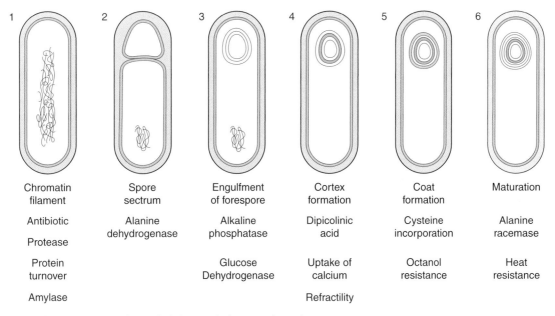

Fig. 14.5 Morphological and biochemical changes during spore formation.

1	2	3	4	5	6
Chromatin filament	Spore sectrum	Engulfment of forespore	Cortex formation	Coat formation	Maturation
Antibiotic	Alanine dehydrogenase	Alkaline phosphatase	Dipicolinic acid	Cysteine incorporation	Alanine racemase
Protease					
Protein turnover		Glucose Dehydrogenase	Uptake of calcium	Octanol resistance	Heat resistance
Amylase			Refractility		

bacteria more permeable to the stain and inhibits lysis. Chemical fixation is commonly carried out using formalin or methyl alcohol; this causes less damage to the specimen but tends to be used principally for blood films and tissue sections.

Differential stains

A large number of differential stains has been developed and the reader is referred to the bibliography for more details. Only a few of those available will be discussed here.

Gram's stain By far the most important in terms of use and application is the Gram stain, developed by Christian Gram in 1884 and subsequently modified. The fixed film of bacteria is flooded initially with a solution of methyl violet. This is followed by a solution of Gram's iodine, which is an iodine–potassium iodine complex acting as a mordant, fixing the dye firmly in certain bacteria and allowing easy removal in others. Decolourization is effected with either alcohol or acetone or mixtures of these. After treatment some bacteria retain the stain and appear a dark purple colour and these are called Gram positive. Others do not retain the stain and appear colourless (Gram negative). The colourless cells may be stained with a counterstain of contrasting colour, such as 0.5% safranin, which is red.

This method, although extremely useful, must be used with caution as the Gram reaction may vary with the age of the cells and the technique of the operator. For this reason, known Gram-positive and Gram-negative controls should be stained alongside the specimen of interest.

Ziehl–Neelsen's acid-fast stain The bacterium responsible for the disease tuberculosis (*Mycobacterium tuberculosis*) contains within its cell wall a high proportion of lipids, fatty acids and alcohols, which render it resistant to normal staining procedures. The inclusion of phenol in the dye solution, together with the application of heat, enables the dye (basic fuchsin) to penetrate the cell and, once attached, to resist vigorous decolourization by strong acids, e.g. 20% sulphuric acid. These organisms are therefore called acid fast. Any unstained material can be counterstained with a contrasting colour, e.g. methylene blue.

Fluorescence microscopy

Certain materials, when irradiated by short-wave illuminations, e.g. UV light, become excited and emit visible light of a longer wavelength. This phenomenon is termed fluorescence and will persist only for as long as the material is irradiated. A number of dyes have been shown to fluoresce and are useful in that they tend to be specific to various tissues, which can then be demonstrated by UV irradiation and subsequent fluorescence of the attached fluorochrome. Coupling antibodies to the fluorochromes can enhance specificity, and this technique has found wide application in microbiology. As with the staining procedures described above, this technique can only be applied to dead cells. The three following techniques have been developed for the examination of living organisms.

Dark-ground microscopy

The usual function of the microscope condenser is to concentrate as much light as possible through the specimen and into the objective. The dark-ground condenser performs the opposite task, producing a hollow cone of light that comes to a focus on the specimen. The rays of light in the cone are at an oblique angle, such that after passing across the specimen they continue without meeting the front lens of the objective, resulting in a dark background. Any objects present at the point of focus scatter the light, which then enters the objective to show up as a bright image against the dark background.

Specimen preparation is more critical, as very dilute bacterial suspensions are required, preferably with all the objects in the same plane of focus. Air bubbles must be absent from both the film and the immersion oil, if used. Dust and grease also scatter light and destroy the uniformly black background required for this technique. With this technique it is not possible to see any real detail but it is useful to study motility.

Phase-contrast microscopy

This technique allows us to see transparent objects well contrasted from the background in clear detail and is the most widely used image enhancement method in microbiology. In essence, an annulus of light is produced by the condenser of the microscope and focused on the back focal plane of the objective where a phase plate, comprising a glass disc containing an annular depression, is situated. The direct rays of the light source annulus pass through the annular groove and any diffracted rays pass through the remainder of the disc. Passage of the diffracted light through this thicker glass layer results in retardation of the light. This alters its phase relationship to the direct rays and increases contrast.

Differential-interference contrast microscopy

This method uses polarized light and has other applications outside the scope of this chapter, such as detecting surface irregularities in opaque specimens. It offers some advantages over phase-contrast microscopy, notably the elimination of haloes around the object edges, and enables extremely detailed observation of specimens. It does, however, tend to be more difficult to set up.

Electron microscopy

The highest magnification available using a light microscope is about 1500 times. This limitation is imposed not by the design of the microscope itself, as much higher magnifications are possible, but by the wavelength of light. An object can only be seen if it causes a ray of light to deflect. If a particle is very small indeed then no deflection is produced and the object is not seen. Visible light has a wavelength between 0.3 and 0.8 μm and objects less than 0.3 μm will not be clearly resolved, i.e. even if the magnification were increased no more detail would be seen. In order to increase the resolution it is necessary to use light of a shorter wavelength, such as UV light. This has been done and resulted in some useful applications but generally, for the purposes of increased definition, electrons are now used and they can be thought of as behaving like very short wavelength light. Transmission electron microscopy requires the preparation of ultrathin (50–60 nm) sections of material mounted on copper grids for support. Because of the severe conditions applied to the specimen during preparation, and the likelihood of artefacts, care must be taken in the interpretation of information from electron micrographs.

Growth and reproduction of bacteria

The growth and multiplication of bacteria can be examined in terms of individual cells or populations of cells. During the cell division cycle a bacterium assimilates nutrients from the surrounding medium and increases in size. When a predetermined size has been reached the DNA duplicates itself and a cross-wall will be produced, dividing the large cell into two daughter cells, each containing a copy of the parent chromosome. This process is known as binary fission. In a closed environment, such as a culture in a test tube, the rate at which cell division occurs varies according to the conditions, and this manifests itself in characteristic changes in the population concentration. When fresh medium is inoculated with a small number of bacterial cells, the number remains static for a short time while the cells undergo a period of metabolic adjustment. This period is called the lag phase (Fig. 14.6) and its length depends on the degree of readjustment necessary. Once the cells are adapted to the environment, they begin to divide in the manner described above, and this division occurs at regular intervals. The numbers of bacteria during this period increase in an exponential fashion, i.e. 2, 4, 8, 16, 32, 64, 128, etc., and this is therefore termed the exponential or logarithmic phase. When cell numbers are plotted on a log scale against time, a straight line results for this phase.

During exponential growth (Fig. 14.6) the medium undergoes continuous change, as nutrients are consumed and metabolic waste products excreted. The fact that the cells continue to divide exponentially during this period is a tribute to their physiological adaptability. Eventually, the medium becomes so changed, due to either substrate exhaustion or excessive concentrations of toxic products, that it is unable to support further growth. At this stage cell division slows and eventually stops, leading to the stationary phase. During this period some cells lyse and die whereas others sporadically divide, but the cell numbers remain more or less constant. Gradually all the cells lyse and the culture enters the phase of decline.

It should be appreciated that this sequence of events is not a characteristic of the cell but a consequence of the interaction of the organisms with the nutrients in a closed environment. It does not necessarily reflect the way in which the organism would behave in vivo.

Genetic exchange

In addition to mutations, bacteria can alter their genetic make-up by transferring information from one cell to another, either as fragments of DNA or in the form of small extrachromosomal elements (plasmids). Transfer can be achieved in three ways: by transformation, transduction or conjugation.

Transformation When bacteria die they lyse and release cell fragments, including DNA, into the environment. Several bacterial genera (*Bacillus, Haemophilus, Streptococcus,* etc.) are able to take up these DNA fragments and incorporate them into their own chromosome, thereby inheriting the characteristics carried on that fragment. Cells able to participate in transformation are called competent. The development of competence has

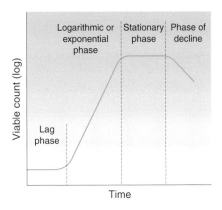

Fig. 14.6 Phases of bacterial growth.

been shown in some cases to occur synchronously in a culture under the action of specific inducing proteins.

Transduction Some bacteriophages infect a bacterial cell and incorporate their nucleic acid into the host cell chromosome, with the result that the viral genes are replicated along with the bacterial DNA. In many instances this is a dormant lysogenic state for the phage but sometimes it is triggered into action and lysis of the cell occurs with liberation of phage particles. These new phage particles may have bacterial DNA incorporated into the viral genome and this will infect any new host cell. On entering a new lysogenic state, the new host cell will replicate the viral nucleic acid in addition to that portion received from the previous host. Bacteria in which this has been shown to occur include *Mycobacterium*, *Salmonella*, *Shigella* and *Staphylococcus*.

Conjugation Gram-negative bacteria such as *Salmonella*, *Shigella* and *Escherichia coli* have been shown to transfer genetic material conferring antibiotic resistance by cellular contact. This process is called conjugation and is controlled by an R-factor plasmid, which is a small circular strand of duplex DNA replicating independently from the bacterial chromosome. R factor comprises a region containing resistance transfer genes that control the formation of sex pili, together with a variety of genes that code for the resistance to drugs. Conjugation is initiated when the resistance transfer genes stimulate the production of a sex pilus and random motion brings about contact with a recipient cell. One strand of the replicating R factor is nicked and passes through the sex pilus into the recipient cell. Upon receipt of this single strand of plasmid DNA, the complementary strand is produced and the free ends are joined. For a short time afterwards this cell has the ability to form a sex pilus itself and so transfer the R factor further.

This is by no means an exhaustive discussion of genetic exchange in bacteria and the reader is referred to the bibliography for further information.

Bacterial nutrition

Bacteria require certain elements in fairly large quantities for growth and metabolism, including carbon, hydrogen, oxygen and nitrogen. Sulphur and phosphorus are also required but not in such large amounts. Only low concentrations of iron, calcium, potassium, sodium, magnesium and manganese are needed. Some elements, such as cobalt, zinc and copper, are required only in trace amounts and an actual requirement may be difficult to demonstrate.

The metabolic capabilities of bacteria differ considerably and this is reflected in the form in which nutrients may be assimilated. Bacteria can be classified according to their requirements for carbon and energy.

Lithotrophs (synonym: autotrophs) These utilize carbon dioxide as their main source of carbon. Energy is derived from different sources within this group:

- chemolithotrophs (chemosynthetic autotrophs) obtain their energy from the oxidation of inorganic compounds
- photolithotrophs (photosynthetic autotrophs) obtain their energy from sunlight.

Organotrophs (synonym: heterotrophs) Organotrophs utilize organic carbon sources and can similarly be divided into:

- chemoorganotrophs, which obtain their energy from oxidation or fermentation of organic compounds
- photoorganotrophs, which utilize light energy.

Oxygen requirements

As mentioned above, all bacteria require elemental oxygen in order to build up the complex materials necessary for growth and metabolism, but many organisms also require free oxygen as the final electron acceptor in the breakdown of carbon and energy sources. These organisms are called aerobes. If the organism will only grow in the presence of air it is called a strict aerobe, but most organisms can either grow in its presence or its absence and are called facultative anaerobes. A strict anaerobe cannot grow and may even be killed in the presence of oxygen, because some other compound replaces oxygen as the final electron acceptor in these organisms. A fourth group of microaerophilic organisms has also been recognized which grow best in only trace amounts of free oxygen and usually prefer an increased carbon dioxide concentration.

Influence of environmental factors on the growth of bacteria

The rate of growth and metabolic activity of bacteria is the sum of a multitude of enzyme reactions. It follows that those environmental factors that influence enzyme activity will also affect growth rate. Such factors include temperature, pH and osmolarity.

Temperature Bacteria can survive wide limits of temperature but each organism will exhibit minimum, optimum and maximum growth temperatures and on this basis fall into three broad groups.

- Psychrophils – grow best below 20°C but have a minimum about 0°C and a maximum of 30°C. These organisms are responsible for low-temperature spoilage.
- Mesophils – exhibit a minimum growth temperature of 5–10°C and a maximum of 45–50°C. Within this

group two populations can be identified: saprophytic mesophils, with an optimum temperature of 20–30°C, and parasitic mesophils with an optimum temperature of 37°C. The vast majority of pathogenic organisms are in this latter group.

- Thermophils – can grow at temperatures up to 70–90°C but have an optimum of 50–55°C and a minimum of 25–40°C.

Organisms kept below their minimum growth temperature will not divide but can remain viable. As a result, very low temperatures (−70°C) are used to preserve cultures of organisms for many years. Temperatures in excess of the maximum growth temperature have a much more injurious effect and will be dealt with in more detail later (in Chapter 16).

pH   Most bacteria grow best at around neutrality, in the pH range 6.8–7.6. There are, however, exceptions, such as the acidophilic organism lactobacillus, a contaminant of milk products, which grows best at pHs between 5.4 and 6.6. Yeasts and moulds prefer acid conditions with an optimum pH range of 4–6. The difference in pH optima between fungi and bacteria is used as a basis for the design of media permitting the growth of one group of organisms at the expense of others. Sabouraud medium, for example, has a pH of 5.6 and is a fungal medium, whereas nutrient broth, which is used routinely to cultivate bacteria, has a pH of 7.4. The adverse effect of extremes of pH has for many years been used as a means of preserving foods against microbial attack, for example by pickling in acidic vinegar.

Osmotic pressure   Bacteria tend to be more resistant to extremes of osmotic pressure than other cells owing to the presence of a very rigid cell wall. The concentration of intracellular solutes gives rise to an osmotic pressure equivalent to between 5 and 20 bar, and most bacteria will thrive in a medium containing around 0.75% w/v sodium chloride. Staphylococci have the ability to survive higher than normal salt concentrations. This has enabled the formulation of selective media, such as mannitol salt agar containing 7.5% w/v sodium chloride, which will support the growth of staphylococci but restrict other bacteria. Halophilic organisms can grow at much higher osmotic pressures but these are all saprophytic and are non-pathogenic to humans. High osmotic pressures generated by either sodium chloride or sucrose have for a long time been used as preservatives. Syrup BP contains 66.7% w/w sucrose and is of sufficient osmotic pressure to resist microbial attack. This is used as a basis for many oral pharmaceutical preparations.

Handling and storage of microorganisms

Because microorganisms have such a diversity of nutritional requirements there has arisen a bewildering array of media for the cultivation of bacteria, yeasts and moulds. Media are produced either as liquids or solidified with agar. Agar is an extract of seaweed, which at concentrations of between 1% and 2% sets to form a firm gel below 45°C. Unlike gelatin, bacteria cannot use agar as a nutrient and so even after growth the gel remains firm. Liquid media are stored routinely in test tubes or flasks, depending upon the volume, both secured with either loose-fitting caps or plugs of sterile cotton wool. Small amounts of solid media are stored in Petri dishes or slopes (also known as slants), whereas larger volumes may be incorporated in Roux bottles or Carrell flasks.

Bacteria may only be maintained on agar in Petri dishes for a short time (days) before the medium dries out. For longer storage periods the surface of an agar slope is inoculated and after growth the culture may be stored at 4°C for several weeks. If even longer storage periods are required then the cultures may be stored at low temperatures (−70°C), usually in the presence of a cryoprotectant such as glycerol. Alternatively they may be freeze-dried (lyophilized) before being stored at 4°C. Some vegetative cells can survive lyophilization and may retain their viability for many years.

When a single cell is placed on the surface of an overdried agar plate, it becomes immobilized but can still draw nutrients from the substrate, and consequently grows and divides. Eventually the numbers of bacterial cells are high enough to become visible and a colony is formed. Each of the cells in that colony is a descendant from the initial single cell or group of cells, and so the colony is assumed to be a pure culture with each cell having identical characteristics. The formation of single colonies is one of the primary aims of surface inoculation of solid media and allows the isolation of pure cultures from specimens containing mixed flora.

Inoculation of agar surfaces by streaking

The agar surface must be smooth. The surface should also be without moisture as this could cause the bacteria to become motile and the colonies to merge together. To dry the surface of the agar, the plates are placed in an incubator or drying cabinet until the surface appears wrinkled. An inoculating loop is made of either platinum or nichrome wire twisted along its length to form a loop 2–3 mm in diameter at the end. Nichrome wire is cheaper than platinum but has similar thermal properties. The wire is held in a handle with an insulated grip and the entire length of the wire is heated in a Bunsen flame to red heat to sterilize it. The first few centimetres of the holder are also flamed before the loop is set aside in a rack to cool.

When cool, the loop is used to remove a small portion of liquid from a bacterial suspension and this is then drawn across the agar surface from A to B, as indicated in Figure 14.7. The loop is then resterilized and again allowed to cool. At this stage the loop is not reinoculated but streaked over the surface again, ensuring a small area of overlap with the previous streak line. The procedure is repeated as necessary. The pattern of streaking (other examples are shown in Fig. 14.7) is dictated largely by the concentration of the original bacterial suspension. The object of the exercise is to dilute the culture such that, after incubation, single colonies will arise in the later streak lines where the cells were sufficiently separated. All plates are incubated in an inverted position to prevent condensation from the lid falling on the surface of the medium and spreading the colonies.

Inoculation of slopes

A wire needle may be used to transfer single colonies from agar surfaces to the surface of slopes for maintenance purposes. The needle is similar to the loop except that the wire is single and straight, not terminating in a closed end. This is flamed and cooled as before and a portion of a single colony picked off the agar surface. The needle is then drawn upwards along the surface of the slant. Before incubation the screw cap of the bottle should be loosened slightly to prevent oxygen starvation during growth. Some slopes are prepared with a shallower slope and a deeper butt to allow the needle to be stabbed into the agar when testing for gas production.

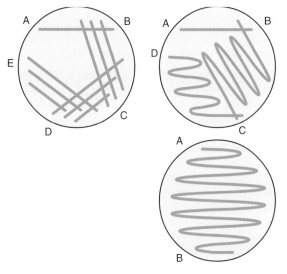

Fig. 14.7 Typical streaking methods for obtaining isolated colonies.

Transference of liquids

Graduated pipettes and Pasteur pipettes may be used for this purpose, the latter being short glass tubes one end of which is drawn into a fine capillary. Both types should be plugged with sterile cotton wool and filled via pipette fillers of appropriate capacity. Mouth pipetting should *never* be permitted. Automatic pipettes have generally replaced glass graduated pipettes in most areas of science for the measurement of small volumes of liquid. Provided they are properly maintained and calibrated, they have the advantage of being easy to use and reliable in performance.

Release of infectious aerosols

During all of these manipulations two considerations must be borne in mind. First, the culture must be transferred with the minimum risk of contamination from outside sources. To this end all pipettes, tubes, media, etc., are sterilized and the manipulations carried out under aseptic conditions. Second, the safety of the operator is paramount. During operations with microorganisms, it must be assumed that all organisms are capable of causing disease and that any route of infection is possible.

Most infections acquired in laboratories cannot be traced to a given incident but arise from the inadvertent release of infectious aerosols. Two types of aerosols may be produced. The first kind produces large droplets (>5 μm), containing many organisms, which settle locally and contaminate surfaces in the vicinity of the operator. These may initiate infections if personnel touch the surfaces and subsequently transfer the organisms to eyes, nose or mouth. The second type of aerosol contains droplets less than 5 μm in size, which dry instantly to form droplet nuclei that remain suspended in the air for considerable periods. This allows them to be carried on air currents to situations far removed from the site of initiation. These particles are so small that they are not trapped by the usual filter mechanisms in the nasal passages and may be inhaled, giving rise to infections of the lungs.

The aerosols described above may be produced by a variety of means, such as heating wire loops, placing hot loops into liquid cultures, splashing during pipetting, rattling loops and pipettes inside test tubes, opening screw-capped tubes and ampoules, etc. All microbiologists should have an awareness of the dangers of aerosol production and learn the correct techniques to minimize them.

Cultivation of anaerobes

Anaerobic microbiology is a much-neglected subject owing principally to the practical difficulties involved in growing organisms in the absence of air. However, with the increasing implication of anaerobes in certain disease states and improved cultivation systems, the number of workers in this field is growing.

The most common liquid medium for cultivation of anaerobes is thioglycollate medium. In addition to sodium thioglycollate, the medium contains methylene blue as a redox indicator, and it permits the growth of aerobes, anaerobes and microaerophilic organisms. When in test tubes, the medium may be used after sterilization until not more than one-third of the liquid is oxidized, as indicated by the colour of the methylene blue indicator. Boiling and cooling of the medium just prior to inoculation are recommended for maximum performance. In some cases the presence of methylene blue poses toxicity problems and under these circumstances the indicator may be removed.

Anaerobic jars have improved considerably in recent years, making the cultivation of even strict anaerobes now relatively simple. The most common ones consist of a clear polycarbonate jar with a lid housing a cold catalyst in a mesh container, and are designed to be used with disposable H_2/CO_2 generators. The agar plates, which may need to be pre-reduced prior to inoculation, are placed in the jar together with a gas generator and an anaerobic indicator. A measured amount of water is added to the gas generator sachet and the lid sealed. Hydrogen and carbon dioxide are evolved and the hydrogen combines with any oxygen present under the action of the cold catalyst to form a light mist of water vapour. Carbon dioxide is produced in sufficient quantities to allow the growth of many fastidious anaerobes, which fail to grow in its absence. The absence of oxygen will be demonstrated by the action of the redox indicator, which in the case of methylene blue will be colourless.

Counting bacteria

Estimates of bacterial numbers in a suspension can be evaluated from a number of standpoints, each equally valid depending upon the circumstances and the information required. In some cases it may be necessary to know the total amount of biomass produced within a culture, irrespective of whether the cells are actively metabolizing. In other instances only an assessment of living bacteria may be required. Bacterial counts can be divided into total counts and viable counts.

Total counts

These counts estimate the total number of bacteria present within a culture, both dead and living cells. A variety of methods is available for the determination of total counts and the one chosen will depend largely upon the

characteristics of the cells being studied, i.e. whether they aggregate together.

Microscopic methods   Microscopic methods employ a haemocytometer counting chamber (Fig. 14.8), which has a platform engraved with a grid of small squares each $0.0025 \ mm^2$ in area. The platform is depressed 0.1 mm and a glass coverslip is placed over the platform, enclosing a space of known dimensions. The volume above each square is $0.00025 \ mm^3$. For motile bacteria the culture is fixed by adding two to three drops of 40% formaldehyde solution per 10 mL of culture to prevent the bacteria from moving across the field of view. A drop of the suspension is then applied to the platform at the edge of the coverslip. The liquid is drawn into the space by capillary action. It is important to ensure that liquid does not enter a trench that surrounds the platform; the liquid must fill the whole space between the coverslip and the platform. This slide is examined using phase-contrast or dark-ground microscopy and, if necessary, the culture is diluted to give 2–10 bacteria per small square. A minimum of 300 bacterial cells should be counted to give statistically significant results.

Another microscopic technique is Breed's method. A microscope slide is marked with a square of known area (usually $1 \ cm^2$), and 0.01 mL of bacterial suspension is spread evenly over the square. This is allowed to dry and is then fixed and stained. A squared-eyepiece

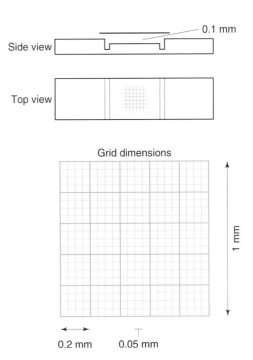

Fig. 14.8   Counting chamber for microscopic estimation of cell numbers.

micrometer is then used to determine the original count, knowing the dilution and the size of each square.

Example calculation of haematocytometer method
Assume the mean cell count per small square was 6. The area of each small square $= 2.5 \times 10^{-4}$ mm^3
$$= 2.5 \times 10^{-7} \text{ cm}^3.$$
If the volume above each square contains 6 cells then there are:

$$\frac{6 \text{ cells/mL}}{2.5 \times 10^{-7}} = 2.4 \times 10^7 \text{ cells/mL}.$$

Spectroscopic methods These methods are simple to use and very rapid but require careful calibration if meaningful results are to be obtained. Either opacity or light scattering may be used but both methods may only be used for dilute, homogeneous suspensions as at higher concentrations the cells obscure each other in the light path and the relationship between optical density and concentration is not linear. Simple colorimeters and nephelometers can be used but more accurate results are obtained using a spectrophotometer.

Electronic methods A variety of automated methods is available for bacterial cell counting, including electronic particle counting, microcalorimetry, changes in impedance or conductivity, and radiometric and infrared systems for monitoring CO_2 production.

Other methods If an organism is prone to excessive clumping, or if a measure of biomass is needed rather than numbers, then estimates may be made by performing dry weight or total nitrogen determinations. For dry weight determinations, a sample of suspension is centrifuged and the pellet washed free of culture medium by further centrifugation in water. The pellet is collected and dried to a constant weight in a desiccator. Total nitrogen measures the total quantity of nitrogenous material within a cell population. A known volume of suspension is centrifuged and washed as before and the pellet digested using sulphuric acid in the presence of a $CuSO_4$-K_2SO_4-selenium catalyst. This produces ammonia, which is removed using boric acid and estimated either by titration or colorimetrically.

Viable counts

These are counts to determine the number of bacteria in a suspension that are capable of division. In all these methods the assumption is made that a colony arises from a single cell, although clearly this is often not the case, as cells frequently clump or grow as aggregates, e.g. *Staphylococcus aureus*. In these cases the count is usually given as colony-forming units (cfu) per mL rather than cells per mL.

Spread plates A known volume, usually no more than 0.2 mL, of a suitably diluted culture is pipetted on to an overdried agar plate and distributed evenly over the surface using a sterile spreader made of wire or glass capillary. All the liquid must be allowed to soak in before the plates are inverted. A series of 10-fold dilutions should be made in a suitable sterile diluent and replicates plated out at each dilution in order to ensure that countable numbers of colonies (30–300) are obtained per plate.

The viable count is calculated from the average colony count per plate, knowing the dilution and the volume pipetted onto the agar.

Example calculation of a serial dilution scheme

Stock bacterial suspension, 1 mL added to 99 mL of sterile diluent – *call dilution A*. At this point the stock solution has therefore been diluted by a factor of 100 (10^2).

1 mL of dilution A added to 99 mL of sterile diluent – *call dilution B* (dilution B has been diluted by a factor of 10^4).

1 mL of dilution B added to 9 mL of sterile diluent – *call dilution C* (dilution C has been diluted by a factor of 10^5).

1 mL of dilution C added to 9 mL of sterile diluent – *call dilution D* (dilution D has been diluted by a factor of 10^6).

1 mL of dilution D added to 9 mL of sterile diluent – *call dilution E* (dilution E has been diluted by a factor of 10^7).

0.2 mL of each dilution plated in triplicate.

Mean colony counts for each dilution after incubation at 37°C are as follows:

Dilution A	too many to count
Dilution B	too many to count
Dilution C	400 colonies
Dilution D	45 colonies
Dilution E	5 colonies.

The result for dilution C is unreliable, as the count is too high. If the colony count exceeds 300, errors arise because the colonies become very small and some may be missed. This is why the colony count for dilution C does not exactly correspond to 10× that found for dilution D. Similarly, the count for dilution E is unreliable because at counts below about 30 small variations introduce high percentage errors.

The result from dilution D is therefore taken for calculation, as the colony count lies between 30 and 300.

45 colonies in 0.2 mL, therefore
$= 45 \times 5$ colonies per mL
$= 225$ cfu/mL in dilution D.

This was diluted by a factor of 10^6 $(100 \times 100 \times 10 \times 10)$ and so the count in the stock suspension was $225 \times 10^6 = 2.25 \times 10^8$ cfu/mL.

Pour plates

A series of dilutions of original culture is prepared as before, ensuring that at least one is in the range 30–300 organisms/mL. One-millilitre quantities are placed into empty sterile Petri dishes. Molten agar, cooled to 45°C, is poured on to the suspension and mixed by gentle swirling. After setting, the plates are inverted and incubated. Because the colonies are embedded within the agar they do not exhibit the characteristic morphology seen with surface colonies. In general, they assume a lens shape and are usually smaller. Because the oxygen tension below the surface is reduced this method is not suitable for strict aerobes. Calculations are similar to that given above, except that no correction is necessary for volume placed upon the plate.

Membrane filtration This method is particularly useful when the level of contamination is very low, such as in water supplies. A known volume of sample is passed through a membrane filter, typically made of cellulose acetate/nitrate, of sufficient pore size to retain bacteria (0.2–0.45 μm). The filtrate is discarded and the membrane placed bacteria uppermost on the surface of an overdried agar plate, avoiding trapped air between membrane and surface. Upon incubation the bacteria draw nutrients through the membrane and form countable colonies.

ATP determination There are sometimes instances when viable counts are required for clumped cultures or for bacteria adhered to surfaces, for example in biofilms. Conventional plate count techniques are not appropriate here and ATP determinations can be used. The method assumes that viable bacteria contain a relatively constant level of ATP, but this falls to zero when the cells die. ATP is extracted from the cells using a strong acid such as trichloroacetic acid, and the extract is then neutralized by dilution with buffer. The ATP assay is based upon the quantitative measurement of a stable level of light produced as a result of an enzyme reaction catalysed by firefly luciferase.

$$ATP + luciferin + O_2 \xrightarrow{\text{luciferase}} oxyluciferin + AMP + PPi + CO_2 + light$$

The amount of ATP is calculated by reference to light output from known ATP concentrations and the number of bacterial cells is calculated by reference to a previously constructed calibration plot.

Isolation of pure bacterial cultures

Mixed bacterial cultures from pathological specimens or other biological materials are isolated first on solid media to give single colonies. The resultant pure cultures can then be subjected to identification procedures. The techniques used for isolation depend upon the proportion of the species of interest compared to the background contamination. Direct inoculation can only be used when an organism is found as a pure culture in nature. Examples include bacterial infections of normally sterile fluids such as blood or cerebrospinal fluid.

Streaking is the most common method employed. If the proportions of bacteria in the mixed culture are roughly equal then streaking on an ordinary nutrient medium should yield single colonies of all microbial types. More usually, the organism of interest is present only as a very small fraction of the total microbial population, necessitating the use of selective media.

A selective enrichment broth is initially inoculated with the mixed population of cells and this inhibits the growth of the majority of the background population. At the same time the growth of the organism of interest is encouraged. After incubation in these media the cultures are streaked out on to solid selective media, which frequently contain indicators to further differentiate species on the basis of fermentation of specific sugars.

Classification and identification

Taxonomy is the ordering of living organisms into groups on the basis of their similarities. In this way we can construct a hierarchy of interrelationships such that species with similar characteristics are grouped within the same genus, genera which have similarities are grouped within the same family, families grouped into orders, orders into classes and classes into divisions. The classification of bacteria does pose a problem because a species is defined as a group of closely related organisms that reproduce sexually to produce fertile offspring. Of course, bacteria do not reproduce sexually and so a bacterial species is simply defined as a population of cells with similar characteristics.

Nomenclature

Bergey's Manual of Determinative Bacteriology (Holt et al 1994) lists over 500 bacterial genera and each of these contains many species. It is therefore extremely important to be sure there is no confusion when describing any one particular bacterial species. Although we are familiar with the use of trivial names in ornithology and botany (we understand what we mean when we describe a sparrow or a daffodil), such an approach could have disastrous consequences in clinical microbiology. For this reason, we use the binomial system of nomenclature developed by Carolus Linnaeus in the 18th century. In this system every bacterium is given two names, the first being the genus name and the second the species name. By convention, the name is italicized or underlined, and the genus name always begins with a capital letter whereas the species name begins in lower case.

Identification

The organization of bacteria into groups of related microorganisms is based upon the similarity of their chromosomal DNA. Although this provides a very accurate indicator of genetic relatedness it is far too cumbersome a tool to use for the identification of an unknown bacterium isolated from a sample. In this instance a series of rapid and simple tests is required that probe the phenotypic characteristics of the microorganism. The tests are conducted in a logical series of steps, the results from each test providing information for the next stage of the investigation. An example of such a procedure is given below:

Morphology:	microscopical investigations using a wet mount to determine cell size, shape, formation of spores, aggregation, motility, etc.
Staining reactions:	Gram stain, acid-fast stain, spore stain
Cultural reactions:	appearance on solid media (colony formation, shape, size, colour, texture, smell, pigments, etc.); aerobic/anaerobic growth, temperature requirements, pH requirements
Biochemical reactions:	enzymatic activities are probed to distinguish between closely related bacteria. Can be performed in traditional mode or using kits

Biochemical tests These are designed to examine the enzymatic capabilities of the organism. As there is a large number of biochemical tests that can be performed, the preliminary steps help to narrow down the range to those that will be most discriminatory. Given below are a few examples of commonly used biochemical tests.

Sugar fermentation is very frequently used and examines the ability of the organism to ferment a range of sugars. A number of tubes of peptone water are prepared, each containing a different sugar. An acid–base indicator is incorporated into the medium that also contains a

Durham tube (a small inverted tube filled with medium) capable of collecting any gas produced during fermentation. After inoculation and incubation, the tubes are examined for acid production (as indicated by a change in the colour of the indicator) and gas production (as seen by a bubble of gas collected in the inverted Durham tube).

Proteases are produced by a number of bacteria, e.g. *Bacillus* species and *Pseudomonas*, and they are responsible for the breakdown of protein into smaller units. Gelatin is a protein that can be added to liquid media to produce a stiff gel similar to agar. Unlike agar, which cannot be utilized by bacteria, those organisms producing proteases will destroy the gel structure and liquefy the medium. A medium made of nutrient broth solidified with gelatin is normally incorporated in boiling tubes or small bottles and inoculated by means of a stab wire. After incubation it is important to refrigerate the gelatin prior to examination, otherwise false positives may be produced. Proteases can also be detected using milk agar, which is opaque. Protease producers form colonies with clear haloes around them where the enzyme has diffused into the medium and digested the casein.

Oxidase is produced by *Neisseria* and *Pseudomonas* and can be detected using 1% tetramethylparaphenylene diamine. The enzyme catalyses the transport of electrons between electron donors in the bacteria and the redox dye. A positive reaction is indicated by a deep purple colour in the reduced dye. The test is carried out by placing the reagent directly on to an isolated colony on an agar surface. Alternatively, a filter paper strip impregnated with the dye is moistened with water and, using a platinum loop, a bacterial colony spread across the surface. If positive, a purple colour will appear within 10 seconds. Note that the use of iron loops may give false-positive reactions.

The indole test distinguishes those bacteria capable of decomposing the amino acid tryptophan to indole. Any indole produced can be tested by a colorimetric reaction with *p*-dimethylaminobenzaldehyde. After incubation in peptone water, 0.5 mL Kovacs reagent is placed on the surface of the culture, shaken, and a positive reaction is indicated by a red colour. Organisms giving positive indole reactions include *E. coli* and *Proteus vulgaris*.

Catalase is responsible for the breakdown of hydrogen peroxide into oxygen and water. The test may be performed by adding 1 mL of 10-vol hydrogen peroxide directly to the surface of colonies growing on an agar slope. A vigorous frothing of the surface liquid indicates the presence of catalase. *Staphylococcus* and *Micrococcus* are catalase positive, whereas *Streptococcus* is catalase negative.

Urease production enables certain bacteria to break down urea to ammonia and carbon dioxide:

$$NH_2 - CO - NH_2 + H_2O \xrightarrow{\text{Urease}} 2NH_3 + CO_2$$

This test is readily carried out by growing the bacteria on a medium containing urea and an acid–base indicator. After incubation the production of ammonia will be shown by the alkaline reaction of the indicator. Examples of urease-negative bacteria include *E. coli* and *Enterococcus faecalis*.

Simmons citrate agar was developed to test for the presence of organisms that could utilize citrate as the sole source of carbon and energy and ammonia as the main source of nitrogen. It is used to differentiate members of the Enterobacteriaceae. The medium, containing bromothymol blue as indicator, is surface inoculated on slopes and citrate utilization demonstrated by an alkaline reaction and a change in the indicator colour from a dull green to a bright blue. *E. coli, Shigella, Edwardsiella* and *Yersinia* do not utilize citrate, whereas *Serratia, Enterobacter, Klebsiella* and *Proteus* do and so give a positive result.

The methyl red test is used to distinguish organisms that produce and maintain a high level of acidity from those that initially produce acid but restore neutral conditions with further metabolism. The organism is grown on glucose phosphate medium and, after incubation, a few drops of methyl red are added and the colour immediately recorded. A red colour indicates acid production (positive), whereas a yellow colour indicates alkali (negative).

Some organisms can convert carbohydrates to acetyl methyl carbinol (CH_3-CO-CHOH-CH_3). This may be oxidized to diacetyl (CH_3-CO-CO-CH_3), which will react with guanidine residues in the medium under alkaline conditions to produce a colour. This is the basis of the Voges Proskauer test, which is usually carried out at the same time as the methyl red test. The organism is again grown in glucose phosphate medium and, after incubation, 40% KOH is added together with 5% α-naphthol in ethanol. After mixing, a positive reaction is indicated by a pink colour in 2–5 minutes, gradually becoming darker red up to 30 minutes. Organisms giving positive Voges Proskauer reactions usually give negative methyl red reactions, as the production of acetylmethyl carbinol is accompanied by low acid production. *Klebsiella* species typically give a positive Voges Proskauer reaction.

Rapid identification systems With the increasing demand for quick and accurate identification of bacteria, a number of micromethods have been developed combining a variety of biochemical tests selected for their rapidity of reading and high discrimination. The API bacterial identification system is an example of such a micromethod and comprises a plastic tray containing dehydrated substrates in a number of wells. Culture is added to the wells, dissolving the substrate and allowing the fermentation of carbohydrates or the presence of enzymes similar to those just described to be demonstrated. In some cases incubation times of 2 hours are sufficient for accurate identification. Kits are available with different reagents, permitting the identification of Enterobacteriaceae, Streptococcaceae, staphylococci, anaerobes, yeasts and moulds. Accurate identification is made by reference to a table of results.

The tests described so far will enable differentiation of an unknown bacterium to species level. However, it is apparent that not all isolates of the same species behave in an identical manner. For example, *E. coli* isolated from the intestines of a healthy person is relatively harmless compared to the well-publicized *E. coli* O157.H7, which causes intense food poisoning and haemolytic uraemic syndrome. On occasions it is therefore necessary to distinguish further between isolates from the same species. This can be performed using, among other things, serological tests and phage typing.

Serological tests Bacteria have antigens associated with their cell envelopes (O-antigens), with their flagella (H-antigens) and with their capsules (K-antigens). When injected into an animal, antibodies will be produced directed specifically towards those antigens and able to react with them. Specific antisera are prepared by immunizing an animal with a killed or attenuated bacterial suspension and taking blood samples. Serum containing the antibodies can then be separated. If a sample of bacterial suspension is placed on a glass slide and mixed with a small amount of specific antiserum, then the bacteria will be seen to clump when examined under the microscope. The test can be made more quantitative by using the tube dilution technique, where a given amount of antigen is mixed with a series of dilutions of specific antisera. The highest dilution at which agglutination occurs is called the agglutination titre.

Phage typing Many bacteria are susceptible to lytic bacteriophages whose action is very specific. Identification may be based on the susceptibility of a culture to a set of such type-specific lytic bacteriophages. This method enables very detailed identification of the organisms to be made, e.g. one serotype of *Salmonella typhi* has been further subdivided into 80 phage types using this technique.

FUNGI

Fungus is a general term used to describe all yeasts and moulds, whereas a mould is a filamentous fungus exhibiting a mycelial form of growth. The study of fungi is called mycology. Yeasts and moulds are eukaryotic microorganisms possessing organized demonstrable nuclei enclosed within an outer membrane, a nucleolus and chromatin strands that become organized into chromosomes during cell division. Fungal cell walls are composed predominantly of polysaccharide. In most cases this is chitin mixed with cellulose, glucan and mannan. Proteins and glycoproteins are also present but peptidoglycan is absent. The polysaccharide polymers are crosslinked to provide a structure of considerable strength which gives the cell osmotic stability. The fungal membrane contains sterols such as ergosterol and zymosterol not found in mammalian cells, and this provides a useful target for antifungal antibiotics. The role of fungi in nature is predominantly a scavenging one and in this respect they are vital for the decomposition and recycling of organic materials. Of the more than 100 000 species of known fungi, fewer than 100 are human pathogens and most of these are facultative and not obligate parasites.

Fungal morphology

The fungi can be divided into five broad groups on the basis of their morphology.

Yeasts

These are spherical or ovoid unicellular bodies 2–4 μm in diameter which typically reproduce by budding. In liquid cultures and on agar they behave very much like bacteria. Examples include *Saccharomyces cerevisiae*, strains of which are used in baking and in the production of beers and wines. *Cryptococcus neoformans* is the only significant pathogen and this gives rise to a respiratory tract disease called cryptococcosis, which in most cases is relatively mild. However, the microorganism may disseminate, leading to multiorgan disease, including meningitis. Cryptococcosis is of particular significance in immune-compromised patients. If left untreated, 80% of patients with disseminated cryptococcosis will die within 1 year.

Yeast-like fungi

These organisms normally behave like typical budding yeasts but under certain circumstances the buds do not separate and become elongated. The resulting structure resembles a filament and is called a pseudomycelium. It differs from a true mycelium in that there are no interconnecting pores between the cellular compartments comprising the hyphae.

The most important member of this group is *Candida albicans*, which is usually resident in the mouth, intestines and vagina. Under normal conditions *Candida* does not cause problems but if the environmental balance is disturbed then problems can arise. These include vaginal thrush (vaginitis) and oral thrush. Overgrowth of *Candida albicans* within the gut can lead to symptoms of inexplicable fatigue and malaise that is difficult to diagnose. Predisposing factors may include poor diet, diabetes, alcoholism and long-term treatment with steroids.

Dimorphic fungi

These grow as yeasts or as filaments depending upon the cultural conditions. At 22°C, either in the soil or in culture media, filamentous mycelial forms and reproductive spores are produced, whereas at 37°C in the body, the microorganisms assume a yeast-like appearance. *Histoplasma capsulatum* is an important pathogen that gives rise to respiratory illness. The infectious form is the spore that is borne on the wind and is inhaled. It has been postulated that a single spore can elicit an infection. On entering the body, the spores germinate to give rise to the yeast form. Primary infections are often mild but progressive disseminated histoplasmosis is a very severe disease that can affect many organs of the body.

Filamentous fungi

This group comprises those multicellular moulds that grow in the form of long, slender filaments 2–10 μm in diameter called hyphae. The branching hyphae, which constitute the vegetative or somatic structure of the mould, intertwine and gradually spread over the entire surface of the available substrate, extracting nutrients and forming a dense mat or mycelium. The hyphae may be non-septate (coenocytic) or septate but in each case the nutrients and cellular components are freely diffusible along the length of the filament. This is facilitated by the presence of pores within the septa.

Mushrooms and toadstools

This group is characterized by the production of large reproductive fruiting bodies of complex structure. They also possess elaborate propagation mechanisms. Some of these fungi are edible and are used in cooking but others, such as *Amanita phalloides* (death angel), produce potent mycotoxins that may result in death if eaten.

Reproduction of fungi

In the somatic portion of most fungi the nuclei are very small and the mechanism of nuclear division is uncertain. Under the correct environmental conditions the organisms will switch from the somatic or vegetative growth phase to a reproductive form, so that the fungus may propagate the species by producing new mycelia on fresh food substrates. Two types of reproduction are found: asexual and sexual.

Asexual reproduction

Asexual reproduction is in general more important for the propagation of the species. Mechanisms include binary fission, budding, hyphal fragmentation and spore formation. Each progeny is an exact replica of the parent and no species variation can occur. Some yeasts (e.g. *Schizosaccharomyces rouxii*) reproduce by binary fission in the same way as bacteria. The parent cell enlarges, its nucleus divides and, when a cross-wall is produced across the cell, two identical daughter cells form.

Budding occurs in the majority of yeasts and is the production of a small outgrowth or bud from the parent cell. As the bud increases in size, the nucleus divides and one of the pair migrates into the bud. The bud eventually breaks off from the parent to form a new individual. A scar is left behind on the parent cell and each parent can produce up to 24 buds.

Fungi growing in a filamentous form may employ hyphal fragmentation as a means of asexual propagation. The hyphal tips break up into component segments (called arthroconidia or arthrospores), each of which can disperse on the wind to other environments and fresh food substrates.

The formation of specialized spore-bearing structures containing reproductive spores is the most common method of asexual reproduction (Fig.14.9). The spores can be borne in a sporangium, supported on a sporangiophore. A limiting membrane surrounds the sporangium and the spores contained within it are called sporangiospores. The spores are released when the sporangium ruptures. This type of reproduction is found in the lower fungi possessing non-septate hyphae (e.g. *Mucor* and *Rhizopus*). Separate spores produced at the tips of specialized conidiophores are called conidiospores. A diverse range of structures is found in nature and Figure 14.9 illustrates some of the different types of asexual spores found in fungi.

Sexual reproduction

Sexual reproduction involves the union of two compatible nuclei and allows variation of the species. Mycology is made much more complex because individual fungi are given different names depending upon whether they are in the sexual or the asexual stage. Not all fungi have been observed to carry out sexual reproduction. Some species produce distinguishable male and female sex organs on the same mycelium and are therefore hermaphroditic, i.e. a single colony can reproduce sexually by itself. Others produce mycelia which are either male or female (called dioecious) and can therefore only reproduce when two dissimilar organisms come together.

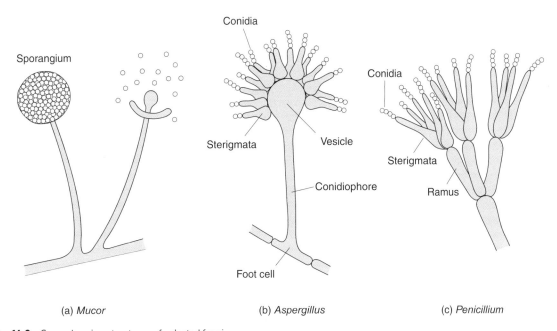

(a) *Mucor* (b) *Aspergillus* (c) *Penicillium*

Fig. 14.9 Spore-bearing structures of selected fungi.

Fungal classification

The pharmaceutically important fungi can be found within four main taxonomic classes.

Zygomycetes

These are terrestrial saprophytes possessing non-septate hyphae and are sometimes referred to as the lower fungi. Apart from their hyphae, they can be distinguished from other filamentous fungi by the presence of sporangia. Examples are *Mucor* and *Rhizopus*, which are important in the manufacture of organic acids and the biotransformation of steroids. They are also common spoilage organisms.

Ascomycetes

Ascomycetes possess septate hyphae and the sexual or perfect stage is characterized by the presence of a sac-like reproductive structure called an ascus. This typically contains eight ascospores. The asexual or imperfect stage involves conidiospores. An example is *Claviceps purpurea*, which is a parasite of rye and is important as a source of ergot alkaloids used to control haemorrhage and in treating migraine. A subclass of the Ascomycetes is the Hemiascomycetes. This includes the yeasts such as *Saccharomyces* and *Cryptococcus*, together with *Torulopsis* and *Candida*.

Deuteromycetes

Sometimes called the Fungi Imperfecti, this group includes those fungi in which the sexual stage of reproduction has not been observed. *Penicillium* and *Aspergillus* are Ascomycetes but classified among the Deuteromycetes as the perfect stage is apparently absent. *Penicillium chrysogenum* is important in the production of the antibiotic penicillin, whereas *Aspergillus* species have found widespread industrial usage owing to their extensive enzymic capabilities. Some *Aspergillus* species also produce mycotoxins and can cause serious infections in humans. The Deuteromycetes contains most of the human pathogens, such as *Blastomyces* and *Coccidioides*, and some of the dermatophyte fungi.

Basidiomycetes

This is the most advanced group, containing the mushrooms and toadstools. Sexual reproduction is by basidiospores. The group also includes the rusts (cereal parasites) and smuts.

REFERENCE

Holt, J.G., Krieg, N.R., Sneath, P.H.A., Stanley, T., Williams, S.T. (eds) (1994) *Bergey's Manual of Determinative Bacteriology,* 9th edn. Williams and Wilkins, Baltimore.

BIBLIOGRAPHY

Bannister, B.A., Begg, N.T., Gillespie, S.H. (2000) *Infectious Disease,* 2nd edn. Blackwell Science, Oxford.
Collins, C.H., Lyne, P.M., Grange, J.M., Falkinham, J. (2004) *Microbiological Methods,* 8th edn. Hodder Arnold, London.
Davies, B.D., Dulbecco, R., Eisen H.N., Ginsberg H.S. (eds) (1990) *Microbiology,* 4th edn. J.B. Lippincott, Philadelphia.
Denyer, S.P., Hodges, N.A., Gorman, S.P. (2004) *Hugo and Russell's Pharmaceutical Microbiology,* 7th edn. Blackwell Publishing, Oxford.
Mims, C., Playfair, J., Roitt, I., Wakelin, D., R. Williams (eds) (2004) *Medical Microbiology,* 3rd edn. Mosby International, London.
Neidhardt, F., Ingraham, J.L., Schaechter, M. (1990) *Physiology of the Bacterial Cell: A Molecular Approach.* Sinauer Associates, Massachusetts.
Russell, A.D., Chopra, I. (1996) *Understanding Antibacterial Action and Resistance,* 2nd edn. Ellis Horwood, London.
Stryer, L., Berg, J., Tymoczko, J. (2002) *Biochemistry,* 5th edn. Freeman, New York.

Pharmaceutical applications of microbiological techniques

N. A. Hodges

INTRODUCTION

The purpose of this chapter is to bring together those
microbiological methods and procedures that are relevant
to the design and production of medicines and medical
devices. These are methods used (a) to determine the
potency or activity of antimicrobial chemicals, e.g. antibiotics, preservatives and disinfectants, and (b) as part of
the microbiological quality control of manufactured sterile and non-sterile products. The chapter describes the
experimental procedures that are unique or particularly
relevant to pharmacy, rather than those that are common
to microbiology as a whole. In the latter category, for
example, are procedures used to identify and enumerate
microorganisms. These, together with staining and micro-
scopical techniques, are described in Chapter 14.

   Several of the methods and tests discussed here are the
subject of monographs or appendices in pharmacopoeias
or they are described in national and international standards or other recognized reference works. It is not the
intention to reproduce these official testing procedures in
detail but rather to explain the principles of the tests, to
draw attention to difficult or important aspects, and to
indicate the advantages, problems or shortcomings of the
various methods.

MEASUREMENT OF ANTIMICROBIAL ACTIVITY

In most of the methods used to assess the activity of
antimicrobial chemicals, an inoculum of the test organism is added to a solution of the chemical under test,
samples are removed over a period of time, the chemical
is inactivated and the proportion of surviving cells determined. Alternatively, culture medium is present together
with the chemical and the degree of inhibition of growth
of the test organism is measured. In each case it is
necessary to standardize and control such factors as the

concentration of the test organism, its origin, i.e. the species and strain employed, together with the culture medium in which it was grown, the phase of growth from which the cells were taken, and the temperature and time of incubation of the cells after exposure to the chemical. Because such considerations are common to several of the procedures described here, e.g. antibiotic assays, preservative efficacy (challenge) tests and determinations of minimum inhibitory concentration (MIC), it is appropriate that they should be considered first, both to emphasize their importance and to avoid repetition.

Factors to be controlled in the measurement of antimicrobial activity

Origin of the test organism

Although two cultures may bear the same generic and specific name, i.e. they may both be called *Escherichia coli*, this does not mean that they are identical. Certainly, they would normally be similar in many respects, e.g. morphology (appearance), cultural requirements and biochemical characteristics, but they may exhibit slight variations in some of these properties; such variants are described as strains of *E. coli*. A variety of strains of a single species may normally be obtained from a culture collection, e.g. the National Collection of Industrial and Marine Bacteria or the National Collection of Type Cultures. Different strains may also occur in hospital pathology laboratories by isolation from swabs taken from infected patients or by isolation from contaminated food, cosmetic or pharmaceutical products, and from many other sources. Strains obtained in these ways are likely to exhibit variations in resistance to antimicrobial chemicals. Strains from human or animal infections are frequently more resistant to antimicrobial chemicals, particularly antibiotics, than those from other sources. Similarly, strains derived from contaminated medicines may be more resistant to preservative chemicals than those obtained from culture collections. Therefore, in order to achieve results that are reproducible by a variety of laboratories, it is necessary to specify the strain of the organism used for the determination.

It is becoming increasingly common, too, for official testing methods to limit the number of times the culture collection specimen may be regrown in fresh medium (called the number of subcultures or passages) before it must be replaced. This is because the characteristics of the organism (including its resistance to antimicrobial chemicals) may progressively change as a result of mutation and natural selection through the many generations that might arise during months or years of laboratory cultivation.

Composition and pH of the culture medium

There are several methods of assessing antimicrobial activity which all have in common the measurement of inhibition of growth of a test organism when the antimicrobial chemical is added to the culture medium. In such cases the composition and pH of the medium may influence the result. The medium may contain substances that antagonize the action of the test compound, e.g. high concentrations of thymidine or paraaminobenzoic acid will interfere with sulfonamide activity.

The antimicrobial activities of several groups of chemical are influenced by the ease with which they cross the cell membrane and interfere with the metabolism of the cell. This, in turn, is influenced by the lipid solubility of the substance, because the membrane contains a high proportion of lipid and tends to permit the passage of lipid-soluble substances. Many antimicrobial chemicals are weak acids or weak bases, which are more lipid soluble in the unionized form. The pH of the environment therefore affects their degree of ionization, hence their lipid solubility and so, ultimately, their antimicrobial effect. Benzoic acid, for example, is a preservative used in several oral mixtures which has a much greater activity in liquids buffered to an acid pH value than those which are neutral or alkaline. Conversely, weak bases such as the aminoglycoside antibiotics, e.g. streptomycin, neomycin and gentamicin, are more active at slightly alkaline pH values. The presence of organic matter, e.g. blood, pus or serum, is likely to have a marked protective effect on the test organism and so antimicrobial chemicals may appear less active in the presence of such material.

The activity of several antibiotics, notably tetracyclines and aminoglycosides, is reduced by the presence of high concentrations of di- or trivalent cations in the medium.

Exposure and incubation conditions

The temperature, duration and redox conditions of exposure to the antimicrobial chemical (or incubation of survivors after exposure) may all have a significant effect on its measured activity. Increasing the temperature of exposure of the test organism to the chemical increases the antimicrobial activity by a factor which is quantified by the temperature coefficient (Q_{10} value: the number of times increase in activity for a 10°C rise in temperature). Phenols and alcohols, for example, may respectively exhibit Q_{10} values of 3–5 and >10, and so a variation of 5°C in the temperature of exposure (which is permitted by pharmacopoeial preservative efficacy tests, for example) may lead to a markedly different rate of kill of the organism in question.

The period of time for which the test organism is exposed to the antimicrobial chemical may influence the recorded result because it is possible for the organism to adapt and become resistant to the presence of the chemical. In preservative efficacy tests, the exposure period is normally 28 days, which is sufficient time for any cells that are not killed during the first 24–48 hours to recover and start to reproduce, so that the final bacterial concentration may be much higher than that at the start. This is illustrated in Figure 15.1, which shows the effect of the quaternary ammonium preservative benzethonium bromide on *Pseudomonas aeruginosa*. The concentration of bacteria was reduced to approximately 0.01% of the initial value during the first 6 hours but the bacteria that survived this early period recovered to the original level within 2 days. There is the potential for a similar phenomenon to arise in other situations, e.g. in minimum inhibitory concentration (MIC) determinations of bacteriostatic agents (those that do not kill but merely inhibit the growth of the test organism), although it is not common in MICs because the exposure (incubation) time is much shorter than that in preservative testing.

The effect of some antibiotics may be influenced by the redox conditions during their period of contact with the test organism. Aminoglycosides, for example, are far less active, and metronidazole is far more active, under conditions of low oxygen availability. Such effects may even be seen during agar diffusion antibiotic assays, in which the antibiotic diffuses from a well into an agar gel inoculated with the test organism; the diameter of the zone of growth inhibition that surrounds a well filled with neomycin solution, for example, may be significantly greater at the surface of the agar (where there is abundant oxygen) than at its base, where the oxygen concentration is limited by its poor diffusion through the gel.

Inoculum concentration and physiological state

It is perhaps not surprising that the concentration of the inoculum can markedly affect antimicrobial action, with high inoculum levels tending to result in reduced activity. There are two main reasons for this. First, there is the phenomenon of drug adsorption on to the cell surface or absorption into the interior of the cell. If the number of drug molecules in the test tube is fixed yet the number of cells present is increased, this obviously results in fewer molecules available per cell and consequently the possibility of a diminished effect. In addition to this there is the second, more specialized case, again concerning antibiotics, where it is frequently observed that certain species of bacteria can synthesize antibiotic-inactivating enzymes, the most common of which are the various types of β-lactamases (those destroying penicillin, cephalosporin and related antibiotics). Thus a high inoculum means a high carryover of enzyme with the inoculum cells, or at least a greater potential synthetic capacity.

Perhaps less predictable than the inoculum concentration effect is the possibility of the inoculum history influencing the result. There is a substantial amount of evidence to show that the manner in which the inoculum of the test organism has been grown and prepared can significantly influence its susceptibility to toxic chemicals. Features such as the nature of the culture medium, e.g. nutrient broth or a defined glucose-salts medium, the metal ion composition of the medium and hence of the cells themselves, and the physiological state of the cells, i.e. 'young' actively growing cells from the logarithmic growth phase or 'old' non-dividing cells from the stationary phase, all have the potential to influence the observed experimental values.

Antibiotic assays

Methods of assaying antibiotics may be broadly divided into three groups.
- Conventional chemical assays, e.g. titrations, spectrophotometry and high-performance liquid chromatography (HPLC).
- Enzyme-based and immunoassays, where the antibiotic is, respectively, the substrate for a specific enzyme or the antigen with which a specific antibody combines.
- Biological assays in which biological activity, in this case bacterial growth inhibition, of the 'test' solution is compared with that of a reference standard.

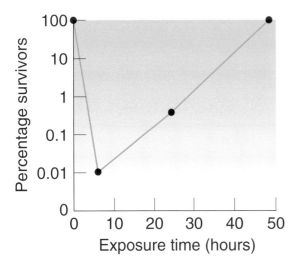

Fig. 15.1 The survival and recovery of *Pseudomonas aeruginosa* exposed to benzethonium chloride during a preservative efficacy test.

Biological methods offer the advantage that the parameter being measured in the assay (growth inhibition) is the property for which the drug is used, and so inactive impurities or degradation products will not interfere and lead to an inaccurate result. Biological methods also offer other advantages (Table 15.1) but they have several significant limitations and non-biological methods are now generally preferred.

Enzyme-based and immunoassay kits are used in hospitals, notably for therapeutic monitoring of toxic antibiotics (e.g. aminoglycosides and vancomycin), whereas HPLC tends to be preferred in the pharmaceutical industry, particularly for quality assurance applications. Biological assays are most likely to be used when the alternatives are inappropriate, especially when the active antibiotic cannot readily be separated from inactive impurities, degradation products or interfering substances, or it cannot easily be assayed by HPLC without derivatization to enhance ultraviolet absorption (e.g. aminoglycosides). These situations may arise:

- when the antibiotic is present in a solution containing a wide variety of complex substances that would interfere with a chemical assay, e.g. fermentation broth, serum or urine
- when the antibiotic is present together with significant concentrations of its breakdown products, e.g. during stability studies as part of product development
- when it has been extracted from a formulated medicine, for example a cream or linctus, when excipients might cause interference
- where the commercially available product is a mixture of isomers that have inherently different antimicrobial activities, which cannot easily be distinguished chemically and which may differ in proportion from batch to batch (e.g. neomycin and gentamicin).

Biological antibiotic assays, or bioassays as they are frequently known, may be of two main types: agar diffusion and turbidimetric. The *European Pharmacopoeia* (EP) (2004) describes experimental details for both methods, e.g. test microorganisms, solvents, buffers, culture media and incubation conditions. In each case a reference material of known activity must be available. When antibiotics were in their infancy few could be produced in the pure state free from contaminating material and specific chemical assays were rarely available. Thus the potency or activity of reference standards was expressed in terms of (international) units of activity. There are few antibiotics for which dosage is still normally expressed in units: nystatin and polymyxin are two of the remaining examples. More commonly, potencies are recorded in terms of $\mu g\ mL^{-1}$ of solution or μg antibiotic mg^{-1} of salt, with dosages expressed in mg. Antibiotic assay results are usually in the form of a potency ratio of the activity of the unknown or test solution divided by that of the standard.

Agar diffusion assays

In this technique the agar medium in a Petri dish or a larger assay plate is inoculated with the test organism, wells are created by removing circular plugs of agar, and these wells are filled with a solution of the chemical under test (Fig. 15.2).

The chemical diffuses through the gel from A towards B and the concentration falls steadily in that direction. The concentration in the region A to X is sufficiently high to prevent growth, i.e. it is an inhibitory concentration. Between X and B the concentration is subinhibitory and growth occurs. The concentration at X at the time the zone edge is formed is known as the critical inhibitory concentration (CIC). After incubation, the gel between A

Table 15.1 Relative merits of alternative antibiotic assay methods

Assay method	Advantages	Disadvantages
Biological methods	Inactive impurities or degradation properties do not interfere Easily scaled up for multiple samples Do not require expensive equipment	Slow, usually requiring overnight incubation Relatively labour-intensive Relatively inaccurate and imprecise, particularly with inexperienced operators
Non-biological methods	Usually rapid, accurate and precise May be more sensitive than biological assays Enzyme and immunological methods are usually assay kits, which give reliable results with inexperienced operators	May require expensive equipment (e.g. HPLC) or expensive reagents or assay kits (enzyme and immunological methods) HPLC can only assay samples sequentially, so unusually large sample numbers may cause problems

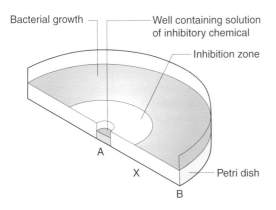

Fig. 15.2 Assessment of antimicrobial activity by agar diffusion.

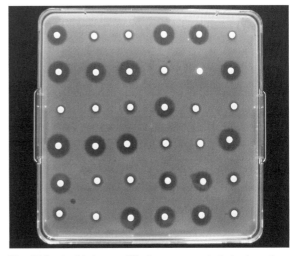

Fig. 15.4 Antibiotic agar diffusion assay conducted using a 6 × 6 assay design in a 30 cm square assay plate.

and X is clear and that between X and B is opaque as a result of microbial growth which, with the common test organisms, is usually profuse. A zone of inhibition is therefore created, the diameter of which will increase as the concentration of chemical in the well increases.

A graph may be constructed which relates zone diameter to the logarithm of the concentration of the solution in the well (Fig. 15.3). It is normally found to be linear over a small concentration range but the square of the diameter must be plotted to achieve linearity over a wide range. A plot such as that in Figure 15.3 may, quite correctly, be used to calculate the concentration of a test solution of antibiotic. In practice, however, it is found to be more convenient to obtain reliable mean zone diameters for the standard at just two or three concentrations, rather than somewhat less reliable values for six or seven concentrations. There is no reason why an assay should not be based upon a two- or three-point line, provided that those points are reliable and that preliminary experiments have shown that the plotted relationship over the concentration range in question is linear.

It is not common to conduct antibiotic assays in Petri dishes because too few zones may be accommodated on a standard-sized dish to permit the replication necessary to obtain the required accuracy and precision. Antibiotic

assays, when performed on a large scale, are more often conducted using large assay plates 300 mm or more square (Fig. 15.4). The wells are created in a square design and the number that may be accommodated will depend upon the anticipated zone diameters: 36 or 64 wells are common (6 × 6 or 8 × 8, respectively). The antibiotic standard material may be used in solution at three known concentrations (frequently referred to as 'doses') and the antibiotic solution of unknown concentration treated likewise; alternatively, each may be employed at two concentrations. A randomization pattern known as a Latin square is used to ensure that there is a suitable distribution of the solutions over the plate, thereby minimizing any errors due to uneven agar thickness.

In the case of an assay based upon standard solutions used at two concentrations, the potency ratio may be calculated directly from the graph (as shown in Fig. 15.5) or by using the formula below:

$$\mathrm{Log}\,X = \mathrm{LDR} \times \frac{(\mathrm{UH}+\mathrm{UL})-(\mathrm{SH}+\mathrm{SL})}{(\mathrm{SH}-\mathrm{SL})+(\mathrm{UH}-\mathrm{UL})} \quad (15.1)$$

where X is the potency ratio, LDR is the logarithm of the dose ratio (i.e. ratio of concentrations of standard solutions), UH, UL, SH and SL are the mean zone diameters for the unknown and standard high and low doses. The derivation of this is described in detail by Wardlaw (1999), who deals extensively with the subject of antibiotic assays. The tests for acceptable limits of parallelism between the line joining the standards and that joining the test points, together with confidence limits applicable to the calculated potency ratios, are described in the current EP.

In calculating the potency ratio directly from Figure 15.5, the zone diameters for the standard and unknown

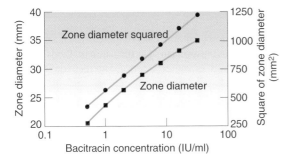

Fig. 15.3 Calibration plots for agar diffusion assays.

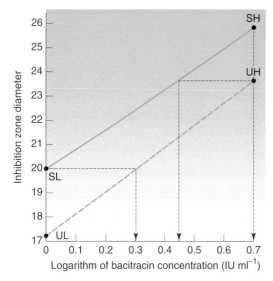

Fig. 15.5 Four-point agar diffusion assay for bacitracin.

high concentrations are plotted at the same abscissa values, and those for the low concentrations similarly. Two zone diameters are considered which are as widely separated on the ordinate as possible while still being covered by the standard and the test lines. The ratio of the concentrations required to achieve the selected diameter is thus an estimate of the potency ratio. The mean of the two estimates taken at the extremes of the range of common zone diameters should be identical to the value by calculation from the formula. Thus, in Figure 15.5, at a zone diameter of 23.75 mm the first estimate of potency ratio is 0.557 (antilog of 0.445 divided by antilog of 0.699); the second is 0.507 (antilog of zero divided by the antilog of 0.295). The mean value of 0.53 indicates the unknown solution to have approximately half the activity of the standard.

Practical aspects of the conduct of agar diffusion assays The agar may be surface inoculated or inoculated throughout while in the molten state prior to pouring. In the latter case zones may arise which are different in diameter at the agar surface than at the base of the Petri dish; this may complicate the recording of zone diameters. Zones which are not perfectly circular may be disregarded, although it may be appropriate to record the mean of the long and short axes. Such zones may result from non-circular wells, careless filling or uneven drying of the agar gel owing to a poorly fitting plate cover. The zones may be read directly with callipers or, more conveniently, after enlargement by projection onto a screen. Automatic zone readers incorporating a series of photocells that detect opacity changes at the zone edge are available, and may be linked to a personal computer which rapidly calculates the

result together with the appropriate statistical analyses. The size of the zone is determined by the relative rates of diffusion of the drug molecule and growth of the test organism. If the assay plates are left at room temperature for 1–4 hours prior to incubation, growth is retarded whereas diffusion proceeds. This may result in larger zones and improved precision.

The zone diameter is affected by most of the factors previously stated to influence antimicrobial activity and, in addition, gel strength and the presence of other solutes in the antibiotic solution, e.g. buffer salts. If the antibiotic has been extracted from a formulated medicine, e.g. cream, lotion or mixture, excipients may be simultaneously removed and influence the diffusion of the antibiotic in the gel; sugars are known to have this effect. Because antibiotic assays involve a comparison of two solutions that are similarly affected by changes in experimental conditions, day-to-day variations in, for example, inoculum concentration will not have a great effect on the accuracy of the potency ratio obtained. However, the precision may be affected. The volume of liquid in the well is of minimal importance; it is usually of the order of 0.1 mL and is delivered by semi-automatic pipette. As an alternative to wells, the antibiotic may be introduced on to the agar using absorbent paper discs, metal cylinders or 'fish spine' beads (beads having a hole drilled in them which contains the liquid).

For many antibiotics, the test organism is a *Bacillus* species and the inoculum is in the form of a spore suspension, which is easy to prepare, standardize and store. Alternatively, frozen inocula from liquid nitrogen may be used as a means of improving reproducibility.

Careful storage and preparation of the reference standards are essential. The reference antibiotic is usually stored at low temperature in a freeze-dried condition.

Turbidimetric assays

In this case antibiotic standards at several concentrations are incorporated into liquid media and the extent of growth inhibition of the test organism is measured turbidimetrically using a nephelometer or spectrophotometer. The unknown or test antibiotic preparation is run simultaneously, again at several concentrations, and the degree of growth inhibition compared. Such assays are less commonly used than agar diffusion methods because their precision is rather inferior but they do have the advantage of speed: the result may be available after an incubation period as short as 3–4 hours. They are also more sensitive than diffusion assays and consequently may be applied to low-activity preparations.

The shape and slope of the dose–response plot for a turbidimetric assay may be more variable than that for agar diffusion, and non-linear plots are common. Typical dose–response plots are shown in Hewitt & Vincent (1989). The plotted points are usually the mean turbidity values obtained from replicate tubes and the assay may be conducted using a Latin square arrangement of tubes incubated in a shaker, which is necessary to ensure adequate aeration and uniform growth throughout the tube.

Practical aspects of the conduct of turbidimetric assays Incubation time is critical in two respects. First, it is necessary to ensure that the culture in each of the many tubes in the incubator has exactly the same incubation period, because errors of a few minutes become significant in a total of only 3–4 hours' incubation. Care must therefore be taken to ensure that the tubes are inoculated in a precise order, and that growth is stopped in the same order by the addition of formalin, heating or other means.

The incubation period must be appropriate to the inoculum level so that the cultures do not achieve maximal growth. At the concentrations used for such assays, the antibiotics usually reduce growth rate but do not limit total growth. Therefore, if the incubation period is sufficiently long, all the cultures may achieve the same cell density regardless of the antibiotic concentration.

There are certain other limitations to the use of turbidimetric assays. Because it is the 'cloudiness' of the culture that is measured, standard and test solutions in which the organisms are suspended should, ideally, be clear before inoculation. Cloudy or hazy solutions which may result from the extraction of the antibiotic from a cream, for example, can only be determined after similarly compensating the standards or otherwise eliminating the error. Test organisms that produce pigments during the course of the incubation period should be avoided; so too should those that normally clump in suspension.

The rate of growth of the test organism may vary significantly from one batch of medium to another. Thus it is important to ensure that all the tubes in the assay contain medium from the same batch, and were prepared and sterilized at the same time. Many liquid media become darker brown on prolonged heating, and so samples from the same batch may differ in colour if the sterilizing time is not strictly controlled.

Minimum inhibitory concentration determinations (MICs)

The MIC is the lowest concentration of an antimicrobial chemical found to inhibit the growth of a particular test organism. It is therefore a fundamental measure of the intrinsic antimicrobial activity (potency) of a chemical, which may be an antiseptic, disinfectant, preservative or antibiotic. MIC determinations are applied to chemicals in the pure state, i.e. they are particularly relevant to raw materials rather than to the final formulated medicines;

the latter are usually subject to preservative efficacy (challenge) tests to assess their antimicrobial activity. MIC values are usually expressed in terms of $\mu g\ mL^{-1}$ or, less commonly, as in the case of some antibiotics, units mL^{-1}. It is important to recognize that the test organism is not necessarily killed at the MIC. Whether or not the cells die or merely cease growing depends upon the mode of action of the antimicrobial agent in question.

An MIC is an absolute value which is not based upon a comparison with a standard/reference preparation, as in the case of antibiotic assays and certain disinfectant tests. For this reason inadequate control of experimental conditions is particularly likely to have an adverse effect on results. Discrepancies in MIC values measured in different laboratories are often attributable to slight variations in such conditions, and care must be taken to standardize all the factors previously stated to influence the result. It is important also to state the experimental details concerning an MIC determination. A statement such as 'the MIC for phenol against *E. coli* is 0.1% w/v' is not, by itself, very useful. It has far more value if the strain of *E. coli*, the inoculum concentration, the culture medium, etc., are also stated.

MIC test methods

The most common way to conduct MIC determinations is to incorporate the antimicrobial chemical at a range of concentrations into a liquid medium, the containers of which are then inoculated, incubated and examined for growth.

Test tubes may be used but microtitre plates (small rectangular plastic trays with, usually, 96 wells each holding approximately 0.1 mL liquid) and other miniaturized systems are common. It is possible to incorporate the chemical into molten agar, which is then poured into Petri dishes and allowed to set. Two advantages of using a series of agar plates are that several organisms can be tested at the same time using a multipoint inoculator, and there is a greater chance of detecting contaminating organisms (as uncharacteristic colonies) on the agar surface than in liquid media. Usually the presence or absence of growth is easier to distinguish on the surface of agar than in liquid media. In tubes showing only faint turbidity, it is often difficult to decide whether growth has occurred or not. Regardless of the method used, the principle is the same and the MIC is the lowest concentration at which growth is inhibited.

In addition to the other experimental details that should be described in order to make the measured result meaningful, it is necessary to specify the increment by which the concentration of test chemical changes from one container to the next. The operator could, for example, change the concentration 10-fold from one tube to the next in the rare circumstance where even the likely order of magnitude of the MIC is not known. Far more commonly, however, the concentration changes by a factor of 2, and this is almost invariably the case when antibiotic MIC values are determined; thus, reference is made to 'doubling dilutions' of the antibiotic. If, for example, an MIC was to be measured using test tubes, an aqueous solution of the chemical would normally be mixed with an equal volume of *double*-strength growth medium in the first tube in the series, then half the contents of the first tube added to an equal volume of *single*-strength medium in the second, and so on. In this case half the contents of the last tube in the series would have to be discarded prior to inoculation in order to maintain the same volume in each tube. Control tubes may be included to demonstrate (a) that the inoculum culture was viable and that the medium was suitable for its growth (a tube containing medium and inoculum but no test chemical) and (b) that the operator was not contaminating the tubes with other organisms during preparation (a tube with no test chemical or added inoculum). It is possible to use an arithmetic series of concentrations of test chemical, e.g. 0.1, 0.2, 0.3, 0.4 ... rather than 0.1, 0.2, 0.4, 0.8 ... $\mu g\ mL^{-1}$. The potential problem with this approach is that there may be merely a gradation in growth inhibition, rather than a sharp point of demarcation, with obvious growth in one tube in the series and no growth in the next.

All the solutions used must be sterilized; it must not be assumed that the test chemical is self-sterilizing. Most disinfectants, antiseptic and preservative chemicals are bactericidal but they are unlikely to kill bacterial spores. Also, several antibiotics act by inhibiting growth and so would not necessarily kill vegetative cells with which they might be contaminated. If the experiment is conducted in tubes, all the tube contents must be mixed before inoculation as well as after, otherwise there is the possibility of the inoculum cells being killed by an artificially high concentration of the test chemical towards the top of the tube. If there is any risk of precipitation of the test chemical or the medium components during incubation, a turbidity comparison must be available for each concentration (same tube contents without inoculum); alternatively, in the case of bactericidal chemicals, the liquid in each tube may be subcultured into pure medium to see whether the inoculum has survived. Each of the tubes in the series may be prepared in duplicate or triplicate if it is considered desirable. This is the case where the incremental change in concentration is small.

Distinction between MICs conducted in agar and the assessment of sensitivity using agar diffusion methods

It is important to understand that when MICs are determined in Petri dishes the antimicrobial chemical is *dissolved* in the agar and is uniformly distributed through the gel when the test organism is inoculated onto the surface. This is a fundamental difference from the test procedure used for antibiotic bioassays where the antibiotic *diffuses* through the agar to create a growth inhibition zone. When MICs are conducted in agar there is no diffusion and no zones of growth inhibition; the result merely depends on the presence or absence of growth of the test organism.

If the agar diffusion method were used to measure the size of the inhibition zones from a series of solutions of progressively decreasing concentration, it would obviously be possible to identify the concentration that just fails to produce an inhibition zone. This is sometimes incorrectly described as the MIC value for the chemical in question; such a procedure, however, gives the critical inhibitory concentration (CIC), not the MIC. CIC values usually exceed MIC values by a factor of 2–4. Not only is this misconception about agar diffusion methods giving MIC values commonly found in the pharmaceutical and chemical literature but misinterpretations of agar diffusion *data* are, unfortunately, also common. The diameter of a growth inhibition zone depends upon several factors. Whilst the sensitivity of the test organism, its concentration and that of the chemical are paramount, the incubation conditions, the physicochemical composition of the gelled culture medium and the properties of the diffusing molecule are also important. It is tempting to take the simplistic view that if two chemicals are used at the same concentration and one produces a larger zone of growth inhibition than the other, that is a direct reflection of their intrinsic antimicrobial activities. Unfortunately, that is often not the case because it fails to take into account the diffusion coefficients of the different molecules. To diffuse well in agar, a molecule should be small, water soluble and of a charge that does not interact with the components of the gel. There are several very effective antimicrobial chemicals that do not diffuse well in agar and if this ability were to be used to assess their antimicrobial activity, they would be incorrectly dismissed as worthless. Parabens are a prime example. Even saturated solutions of parabens in water can fail to give inhibition zones by agar diffusion (Fig. 15.6) but they are, nevertheless, amongst the most effective and widely used antimicrobial preservatives. This fundamental limitation of agar diffusion as a method of assessing antimicrobial potency is all too frequently overlooked.

Preservative efficacy tests (challenge tests)

These are tests applied to the formulated medicine in its final container to determine whether it is adequately protected against microbial spoilage. Preservative efficacy tests are used for this purpose (rather than chemical assays of preservatives) because it is not normally possible

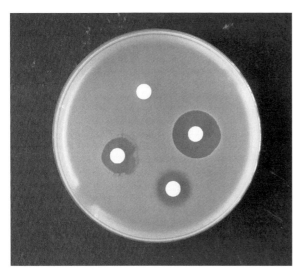

Fig. 15.6 Zones of growth inhibition resulting from preservative chemicals. The disc at the top was soaked in a saturated solution of parabens but failed to produce an inhibition zone because parabens diffuse poorly in agar.

to predict how the activity of a preservative chemical will be influenced by the active ingredients, the excipients and the container itself.

Certain products may contain no added preservative, either because the active ingredients have sufficient antimicrobial activity themselves or because they already contain high concentrations of sugar or salts which restrict the growth of microorganisms. However, such products are rare; multidose injections or eye drops, the majority of oral mixtures, linctuses and similar preparations, together with creams and lotions, all contain preservatives. They are not normally required in anhydrous products, e.g. ointments, or in single-dose injections.

Again, it must not be assumed that products containing antimicrobial agents as the active ingredients are self-sterilizing, It is quite possible for an antibiotic cream, for example, to be active against certain bacteria yet fail to restrict the growth of contaminating yeasts or moulds in the cream itself.

The basic principle of a preservative test is to inoculate separate containers of the product with known concentrations of a variety of test organisms, then remove samples from each container over a period of time and determine the proportion of the inoculum that has survived. When first introduced into national pharmacopoeias, preservative efficacy tests differed to some extent in experimental detail and differed markedly in the required performance criteria for preservatives to be used in different product categories. In the late 1990s moves towards international harmonization of preservative testing procedures in the European, United States and

Japanese pharmacopoeias (EP, USP and JP, respectively) meant that many (but not all) of the discrepancies in experimental detail were eliminated. The differences in performance criteria remain, however, with the EP generally requiring a greater degree of microbial inactivation for the preservative to be considered satisfactory than the USP and JP which, in this respect, are very similar.

The EP (2004) recommends the routine use of four test organisms, each at a final concentration of 10^5–10^6 cells mL^{-1} or g^{-1} in the product. Counts are performed on samples removed at 0h, 6h, 24h, 48h, 7 days, 14 days and 28 days. Various aspects of the test are considered in more detail below.

Choice of test organisms and inoculum concentration

The test organisms used are the bacteria *Staphylococcus aureus*, *Pseudomonas aeruginosa* and *E. coli* (which is used for testing all product types in the USP test but for oral products only in the EP test), together with the yeasts/moulds *Candida albicans* and *Aspergillus niger* (plus the osmophilic *Zygosaccharomyces rouxii* in the EP test for oral syrups). The current EP recommends that the designated organisms be supplemented, where appropriate, by other strains or species that may represent likely contaminants to the preparation. A similar recommendation was contained in earlier versions of the USP preservative test but this has been deleted from the current test (2005).

One problem with adding other organisms (such as those isolated from the manufacturing environment) is that they are not universally available and so a particular product could be tested at different manufacturing sites of the same company and pass in one location yet fail in another simply because the organisms used locally were not the same. The possibility of using resistant strains isolated from previous batches of spoilt product has been advocated but this too may pose problems, in that organisms may rapidly lose their preservative resistance unless routinely grown on media supplemented with the preservative in question.

Previous versions of the British Pharmacopoeial test have recommended consideration of extending the sampling period beyond 28 days and reinoculating the product after the first 28-day sampling period is complete. Both of these practices, however, militate against the development of an international standardized test which is capable of providing reproducible results in different laboratories; consequently, these two procedures are no longer part of the current EP or USP tests.

The inoculum concentration of 10^5–10^6 microorganisms mL^{-1} or g^{-1} of the preparation under test has been criticized as being unrealistic, as it is much higher than that which would be acceptable in a freshly manufactured product. It is adopted, however, in order for the

1000-fold fall in microbial concentration that would be required from an effective parenteral or ophthalmic preservative to be easily measured. The test organisms are added separately to different containers rather than as a mixed inoculum.

Inactivation of preservative

It is quite possible for sufficient of the preservative to be contained in, and carried over with, the sample removed from the container to prevent or retard growth of colonies on the Petri dishes. If the inoculum level of the test organism initially is about 10^6 cells mL^{-1} or g^{-1} of product, the problem of carryover may not arise because a dilution factor of 10^3 or 10^4 would be required to achieve a countable number of colonies on a plate; at this dilution most preservatives would no longer be active. When a high proportion of the cells in the product has died, however, little or no such dilution is required, so preservative carryover is a real problem which may artificially depress the count even more. To avoid this, preservative inhibitors or antagonists may be used. There are several of these; common examples being glycine for aldehydes, thioglycollate or cysteine for heavy metals, and mixtures of lecithin and polysorbate-80 with or without Lubrol W for quaternary ammonium compounds, chlorhexidine and parabens. The use of these and other inactivators has been tabulated by Russell (2004).

An alternative method of removing residual preservative is to pass the sample of inoculated product through a bacteria-proof membrane, so that surviving organisms are retained and washed on the surface of the membrane and the preservative is thus physically separated from them. After washing, the membrane is transferred to the surface of a suitable agar medium and colonies of microorganisms develop on it in the normal way. It is necessary to incorporate controls (validate the method) to demonstrate both that the inactivator really works and that it is not, itself, toxic. The former usually involves mixing the inactivator with the concentrations of preservative likely to be carried over, then inoculating and demonstrating no viability loss. Details of these validation procedures and other aspects of the test are described more fully elsewhere (Hodges 1999).

One further control is a viable count of the inoculum performed by dilution in peptone water to check the actual number of cells introduced into the product. This is necessary because even a 'zero time sample' of the product will contain cells that have been exposed to the preservative for a short period, as it usually takes 15–45 seconds or more to mix the inoculum with the product and then remove the sample. Some of the cells may be killed even in such a short time and so a viable count of the inoculum culture will reflect this.

Interpretation of results

The extent of microbial killing required at the various sampling times for a preservative to be considered acceptable for use in parenteral or ophthalmic products is greater than that required for a preservative to be used in topical products, which in turn exceeds that for an oral product preservative (Table 15.2).

In the case of the first two product categories, the EP specifies two alternative performance criteria, designated A and B. The A criteria express the recommended efficacy to be achieved, whereas the B criteria must be satisfied in justified cases where the A criteria cannot be attained, for example because of an increased risk of adverse reactions. The baseline used as the reference point to assess the extent of killing is the concentration of microorganisms expected to arise in the product after addition and mixing of the inoculum, as calculated from a viable count performed on the concentrated inoculum suspension prior to its addition to the product. The viable count on the time-zero samples removed from the inoculated product is not the baseline.

Disinfectant evaluation

A variety of tests have been described over many years for the assessment of disinfectant activity. Those developed during the early part of the 20th century, e.g. the Rideal–Walker and Chick–Martin tests, were primarily intended for testing phenolic disinfectants against pathogenic organisms such as *Salmonella typhi*. Such phenol coefficient tests are now outmoded because *S. typhi* is no longer endemic in Britain and phenolics are no longer preeminent; indeed, they now represent a minor fraction of the total biocides used for floor disinfection in aseptic dispensing areas in British hospital pharmacies (Murtough et al 2000).

In the second half of the 20th century several other testing procedures were described for use in the UK which reduced the sampling or other problems associated with the early phenol coefficient tests; these included the Berry and Bean method, the British Standard 3286 test for quaternary ammonium compounds and the Kelsey– Sykes test. Other countries adopted procedures that were similar in concept but which differed in experimental detail; these and other tests used in the UK, Europe and the USA are described by Reybrouck (2004). At present there is no internationally applicable and officially recommended disinfectant testing procedure, although a measure of uniformity has emerged in Europe with the establishment by the European Committee for Standardization in 1990 of Technical Committee (TC) 216 that has a responsibility for chemical disinfectants and antiseptics. The European Standard BS EN 1276 (1997) was the first result of the

Table 15.2 Log reductions required in viable counts of microorganisms used in EP (2004) preservative efficacy tests

Product type	Microorganism	Criteria	6 h	24 h	48 h	7 d	14 d	28 d
Parenteral and opthalmic	Bacteria *Pseudomonas aeruginosa* *Staphylococcus aureus* *Escherichia coli**	A B	2	3 1		3 3		NR NI
	Fungi *Aspergillus niger* *Candida albicans*	A B				2	1	NI NI
Topical	Bacteria	A B			2	3	3	NI NI
	Fungi	A B					2 1	NI NI
Oral	Bacteria						3	NI
	Fungi						1	NI
Ear preparations BP 2004 only	Bacteria		2	3				NR
	Fungi						2	NI

*In oral products only
NR, no recovery;
NI, no increase (see text).

work of TC 216; this deals with assessment of bactericidal activity of disinfectants on bacteria in aqueous suspension. Other procedures applicable to more specialized situations, e.g. disinfection of solid surfaces, are currently under development by TC 216.

A confusing variety of methods for describing and categorizing test procedures is in use. Thus, some schemes classify tests according to the organisms to be killed (bactericidal, fungicidal, virucidal, etc.) but classification based upon test design is more common, for example:

- suspension tests
- capacity tests which measure the extent to which the disinfectant can withstand repeated additions of test organisms
- carrier tests, where the organism is loaded or dried on to a carrier
- in-use tests, which are intended to simulate actual conditions of use as closely as possible.

Although most suspension tests of disinfectants have in common the addition of a defined concentration of test organism to the disinfectant solution at a specified temperature, followed by assessment of viability in samples removed after suitable time periods, there are four aspects of disinfectant testing that merit special note.

1. Because disinfectants are normally used in circumstances where there is a significant amount

of organic 'dirt' present, modern testing procedures invariably attempt to take this into consideration. Thus, yeast, albumin or other material is added in known concentration to the disinfectant/microorganism mixture.

2. Regardless of the method by which the antimicrobial activity is assessed (see below), it is a fundamental principle of disinfectant testing, just as it is with preservative efficacy tests, that the antimicrobial activity of the disinfectant must be halted (also referred to as neutralized, inactivated or quenched) in the sample when it is removed from the disinfectant/organism mixture. Clearly, meaningful results cannot be obtained if it is impossible to distinguish what fraction of the microbial killing occurred during the timed period of exposure to the disinfectant from that arising due to carryover of disinfectant into the incubation step that follows exposure. Verification that the disinfectant inactivation method is effective and that any chemical neutralizers used are, themselves, non-toxic to the test organisms is an integral part of the test.

3. It is in viability assessment that there is a fundamental difference of approach between recently developed tests (exemplified by BS EN 1276) and many of the tests that originated before the 1980s. The simplest method of viability

assessment, which was employed in the Rideal–Walker and Kelsey–Sykes tests, for example, is to transfer the sample from the disinfectant/microorganism mixture to a known volume of neutralizing broth, incubate and examine for growth (manifest as turbidity). This procedure contains the inherent defect that any growth in the tubes of broth may result from the transfer of very few surviving cells, or from many. Thus, it is possible for the disinfectant to kill a high proportion of the inoculum within a short period yet fail to kill a small fraction of the cells, possibly mutants, which have atypically high resistance. In this case there is the risk that the disinfectant may be dismissed as insufficiently active despite the fact that it achieved a rapid and extensive initial kill. For this reason it has become common for disinfectant and preservative efficacy tests to be very similar in design, in that both employ viable counting methods to assess microorganism survival but the former utilize a sampling period of minutes or hours, whereas the latter use a 28-day period.

4. When viable counting is used to assess the survival of test organisms, the adoption of disinfection performance criteria based upon a required reduction in the number of surviving organisms is a logical strategy, just as it is in preservative testing. Thus, the so-called 5-5-5 testing principle has found much favour. Here, five test organisms are (separately) exposed for 5 minutes to the disinfectant, which is considered satisfactory if a 5-log reduction in viable numbers (a 10^5 fall in viable cells mL^{-1}) is recorded in each case. This principle is adopted in the BS EN 1276, although only four bacterial strains are recommended for routine use; there is, however, the option to supplement the standard organisms with others more relevant to the intended use of the disinfectant in question.

MICROBIOLOGICAL QUALITY OF PHARMACEUTICAL MATERIALS

Non-sterile products

Non-sterile pharmaceutical products obviously differ from sterile products in that they are permitted to contain some microorganisms but the EP (2004) specifies the maximum concentrations acceptable in different types of product and the species of organism that are not permitted at all (Table 15.3). Similar specifications arise in the US and other pharmacopoeias.

Table 15.3 European Pharmacopoeia (2004) specifications for the microbiological quality of pharmaceutical products*

Product category	Quantitative specification	Organisms which must be absent
Topical and non-sterile respiratory products	• Not more than 10^2 aerobic bacteria and fungi per g or mL • Not more than 10^1 enterobacteria and certain other Gram-negative bacteria per g or mL	• *Pseudomonas aeruginosa* • *Staphylococcus aureus*
Oral and rectal products	• Not more than 10^3 aerobic bacteria per g or mL • Not more than 10^2 fungi per g or mL	• *Escherichia coli*
Oral products containing raw materials of natural origin foe which antimicrobial pretreatment is not feasible	• Not more than 10^4 aerobic bacteria and not more than 10^2 fungi per g or mL • No more than 10^2 enterobacteria and certain other Gram-negative bacteria per g or mL	• *Salmonella* • *Escherichia coli* • *Staphylococcus aureus*
Herbal remedies made with boiling water	• Not more than 10^7 aerobic bacteri and not more than 10^5 fungi per g or mL • Not more than 10^2 *Escherichia coli* per g or mL	
Other herbal remedies	• Not more than 10^5 aerobic bacteria and not more than 10^4 fungi per g or mL • Not more than 10^3 enterobacteria and certain other Gram-nagetive bacteria per go or mL	• *Escherichia coli* • *Salmonella*

*Excluding transdermal patches.

The required microbiological quality of the manufactured medicine cannot be achieved by the application of an antimicrobial process (heating, radiation, etc.) as the final production step for two reasons: first, an approach that uses poor-quality raw materials and manufacturing procedures and then attempts to 'clean up' the product at the end is not acceptable to the licensing authorities; and second, some products would not withstand such antimicrobial treatment, e.g. heating an emulsion may cause cracking or creaming. Thus, the most reliable approach to ensure that the manufactured medicine complies with the pharmacopoeial specification is to ensure that the raw materials are of good quality and that the manufacturing procedures conform to the standards laid down in the latest edition of *Rules and Guidance for Pharmaceutical Manufacturers and Distributors*.

Implicit in these standards is the principle that the extent of product contamination originating from the manufacturing environment and production personnel should be subject to regular monitoring and control.

Environmental monitoring

Environmental monitoring is normally taken to mean regular monitoring of the levels of microbial contamination of the atmosphere, of solid surfaces and, less frequently, of the personnel in the production areas. Water used to clean floors, benches and equipment (as distinct from water incorporated in the product) may be considered as part of environmental monitoring but will not be considered here as the procedures for counting microorganisms in water are described below.

Atmospheric monitoring is most commonly undertaken by means of settle plates, which are simply Petri dishes containing media suitable for the growth of bacteria and/or yeasts and moulds, e.g. tryptone soya agar, which are exposed to the atmosphere for periods of, typically, 1–4 hours. Microorganisms in the air may exist as single cells, e.g. mould spores, but more commonly they are attached to dust particles, so that any organisms in the latter category (for which the culture medium is suitable) will grow into visible colonies during incubation after dust particles have settled on the agar surface. The colony counts recorded on the plates are obviously influenced by:

- the duration of exposure
- the degree of air turbulence, which determines the volume of air passing over the plate
- the intrinsic level of atmospheric contamination (microorganisms per litre of air), which in turn is often a reflection of the number and activity level of the operating personnel, as skin scales shed by the operators are usually the most potent source of atmospheric contaminants.

The disadvantage of settle plates is that it is not possible to relate colony counts directly to air volume. This limitation is overcome in active sampling methods, whereby a known volume of air is drawn over, or caused to impact upon, the agar surface. These methods and the equipment available for active sampling have been reviewed by Johnson (2003).

Surface and equipment sampling is most frequently undertaken by swabbing or the use of contact plates (also known as RODAC – replicate organism detection and counting – plates). Swabbing a known area of bench, floor or equipment with a culture medium-soaked swab is convenient for irregular surfaces. The organisms on the swab may be counted after they have been dispersed by agitation into a fixed volume of suspending medium but it is not easy to quantify either the proportion of total organisms removed from the swabbed surface or the proportion dispersed in the diluent. This second limitation is overcome using contact plates, which are simply specially designed Petri dishes slightly overfilled with molten agar which, on setting, present a convex surface that projects above the rim of the plate. When the plate is inverted on to the surface to be sampled, microorganisms are transferred directly on to the agar (Fig. 15.7).

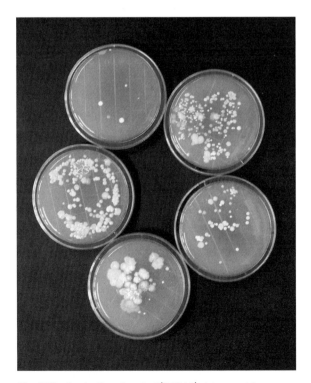

Fig. 15.7 A selection of contact (RODAC) plates used for sampling the following surfaces (from the top left clockwise): laminar flow cabinet; book cover; computer keyboard; tap handle; reagent bottle.

Sampling of manufacturing personnel usually consists of sampling clothing, face masks or, more commonly, gloves. 'Finger dabs' is the phrase used to describe the process whereby an operator rolls the gloved surface of each finger over a suitable solid medium in a manner similar to that in which fingerprints are taken. Operator sampling by any means other than finger dabs is rare, particularly outside aseptic manufacturing areas.

Counting of microorganisms in pharmaceutical products

Most pharmaceutical raw materials are contaminated with microorganisms. The levels of contamination are often a reflection of the source of the raw material in question, with 'natural' products derived from vegetable or animal sources, or mined minerals such as kaolin and talc, being more heavily contaminated than synthetic materials whose microbial burden has been reduced by heat, extremes of pH or organic solvents during the course of manufacture. Determining the bioburden in these materials is often straightforward, utilizing without modification the viable counting procedures described in Chapter 14. Occasionally the physical nature of the raw material makes this difficult or impossible, and this is often found to be the case with the finished manufactured medicine, where problems of dispersibility, sedimentation or viscosity cause complications. As a consequence, modifications to the standard viable counting procedures are necessary to reduce errors. Some of modifications and the circumstances that necessitate them are considered below.

Very low concentrations of microorganisms in aqueous solutions The reliability of calculated viable cell concentrations becomes much reduced when they are based upon colony counts much lower than about 10–15 per Petri dish. Using a surface-spread method, it is rarely possible to place more than about 0.5 mL of liquid on to the agar surface in a standard Petri dish because it will not easily soak in. By a pour-plate method, 1 mL or more may be used but a point is reached where the volume of sample significantly dilutes the agar and nutrients. Thus, using a conventional plating technique, the lowest concentration conveniently detectable is of the order of 10–50 cells mL^{-1}. When the cell concentration is below this value it is necessary to pass a known quantity of the liquid – 10–100 mL or more – through a filter membrane having a pore size sufficiently small to retain bacteria. The membrane is then placed with the organisms uppermost on to the agar surface in a Petri dish, which is incubated without inversion. As a result of diffusion of nutrients through the membrane, colonies grow on the surface in the normal way (Fig. 15.8). Diffusion may be assisted by the inclusion of a medium-soaked pad between the membrane and the agar. It is important to ensure that all the membrane is in

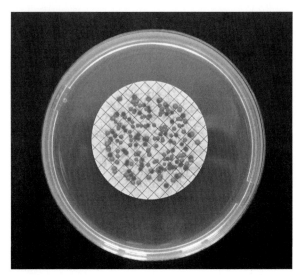

Fig. 15.8 Membrane filter counting: colonies of the red pigmented bacterium *Serratia marcescens* growing on the surface of a cellulose nitrate filter membrane on agar in a Petri dish.

contact with the pad or agar, otherwise elevated areas may become dry and no colonies will appear upon them.

Insoluble solids It is necessary to suspend an insoluble solid in a medium that will permit uniform dispersion and adequate wetting of the suspended material. Nutrient broth, peptone water or a buffered salt solution is frequently used and a low concentration of a surfactant incorporated to promote wetting, e.g. polysorbate 80 (0.01–0.05%). Suspension in distilled water alone carries the risk of osmotic damage to sensitive cells, with a consequently low count; for this reason it is best avoided. Having obtained the suspension, there are two options available depending upon the nature and concentration of the suspended material.

The first is to remove a sample of the mixed suspension, dilute if necessary, and plate in or on a suitable medium using a pour- or spread-plate method. If the concentration of suspended material is low it may still be possible to see clearly the developing colonies. High concentrations may obscure the colonies and make counting impossible. The alternative is to dislodge the microbial cells from the solid to which they are attached, allow the solid to sediment out and then sample the supernatant. Methods of removal include vigorous manual shaking, use of a vortex mixer or equipment designed for the purpose, e.g. the Colworth 'stomacher' in which the aqueous suspension is placed in a sealed sterile bag which is repeatedly agitated by reciprocating paddles. The use of ultrasonics to dislodge the cells carries the risk of damage to or lysis of the cells themselves.

Assuming the suspended material has no antimicrobial activity, plating the 'whole suspension' is probably the easiest and most reliable method. The alternative strategy of sampling the supernatant involves the assumption that all the cells have been removed from the solid but this would have to be confirmed by control (validation) experiments in which a known quantity of similar organisms was artificially dried on to sterile samples of the material. The second method also relies upon the solid sedimenting sufficiently rapidly for it to be separated from the bacteria in aqueous suspension above. If all or part of the sample has a particle size similar to that of bacteria, yeasts or mould spores, i.e. approximately 1–5 μm, then a separation cannot easily be achieved.

Oils and hydrophobic ointments These materials are usually not heavily contaminated because they are anhydrous and microorganisms will not multiply without water. Thus the microorganisms contained in oily products have usually arisen by contamination from the atmosphere, equipment used for manufacture and from storage vessels. To perform a viable count the oil sample must be emulsified or solubilized without the aid of excessive heat or any other agent that might kill the cells.

An oil-in-water emulsion must be produced using a suitable surfactant; non-ionic emulsifiers generally have little antimicrobial activity. The proportion of surfactant to use must be determined experimentally and validation experiments conducted to confirm that the surfactant is not, itself, toxic to the species that typically arise as contaminants of the sample in question; Millar (2000) has described the use of up to 5 g of polysorbate 80 added to a 10 g sample. Such an emulsion may be diluted in water or buffered salts solution if necessary, and aliquots placed on or in the agar medium in the usual way. Alternatively, the oil may be dissolved in a sterile non-toxic solvent and passed through a membrane filter. Isopropyl myristate, for example, is recommended in pharmacopoeial sterility testing procedures as a solvent for anhydrous materials but it may kill a significant fraction of the cells of some sensitive species, even during an exposure period of only a few minutes.

Creams and lotions Oil-in-water emulsions do not usually represent a problem because they are miscible with water and thus easily diluted. Water-in-oil creams, however, are not miscible and cannot be plated directly because bacteria may remain trapped in a water droplet suspended in a layer of oil on the agar surface. Such bacteria are unlikely to form colonies because the diffusion of nutrients through the oil would be inadequate. These creams are best diluted, dispersed in an aqueous medium and membrane filtered or converted to an oil-in-water type, and then counted by normal plating methods.

Dilution and emulsification of the cream in broth containing Lubrol W, polysorbate 80 or Triton X 100 is probably the best procedure, although the addition of approximately 0.1 g of the w/o emulsion sample to 25 g of isopropyl myristate followed by membrane filtration may be satisfactory.

Detection of specific hazardous organisms

In addition to placing limits on the maximum concentration of microorganisms that is acceptable in different materials, pharmacopoeias usually specify certain organisms that must not be present at all. In practice, this means that detection methods which are described in the pharmacopoeia must be applied to a known weight of material (typically 1–50 g), and the sample passes the test if, on the culture plates, no organisms arise that conform to the standard textbook descriptions of those to be excluded. Typically the pharmacopoeial methods involve preliminary stages using selective liquid culture media; these are designed to increase the concentration of the organism that is the subject of the test ('target' organism) and so render it more readily detectable. Supplementary biochemical tests are also used to confirm the identity of any isolates having the typical appearance of the target organisms.

Both the EP (2004) and the USP (2005) describe detection tests for *Staphylococcus aureus*, *Pseudomonas aeruginosa*, *Escherichia coli* and salmonellae. In addition, the EP describes a test for clostridia but this is unlikely to be applied to any material other than mined minerals, e.g. talc and bentonite. The four organisms common to both pharmacopoeias are the subject of these tests primarily because of their potential to cause infections. However, they may also represent common contaminants of the products to which the tests are applied, or their presence may be indicative of the quality of the raw material or finished manufactured product. *E. coli*, for example, is a natural inhabitant of mammalian intestines and so its presence in a material such as gelatin (which originates in the slaughterhouse) would indicate unacceptable quality. The most likely source of *Staphylococcus aureus* in a manufactured medicine is the production personnel, so that if this origin were confirmed it would indicate the need for higher manufacturing standards. In general the tests are applied to pharmaceutical raw materials of 'natural' origin, e.g. carbohydrates, cellulose derivatives, gums and vegetable drugs. In addition, there is a requirement that topical products should be free of both *Pseudomonas aeruginosa* and *Staphylococcus aureus*. Table 15.4 summarises the EP (2004) testing schemes for the four principal organisms of interest. These schemes are described in more detail elsewhere, together with photographs of the typical appearance of the organisms in question (Hodges 2000).

Microbiological assays of B-group vitamins

Microbiological assays of B-group vitamins employ similar techniques to turbidimetric assays of antibiotics (see earlier in this chapter). A culture medium is used which is suitable for the assay organism, except for the omission of the vitamin in question. The extent of bacterial growth in

Table 15.4   Procedures recommended by the EP (2004) in tests for specified microorganisms

Medium	Organism				
	Escherichia coli	Salmonellae		Pseudomonas aeruginosa	Staphylococcus aureus
Liquid enrichment	MacConkey broth	Tetrathionate bile brilliant green broth		Casein soya bean digest broth (troptone soya broth)	Casein soya bean digest broth (tryptone soya broth)
			Appearance		
Agar media (primary test)	MacConkey agar (appearance: pink colonies with precipitation of bile due to acid production)	Deoxycholate citrate agar. Xylose lysine deoxycholate (XLD) agar and Brilliant green agar	Yellow colonies with grey or black centre Red colonies with black centres Pink colonies	Growth on cetrimide agar	Baird–Parker agar (black colonies immediately surrounded by zones of opacity beyond which are zones of clearing)
Result(s) of secondary tests which confirm the presence of organism in question	Production of indole at 44°C	Reactions characteristic of Salmonella on triple sugar iron agar and other biochemical or serological tests	Black precipitate of iron sulphide Yellow (acid) butt (i.e. subsurface), with pink (alkaline) slope (i.e. surface)	Absence of growth at 41–43°C	Positive coagulase or deoxyribonuclease tests

the medium is thus directly proportional to the amount of reference standard or test vitamin added. It is important to select an assay organism that has an absolute requirement for the substance in question and is unable to obtain it by metabolism of other medium components; species of *Lactobacillus* are often used for this purpose. 'Carryover' of the vitamin with the inoculum culture must be avoided because this results in some growth even when none of the test material has been added. Growth may be determined turbidimetrically or by acid production from sugars.

Just as HPLC has become the favoured method of antibiotic assay, so too has it become the method of choice for assaying B-group vitamins. Turbidimetric assays are still occasionally used, however, for example when insurmountable problems arise in resolving the many peaks that might arise on an HPLC chromatogram from a multivitamin product (which might contain 10 or more active ingredients plus excipients, all of which may cause assay interference).

Sterile products

Sterile products must, by definition, be free of microorganisms and it is important to understand that this is an absolute requirement. Thus, the presence of one single surviving microbial cell is sufficient to render the product non-sterile. There is not a level of survivors which is so small as to be regarded as negligible and therefore acceptable.

The principal component of microbiological quality assurance which has traditionally been applied to sterile products is, of course, the test for sterility itself. In essence, this is quite simple: a sample of the material to be tested is added to culture medium which is incubated and then examined for signs of microbial growth. If growth occurs the assumption is made that the contamination arose from the sample, which consequently fails the test. However, the limitations of this simplistic approach became more widely recognized in the second half of the 20th century, and there was an increasing awareness of the fact that contaminated products could pass the test and sterile ones apparently fail it (because of contamination introduced during the testing procedure itself). For these reasons the sterility test alone could no longer be relied upon to provide an assurance of sterility, and that assurance is now derived from a strict adherence to high-quality standards throughout the manufacturing process. These encompass:

- the adoption of the highest possible specifications for the microbiological quality of the raw materials. The rationale here is that sterilization processes are more likely to be effective when the levels of microorganisms to be killed or removed (bioburdens) are as low as possible to begin with. Procedures used to determine bioburdens are described in Chapter 14 and earlier in this chapter
- the rigorous application of environmental monitoring procedures (as described above) during the course of manufacture, with more stringent limits for acceptable levels of microorganisms than those applicable during the manufacture of non-sterile products
- comprehensive validation procedures when sterilization processes are designed, together with regular in-process monitoring when those processes are in operation for product manufacture. Initial validation seeks to demonstrate that adequate sterilizing conditions are achieved throughout the load, and entails extensive testing with thermocouples, radiation dosimeters and biological indicators (see below) as appropriate.

The pharmacopoeias and regulatory authorities require a sterility assurance level for terminally sterilized products of 10^{-6} or better. This means that the probability of non-sterility in an item selected at random from a batch should be no more than 1 in 1 million. This sterility assurance level (SAL) may be demonstrated in the case of some terminally sterilized products simply by reference to data derived from bioburdens, environmental monitoring and in-process monitoring of the sterilization procedure itself. In this case the sterility test is unnecessary and omitted; the term 'parametric release' is used to describe the release of products for sale or use under these circumstances.

Sterilization monitoring

Sterilization processes may be monitored physically, chemically or biologically. Physical methods are exemplified by thermocouples, which are routinely incorporated at different locations within an autoclave load, whereas chemical indicators usually exhibit a colour change after exposure to a heat sterilization process. Biological indicators consist of preparations of spores of the *Bacillus* species that exhibits the greatest degree of resistance to the sterilizing agent in question. The principle of their use is simply that if such spores are exposed to the sterilization process and fail to survive, it can be assumed that all other common organisms will also have been killed and the process is safe. Spores of *Bacillus stearothermophilus* (strictly speaking now *Geobacillus*

stearothermophilus, although this name is not yet in common use in pharmaceutical literature) are used to monitor autoclaves and gaseous hydrogen peroxide or peracetic acid sterilization processes, whereas *Bacillus subtilis* var. *niger* is the organism normally employed for dry heat, ethylene oxide and low-temperature steam-formaldehyde methods; *Bacillus pumilus* is used in radiation sterilization procedures.

Such biological indicators are regularly employed for validation of a sterilization process which is under development for a new product, or when a new autoclave is being commissioned; they are less commonly used for routine monitoring during product manufacture. Spores possess the advantage that they are relatively easy to produce, purify and dry on to an inert carrier, which is frequently an absorbent paper strip or disc, or a plastic or metal support. Spore resistance to the sterilizing agent must be carefully controlled and so rigorous standardization of production processes followed by observance of correct storage conditions and expiry dates are essential.

Tests for sterility

It is sufficient here to repeat that the test is really one of the absence of gross contamination with readily grown microorganisms, and is not capable of affording a guarantee of sterility in any sample that passes.

The experimental details of these procedures are described in the EP (2004). This section is therefore restricted to an account of the major features of the test and a more detailed consideration of those practical aspects that are important or problematical.

It is obviously important that materials to be tested for sterility are not subject to contamination from the operator or the environment during the course of the test. For this reason it is essential that sterility tests are conducted in adequate laboratory facilities by competent and experienced personnel. Clearly, the consequences of recording an incorrect sterility result may be very severe. If a material which was *really* sterile were to fail the test it would need to be resterilized or, more probably, discarded. This would have significant cost implications. If, on the other hand, a contaminated batch were to pass a test for sterility and be released for use this would obviously represent a significant health hazard. For these reasons sterility testing procedures have improved significantly in recent years and failures are now viewed very seriously by the regulatory authorities. If a product does fail, it means either that the item in question was *really* contaminated, in which case the manufacturing procedures are seriously inadequate, or that the item was in fact sterile but the testing procedure was at fault. Either way, it is not possible to dismiss a failure lightly.

Sterility tests may be conducted in clean rooms or laminar flow cabinets which provide a grade A atmosphere as defined by the *Rules and Guidance for Pharmaceutical Manufacturers and Distributors* (2002). However, it is becoming increasingly common for testing to be undertaken in an isolator that physically separates the operator from the test materials and so reduces the incidence of false-positive test results due to extraneous contamination introduced during the test itself. Such isolators are similar in principle to a glove box, and typically consist of a cabinet (supported on legs or a frame) that is sufficiently large for the operator, who is covered by a transparent hood of moulded flexible plastic forming the cabinet base, to sit or stand within it.

A sterility test may be conducted in two ways. The direct inoculation method involves the removal of samples from the product under test and their transfer to a range of culture media that might be expected to support the growth of contaminating organisms. After incubation the media are examined for evidence of growth which, if present, is taken to indicate that the product may not be sterile. It is not certain that the product is contaminated because the organisms responsible for the growth may have arisen from the operator or have been already present in the media to which the samples were transferred, i.e. the media used for the test were not themselves sterile. Thus, in conducting a sterility test it is necessary to include controls that indicate the likelihood of the contaminants arising from these sources. The size and number of the samples to be taken are described in the EP (2004).

Again it is necessary to inactivate any antimicrobial substances contained in the sample. These may be the active drug, e.g. antibiotic, or a preservative in an eye drop or multidose injection. Suitable inactivators may be added to the liquid test media to neutralize any antimicrobial substances but in the case of antibiotics particularly, no such specific inactivators are available (with the exception of β-lactamases which hydrolyse penicillins and cephalosporins). This problem may be overcome using a membrane filtration technique. This alternative method of conducting sterility tests is obviously only applicable to aqueous or oily solutions that will pass through a membrane having a pore size sufficiently small to retain bacteria. The membrane, and hence the bacteria retained on it, is washed with isotonic salts solution, which should remove any last traces of antimicrobial substances. It is then placed in a suitable liquid culture medium. This method is certainly to be preferred to direct inoculation because there is a greater chance of effective neutralization of antimicrobial substances.

Solids may be dissolved in an appropriate solvent. This is almost invariably water because most other common solvents have antimicrobial activity. If no suitable solvent can be found the broth dilution method is the only one available. If there is no specific inactivator available for antimicrobial substances that may be present in the solid then their dilution to an ineffective concentration by use of a large volume of medium is the only course remaining.

The controls associated with a sterility test are particularly important because incomplete control of the test may lead to erroneous results. Failure to neutralize a preservative completely may lead to contaminants in the batch going undetected and subsequently initiating an infection when the product is introduced into the body.

The EP (2004) recommends that four controls are incorporated. The so-called growth promotion test simply involves the addition of low inocula (10–100 cells or spores per container) of suitable test organisms into the media used in the test to show that they do support the growth of the common contaminants for which they are intended. *Staphylococcus aureus, Bacillus subtilis* and *Pseudomonas aeruginosa* are the three aerobic bacteria used, *Clostridium sporogenes* the anaerobic bacterium and *Candida albicans* and *Aspergillus niger* the fungi. Organisms having particular nutritional requirements, such as blood, milk or serum, are not included; therefore they, in addition to the more obvious omissions such as viruses, may not be detected in a routine sterility test because suitable cultural conditions are not provided. On the other hand, it is impossible to design an all-purpose medium and sterilization processes that kill the spore-forming bacteria and other common contaminants are likely also to eradicate the more fastidious pathogens such as streptococci and *Haemophilus* species, which would be more readily detected on blood-containing media. This argument does not, however, cover the possibility of such pathogens entering the product, perhaps via defective seals or packaging, after the sterilization process itself and then going undetected in the sterility test.

The second control (validation test) is intended to demonstrate that any preservative or antimicrobial substance has been effectively neutralized. This requires the addition of test organisms to containers of the various media as before but, in addition, samples of the material under test must also be added to give the same concentrations as those arising in the test itself. For the sterility test as a whole to be valid, growth must occur in each of the containers in these controls.

It is necessary also to incubate several tubes of the various media just as they are received by the operator. If the tubes are not opened but show signs of growth after incubation this is a clear indication that the medium is itself contaminated. This should be an extremely rare occurrence but, in view of the small additional cost or effort, the inclusion of such a control is worthwhile.

A control to check the likelihood of contamination being introduced during the test may be included in the programme of regular monitoring of test facilities. The EP 2004 recommends the use of negative controls, which may be employed to check the adequacy of facilities and operator technique. These items, identical to the sample to be tested, are manipulated in exactly the same way as the test samples. If, after incubation, there are signs of microbial growth in the media containing these negative controls, the conclusion is drawn that the contamination arose during the testing process itself.

Some items present particular difficulties in sterility testing because of their shape or size, e.g. surgical dressings and medical devices. These problems are most conveniently overcome simply by testing the whole sample rather than attempting to withdraw a portion of it. So, for example, large clear plastic bags which have been radiation sterilized may be used to hold the entire medical device or complete roll or pack of dressings, which would then be totally immersed in culture medium. This method would only be valid if the culture medium gained access to the entire sample; otherwise the possibility exists, for example, of aerobic bacterial spores trapped within it failing to grow owing to insufficient diffusion of oxygen. This approach has the advantage of imposing a more rigorous test because a much larger sample is used. In the case of dressings, it may also reduce the risk of operator-induced contamination compared to the alternative approach, which would require the withdrawal of representative samples for testing from different areas of the roll or pack.

The final aspect of the test which is worthy of comment is the interpretation of results. If there is evidence that any of the test samples are contaminated, the batch fails the test. If, however, there is convincing evidence that the test was invalid because the testing facility, procedure or media were inadequate, a single retest is permitted; this contrasts with earlier pharmacopoeial protocols, which under certain circumstances permitted two retests.

Endotoxin and pyrogen testing

This is an aspect of microbial contamination of medicines which is not normally considered part of microbiology but is discussed here because pyrogens are normally the products of microbial growth. A pyrogen is a material which when injected into a patient will cause a rise in body temperature (pyrexia). The lipopolysaccharides that comprise a major part of the cell wall of Gram-negative bacteria are called endotoxins, and it is

these that are the most commonly encountered pyrogens (although any other substance that causes a rise in body temperature may be classified under the same heading). Bacterial cells may be pyrogenic even when they are dead and when they are fragmented, and so a solution or material that passes a test for sterility will not necessarily pass a pyrogen test. It follows from this that the more heavily contaminated with bacteria an aqueous injection becomes during manufacture, the more pyrogenic it is likely to be at the end of the process.

Two main procedures are used for the detection of pyrogens. The traditional method requires the administration of the sample to laboratory rabbits, whose body temperature is monitored for a period of time thereafter. The alternative procedure, which is now by far the most common, is to use the Limulus Amoebocyte Lysate Test (LAL), in which the pyrogen-containing sample causes gel formation in the lysis product of amoebocyte cells of the giant horseshoe crab *Limulus polyphemus*. A detailed account of endotoxin testing is outside the scope of this chapter but the review by Baines (2000) provides a comprehensive account of the practicalities of the method.

REFERENCES

Baines, A. (2000) Endotoxin testing. In: Baird, R.M., Hodges, N.A., Denyer, S.P. (eds) *Handbook of Microbiological Quality Assurance*. Taylor and Francis, London.

BS EN 1276 (1997) *Quantitative suspension test for the evaluation of bactericidal activity of chemical disinfectants and antiseptics used in food, industrial, domestic and institutional areas*. British Standards Institute, London.

European Pharmacopoeia (2004) 5th edn. Council of Europe, Strasbourg.

Hewitt, W., Vincent, S. (1989) *Theory and Application of Microbiological Assay*. Academic Press. London.

Hodges, N.A. (1999) Assessment of preservative activity during stability studies. In: Mazzo D.J. (ed.) *International Stability Testing*. Interpharm Press, Buffalo Grove, US.

Hodges, N.A. (2000) Pharmacopoeial methods for the detection of specified microorganisms In: Baird, R.M., Hodges, N.A., Denyer, S.P. (eds) *Handbook of Microbiological Quality Assurance*. Taylor and Francis, London.

Johnson, S.M. (2003) Microbiological environmental monitoring. In: Hodges, N.A., Hanlon G.W. (eds.) *Industrial Pharmaceutical Microbiology: Standards and Controls*. Euromed Communications, Haslemere, UK.

Millar, R. (2000) Enumeration In: Baird, R.M., Hodges, N.A., Denyer, S.P. (eds) *Handbook of Microbiological Quality Assurance*. Taylor and Francis, London.

Murtough, S.M., Hiom, S.J., Palmer, M., Russell, A.D. (2000) A survey of disinfectant use in hospital pharmacy aseptic preparation areas. *Pharmaceutical Journal,* **264**, 446-448.

Reybrouck, G. (2004) Evaluation of the antibacterial and antifungal activity of disinfectants. In: Fraise, A.P., Lambert, P.A., Maillard J-Y. (eds) *Principles and Practice of Disinfection Preservation and Sterilization*, 4th edn. Blackwell Science, Oxford.

Rules and Guidance for Pharmaceutical Manufacturers and Distributors (Latest edition). Pharmaceutical Press, London.

Russell, A.D. (2004) Factors influencing the efficacy of antimicrobial agents. In: Fraise, A.P., Lambert, P.A., Maillard J-Y. (eds) *Principles and Practice of Disinfection Preservation and Sterilization*, 4th edn. Blackwell Science, Oxford.

United States Pharmacopoeia (2005) 28th edn. US Pharmacopoeial Convention Inc., Rockville, Maryland.

Wardlaw, A.C. (1999) *Practical Statistics for Experimental Biologists*, 2nd edn. Wiley, Chichester.

Action of physical and chemical agents on microorganisms

G. W. Hanlon, N. A. Hodges

CHAPTER CONTENTS

INTRODUCTION

The subject of this chapter is of importance because pharmaceutical scientists have a responsibility for:

- the production of medicines having as their prime function the destruction of microorganisms, e.g. antiseptic liquids and antibiotic formulations
- the production of sterile medicaments having no living microorganisms, e.g. injections and eye drops
- the production of a wide range of medicines which must be effectively protected against microbial spoilage.

Thus the major pharmaceutical interest in microorganisms is that of killing them, or at least preventing their growth. Consequently it is necessary to have both an understanding of the physical processes, e.g. heating and irradiation, that are used to kill microorganisms and knowledge of the more diverse subject of antimicrobial chemicals.

This background knowledge must therefore include an understanding of the kinetics of cell inactivation, the calculation of parameters by which microbial destruction and growth inhibition are measured, and an appreciation of the factors that influence the efficiency of the physical and chemical processes used. These aspects, together with a synopsis of the major groups of antimicrobial chemicals, are the subject of this chapter.

KINETICS OF CELL INACTIVATION

The death of a population of cells exposed to heat or radiation is often found to follow or approximate to first-order kinetics. In this sense it is similar to bacterial growth during the logarithmic phase of the cycle, the graphs representing these processes being similar but of opposite slope. Assuming first-order kinetics (the exceptions will be considered later), an initial population of N_o cells per mL will, after a time t minutes, be reduced to N_t cells per mL, according to the following equations in which k is the inactivation rate constant:

$$N_t = N_0 \, e^{-kt} \qquad (16.1)$$

$$\ln N_t = \ln N_0 - kt \qquad (16.2)$$

$$\log_{10} N_t = \log_{10} N_0 \frac{-kt}{2.303} \qquad (16.3)$$

Thus the data in Table 16.1 may be used to produce a plot of logarithm of cell concentration against exposure time (Fig. 16.1), where the intercept is $\log N_0$ and the slope is $-k/2.303$. This may be plotted with the logarithm of the percentage of survivors as the ordinate; thus the largest

Table 16.1 Death of *B. megaterium* spores in pH 7.0 buffer at 95°C

Time (minutes)	Viable cell concentration mL^{-1}	Percent survivors	Log$_{10}$% survivors
0	2.50×10^6	100	2.000
5	5.20×10^5	20.8	1.318
10	1.23×10^5	4.92	0.692
15	1.95×10^4	0.78	−0.108
20	4.60×10^3	0.18	−0.745
25	1.21×10^3	0.048	−1.319
30	1.68×10^2	0.0067	−2.174

numerical value on this axis is 2.0 (100%). An important feature of Figure 16.1 is the fact that there is no lower endpoint to the ordinate scale – it continues indefinitely. If the initial population was 1000 cells mL^{-1} the logarithmic value would be 3.0; at 100 cells mL^{-1} the value would be 2.0; at 10 cells mL^{-1} 1.0, and at 1 cell mL^{-1} zero. The next incremental point on the logarithmic scale would be −1, which corresponds to 0.1 cells mL^{-1}. It is clearly nonsense to talk of a fraction of a viable cell per mL but this value corresponds to one whole cell in 10 mL of liquid. The next point, −2.0, corresponds to one cell in 100 mL, and so on. Sterility is the complete absence of life, i.e. zero cells mL^{-1}, which has a log value of −∞.

Guaranteed sterility would therefore require an infinite exposure time.

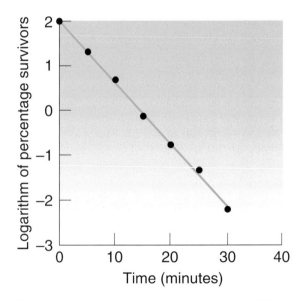

Fig. 16.1 Heat inactivation of *B. megaterium* spores at 95°C.

D value, or decimal reduction time

It is characteristic of first-order kinetics that the same percentage change in concentration occurs in successive time intervals. Thus in Figure 16.1 it can be seen that the viable population falls to 10% of its initial value after 7.5 minutes; in the next 7.5-minute period the population again falls to 10% of its value at the start of that period. This time period for a 90% reduction in count is related to the slope of the line and is one of the more useful parameters by which the death rate may be indicated. It is known as the decimal reduction time, or *D* value, and usually has a subscript showing the temperature at which it was measured, e.g. D_{121} or D_{134}. It is quite possible to indicate the rate of destruction by the inactivation rate constant calculated from the slope of the line but the significance of this value cannot be as readily appreciated during conversation as that of a *D* value, and so the former is rarely used.

Z values

When designing steam sterilization processes, it is necessary to know both the *D* value, which is a measure of the effectiveness of heat at any given temperature, and the extent to which a particular increase in temperature will reduce the *D* value, i.e. it is necessary to have a measure of the effect of temperature change on death rate. One such measure is the *Z* value, which is defined as the number of degrees of temperature change required to achieve a 10-fold change in *D* value, e.g. if the *D* value for *Bacillus stearothermophilus* spores at 110°C is 20 minutes and they have a *Z* value of 9°C, this means that at 119°C the *D* value would be 2.0 minutes and at 128°C the *D* value would be 0.20 minutes. The relationship between *D* and *Z* values is shown in Figure 16.2. The *Z* value is one of several parameters that relate change in temperature to change in death rate, and is probably the most commonly used and readily understood.

The activation energy obtained from an Arrhenius plot (see Chapter 7) or a temperature coefficient, a Q_{10} value (change in rate for a 10°C change in temperature, Chapter 15), do the same but are less commonly used.

Alternative survivor plots

It was stated earlier that bacterial death often approximates to first-order kinetics, although exceptions do arise. Some of the more common are illustrated in Figure 16.3. The plot labelled A is that conforming to first-order kinetics, which has already been described. A shoulder on the curve, as in case B, is not uncommon and various explanations have been offered. Cell aggregation or clumping may be responsible for such a shoulder, because it would

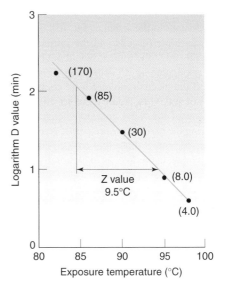

Fig. 16.2   Relationship between logarithm of *D* value and exposure temperature for heated *B. megaterium* spores. Individual *D* values (minutes) are shown in parentheses.

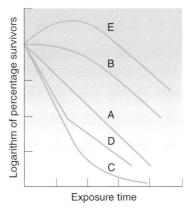

Fig. 16.3   Alternative survivor plots for cells exposed to lethal agents.

be necessary to apply sufficient heat to kill all the cells in the clump, not merely the most sensitive, before a fall is observed in the number of colonies appearing on the agar. Under normal circumstances one single colony could arise both from one cell alone or, say, from 100 cells aggregated together. In the latter case, if sufficient heat was applied to kill the 99 most sensitive cells in the clump, the colony count would be unaltered. Clumping is not the only explanation, because substantial shoulders may arise using suspensions where the vast majority of cells exist individually.

Tailing of survivor curves, as in plot C, is often observed if the initial cell concentration is high. This has been attributed to the presence of mutants that are exceptionally resistant to the lethal agent. If the proportion of mutants was 1 in 10^6 cells and the initial concentration only 10^5 cells mL^{-1} the mutant would not be detected but an initial population of 10^9 cells mL^{-1} would permit easy detection if the inactivation plot were continued down to low levels of survivors. Again there are alternative explanations, one of the most common being that the cells dying during the early exposure period release chemicals which help to protect those that are still alive.

A sharp break in the line, as in D, usually indicates that there are two distinct populations of cells present which have markedly different resistances. Contamination of a cell suspension or culture is a possible explanation or it may be that a mutant has arisen naturally and the cultural conditions are such that it has a selective advantage and its numbers have increased until it is a substantial proportion of the population.

Plot E is uncommon and is usually only seen as a result of 'heat activation' of bacterial spores. This is a situation in which a significant proportion of a population of spores (usually a thermophil) remain dormant and fail to germinate and produce colonies under 'normal' conditions. If the suspension receives a heat stimulus or shock which is insufficient to kill the spores, some or all of those that would otherwise remain dormant become activated, germinate and thus produce a rise in the colony count.

Killing of microorganisms by chemicals results in first-order kinetics less commonly than heat- or radiation-induced killing. This is because the chemical must interact with a target molecule within the cell, and the concentration of both the chemical and the intracellular target might influence death rate and so result in second-order kinetics. In practice, however, the antimicrobial chemical is often present in such a high concentration that the proportion of it that is 'used up' by interaction with the cell is negligible; this means its concentration is effectively constant and pseudo first-order kinetics result.

ANTIMICROBIAL EFFECTS OF MOIST AND DRY HEAT

Moist heat (steam) and dry heat (hot air) both have the potential to kill microorganisms but their efficiencies and their mechanisms of action differ. In autoclaves dry, saturated steam, i.e. 100% water vapour with no liquid water present, is used at temperatures between 121 and 135°C, at which it rapidly kills microorganisms. An advantage of using steam is that it possesses a large latent heat of vaporization, which it transfers to any object upon which it condenses (see Chapter 46). It is essential to use dry saturated steam if maximal autoclaving efficiency is to be achieved. If the steam is wet, i.e. contains liquid

water, penetration of vapour-phase steam into dressings may be retarded. If the steam is superheated, i.e. its temperature has been raised while the pressure remains constant or the pressure fell while the temperature remains constant, it contains less moisture and latent heat than dry saturated steam at the same temperature. In this case the effect is similar to using a steam–air mixture at that temperature. The process by which steam kills cells is hydrolysis of essential proteins (enzymes) and nucleic acids. In contrast, dry heat causes cell death by oxidative processes, although again it is the proteins and nucleic acids that are the vulnerable targets. Dry heat is much less effective at killing microorganisms than steam at the same temperature. Exposures of not less than 2 hours at 160°C (or an equivalent temperature/time combination) are recommended in the EP for sterilization by dry heat methods. The state of hydration of a cell is thus an important factor determining its resistance to heat.

Resistance of microorganisms to moist and dry heat

Numerous factors influence the observed heat resistance of microbial cells and it is difficult to make comparisons between populations unless these factors are controlled. Not surprisingly, marked differences in resistance exist between different genera, species and strains, and between the spore and vegetative cell forms of the same organism. The resistance may be influenced, sometimes extensively, by the age of the cell, i.e. lag, exponential or stationary phase; its chemical composition, which in turn is influenced by the medium in which the cell is grown; and by the composition and pH of the fluid in which the cell is heated. It is difficult to obtain strictly comparable heat resistance data for grossly dissimilar organisms but the values quoted in Table 16.2 indicate the relative order of heat resistance of the various microbial groups. Tabulation of D values at a designated temperature is perhaps the most convenient way of comparing resistance but this is only suitable for first-order kinetics. Alternative methods of comparison include the time to achieve a particular percentage kill or the time required to achieve no survivors; the latter is, of course, dependent upon the initial population level.

The most heat-resistant infectious agents (as distinct from microbial cells) are prions, which are proteins rather than living cells and the cause of spongiform encephalopathies, e.g. Creutzfeldt–Jakob disease (CJD) and bovine spongiform encephalopathy (BSE or 'mad cow disease'). Prion proteins are so resistant to heat inactivation that an autoclave cycle of 134–138°C for 18 minutes has been recommended for the decontamination of prion-contaminated materials, and the efficacy of even this extreme heat treatment has been questioned.

Table 16.2   A 'league table' of heat resistances of different microorganisms and infectious agents

Organism or agent	Heat resistance (values are for fully hydrated organisms unless otherwise stated)
Prions	The most heat-resistant infectious agent. May survive steam sterilization at 134–138°C for 1 hour
Bacterial spores (endospores)	Little or no inactivation at <80°C. Some species survive boiling for several hours
Fungal spores	Ascospores of *Byssochlamys* species may survive 88°C for 60 minutes but most fungal spores are less resistant
Actinomycete spores	Spores of *Nocardia sebivorans* reported to survive for 10 minutes at 90°C but the majority of species are less resistant
Mycobacterium tuberculosis	May survive for 30 minutes at 100°C in the dry state but when hydrated is killed by pasteurization (63°C for 30 minutes or 72°C for 15 seconds)
Yeasts	Ascospores and vegetative cells show little difference in resistance. Survival for 20 minutes at 60°C is typical
Most non-sporing bacteria of pharmaceutical or medical importance	D_{60} of 1–5 minutes is typical of staphylococci and many Gram-negative enteric organisms. Enterococci may be more resistant, and pneumococci may survive for 30 minutes at 110°C when dry
Fungi and actinomycetes	Vegetative mycelia exhibit similar resistance to that of non-sporing bacteria described above
Viruses	Rarely survive for >30 minutes at 55–60°C except perhaps in blood or tissues, but papovaviruses and hepatitis viruses are more resistant
Protozoa and algae	Most are no more resistant than mammalian cells and survive only a few hours at 40–45°C, but cysts of *Acanthamoeba* species are more resistant

Bacterial endospores are invariably found to be the most heat-resistant *cell* type, and those of certain species may survive boiling water for many hours. The term 'endospore' refers to the spores produced by *Bacillus* and *Clostridium* species and is not to be confused with the spores produced by other bacteria, such as actinomycetes, which do not develop within the vegetative cell. The majority of *Bacillus* and *Clostridium* species normally form spores which survive in water for 15–30 minutes at 80°C without significant damage or loss of viability. Because endospores are more resistant than other cells, they have been the subject of a considerable amount of research in the food and pharmaceutical industries and much of the earlier work has been reviewed by Russell (1999).

Mould spores and those of yeasts and actinomycetes usually exhibit a degree of moist heat resistance intermediate between endospores and vegetative cell forms; survival at 60°C for several hours but death at 80°C or higher would be typical of such cells. Bacterial and yeast vegetative cells and mould mycelia all vary significantly in heat resistance: mycobacteria, which possess a high proportion of lipid in their cell wall, tend to be more resist-

ant than others. Protozoa and algae are, by comparison, susceptible to heat and when in the vegetative (uncysted) state, like mammalian cells, they rapidly die at temperatures much in excess of 40°C. Information on the heat resistance of viruses is limited but the available data suggest that they may vary significantly between types. The majority of viruses are no more heat resistant than vegetative bacteria but hepatitis viruses have been reported to be less susceptible than others.

Resistance to dry heat by different groups of infectious agents and microorganisms usually follows a pattern similar to that in aqueous environments. Again, prions head the 'league table' by exhibiting extreme heat resistance and endospores are substantially more resilient than other cell types, with those of *B. stearothermophilus* and *B. subtilis* usually more resistant than other species. Exposures of 2 hours at 160°C are required by the *European Pharmacopoeia* (2004) to achieve an acceptable level of sterility assurance for materials sterilized by dry heat.

Cells of pneumococci have been reported to survive dry heat at 110°C for 30 minutes but this represents exceptional resistance for vegetative cells, most of which may be expected to die after a few minutes heating at 100°C or less.

Valid comparisons of dry heat resistance among dissimilar organisms are even less common than those for aqueous environments because there is the additional problem of distinguishing the effects of drying from those of heat. For many cells desiccation is itself a potentially lethal process, even at room temperature, so that experiments in which the moisture content of the cells is uncontrolled may produce results that are misleading or difficult to interpret. This is particularly so when the cells are heated under conditions where their moisture content is changing and they become progressively drier during the experiment.

Factors affecting heat resistance and its measurement

The major factors affecting heat resistance are listed in the previous section and will be considered in some detail here. The subject has been extensively studied and again, many of the experimental data and consequently many of the examples quoted in this section come from the field of spore research.

The measurement of heat resistance in fully hydrated cells, i.e. those suspended in aqueous solutions or exposed to dry saturated steam, does not normally represent a problem when conducted at temperatures less than 100°C but errors may occasionally arise when spore heat resistance is measured at higher temperatures. In these circumstances it is necessary to heat suspensions sealed in glass ampoules immersed in glycerol or oil baths or to expose the spores to steam in a modified autoclave. Monitoring and control of heat-up and cool-down times become important, and failure to pay adequate attention to these aspects may lead to apparent differences in resistance, which may be due simply to factors such as variations in the thickness of glass in two batches of ampoules.

Species and strain differences

Variations in heat resistance between the species within a genus are very common, although it is difficult to identify from the published reports the precise magnitude of these differences because different species may require different growth media and incubation conditions which, together with other factors, might influence the results. One report in the 1960s described a 700-fold variation in spore heat resistance within 13 *Bacillus* species but to produce the spore crops for testing, the authors necessarily had to use eight culture media, three incubation temperatures and six procedures for cleaning the spores. Differences between strains of a single species are, not surprisingly, more

limited; D_{90} values ranging from 4.5 to 120 minutes have been reported for five strains of *Clostridium perfringens* spores.

Cell form

Whether or not the heated cells exist in the vegetative or the spore form may in some cases be related to the age of the culture or the cell population being heated. In cultures of *Bacillus* and *Clostridium* species, the proportion of spores usually increases as the incubation period is extended and the culture ages. This may be due to more and more of the vegetative cells producing spores, in which case the spore count increases. Alternatively, the spore count may remain unchanged but the vegetative cell count falls as a result of the action of lytic enzymes produced by the cells themselves. Among the common mesophilic *Bacillus* species, spore formation is largely complete 6–10 hours after the end of exponential growth under optimal cultural conditions. The degree of heat resistance and the concentration of spores would not be expected to rise much after this time. Conducting heat resistance studies on a mixture of spores and vegetative cells is undesirable because the likely result is a rapid initial fall in count due to killing of the vegetative cells, and a subsequent slower rate due to death of spores. If necessary, the vegetative cells can usually be removed by addition of the enzymes lysozyme and trypsin.

The degree of heat resistance shown by vegetative cells may also be influenced by the stage of growth from which the cells were taken. It is normally found that stationary-phase cells are more heat resistant than those taken from the logarithmic phase of growth, although several exceptions have been reported.

Cultural conditions

The conditions under which the cells are grown is another factor that can markedly affect heat resistance. Insufficient attention has been paid to this potential source of variation in a substantial part of the research conducted. Not infrequently, insufficient details of the cultivation procedures are described in the scientific reports, or materials of variable composition, e.g. tap water or soil extracts, were used in media without regard to the possible differences that might have arisen between successive batches or populations of cells.

Factors such as growth temperature, medium pH and buffering capacity, oxygen availability and concentrations of culture medium components may all affect resistance.

Thermophilic organisms are generally more heat resistant than mesophils, which in turn tend to be more resistant than psychrophils. If a 'league table' of spore heat resistance were to be constructed, it is probable that *B. stearothermophilus*, *B. coagulans* and *Cl. thermosaccharolyticum* would head the list; all three have growth optima of 50–60°C. Variable results have arisen when single species have been grown at a variety of temperatures. *Escherichia coli* and *Streptococcus faecalis* have both been the subject of conflicting reports on the influence of growth temperature on heat resistance, whereas spores of *B. cereus* produced at temperatures between 20 and 41°C showed maximal resistance at 30°C.

The effects of medium pH, buffering capacity, oxygen availability and the concentrations of culture medium components are often complex and interrelated. An unsuitable pH, inadequate buffer or insufficient aeration may all limit the extent of growth, with the result that the cells that *do* grow each have available to them a higher concentration of nutrients than would be the case if a higher cell density had been achieved. The levels of intracellular storage materials and metal ions may therefore differ and so influence resistance to heat and other lethal agents. Cells existing in or recently isolated from their 'natural' environment, e.g. water, soil, dust or pharmaceutical raw materials, have often been reported to have a greater heat resistance than their progeny that have been repeatedly subcultured in the laboratory and then tested under similar conditions.

pH and composition of heating menstruum

It is frequently found that cells survive heating more readily when they are at neutrality (or their optimum pH for growth if this differs from neutrality). The combination of heat and an unfavourable pH may be additive or even synergistic in killing effects; thus *B. stearothermophilus* spores survive better at 110°C in dilute pH 7.0 phosphate buffer than at 85°C in pH 4.0 acetate buffer. Differences in heat resistance may also result merely from the presence of the buffer, regardless of the pH it confers. Usually an apparent increase in resistance occurs when cells are heated in buffer rather than in water alone. A similar increase is often found to occur on the addition of other dissolved or suspended solids, particularly those of a colloidal or proteinaceous nature, e.g. milk, nutrient broth and serum.

Because dissolved solids can have such a marked effect on heat resistance, great care must be taken in attempting to use experimental data from simple solutions to predict the likely heat treatment required to kill the same cells in a complex formulated medicine or food material. An extreme case of protection of cells from a lethal agent is the occlusion of cells within crystals. When spores of *B. subtilis* var. *niger* were occluded within crystals of calcium carbonate, their resistances to

inactivation were approximately 900 times and nine times higher than for unoccluded spores when subjected to steam and dry heat, respectively; an exposure period of 2.5 hours at 121°C (moist heat) was required to eliminate survivors within the crystals. It is to minimize the risk of such situations arising that there is a requirement in the latest edition of *Rules and Guidance for Pharmaceutical Manufacturers and Distributors* that medicines be prepared in clean conditions.

The solute concentrations normally encountered in dilute buffer solutions used as suspending media for heat resistance experiments cause no significant reduction in the vapour pressure of the solution relative to that of pure water, i.e. they do not reduce the water activity, A_w, of the solution (which has a value of 1.0 for water). If high solute concentrations are used or the cells are heated in a 'semi-dry' state the A_w is significantly lower and the resistance is increased, e.g. a 1000-fold increase in D value has been reported for *B. megaterium* spores when the water activity was reduced from 1.0 to between 0.2 and 0.4.

Recovery of heat-treated cells

The recovery conditions available to cells after exposure to heat may influence the proportion of cells that produce colonies. A heat-damaged cell may require an incubation time longer than normal to achieve a colony of any given size, and the optimum incubation temperature may be several degrees lower. The composition of the medium may also affect the colony count, with nutritionally rich media giving a greater percentage survival than a 'standard' medium, whereas little or no difference can be detected between the two when unheated cells are used. Adsorbents such as charcoal and starch have been found to have beneficial effects in this context.

IONIZING RADIATIONS

Ionizing radiations can be divided into electromagnetic and particulate (corpuscular) types. Electromagnetic radiations include γ-rays and X-rays, whereas particulate radiation includes α and β particles, positrons and neutrons.

Particulate radiation

The nuclear disintegration of radioactive elements results in the production of charged particles. α particles are heavy and positively charged, being equivalent to the nuclei of helium atoms. They travel relatively slowly in air and although they cause a great deal of ionization along their paths, they have very little penetrating power, their range being just a few centimetres in air. α particles have no application in this aspect of pharmacy and will not be considered further. β particles are negatively charged and have the same mass as an electron. In air the penetrating power of these particles is a few metres but they will be stopped by a thin sheet of aluminium. β particles resulting from radioactive decay are therefore not sufficiently penetrative for use in sterilization processes but the production of accelerated electrons from man-made machines (cathode rays) results in particles of great energy with enhanced penetrating power.

Electromagnetic radiation

γ radiation results when the nucleus still has too much energy even after the emission of α or β particles. This energy is dissipated in the form of very short wavelength radiation which, as it has no mass or charge, travels with the speed of light, penetrating even sheets of lead. Although travelling in a wave form, γ radiation behaves as if composed of discrete packets of energy called quanta (photons). A ^{60}Co source emits γ-rays with photons of 1.17 and 1.33 MeV and the source has a half-life of 5.2 years. X-rays are generated when a heavy metal target is bombarded with fast electrons. They have similar properties to γ-rays despite originating from a shift in electron energy rather than from the nucleus.

Units of radioactivity

The unit of activity is the becquerel (Bq), which is equal to one nuclear transformation per second. This replaces the term 'curie' (Ci); 3.7×10^{10} becquerels = 1 curie. The unit of absorbed dose according to the SI system is the gray (Gy), which is equal to one joule per kilogram. However, the old term 'rad' is still used occasionally and is equivalent to 100 ergs per gram of irradiated material.

$$1 \text{ gray} = 100 \text{ rads}$$

The energy of radiation is measured in electron volts (eV) or millions of electron volts (MeV). An electron volt is the energy acquired by an electron falling through a potential difference of 1 volt.

Effect of ionizing radiations on materials

Ionizing radiations are absorbed by materials in a variety of ways, depending upon the energy of the incident photons:

1. *Photoelectric effect*: low-energy radiation (<0.1 MeV) is absorbed by the atom of the material, resulting in the ejection or excitation of an electron.

2. *Compton effect*: incident photons of medium energy 'collide' with atoms and a portion of the energy is absorbed with the ejection of an electron. The remaining energy carries on impacting with further atoms and emitting further electrons until all the energy is scattered.

3. *Pair production*: radiations of very high energy are converted on impact into negatively charged electrons and positively charged particles called positrons. The positron has an extremely short life and quickly annihilates itself by colliding with an orbital electron.

The ionization caused by the primary radiation results in the formation of free radicals, excited atoms, etc., along a discrete track through the material. However, if secondary electrons contain sufficient energy they may cause excitation and ionization of adjacent atoms, thereby effectively widening the track. Accelerated electrons used in electron beam sterilizers are essentially equivalent to the secondary electrons arising from γ irradiation – they cause direct ionization of molecules within materials. Temperature rise during irradiation is very small and even high-energy radiation resulting in pair production is only accompanied by an increase of approximately 2°C but nevertheless, the chemical changes that occur in irradiated materials are very widespread. Of particular significance here are the deleterious changes that may occur in packaging materials at normal dosage levels. Such effects may include changes in tensile strength, colour, odour and gas formation of polymers. Materials most affected include acetal, FEP, PTFE and PVA. Total absorbed energy determines the extent of physical and chemical reactions that occur, and so damage is cumulative. For sterilization purposes, exposure times can be long but the process is predictable and delivers a reproducible level of lethality.

The lethal effect of irradiation on microorganisms can occur in two ways:

1. *Direct effect*. In this case the ionizing radiation is directly responsible for the damage by causing a direct hit on a sensitive target molecule. It is generally accepted that cellular DNA is the principal target for inactivation, and that the ability to survive irradiation is attributable to the organism's ability to repair damaged DNA rather than to any intrinsic resistance of the structure. Further damage may be caused by free radicals produced within the cell but not directly associated with DNA. These radicals can diffuse to a sensitive site and react with it, causing damage.

2. *Indirect effect*. The passage of ionizing radiation through water causes ionization along and immediately next to the track and the formation of free radicals and peroxides. These peroxides and

free radicals are highly reactive and destructive and are responsible for both killing capability and the ability to modify the properties of polymers.

Some of the possible reactions are as follows:

radiation

$$H_2O \rightarrow H_2O^+ + e^-$$

$$H_2O^+ \rightarrow \cdot OH + H^+$$

$$e^- + H_2O \rightarrow OH^- + H\cdot$$

$$2H\cdot \rightarrow H_2$$

$$2\cdot OH \rightarrow H_2O_2$$

The presence of oxygen has a significant effect on the destructive properties of ionizing radiation owing to the formation of hydroperoxyl radicals.

$$H\cdot + O_2 \rightarrow \cdot HO_2$$

Peroxides and free radicals can act as both oxidizing and reducing agents according to the conditions.

Factors affecting the radiation resistance of microorganisms

Across the spectrum of microorganisms, viruses are the forms most resistant to the effects of radiation, followed by bacterial endospores, then Gram-positive cells and finally Gram-negative cells. Resistance to radiation is genetically determined and a particularly resistant bacterium called *Deinococcus radiodurans* can withstand a radiation dose up to three times that which would kill a normal bacterium. Fortunately, this organism does not have any clinical significance. It is worth noting that microbial products such as endotoxins will not be inactivated by normal doses of ionizing radiations. Consequently it is important to ensure that initial bioburden levels are low.

Oxygen has already been mentioned as having a significant effect on radiation resistance as the increased levels of hydroperoxyl radicals lead to marked increases in sensitivity. Vegetative cells such as *E. coli* and *Pseudomonas aeruginosa* are 3–4 times more sensitive in the presence of oxygen than in its absence. The presence of moisture will influence sensitivity. Dehydration also increases resistance owing to an indirect effect on the formation and mobility of free radicals. Freezing also increases radiation resistance owing to the reduction of mobility of free radicals in the menstruum, preventing them from diffusing to sites of action at the cell membrane. Above the freezing point there is very little effect of temperature.

A variety of organic materials provide a protective environment for microorganisms, and comparison of radiation resistance is greatly complicated by different complexities of the media used. Sulphydryl groups, such as may be found in amino acids and proteins, have a protective effect on microorganisms owing to their interaction with free radicals. In contrast, compounds that combine with -SH groups, such as halogenated acetates, tend to increase sensitivity. Some naturally occurring materials, particularly foods, may have a profound protective effect on contaminant bacteria. This is of concern to the food-processing industry.

ULTRAVIOLET RADIATION

Although UV radiation has a range of wavelength of approximately 15–330 nm, its range of maximum bactericidal activity is much narrower (220–280 nm), with an optimum of about 265 nm. Whereas ionizing radiations cause electrons to be ejected from atoms in their path, UV radiation does not possess sufficient energy for this and merely causes the electrons to become excited. It has much less penetrating power than ionizing radiations and tends to be used for the destruction of microorganisms in air and on surfaces.

The bactericidal effect of UV light is due to the formation of linkages between adjacent pyrimidine bases in the DNA molecule to form dimers. These are usually thymine dimers, although other types have been identified. The presence of thymine dimers alters the structural integrity of the DNA chain, thereby hindering chromosome replication. Certain cells can repair damaged DNA in a variety of ways, enhancing their radiation resistance.

Exposure of UV-damaged cells to visible light (photoreactivation) enables a light-dependent photoreactivating enzyme to split the thymine dimers into monomers. A second mechanism is not light dependent and is called dark recovery. In this case the thymine dimers are removed by a specific endonuclease enzyme that nicks the damaged DNA strand either side of the dimer. DNA polymerase then replaces the missing nucleotides and the ends are joined by a ligase enzyme.

Factors affecting resistance to UV light

As already mentioned, UV light has very little penetrating power and anything that acts as a shield around the cells will afford a degree of protection. The formation of aggregates of cells will result in those cells at the centre of the aggregate surviving an otherwise lethal dose of radiation. Similarly, microorganisms suspended in water withstand considerably higher doses of radiation than in the dry state owing to lack of penetration of the radiation.

Suspension of bacteria in broth containing organic matter such as proteins increases the resistance of the cells still further. The stage of growth of the culture will affect the sensitivity of the cells, with maximum sensitivity being shown during the logarithmic phase.

Other factors shown to influence radiation resistance include pH, temperature and humidity, although the effect of the last parameter is still somewhat confused.

GASES

The use of gases as antimicrobial agents has been documented for centuries, although it is only recently that their mechanisms of action and factors affecting activity have been elucidated. A wide variety of gaseous agents has been used for their antimicrobial properties and a few of the major ones will be dealt with here.

Ethylene oxide

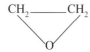

Ethylene oxide is a gas at room temperature (with a boiling point at 10.7°C) that readily permeates a variety of materials (plastics, cardboard, cloth, etc.) but not crystals. Its odour is reported as being rather pleasant, although the levels at which it is detected in the atmosphere (700 ppm) greatly exceed the 5 ppm maximum safety limit for humans. Toxicity problems include burns and blistering if the material comes into contact with the skin, whereas inhalation results in lachrymation, headache, dizziness and vomiting. Great care must be taken to ensure the removal of residual ethylene oxide from treated products (e.g. rubber gloves) to avoid the risk of skin reactions. Explosive mixtures are formed when ethylene oxide is mixed with air at any concentration above 3% and this is especially dangerous if the gas mixture is confined. The addition of carbon dioxide or fluorinated hydrocarbons will eliminate this risk, and for sterilization purposes gas mixtures of 10% ethylene oxide/90% carbon dioxide are typically used.

Ethylene oxide is extremely effective at killing microorganisms and its activity is related to its action as an alkylating agent. Reactive hydrogen atoms on hydroxyl, carboxyl, sulphydryl and amino groups can all be replaced with hydroxyethyl groups, thereby interfering with a wide range of metabolic activities. Ethylene oxide inactivates the complete spectrum of microorganisms, including endospores and viruses. The difference in resistance between endospore-forming bacteria and vegetative cells is only of the order of 5–10 times, compared to several thousand-fold differences with other physical and chemical processes. In addition, no microorganism of genetically determined high resistance has been found. Spores of *B. subtilis* var. *niger* are among the most resistant to the effect of ethylene oxide. The moist heat-resistant spore former *B. stearothermophilus* and spores of *Clostridium sporogenes* are no more resistant than a number of vegetative organisms, such as *Staph. aureus* and *Micrococcus luteus*. Fungal spores exhibit the same order of resistance as vegetative cells.

Factors affecting the activity of ethylene oxide

The bactericidal activity of ethylene oxide is proportional to the partial pressure of gas in the reaction chamber, time of exposure, temperature of treatment and level and type of contamination. At room temperature the time taken to reduce the initial concentration of cells by 90% can be very slow. For this reason elevated temperatures of 50–60°C are recommended and these result in greatly increased rates of kill. Concentrations of ethylene oxide between 500 and 1000 mg L^{-1} are usually employed. Relative humidity has a most pronounced effect, as at very high humidities ethylene oxide may be hydrolysed to the much less active ethylene glycol. This is borne out by the observation that the gas is 10 times more active at 30% RH than at 97% RH. The optimum value for activity appears to be between 28% and 33% RH. Below 28% RH the alkylating action of ethylene oxide is inhibited due to lack of water. The degree of dehydration of cells greatly influences activity and it may not be possible to rehydrate very dry organisms simply by exposure to increased RH. The RH value chosen in practice is usually between 40% and 70%.

Microorganisms may be protected from the action of ethylene oxide by occlusion within crystalline material or when coated with organic matter or salts. *B. subtilis* var. *niger* spores dried from salt-water solutions are much more resistant to the gas than are suspensions dried from distilled water.

Biological indicators used to test the efficacy of ethylene oxide treatment employ spores of *B. subtilis* dried on to suitable carriers, such as pieces of aluminium foil.

Formaldehyde

Formaldehyde (H.CHO) in its pure form is a gas at room temperature, with a boiling point of −19°C but readily polymerizes at temperatures below 80°C to form a white solid. The vapour, which is extremely irritating to the eyes, nose and throat, can be generated either from solid polymers such as paraformaldehyde or from a solution of 37% formaldehyde in water (formalin). Formalin usually contains about 10% methanol to prevent polymerization.

As with ethylene oxide, formaldehyde is a very reactive molecule and there is only a small differential in resistance between bacterial spores and vegetative cells. Its bactericidal powers are superior to those of ethylene oxide (concentrations of 3–10 mg L^{-1} are effective) but it has weak penetrating power and is really only a surface bactericide. It is also more readily inactivated by organic matter. Adsorbed gas is very difficult to remove and long airing times are required. Its mechanism of action is thought to involve the production of intramolecular crosslinks between proteins, together with interactions with RNA and DNA. It acts as a mutagenic agent and an alkylating agent, reacting with carbonyl, thiol and hydroxyl groups. In order to be effective, the gas must dissolve in a film of moisture surrounding the bacteria. For this reason relative humidities in the order of 75% are required. Formaldehyde used in conjunction with low-temperature steam is a very effective sterilization medium.

Peracetic acid

The toxic nature of ethylene oxide and formaldehyde has prompted the search for further gaseous sterilants. Peracetic acid has been widely used as an aqueous solution but its use in the gaseous phase is more limited. It is a liquid at room temperature, requiring heat treatment to vaporize. Although it is highly active against bacteria (including mycobacteria and endospores), fungi and viruses, it is rather unstable and is damaging to certain materials such as metals and rubber.

Hydrogen peroxide

Hydrogen peroxide is similar to peracetic acid in that it is a solution at room temperature and must be heated to generate the gaseous phase. The main attraction of hydrogen peroxide as an antimicrobial agent is the fact that its decomposition products are oxygen and water. Most work on the antimicrobial properties of hydrogen peroxide has been carried out on aqueous solutions where it has been shown to have a good range of activity, including against bacterial spores. The biocidal efficacy of the vapour phase is less than that in solution and is influenced by environmental conditions.

Chlorine dioxide

Chlorine dioxide is a gas at room temperature but is primarily used in aqueous solution where it has good broad-spectrum activity. If it is to be employed in the gaseous phase then it must be generated at the point of use and in this form it is highly effective and relatively safe.

Propylene oxide

Propylene oxide is a liquid (boiling point = 34°C) at room temperature which requires heating to volatilize. It is inflammable between 2.1% and 21.5% by volume in air but this can be reduced by mixing with CO_2. Its mechanism of action is similar to that of ethylene oxide and involves the esterification of carbonyl, hydroxyl, amino and sulphydryl groups present on protein molecules. It is, however, less effective than ethylene oxide in terms of its antimicrobial activity and its ability to penetrate materials. Whereas ethylene oxide breaks down to give ethylene glycol or ethylene chlorohydrin, both of which are toxic, propylene oxide breaks down to propylene glycol, which is much less so.

Methyl bromide

Methyl bromide boils at 3.46°C and so is a gas at room temperature. It is used as a disinfectant and a fumigant at concentrations of 3.5 mg L^{-1} with a relative humidity between 30% and 60%. It has inferior antimicrobial properties compared to the previous compounds but has good penetrating power.

Gas plasmas

A plasma is formed by applying energy to a gas or vapour under vacuum. Natural examples are lightning and sunlight but plasmas can also be generated under low energy such as in fluorescent strip lights. Within a plasma, positive and negative ions, electrons and neutral molecules collide to produce free radicals. The destructive power of these entities has already been described and so plasmas can be used as biocidal agents in a variety of applications. This type of system can be produced at temperatures below 50°C using vapours generated from hydrogen peroxide or peracetic acid. Dusseau et al (2004) have produced a useful review of the applications of gas plasmas in the sterilization of medical devices.

ANTIMICROBIAL EFFECTS OF CHEMICAL AGENTS

Chemical agents have been used since very early times to combat such effects of microbial proliferation as spoilage of foods and materials, infection of wounds and decay of bodies. Thus, long before the role of microorganisms in disease and decay was recognized, salt and sugar were used in food preservation, a variety of oils and resins were applied to wounds and employed for embalming, and sulphur was burned to fumigate sick rooms.

The classic researches of Pasteur, which established microorganisms as causative agents of disease and spoilage, paved the way for the development and rational use of chemical agents in their control. Traditionally, two definitions have been established describing the antimicrobial use of chemical agents. Those used to destroy microorganisms on inanimate objects are described as *disinfectants*, and those used to treat living tissues, as in wound irrigation, cleansing of burns or eye washes, are called *antiseptics*. Other definitions have been introduced to give more precise limits of meaning, namely, *bactericide* and *fungicide* for chemical agents that kill bacteria and fungi, respectively, and *bacteriostat* and *fungistat* for those that prevent the growth of a bacterial or fungal population. The validity of drawing a rigid demarcation line between those compounds that kill and those that inhibit growth without killing is doubtful. In many instances concentration and time of contact are the critical factors. The term *preservative* describes those antimicrobial agents used to protect medicines, pharmaceutical formulations, cosmetics, foods and general materials against microbial spoilage. *Biocide* is a general term for antimicrobial chemicals but it excludes antibiotics and other agents used for systemic treatment of infections.

The mechanisms by which biocides exert their effects have been intensively investigated and the principal sites of their attack upon microbial cells identified. These are the cell wall, the cytoplasmic membrane and the cytoplasm. Chemical agents may weaken the cell wall, thereby allowing the extrusion of cell contents, distortion of cell shape, filament formation or complete lysis. The cytoplasmic membrane, controlling as it does permeability and being a site of vital enzyme activity, is vulnerable to a wide range of substances that interfere with reactive groups or can disrupt its phospholipid layers. Chemical and electrical gradients exist across the cell membrane and these represent a proton-motive force which drives such essential processes as oxidative phosphorylation, adenosine triphosphate (ATP) synthesis and active transport; several agents act by reducing the proton-motive force. The cytoplasm, which is the site of genetic control and protein synthesis, presents a target for those chemical agents that disrupt ribosomes, react with nucleic acids or generally coagulate protoplasm.

Principal factors affecting activity

The factors most easily quantified are temperature and concentration. In general, an increase in temperature increases the rate of kill for a given concentration of agent and inoculum size. The commonly used nomenclature is Q_{10} (temperature coefficient), which is the change in activity of the agent per $10°C$ rise in temperature (e.g. Q_{10} phenol = 4).

The effect of change in concentration of a chemical agent upon the rate of kill can be expressed as:

$$\eta = \frac{\log t_2 - \log t_1}{\log C_1 - \log C_2} \qquad (16.4)$$

where C_1 and C_2 represent the concentrations of agent required to kill a standard inoculum in times t_1 and t_2. The concentration exponent η represents the slope of the line when log death time (t) is plotted against log concentration (C).

When values of η are greater than 1, changes of concentration will have a pronounced effect. Thus, in the case of phenol, when $\eta = 6$, halving the concentration will decrease its activity by a factor of 2^6 (i.e. 64-fold), whereas for a mercurial compound, $\eta = 1$, the same dilution would only reduce activity twofold (2^1). Further details and tabulations of both temperature coefficients and concentration exponents may be found in Denyer & Wallhaeusser (1990).

Range of chemical agents

The broad categories of antibacterial chemical compounds have remained surprisingly constant over the years, with phenolics and hypochlorites comprising the major disinfectants and quaternary ammonium compounds widely used as antiseptics. The compounds capable of use as preservatives in preparations for oral, parenteral or ophthalmic administration are obviously strictly limited by toxicity requirements. As concerns over toxicity have intensified, the range of available preservatives has diminished: mercury-containing compounds, for example, are now very little used for the preservation of parenteral and ophthalmic products. The high cost of research and testing coupled with the poor prospects for an adequate financial return militate against the introduction of new agents. For this reason there is a tendency towards the use of existing preservatives in combination, with a view to achieving one or more of the following benefits: synergy, a broader antimicrobial spectrum or reduced human toxicity resulting from the use of lower concentrations. The subjects of preservative toxicity and their potentiation and synergy are reviewed by Denyer & Wallhaeusser (1990), and Moore & Payne (2004) have described in detail characteristics of the commonly used biocides. Table 16.3 summarizes the properties and uses of the major groups of biocides.

Phenolics

A limited selection of phenolic compounds is shown in Figure 16.4.

Various distillation fractions of coal tar yield phenolic compounds, including cresols, xylenols and phenol

Table 16.3 Properties and uses of the major groups of antimicrobial chemicals (biocides)

Chemical group	Examples	Mode(s) of action	Principal uses	Advantages	Disadvantages
Alcohols and phenols	Ethanol, isopropanol, benzyl alcohol, chlorbutanol, phenylethyl alcohol, phenoxyethanol, phenol, chlorocresol, chloroxylenol	Membrane damage, protein denaturation, cell lysis	Ethanol and isopropanol as skin antiseptics and disinfectants; other agents variously used as antiseptics, disinfectants and preservatives for injections, and some oral and topical products	Ethanol, isopropanol and phenol are very water soluble and have good cleansing properties. Relatively low toxicity. Broad antimicrobial activity	Several alcohols are flammable. Activity much reduced on dilution, by organic matter and, for phenolics, by high pH. Phenolics absorbed by rubber and plastics. Little or no sporicidal activity at room temperature
Aldehydes	Formaldehyde, glutaraldehyde, orthophthalaldehyde	React with amino and other groups causing protein cross-linking and denaturation	Glutaraldehyde has limited use as a chemosterilant for surgical instruments, and formaldehyde as a gaseous sterilant	Little affected by organic matter. Broad antimicrobial spectrum including spores. Non-corrosive sterilants	Relatively high toxicity: may cause respiratory distress and dermatitis
Biguanides	Chlorhexidine	Membrane disruption and cytoplasmic coagulation at high concentration	Antiseptic	Relatively non-toxic. Good activity against. Gram-positive bacteria	Less active against Gram negative bacteria and fungi. Incompatible with many negatively charged materials
Halogens	Hypochlorites, iodine and iodophors	Interaction with thiol and amino groups causing enzyme and protein damage	Disinfectants	Broad antimicrobial spectrum including spores	Chlorine liberated from hypochlorite is irritant to skin, eyes and lungs. Hypochlorites are corrosive. Iodine stains
Organic acids	Benzoic acid, sorbic acid	Uncoupling agents that prevent the uptake of substrates requiring a proton-motive force to enter the cell	Preservatives in oral products	Sufficiently low toxicity for oral use.	Activity much diminished with rising pH. Only useful for products with pH lower than approx 5
Organic acid esters (parabens)	Methyl, ethyl, butyl, propyl, benzyl parabens and their salts		Preservatives used principally in topical and oral products and in some injections	Relatively good activity against fungi. Activity little changed with rising pH. Relatively low toxicity	Poor water solubility and a tendency to partition into the oily phase of emulsions. Relatively weak activity against Gram-negative bacteria

Continued

Table 16.3 Properties and uses of the major groups of antimicrobial chemicals (biocides)—Cont'd					
Chemical group	Examples	Mode(s) of action	Principal uses	Advantages	Disadvantages
Oxidizing agents	Hydrogen peroxide, peracetic acid	Oxidation of protein functional groups	Disinfectants and gaseous phase sterilants for isolators and equipment	Broad antimicrobial spectrum including spores	Peracetic acid has pungent smell and is corrosive. Hydrogen peroxide is unstable
Quaternary ammonium compounds	Benzalkonium chloride, benzethonium chloride, cetrimide, cetyl pyridinium chloride	Cell membrane damage and loss of essential chemicals from the cell. Cytoplasmic coagulation in high concentration	Disinfectants and antiseptics Preservatives in ophthalmic, topical and some injectable products	Very water soluble and effective at neutral and alkaline pH. Good stability, non-corrosive and generally non-hazardous	Benzalkonium chloride causes skin and ophthalmic sensitization. Incompatible with many negatively charged materials

itself, all of which are toxic and caustic to skin and tissues. Disinfectant formulations traditionally described as 'black fluids' and 'white fluids' are prepared from higher-boiling coal tar fractions. The former make use of soaps to solubilize the tar fractions in the form of stable homogeneous solutions, whereas the latter are emulsions of the tar products and unstable on dilution.

Remarkable success has been achieved in modifying the phenol molecule by the introduction of chlorine and methyl groups, as in chlorocresol and chloroxylenol. This has the dual effect of eliminating toxic and corrosive properties while at the same time enhancing and prolonging antimicrobial activity. Thus, chlorocresol is used as a bactericide in injections and to preserve oil-in-water creams, whereas chloroxylenol is employed as a household and hospital antiseptic. Phenol may itself be rendered less caustic by dilution to 1% w/v or less for lotions and gargles, or by dissolving in glycerol for use as ear drops. Bisphenols, such as hexachlorophane and triclosan (Irgasan), share the low solubility and enhanced activity of the other phenol derivatives described but have a substantive effect which makes them particularly

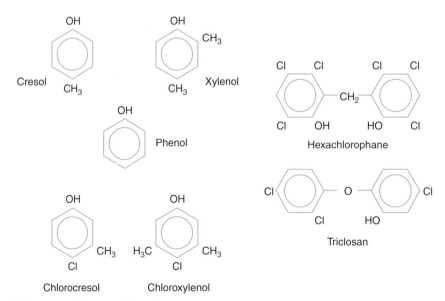

Fig. 16.4   Chemical structures of a range of phenols.

useful as skin antiseptics. Formulated as creams, cleansing lotions or soaps, they have proved valuable in reducing postoperative and cross-infection. Again toxicity concerns have emerged. Consequently, hexachlorophane, for example, is restricted in the UK both in respect of the concentrations that may be employed and the type of product in which it may be used.

Phenols generally are active against vegetative bacteria and fungi, are readily inactivated by dilution and organic matter and are most effective in acid conditions. Depending on concentration, phenols may cause cell lysis at low concentrations or general coagulation of cell contents at higher concentrations.

Alcohols, aldehydes, acids and esters

Ethyl alcohol has long been used, usually as 'surgical spirit' for rapid cleansing of preoperative areas of skin before injection. It is most effective at concentrations of 60–70%. It is rapidly lethal to bacterial vegetative cells and fungi but has no activity against bacterial endospores and little effect on viruses. The effect of aromatic substitution is to produce a range of compounds which are less volatile and less rapidly active and find general use as preservatives, e.g. phenylethanol for eye drops and contact lens solutions, benzyl alcohol in injections, Bronopol (2-bromo-2-nitropropane-1,3-diol) in shampoos and other toiletries. Phenoxyethanol, which has good activity against *Ps. aeruginosa*, has been used as an antiseptic. In general the alcohols act by disrupting the bacterial cytoplasmic membrane and can also interfere with the functioning of specific enzyme systems contained within the membrane.

Formaldehyde and glutaraldehyde are both powerful disinfectants, denaturing protein and destroying vegetative cells and spores. Formaldehyde is used in sterilization procedures both as a gas and as a solution in ethyl alcohol. Glutaraldehyde solutions are also used to sterilize surgical instruments.

The organic acids, sorbic and benzoic and their esters, because of their low toxicity, are well established as preservatives for food products and medicines (see Chapter 43). The exact mode of action of these agents on microorganisms is still uncertain but they have been shown to influence the pH gradient across the cell membrane. At higher concentrations the parabens induce leakage of intracellular constituents.

Quaternary ammonium compounds

The chemical formula for quaternary ammonium compounds is shown in Figure 16.5.

These cationic surface-active compounds are, as their name implies, derivatives of an ammonium halide in

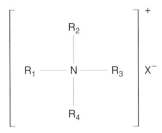

Cetrimide
$R_1R_2R_3$ — CH_3
R_4 — mainly $C_{14}H_{29}$
X — Br

Benzalkonium chloride
R_1R_2 — CH_3
R_3 — $C_6H_5CH_2$
R_4 — mainly $C_{13}H_{27}$
X — Cl

Fig. 16.5 Chemical structure of cetrimide and benzalkonium chloride.

which the hydrogen atoms are substituted by at least one lipophilic group, a long-chain alkyl or aryl-alkyl radical containing C_8–C_{18} carbon atoms. In marked contrast to phenol and the cresols, these compounds are mild in use and active at such high dilutions as to be virtually non-toxic. Their surface-active properties make them powerful cleansing agents, a useful adjunct to their common use as skin antiseptics and preservatives in contact lens cleansing and soaking solutions. They are also safe for formulating into eye drops and injections and are widely used in gynaecology and general surgery. Active as cations, ambient pH is important, as is interference caused by anions. Thus, alkaline conditions promote activity and it is important that all traces of soap, which is anion active, are removed from the skin prior to treatment with a quaternary ammonium compound. Foreign organic matter and grease also cause inactivation.

One effect of the detergent properties of these compounds is to interfere with cell permeability such that susceptible bacteria, mainly the Gram-positive groups, leak their contents and eventually undergo lysis. Gram-negative bacteria are less susceptible and, to widen the spectrum to include these, mixtures of quaternary ammonium compounds with other antimicrobial agents such as phenoxyethanol or chlorhexidine are used.

Biguanides and amidines

Chlorhexidine (Fig. 16.6) is a widely used biocide which has activity against Gram-positive and Gram-negative bacteria but little activity against endospores or viruses. It is widely used in general surgery, both

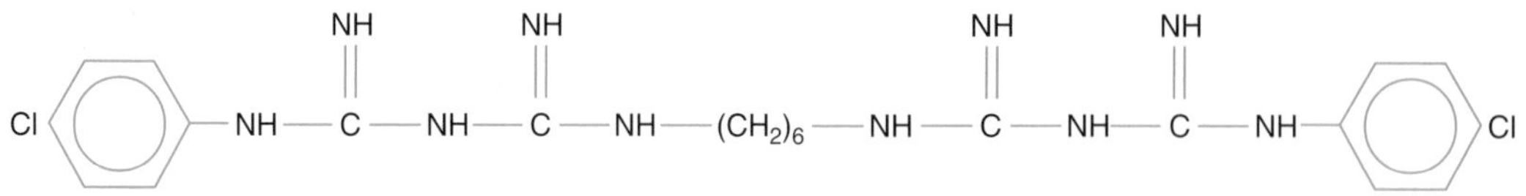

Fig. 16.6 Chemical structure of chlorhexidine.

alone and in combination with cetrimide, and can also be used as a preservative in eye drops. Polyhexamethylene biguanide (PHMB) is a polymeric biguanide used widely in the food, brewing and dairy industries. It has also found application as a disinfectant in contact lens cleaning solutions. The biguanides act on the cytoplasmic membrane, causing leakage of intracellular constituents.

The aromatic diamidines, propamidine and dibromopropamidine, are non-toxic antiseptics mainly active against Gram-positive bacteria and fungi. However, resistance to these agents can develop quickly during use.

Halogens and their compounds

Chlorine gas is a powerful disinfectant used in the municipal treatment of drinking water and in swimming baths. Solutions of chlorine in water may be made powerful enough for use as general household bleach, and disinfectant and dilute solutions are used for domestic hygiene. The high chemical reactivity of chlorine renders it lethal to bacteria, fungi and viruses, and to some extent spores. This activity is optimal at acid pH levels around 5.0. Unionized hypochlorous acid (HOCl) is an extremely potent and widely used bactericidal agent that acts as a non-selective oxidant, reacting readily with a variety of cellular targets. Salt solutions subjected to electrolysis in an electrochemical cell yield a mixture of biocidal species of which the predominant one is hypochlorous acid. This system is available commercially for use in endoscope washers.

Two traditional chlorine-containing pharmaceutical formulations, which are used much less frequently now, are Eusol (Edinburgh University solution of lime, also known as Chlorinated Lime and Boric Acid Solution BPC 1973) and Dakin's Solution (Surgical Chlorinated Soda Solution BPC 1973), both of which are designed to provide slow release of chlorine.

An alternative method of obtaining more prolonged release of chlorine is by the use of organic chlorine compounds such as Chloramine T (sodium *p*-toluenesulphonchloramide) and Halazone BPC 1973 (*p*-sulphondichloramide benzoic acid). These are used in pharmaceutical products much less frequently now but

have retained some application in the disinfection of water such as whirlpool spas and in fish farms.

Iodine, which, like chlorine, is a highly reactive element, denatures cell proteins and essential enzymes by its powerful oxidative effects. Traditionally it has been used in alcoholic solutions such as Tincture of Iodine (BP 1973) or complexed with potassium iodide to form an aqueous solution (Lugol's Iodine BP 1973). The latter product, although highly effective as a bactericide, probably fell out of favour because of the tendency to stain both the clothes and skin.

The staining and irritant properties of iodine have resulted in the development of iodophores, mixtures of iodine with surface-active agents, which hold the iodine in micellar combination from which it is released slowly. Such a preparation is Betadine (polyvinylpyrrolidone-iodine formulated as 10% povidone iodine), used as a non-staining, non-irritant antiseptic.

Metals

Many metallic ions are toxic to essential enzyme systems, particularly those utilizing thiol (-SH) groups, but those used medically are restricted to mercury, silver and aluminium. The extreme toxicity of mercury has rendered its use obsolete apart from in organic combination. The organic compounds that still have a limited use in pharmacy are phenylmercuric nitrate (and acetate) as a bactericide in eye drops and injections, and thiomersal (sodium ethylmercurithiosalicylate) as a preservative in biological products and certain eye drops.

Silver, in the form of the nitrate, has been used to treat infections of the eyes, as have silver protein solutions. Aluminium foil has been used as a wound covering in the treatment of burns and venous ulcers. It has been shown to adsorb microorganisms and inhibit their growth.

The acridines

This group of compounds interferes specifically with nucleic acid function and has some ideal antiseptic properties. Thus aminacrine hydrochloride is non-toxic, non-irritant, non-staining and active against Gram-positive and Gram-negative bacteria even in the presence of serum.

SUMMARY

This brief survey has given some indication of the variety of antimicrobial compounds available. Each of these has a defined spectrum of utility and in the correct conditions of use can substantially contribute to the control of microbial proliferation and infection.

REFERENCES

Denyer, S.P., Wallhaeusser, K.H. (1990) Antimicrobial preservatives and their properties. In: Denyer, S.P., Baird, R. (eds) *Guide to Microbiological Control in Pharmaceuticals*. Ellis Horwood, Chichester.

Dusseau, J-Y., Duroselle, P., Freney, J. (2004) Gaseous sterilization. In: Fraise, A.P., Lambert, P.A., Maillard, J-Y. (eds) *Principles and Practice of Disinfection, Preservation and Sterilisation*, 4th edn. Blackwell Science, Oxford.

European Pharmacopoeia (2004) 5th edn. Council of Europe, Strasbourg.

Moore, S.L., Payne, D.N. (2004) Types of antimicrobial agents. In: Fraise, A.P., Lambert, P.A., Maillard, J-Y. (eds) *Principles and Practice of Disinfection, Preservation and Sterilisation*, 4th edn. Blackwell Science, Oxford.

Rules and Guidance for Pharmaceutical Manufacturers and Distributors (Latest edition) Pharmaceutical Press, London.

Russell, A.D. (1999) Destruction of bacterial spores by thermal methods. In: Russell, A.D., Hugo, W.B., Ayliffe, G.A.J. (eds) *Principles and Practice of Disinfection, Preservation and Sterilisation*, 3rd edn. Blackwell Science, Oxford.

17

Principles of sterilization

S. E. Walsh, J-Y. Maillard

INTRODUCTION

Previous chapters in this Part have described the types and properties of microorganisms (Chapter 14) and the action of heat and chemical agents upon them (Chapter 16). This chapter will build on those fundamentals and describe the principles underlying the different methodologies available to achieve sterility. These will be described both for pharmaceutical preparations and also for other products and devices. This chapter will also describe the criteria used to measure sterility. The practicalities associated with the processes of sterilization are described in Chapter 18.

By definition, a sterile preparation is described as the absolute absence of microbial contaminants. In practice, this definition is not achievable as a preparation cannot be *guaranteed* to be sterile. This remark is discussed further in Chapter 18.

Certain pharmaceutical preparations, medical devices and items for which usage involves contact with broken skin, mucosal surfaces or internal organs are required to be sterile. These are frequently referred to in pharmacopoeias as Category One products. Microbiological materials, such as soiled dressings and other contaminated items, also need to be sterilized before disposal or reuse.

Sterilization is the process by which a product is rendered sterile, i.e. the destruction or removal of microorganisms. Most preparations can be sterilized in their final container or packaging. Certain processes will achieve terminal sterilization through the destruction of the microorganisms, for example by physical means such as heat and radiation or a combination of physical and chemical means (e.g. gaseous sterilization). However, such processes can be detrimental for the chemical composition of certain preparations. For these sensitive preparations or for preparations to which an additional component is added aseptically, the process of non-terminal sterilization, which is based on aseptic filtration, is used.

NEED FOR STERILITY

As mentioned in the introduction, certain pharmaceutical preparations, medical products and devices are required to be sterile (further information is given in Chapter 18, Table 18.1). Briefly, these include:

- injections – intravenous infusion, total parenteral nutrition (TPN), small-volume injections and small-volume oily injections
- non-injectable sterile fluids – non-injectable water, urological irrigation solutions, peritoneal dialysis and haemodialysis solutions, inhaler solutions
- ophthalmic preparations – eye drops, lotions and ointments and some contact lens solutions
- dressings
- implants
- absorbable haemostats
- surgical ligatures and sutures (absorbable and non-absorbable)
- instruments and equipment – syringes, metal instruments, respirator parts.

Failure to achieve sterility can result in serious consequences. In the best case scenario, surviving microorganisms induce spoilage of the product (i.e. chemical and physical degradation) that might be identified before the preparation is used. The product (or batch of product) is then removed from consumption and destroyed. In the worst case scenario, where microbial survival cannot be identified through deleterious effects to the product, infection (sometimes deadly) might result from the use of the contaminated preparation. There have been many reports in the literature of such incidents over the years. For example, in the Devonport incident (1971–1972) the death of five patients (from acute endotoxic shock) was traced to dextrose 5% infusion bottles sterilized with a faulty autoclave. In 1996, in Romaira (Brazil), 35 newborn infants died of sepsis attributed to locally produced i.v. solutions (Editorial 1998). More recently, a contaminated heparin i.v. flush was responsible for infecting several patients in different states in the USA (Editorial 2005). In these cases inappropriate quality control procedures were implicated. These incidents emphasize that not only must an appropriate sterilization regimen be used but appropriate monitoring and control must be performed. This requires an understanding of the principles of sterilizing processes and their validation.

STERILIZATION PARAMETERS

The inactivation kinetics of a pure culture of microorganisms exposed to a physical or chemical sterilization process is generally described by an exponential relationship between the number of organisms surviving and the extent of treatment (ISO 2000), although variations from this are likely (Chapter 16 gives more details). Survivor curves have been used to generate inactivation data for specific sterilization processes using specific biological indicators (see Chapter 18). These data are important for calculating a number of sterilization parameters which help to establish a sterilizing regimen adapted to a specific preparation or product.

D value and *Z* value

One of the important concepts in sterilization is the D value (Fig. 17.1). This parameter is calculated as the time taken for a one log (90%) reduction in the number of microorganisms. Another important concept is the Z value, which calculates the temperature (or dose for radiation sterilization) required to produce a one log (90%) reduction in D value for a particular microorganism. This parameter is used to compare the heat (or dose) resistance of different biological indicators following alterations in temperature or radiation. Chapter 16 provides more information on both these parameters.

Inactivation factor and most probable effective dose

The inactivation factor is the reduction in number of microorganisms brought about by a defined sterilization process. This parameter can be calculated from the D value but only if the destruction curve follows the linear

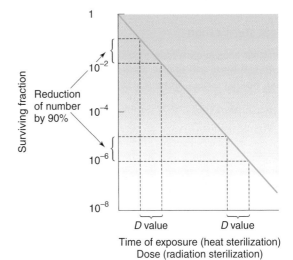

Fig. 17.1 Calculation of D value and Z value. Note that the D value remains the same although calculated with different surviving fractions.

logarithmic model. To overcome problems caused by variations from this model, a most probable effective dose value can be used. This is the dose needed to achieve n decimal reductions in the number of microorganisms. These concepts are further developed in Chapter 18.

F value

The F value is used to compare the lethality of different heat sterilization processes. A reference value (F_o) of *Geobacillus stearothermophilus* (formerly *Bacillus stearothermophilus*) spores at 121°C is often used with a Z value of 10°C. The total F_o of a process includes the heating up and cooling down phases of the sterilization cycle.

For dry heat sterilization the F value concept has some limited application. The F_H value is used and corresponds to the lethality of a dry heat process in terms of the equivalent number of minutes exposure at 170°C. A Z value of 20°C is used for the calculation.

PRINCIPLES OF STERILIZATION PROCESSES

Five main types of sterilization processes are usually recommended for pharmaceutical products (*British Pharmacopoeia* 2004, *European Pharmacopoeia* 2004). Among these, heat sterilization still represents the gold standard. Novel sterilization processes are being developed and have already been applied in the food industry. These are mentioned in the 'New Technologies' section later in this chapter.

Heat sterilization

Heat has been employed as a purifying agent since early historical times and is now used worldwide in sterilization. Boiling is not a form of sterilization as higher temperatures are needed to ensure the destruction of all microorganisms.

Microorganisms vary in their response to heat. Species of bacterial spores are thought to be some of the most heat-resistant forms of life and can survive temperatures above 100°C. Non-sporulating bacteria are destroyed at lower temperatures (50–60°C) and vegetative forms of yeasts and moulds have a similar response. Cysts of amoeba (e.g. *Acanthamoeba polyphaga*) are less sensitive than their vegetative cells which are inactivated at 55–60°C. It is generally thought that viruses are less resistant than bacterial spores (Gould 2004). The agents responsible for spongiform encephalopathies, the prions, are worth mentioning due to their infectious nature and high resistance to heat (current thermal sterilization procedures are probably not effective in inactivating prions).

Despite the widespread use of heat sterilization, the exact mechanisms and target sites involved are still uncertain. It is likely that several mechanisms and targets are implicated and those proposed include damage to the outer membrane (Gram-negative bacteria), cytoplasmic membrane, RNA breakdown and coagulation, damage to DNA and denaturation of proteins, probably as a result of an oxidation process. For hydrated cells (moist heat sterilization), it is likely that the chemical lethal reactions occur more rapidly with the presence of water. The denaturation and coagulation of key enzymes and structural proteins probably result from a hydrolytic reaction.

The thermal death of bacterial cells and spores is usually thought to have a first-order reaction kinetic. Although some controversy over this does exist, the use of an exponential inactivation model for the kinetics of spores is unlikely to be underestimating the heat required (Gould 2004, Joslyn 2001a). One way to express the order of death as a first-order reaction is:

$$N_t = N_0 e^{-kt}$$

This relationship is discussed further in Chapter 16.

Heat sterilization processes usually occurs in three phases:

- the heating up phase, where the temperature within the chamber is brought to the appropriate level
- the holding phase – when the optimal temperature is reached, the holding time is maintained for the required length (e.g. 15 minutes at 121°C).
- the cooling down phase, where the chamber temperature is brought down before the preparation/product can be removed safely from the autoclave.

Principles of moist heat sterilization

Moist heat sterilization relies on a combination of steam, temperature and pressure. Steam is used to deliver heat to the product to be sterilized. There are different types of steam but only steam at the phase boundary has the appropriate characteristics for maximum effectiveness (Fig. 17. 2). Steam at the phase boundary between itself and its condensate has the same temperature as the boiling water that produced it but holds much more latent heat. This latent heat is available for transfer (without a decrease in temperature) when it condenses on to a cooler surface. This rapid transfer of latent heat is responsible for the rapid rise in temperature (to the sterilization temperature) of any items it touches (Chapters 16 and 46 provide more information). The condensed

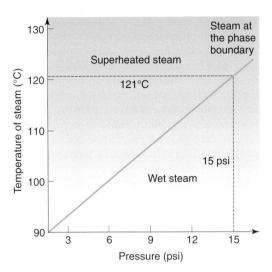

Fig. 17. 2 Steam for moist heat sterilization.

Table 17.1 Time temperature combinations used for moist and dry heat sterilization

Process	Minimum temperature (°C)	Minimum holding period (minutes)
Moist heat (autoclaving)	115	30
	121	15
	126	10
	134	3
Dry heat	140	180
	150	150
	160	120
	170	60
	180	30

water also aids the process by hydrating microorganisms and making them more sensitive.

Principles of dry heat sterilization

Sterilization using dry heat is less efficient than moist heat but is the preferred method for items that are thermostable but moisture sensitive or impermeable to steam (Sharp 2000). This includes some metal items (e.g. metal instruments and scalpels), glassware, oils/oily injections and some powders (see Chapter 18, Table 18.1). In addition, temperatures greater than 220°C are used for depyrogenation of glassware (in this case the process needs to demonstrate a three log reduction in heat-resistant endotoxin). The main advantage of dry heat over moist heat is its ability to penetrate items and kill microorganisms via oxidation. The process is generally slower and holding times for dry heat are much longer than those needed for moist heat sterilization (Table 17.1).

Combination treatments

The amount of heat required for sterilization can be reduced by using combination treatment of heat plus a reduced pH (below 4.5) or low water potential (A_w). Although some spores may survive the initial treatment, they then germinate and die, reducing the numbers of organisms present as time passes (a process called autosterilization). This technique has been used in the food industry with meat-based canned foods to avoid high-temperature sterilization. In addition, the combination of heat hydrostatic pressure is thought to be synergistic. This is further discussed in the 'Ultrahigh pressure' section below.

In the pharmaceutical industry, another type of combination treatment involves low-temperature steam formaldehyde (LTSF). The steam is below atmospheric pressure (70–80°C) and formaldehyde gas provides the sporicidal effect. Formaldehyde has been used to sterilize medical devices but care must be taken with its use as it is acutely toxic to humans and is also mutagenic and possibly carcinogenic (Sharp 2000). Some caution should be attached to the sterility assurance level (see Chapter 18) of the process, as it has been suggested that revival of spores after LTSF treatment is possible (Gould 2004). Finally, the processing of thermolabile medical equipment such as endoscopes is conducted in automated washer disinfectors. These make use of high-level disinfectants and slightly raised temperature. This is further discussed in the 'High-level disinfection' section below.

Alternative means for heat delivery and control

Systems for the delivery of heat via direct application of flame, heating using alternating electric currents and microwave energy have been developed and adopted in some parts of the world. The use of infrared radiation allows the rapid elevation in temperature. Advances in packaging have improved heat penetration and made it more uniform. These include flexible pouches, polypropylene rigid containers, thermoformed containers, tin-free steel and foil-plastic combinations.

Gaseous sterilization

When sterilization by heat is not possible, one alternative is to use a sterilizing gas. Not many gases are used in the pharmaceutical industry for sterilization and it is important to note that some of these gases are also used for disinfection (as either a liquid or a gas) under different conditions. Pharmacopoeias usually recommend the use of ethylene oxide for gaseous sterilization, although other chemicals are available, such as formaldehyde, hydrogen peroxide, chlorine dioxide, peracetic acid and ozone. The chemical biocides are generally separated, according to their mode of action, into alkylating and oxidizing agents.

Alkylating gases

Some alkylating gases can permeate through many polymeric materials and are therefore not limited to just surface applications.

In the past, ethylene oxide was used in hospitals but this is now less common. However, it is still widely used in pharmaceutical manufacturing. It occurs in gaseous form at room temperature (boiling point 10.7°C) and penetrates narrow spaces well. Ethylene oxide has been shown to possess bactericidal, fungicidal, virucidal, sporicidal and antiprotozoan properties (Dusseau et al 2004). Propylene oxide also has sterilization and penetration properties but it is not as widely used as ethylene oxide as it requires a longer sterilization cycle (Joslyn 2001b).

The use of low-temperature steam formaldehyde (LTSF) sterilization has been mentioned already. Formaldehyde is a surface sterilant only and cannot be used to sterilize occluded areas. Penetration into porous materials can be inhibited by the formation of polymers that crosslink, preventing further sterilant access (Chapter 16 provides more information).

Oxidizing gases

Oxidizing gases are relatively unstable and their decomposition can lead to microenvironments within the load that are not exposed to the full concentration of the agent.

Hydrogen peroxide gas has been shown to be effective against spores at a range of temperatures. Its action is greatest when used at near-saturation levels on clean dry surfaces and it does not leave a toxic residue (Joslyn 2001b). The vapour is usually obtained via evaporation of a heated stock solution. Water condensation on surfaces that are being sterilized can reduce local concentrations of hydrogen peroxide and hence its activity, and decomposition by catalytic activity and absorption by cellulosic materials (e.g. paper) can also reduce its effectiveness. The combination of hydrogen peroxide with cold plasma, cupric or ferric ions, ozone or UV has been shown to enhance activity (Dusseau et al 2004).

Ozone has been demonstrated to be an effective sterilant but the complex control of humidity required and corrosion problems have limited its applications and it is not routinely used. Ozone as a disinfectant for water

currently shows more promise and commercial systems are available for several applications.

Chlorine dioxide has sporicidal activity and is currently under commercial development, although its applications are limited due to its effect on materials such as uncoated aluminium foil, uncoated copper, polycarbonate and polyurethane (Joslyn 2001b).

Peracetic acid exists as a liquid at room temperature and is used for high-level disinfection (discussed below). However, vaporized peracetic acid is used to sterilize isolators, although a long contact time is required. Peracetic acid can cause corrosion of certain metals and rubbers and has low penetrating power.

Radiation sterilization

There are two main types of radiation: electromagnetic and particulate.

- Electromagnetic radiation – γ-rays, X-rays, ultraviolet (UV), infrared (IR), microwave energy and visible light.
- Particulate radiation – α-rays, β-rays (high-speed electrons), neutrons and protons.

Of these, only γ-rays and high-speed electron beams are used for sterilization of pharmaceutical products, since other forms of radiation have not been shown to be effective as sterilants and/or are not suitable (Lambert 2004). Both γ- and β-rays are forms of ionizing radiation (Chapter 16 provides more information on mode of action and resistance). One advantage of irradiation is that it does not cause a significant rise in temperature and hence has been called 'cold sterilization'. The main target site for radiation is DNA but damage to other vital components such as RNA, enzymes and cell membranes is also involved. Single-strand or double-strand DNA breaks will inhibit DNA synthesis or cause errors in protein synthesis. Damage to the sugars and bases may also occur (Hansen & Shaffer 2001).

Ionizing radiation can be used to sterilize items that cannot be sterilized with heat (see Chapter 18, Table 18.1). This is not a process that is normally carried out in a standard pharmaceutical manufacturing facility; instead specialized plants are used (Sharp 2000).

D values are used in radiation sterilization (see Fig. 17.1) and can be calculated from the formula:

$$D = \text{radiation dose}/\log N_0 - \log N$$

where N_0 and N represent a one log difference in numbers.

As with heat sterilization, the dose–response curve to radiation can vary (shoulders and tailing off can occur) but in general the exponential model holds. The initial lag that causes a shoulder is thought to result from multiple targets being hit before death or from DNA repair taking place. More details and equations are given by Lambert (2004).

Despite having been shown to have activity against bacterial spores, viruses and vegetative cells, UV radiation is not used for sterilization of pharmaceutical products because of its low penetrative power and absorption by glass and plastics. It is used for disinfection of surfaces, including isolators and safety cabinets, and can be used as part of the treatment for drinking water (Lambert 2004).

Filtration sterilization

Thermolabile solutions can be sterilized by filtration through filters that remove bacteria. Filtration sterilization is the complete removal of microorganisms within a specific size range from liquids or gases. It is a non-terminal process and strict aseptic techniques need to be observed. Because of their small size, viruses are not removed by sterilization filtration and therefore, where possible, terminal sterilization processes should be preferred. Items that might be filter sterilized include heat-sensitive injections and ophthalmic solutions, biological products and air and other gases for supply to aseptic areas (Denyer & Hodges 2004).

There are two main types of filtration mechanisms:

- sieving, which makes use of synthetic membrane filters. This is an absolute mechanism since it ensures the exclusion of all particles above a defined size
- adsorption and trapping, which make use of depth filters. Depth filters have a high dirt-handling capacity and are often used as prefilters.

Generally, only membrane filters are thought to be suitable for the removal of microorganisms. The types used for pharmaceutical applications are usually made from cellulose esters or other polymers and are highly uniform with regular spaces or holes. When a liquid passes through the filter, all particles and microorganisms larger than the holes are retained. Membrane filters have the advantage of removing particles and microorganisms efficiently while retaining very little of the product in their holder or housing. However, they can become blocked quickly if the liquid being sterilized contains a lot of particles and smaller particles can become trapped in the holes, causing a pressure differential (Levy 2001). Because of this, prefilters are often used.

High-level disinfection

The term 'high-level' disinfection is often employed with chemical biocides that have demonstrated a high sporicidal activity. Hence they are sometimes described as 'chemosterilants'. High-level disinfectants can be generally divided into two main groups of highly reactive biocides: alkylating and oxidizing agents (Table 17.2). Among the former, the aldehydes, and notably formaldehyde (gas), glutaraldehyde but also *ortho*-phthalaldehyde are the most important. Oxidizing agents are composed of a wider family, such as peroxygen compounds (e.g. peracetic acid, hydrogen peroxide and accelerated hydrogen peroxide) and also chlorine dioxide and superoxidized water (Babb & Bradley 1995). Peracetic acid has also been used for the cold sterilization of some pharmaceutical preparations such as emulsions, hydrogels, ointments and powders.

Oxidizing agents, as their name suggests, owe their antimicrobial property to their oxidizing effects against proteins, notably against thiol groups of cysteine residues. In short, these agents damage many important microbial enzymes that possess these groups, which often results in metabolic inhibition in the cells. Structural proteins but also other components such as nucleic acid and ribosomes (in eukaryotes) are also affected. On the other hand, alkylating agents react with cell components such as nucleic acid and protein by alkylation, which also results in a metabolic inhibition of the cell. Aldehydes, in particular, will react with several groups including amino, carboxyl, thiol, hydroxyl, imino and amide substituents. The crosslinking property of aldehydes is important for their microbicidal action.

On occasion, the use of chemical biocides has been combined with a physical process, such as temperature

Table 17.2 Sterilization and high-level disinfection using chemical biocides

Chemical agents	Usage
Hydrogen peroxide	Gas plasma sterilization (endoscopes)
Peracetic acid	Endoscopes, pharmaceutical preparations
Chlorine dioxide	Gas-phase chlorine dioxide sterilization (medical equipment)
Glutaraldehyde	High-level disinfection (endoscopes)
Ortho-phthalaldehyde	High-level disinfection (endoscopes)
Formaldehyde	Gaseous sterilization (LTSF)[*]
Ethylene oxide	Liquid and gaseous sterilization

[*]LTSF: low-temperature steam formaldehyde

(e.g. low-temperature steam formaldehyde (LTSF), discussed earlier in this chapter). High-level disinfectants are often used in automated machines. For example, for endoscopes, high-level disinfection is conducted in specially designed automated washer disinfectors, which clean, disinfect and rinse the lumens and external surfaces of the flexible endoscopes.

NEW TECHNOLOGIES

Although only five sterilization procedures are usually recommended in pharmacopoeias, there has been an interest in developing alternative methodologies to palliate the disadvantages of existing ones (see Chapter 18). It has to be noted that most of the progress has been made in the food area. These technologies include ultrahigh pressure, high-voltage electric pulse, high-intensity light pulse, ultrasonication and gas plasma, and offer full or partial alternatives to heat sterilization (for further information see Gould 2004). The principles of these new sterilization processes, although they are not used for pharmaceutical preparations, are worth mentioning briefly.

Ultrahigh pressure

The principle in using high pressure is that vegetative microorganisms are inactivated at pressures above 100 MPa and bacterial spores at pressures above 1200 MPa. The use of high pressure for food preservation has been combined with the chemical effect of the preservative system, such as a low pH in certain foodstuff (e.g. jams, fruit juices, etc.). The low pH ensures the prevention of outgrowth of bacterial spores. The use of high pressure has now been applied to other foodstuffs and such technology has been evaluated for the production of vegetative bacterial vaccine (Larson et al 1918). The advantage of this process is that the quality and taste of products tend not to be affected by such a system. Indeed, high pressure tends to denature preferably macromolecules rather than low molecular weight flavour and odour compounds. Hence, the microbial cell offers multiple pressure-sensitive target sites (e.g. enzymes, membranes, genomic material, etc.). Bacterial spores are more resilient to high pressures. However, the combination of high pressure with elevated temperature has been shown to be synergistic, although the process varies depending upon the combination and the type of spores.

Another advantage of using high pressure is the rapid control of thermal processes. Indeed, the application of pressure raises the temperature but conversely the temperature decreases as the pressure is reduced. Hence,

rapid temperature changes following a rapid change in pressure can help in controlling a thermal process and reduce heat-induced damage to a product (Heinz & Knorr 2001).

High-voltage electric pulse (high-intensity pulsed electric fields)

The use of electricity to heat foods is well established (e.g. microwave heating). The process of high-voltage electric pulse relies on a non-thermal microbial inactivation through the leakage of cell content following a potential difference across the membrane. Typical field intensities ranged from 12 to 25 kV/cm for periods from 1 to 100 μs (Qin et al 1995). Although this process is effective against vegetative microorganisms, bacterial spores and ascospores (yeast) are highly resistant even at high-voltage gradients (>30 kV/cm).

High-intensity light pulse

The application of intense light, such as high-intensity laser, has been known to inactivate microorganisms, principally through a combination of UV irradiation and heat treatment. This principle already has applications in the food industry and also in the medical area, notably in dentistry. Such processes have been shown to inactivate vegetative microorganisms and bacterial spores (Dunn et al 1988). In the food industry, broad-spectrum light with pulse durations from 10^{-6} to 10^{-1} seconds and with energy densities ranging from 0.1 to 50 J/cm^2 is used in commercially available machines. In the dental field, such technology has been combined with the use of dyes (e.g. toluidine blue) to achieve a better inactivation of microorganisms, for example in the treatment of root canal infection (Wilson 2004).

For pharmaceutical preparations, a potential application is the terminal sterilization of clear solutions such as water, saline, dextrose and ophthalmic products. The type of container is of prime importance since it must not hinder the transmission of light.

Ultrasonication

The use of sonication to inactivate microorganisms was first reported over 30 years ago. The principle is based on cavitation through the material exposed, resulting in the formation and collapse of small bubbles. The ensuing shock waves associated with high temperatures and pressures can be sufficiently intense to disrupt the microbial cell; however, spores are highly resistant. A synergistic effect has been reported by combining ultrasound and heat to a certain extent; the effect of ultrasound becomes less with high temperature (near boiling point).

Interestingly, such a combination has been reported to reduce the heat resistance of microorganisms.

Gas plasma

Gas plasma is generated with the application of a strong magnetic field to a gaseous phase compound (e.g. hydrogen peroxide). This process creates free radicals that can then damage cellular components (e.g. membrane, nucleic acid), a mechanism of action similar to that of oxidizing agents. This dry sterilization process is effective against vegetative microorganisms but also bacterial spores and has the advantage of being non-thermal. The gas plasma of hydrogen peroxide has been shown to have sporicidal activity and sterilizers are available commercially (Joslyn 2001b).

SUMMARY

Sterilization is an important process for pharmaceutical and medical areas. There are several processes that can be used to achieve appropriate sterilization for a given preparation or product/device. Each of these processes presents advantages and disadvantages, although moist heat sterilization remains the reference standard. The advances in non-thermal sterilization and the coming new technologies, although mainly applied to the food industry to date, offer potentially valuable alternatives. The demonstration of sporicidal activity of a new technology, as well as its control and reproducibility, remains essential.

Common to all these processes is the need for the user to understand the technology, its activity and limitations, to follow the appropriate guidelines but also, importantly, to ensure the validation of the process. Failure to provide the appropriate documentation and to control a sterilization process adequately might result in failure of the process, with potentially fatal consequences.

It is important to note at this point that although terminal sterilization ensures the destruction of possible microbial contaminants, it needs to be operated alongside good manufacturing practice. Therefore, suitable measures must be taken to ensure the microbiological quality of pharmaceutical preparations during manufacture but also during packaging, storage and distribution. These important aspects are discussed in more depth in Chapter 18.

REFERENCES

Babb, J.R., Bradley, C.R. (1995) A review of glutaraldehyde alternatives. *British Journal of Theatre Nursing*, **5**, 20-41.

British Pharmacopoeia (2004) *Appendix XVII Methods of sterilization (methods of preparation of sterile products).* Pharmaceutical Press, London.

Denyer, S.P., Hodges, N.A. (2004) Sterilization: filtration sterilization. In: Fraise, A.P., Lambert, P.A., Maillard, J-Y. (eds) *Principles and Practice of Disinfection, Preservation and Sterilization*, 4th edn. Blackwell Science, Oxford.

Dunn, J.E., Clark, R.W., Asmus, J.E. et al (1988) *Method and apparatus for preservation of foodstuffs*. International Patent WO88/03369.

Dusseau, J-Y., Duroselle, P., Freney, J. (2004) Sterilization: gaseous sterilization. In: Fraise, A.P., Lambert, P.A., Maillard, J-Y. (eds) *Principles and Practice of Disinfection, Preservation and Sterilization*, 4th edn. Blackwell Science, Oxford.

Editorial 1998 *Morbidity and Mortality Weekly Report*, **47**, 610-612.

Editorial 2005 *Morbidity and Mortality Weekly Report*, **54**, 269-272.

European Pharmacopoeia 2004 *Methods of Preparation of Sterile Products. 5.1.1*, 5th Council of Europe, Strasbourg.

International Standards Organization (ISO) (2000) *Sterilization of health care products -general requirements for characterization of a sterilizing agent and the development, validation and routine control of a sterilization process for medical devices.* ISO 14937. ISO, Geneva.

Gould, G.W. (2004) Sterilization: heat sterilization. In: Fraise, A.P., Lambert, P.A., Maillard, J-Y. (eds) *Principles and Practice of Disinfection, Preservation and Sterilization*, 4th edn. Blackwell Science, Oxford.

Hansen, J.M., Shaffer, H.L. (2001) Sterilization and preservation by radiation sterilization. In: Block, S.S. (ed.) *Disinfection, Sterilization, and Preservation*, 5th edn. Lippincott Williams and Wilkins, Philadelphia.

Heinz, V., Knorr, D. (2001) Effects of high pressure on spores. In: Hendrickx, M.E.G., Knorr, D. (eds) *Ultra High Pressure Treatments of Foods*. Kluwer Academic/Plenum Publishers, New York.

Joslyn, L.J. (2001a) Sterilization by heat. In: Block, S.S. (ed.) *Disinfection, Sterilization, and Preservation*, 5th edn. Lippincott Williams and Wilkins, Philadelphia.

Joslyn, L.J. (2001b) Gaseous chemical sterilization. In: Block, S.S. (ed.) *Disinfection, Sterilization, and Preservation*, 5th edn. Lippincott Williams and Wilkins, Philadelphia.

Lambert, P. (2004) Sterilization: radiation sterilization. In: Fraise, A.P., Lambert, P.A., Maillard, J-Y. (eds) *Principles and Practice of Disinfection, Preservation and Sterilization*, 4th edn. Blackwell Science, Oxford.

Larson, W.P., Hartzell, T.B., Diehl, H. S. (1918) The effect of high pressure on bacteria. *Journal of Infectious Diseases*, **22**, 271-279.

Levy, R.V. (2001) Sterile filtration of liquids and gases. In: Block, S.S. (ed.) *Disinfection, Sterilization, and Preservation*, 5th edn. Lippincott Williams and Wilkins, Philadelphia.

Qin, B., Pothakamury, U., Vega, H. et al (1995) Food pasteurisation using high intensity pulsed electric fields. *Journal of Food Technology*, **49**, 55-60.

Sharp, J. (2000) Sterile products: basic concepts and principles. In: *Quality in the Manufacture of Medicines and Other Healthcare Products*. Pharmaceutical Press, London.

Wilson, M. (2004) Lethal photosensitisation of oral bacteria and its potential application in the photodynamic therapy of oral infections. *Photocemical and Photobiological Sciences*, **3**, 412-418.

BIBLIOGRAPHY

Block, S.S. (ed.) (2001) *Disinfection, Sterilization, and Preservation*, 5th edn. Lippincott Williams and Wilkins, Philadelphia.

British Society for Gastroenterology Working Party 1998 Cleaning and disinfection of equipment for gastrointestinal endoscopy. *Gut*, **42**, 585-593.

Fraise, A.P., Lambert, P.A., Maillard, J-Y. (eds) (2004) *Principles and Practice of Disinfection, Preservation and Sterilization*, 4th edn. Blackwell Science, Oxford.

The appropriate pharmacopoeias relevant to your area of work.

J-Y. Maillard, S. E. Walsh

STERILE PRODUCTS

Sterilization is an essential part of the processing of some pharmaceutical preparations (defined as Category One in some pharmacopoeias). By definition, a sterile product is completely free of microorganisms. As briefly described in Chapter 17, a number of pharmaceutical preparations are required to be sterile. In addition, a number of other items mainly used in the medical field need to be sterilized as they generally come into contact with sterile parts of the body or are reused (Table 18.1). The range of preparations or products to be sterilized necessitates the use of a number of different sterilization processes. Regardless of the sterilization technology used, it is important that the process itself is appropriately validated, as failure to control and/or document a sterilization process adequately can lead to serious incidents. This chapter will consider the recommended sterilization processes, their control and validation.

DETERMINATION OF STERILIZATION PROTOCOLS

There are various technologies available to achieve sterility in a preparation or device (Table 18.2). Sterilization processes can be separated into terminal and non-terminal sterilization. These processes have distinct characteristics and can involve the use of high temperature, high pressure, a reactive gas, irradiation or filtration. Combinations of different processes are also employed, for example a combination of reactive gas and slightly elevated temperature and pressure, or high temperature and steam. In the selection of an appropriate process, the choice of terminal or non-terminal sterilization is of paramount importance. The selected sterilization process must be suitable for its purpose, i.e. the sterilization of a given product, device and preparation, which means that the product and its container have to be rendered safe and must not be damaged by the process or post process.

Table 18.1 Examples of sterile preparations and devices

Preparation/product/item	Typical volume	Typical container	Sterilization process
Injections			
Intravenous infusion, e.g. blood products	0.5 L	Plastic, glass	Moist heat Filtration (e.g. addition of additives)
Total parenteral nutrition (TPN)	>3 L	Plastic, glass	Moist heat Filtration (e.g. addition of vitamins)
Small volume injections, e.g. insulin, vaccine	1–50 mL	Plastic, glass	Moist heat[a] Filtration
Small-volume oily injections		Glass	Dry heat
Non-injectable sterile fluids			
Non-injectable water, e.g. surgery, irrigation	0.5–1 L	Plastic (polyethylene or polypropylene)	Moist heat
Urological irrigation solution	>3 L	Plastic (rigid)	Moist heat Filtration
Peritoneal dialysis and haemodialysis solutions	2.5 L	Plastic	Moist heat
Inhaler solutions	Diluted in WFI[a]	Plastic (polyethylene nebulas)	Dry heat
Ophthalmic preparations			
Eye drops	0.3–0.5 mL	Plastic, glass	Moist heat[b] Filtration
Eye lotions	>0.1 L	Plastic, glass	Moist heat
Eye ointments	–	Plastic, aluminium	Dry heat Filtration
Contact lens solutions	Small	Plastic	Chemical disinfection
Dressings			
Chlorhexidine gauze dressing	Different wrapping[c]	Moist heat[d]	
Polyurethane foam dressing		Dry heat	
Elastic adhesive dressing		Ethylene oxide	
Plastic wound dressings		Ionizing radiation	
		Other effective method	
Implants	Small, sterile cylinders of drug	Dry heat Chemical (0.02% PMN, 12h 75°C)	
Absorbable haemostats,			
Oxidized cellulose, human fibrin foam		Dry heat	
Surgical ligatures and sutures			
Sterilized surgical catgut		γ-radiation Chemical (96% ethanol + 0.002% PMN + formaldehyde in ethanol 24h prior use; naphthalene or toluene at 160°C for 2 h)	
Non-absorbable type		γ-radiation Moist heat	
Instruments and equipment			
Syringes	Glass, plastic	Dry heat Moist heat	

Table 18.1   Examples of sterile preparations and devices–Cont'd

Preparation/product/item	Typical volume	Typical container	Sterilization process
		γ-radiation	
		Ethylene oxide	
Metal instruments		Moist heat	
Rubber gloves		γ-radiation	
		Ethylene oxide	
Respirator parts		Moist heat	
Fragile heat-sensitive devices		Chemical disinfection	

[a] Water for injection.
[b] Depends upon the preparations (thermostable or thermolabile).
[c] Dressings must be appropriately wrapped (aseptic handling) for their specific usage.
[d] Sterilization process depends upon the stability of the dressing constituents (e.g. dressings containing waxes cannot be sterilized by moist heat) and the nature of their components.

Table 18.2   Sterilization technologies (for pharmaceutical preparations and medical devices)

Type	Principle	Examples
Terminal sterilization		
Physical	Heat	Moist heat
		Dry heat
	Radiation	γ-radiation
		Accelerated electron (particle radiation)
Chemical	Gaseous	Ethylene oxide
		LTSF
		Gas plasma
	Liquid	GTA, OPA, PAA
Non-terminal sterilization		
Filtration	Aseptic procedure	

The choice of an appropriate sterilization process depends on a number of factors (Table 18.3) related to the product to be sterilized, such as type and composition of product and also the quantity to be sterilized. Additionally, the composition and the packaging of the product are significant factors that rule out some sterilization processes. For example, a heat-labile preparation would not be sterilized by heat and a small oily injection would not be sterilized by moist heat (further examples are given in Table 18.1). For specific types of products such as dressings, although moist heat sterilization is generally the method of choice, only certain types of autoclave such as high-prevacuum (HPV) autoclave or similar are appropriate.

For any given preparation or product, it is difficult to predict the microbial bioburden prior to sterilization. It is assumed that the bioburden of pharmaceutical preparations will be minimal as the manufacturing process should adhere to good manufacturing practice (GMP) (Table 18.4). However, a sterilization process should be able to deal with a worst case scenario. This is usually exemplified by the use of biological indicators (see the `Process indicators' section later in this chapter) such as bacterial spores, which are considered as the most resistant microorganisms (with the exception of prions, the agents responsible for spongiform encephalopathies). This is usually the situation for official sterilization methods. Modern pharmacopoeial recommendations are derived from data generated from use of bacterial spores (biological indicators) for a given sterilization process.

RECOMMENDED PHARMACOPOEIAL STERILIZATION PROCESSES

Five main sterilization processes which possess different characteristics are usually recommended by pharmacopoeias.

- Moist heat sterilization (terminal)
- Dry heat sterilization (terminal)
- Ionizing radiation sterilization (terminal)
- Gaseous (ethylene oxide) sterilization (terminal)
- Sterilization by filtration (non-terminal)

Although the use of other sterilization methodologies is not necessarily precluded, appropriate validation documentations per product need to be provided. More information can be found in Chapters 16 and 17 or by consulting the relevant pharmacopoeia. At the time of writing, examples of these include the *European Pharmacopoeia* (2004), the *United States Pharmacopeia* (2005) and the *British Pharmacopoeia* (2004a) but it is always important to consult the most up-to-date texts and guidelines.

Table 18.3   Selection of a sterilization process

Type of product/preparation		
Pharmaceutical preparations	Volume	Large, small injection
	Composition	Water, oil, powder
Medical devices	Size	Small, large, complex devices (e.g. endoscopes, respirator parts)
	Composition	Plastic, glass, metal, porous (e.g. dressing)

Possible damage to the preparation/product	
	Heat (heat-sensitive preparations)
	Radiation (water)
	Corrosiveness (oxidizing agents)

Possible damage to the product/container	
	Water ballasting
	Moisture
	Glass breaking (upon cooling)
	Change in composition (irradiation)
	Corrosiveness
Toxicity/safety	Gas sterilization (ethylene oxide, formaldehyde)
	Liquid sterilants: aldehydes
	Radiation sterilization: radioactive source
Level of bioburden	Expected heavy contamination
	Surgical instruments
Sterilization regimen	Local sterilization (portable autoclave)
	Large quantity of items to be sterilized
	Need for quarantine (desorption)
Cost of sterilization process	Equipment, e.g. autoclave, electron accelerator
	Facility, e.g. irradiation plant
	Running cost: gas, ^{60}Co
	Training of end users
	Documentation, audit, etc.

Table 18.4   Key points to achieve good manufacturing practice

- Qualified personnel with appropriate training
- Adequate premises
- Suitable production equipment, designed for easy cleaning and sterilization
- Adequate precautions to minimize the bioburden prior to sterilization (starting material, etc.)
- Validated procedures for all critical production steps
- Environmental monitoring and in-process testing procedures

Moist heat sterilization

Moist heat sterilization is the most reliable, versatile and universally used form of sterilization. The typical cycle consists of a holding time of 15 minutes at a temperature of 121°C (Table 18.5). Steam under pressure is commonly used for moist heat sterilization unless prohibited by lack of load penetration or heat and/or moisture damage. Steam can only kill microorganisms if it makes direct contact, so it is very important to avoid air pockets in the sterilizer during a sterilization process. Air can reduce the partial pressure of the steam so that the temperature reached will be less than that expected with the pressure used. To remove the air present when an autoclave is loaded, autoclaves are equipped with air removal/displacement systems (e.g. vacuum systems, gravity displacement systems, etc., further discussed in Chapter 46). For porous loads, gravity displacement systems are no longer considered adequate and high-vacuum autoclaves are the method of choice (Gould 2004). Non-condensable gases must also be removed and monitored; these are atmospheric gases like nitrogen and oxygen that form part of the initial atmosphere of the chamber.

Steam under pressure is generated in autoclaves which can vary greatly in size and shape from portable bench-top units to industrial production facilities (Fig. 18.1). A cross-section through an autoclave is illustrated in Figure 18.2. The aim is to deliver steam at the phase boundary (dry saturated steam; see Chapter 17, Fig. 17.2) to all areas of the load. This is achieved using a combination of steam and pressure (Table 18.6).

Table 18.5 Typical terminal sterilization cycles

Sterilization process	Temperature (°C)	Pressure (psi) ((kPa))	Holding time/dose	Concentration	Parametric release	Desorption
Heat						
Moist heat	121	15 (103)	15 min	–	yes	no
	134	30 (207)	3 min	–	yes	no
Dry heat	160	–	≥2 h	–	yes	no
Radiation						
γ-radiation	Room	–	25 kGy[a]	–	yes	no
Particle radiation	Room	–	25 kGy	–	no	no
Gaseous	**Temperature (°C)**	**Humidity (%)**	**Holding time**	**Concentration**	**Parametric release**	**Desorption**
Ethylene oxide[b]	40–50	40–80	30 min–10 h	400–1000 mg/L	no	yes[c]
LTSF[d]	70–80[e]	75–100	90 min	6–50 mg/L	no	yes

[a] Standard dose. Time necessary to achieve this dose depends upon the source. For γ-ray irradiation, the process can take up to 20 h, whereas for high-energy electron (particle radiation) only few minutes may be required.

[b] Vacuum cycle; pretreatment of the load: preheating and humidification of the load. Pressurized cycle: always higher than atmospheric pressure; allows shorter contact time.

[c] Desorption could take up to 15 days; maximum threshold of ethylene oxide residues and evaluation documented in ISO 10993-7 (1996).

[d] Low temperature steam formaldehyde; values can differ slightly depending upon the literature.

[e] Lower temperature of 55–56°C can be used depending upon the thermotolerance of the preparation.

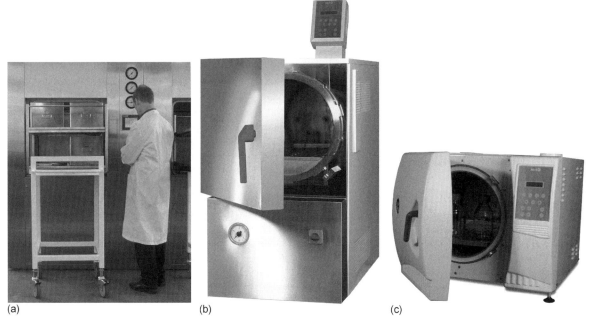

(a)   (b)   (c)

Fig. 18.1 Examples of autoclaves. (a) Square section. (b) Swiftlock. (c) Swiftlock Compact autoclaves (photographs provided by Astell).

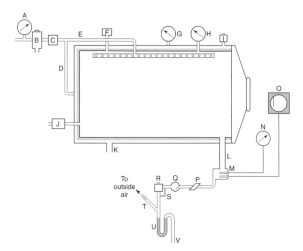

Fig. 18.2 Diagrammatic representation of the features of a large steam sterilizer (for simplicity, the control valves have been omitted). A, Mains pressure guage; B, separator; C, reducing valve; D, steam supply to jacket; E, steam supply to chambers; F, air filter; G, jacket pressure guage; H, chamber pressure guage; I, jacket air vent; J, vacuum pump; K, jacket discharge channel (detail not shown); L, chamber discharge channel; M, thermometer pocket; N, direct-reading thermometer; O, recording thermometer; P, strainer; Q, check valve; R, balanced-pressure thermostatic trap; S, bypass; T, vapour escape line; U, water seal; V, air-break.

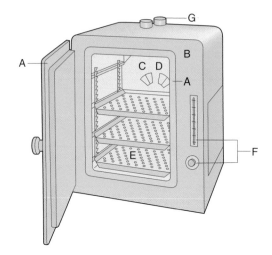

Fig. 18.3 Hot air oven. A, Asbestos gasket; B, outer case containing glass-fibre insulation, and heaters in chamber wall; C, false wall; D, fan; E, perforated shelf; F, regulator; G, vents.

Table 18.6 Examples of temperature and pressure combinations used for moist heat sterilization. Steam pressures are expressed in kPa and pounds per square inch (psi), the latter still finding continuing usage

Temperature °C	Steam pressure	
	kPa	psi
115	69	10
121	103	15
126	138	20
134	207	30

Dry heat sterilization

The most common dry heat sterilization method uses hot air ovens (Fig. 18.3). Other procedures, such as sterilizing tunnels utilizing high-temperature filtered laminar air flow or infrared irradiation to achieve rapid heat transfer, are also available. Hot air ovens are usually heated electrically and often have heaters under a perforated bottom plate to provide convection currents (gravity convection type). Mechanical convection hot air ovens are equipped with

a fan to assist air circulation and increase heat transfer by convection (Joslyn 2001). Overloading should be avoided, wrappings and other barriers minimized and the load positioned to allow optimal air circulation. Other problems include long heating up times (e.g. with large loads of instruments) and the charring or baking of organic matter onto items. Dry heat sterilization cycles are generally longer than for moist heat sterilization, typically 2 hours at 160°C (see Table 18.5). The process is thermostatically controlled and monitored using thermocouples.

Integrated lethality in sterilization practice

All heat sterilization processes must include heating up and cooling down time periods. These prolonged time periods at a raised temperature may increase the degradation of the product. Integrated lethality attempts to examine the effects of heat on the inactivation process during these time periods.

For moist heat sterilization, the F_o concept is used. This takes into account the heating up and cooling down stages of the cycle and is expressed as the equivalent time in minutes at a temperature of 121°C delivered by the process to the product in its final container with reference to microorganisms possessing a Z value of 10. Its calculation is complex and further information can be found in the relevant pharmacopoeia. In practice, computer programs can be used to calculate the combined effect of whole processes, allowing a reduction in the total process time. It is important that the appropriate sterility assurance level is consistently achieved and the routine use of biological indicators is recommended.

Gaseous sterilization

The gaseous sterilization method recommended by pharmacopoeias usually employs ethylene oxide. It is mainly used on a commercial scale for the sterilization of catheters, infusion giving sets, syringes, prostheses and some plastic containers and thermolabile powders (if humidity is not a problem; Sharp 2000). The ethylene oxide sterilization cycle is complex, as many factors need to be controlled over a long period of time (see Table 18.5). The control of the temperature, concentration and relative humidity is critical. In addition, ethylene oxide is very inflammable and can form explosive mixtures in air. It is therefore combined with an inert gas carrier (e.g. carbon dioxide, nitrogen or chlorofluorocarbon). Ethylene oxide is also toxic, mutagenic and a possible human carcinogen. The sterilization procedure is usually carried out in a purpose-built, gas-tight stainless steel chamber which can withstand high pressures and vacuum (Sharp 2000). However, systems utilizing a slight negative pressure rather than drawing a full vacuum are available (Fig. 18.4) and these are suitable for smaller, vacuum-sensitive loads.

Packaging should be permeable to air, water vapour and ethylene oxide. The sterilized products need to be quarantined post process to allow the removal of gas. The *European Pharmacopoeia* and other international standards set limits for ethylene oxide residue levels (e.g. a maximum of 10 ppm for plastic syringes).

Low-temperature steam formaldehyde (LTSF, discussed in Chapter 17), although not included in this chapter's list of recommended methods, is used for the sterilization of certain preparations. As with ethylene oxide, its sterilization cycle is rather complex as several parameters have to be controlled (see Table 18.5).

Radiation sterilization

There are two types of radiation unit. The becquerel (Bq) measures the activity of a source of radiation (physical radiation). One Bq equates to a source that has one nuclear disintegration per second). The gray (Gy) measures the effect of radiation on living tissue. One Gy is equal to the transfer of 1 J of energy to 1 kg of living tissue. The gray has replaced the rad that quantified radiation absorbed dose.

The source of γ-rays for sterilization is usually cobalt 60. Caesium 137 can also be used but has less penetrating power. Cobalt 60 decays with the emission of two high-energy γ-rays (1.17 and 1.33 MeV) and a lower energy (0.318 MeV) β particle. Gamma radiation is highly penetrative, causes negligible heating of the sterilized product at normal doses and induces no radioactivity in the final product.

Irradiation of product can be carried out in batches but is more commonly a continuous process using a conveyor system. The products pass through the irradiation chamber and are irradiated from one or two sides. The source is shielded with concrete to protect the operators and the environment. The intensity of radiation decreases as it penetrates. For example, 100 mm of a product with

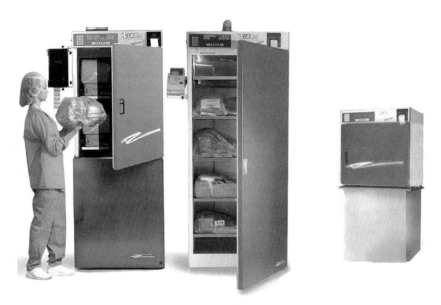

Fig. 18.4 Examples of ethylene oxide sterilizers utilizing slight negative pressure rather than the conventional vacuum system. Suitable for smaller loads, e.g. hospital reprocessing loads, research and development work, short production runs and low-volume production (courtesy of Andersen Caledonia).

a density of 1 g/cm^3 would reduce the cobalt 60 intensity by 50%. A cobalt 60 source of 1–4 ×10^{16} Bq is used for industrial irradiation and this provides a radiation dose in excess of 25 kGy. In most of Europe 25 kGy is the standard dose (e.g. *European Pharmacopoeia* 2004) but in Scandinavia doses of up to 45 kGy are recommended (Lambert 2004). When not in use, the radioactive source is submerged in water for shielding and cooling.

Particle radiation sterilization utilizes β particles that are accelerated to a high energy level by application of high-voltage potentials (no radioactivity required). Their low energy means that beams from particle accelerators are less penetrating than γ-rays, with only 10 mm of a 1 g/cm^3 material being penetrated per million electron volts (MeV). However, an important advantage of particle radiation is that the source can be turned off and is directional (Lambert 2004). The design of an accelerator can be customized to applications by including different energy and power requirements. The beam source is shielded with concrete and products are conveyed through the exposure area and irradiated. Another advantage is that shorter exposure times are required than those needed for γ irradiation. High-energy beams with energies of 5–10 MeV are used for sterilization, the accelerating field being generated using radiofrequency or microwave energy. Once it has been accelerated to the required energy, the beam of electrons is managed by magnetic fields which can alter its size, shape or direction (Hansen & Shaffer 2001).

Radiation can affect the product (e.g. through the process of water radiolysis) (Denyer & Hodges 1998) and its packaging (Sharp 2000) (discussed further in the 'Limitation of sterilization methods' section later in this chapter).

Resterilization of previously irradiated items can cause their degradation (repeated irradiation or autoclaving) or even cause them to become toxic (can occur with ethylene oxide; Richards 2004). Therefore any proposed resterilization must be carefully investigated.

Validation of radiation sterilization involves the use of *Bacillus pumilis* as a biological indicator and dosimetric analysis (discussed later in this chapter). Routine monitoring involves measurements to ensure that all products are receiving the required dose (Lambert 2004).

Filtration

Filtration is employed for non-terminal sterilization and has to be used under strict aseptic conditions. It is used for those preparations that cannot be sterilized by a terminal process or to which an agent (e.g. additive, heparin, vitamin, etc.) is added post sterilization. Filtration is used to sterilize aqueous liquid, oils and organic solutions, and also air and other gases. Membrane filtration is an absolute process which ensures the exclusion of all particles above a defined size. Although many materials have been used to make filters, only a few are suitable for sterilization of pharmaceutical products.

Depth and surface filtration are suitable for prefiltration of pharmaceutical products as they can retain large amounts of particles. Depth filters can be made of fibrous, granular or sintered material that is bonded into a maze of channels that trap particles throughout their depth. Surface filters are made of multiple layers of a substance such as glass or polymeric microfibres. Any particles that are larger than the spaces between the fibres are retained and smaller particles may be trapped in the matrix (Levy 2001). A membrane filter downstream is needed to retain any fibres shed from these filters as well as small particles and microorganisms.

To sterilize a product, it is often necessary to combine several types of filtration (e.g. depth, surface and membrane filters) to achieve the removal of microorganisms. Depth and surface filtration are used to remove the majority of particles by acting as prefilters. The final filtration step is accomplished using a membrane filter. This combined approach removes particles and microorganisms without the membrane filter blocking up rapidly with large particles.

CHEMOSTERILANTS

In addition to the processes described above, high-level disinfectants (chemical biocides) have to be mentioned, since they are used for the *chemosterilization* of medical devices, particularly high-risk items that come into contact with sterile parts of the body, such as surgical instruments, intrauterine devices, endoscopes (which are used for a wide range of diagnostic and therapeutic procedures) (see Table 18.1).

Like the gaseous biocides, the activity of high-level liquid disinfectants depends upon a number of factors (Russell 2004). Consequently, the training of the end user is of prime importance. Indeed, very often guidelines are available from professional societies regarding their appropriate use; for example, the sterilization procedure and risk assessment for gastroscopes is published by the British Society of Gastroenterology (1998). There have been reports describing the survival of microbial contaminants after a high-level disinfection process; however, contamination resulted from the use of a biocide at an inappropriate (i.e. low) concentration or the presence of a biofilm (i.e. inappropriate cleaning).

To ensure the efficacy of these high-level disinfectants, certain conditions are necessary such as knowledge of the chemical biocide (e.g. its activity and limitation), appropriate training of end users and compliance with the manufacturer's instructions. Although the use of high-level disinfectants offers some advantages, where possible physical processing (e.g. heat sterilization) should be the method of choice (Fraise 2004).

STATISTICAL CONSIDERATIONS OF STERILITY TESTING AND STERILITY ASSURANCE LEVEL

The strict definition of sterility is the complete absence of microorganisms. In other words, after a successful sterilization process, the number of microbial survivors should be zero. When one looks at microbial inactivation following, for example, exposure to heat or radiation, the inactivation usually follows first-order kinetics (see Chapters 16 and 17). This implies that the process depends upon its dose or duration and the original number of microbial contaminants. To achieve a total kill, mathematically an infinite dose or infinite exposure time is required. Clearly, the complete elimination of microbial contaminants and thus sterility cannot be *guaranteed*.

Therefore, caution must be applied when the sterility of a product is considered. Instead of defining sterility in a strict microbiological sense, it is more appropriate to consider the likelihood of a preparation being free of microorganisms. This is best expressed as the probability of a product containing a surviving microorganism after a given sterilization process. Survival depends upon the number and the type of microorganisms, soiling and the environmental conditions within sterilizing equipment. The concept of a sterility assurance level (SAL) or microbial safety index provides a numerical value to the probability of survival of a single microorganism. The SAL is therefore the degree of assurance for a sterilizing process to render a population of products sterile. For pharmaceutical preparations a SAL of $\leq 10^{-6}$ is required. This equates to not more than one viable microorganism per million items/units processed. Practically, the lethality of a sterilization process and in particular the number of log cycles required need to be calculated.

The inactivation factor (IF) which measures the reduction in the number of microorganisms (of a known D value; see Chapters 16 and 17) brought about by a defined sterilization process can be calculated as follows:

$$IF = 10^{t/D} \tag{18.1}$$

where t is the contact time (for heat or gaseous process) or radiation dose and D is the D value appropriate to the process employed. For example, if we consider moist heat sterilization, for an initial bioburden of 10^4 spores of *Geobacillus stearothermophilus*, an IF of 10^{10} will be required to achieve a SAL of 10^{-6}. *G. stearothermophilus* has a D value of 1.5 for moist heat sterilization. Thus according to Eqn 18.1, a 15-minute sterilization process

(i.e. holding time) at 121°C will be required to achieve an IF of 10^{10} (i.e. $10^{15/1.5}$). The process will therefore reduce the level of microorganisms by 10 log cycles.

Calculation of IF is based on obtaining an inactivation kinetic that follows a first-order kinetic. In reality, this is not always the case. In the food industry, the calculation of the most probable effective dose (MPED) is preferred as it is independent of the slope of the survivor curve for the process. However, to establish a MPED that will achieve the required reduction in a number of microorganisms, complex calculations are required.

TEST FOR STERILITY OF THE PRODUCT

Sterility testing assesses whether a sterilized pharmaceutical or medical product is free from microorganisms by incubating all or part of the product with a nutrient medium (Denyer 1998). Due to the destructive nature of the test and the probabilities involved in sampling only a portion of a batch, it is only possible to say that no contaminating microorganisms have been found in the sample examined in the conditions of the test (*British Pharmacopoeia* 2004b). In other words, it is impossible to prove sterility since sampling may fail to select non-sterile containers and culture techniques have limited sensitivity.

Testing for sterility is a destructive process. For an item to be shown not to contain organisms, unfortunately it has to be destroyed. Hence an item that is sterility tested cannot then be sold or used. This is another reason why measurements of sterility rely on statistical probability. To make matters even more complicated, it is quite possible/probable that not all types of microorganism that might be present can be detected. Some microorganisms may not have been identified and/or may undetectable using current culture techniques. As not all microorganisms are affected by a sterilization process in the same way, it is possible that some may not be killed or removed. This is more likely when a non-terminal sterilization method like filtration is used, as many processes use a filter pore size of 0.22 μm, which could potentially allow the small organisms through (e.g. viruses).

Detailed sampling and testing procedures are given in pharmacopoeias and further details can be found in Chapter 15. For terminally sterilized products, biologically based and automatically documented physical proofs that show correct treatment during sterilization are of greater assurance than the sterility test. This method of assuring sterility is termed parametric release and is defined as the release of a sterile product based on process compliance to physical specification. Parametric release is currently acceptable for moist and dry heat and radiation sterilization (Baird 2004).

VALIDATION OF A STERILIZATION PROCESS

The *British Pharmacopoeia* (2004a) states:

> The sterility of a product cannot be guaranteed by testing; it has to be assured by the application of a suitably validated production process. It is essential that the effect of the chosen sterilization procedure on the product (including its final container or package) is investigated to ensure effectiveness and the integrity of the product and that the procedure is validated before being applied in practice.

Clearly this statement points out that testing for sterility is not enough and a suitable production process should be appropriately validated. Any changes in the sterilization procedure (i.e. change in sterilization process, product packaging or load) require revalidation. For pharmaceutical preparations, good manufacturing practices (GMP) have to be observed for the entire manufacturing process, not just the sterilization procedure.

The process of validation requires that the appropriate documentation is obtained to show that a process is consistently complying with predetermined specifications. International organizations such as the International Standards Organization (www.ISO.org) and the Food and Drug Administration in the USA (www.FDA.gov) provide detailed documentation for the validation of sterilization of health-care products or medical devices with various processes (e.g. moist heat, radiation and gaseous). For the validation of sterilization processes, two types of data are required: commissioning data and performance qualification data (Table 18.7). Commissioning data refer mainly to the installation and characteristics of the equipment and the performance data ensure that the equipment will produce the required sterility assurance level. The performance qualification data can be divided into physical and biological performance data (Table 18.7).

Obtaining biological performance data is only required if the sterilization conditions are not well defined (e.g. gaseous sterilization; non-standard methods). The use of biological indicators (discussed below) requires a good knowledge of the inactivation kinetics (e.g. D value) for a given process. Performance qualification data must be reevaluated following a change to the preparation or product and its packaging, the loading pattern or the sterilization cycle.

Process indicators

For all methods of sterilization it is essential that the equipment used works correctly. Routine tests are carried out to demonstrate that all parts of the sterilizer have

---

Table 18.7 Information required for the validation of a sterilization process

Commissioning data
- Evidence that the equipment has been installed in accordance with specifications
- Equipment is safe to use
- Equipment functions within predetermined limits

Performance qualification data
- Evidence that equipment will produce a product with an acceptable assurance of sterility
- Physical performance qualification – evidence that the specified sterilization conditions have been met throughout the sterilization cycle
  - tests performed depends upon the sterilization process
  - data should be generated from the worst spot in sterilizer
  - data generated should also show no detrimental effect on the product and its packaging
- Biological performance qualification – evidence that the specified sterilizing conditions deliver the required microbiological lethality to the preparation/product
  - makes use of biological indicators
  - data not required if the process is well defined (e.g. use of F value)

---

been correctly installed (installation qualification) and that they operate properly, with sterilizing conditions reaching every part of the load (operation qualification; Baird 2004). The test methods used vary according to the sterilization method and may involve the use of physical indicators, chemical indicators and biological indicators.

Physical indicators measure parameters such as heat distribution (i.e. temperature) by thermocouples, pressure variation by gauges or transducers, gas concentration, steam purity, relative humidity by hygrometers or direct calorimetry, delivered dose and time exposure. Sensors must be maintained and calibrated regularly. They are usually the first indicator of a problem with a sterilization process and if documented correctly can be sufficient to meet the requirements for parametric release (Berube et al 2001).

Chemical indicators vary depending on the sterilization method but essentially they all change in physical or chemical nature in response to one or more parameters. There are several types of chemical indicators (Fig. 18.5); temperature-specific indicators just show whether a specific temperature has been reached (single variable indicators) whereas multiparameter/multivariable indicators can measure more than one variable at a time, for example heat and time or gas concentration and time or time, steam and temperature.

Process indicators demonstrate that an indicator has gone through a process but they do not guarantee that sterilization was satisfactory. A common example is autoclave tape (single end-point indicator), which reflects the

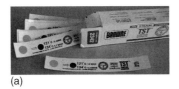

(a)

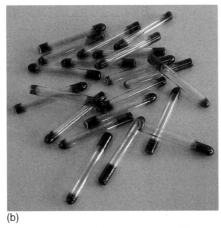

(b)

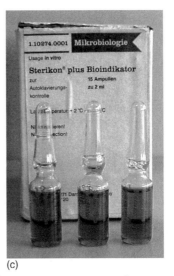

(c)

Fig. 18.5 Examples of chemical and biological indicators. (a) Multiparameter (time, steam and temperature) indicators. (b) Sterilization control tubes. (c) *Bacillus stearothermophilis* biological indicators.

conditions inside the chamber environment but is not able to demonstrate that an item has been sterilized. Another example is Temptubes®, which are glass tubes containing chemical with a specific melting point indicated by a colour change. More specific indicators, such as the 'Bowie Dick tests', are used to monitor air removal from autoclaves. They must be used in the first cycle of the day as an equipment function test (Baird 2004). The standardized test pack is placed in the centre of porous load sterilizers and if the process is correct (i.e. air removal is appropriate), uniform colour change occurs across the test package.

A common example of multivariable indicators is sterilization control tubes (e.g. Browne's tubes), which produce a colour change when the appropriate temperature and exposure time have been achieved. Other chemical indicators are quantitative and indicate a combination of critical variables within a process. This is the case with dosimeters (e.g. Perspex®), which gradually change colour upon exposure to radiation sterilization. It should be noted that the performance of chemical indicators can be altered by storage conditions before and after use and by the method of use.

Biological indicators consist of a carrier or package containing a standardized preparation of defined microorganisms of a known resistance to a specific mode of sterilization (Berube et al 2001; see Fig. 18.5). The carriers used are usually made of filter paper, a glass slide, stainless steel or a plastic tube. Some new versions incorporate ampoules containing a growth medium. The carrier is covered to prevent deterioration or contamination while still allowing entry of the sterilizing agent (*British Pharmacopoeia* 2004b). Different organisms are used for different processes (Table 18.8) but biological indicators usually consist of bacterial spores ($\leq 10^6$). After exposure to the sterilization process, the indicators are removed aseptically and incubated in suitable media to detect the presence of surviving microorganisms. If no growth occurs, the sterilization process is said to have had sufficient lethality (Berube et al 2001).

Testing filtration efficacy

Compared to other sterilization methods, the potential risk of failure is higher for filtration sterilization. This means that it may be advisable to add an extra prefiltration stage using a bacteria-retentive filter. Confidence in the filters used is of prime importance during filtration sterilization. Each batch of filters is tested to ensure that they meet the specifications for release of particulate materials, mechanical strength, chemical characteristics (e.g. oxidizable materials and leaching of materials) and filtration performance. The methods for testing filtration

Table 18.8 Organisms used as biological indicators for sterilization

Sterilization process	Spores used as a biological indicator
Dry heat	*Bacillus subtilis* var. *niger* ATCC 9372, NCIMB 8058 or CIP 77.18
Moist heat	*Geobacillus stearothermophilius* ATCC 7953, NCTC 10007, NCIMB 8157 or CIP 52.81
Ethylene oxide	*Bacillus subtilis* var. *niger* ATCC 9372, NCIMB 8058 ou CIP 77.18
Radiation	*Bacillus pumilius* ATCC 27.142, NCTC 10327, NCIMB 10692 or CIP 77.25

performance involve either a challenge test (which is destructive so cannot be carried out on every filter in a batch) or an integrity test (Denyer & Hodges 2004).

The microbial challenge test is used to demonstrate that a filter is capable of retaining microorganisms. This is normally carried out using a suspension of at least 10^7 cfu (colony-forming units; see Chapter 15) of *Brevundimonas diminuta* (formerly known as *Pseudomonas diminuta*) per cm^2 of active filter surface. *Brevundimonas diminuta* is a small (0.2–0.9 µm) Gram-negative short rod that is a natural choice for this test due to its size and because it was originally isolated from contaminated filtered solutions (Levy 2001). After filtration of a bacterial suspension prepared in tryptone soya broth, the filtrate is collected and incubated at 32°C.

Integrity tests are used to verify the integrity of an assembled sterilizing filter before use and confirmed integrity after use. The tests used must be appropriate to the filter type and the stage of testing and may include bubble point tests, pressure hold tests and diffusion rate tests. The bubble point test is the oldest and one of the most widely used non-destructive tests. It measures the pressure (bubble point pressure) needed to pass gas through the largest pore of a wetted filter. In practice, the pressure required to produce a steady stream of gas bubbles through a wetted filter is often used as the bubble point. The basis of the test relies on the holes through the filter resembling uniform capillaries passing from one side to another. If these capillaries become wet then they will retain liquid via surface tension and the force needed to expel the liquid using a gas is proportional to the diameter of the capillaries (pore diameter). The main limitations of this technique are that it is reliant on operator judgement and on the holes in the filter being perfect uniform capillaries (Denyer & Hodges 2004).

Diffusion rate tests are especially useful for large area filters. They measure the rate of flow of a gas as it diffuses through the water in a wetted filter. The pressure required to cause migration of the gas through the liquid in the pores can be compared to data specified by the filter's manufacturer to establish if the filter has defects (Levy 2001).

LIMITATIONS OF STERILIZATION METHODS

Sterilization processes can involve some extreme conditions such as high temperatures, the use of toxic substances, etc. that can damage the products and/or its packaging. The alteration of a pharmaceutical preparation might lead to a reduced therapeutic efficacy or patient acceptability and damage to the container might lead to the post-sterilization contamination of the product. Therefore, there needs to be a balance between acceptable sterility assurance and acceptable damage to the product and container. Knowledge of the preparations and packaging design and the choice and understanding of the sterilization technologies help in making the appropriate selection to achieve maximum kill while decreasing the risk of product and packaging deterioration.

Nevertheless, each sterilization technology is associated with its own limitations (Table 18.9). Limitations associated with established and recommended procedures are usually linked to the nature of the process (e.g. heat, irradiation), whereas newer technologies tend to suffer from a lack of reproducibility.

SUMMARY

The achievement of sterility is a complex process that requires proper documentation. Sterility in the microbiological sense cannot be guaranteed. Therefore the sterility of a product has to be assured by the application of an appropriate validation process. It is important that the sterilization methodology is compatible with the preparation or product, including its final container or packaging, and combines effectiveness and the absence of detrimental effects. Although not described in detail, the choice of the container/packaging must allow the optimum sterilization to be applied and assure that sterility is maintained post process. Sterilization occurs at the end of manufacturing but it does not replace or permit a relaxation of the principles of good manufacturing practice. In particular, the microbiological quality of ingredients for pharmaceutical preparations and the removal of bioburden must be monitored. Monitoring the critical parameters of the sterilization process will ensure

Table 18.9 Limitations of sterilization processes

Sterilization processes	Limitations
Heat sterilization	
Moist heat	Heat: damage to preparation
	Vapour: damage to the container (wetting of final product, risk of contamination post sterilization)
	Pressure: air ballasting; damage to the container
Dry heat	Heat: damage to preparation
	Potentially longer exposure time needed
Gaseous sterilization	
Ethylene oxide	High toxicity: risk to the operator
	Decontamination required post process
	Explosive: risk to the operator
	Slow process[a]
	Many factors to control
Formaldehyde	High toxicity: risk to the operator
	Damage to some materials (e.g. cellulose-made materials)
	Decontamination required post process
	Slow process[a]
	Many factors to control
Radiation sterilization	
γ-radiation	Risk to the operator
	Water radiolysis: damage to the product
	Discolouration of some glasses and plastics (including PVC), destructive process may continue after sterilization finished
	Liberation of gases (e.g. hydrogen chloride from PVC)
	Hardness and brittleness properties of metals may change
	Butyl and chlorinated rubber are degraded
	Changes in potency can occur
	High costs
Particle radiation	β-radiation: risk to the operator
	Water radiolysis: damage to the product
	Poor penetration of electrons exacerbated by density of product
	Significant product heating may take place at high doses
	High costs
Chemosterilants	
Glutaraldehyde and OPA	Toxicity: risk to the operator
	Activity: reports of microbial resistance[b]
Peracetic acid	Corrosiveness: damage to the product/device
	Activity: reports of microbial resistance[b]
Filtration sterilization	Not efficient for small particles (viruses, prions)
	Require strict aseptic techniques
	Integrity of membrane filter
	Growth of microbial contaminants in depth filter
	Shedding of materials from depth filter

[a] Relative to moist heat sterilization.
[b] Reports of resistance when the concentration falls below the recommended in-use concentration. No report of emerging resistance to OPA to date.

that the predetermined conditions (during validation) are met. The lack of validation or failure to follow a validated process carries the risk of a non-sterile product, deterioration and possible infection.

Where possible, terminal sterilization is the method of choice. Those processes that are fully validated, such as moist and dry heat sterilization and ionizing radiation sterilization, allow the parametric release of the preparation/product and hence their rapid commercialization, since sterility testing and the delay it incurs might not be necessary.

A clear understanding of the methodology, the product to be sterilized (including its packaging), the validation process and the overall documentation required is therefore necessary to carry out a successful sterilization.

REFERENCES

Baird, R.M. (2004) Sterility assurance: concepts, methods and problems. In: Fraise, A.P., Lambert, P.A., Maillard, J-Y. (eds) *Principles and Practice of Disinfection, Preservation and Sterilization*, 4th edn. Blackwell Science, Oxford.

Berube, R., Oxborrow, G.S., Gaustad, J.W. (2001) Sterility testing: validation of sterilization processes and sporicide testing. In: Block, S.S. (ed.) *Disinfection, Sterilization, and Preservation*, 5th edn. Lippincott Williams and Wilkins, Philadelphia.

British Pharmacopoeia (2004a) *Appendix XVII Methods of sterilization (methods of preparation of sterile products)*. Pharmaceutical Press, London.

British Pharmacopoeia (2004b) *Appendix XVI A. Test for sterility*. Pharmaceutical Press, London.

British Society for Gastroenterology Working Party (1998) Cleaning and disinfection of equipment for gastrointestinal endoscopy. *Gut*, **42**, 585-593.

Denyer S.P. (1998) Factory and hospital hygiene and good manufacturing practice. In: Hugo, W.B., Russell, A.D. (eds) *Pharmaceutical Microbiology*, 5th edn. Blackwell Science, Oxford.

Denyer, S.P., Hodges, N.A. (1998) Principles and practice of sterilization. In: Hugo, W.B., Russell, A.D. (eds) *Pharmaceutical Microbiology*, 5th edn. Blackwell Science, Oxford.

Denyer, S.P., Hodges, N.A. (2004) Sterilization: filtration sterilization. In: Fraise, A.P., Lambert, P.A., Maillard, J-Y. (eds) *Principles and Practice of Disinfection, Preservation and Sterilization*, 4th edn. Blackwell Science, Oxford.

European Pharmacopoeia 2004 *Methods of Preparation of Sterile Products. 5.1.1*, 5th Council of Europe, Strasbourg.

Fraise, A.P. (2004) Decontamination of the environment and medical equipment in hospitals. In: Fraise, A.P., Lambert, P.A., Maillard, J-Y. (eds) *Principles and Practice of Disinfection, Preservation and Sterilization*, 4th edn. Blackwell Science, Oxford.

Gould, G.W. (2004) Sterilization: heat sterilization. In: Fraise, A.P., Lambert, P.A., Maillard, J-Y. (eds) *Principles and Practice of Disinfection, Preservation and Sterilization*, 4th edn. Blackwell Science, Oxford.

Hansen, J.M., Shaffer, H.L. (2001) Sterilization and preservation by radiation sterilization. In: Block, S.S. (ed.) *Disinfection, Sterilization, and Preservation*, 5th edn. Lippincott Williams and Wilkins, Philadelphia.

International Standards Organization (ISO) (1996) *Biological evaluation of medical devices - part 7: ethylene oxide sterilization residuals*. ISO 10993-7. ISO, Geneva.

Joslyn, L.J. (2001) Sterilization by heat. In: Block, S.S. (ed.) *Disinfection, Sterilization, and Preservation*, 5th edn. Lippincott Williams and Wilkins, Philadelphia.

Lambert, P. (2004) Sterilization: radiation sterilization. In: Fraise, A.P., Lambert, P.A., Maillard, J-Y. (eds) *Principles and Practice of Disinfection, Preservation and Sterilization*, 4th edn. Blackwell Science, Oxford.

Levy, R.V. (2001) Sterile filtration of liquids and gases. In: Block, S.S. (ed.) *Disinfection, Sterilization, and Preservation*, 5th edn. Lippincott Williams and Wilkins, Philadelphia.

Richards, R.M.E. (2004) Principles and methods of sterilization. In: Winfield, A.J., Richards, R.M.E. (eds) *Pharmaceutical Practice*. Churchill Livingstone, London.

Russell, A.D. (2004) Factors influencing the activity of antimicrobial agents. In: Fraise, A.P., Lambert, P.A., Maillard, J-Y. (eds) *Principles and Practice of Disinfection, Preservation and Sterilization*, 4th edn. Blackwell Science, Oxford.

Sharp, J. (2000) Sterile products: basic concepts and principles. In: *Quality in the Manufacture of Medicines and Other Healthcare Products*. Pharmaceutical Press, London.

United States Pharmacopeia (2005) USP 28, NF 23. United States Pharmacopeial Convention, Maryland.

BIBLIOGRAPHY

Block, S.S. (ed.) (2001) *Disinfection, Sterilization, and Preservation*, 5th edn. Lippincott Williams and Wilkins, Philadelphia.

Fraise, A.P., Lambert, P.A., Maillard, J-Y. (eds) (2004) *Principles and Practice of Disinfection, Preservation and Sterilization*, 4th edn. Blackwell Science, Oxford.

The appropriate pharmacopoeias relevant to your area of work.

PART 4

BIOPHARMACEUTICAL PRINCIPLES OF DRUG DELIVERY

19

Introduction to biopharmaceutics

M. Ashford

WHAT IS BIOPHARMACEUTICS?

Biopharmaceutics can be defined as the study of how the physicochemical properties of drugs, dosage forms and routes of administration affect the rate and extent of drug absorption.

The relationship between the drug, its dosage form and the route by which it is administered governs how much of the drug and how fast it enters the systemic circulation. For a drug to be effective, enough of it needs to reach its site(s) of action and stay there long enough to be able to exert its pharmacological effect. This depends upon the route of administration, the form in which the drug is administered and the rate at which it is delivered.

Background

Apart from the intravenous route, where a drug is introduced directly into the blood stream, all other routes of administration where a systemic action is required involve the absorption of the drug into the blood from the route of administration. Once the drug reaches the blood stream, it partitions between the plasma and the red blood cells, the erythrocytes. Drug in the plasma partitions between the plasma proteins (mainly albumin) and the plasma water. It is this free or unbound drug in plasma water, and not the drug bound to the proteins, that can pass out of the plasma through the capillary endothelium and reach other body fluids and tissues and hence the site(s) of action.

A dynamic equilibrium exists between the concentration of the drug in the blood plasma and the drug at its site(s) of action. This is termed distribution, the degree of which will depend largely on the physicochemical properties of the drug, in particular its lipophilicity. As it is often difficult to access the drug at its site(s) of action, its concentration in the plasma is often taken as a surrogate for its concentration at its site(s) of action. Even though the unbound drug in the plasma would give a better estimate of the concentration of the drug at its site(s) of action, this requires a much more complex and sensitive assay than a measurement of the total concentration of the drug (i.e. the sum of the bound and unbound drug) within the blood plasma. Thus it is this total drug concentration within the plasma that is usually measured for clinical purposes. Therefore, plasma protein binding is a critical parameter to consider when investigating the therapeutic effect of a drug molecule.

The concentration of the drug in blood plasma depends on numerous factors. These include the amount of an administered dose that is *absorbed* and reaches the systemic circulation; the extent of *distribution* of the drug between the systemic circulation and other tissues and fluids (which is usually a rapid and reversible process); and the rate of *elimination* of the drug from the body. The drug can either be eliminated unchanged or be enzymatically cleaved or biochemically transformed, in which case it is said to have been *metabolized*. The study and characterization of the time course of drug **a**bsorption, **d**istribution, **m**etabolism and **e**limination (ADME) is termed *pharmacokinetics*. Pharmacokinetics is used in the clinical setting to enhance the safe and effective therapeutic management of individual patients.

Figure 19.1 illustrates some of the factors that can influence the concentration of the drug in the blood plasma and also at its site(s) of action. Biopharmaceutics is concerned with the first stage – getting the drug from its route of administration to the blood.

CONCEPT OF BIOAVAILABILITY

If a drug is given intravenously it is administered directly into the blood and therefore we can be sure that all the drug reaches the systemic circulation. The drug is therefore said to be 100% *bioavailable*. However, if a drug is given by another route there is no guarantee that the whole dose will reach the systemic circulation intact. The fraction of an administered dose of the drug that reaches the systemic circulation in the unchanged form is known as the *bioavailable dose*. The relative amount of an administered dose of a particular drug that reaches the systemic circulation intact and the rate at which this occurs is known as the *bioavailability*. Bioavailability is therefore defined as the rate and extent of drug absorption. The bioavailability exhibited by a drug is thus very important in determining whether a therapeutically effective concentration will be achieved at the site(s) of action.

In defining bioavailability in these terms, it is assumed that the administered drug is the therapeutically active form. This definition would not be valid in the case of prodrugs, whose therapeutic action normally depends on their being converted into a therapeutically active form prior to or on reaching the systemic circulation. It should also be noted that, in the context of bioavailability, the term 'systemic circulation' refers primarily to venous blood (excluding the hepatic portal vein, which carries

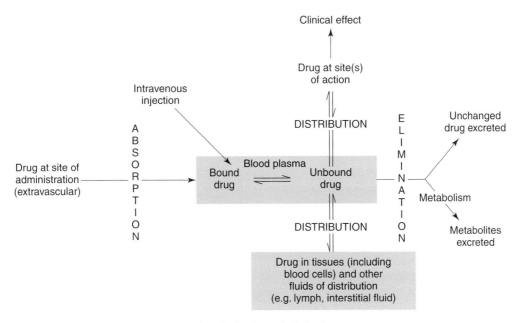

Fig. 19.1 Schematic representation of drug absorption, distribution and elimination.

blood from the gastrointestinal tract to the liver in the absorption phase) and the arterial blood, which carries the intact blood to the tissues.

Therefore, for a drug which is administered orally to be 100% bioavailable, the entire dose must move from the dosage form to the systemic circulation. The drug must therefore:

- be completely released from the dosage form
- be fully dissolved in the gastrointestinal fluids
- be stable in solution in the gastrointestinal fluids
- pass through the gastrointestinal barrier into the mesenteric circulation without being metabolized
- pass through the liver into the systemic circulation unchanged.

Anything which adversely affects either the release of the drug from the dosage form, its dissolution into the gastrointestinal fluids, its permeation through and stability in the gastrointestinal barrier or its stability in the hepatic portal circulation will influence the bioavailability exhibited by that drug from the dosage form in which it was administered.

CONCEPT OF BIOPHARMACEUTICS

Many factors have been found to influence the rate and extent of absorption, and hence the time course of a drug in the plasma and therefore at its site(s) of action. These include the foods eaten by the patient, the effect of the disease state on drug absorption, the age of the patient, the site(s) of absorption of the administered drug, the coadministration of other drugs, the physical and chemical properties of the administered drug, the type of dosage form, the composition and method of manufacture of the dosage form, the size of the dose and the frequency of administration.

Thus, a given drug may exhibit differences in its bioavailability if it is administered:

- in the same type of dosage form by different routes of administration, e.g. an aqueous solution of a given drug administered by the oral and intramuscular routes
- by the same routes of administration but different types of dosage form, e.g. a tablet, a hard gelatin capsule and an aqueous suspension administered by the peroral route
- in the same type of dosage form by the same route of administration but with different formulations of the dosage form, e.g. different formulations of an oral aqueous suspension.

Variability in the bioavailability exhibited by a given drug from different formulations of the same type of dosage form, or from different types of dosage forms, or by different routes of administration, can cause the plasma concentration of the drug to be too high, and therefore cause side-effects, or too low, and therefore the drug will be ineffective. Figure 19.2 shows the plasma concentration–time curve following a single oral dose of a drug, indicating the parameters associated with a therapeutic effect.

Poor biopharmaceutical properties often result in:

- poor and variable bioavailability
- difficulties in toxicological evaluation
- difficulties with bioequivalence of formulations
- multi-daily dosing
- the requirement for a non-conventional delivery system
- long and costly development times.

SUMMARY

The following chapters (Chapters 20 and 21) deal in more detail with the physiological factors, dosage form factors and intrinsic properties of drugs that influence the rate and extent of absorption. Chapter 22 looks at means of assessing the biopharmaceutical properties of compounds.

A thorough understanding of the biopharmaceutical properties of a candidate drug are important both in the

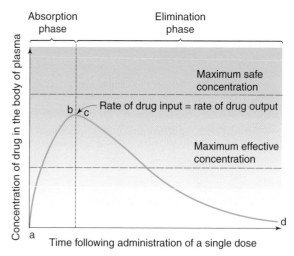

a–b rate of drug absorption > rate of drug elimination
c–d rate of drug elimination > rate of drug absorption

Fig. 19.2 A typical blood plasma concentration–time curve obtained following the peroral administration of a single dose of a drug in a tablet.

discovery setting, where potential drug candidates are being considered, and in the development setting, where it is important to anticipate formulation problems and assess whether the drug is a candidate for a controlled-release formulation.

BIBLIOGRAPHY

Dressman J.B., Lennernäs, H. (2000) *Oral Drug Absorption: Prediction and Assessment*. Marcel Dekker, New York.

Gibaldi, M. (1991) *Biopharmaceutics and Clinical Pharmacokinetics*, 4th edn. Lea and Febiger, Philadelphia.

Johnson, L.R. (1994) *Physiology of the Gastro-intestinal Tract*, vol 2, 3rd edn. Raven Press, New York.

Macheras, P., Reppas, C., Dressman, J.B. (1995) *Biopharmaceutics of Orally Administered Drugs*. Ellis Horwood, London.

Washington, N., Wilson, C. (2000) *Physiological Pharmaceutics*, 2nd edn. Taylor and Francis, London.

Waterbeemd, H. (2003) *Drug Bioavailability: Estimation of Solubility, Permeability, Absorption and Bioavailability*. Wiley-VCH, Weinheim.

20

Gastrointestinal tract – physiology and drug absorption

M. Ashford

INTRODUCTION

The factors that influence the rate and extent of absorption depend upon the route of administration. As stated in Chapter 19, the intravenous route offers direct access to the systemic circulation and the total dose administered via this route is available in the plasma for distribution into other body tissues and the site(s) of action of the drug. Other routes will require an absorption step before the drug reaches the systemic circulation. Factors affecting this absorption will depend on the physiology of the administration site(s) and the membrane barriers present at those site(s) that the drug needs to cross in order to reach the systemic circulation. A summary of some of the properties of each route of administration is given in Chapter 1.

The gastrointestinal tract is discussed in detail in this chapter and a detailed description of the physiology of some of the other more important routes of administration is given in the relevant chapters of Part 5. The oral route of delivery is by far the most popular, mainly because it is natural and convenient for the patient and because it is relatively easy to manufacture oral dosage forms. Oral dosage forms do not need to be sterilized, are compact, and can be produced in large quantities by automated machines. This chapter and the next will therefore be confined to discussing the biopharmaceutical factors (that is, physiological, dosage form and drug factors) that influence oral drug absorption.

PHYSIOLOGICAL FACTORS INFLUENCING ORAL DRUG ABSORPTION

The gastrointestinal tract is complex, as shown in Figure 20.1, which outlines some of the key structures involved in and key physiological parameters that affect oral drug absorption. In order to gain an insight into the numerous factors that can potentially influence the rate and extent of drug absorption into the systemic circulation, a schematic

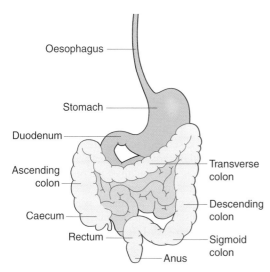

Fig. 20.1 The gastrointestinal tract.

illustration of the steps involved in the release and absorption of a drug from a tablet dosage form is presented in Figure 20.2. It can be seen from this that the rate and extent of appearance of intact drug in the systemic circulation depend on a succession of kinetic processes.

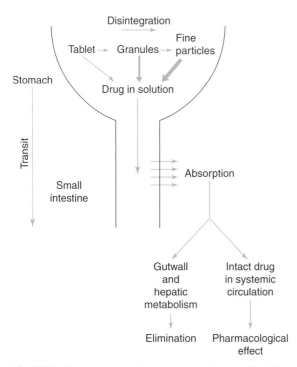

Fig. 20.2 Steps involved prior to a pharmacological effect after administration of a rapidly disintegrating tablet.

The slowest step in this series, which is known as the *rate-limiting step*, controls the overall rate and extent of appearance of intact drug in the systemic circulation. The particular rate-limiting step will vary from drug to drug. For a drug which has a very poor aqueous solubility, the rate at which it dissolves in the gastrointestinal fluids is often the slowest step and the bioavailability of that drug is said to be *dissolution rate limited*. In contrast, for a drug that has a high aqueous solubility, its dissolution will be rapid and the rate at which the drug crosses the gastrointestinal membrane may be the rate-limiting step (*permeability limited*). Other potential rate-limiting steps include the rate of drug release from the dosage form (this can be by design in the case of controlled-release dosage forms), the rate at which the stomach empties the drug into the small intestine, the rate at which the drug is metabolized by enzymes in the intestinal mucosal cells during its passage through them into the mesenteric blood vessels, and the rate of metabolism of drug during its initial passage through the liver, often termed the *'first-pass' effect*.

PHYSIOLOGY OF THE GASTROINTESTINAL TRACT

The gastrointestinal tract is a muscular tube approximately 6 m in length with varying diameters. It stretches from the mouth to the anus and consists of four main anatomical areas: the oesophagus, the stomach, the small intestine and the large intestine or colon. The luminal surface of the tube is not smooth but very rough, thereby increasing the surface area for absorption.

The wall of the gastrointestinal tract is essentially similar in structure along its length, consisting of four principal histological layers (Fig. 20.3):

1. The serosa, which is an outer layer of epithelium and supporting connective tissue
2. The muscularis externa, which contains two layers of smooth muscle tissue, a thinner outer layer, which is longitudinal in orientation, and a thicker inner layer, whose fibres are oriented in a circular pattern. Contractions of these muscles provide the forces for movement of gastrointestinal contents
3. The submucosa, which is a connective tissue layer containing some secretory tissue and which is richly supplied with blood and lymphatic vessels. A network of nerve cells, known as the submucous plexus, is also located in this layer
4. The mucosa, which is essentially composed of three layers: the muscularis mucosa, which can alter the local conformation of the mucosa, a layer of connective tissue known as the lamina propria and the epithelium.

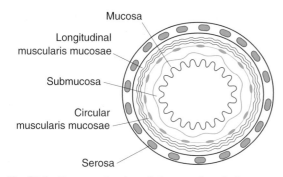

Fig. 20.3 Cross-section through the gastrointestinal tract.

The majority of the gastrointestinal epithelium is covered by a layer of mucus. This is a viscoelastic translucent aqueous gel that is secreted throughout the gastrointestinal tract, acting as a protective layer and a mechanical barrier. Mucus is a constantly changing mix of many secretions and exfoliated epithelial cells. It has a large water component (~95%). Its other primary components, which are responsible for its physical and functional properties, are large glycoproteins called mucins. Mucins consist of a protein backbone approximately 800 amino acids long and oligosaccharide side chains that are typically up to 18 residues in length.

The mucus layer ranges in thickness from 5 μm to 500 μm along the length of the gastrointestinal tract, with average values of around 80 μm. The layer is thought to be continuous in the stomach and duodenum but may not be so in the rest of the small and large intestines.

Mucus is constantly being removed from the luminal surface of the gastrointestinal tract through abrasion and acidic and enzymatic breakdown, and is continually replaced from beneath. Turnover time has been estimated at 4–5 hours but this may well be an underestimate and is liable to vary along the length of the tract.

Oesophagus

The mouth is the point of entry for most drugs (so-called peroral – via the mouth – administration). At this point contact with the oral mucosa is usually brief. Linking the oral cavity with the stomach is the oesophagus. This is composed of a thick muscular layer approximately 250 mm long and 20 mm in diameter. It joins the stomach at the gastrooesophageal junction, or cardiac orifice as it is sometimes known.

The oesophagus, apart from the lowest 20 mm which is similar to the gastric mucosa, contains a well-differentiated squamous epithelium of non-proliferative cells. Epithelial cell function is mainly protective: simple mucous glands secrete mucus into the narrow lumen to lubricate food and protect the lower part of the oesophagus from gastric acid. The pH of the oesophageal lumen is usually between 5 and 6.

Materials are moved down the oesophagus by the act of swallowing. After swallowing, a single peristaltic wave of contraction, its amplitude linked to the size of the material being swallowed, passes down the length of the oesophagus at the rate of 20–60 mm per second, speeding up as it progresses. When swallowing is repeated in quick succession, the subsequent swallows interrupt the initial peristaltic wave and only the final wave proceeds down the length of the oesophagus to the gastrointestinal junction, carrying material within the lumen with it. Secondary peristaltic waves occur involuntarily in response to any distension of the oesophagus and serve to move sticky lumps of material or refluxed material to the stomach. In the upright position, the transit of materials through the oesophagus is assisted by gravity. The oesophageal transit of dosage forms is extremely rapid, usually of the order of 10–14 seconds.

Stomach

The next part of the gastrointestinal tract to be encountered by both food and pharmaceuticals is the stomach. The two major functions of the stomach are:

- to act as a temporary reservoir for ingested food and to deliver it to the duodenum at a controlled rate
- to reduce ingested solids to a uniform creamy consistency, known as chyme, by the action of acid and enzymatic digestion. This enables better contact of the ingested material with the mucous membrane of the intestines and thereby facilitates absorption.

Another, perhaps less obvious, function of the stomach is its role in reducing the risk of noxious agents reaching the intestine.

The stomach is the most dilated part of the gastrointestinal tract and is situated between the lower end of the oesophagus and the small intestine. Its opening to the duodenum is controlled by the pyloric sphincter. The stomach can be divided into four anatomical regions (Fig. 20.4), namely the fundus, the body, the antrum and the pylorus.

The stomach has a capacity of approximately 1.5 L, although under fasting conditions it usually contains no more than 50 mL of fluid, which is mostly gastric secretions. These include:

- acid secreted by the parietal cells, which maintains the pH of the stomach between 1 and 3.5 in the fasted state

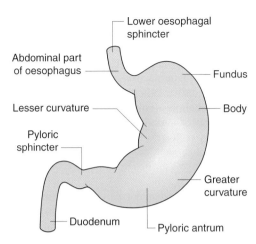

Fig. 20.4 The anatomy of the stomach.

- the hormone gastrin, which itself is a potent stimulator of gastric acid production. The release of gastrin is stimulated by peptides, amino acids and distension of the stomach
- pepsins, which are secreted by the peptic cells in the form of its precursor pepsinogen. Pepsins are peptidases which break down proteins to peptides at low pH. Above pH 5, pepsin is denatured
- mucus, which is secreted by the surface mucosal cells and lines the gastric mucosa. In the stomach, the mucus protects the gastric mucosa from autodigestion by the pepsin–acid combination.

Contrary to popular belief, very little drug absorption occurs in the stomach owing to its small surface area compared to the small intestine. The rate of gastric emptying can be a controlling factor in the onset of drug absorption from the major absorptive site, the small intestine. Gastric emptying will be discussed under gastrointestinal transit later in this chapter.

Small intestine

The small intestine is the longest (4–5 m) and most convoluted part of the gastrointestinal tract, extending from the pyloric sphincter of the stomach to the ileocaecal junction where it joins the large intestine. Its main functions are:

- *digestion* – the process of enzymatic digestion, which began in the stomach, is completed in the small intestine
- *absorption* – the small intestine is the region where most nutrients and other materials are absorbed.

The small intestine is divided into the duodenum, which is 200–300 mm in length, the jejunum, which is approximately 2 m in length, and the ileum, which is approximately 3 m in length.

The wall of the small intestine has a rich network of both blood and lymphatic vessels. The gastrointestinal circulation is the largest systemic regional vasculature and nearly a third of the cardiac output flows through the gastrointestinal viscera. The blood vessels of the small intestine receive blood from the superior mesenteric artery via branched arterioles. The blood leaving the small intestine flows into the hepatic portal vein that carries it via the liver to the systemic circulation. Drugs that are metabolized by the liver are degraded before they reach the systemic circulation, this is termed hepatic presystemic clearance or first-pass metabolism.

The wall of the small intestine also contains lacteals, which contain lymph and are part of the lymphatic system. The lymphatic system is important in the absorption of fats from the gastrointestinal tract. In the ileum are areas of lymphoid tissue close to the epithelial surface which are known as Peyer's patches. These cells play a key role in the immune response as they transport macromolecules and are involved in antigen uptake.

The surface area of the small intestine is increased enormously, by about 600 times that of a simple cylinder, to approximately 200 m² in an adult, by several adaptations which make the small intestine such a good absorption site.

- *Folds of Kerckring* – these are submucosal folds which extend circularly most of the way around the intestine and are particularly well developed in the duodenum and jejunum. They are several millimetres in depth.
- *Villi* – these have been described as finger-like projections into the lumen (approximately 0.5–1.5 mm in length and 0.1 mm in diameter). They are well supplied with blood vessels. Each villus contains an arteriole, a venule and a blind-ending lymphatic vessel (lacteal). The structure of a villus is shown in Figure 20.5.
- *Microvilli* – approximately 600–1000 of these brush-like structures (~1 μm in length and 0.1 μm in width) cover each villus, providing the largest increase in surface area. These are covered by a fibrous substance known as glycocalyx.

The luminal pH of the small intestine increases to between about 6 and 7.5. The sources of the secretions that produce these pH values in the small intestine are as follows:

- *Brunner's glands* – these are located in the duodenum and are responsible for the secretion of

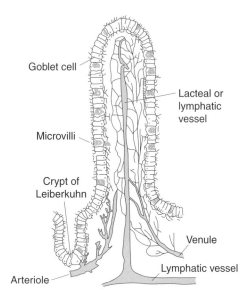

Fig. 20.5 Structure of a villus.

bicarbonate, which neutralizes the acid emptied from the stomach.

- *Intestinal cells* – these are present throughout the small intestine and secrete mucus and enzymes. The enzymes, hydrolases and proteases, continue the digestive process.
- *Pancreatic secretions* – the pancreas is a large gland that secretes about 1–2 L of pancreatic juice per day into the small intestine via a duct. The components of pancreatic juice are sodium bicarbonate and enzymes. The enzymes consist of proteases, principally trypsin, chymotrypsin and carboxypeptidases, which are secreted as inactive precursors or zymogens and converted to their active forms in the lumen by the enzyme enterokinase. Lipase and amylase are both secreted in their active forms. The bicarbonate component is largely regulated by the pH of chyme delivered into the small intestine from the stomach.
- *Bile* – bile is secreted by hepatocytes in the liver into bile canaliculi, concentrated in the gallbladder and hepatic biliary system by the removal of sodium ions, chloride and water, and delivered to the duodenum. Bile is a complex aqueous mixture of organic solutes (bile acids, phospholipids, particularly lecithin, cholesterol and bilirubin) and inorganic compounds (plasma electrolytes: sodium and potassium). Bile pigments, the most important of which is bilirubin, are excreted in the faeces but the bile acids are absorbed by an active process in the

terminal ileum. They are returned to the liver via the hepatic portal vein and, as they have a high hepatic clearance, are resecreted in the bile. This process is known as enterohepatic recirculation. The main functions of the bile are promoting the efficient absorption of dietary fat, such as fatty acids and cholesterol, by aiding its emulsification and micellar solubilization, and the provision of excretory pathways for degradation products.

Colon

The colon is the final major part of the gastrointestinal tract. It stretches from the ileocaecal junction to the anus and makes up approximately the last 1.5 m of the 6 m of the gastrointestinal tract. It is composed of the caecum (~85 mm in length), the ascending colon (~200 mm), the hepatic flexure, the transverse colon (usually greater than 450 mm), the splenic flexure, the descending colon (~300 mm), the sigmoid colon (~400 mm) and the rectum, as shown in Figure 20.6. The ascending and descending colons are relatively fixed, as they are attached via the flexures and the caecum. The transverse and sigmoid colons, however, are much more flexible.

The colon, unlike the small intestine, has no specialized villi. However, the microvilli of the absorptive epithelial cells, the presence of crypts and the irregularly folded mucosae serve to increase the surface area of the colon by 10–15 times that of a simple cylinder. The surface area nevertheless remains approximately 1/30th that of the small intestine.

The main functions of the colon are:

- the absorption of sodium ions, chloride ions and water from the lumen in exchange for bicarbonate

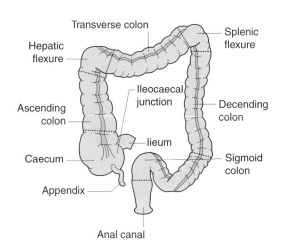

Fig. 20.6 The anatomy of the colon.

and potassium ions. Thus the colon has a significant homeostatic role in the body
* the storage and compaction of faeces.

The colon is permanently colonized by an extensive number (about 10^{12} per gram of contents) and variety of bacteria. This large bacterial mass is capable of several metabolic reactions, including hydrolysis of fatty acid esters and the reduction of inactive conjugated drugs to their active form. The bacteria rely upon undigested polysaccharides in the diet and the carbohydrate components of secretions such as mucus for their carbon and energy sources. They degrade the polysaccharides to produce short-chain fatty acids (acetic, proprionic and butyric acids), which lower the luminal pH, and the gases hydrogen, carbon dioxide and methane. Thus the pH of the caecum is around 6–6.5. This increases to around 7–7.5 towards the distal parts of the colon.

Recently there has been much interest in the exploitation of the enzymes produced by these bacteria with respect to targeted drug delivery to this region of the gastrointestinal tract.

TRANSIT OF PHARMACEUTICALS IN THE GASTROINTESTINAL TRACT

As the oral route is the one by which the majority of pharmaceuticals are administered, it is important to know how these materials behave during their passage through the gastrointestinal tract. It is known that the small intestine is the major site of drug absorption, and thus the time a drug is present in this part of the gastrointestinal tract is extremely significant. If sustained- or controlled-release drug delivery systems are being designed, it is important to consider factors that will affect their behaviour and, in particular, their transit times through certain regions of the gastrointestinal tract.

In general, most dosage forms, when taken in an upright position, transit through the oesophagus quickly, usually in less than 15 seconds. Transit through the oesophagus is dependent upon both the dosage form and posture.

Tablets/capsules taken in the supine position, especially if taken without water, are liable to lodge in the oesophagus. Adhesion to the oesophageal wall can occur as a result of partial dehydration at the site of contact and the formation of a gel between the formulation and the oesophagus. The chances of adhesion will depend on the shape, size and type of formulation. Transit of liquids, for example, has always been observed to be rapid, and in general faster than that of solids. A delay in reaching the stomach may well delay a drug's onset of action or cause

damage or irritation to the oesophageal wall, e.g. potassium chloride tablets.

Gastric emptying

The time a dosage form takes to traverse the stomach is usually termed the *gastric residence time, gastric emptying time* or *gastric emptying rate*.

Gastric emptying of pharmaceuticals is highly variable and is dependent on the dosage form and the fed/fasted state of the stomach. Normal gastric residence times usually range between 5 minutes and 2 hours, although much longer times (over 12 hours) have been recorded, particularly for large single units.

In the fasted state the electrical activity in the stomach – the interdigestive myoelectric cycle or migrating myoelectric complex (MMC), as it is known – governs its activity and hence the transit of dosage forms. It is characterized by a repeating cycle of four phases. Phase I is a relatively inactive period of 40–60 minutes with only rare contractions occurring. Increasing numbers of contractions occur in phase II, which has a similar duration to phase I. Phase III is characterized by powerful peristaltic contractions which open the pylorus at the base and clear the stomach of any residual material. This is sometimes called the *housekeeper wave*. Phase IV is a short transitional period between the powerful activity of phase III and the inactivity of phase I.

The cycle repeats itself every 2 hours until a meal is ingested and the fed state or motility is initiated. In this state, two distinct patterns of activity have been observed. The proximal stomach relaxes to receive food and gradual contractions of this region move the contents distally. Peristalsis – contractions of the distal stomach – serve to mix and break down food particles and move them towards the pyloric sphincter. The pyloric sphincter allows liquids and small food particles to empty while other material is retropulsed into the antrum of the stomach and caught up by the next peristaltic wave for further size reduction before emptying.

Thus in the fed state, liquids, pellets and disintegrated tablets will tend to empty with food yet large sustained- or controlled-release dosage forms can be retained in the stomach for long periods of time. In the fasted state, the stomach is less discriminatory between dosage form types, with emptying appearing to be an exponential process and being related to the point in the MMC at which the formulation is ingested.

Many factors influence gastric emptying, as well as the type of dosage form and the presence of food. These include postural position, the composition of the food and the effect of drugs and disease state. In general, food, particularly fatty foods, delays gastric emptying and hence the absorption of drugs. Therefore, a drug will reach the small intestine most rapidly if it is administered with water to a patient whose stomach is empty.

Small intestinal transit

There are two main types of intestinal movement – propulsive and mixing. The propulsive movements primarily determine the intestinal transit rate and hence the residence time of the drug or dosage form in the small intestine. As this is the main site of absorption in the gastrointestinal tract for most drugs, the small intestinal transit time (that is, the time of transit between the stomach and the caecum) is an important factor with respect to drug bioavailability.

Small intestinal transit has been found to be relatively constant, at around 3 hours. In contrast to the stomach, the small intestine does not discriminate between solids and liquids, and hence between dosage forms, or between the fed and the fasted state.

Small intestinal residence time is particularly important for:

- dosage forms that release their drug slowly (e.g. controlled-, sustained- or prolonged-release systems) as they pass along the length of the gastrointestinal tract
- enteric-coated dosage forms which release drug only when they reach the small intestine
- drugs that dissolve slowly in intestinal fluids
- drugs that are absorbed by intestinal carrier-mediated transport systems.

Colonic transit

The colonic transit of pharmaceuticals is long and variable and depends on the type of dosage form, diet, eating pattern and disease state.

Contractile activity in the colon can be divided into two main types:

- propulsive contractions or mass movements that are associated with the aboral (away from the mouth) movement of contents
- segmental or haustral contractions that serve to mix the luminal contents and result in only small aboral movements. Segmental contractions are brought about by contraction of the circular muscle and predominate, whereas the propulsive contractions, which are due to contractions of the longitudinal muscle, occur only 3–4 times daily in normal individuals.

Colonic transit is thus characterized by short bursts of activity followed by long periods of stasis. Movement is mainly aboral, i.e. towards the anus. Colonic transit can vary from anything between 2 and 48 hours. In most individuals mouth-to-anus transit times are longer than 24 hours.

BARRIERS TO DRUG ABSORPTION

Figure 20.7 shows some of the barriers to absorption that a drug may encounter once it is released from its dosage

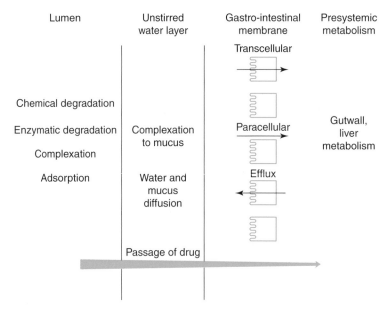

Fig. 20.7 Barriers to absorption.

form and has dissolved into the gastrointestinal fluids. The drug needs to remain in solution and not become bound to food or other material within the gastrointestinal tract. It needs to be chemically stable in order to withstand the pH of the gastrointestinal tract and it must be resistant to enzymatic degradation in the lumen. The drug then needs to diffuse across the mucous layer without binding to it, across the unstirred water layer and subsequently across the gastrointestinal membrane, its main cellular barrier. After passing through this cellular barrier, the drug encounters the liver and all its metabolizing enzymes before it reaches the systemic circulation. Any of these barriers can prevent some or all of the drug reaching the systemic circulation and can therefore have a detrimental effect on its bioavailability.

Environment within the lumen

The environment within the lumen of the gastrointestinal tract has a major effect on the rate and extent of drug absorption.

Gastrointestinal pH

The pH of fluids varies considerably along the length of the gastrointestinal tract. Gastric fluid is highly acidic, normally exhibiting a pH within the range 1–3.5 in healthy people in the fasted state. Following the ingestion of a meal, the gastric juice is buffered to a less acidic pH that is dependent on meal composition. Typical gastric pH values following a meal are in the range 3–7. Depending on the size of the meal, the gastric pH returns to the lower fasted-state values within 2–3 hours. Thus only a dosage form ingested with or soon after a meal will encounter these higher pH values. This may be an important consideration in terms of the chemical stability of a drug or in achieving drug dissolution or absorption.

Intestinal pH values are higher than gastric pH values owing to the neutralization of the gastric acid with bicarbonate ions secreted by the pancreas into the small intestine. There is a gradual rise in pH along the length of the small intestine from the duodenum to the ileum. Table 20.1 summarizes some of the literature values recorded for small intestinal pH in the fed and fasted states. The pH drops again in the colon as the bacterial enzymes, which are localized in the colonic region, break down undigested carbohydrates into short-chain fatty acids; this lowers the pH in the colon to around 6.5.

The gastrointestinal pH may influence the absorption of drugs in a variety of ways. If the drug is a weak electrolyte, pH may influence the drug's chemical stability in the lumen, its rate and extent of dissolution or its absorption characteristics. Chemical degradation due to pH-dependent hydrolysis can occur in the gastrointesti-

Table 20.1 pH in the small intestine in healthy humans in the fasted and fed states

Location	Fasted state pH	Fed state pH
Mid-distal duodenum	4.9	5.2
	6.1	5.4
	6.3	5.1
	6.4	
Jejunum	4.4–6.5	5.2–6.0
	6.6	6.2
Ileum	6.5	6.8–7.8
	6.8–8.0	6.8–8.0
	7.4	7.5

Data from Gray & Dressman 1996

nal tract. The result of this instability is incomplete bioavailability, as only a fraction of the administered dose reaches the systemic circulation in the form of intact drug. The extent of degradation of penicillin G (benzylpenicillin), the first of the penicillins, after oral administration depends on its residence time in the stomach and the gastric pH. This gastric instability has tended to preclude its oral use. The antibiotic erythromycin and proton pump inhibitors (e.g. omeprazole) degrade rapidly at acidic pH values and therefore have to be formulated as enteric-coated dosage forms to ensure good bioavailability (Chapter 21). The effects of pH on the drug dissolution and absorption processes are also discussed in Chapter 21.

Luminal enzymes

The primary enzyme found in gastric juice is pepsin. Lipases, amylases and proteases are secreted from the pancreas into the small intestine in response to ingestion of food. These enzymes are responsible for most nutrient digestion. Pepsins and the proteases are responsible for the degradation of protein and peptide drugs in the lumen. Other drugs that resemble nutrients, such as nucleotides and fatty acids, may also be susceptible to enzymatic degradation. The lipases may also affect the release of drugs from fat/oil-containing dosage forms. Drugs that are esters can also be susceptible to hydrolysis in the lumen.

Bacteria, which are mainly localized within the colonic region of the gastrointestinal tract, also secrete enzymes that are capable of a range of reactions. These enzymes have been utilized when designing drugs or dosage forms to target the colon. Sulfasalazine, for example, is a prodrug of 5-aminosalicylic acid linked via an azo bond to sul-fapyridine. The sulfapyridine moiety makes the drug too large and hydrophilic to be absorbed in the upper gastrointestinal tract, and thus permits its transport intact to the colonic region. Here the bacterial enzymes reduce the azo bond and release the active drug, 5-aminosalycilic acid, for local action in colonic diseases such as inflammatory bowel disease.

Influence of food in the gastrointestinal tract

The presence of food in the gastrointestinal tract can influence the rate and extent of absorption, either directly or indirectly via a range of mechanisms.

Complexation of drugs with components in the diet Drugs are capable of binding to components within the diet. In general this only becomes an issue (with respect to bioavailability) where an irreversible or an insoluble complex is formed. In such cases the fraction of the administered dose that becomes complexed is unavailable for absorption. Tetracycline, for example, forms non-absorbable complexes with calcium and iron, and thus patients are advised not to take products containing calcium or iron, such as milk, iron preparations or indigestion remedies, at the same time of day as the tetracycline. However, if the complex formed is water soluble and readily dissociates to liberate the 'free' drug then there may be little effect on drug absorption.

Alteration of pH In general, food tends to increase stomach pH by acting as a buffer. This is liable to decrease the rate of dissolution and subsequent absorption of a weakly basic drug and increase that of a weakly acidic one.

Alteration of gastric emptying As already mentioned, some foods, particularly those containing a high proportion of fat, and some drugs tend to reduce gastric emptying and thus delay the onset of action of certain drugs.

Stimulation of gastrointestinal secretions Gastrointestinal secretions (e.g. pepsin) produced in response to food may result in the degradation of drugs that are susceptible to enzymatic metabolism and hence in a reduction in their bioavailability. The ingestion of food, particularly fats, stimulates the secretion of bile. Bile salts are surface-active agents and can increase the dissolution of poorly soluble drugs, thereby enhancing their absorption. However, bile salts have been shown to form insoluble and hence non-absorbable complexes with some drugs such as neomycin, kanamycin and nystatin.

Competition between food components and drugs for specialized absorption mechanisms In the case of those drugs that have a chemical structure similar to nutrients required by the body for which specialized absorption mechanisms exist, there is a possibility of competitive inhibition of drug absorption.

Increased viscosity of gastrointestinal contents The presence of food in the gastrointestinal tract provides a viscous environment which may result in a reduction in the rate of drug dissolution. In addition, the rate of diffusion of a drug in solution from the lumen to the absorbing membrane lining the gastrointestinal tract may be reduced by an increase in viscosity. Both of these effects tend to decrease the bioavailability of drug.

Food-induced changes in presystemic metabolism Certain foods may increase the bioavailability of drugs that are susceptible to presystemic intestinal metabolism by interacting with the metabolic process. Grapefruit juice, for example, is capable of inhibiting the intestinal cytochrome P450 (CYP3A family) and thus, when taken with drugs that are susceptible to CYP3A metabolism, is likely to result in their increased bioavailability. Clinically relevant interactions exist between grapefruit juice and the antihistamine terfenadine, the immunosuppresant ciclosporin, the protease inhibitor saquinavir and the calcium channel blocker verapamil.

Food-induced changes in blood flow Blood flow to the gastrointestinal tract and liver increases shortly after a meal, thereby increasing the rate at which drugs are presented to the liver. The metabolism of some drugs (e.g. propranolol, hydralazine, dextropropoxyphene) is sensitive to their rate of presentation to the liver; the faster the rate of presentation, the larger the fraction of drug that escapes first-pass metabolism. This is because the enzyme systems responsible for their metabolism become saturated by the increased rate of presentation of the drug to the site of biotransformation. For this reason, the effects of food serve to increase the bioavailability of some drugs that are susceptible to first-pass metabolism.

It is evident that food can influence the absorption of many drugs from the gastrointestinal tract by a variety of mechanisms. Drug–food interactions are often classified into five categories: those that cause reduced, delayed, increased and accelerated absorption, and those on which food has no effect. The reader is referred to reviews by Fleischer et al (1999), Welling (1996), Evans (2000) and Schmidt & Dalhoff (2002) for more detailed information on the effect of food on the rate and extent of drug absorption.

Disease state and physiological disorders

Disease states and physiological disorders associated with the gastrointestinal tract are likely to influence the absorption and hence the bioavailability of orally administered drugs. Local diseases can cause alterations in gastric pH that can affect the stability, dissolution and/or absorption of the drug. Gastric surgery can cause drugs to exhibit differences in bioavailability from that in normal individuals. For example, partial or total gastrectomy results in drugs reaching the duodenum more rapidly than in normal individuals. This increased rate of presentation to the small intestine may result in an increased overall rate of absorption of drugs that are primarily absorbed in the small intestine. However, drugs that require a period of time in the stomach to facilitate their dissolution may show reduced bioavailability in such patients.

Unstirred water layer

The unstirred water layer or aqueous boundary layer is a more or less stagnant layer of water, mucus and glycocalyx adjacent to the intestinal wall. It is thought to be created by incomplete mixing of the luminal contents near the intestinal mucosal surface. This layer, which is around 30–100 μm in thickness, can provide a diffusion barrier to drugs. Some drugs are also capable of complexing with mucus, thereby reducing their availability for absorption.

Gastrointestinal membrane

Structure of the membrane

The gastrointestinal membrane separates the lumen of the stomach and intestines from the systemic circulation. It is the main cellular barrier to the absorption of drugs from the gastrointestinal tract. The membrane is complex in nature, being composed of lipids, proteins, lipoproteins and polysaccharides. It has a bilayer structure, as shown in Figure 20.8. The barrier has the characteristics of a semi-permeable membrane, allowing the rapid transit of some materials and impeding or preventing the passage of others. It is permeable to amino acids, sugars, fatty acids and other nutrients and is impermeable to

plasma proteins. The membrane can be viewed as a semi-permeable lipoidal sieve, which allows the passage of lipid-soluble molecules across it and the passage of water and small hydrophilic molecules through its numerous aqueous pores. In addition, there are a number of transporter proteins or carrier molecules that exist in the membrane and which, with the help of energy, transport materials back and forth across it.

Mechanisms of transport across the membrane

There are two main mechanisms of drug transport across the gastrointestinal epithelium: transcellular (i.e. across the cells) and paracellular (i.e. between the cells). The transcellular pathway is further divided into simple passive diffusion, carrier-mediated transport (active transport and facilitated diffusion) and endocytosis. These pathways are illustrated in Figure 20.9.

Transcellular pathways

Passive diffusion   This is the preferred route of transport for relatively small lipophilic molecules and thus many drugs. In this process, drug molecules pass across the lipoidal membrane via passive diffusion from a region of high concentration in the lumen to a region of lower concentration in the blood. This lower concentration is maintained primarily by blood flow. The rate of transport is determined by the physicochemical properties of the drug, the nature of the membrane and the concentration gradient of the drug across the membrane. The process initially involves the partitioning of the drug between the aqueous fluids within the gastrointestinal tract and the lipoidal-like membrane of the lining of the epithelium. The drug in solution in the membrane then diffuses across the epithelial cell/cells within the gastrointestinal barrier to blood in the capillary network in the lamina propria. Upon reaching the blood, the drug

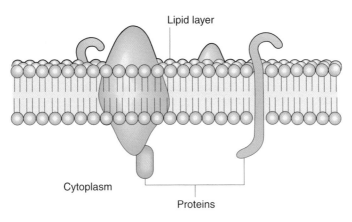

Fig. 20.8   Structure of the membrane.

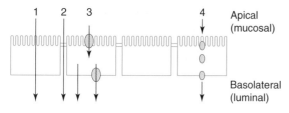

1 – Transcellular   3 – Carrier mediated
2 – Paracellular   4 – Transcytosis

Fig. 20.9   Mechanisms of permeability (absorptive).

will be rapidly distributed, so maintaining a much lower concentration than that at the absorption site. If the cell membranes and fluid regions making up the gastrointestinal–blood barrier can be considered as a single membrane, then the stages involved in gastrointestinal absorption could be represented by the model shown in Figure 20.10.

Passive diffusion of drugs across the gastrointestinal–blood barrier can often be described mathematically by Fick's First Law of Diffusion (see Chapter 2). When considered in the context of bioavailability, this indicates that the rate of diffusion across a membrane (dC/dt) is proportional to the difference in concentration on each side of that membrane. Therefore, the rate of appearance of drug in the blood at the absorption site is given by:

$$dC/dt = k(C_g - C_b) \qquad (20.1)$$

where dC/dt is the rate of appearance of drug in the blood at the site of absorption, k is the proportionality constant, C_g is the concentration of drug in solution in the gastrointestinal fluid at the absorption site and C_b is the concentration of drug in the blood at the site of absorption.

The proportionality constant k incorporates the diffusion coefficient of the drug in the gastrointestinal membrane (D), and the thickness (h) and surface area of the membrane (A).

In

$$k = \frac{DA}{h} \qquad (20.2)$$

These equations indicate that the rate of gastrointestinal absorption of a drug by passive diffusion depends on the surface area of the membrane that is available for drug absorption. Thus the small intestine, primarily the duodenum, is the major site of drug absorption, owing principally to the presence of villi and microvilli which provide such a large surface area for absorption (discussed earlier in this chapter).

Equation 20.1 also indicates that the rate of drug absorption depends on a large concentration gradient of drug existing across the gastrointestinal membrane. This concentration gradient is influenced by the apparent partition coefficients exhibited by the drug with respect to the gastrointestinal membrane–fluid interface and the gastrointestinal membrane–blood interface. It is important that the drug has sufficient affinity (solubility) for the membrane phase so that it can partition readily into the gastrointestinal membrane. In addition, after diffusing across the membrane, the drug should exhibit sufficient solubility in the blood such that it can partition readily out of the membrane phase into the blood.

On entering the blood in the capillary network in the lamina propria, the drug will be carried away from the site of absorption by the rapidly circulating gastrointestinal blood supply. It will then become diluted by distribution into a large volume of blood (i.e. the systemic circulation), by distribution into body tissues and other fluids, and by subsequent metabolism and excretion. In addition,

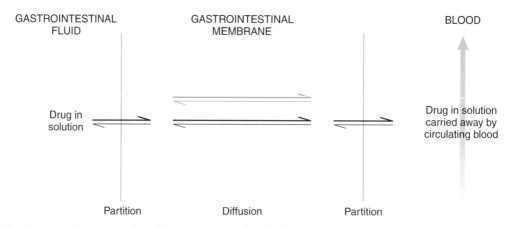

Fig. 20.10   Diagrammatic representation of absorption via passive diffusion.

the drug may bind to plasma proteins in the blood which will further lower the concentration of free (i.e. diffusible) drug in the blood. Consequently, the blood acts as a 'sink' for absorbed drug and ensures that the concentration of drug in the blood at the site of absorption is low in relation to that in the gastrointestinal fluids at the site of absorption, i.e. $C_g \gg C_b$. The 'sink' conditions provided by the systemic circulation ensure that a large concentration gradient is maintained across the gastrointestinal membrane during the absorption process.

The passive absorption process is driven solely by the concentration gradient of the diffusible species of the drug that exists across the gastrointestinal–blood barrier. Thus Eqns 20.1 and 20.2 can be combined and written as:

$$dC/dt = \frac{DAC_g}{h} \qquad (20.3)$$

and because for a given membrane D, A and h can be regarded as constants, Eqn 20.3 becomes:

$$dC/dt = kC_g \qquad (20.4)$$

Equation 20.4 is an expression for a first-order kinetic process (discussed in Chapter 7) and indicates that the rate of passive absorption will be proportional to the concentration of absorbable drug in solution in the gastrointestinal fluids at the site of absorption and therefore that the gastrointestinal absorption of most drugs follows first-order kinetics.

It has been assumed in this description that the drug exists solely in one single absorbable species. Many drugs, however, are weak electrolytes that exist in aqueous solution as two species, namely the unionized species and the ionized species. Because it is the unionized form of a weak electrolyte drug that exhibits greater lipid solubility compared to the corresponding ionized form, the gastrointestinal membrane is more permeable to the unionized species. Thus the rate of passive absorption of a weak electrolyte is related to the fraction of total drug that exists in the unionized form in solution in the gastrointestinal fluids at the site of absorption. This fraction is determined by the dissociation constant of the drug (i.e. its pK_a value) and by the pH of the aqueous environment, in accordance with the Henderson–Hasselbalch equations for weak acids and bases (discussed in Chapter 3). The gastrointestinal absorption of a weak electrolyte drug is enhanced when the pH at the site of absorption favours the formation of a large fraction of the drug in aqueous solution that is unionized. This forms the basis of the pH-partition hypothesis (see Chapter 21).

Carrier-mediated transport As already stated, the majority of drugs are absorbed across cells (i.e. transcellularly) via passive diffusion. However, certain compounds and many nutrients are absorbed transcellularly by a carrier-mediated transport mechanism of which there are two main types: *active transport* and *facilitated diffusion* or *facilitated transport*.

Active transport In contrast to passive diffusion, active transport involves the active participation by the apical cell membrane of the columnar absorption cells. A carrier or membrane transporter is responsible for binding a drug and transporting it across the membrane by a process illustrated in Figure 20.11.

Carrier-mediated absorption is often explained by assuming a shuttling process across the epithelial membrane. The drug molecule or ion forms a complex with the carrier/transporter in the surface of the apical cell membrane of a columnar absorption cell. The drug–carrier complex then moves across the membrane and liberates the drug on the other side of the membrane. The carrier (now free) returns to its initial position in the surface of the cell membrane adjacent to the gastrointestinal tract to await the arrival of another drug molecule or ion.

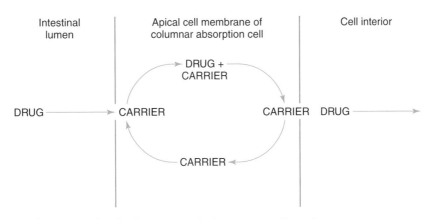

Fig. 20.11 Diagrammatic representation of active transport of a drug across a cell membrane.

Active transport is a process whereby materials can be transported against a concentration gradient across a cell membrane, i.e. transport can occur from a region of lower concentration to one of higher concentration. Therefore, active transport is an energy-consuming process. The energy arises either from the hydrolysis of ATP or from the transmembranous sodium gradient and/or electrical potential.

There are a large number of carrier-mediated active transport systems or membrane transporters in the small intestine. These can be present either on the apical (brush border) or on the basolateral membrane. They include the peptide transporters, the nucleoside transporters, the sugar transporters, the bile acid transporters, the amino acid transporters, the organic anion transporters and the vitamin transporters.

Many nutrients, such as amino acids, sugars, electrolytes (e.g. sodium, potassium, calcium, iron, chloride, bicarbonate), vitamins (thiamine (B_1), nicotinic acid, riboflavin (B_2), pyroxidine (B_6) and cobalamin (B_{12})) and bile salts, are actively transported. Each carrier system is generally concentrated in a specific segment of the gastrointestinal tract. The substance that is transported by that carrier will thus be absorbed preferentially in the location of highest carrier density. For example, the bile acid transporters are only found in the lower part of the small intestine, the ileum. Each carrier/transporter has its own substrate specificity with respect to the chemical structure of the substance that it will transport. Some carriers/transporters have broader specificity than others. Thus if a drug structurally resembles a natural substance which is actively transported then the drug is also likely to be transported by the same carrier mechanism.

Many peptide-like drugs, such as the penicillins, cefalosporins, angiotensin-converting enzyme (ACE) inhibitors and renin inhibitors, rely on the peptide transporters for their efficient absorption. Nucleosides and their analogues for antiviral and anticancer drugs depend on the nucleoside transporters for their uptake. *L*-dopa and α-methyldopa are transported by the carrier-mediated process for amino acids. *L*-dopa has a much faster permeability rate than methyldopa, which has been attributed to the lower affinity of methyldopa for the amino acid carrier.

Unlike passive absorption, where the rate of absorption is directly proportional to the concentration of the absorbable species of the drug at the absorption site, active transport proceeds at a rate that is proportional to the drug concentration only at low concentrations. At higher concentrations, the carrier mechanism becomes saturated and further increases in drug concentration will not increase the rate of absorption, i.e. the rate of absorption remains constant. Absorption rate–concentration

relationships for active and passive processes are compared in Figure 20.12.

Competition between two similar substances for the same transfer mechanism, and the inhibition of absorption of one or both compounds, are other characteristics of carrier-mediated transport. Inhibition of absorption may also be observed with agents that interfere with cell metabolism. Some substances may be absorbed by simultaneous carrier-mediated and passive transport processes. The contribution of the carrier-mediated process to the overall absorption rate decreases with concentration, and at a sufficiently high concentration is negligible.

In summary, active transport mechanisms:

- must have a carrier molecule
- must have a source of energy
- can be inhibited by metabolic inhibitors such as dinitrophenol
- show temperature dependence
- can be competitively inhibited by substrate analogues.

Active transport also plays an important role in the intestinal, renal and biliary excretion of many drugs.

Facilitated diffusion or transport This carrier-mediated process differs from active transport in that it cannot transport a substance against a concentration gradient of that substance. Therefore, facilitated diffusion does not require an energy input but does require a concentration gradient for its driving force, as does passive diffusion. When substances are transported by facilitated diffusion, they are transported down the concentration gradient but at a much faster rate than would be anticipated based on the molecular size and polarity of the molecule. The process, like active transport, is saturable and is subject to inhibition

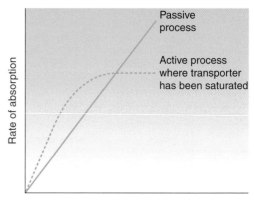

Fig. 20.12 Relationship between rate of absorption and concentration at the absorption site for active and passive processes.

by competitive inhibitors. In terms of drug absorption, facilitated diffusion seems to play a very minor role.

More information on carrier-mediated transport of drugs within the intestines can be obtained from reviews by Oh et al (1999), Tsuji & Tamia (1996) and Yang et al (1999).

Endocytosis Endocytosis is the process by which the plasma membrane of the cell invaginates and the invaginations become pinched off, forming small intracellular membrane-bound vesicles that enclose a volume of material. Thus material can be transported into the cell. After invagination, the material is often transferred to other vesicles or lysosomes and digested. Some material will escape digestion and migrate to the basolateral surface of the cell where it is exocytosed. This uptake process is energy dependent. Endocytosis can be further subdivided into four main processes: fluid-phase endocytosis or pinocytosis; receptor-mediated endocytosis; phagocytosis; and transcytosis. Endocytosis is thought to be the primary mechanism of transport of macromolecules. The process and pathways of endocytosis are complex.

Pinocytosis Fluid-phase endocytosis or pinocytosis is the engulfment of small droplets of extracellular fluid by membrane vesicles. The cell will internalize material regardless of its metabolic importance to that cell. The efficiency of this process is low. The fat-soluble vitamins A, D, E and K are absorbed via pinocytosis.

Receptor-mediated endocytosis Many cells within the body have receptors on their cell surfaces that are capable of binding with suitable ligands to form ligand–receptor complexes. These complexes cluster on the cell surface and then invaginate and break off from the membrane to form coated vesicles. The binding process between the ligand and the receptor on the cell surface is thought to trigger a conformational change in the membrane to allow this process to occur. Once within the cytoplasm of the cell, the coated vesicles rapidly lose their coat and the resulting uncoated vesicles will promptly deliver their contents to early endosomes. Within the endosomes, the ligands usually dissociate from their receptors, many of which are then recycled to the plasma membrane. The dissociated ligands and solutes are next delivered to prelysosomes and finally to lysosomes, the end-stage of the endocytic pathway. Lysosomes are spherical or oval cell organelles surrounded by a single membrane. They contain digestive enzymes which break down bacteria and large molecules, such as protein, polysaccharides and nucleic acids, which have entered the cell via endocytosis.

Phagocytosis Phagocytosis can be defined as the engulfment by the cell membrane of particles larger than 500 nm. This process is important for the absorption of polio and other vaccines from the gastrointestinal tract.

Transcytosis Transcytosis is the process by which the material internalized by the membrane domain is transported through the cell and secreted on the opposite side.

Paracellular pathway The paracellular pathway differs from all the other absorption pathways as it is the transport of materials in the aqueous pores between the cells rather than across them. The cells are joined together via closely fitting tight junctions on their apical side. The intercellular spaces occupy only about 0.01% of the total surface area of the epithelium. The tightness of these junctions can vary considerably between different epithelia in the body. In general, absorptive epithelia, such as that of the small intestine, tend to be leakier than other epithelia. The paracellular pathway decreases in importance down the length of the gastrointestinal tract and as the number and size of pores between the epithelial cells decrease.

The paracellular route of absorption is important for the transport of ions such as calcium and for the transport of sugars, amino acids and peptides at concentrations above the capacity of their carriers. Small hydrophilic and charged drugs that do not distribute into cell membranes cross the gastrointestinal epithelium via the paracellular pathway. The molecular weight cut-off for the paracellular route is usually considered to be 200 Da, although some larger drugs have been shown to be absorbed via this route.

The paracellular pathway can be divided into convective ('solvent drag') and diffusive components. The convective component is the rate at which the compound is carried across the epithelium via the water flux.

Efflux of drugs from the intestine It is now known that there are countertransport efflux proteins that expel specific drugs back into the lumen of the gastrointestinal tract after they have been absorbed. One of the key countertransport proteins is P-glycoprotein. P-glycoprotein is expressed at high levels on the apical surface of columnar cells (brush border membrane) in the jejunum. It is also present on the surface of many other epithelia and endothelia in the body, and on the surface of tumour cells. P-glycoproteins were originally discovered because of their ability to cause multidrug resistance in tumour cells by preventing the intracellular accumulation of many cytotoxic cancer drugs by pumping the drugs back out of the tumours. Certain drugs with wide structural diversity (Table 20.2) are susceptible to efflux from the intestine via P-glycoprotein. Such efflux may have a detrimental effect on drug bioavailability. These countertransport efflux proteins pump drugs out of cells in a similar way to which nutrients, and drugs are actively absorbed across the gastrointestinal membrane. This process therefore requires energy, can work against a concentration

Table 20.2 Examples of transport mechanisms of commonly used drugs across the gastrointestinal absorptive epithelia (adapted from Brayden 1997)

Route	Examples	Therapeutic class
Transcellular passive diffusion	Propranolol	β-blocker
	Testosterone	Steroid
	Ketoprofen	Non-steroidal antiinflammatory
	Cisapride	Antispasmodic
	Oestradiol	Sex hormone
	Naproxen	Non-steroidal antiinflammatory
Paracellular	Cimetidine	H2 antagonist
	Loperamide	Antidiarrhoeal
	Atenolol	β-blocker
	Mannitol	Sugar used as paracellular marker
	Tiludronate	Bisphosphonate
Carrier mediated	Cefalexin	Antibacterial
	Captopril	ACE inhibitor
	Bestatin	Anticancer
	Levodopa	Dopaminergic
	Foscarnet	Antiviral
Transcellular diffusion subject to P-glycoprotein efflux	Ciclosporin	Immunosuppressant
	Nifedipine	Calcium channel blocker
	Verapamil	Calcium channel blocker
	Paclitaxel	Anticancer
	Celiprolol	β-blocker
	Digoxin	Cardiac glycoside

gradient, can be competitively inhibited by structural analogues or by inhibitors of cell metabolism and is a saturable process.

Table 20.2 summarizes the main mechanisms of drug transport across the gastrointestinal epithelia for a number of commonly used drugs.

Presystemic metabolism

As well as having the ability to cross the gastrointestinal membrane by one of the routes described, drugs also need to be resistant to degradation/metabolism during this passage. All drugs that are absorbed from the stomach, small intestine and upper colon pass into the hepatic portal system and are presented to the liver before reaching the systemic circulation. Therefore, if the drug is going to be available to the systemic circulation, it must also be resistant to metabolism by the liver. Hence, an

oral dose of drug could be completely absorbed but incompletely available to the systemic circulation because of *first-pass* or *presystemic* metabolism by the gut wall and/or liver.

Gut wall metabolism

The gut walls contain a number of metabolizing enzymes that can degrade drugs before they reach the systemic circulation. For example, the major cytochrome P450 enzyme CYP3A, present in the liver and responsible for the hepatic metabolism of many drugs, is present in the intestinal mucosa and intestinal metabolism may be important for substrates of this enzyme. This effect can also be known as *first-pass metabolism by the intestine*.

Hepatic metabolism

The liver is the primary site of drug metabolism and thus acts as a final barrier for oral absorption. This first pass of absorbed drug through the liver may result in extensive metabolism of the drug, and a significant portion may never reach the systemic circulation, resulting in a low bioavailability of those drugs which are rapidly metabolized by the liver. The bioavailability of a susceptible drug may be reduced to such an extent as to render the gastrointestinal route of administration ineffective or to necessitate an oral dose which is many times larger than the intravenous dose, e.g. propranolol. Although propranolol is well absorbed, only about 30% of an oral dose is available to the systemic circulation owing to the first-pass effect. The bioavailability of sustained-release propranolol is even less as the drug is presented via the hepatic portal vein more slowly than from an immediate-release dosage form, and the liver is therefore capable of extracting and metabolizing a larger portion. Other drugs which are susceptible to a large first-pass effect are the anaesthetic lidocaine (lignocaine), the tricyclic antidepressant imipramine and the analgesic pentazocine.

First-pass metabolism can be avoided by drug administration to the mouth (buccal or sublingual; see Chapter 31) or to the rectum (see Chapter 40). The arrangement of the blood vessels in this region means that absorbed drug does not pass through the liver first, prior to entering the systemic circulation.

SUMMARY

There are many physiological factors that influence the rate and extent of drug absorption; these are initially dependent on the route of administration. For the oral route, the physiological and environmental factors of the gastrointestinal tract, the gastrointestinal membrane and presystemic metabolism can all influence drug bioavailability.

REFERENCES

Brayden, D. (1997) Human intestinal epithelial monolayers as prescreens for oral drug delivery. *Pharmaceutical News*, **4** (1), 11-13.

Evans A.M. (2000) Influence of dietary components on the gastrointestinal metabolism and transport of drugs. *Therapeutic Drug Monitoring,* **22**, 131-136.

Fleisher, D., Cheng, L., Zhou, Y., Li-Heng, P., Karim, A. (1999) Drug, meal and formulation interactions influencing drug absorption after oral administration. *Clinical Pharmacokinetics*, **36**, 233-254.

Gray, V., Dressman, J. (1996) Change of pH requirements for simulated intestinal fluid TS. *Pharmacopeial Forum,* **22**, 1943-1945.

Oh, D.M., Han, H.K., Amidon, G.L. (1999) Drug transport and targeting. *Pharmaceutical Biotechnology,* **12**, 59-88.

Schmidt, L.E., Dalhoff, K. (2002) Food–drug interactions. *Drugs,* **62**, 1481-1502.

Tsuji, A., Tamia, I. (1996) Carrier-mediated intestinal transport of drugs. *Pharmaceutical Research,* **13**, 963-977.

Welling, P.G. (1996) Effects of food on drug absorption. *Annual Review of Nutrition*, **16**, 383-414.

Yang, C.Y., Dantzig, A.H., Pidgeon, C. (1999) Intestinal peptide transporter systems and oral drug availability. *Pharmaceutical Research,* **16**, 1331-1343.

BIBLIOGRAPHY

Lennernas, H. (1998) Human intestinal permeability. *Journal of Pharmaceutical Science,* **87**, 403-410.

Bioavailability – physicochemical and dosage form factors

M. Ashford

INTRODUCTION

As discussed in Chapter 20, the rate and extent of absorption are influenced by the physiological factors associated with the structure and function of the GI tract. This chapter discusses the physicochemical properties of the drug and dosage form factors that influence bioavailability. For a drug to be absorbed, it needs to be in solution and to be able to pass across the membrane. In the case of orally administered drugs, this is the gastrointestinal epithelium. The physicochemical properties of the drug that will influence its passage into solution and transfer across membranes include its dissolution rate, pK_a, lipid solubility, chemical stability and complexation potential.

PHYSICOCHEMICAL FACTORS INFLUENCING BIOAVAILABILITY

Dissolution and solubility

Solid drugs need to dissolve before they can be absorbed. The dissolution of drugs can be described by the Noyes–Whitney equation (Eqn 21.1). This equation, first proposed in 1897, describes the rate of dissolution of spherical particles when the dissolution process is diffusion controlled and involves no chemical reaction:

$$dC/dt = \frac{DA\,(C_S - C)}{h} \qquad (21.1)$$

where dC/dt is the rate of dissolution of the drug particles, D is the diffusion coefficient of the drug in solution in the gastrointestinal fluids, A is the effective surface area of the drug particles in contact with the gastrointestinal fluids, h is the thickness of the diffusion layer around each drug particle, C_S is the saturation solubility of the drug in solution in the diffusion layer and C is the concentration of the drug in the gastrointestinal fluids.

The limitations of the Noyes–Whitney equation in describing the dissolution of drug particles are discussed

Table 21.1 Physicochemical and physiological factors affecting drug dissolution in the gastrointestinal tract (adapted from Dressman et al 1998)

Factor	Physicochemical parameter	Physiological parameter
Effective surface area of drug	Particle size, wettability	Surfactants in gastric juice and bile, pH, buffer capacity, bile, food components
Solubility in diffusion layer	Hydrophilicity, crystal structure, solubilization	
Amount of drug already dissolved		Permeability, transit
Diffusivity of drug	Molecular size	Viscosity of luminal contents
Boundary layer thickness		Motility patterns and flow rate
Volume of solvent available		Gastrointestinal secretions, co-administered fluids

in Chapter 2. Despite these limitations, the equation serves to illustrate and explain how various physico-chemical and physiological factors can influence the rate of dissolution in the gastrointestinal tract. These are summarized in Table 21.1 and are discussed in more detail in the next section.

Figure 21.1 illustrates the dissolution of a spherical drug particle in the gastrointestinal fluids.

Physiological factors affecting the dissolution rate of drugs

The environment of the gastrointestinal tract can affect the parameters of the Noyes–Whitney equation (Eqn 21.1) and hence the dissolution rate of a drug. For instance, the diffusion coefficient, D, of the drug in the gastrointestinal fluids may be decreased by the presence of substances that increase the viscosity of the fluids.

Hence the presence of food in the gastrointestinal tract may cause a decrease in dissolution rate of a drug by reducing the rate of diffusion of the drug molecules away from the diffusion layer surrounding each undissolved drug particle. Surfactants in gastric juice and bile salts will affect both the wettability of the drug, and hence the effective surface area, A, exposed to gastrointestinal fluids, and the solubility of the drug in the gastrointestinal fluids via micellization. The thickness of the diffusion layer, h, will be influenced by the degree of agitation experienced by each drug particle in the gastrointestinal tract. Hence an increase in gastric and/or intestinal motility may increase the dissolution rate of a sparingly soluble drug by decreasing the thickness of the diffusion layer around each drug particle.

The concentration, C, of drug in solution in the bulk of the gastrointestinal fluids will be influenced by such factors as the rate of removal of dissolved drug by absorption

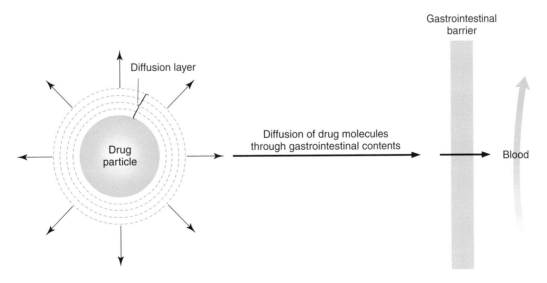

Fig. 21.1 Schematic representation of the dissolution of a drug particle in the gastrointestinal fluids.

through the gastrointestinal–blood barrier and by the volume of fluid available for dissolution, which in turn will be dependent on the position of the drug in the gastrointestinal tract and the timing with respect to meal intake. In the stomach, the volume of fluid will be influenced by the intake of fluid in the diet. According to the Noyes–Whitney equation, a low value of C will favour more rapid dissolution of the drug by virtue of increasing the value of the term $(C_S - C)$. In the case of drugs whose absorption is dissolution rate limited, the value of C is normally kept very low by absorption of the drug. Hence dissolution occurs under sink conditions; that is, under conditions such that the value of $(C_S - C)$ approximates to C_S. Thus for the dissolution of a drug from the gastrointestinal tract under sink conditions, the Noyes–Whitney equation can be expressed as:

$$dC/dt = \frac{DAC_S}{h} \qquad (21.2)$$

Drug factors affecting dissolution rate

Drug factors that can influence the dissolution rate are the particle size, the wettability, the solubility and the form of the drug (whether a salt or a free form, crystalline or amorphous).

Surface area and particle size According to Eqn 21.1, an increase in the total surface area of drug in contact with the gastrointestinal fluids will cause an increase in dissolution rate. Provided that each particle of drug is intimately wetted by the gastrointestinal fluids, the effective surface area exhibited by the drug will be directly proportional to the particle size of the drug. Hence the smaller the particle size, the greater the effective surface area exhibited by a given mass of drug and the higher the dissolution rate. Particle size reduction is thus likely to result in increased bioavailability, provided that the absorption of the drug is dissolution rate limited.

One of the classic examples of particle size effects on the bioavailability of poorly soluble compounds is that of griseofulvin, where a reduction of particle size from about 10 μm (specific surface area = 0.4 m² g⁻¹) to 2.7 μm (specific surface area = 1.5 m² g⁻¹) was shown to produce approximately double the amount of drug absorbed in humans. Many poorly soluble, slowly dissolving drugs are routinely presented in micronized form to increase their surface area.

Examples of drugs where a reduction in particle size has been shown to improve the rate and extent of oral absorption and hence bioavailability are shown in Table 21.2. Such improvements in bioavailability can result in an increased incidence of side-effects; thus for certain drugs it is important that the particle size is well controlled, and many pharmacopoeia state a requirement for particle size.

Table 21.2 Examples of drugs where a reduction in particle size has led to improvements in bioavailability

Drug	Therapeutic class
Digoxin	Cardiac glycoside
Nitrofurantoin	Antifungal
Medroxyprogesterone	Hormone acetate
Danazol	Steroid
Tolbutamide	Antidiabetic
Aspirin	Analgesic
Sulfadiazine	Antibacterial
Naproxen	Non-steroidal antiinflammatory
Ibuprofen	Non-steroidal antiinflammatory
Phenacetin	Analgesic

For some drugs, particularly those that are hydrophobic in nature, micronization and other dry particle size reduction techniques can result in aggregation of the material. This will cause a consequent reduction in the effective surface area of the drug exposed to the gastrointestinal fluids and hence a reduction in its dissolution rate and bioavailability. Aspirin, phenacetin and phenobarbital are all prone to aggregation during particle size reduction. One approach that may overcome this problem is to micronize or mill the drug with a wetting agent or hydrophilic carrier. To overcome aggregation and to achieve particle sizes in the nano-size region, wet milling in the presence of stabilizers has been used. The relative bioavailability of danazol has been increased 400% by administering particles in the nanometer rather than the micrometre size range.

As well as milling with wetting agents, the effective surface area of hydrophobic drugs can be increased by the addition of a wetting agent to the formulation. The presence of polysorbate 80 in a fine suspension of phenacetin (particle size less than 75 μm) greatly improved the rate and extent of absorption of the phenacetin in human volunteers compared to the same-size suspension without a wetting agent. Polysorbate 80 helps by increasing the wetting and solvent penetration of the particles and by minimizing aggregation of suspended particles, thereby maintaining a large effective surface area. Wettability effects are highly drug specific.

If an increase in the effective surface area of a drug does not increase its absorption rate, it is likely that the dissolution process is not rate limiting. For drugs such as penicillin G and erythromycin, which are unstable in gastric fluids, their chemical degradation will be minimized if they remain in the solid state. Thus particle size reduction would not only serve to increase their dissolution rate but would simultaneously increase chemical degradation and therefore reduce the amount of intact drug available for absorption.

Solubility in the diffusion layer, C_S The dissolution rate of a drug under sink conditions, according to the Noyes–Whitney equation, is directly proportional to its intrinsic solubility in the diffusion layer surrounding each dissolving drug particle, C_S. The aqueous solubility of a drug is dependent on the interactions between molecules within the crystal lattice, intermolecular interactions with the solution in which it is dissolving, and the entropy changes associated with fusion and dissolution. In the case of drugs that are weak electrolytes, their aqueous solubilities are dependent on pH (discussed in Chapter 2). Hence in the case of an orally administered solid dosage form containing a weak electrolyte drug, the dissolution rate of the drug will be influenced by its solubility and the pH in the diffusion layer surrounding each dissolving drug particle. The pH in the diffusion layer – the microclimate pH – for a weak electrolyte will be affected by the pK_a and solubility of the dissolving drug and the pK_a and solubility of the buffers in the bulk gastrointestinal fluids. Thus differences in dissolution rate will be expected in different regions of the gastrointestinal tract.

The solubility of weakly acidic drugs increases with pH and so as a drug moves down the gastrointestinal tract from the stomach to the intestine, its solubility will increase. Conversely, the solubility of weak bases decreases with increasing pH, i.e. as the drug moves down the gastrointestinal tract. It is important therefore for poorly soluble weak bases to dissolve rapidly in the stomach, as the rate of dissolution in the small intestine will be much slower. The antifungal drug ketoconazole,

a weak base, is particularly sensitive to gastric pH. Dosing ketoconazole 2 hours after the administration of the H_2 blocker cimetidine, which reduces gastric acid secretion, results in a significantly reduced rate and extent of absorption (van der Meer et al 1980). Similarly, in the case of the antiplatelet drug dipyrimidole, pretreatment with the H_2 blocker famotidine reduces the peak plasma concentration by a factor of up to 10 (Russell et al 1994).

Salts The dissolution rate of a weakly acidic drug in gastric fluid (pH 1–3.5) will be relatively low. If the pH in the diffusion layer could be increased, then the solubility, C_S, exhibited by the acidic drug in this layer, and hence its dissolution rate in gastric fluids, would be increased even though the bulk pH of gastric fluids remained at the same low value. The pH of the diffusion layer would be increased if the chemical nature of the weakly acidic drug were changed from that of the free acid to a basic salt, for example the sodium or potassium form of the free acid. The pH of the diffusion layer surrounding each particle of the salt form would be higher (e.g. 5–6) than the low bulk pH (1–3.5) of the gastric fluids because of the neutralizing action of the strong anions (Na^+ or K^+) ions present in the diffusion layer (Fig. 21.2).

Because the salt form of the weakly acidic drug has a relatively high solubility at the elevated pH in the diffusion layer, dissolution of the drug particles will take place at a faster rate. When dissolved drug diffuses out of the diffusion layer into the bulk of the gastric fluid, where the pH is lower than that in the diffusion layer, precipitation of the free acid form is likely to occur. This will be a result of the overall solubility exhibited by the drug at the lower bulk pH. Thus the free acid form of the

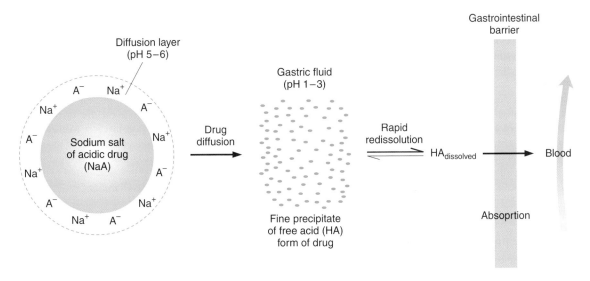

Fig. 21.2 Schematic representation of the dissolution process of a salt form of a weakly acidic drug in gastric fluid.

drug in solution, which is in excess of its solubility at the bulk pH of gastric fluid, will precipitate out, leaving a saturated (or near-saturated) solution of free acid in gastric fluid. Often this precipitated free acid will be in the form of very fine, non-ionized wetted particles which exhibit a very large total effective surface area in contact with gastric fluids. This large total effective surface area will facilitate rapid redissolution of the precipitated particles of free acid when additional gastric fluid becomes available as a consequence of either dissolved drug being absorbed, additional fluid accumulating in the stomach or the fine precipitated particles being emptied from the stomach to the intestine. This rapid redissolution will ensure that the concentration of free acid in solution in the bulk of the gastric fluids will be at or near to saturation.

Thus the oral administration of a solid dosage form containing a strong basic salt of a weakly acidic drug would be expected to give a more rapid rate of drug dissolution and (in the case of drugs exhibiting dissolution rate-limited absorption) a more rapid rate of drug absorption than the free acid form of the drug.

Many examples can be found of the effects of salts improving the rate and extent of absorption. The dissolution rate of the oral hypoglycaemic tolbutamide sodium in 0.1 M HCl is 5000 times faster than that of the free acid. Oral administration of a non-disintegrating disc of the more rapidly dissolving sodium salt of tolbutamide produced a very rapid decrease in blood sugar level (a consequence of the rapid rate of drug absorption), followed by a rapid recovery. In contrast, a non-disintegrating disc of the tolbutamide free acid produces a much slower rate of decrease of blood sugar (a consequence of the slower rate of drug absorption) that is maintained over a longer period of time. The barbiturates are often administered in the form of sodium salts to achieve a rapid onset of sedation and provide more predictable effects.

The non-steroidal antiinflammatory drug naproxen was originally marketed as the free acid for the treatment of rheumatoid and osteoarthritis. However, the sodium salt (naproxen sodium) is absorbed faster and is more effective in newer indications, such as mild to moderate pain (Sevelius et al 1980).

Conversely, strongly acidic salt forms of weakly basic drugs, for example chlorpromazine hydrochloride, dissolve more rapidly in gastric and intestinal fluids than do the free bases (e.g. chlorpromazine). The presence of strongly acidic anions (e.g. Cl^- ions) in the diffusion layer around each drug particle ensures that the pH in that layer is lower than the bulk pH in either the gastric or the intestinal fluid. This lower pH will increase the solubility of the drug in the diffusion layer.

The oral administration of a salt form of a weakly basic drug in a solid oral dosage form generally ensures that dissolution occurs in the gastric fluid before the drug passes into the small intestine where pH conditions are unfavourable. Thus the drug should be delivered to the major absorption site, the small intestine, in solution. If absorption is fast enough, precipitation of the dissolved drug is unlikely to significantly affect bioavailability. It is important to be aware that hydrochloride salts may experience a common ion effect owing to the presence of chloride ions in the stomach (also discussed in Chapter 24). The in vitro dissolution of a sulfate salt of an HIV protease inhibitor analogue is significantly greater in hydrochloric acid than that of the hydrochloride salt. The bioavailability of the sulfate salt is more than three times greater than that of the hydrochloride salt. These observations are attributed to the common ion effect of the hydrochloride (Loper et al 1999).

The sodium salts of acidic drugs and the hydrochloride salts of basic drugs are by far the most common. However, many other salt forms are increasingly being employed (there is further information in Chapter 24). Some salts have a lower solubility and dissolution rate than the free form, for example aluminium salts of weak acids and palmoate salts of weak bases. In these cases insoluble films of either aluminium hydroxide or palmoic acid are found to coat the dissolving solids when the salts are exposed to a basic or an acidic environment, respectively. In general, poorly soluble salts delay absorption and may therefore be used to sustain the release of the drug. A poorly soluble salt form is generally employed for suspension dosage forms.

Although salt forms are often selected to improve bioavailability, other factors such as chemical stability, hygroscopicity, manufacturability and crystallinity will all be considered during salt selection and may preclude the choice of a particular salt. The sodium salt of aspirin, sodium acetylsalicylate, is much more prone to hydrolysis than is aspirin, acetylsalicylic acid, itself. One way to overcome chemical instabilities or other undesirable features of salts is to form the salt in situ or to add basic/acidic excipients to the formulation of a weakly acidic or weakly basic drug. The presence of the basic excipients in the formulation of acidic drugs ensures that a relatively basic diffusion layer is formed around each dissolving particle. The inclusion of the basic ingredients aluminium dihydroxyaminoacetate and magnesium carbonate in aspirin tablets was found to increase their dissolution rate and bioavailability.

Crystal form

Polymorphism Many drugs can exist in more than one crystalline form, e.g. chloramphenicol palmitate, cortisone acetate, tetracyclines and sulfathiazole. This property is referred to as *polymorphism* and each crystalline form is known as a polymorph (discussed further in Chapter 8). As discussed in Chapter 2, a metastable polymorph usually exhibits a greater dissolution rate than the corresponding stable polymorph. Consequently, the metastable polymorphic form of a poorly soluble drug may exhibit an increased bioavailability compared to the stable polymorphic form.

A classic example of the influence of polymorphism on drug bioavailability is provided by chloramphenicol palmitate. This drug exists in three crystalline forms designated A, B and C. At normal temperature and pressure, A is the stable polymorph, B is the metastable polymorph and C is the unstable polymorph. Polymorph C is too unstable to be included in a dosage form but polymorph B, the metastable form, is sufficiently stable. The plasma profiles of chloramphenicol from orally administered suspensions containing varying proportions of the polymorphic forms A and B were investigated. The extent of absorption of chloramphenicol increases as the proportion of the polymorphic form B of chloramphenicol palmitate is increased in each suspension. This was attributed to the more rapid in vivo rate of dissolution of the metastable polymorphic form, B, of chloramphenicol palmitate. Following dissolution, chloramphenicol palmitate is hydrolysed to give free chloramphenicol in solution, which is then absorbed. The stable polymorphic form A of chloramphenicol palmitate dissolves so slowly and consequently is hydrolysed so slowly to chloramphenicol in vivo that this polymorph is virtually ineffective. The importance of polymorphism to the gastrointestinal bioavailability of chloramphenicol palmitate is reflected by a limit being placed on the content of the inactive polymorphic form, A, in chloramphenicol palmitate mixture.

Amorphous solids   In addition to different polymorphic crystalline forms, a drug may exist in an amorphous form (see Chapter 8). Because the amorphous form usually dissolves more rapidly than the corresponding crystalline form(s), the possibility exists that there will be significant differences in the bioavailabilities exhibited by the amorphous and crystalline forms of drugs that show dissolution rate-limited bioavailability.

A classic example of the influence of amorphous versus crystalline forms of a drug on its gastrointestinal bioavailability is provided by the antibiotic novobiocin. The more soluble and rapidly dissolving amorphous form of novobiocin was readily absorbed following oral administration of an aqueous suspension to humans and dogs. However, the less soluble and slower dissolving crystalline form was not absorbed to any significant extent. The crystalline form was thus therapeutically ineffective. A further important observation was made in the case of aqueous suspensions of novobiocin. The amorphous form slowly converts to the more thermodynamically stable crystalline form, with an accompanying loss of therapeutic effective-

ness. Thus unless adequate precautions are taken to ensure the stability of the less stable, more therapeutically effective amorphous form of a drug in a dosage form, then unacceptable variations in therapeutic effectiveness may occur.

Several delivery technologies for poorly soluble drugs rely on stabilizing the drug in its amorphous form to increase its dissolution and bioavailability.

Solvates   Another variation in the crystalline form of a drug can occur if the drug is able to associate with solvent molecules to produce crystalline forms known as solvates. When water is the solvent, the solvate formed is called a hydrate. Generally, the greater the solvation of the crystal, the lower are the solubility and dissolution rate in a solvent identical to the solvation molecules. As the solvated and non-solvated forms usually exhibit differences in dissolution rates, they may also exhibit differences in bioavailability, particularly in the case of poorly soluble drugs that exhibit dissolution rate-limited bioavailability.

A valuable example is that of the antibiotic ampicillin. The faster dissolving anhydrous form of ampicillin was absorbed to a greater extent from both hard gelatin capsules and an aqueous suspension than was the slower dissolving trihydrate form. The anhydrous form of the hydrochloride salt of an HIV protease inhibitor, an analogue of indinavir, has a much faster dissolution rate than the hydrated form in water. This is reflected by a significantly greater rate and extent of absorption and overdoubling of the bioavailability of the anhydrous form (Loper et al 1999).

Factors affecting the concentration of drug in solution in the gastrointestinal fluids

The rate and extent of absorption of a drug depend on the effective concentration of that drug, i.e. the concentration of drug in solution in the gastrointestinal fluids which is in an absorbable form. Complexation, micellar solubilization, adsorption and chemical stability are the principal physicochemical properties that can influence the effective drug concentration in the gastrointestinal fluids.

Complexation   Complexation of a drug may occur within the dosage form and/or in the gastrointestinal fluids, and can be beneficial or detrimental to absorption.

Mucin, a normal component of gastrointestinal fluids, complexes with some drugs. The antibiotic streptomycin binds to mucin, thereby reducing the available concentration of the drug for absorption. It is thought that this may contribute to its poor bioavailability. Another example of complexation is that between drugs and dietary components, as in the case of the tetracyclines, which is discussed in Chapter 20.

The bioavailability of some drugs can be reduced by the presence of some excipients within the dosage forms. The presence of calcium (e.g. from the diluent dicalcium phosphate) in the dosage form of tetracycline reduces its bioavailability via the formation of a poorly soluble complex. Other examples of complexes that reduce drug bioavailability are those between amfetamine and sodium carboxymethylcellulose, and between phenobarbital and polyethylene glycol 4000. Complexation between drugs and excipients probably occurs quite often in liquid dosage forms.

Complexation is sometimes used to increase drug solubility, particularly of poorly water-soluble drugs. One class of complexing agents that is increasingly being employed is the cyclodextrin family. Cyclodextrins are enzymatically modified starches composed of glucopyranose units which form a ring of either six (α-cyclodextrin), seven (β-cyclodextrin) or eight (γ-cyclodextrin) units. The outer surface of the ring is hydrophilic and the inner cavity is hydrophobic. Lipophilic molecules can fit into the ring to form soluble inclusion complexes. The ring of β-cyclodextrin is the correct size for the majority of drug molecules, and normally one drug molecule will associate with one cyclodextrin molecule to form reversible complexes, although other stoichiometries are possible. For example, the antifungal miconazole shows poor oral bioavailability owing to its poor solubility but in the presence of cyclodextrin, the solubility and dissolution rate of miconazole are significantly enhanced (by up to 55- and 255-fold, respectively). This enhancement of dissolution rate resulted in a more than doubling of the oral bioavailability in a study in rats (Terjarla et al 1998). There are numerous examples in the literature of drugs whose solubility, and hence bioavailability, has been increased by the use of cyclodextrins: they include piroxicam, itraconazole, indometacin, pilocarpine, naproxen, hydrocortisone, diazepam and digitoxin. The first product on the UK market containing a cyclodextrin includes the poorly soluble antifungal itraconazole, which has been formulated as a liquid dosage form with the more soluble derivative of β-cyclodextrin, hydroxypropyl-β-cyclodextrin.

Micellar solubilization Micellar solubilization can also increase the solubility of drugs in the gastrointestinal tract. The ability of bile salts to solubilize drugs depends mainly on the lipophilicity of the drug. Further information on solubilization and complex formation can be found in Florence & Attwood (2006).

Adsorption The concurrent administration of drugs and medicines containing solid adsorbents (e.g. antidiarrhoeal mixtures) may result in the adsorbents interfering with the absorption of drugs from the gastrointestinal tract. The adsorption of a drug on to solid adsorbents such as kaolin or charcoal may reduce its rate and/or extent of absorption owing to a decrease in the effective concentration of the drug in solution available for absorption. A consequence of the reduced concentration of free drug in solution at the site of absorption will be a reduction in the rate of drug absorption. Whether there is also a reduction in extent of absorption will depend on whether the drug–adsorbent interaction is readily reversible. If the absorbed drug is not readily released from the solid adsorbent in order to replace the free drug that has been absorbed from the gastrointestinal tract, there will also be a reduction in the extent of absorption from the gastrointestinal tract.

Examples of drug–adsorbent interactions that give reduced extents of absorption are promazine-charcoal and linomycin-kaopectate. The adsorbent properties of charcoal have been exploited as an antidote to drug intoxification.

Care also needs to be taken when insoluble excipients are included in dosage forms to check that the drug will not adsorb to them. Talc, which can be included in tablets as a glidant, is claimed to interfere with the absorption of cyanocobalamin by virtue of its ability to adsorb this vitamin.

Further details of the biopharmaceutical implications of adsorption can be found in Florence & Attwood (2006).

Chemical stability of the drug in the gastrointestinal fluids If the drug is unstable in the gastrointestinal fluids, the amount of drug that is available for absorption will be reduced and its bioavailability reduced. Instability in gastrointestinal fluids is usually caused by acidic or enzymatic hydrolysis. When a drug is unstable in gastric fluid, its extent of degradation would be minimized (and hence its bioavailability improved) if it exhibited minimal dissolution in gastric fluid but still rapid dissolution in intestinal fluid.

The concept of delaying the dissolution of a drug until it reaches the small intestine has been employed to improve the bioavailability of erythromycin in the gastrointestinal tract. Enteric coating of tablets containing the free base erythromycin is one method that has been used to protect this drug from gastric fluid. The enteric coating resists gastric fluid but disrupts or dissolves at the less acid pH range of the small intestine (discussed later in this chapter and in Chapter 33). An alternative method of protecting a susceptible drug from gastric fluid, which has been employed in the case of erythromycin, is the administration of chemical derivatives of the parent drug. These derivatives, or prodrugs, exhibit limited solubility (and hence minimal dissolution) in gastric fluid but once in the small intestine, liberate the parent drug to be absorbed. For instance, erythromycin stearate, after passing through the stomach undissolved, dissolves and dissociates in the intestinal fluid, yielding the free base erythromycin that is absorbed.

Instability in gastrointestinal fluids is one of the reasons why many peptide-like drugs are poorly absorbed when delivered via the oral route.

Poorly soluble drugs

Poorly water-soluble drugs are increasingly becoming a problem in terms of obtaining the satisfactory dissolution within the gastrointestinal tract that is necessary for good bioavailability. It is not only existing drugs that cause problems but it is the challenge of medicinal chemists to ensure that new drugs are not only active pharmacologically but have enough solubility to ensure fast enough dissolution at the site of administration, often the gastrointestinal tract. This is a particular problem for certain classes of drugs, such as the HIV protease inhibitors, the glycoprotein IIb/IIIa inhibitors, and many antiinfective and anticancer drugs. Medicinal chemists are using approaches such as introducing ionizable groups, reducing melting points, changing polymorphs or introducing prodrugs to improve solubility. Further information on these techniques can be obtained from reviews by Lipinski et al (1997) and Panchagnula & Thomas (2000).

Pharmaceutical scientists are also applying a wide range of formulation approaches to improve the dissolution rate of poorly soluble drugs. These include formulating in the nano-size range; formulating in a solid solution or dispersion or self-emulsifying drug delivery system; stabilizing the drug in the amorphous form; or formulating with cyclodextrins. Many drug delivery companies thrive on technologies designed to improve the delivery of poorly soluble drugs.

Drug absorption

Once the drug has successfully passed into solution, it is available for absorption. In Chapter 20, many physiological factors were shown to influence drug absorption. Absorption, and hence the bioavailability of a drug once in solution, is also influenced by many drug factors, in particular its pK_a, lipid solubility, molecular weight, the number of hydrogen bonds in the molecule and its chemical stability.

Drug dissociation and lipid solubility

The dissociation constant and lipid solubility of a drug and the pH at the absorption site often influence the absorption characteristics of a drug throughout the gastrointestinal tract. The interrelationship between the degree of ionization of a weak electrolyte drug (which is determined by its dissociation constant and the pH at the

absorption site) and the extent of absorption is embodied in the pH-partition hypothesis of drug absorption, first proposed by Overton in 1899. Although it is an oversimplification of the complex process of absorption, the pH-partition hypothesis provides a useful framework for understanding the transcellular passive route of absorption, which is that favoured by the majority of drugs.

pH-partition hypothesis of drug absorption According to the pH-partition hypothesis, the gastrointestinal epithelium acts as a lipid barrier to drugs which are absorbed by passive diffusion, and those that are lipid soluble will pass across the barrier. As most drugs are weak electrolytes, the unionized form of weakly acidic or basic drugs (i.e. the lipid-soluble form) will pass across the gastrointestinal epithelium, whereas it is impermeable to the ionized (i.e. poorly lipid-soluble) form of such drugs. Consequently, according to the pH-partition hypothesis, the absorption of a weak electrolyte will be determined chiefly by the extent to which the drug exists in its unionized form at the site of absorption.

The extent to which a weakly acidic or basic drug ionizes in solution in the gastrointestinal fluid may be calculated using the appropriate form of a Henderson–Hasselbalch equation (discussed further in Chapter 3). For a weakly acidic drug having a single ionizable group (e.g. aspirin, phenylbutazone, salicylic acid), the equation takes the form of:

$$\log \frac{[A^-]}{[HA]} = pH - pK_a \qquad (21.3)$$

This is a slightly rearranged form of Eqn 3.16 where pK_a is the negative logarithm of the acid dissociation constant of the drug, and [HA] and [A$^-$] are the respective concentrations of the unionized and ionized forms of the weakly acidic drug, which are in equilibrium and in solution in the gastrointestinal fluid. pH refers to the pH of the environment of the ionized and unionized species, i.e. the gastrointestinal fluids.

For a weakly basic drug possessing a single ionizable group (e.g. chlorpromazine), the analogous equation is:

$$\log \frac{[BH^+]}{[B]} = pK_a - pH \qquad (21.4)$$

This is a slightly rearranged form of Eqn 3.19 where [BH$^+$] and [B] are the respective concentrations of the ionized and unionized forms of the weak basic drug, which are in equilibrium and in solution in the gastrointestinal fluids.

Therefore, according to these equations, a weakly acidic drug, pK_a 3.0, will be predominantly (98.4%) unionized in gastric fluid at pH 1.2 and almost totally (99.98%) ionized in intestinal fluid at pH 6.8, whereas a weakly basic drug, pK_a 5, will be almost entirely (99.98%) ionized at gastric pH of 1.2 and predominantly

(98.4%) unionized at intestinal pH of 6.8. This means that, according to the pH-partition hypothesis, a weakly acidic drug is more likely to be absorbed from the stomach where it is unionized and a weakly basic drug from the intestine where it is predominantly unionized. However, in practice, other factors need to be taken into consideration.

Limitations of the pH-partition hypothesis The extent to which a drug exists in its unionized form is not the only factor determining the rate and extent of absorption of a drug molecule from the gastrointestinal tract. Despite their high degree of ionization, weak acids are still quite well absorbed from the small intestine. In fact, the rate of intestinal absorption of a weak acid is often higher than its rate of absorption in the stomach, even though the drug is unionized in the stomach. The significantly larger surface area that is available for absorption in the small intestine more than compensates for the high degree of ionization of weakly acidic drugs at intestinal pH values. In addition, a longer small intestinal residence time and a microclimate pH (that exists at the surface of the intestinal mucosa and is lower than that of the luminal pH of the small intestine) are thought to aid the absorption of weak acids from the small intestine.

The mucosal unstirred layer is another recognized component of the gastrointestinal barrier to drug absorption that is not accounted for in the pH-partition hypothesis. During absorption, drug molecules must diffuse across this layer and then on through the lipid layer. Diffusion across this layer is liable to be a significant component of the total absorption process for those drugs that cross the lipid layer very quickly. Diffusion across this layer will also depend on the relative molecular weight of the drug.

The pH-partition hypothesis cannot explain the fact that certain drugs (e.g. quaternary ammonium compounds and tetracyclines) are readily absorbed despite being ionized over the entire pH range of the gastrointestinal tract. One suggestion for this is that the gastrointestinal barrier is not completely impermeable to ionized drugs. It is now generally accepted that ionized forms of drugs are absorbed in the small intestine but at a much slower rate than the unionized form. Another possibility is that such drugs interact with endogenous organic ions of opposite charge to form an absorbable neutral species – an *ion pair* – which is capable of partitioning into the lipoidal gastrointestinal barrier and being absorbed via passive diffusion.

A physiological factor that causes deviations from the pH-partition hypothesis is *convective flow* or *solvent drag*. The movement of water molecules into and out of the gastrointestinal tract will affect the rate of passage of small water-soluble molecules across the gastrointestinal barrier. Water movement occurs because of differences in osmotic pressure between blood and the luminal contents and because of differences in hydrostatic pressure between the lumen and the perivascular tissue. The absorption of water-soluble drugs will be increased if water flows from the lumen to the blood, provided that the drug and water are using the same route of absorption. This will have greatest effect in the jejunum, where water movement is at its greatest. Water flow also affects the absorption of lipid-soluble drugs. It is thought that this is because the drug becomes more concentrated as water flows out of the intestine, thereby favouring a greater drug concentration gradient and increased absorption.

Lipid solubility A number of drugs are poorly absorbed from the gastrointestinal tract despite the fact that their unionized forms predominate. For example, the barbiturates barbitone and thiopentone have similar dissociation constants – pK_a 7.8 and 7.6 respectively – and therefore similar degrees of ionization at intestinal pH. However, thiopentone is absorbed much better than barbitone. The reason for this difference is that the absorption of drugs is also affected by the lipid solubility of the drug. Thiopentone, being more lipid soluble than barbitone, exhibits a greater affinity for the gastrointestinal membrane and is thus far better absorbed.

An indication of the lipid solubility of a drug, and therefore whether that drug is liable to be transported across membranes, is given by its ability to partition between a lipid-like solvent and water or an aqueous buffer. This is known as the drug's *partition coefficient* and is a measure of its lipophilicity. The value of the partition coefficient P is determined by measuring the drug partitioning between water and a suitable non-water miscible solvent at constant temperature. As this ratio normally spans several orders of magnitude it is usually expressed as the logarithm, log P. The solvent that is usually selected to mimic the biological membrane, because of its many similar properties, is octanol.

$$\text{Partition coefficient} = \frac{\begin{array}{c}\text{concentration of drug}\\\text{in organic phase}\end{array}}{\begin{array}{c}\text{concentration in}\\\text{aqueous phase}\end{array}} \quad (21.5)$$

The effective partition coefficient, taking into account the degree of ionization of the drug, is known as the *distribution coefficient* and again is normally expressed as the logarithm (log D); it is given by the following equations for acids and bases:

For acids:

$$D = \frac{[\text{HA}]_{\text{org}}}{[\text{HA}]_{\text{aq}} + [\text{A}^-]_{\text{aq}}} \quad (21.6)$$

$$\log D = \log P - [1 + \text{antilog} (\text{pH} - pK_a)] \quad (21.7)$$

For bases:

$$D = \frac{[B]_{org}}{[B]_{aq} + [BH^+]_{aq}} \qquad (21.8)$$

$$\log D = \log P - [1 + \text{antilog}\,(pK_a - pH)] \quad (21.9)$$

The lipophilicity of a drug is critical in the drug discovery process. Polar molecules, i.e. those that are poorly lipid soluble ($\log P < 0$) and relatively large, such as gentamicin, ceftriaxone, heparin and streptokinase, are poorly absorbed after oral administration and therefore have to be given by injection. Smaller molecules that are poorly lipid soluble and hydrophilic in nature, such as the β-blocker atenolol, can be absorbed via the paracellular route. Lipid-soluble drugs with favourable partition coefficients (i.e. $\log P > 0$) are usually absorbed after oral administration. Drugs which are very lipid soluble ($\log P > 3$) tend to be well absorbed but are also more likely to be susceptible to metabolism and biliary clearance. Although there is no general rule that can be applied to *all* drug molecules, within a homologous series drug absorption usually increases as the lipophilicity rises. This has been shown for a series of barbiturates by Schanker (1960) and for a series of β-blockers by Taylor et al (1985).

Sometimes, if the structure of a compound cannot be modified to yield lipid solubility while maintaining pharmacological activity, medicinal chemists may investigate the possibility of making lipid prodrugs to improve absorption. A prodrug is a chemical modification, frequently an ester of an existing drug, which converts back to the parent compound as a result of metabolism by the body. A prodrug itself has no pharmacological activity. Examples of prodrugs which have been successfully used to improve the lipid solubility and hence absorption of their parent drugs are shown in Table 21.3.

Molecular size and hydrogen bonding Two other drug properties that are important in permeability are the number of hydrogen bonds within the molecule and the molecular size:

For paracellular absorption, the molecular weight should ideally be less than 200 Da; however, there are examples where larger molecules (up to molecular weights of 400 Da) have been absorbed via this route. Shape is also an important factor for paracellular absorption.

In general, for transcellular passive diffusion, a molecular weight of less than 500 Da is preferable. Drugs with molecular weights above this may be absorbed less efficiently. There are few examples of drugs with molecular weights above 700 Da being well absorbed.

Too many hydrogen bonds within a molecule are detrimental to its absorption. In general, no more than five hydrogen bond donors and no more than 10 hydrogen bond acceptors (the sum of nitrogen and oxygen atoms in the molecule is often taken as a rough measure of hydrogen bond acceptors) should be present if the molecule is to be well absorbed. The large number of hydrogen bonds within peptides is one of the reasons why peptide drugs are poorly absorbed.

Summary

There are many properties of the drug itself that will influence its passage into solution in the gastrointestinal tract and across the gastrointestinal membrane, and hence its overall rate and extent of absorption.

DOSAGE FORM FACTORS INFLUENCING BIOAVAILABILITY

Introduction

The rate and/or extent of absorption of a drug from the gastrointestinal tract have been shown to be influenced by many physiological factors and by many physicochemical properties associated with the drug itself. The bioavailability of a drug can also be influenced by factors associated with the formulation and production of the dosage form. Increasingly, many dosage forms are being designed to affect the release and absorption of drugs, for example controlled-release systems (see Chapter 32) and delivery systems for poorly soluble drugs. This section summarizes how the type of dosage form and the excipients used in conventional oral dosage forms can affect the rate and extent of drug absorption.

Influence of the type of dosage form

The type of dosage form and its method of preparation or manufacture can influence bioavailability. Thus, whether a particular drug administered in the form of a solution, a suspension or solid dosage form can influence its rate

Table 21.3	Prodrugs with improved lipid solubility and oral absorption	
Prodrug	**Active drug**	**Ester**
Pivampicillin	Ampicillin	Pivaloyloxymethyl
Bacampicillin	Ampicillin	Carbonate
Indanylcarbenicillin	Carbenicillin	Indanyl
Cefuroxime axetil	Cefuroxime	Acetylethyl
Enalapril	Enalaprilat	Ester of 1-carboxylic acid
Ibuterol	Terbutaline	Dibutyl

and/or extent of absorption from the gastrointestinal tract. The type of oral dosage form will influence the number of possible intervening steps between administration and the appearance of dissolved drug in the gastrointestinal fluids, i.e. it will influence the release of drug into solution in the gastrointestinal fluids (Fig. 21.3).

In general, drugs must be in solution in the gastrointestinal fluids before absorption can occur. Thus the greater the number of intervening steps, the greater will be the number of potential obstacles to absorption and the greater will be the likelihood of that type of dosage form reducing the bioavailability exhibited by the drug. Hence the bioavailability of a given drug tends to decrease in the following order of types of dosage form: aqueous solutions > aqueous suspensions > solid dosage forms (e.g. hard gelatin capsules or tablets). Although this ranking is not universal, it does provide a useful guideline. In general, solutions and suspensions are the most suitable for administering drugs intended to be rapidly absorbed. However, it should be noted that other factors (e.g. stability, patient acceptability, etc.) can also influence the type of dosage form in which a drug is administered via the gastrointestinal route.

Aqueous solutions

For drugs that are water soluble and chemically stable in aqueous solution, formulation as a solution normally eliminates the in vivo dissolution step and presents the drug in the most readily available form for absorption. However, dilution of an aqueous solution of a poorly water-soluble drug whose aqueous solubility had been increased by formulation techniques such as cosolvency, complex formation or solubilization can result in precipitation of the drug in the gastric fluids. Similarly, exposure of an aqueous solution of a salt of a weak acidic compound to gastric pH can also result in precipitation of the free acid form of the drug. In most cases the extremely fine nature of the resulting precipitate permits a more rapid rate of dissolution than if the drug had been administered in other types of oral dosage forms, such as aqueous suspension, hard gelatin capsule or tablet. However, for some drugs this precipitation can have a major effect on bioavailability. The same dose of an experimental drug was given to dogs in three different solution formulations: a polyethylene glycol solution and two different concentrations of hydroxypropyl-β-cyclodextrin. Bioavailabilities of 19%, 57% and 89% were obtained for polyethylene glycol, the lower concentration and the higher concentration of hydroxypropyl-β-cyclodextrin, respectively. The difference in bioavailability of the three solutions was attributed to the difference in precipitation rates of the candidate drug from the three solutions on dilution. The experimental drug was observed to precipitate most quickly from the polyethylene glycol solution, and slowest from the most concentrated hydroxypropyl-β-cyclodextrin solution.

Factors associated with the formulation of aqueous solutions that can influence drug bioavailability

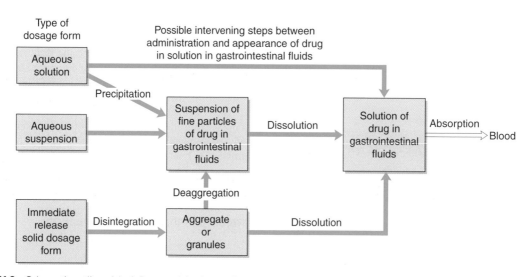

Fig. 21.3 Schematic outline of the influence of the dosage form on the appearance of drug in solution in the gastrointestinal tract.

include:

- the chemical stability exhibited by the drug in aqueous solution and the gastrointestinal fluids
- complexation, i.e. the formation of a chemical complex between the drug and an excipient. The formation of such a complex can increase the aqueous solubility of the drug or increase the viscosity of the dosage form
- solubilization, i.e. the incorporation of the drug into micelles in order to increase its aqueous solubility
- the viscosity of a solution dosage form, particularly if a viscosity-enhancing agent has been included.

Information concerning the potential influence of each of the above factors was given earlier in this chapter. Further details concerning the formulation and uses of oral solution dosage forms are given in Chapter 25.

Aqueous suspensions

An aqueous suspension is a useful dosage form for administering an insoluble or poorly water-soluble drug. Usually the absorption of a drug from this type of dosage form is dissolution rate limited. The oral administration of an aqueous suspension results in a large total surface area of dispersed drug being immediately presented to the gastrointestinal fluids. This facilitates dissolution and hence absorption of the drug. In contrast to powder-filled hard gelatin capsule and tablet dosage forms, dissolution of all drug particles commences immediately on dilution of the suspension in the gastrointestinal fluids. A drug contained in a tablet or hard gelatin capsule may ultimately achieve the same state of dispersion in the gastrointestinal fluids but only after a delay. Thus a well-formulated, finely sub-divided aqueous suspension is regarded as being an efficient oral drug delivery system second only to a non-precipitating solution-type dosage form.

Factors associated with the formulation of aqueous suspension dosage forms that can influence the bioavailabilities of drugs from the gastrointestinal tract include:

- the particle size and effective surface area of the dispersed drug
- the crystal form of the drug
- any resulting complexation, i.e. the formation of a non-absorbable complex between the drug and an excipient such as the suspending agent
- the inclusion of a surfactant as a wetting, flocculating or deflocculating agent
- the viscosity of the suspension.

Information concerning the potential influence of the above factors on drug bioavailability is given in earlier sections of this chapter. Further information concerning

the formulation and uses of suspensions as dosage forms is given in Chapter 27.

Liquid-filled capsules

Liquids can be filled into capsules made from soft or hard gelatin. Both types combine the convenience of a unit dosage form with the potentially rapid drug absorption associated with aqueous solutions and suspensions. Drugs encapsulated in liquid-filled capsules for peroral administration are dissolved or dispersed in non-toxic, non-aqueous vehicles. Such vehicles may be water immiscible (i.e. lipophilic) or water miscible (i.e. hydrophilic). Vegetable oils are popular water-immiscible vehicles, whereas polyethylene glycols and certain non-ionic surfactants (e.g. polysorbate 80) are water miscible. Sometimes the vehicles have thermal properties such that they can be filled into capsules while hot but are solids at room temperature.

The release of the contents of gelatin capsules is effected by dissolution and splitting of the flexible shell. Following release, a water-miscible vehicle disperses and/or dissolves readily in the gastrointestinal fluids, liberating the drug (depending on its aqueous solubility) as either a solution or a fine suspension, which is conducive to rapid absorption. In the case of gelatin capsules containing drugs in solution or suspension in water-immiscible vehicles, release of the contents will almost certainly be followed by dispersion in the gastrointestinal fluids. Dispersion is facilitated by emulsifiers included in the vehicle, and also by bile. Once dispersed, the drug may end up as an emulsion, a solution, a fine suspension or a nano/microemulsion.

Well-formulated liquid-filled capsules are designed to improve the absorption of poorly soluble drugs and will ensure that no precipitation of drug occurs from the nano- or microemulsion formed in the gastrointestinal fluids. If the lipophilic vehicle is a digestible oil and the drug is highly soluble in the oil, it is possible that the drug will remain in solution in the dispersed oil phase and be absorbed (along with the oil) by fat absorption processes. For a drug that is less lipophilic or is dissolved in a non-digestible oil, absorption probably occurs following partitioning of the drug from the oily vehicle into the aqueous gastrointestinal fluids. In this case the rate of drug absorption appears to depend on the rate at which drug partitions from the dispersed oil phase. The increase in interfacial area of contact resulting from dispersion of the oily vehicle in the gastrointestinal fluids will facilitate partition of the drug across the oil/aqueous interface. For drugs suspended in an oily vehicle, release may involve dissolution in the vehicle, diffusion to the oil/aqueous interface and partition across the interface.

Many poorly water-soluble drugs have been found to exhibit greater bioavailabilities from liquid-filled capsule formulations. The cardiac glycoside digoxin, when formulated as a solution in a mixture of polyethylene glycol, ethanol and propylene glycol in a soft gelatin capsule, has been shown to be absorbed faster than from the standard commercial tablets.

More recently, far more complex capsule formulations have been investigated to improve the absorption of poorly soluble drugs. Ciclosporin is a hydrophobic drug with poor solubility in gastrointestinal fluids. It showed low and variable oral bioavailability from its original liquid-filled soft gelatin capsule formulation (Sandimmun) and was particularly sensitive to the presence of fat in diet and bile acids. In its new formulation (Sandimmun Neoral), which is a complex mixture of hydrophilic and lipophilic phases, surfactants, cosurfactants and a cosolvent, it forms a non-precipitating microemulsion on dilution with gastrointestinal fluids. It has a significantly improved bioavailability with reduced variability that is independent of the presence of food (Drewe et al 1992).

Many protease inhibitors (antiviral drugs) are peptidomimetic in nature. They have high molecular weights and low aqueous solubility, are susceptible to degradation in the lumen and extensive hepatic metabolism, and consequently have poor bioavailability (Barry et al 1997). Saquinavir has been reformulated from a powder-filled hard gelatin capsule (Invirase) to a complex soft gelatin formulation (Fortovase). The latter shows a significant improvement in bioavailability (3–4 times) over the standard hard gelatin formulation and, as a consequence, a significantly greater viral load reduction (Perry & Noble 1998).

Factors associated with the formulation of liquid-filled gelatin capsules that can influence the bioavailabilities of drugs from this type of dosage form include:

- the solubility of the drug in the vehicle (and gastrointestinal fluids)
- the particle size of the drug (if suspended in the vehicle)
- the nature of the vehicle, i.e. hydrophilic or lipophilic (and whether a lipophilic vehicle is a digestible or a non-digestible oil)
- the inclusion of a surfactant as a wetting/emulsifying agent in a lipophilic vehicle or as the vehicle itself
- the inclusion of a suspending agent (viscosity-enhancing agent) in the vehicle
- the complexation, i.e. formation, of a non-absorbable complex between the drug and any excipient.

More information on liquid-filled hard gelatin capsules can be found in Chapter 34.

Powder-filled capsules

Generally the bioavailability of a drug from a well-formulated powder-filled hard gelatin capsule dosage form will be better than or at least equal to that from the same drug in a compacted tablet. Provided the hard gelatin shell dissolves rapidly in the gastrointestinal fluids and the encapsulated mass disperses rapidly and efficiently, a relatively large effective surface area of drug will be exposed to the gastrointestinal fluids, thereby facilitating dissolution. However, it is incorrect to assume that a drug formulated as a hard gelatin capsule is in a finely divided form surrounded by a water-soluble shell and that no bioavailability problems can occur. The overall rate of dissolution of drugs from capsules appears to be a complex function of the rates of different processes – such as the dissolution rate of the gelatin shell, the rate of penetration of the gastrointestinal fluids into the encapsulated mass, the rate at which the mass deaggregates (i.e. disperses) in the gastrointestinal fluids and the rate of dissolution of the dispersed drug particles.

The inclusion of excipients (e.g. diluents, lubricants and surfactants) in a capsule formulation can have a significant effect on the rate of dissolution of drugs, particularly those that are poorly soluble and hydrophobic. Figure 21.4 shows that a hydrophilic diluent (e.g. sorbitol, lactose) often serves to increase the rate of penetration of the aqueous gastrointestinal fluids into the contents of the capsule and to aid the dispersion and subsequent dissolution of the drug in these fluids. However, the diluent should exhibit no tendency to adsorb or complex with the drug as either can impair absorption from the gastrointestinal tract.

Both the formulation and the type and process conditions of the capsule-filling process can affect the packing density and liquid permeability of the capsule contents. In general, an increase in packing density (i.e. a decrease in porosity) of the encapsulated mass will probably result in a decrease in liquid permeability and dissolution rate, particularly if the drug is hydrophobic or if a hydrophilic drug is mixed with a hydrophobic lubricant such as magnesium stearate. If the encapsulated mass is tightly packed and the drug is hydrophobic in nature then a decrease in dissolution rate with a concomitant reduction in particle size would be expected unless a surfactant had been included to facilitate liquid penetration.

In summary, formulation factors that can influence the bioavailabilities of drugs from hard gelatin capsules include:

- the surface area and particle size of the drug (particularly the effective surface area exhibited by the drug in the gastrointestinal fluids)

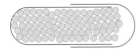

Hard gelatin capsule containing
only hydrophobic drug particles

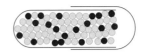

Hard gelatin capsule containing
hydrophobic drug particles (◯)
and hydrophilic diluent particles (●)

In gastrointestinal fluids, hard gelatin capsule shell dissolves, thereby exposing contents to fluids

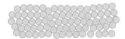

Contents remain as a capsule-shaped
plug. Hydrophobic nature of contents
impedes penetration of gastrointestinal
fluids

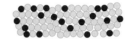

Particles of hydrophilic diluent
dissolve in gastrointestinal fluids
leaving a porous mass of drug

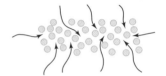

Gastrointestinal fluids can penetrate
porous mass

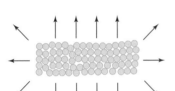

Dissolution of drug occurs only from
surface of plug-shaped mass. Relatively
low rate of dissolution

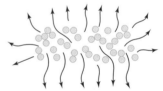

Effective surface area of drug and hence
dissolution rate is increased

Fig. 21.4 Diagrammatic representation of how a hydrophilic diluent can increase the rate of dissolution of a poorly soluble, hydrophobic drug from a hard gelatin capsule.

- the use of the salt form of a drug in preference to the parent weak acid or base
- the crystal form of the drug
- the chemical stability of the drug (in the dosage form and in gastrointestinal fluids)
- the nature and quantity of the diluent, lubricant and wetting agent
- drug–excipient interactions (e.g. adsorption, complexation)
- the type and conditions of the filling process
- the packing density of the capsule contents
- the composition and properties of the capsule shell (including enteric capsules)
- interactions between the capsule shell and its contents.

Tablets

Uncoated tablets   Tablets are the most widely used dosage form. When a drug is formulated as a compacted tablet there is an enormous reduction in the effective surface area of the drug, owing to the granulation and compaction processes involved in tablet making. These processes necessitate the addition of excipients, which serve to return the surface area of the drug back to its original precompacted state. Bioavailability problems can arise if a fine, well-dispersed suspension of drug particles in the gastrointestinal fluids is not generated following the administration of a tablet. Because the effective surface area of a poorly soluble drug is an important factor influencing its dissolution rate, it is especially important that tablets containing such drugs should disintegrate rapidly and completely in the gastrointestinal fluids if rapid release, dissolution and absorption are required. The overall rate of tablet disintegration is influenced by several interdependent factors, which include the concentration and type of drug, diluent, binder, disintegrant, lubricant and wetting agent, as well as the compaction pressure (discussed in Chapter 31).

The dissolution of a poorly soluble drug from an intact tablet is usually extremely limited because of the relatively small effective surface area of drug exposed to the gastrointestinal fluids. Disintegration of the tablet into granules causes a relatively large increase in effective surface area of drug and the dissolution rate may be likened to that of a coarse, aggregated suspension. Further disintegration into small, primary drug particles produces a further large increase in effective surface area and dissolution rate. The dissolution rate is probably comparable to that of a fine, well-dispersed suspension. Disintegration of a tablet into primary particles is thus important, as it ensures that a large effective surface area of a drug is generated in order to facilitate dissolution and subsequent absorption.

However, simply because a tablet disintegrates rapidly, does not necessarily guarantee that the liberated primary drug particles will dissolve in the gastrointestinal fluids and the rate and extent of absorption are adequate. In the case of poorly water-soluble drugs, the rate-controlling step is usually the overall rate of dissolution of the liberated drug particles in the gastrointestinal fluids. The overall dissolution rate and bioavailability of a poorly soluble drug from an uncoated conventional tablet is influenced by many factors associated with the formulation and manufacture of this type of dosage form. These include:

- the physicochemical properties of the liberated drug particles in the gastrointestinal fluids, e.g. wettability, effective surface area, crystal form, chemical stability
- the nature and quantity of the diluent, binder, disintegrant, lubricant and any wetting agent
- drug–excipient interactions (e.g. complexation)
- the size of the granules and their method of manufacture
- the compaction pressure and speed of compaction used in tableting
- the conditions of storage and age of the tablet.

Because drug absorption and hence bioavailability are dependent upon the drug being in the dissolved state, suitable dissolution characteristics can be an important property of a satisfactory tablet, particularly if it contains a poorly soluble drug. On this basis, specific in vitro dissolution test conditions and dissolution limits are included in many pharmacopoeias for tablets (and hard gelatin capsules) for certain drugs. That a particular drug product meets the requirements of a compendial dissolution standard provides a greater assurance that the drug will be released satisfactorily from the formulated dosage form in vivo and be absorbed adequately (also discussed in Chapter 22).

More information on drug release from tablets can be found in Chapter 31.

Coated tablets Tablet coatings may be used simply for aesthetic reasons, to improve the appearance of a tablet or to add a company identity, may be employed to mask an unpleasant taste or odour or to protect an ingredient from decomposition during storage. Currently the most common type of tablet coat is that created with a polymer film. However, several older preparations, such as tablets containing vitamins, ibuprofen and conjugated oestrogens, still have sugar coats.

The presence of a coating presents a physical barrier between the tablet core and the gastrointestinal fluids. Coated tablets therefore not only possess all the potential bioavailability problems associated with uncoated conventional tablets but are subject to the additional potential problem of being surrounded by a physical barrier. In the case of a coated tablet which is intended to disintegrate/dissolve and release drug rapidly into solution in the gastrointestinal fluids, the coating must dissolve or disrupt before these processes can begin. The physicochemical nature and thickness of the coating can thus influence how quickly a drug is released from a tablet.

In the process of sugar coating, the tablet core is usually sealed with a thin continuous film of a poorly water-soluble polymer such as shellac or cellulose acetate phthalate. This sealing coat serves to protect the tablet core and its contents from the aqueous fluids used in the subsequent steps of the sugar-coating process. The presence of this water-impermeable sealing coat can potentially retard drug release from sugar-coated tablets. In view of this potential problem, annealing agents such as polyethylene glycols or calcium carbonate, which do not substantially reduce the water impermeability of the sealing coat during sugar coating but which dissolve readily in gastric fluid, may be added to the sealer coat in order to reduce the barrier effect to rapid drug release.

The film coating of a tablet core by a thin film of a water-soluble polymer, such as hydroxypropyl methycellulose, should have no significant effect on the rate of disintegration of the tablet core and subsequent drug dissolution, provided that the film coat dissolves rapidly and independently of the pH of the gastrointestinal fluids. However, if hydrophobic water-insoluble film-coating materials, such as ethylcellulose or certain acrylic resins, are used (Chapter 33), the resulting film coat acts as a barrier which delays and/or reduces the rate of drug release. Thus these types of film-coating materials form barriers which can have a significant influence on drug absorption. Although the formation of such barriers would be disadvantageous in the case of film-coated tablets intended to provide rapid rates of drug absorption, the concept of barrier coating has been used (along with other techniques) to obtain more precise control over drug release than is possible with conventional uncoated tablets (see Chapter 32). In this context, film coating has been used to provide limited control over the site at which a drug is released from a tablet into the gastrointestinal tract.

Enteric-coated tablets   The use of barrier coating to control the site of release of an orally administered drug is well illustrated by enteric-coated tablets. An enteric coat is designed to resist the low pH of gastric fluids but to disrupt or dissolve when the tablet enters the higher pH of the duodenum. Polymers such as cellulose acetate phthalate, hydroxypropyl methylcellulose phthalate, some copolymers of methacrylic acid and their esters and polyvinyl acetate phthalate can be used as enteric coatings. These materials do not dissolve over the gastric pH range but dissolve rapidly at the less acid pH (about 5) values associated with the small intestine. Enteric coating should preferably begin to dissolve at pH 5 in order to ensure the availability of drugs which are absorbed primarily in the proximal region of the small intestine. Enteric coating thus provides a means of delaying the release of a drug until the dosage form reaches the small intestine. Such delayed release provides a means of protecting drugs which would otherwise be destroyed if released into gastric fluid. Hence, enteric coating serves to improve the oral bioavailability exhibited by such drugs from uncoated conventional tablets. Enteric coating also protects the stomach against drugs which can produce nausea or mucosal irritation (e.g. aspirin, ibuprofen) if released at this site.

In addition to the protection offered by enteric coating, the delayed release of drug also results in a significant delay in the onset of the therapeutic response of a drug. The onset of the therapeutic response is largely dependent on the residence time of the enteric-coated tablet in the stomach. Gastric emptying of such tablets is an all-or-nothing process, i.e. the tablet is either in the stomach or in the duodenum. Consequently, drug is either not being released or being released. The residence time of an intact enteric-coated tablet in the stomach can vary from about 5 minutes to several hours (discussed further in Chapter 20). Hence there is considerable intra- and intersubject variation in the onset of therapeutic action exhibited by drugs administered as enteric-coated tablets.

The formulation of an enteric-coated product in the form of small individually enteric-coated granules or pellets (multiparticulates) contained in a rapidly dissolving hard gelatin capsule or a rapidly disintegrating tablet largely eliminates the dependency of this type of dosage form on the all-or-nothing gastric emptying process associated with intact (monolith) enteric-coated tablets. Provided the coated granules or pellets are sufficiently small (around 1 mm diameter), they will be able to empty from the stomach with liquids. Hence enteric-coated granules and pellets exhibit a gradual but continual release from the stomach into the duodenum. This type of release also avoids the complete dose of drug being released into the duodenum, as occurs with an enteric-coated tablet. The intestinal mucosa is thus not exposed locally to a potentially toxic concentration of drug.

Further information on coated tablets and multiparticulates is given in Chapter 33.

Influence of excipients for conventional dosage forms

Drugs are almost never administered alone but rather in dosage forms that generally consist of a drug (or drugs) together with a varying number of other substances (called *excipients*). Excipients are added to the formulation in order to facilitate the preparation, patient acceptability and functioning of the dosage form as a drug delivery system. Excipients include disintegrating agents, diluents, lubricants, suspending agents, emulsifying agents, flavouring agents, colouring agents, chemical stabilizers, etc. Although historically excipients were considered to be inert in that they themselves should exert no therapeutic or biological action or modify the biological action of the drug present in the dosage form, they are now regarded as having the ability to influence the rate and/or extent of absorption of the drug. For instance, the potential influence of excipients on drug bioavailability has already been illustrated by the formation of poorly soluble, non-absorbable drug–excipient complexes between tetracyclines and dicalcium phosphate, amfetamine and sodium carboxymethylcellulose, and phenobarbital and polyethylene glycol 4000.

Diluents   The classic example of the influence that excipients employed as diluents can have on drug bioavailability is provided by the observed increase in the incidence of phenytoin intoxication which occurred in epileptic patients in Australia as a consequence of the diluent in sodium phenytoin capsules being changed. Many epileptic patients who had been previously stabilized with sodium phenytoin capsules containing calcium sulfate dihydrate as the diluent developed clinical features of phenytoin overdosage when given sodium phenytoin capsules containing lactose as the diluent, even though the quantity of drug in each capsule formulation was identical. The experimental data from this study are shown in Figure 34.6. It was later shown that the excipient calcium sulfate dihydrate had been responsible for decreasing the gastrointestinal absorption of phenytoin, possibly because part of the administered dose of drug formed a poorly absorbable calcium-–phenytoin complex. Hence, although the size of dose and frequency of administration of the sodium phenytoin capsules containing calcium sulfate dihydrate gave therapeutic blood levels of phenytoin in epileptic patients, the efficiency of absorption of phenytoin had been lowered by the incorporation of this excipient in the hard gelatin capsules. Hence, when the calcium sulfate dihydrate was replaced by lactose without any alteration in the quantity of drug in each capsule, or in the frequency of administration, an increased bioavailability of phenytoin was achieved. In many patients the higher plasma levels exceeded the maximum safe concentration for phenytoin and produced toxic side-effects.

Surfactants Surfactants are often used in dosage forms as emulsifying agents, solubilizing agents, suspension stabilizers or wetting agents. However, surfactants in general cannot be assumed to be 'inert' excipients as they have been shown to be capable of increasing, decreasing or exerting no effect on the transfer of drugs across biological membranes.

Surfactant monomers can potentially disrupt the integrity and function of a biological membrane. Such an effect would tend to enhance drug penetration and hence absorption across the gastrointestinal barrier but may also result in toxic side-effects. Inhibition of absorption may occur as a consequence of a drug being incorporated into surfactant micelles. If such surfactant micelles are not absorbed, which appears usually to be the case, then solubilization of a drug may result in a reduction of the concentration of 'free' drug in solution in the gastrointestinal fluids that is available for absorption. Inhibition of drug absorption in the presence of micellar concentrations of surfactant would be expected to occur in the case of drugs that are normally soluble in the gastrointestinal fluids, i.e. in the absence of surfactant. Conversely, in the case of poorly soluble drugs whose absorption is dissolution rate limited, the increase in saturation solubility of the drug by solubilization in surfactant micelles could result in more rapid rates of dissolution and hence absorption.

The release of poorly soluble drugs from tablets and hard gelatin capsules may be increased by the inclusion of surfactants in their formulations. The ability of a surfactant to reduce the solid/liquid interfacial tension will permit the gastrointestinal fluids to wet the solid more effectively and thus enable it to come into more intimate contact with the solid dosage forms. This wetting effect may thus aid the penetration of gastrointestinal fluids into the mass of capsule contents that often remains when the hard gelatin shell has dissolved, and/or reduce the tendency of poorly soluble drug particles to aggregate in the gastrointestinal fluids. In each case the resulting increase in the total effective surface area of drug in contact with the gastrointestinal fluids would tend to increase the dissolution and absorption rates of the drug. It is interesting to note that the enhanced gastrointestinal absorption of phenacetin in humans resulting from the addition of polysorbate 80 to an aqueous suspension of this drug was attributed to the surfactant preventing aggregation and thus increasing the effective surface area and dissolution rate of the drug particles in the gastrointestinal fluids.

The possible mechanisms by which surfactants can influence drug absorption are varied and it is likely that only rarely will a single mechanism operate in isolation. In most cases the overall effect on drug absorption will probably involve a number of different actions of the surfactant (some of which will produce opposing effects on drug absorption) and the observed effect on drug absorption will depend on which of the different actions is the overriding one. The ability of a surfactant to influence drug absorption will also depend on the physicochemical characteristics and concentration of the surfactant, the nature of the drug and the type of biological membrane involved.

Lubricants Both tablets and capsules require lubricants in their formulation to reduce friction between the powder and metal surfaces during their manufacture. Lubricants are often hydrophobic in nature. Magnesium stearate is commonly included as a lubricant during tablet compaction and capsule-filling operations. Its hydrophobic nature often retards liquid penetration into capsule ingredients so that after the shell has dissolved in the gastrointestinal fluids, a capsule-shaped plug often remains, especially when the contents have been machine-filled as a consolidated plug (see Chapter 34). Similar reductions in dissolution rate are observed when magnesium stearate is included in tablets. Alternatively, they can be overcome by the simultaneous addition of a wetting agent (i.e. a water-soluble surfactant) and the use of a hydrophilic diluent (e.g. stearic acid) or minimized by decreasing the magnesium stearate content of the formulation.

Disintegrants Disintegrants are required to break up capsules, tablets and granules into primary powder particles in order to increase the surface area of the drug exposed to the gastrointestinal fluids. A tablet that fails to disintegrate or disintegrates slowly may result in incomplete absorption or a delay in the onset of action of the drug. The compaction force used in tablet manufacture can affect disintegration. In general, the higher the force, the slower the disintegration time. Even small changes in formulation may result in significant effects on dissolution and bioavailability. A classic example is that of tolbutamide where two formulations, the commercial product and the same formulation but containing half the amount of disintegrant, were administered to healthy volunteers. Both tablets disintegrated in vitro within 10 minutes, meeting pharmacopoeial specifications, but the commercial tablet had a significantly greater bioavailability and hypoglycaemic response.

Viscosity-enhancing agents Viscosity-enhancing agents are often employed in the formulation of liquid dosage forms for oral use in order to control such properties as palatability, ease of pouring and, in the case of suspensions, the rate of sedimentation of the dispersed particles. Viscosity-enhancing agents are often hydrophilic polymers.

There are a number of mechanisms by which a viscosity-enhancing agent may produce a change in the gastrointestinal absorption of a drug. Complex formation between a drug and a hydrophilic polymer could reduce the concentration of drug in solution that is available for absorption. The administration of viscous solutions or suspensions may produce an increase in viscosity of the gastrointestinal contents. In turn, this could lead to a decrease in dissolution rate and/or a decrease in the rate of movement of drug molecules to the absorbing membrane.

Normally, a decrease in the rate of dissolution would not be applicable to solution dosage forms unless dilution of the administered solution in the gastrointestinal fluids caused precipitation of the drug.

In the case of suspensions containing drugs with bioavailabilities that are dissolution rate dependent, an increase in viscosity could also lead to a decrease in the rate of dissolution of the drug in the gastrointestinal tract.

SUMMARY

As well as physiological and drug factors, the dosage form can play a major role in influencing the rate and extent of absorption. Often this is by design. However, even with conventional dosage forms, it is important to consider whether changing the dosage form or excipients will affect the bioavailability of the drug. Some drugs will be more susceptible to changes in rate and extent of absorption through dosage form changes than others; this will depend on the biopharmaceutical properties of the drug, which form the basis of the next chapter (Chapter 22).

REFERENCES

Barry, M., Gibbons, S., Back, D., Mulcahy, F. (1997) Protease inhibitors in patients with HIV disease. Clinically important pharmacokinetic considerations. *Clinical Pharmacokinetics,* **32**(3), 194-209.

Dressman, J.B., Amidon, G.L., Reppas, C., Shah, V.P. (1998) Dissolution testing as a prognostic tool for oral drug absorption: immediate release dosage forms. *Pharmaceutical Research,* **15**, 11-22.

Drewe, J., Meier, R., Vonderscher, J. et al. (1992) Enhancement of oral absorption of cyclosporin in man. *British Journal of Clinical Pharmacology,* **34**, 60.

Florence, A.T., Attwood, D. (2006) *Physicochemical Principles of Pharmacy,* 4th edn. Pharmaceutical Press, London.

Lipinski, C.A., Lombardo, F., Dominy, B.W., Feeney, P.J. (1997) Experimental and computational approaches to estimate the solubility and permeability in drug discovery and development settings. *Advanced Drug Delivery Reviews,* **23**, 3-29.

Loper, A., Hettrick, L., Novak, L. et al. (1999) Factors influencing the absorption of an HIV protease inhibitor analogue of indinavir in beagle dogs. *AAPS PharmSciTech* (online), 42-43.

Panchagnula, R., Thomas, N.S. (2000) Biopharmaceutics and pharmacokinetics in drug research. *International Journal of Pharmaceutics,* **201**, 131-150.

Perry, C.M., Noble, S. (1998) Saquinavir soft-gel capsule formulation. A review of its use in patients with HIV infection. *Drugs,* **3**, 461-486.

Russell T.L., Beradi, R.R., Barnet, J.L. et al. (1994) Influence of gastric pH and emptying on dipyridamole absorption. *Pharmaceutical Research,* **11**, 136-143.

Schanker, L.S. (1960) On the mechanism of absorption of drugs from the gastrointestinal tract. *Journal of Medicinal and Pharmaceutical Chemistry,* **2**, 343-359.

Sevelius, H., Runkel, R., Segre, E. et al. (1980) Bioavailability of naproxen sodium and its relationship to clinical analgesic effects. *British Journal of Clinical Pharmacology,* **10**, 259.

Taylor, D.C., Pownall, R., Burke, W. (1985) Absorption of beta-adrenoceptor antagonists in the rat in situ small intestine. *Journal of Pharmacy and Pharmacology,* **37**, 280-283.

Terjarla, S., Puranjoti, P., Kasina, P., Mandal, J. (1998) Preparation, characterisation and evaluation of miconazole–cyclodextrin complexes for improved oral and topical delivery. *Journal of Pharmaceutical Science,* **87**, 425-429.

Van der Meer, J.W., Keuning, J.J., Scheijgrond, H.W., Heykants, J., Van Cutsem, J., Brugmans, J. (1980) The influence of gastric acidity on the bioavailability of ketoconazole. *Antimicrobial Agents and Chemotherapy,* **6**(4), 552-554.

22

Assessment of biopharmaceutical properties

M. Ashford

INTRODUCTION

Biopharmaceutics is concerned with factors that influence the rate and extent of drug absorption. As discussed in Chapters 20 and 21, the factors that affect the release of a drug from its dosage form, its dissolution into physiological fluids, its stability within those fluids, its permeability across the relevant biological membranes and its presystemic metabolism will all influence its rate and extent of absorption (Fig. 22.1). Once the drug is absorbed into the systemic circulation, its distribution within the body tissues (including to its site of action), its metabolism and elimination are described by the *pharmacokinetics* of the compound (discussed in Chapter 19). This in turn influences the length and magnitude of the therapeutic effect or the response of the compound, i.e. its *pharmacodynamics*.

The key biopharmaceutical properties that can be quantified and therefore give an insight into the absorption of a drug are its:

- release from its dosage form into solution at the absorption site
- stability in physiological fluids
- permeability
- susceptibility to presystemic clearance.

As most drugs are delivered via the mouth, these properties will be discussed with respect to the peroral route. The bioavailability of a compound is an overall measure of its availability in the systemic circulation and so the assessment of bioavailability will also be discussed. Other methods of assessing the performance of dosage forms in vivo will also be briefly mentioned. The Biopharmaceutical Classification Scheme, which classifies drugs according to two of their key biopharmaceutical properties, solubility and permeability, is outlined.

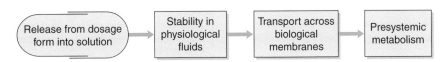

Fig. 22.1 Key biopharmaceutical properties affecting drug absorption.

MEASUREMENT OF KEY BIOPHARMACEUTICAL PROPERTIES

Release of drug from its dosage form into solution

As discussed in Chapter 21 and Part 5 of this book, a dosage form is normally formulated to aid and/or control the release of drug from it. For example, for an immediate-release tablet, the tablet needs to disintegrate to give the primary drug particles. Further, a suspension should not be so viscous that it impedes the diffusion of dissolving drug away from the solid particles.

The solubility of a drug across the gastrointestinal pH range will be one of the first indicators as to whether dissolution is liable to be rate limiting in the absorption process. Knowledge of the solubility across the gastrointestinal pH range can be determined by measuring the equilibrium solubility in suitable buffers or by using an acid or a base titration method.

Methods of measuring the dissolution rate of both a drug itself (intrinsic dissolution rate) and of various dosage forms are discussed in Chapters 2 and 24, and in the relevant chapter of Part 5.

The aim of dissolution testing is to find an in vitro characteristic of a potential formulation that reflects its in vivo performance. Historically, dissolution tests have been used mainly for quality control purposes and as a guide in the development of new formulations, rather than to predict the in vivo performance of the product. The tests tend to be carried out with standard procedures (volumes, agitation rates, etc.) and under sink conditions. These conditions are not representative of physiological conditions and are therefore liable to correlate poorly with the in vivo situation.

When designing a dissolution test to assess drug release from a biopharmaceutical perspective, it is important to mimic as closely as possible the conditions of the gastrointestinal tract. Clinical scientists increasingly want to rely on dissolution tests to establish in vitro/in vivo correlations between the release of drug from the dosage form and its absorption. If this can be successfully achieved, it is possible that the dissolution test could replace some of the in vivo studies that need to be performed during product development and registra-tion. Such correlations should have the benefit of reducing both the use of animals to evaluate formulations and the size and number of costly clinical studies to assess bioavailability.

An in vitro/in vivo correlation may only be possible for those drugs where dissolution is the rate-limiting step in the absorption process. Determining full dissolution profiles of such drugs in a number of different physiologically representative media will aid the understanding of the factors affecting the rate and extent of dissolution. The profiles can also be used to generate an in vitro/in vivo correlation. To achieve this, at least three batches that differ in their in vivo as well as their in vitro behaviour should be available. The differences in the in vivo profiles need to be mirrored by the formulations in vitro. Normally, the in vitro test conditions can be modified to correspond with the in vivo data to achieve a correlation. Very often, a well-designed in vitro dissolution test is found to be more sensitive and discriminating than an in vivo test. From a quality assurance perspective, a more discriminative dissolution method is preferred because the test will indicate possible changes in the product before the in vivo performance is affected.

A dilute hydrochloric acid-based solution at pH 1.2 can simulate gastric fluid quite closely (but obviously not exactly) and phosphate-buffered solution at pH 6.8 can mimic intestinal fluid. However, dissolution media more closely representing physiological conditions may well provide more relevant conditions. Dressman et al (1998) studied in detail a range of physiological parameters and suggested four more appropriate media for simulated gastric and intestinal conditions in the fed and fasted states. Each of these media takes into account not only the pH of the fluids in the different states but their ionic composition, surface tension, buffer capacity and bile and lecithin contents. The proposed compositions for gastric fluid in the fasted state and intestinal fluids in the fed and fasted states are shown in Tables 22.1–22.3.

The conditions within the stomach in the fed state are highly dependent on the composition of the meal eaten and therefore difficult to simulate. In trying to produce an in vitro/in vivo correlation, it has been suggested that a more appropriate way of simulating the fed-state gastric fluids is to homogenize the meal to be used in clinical studies and then dilute it with water. Long-life milk has

Table 22.1 Dissolution medium to simulate gastric conditions in the fasted state (proposed by Dressman et al 1998)

Component	Concentration/amount
Hydrochloric acid	0.01–0.05 M
Sodium lauryl sulfate	2.5 g
Sodium chloride	2 g
Distilled water	qs to 1000 mL

Table 22.3 Dissolution medium to simulate intestinal conditions in the fed state (proposed by Dressman et al 1998)

Component	Concentration/amount
Acetic acid	0.144 M
Sodium hydroxide	qs to pH 5
Sodium taurocholate (bile salt)	15 mM
Lecithin	4 mM
Potassium chloride	0.19 M
Distilled water	qs to 1000 mL

pH = 5
Osmolarity = 485–535 mOsmol
Buffer capacity = 76 ± 2 mEq/L/pH

also been used to simulate gastric conditions in the fed state.

It has been proposed that the duration of the dissolution test should depend on the site of absorption of the drug and its timing of administration. Thus, in designing a dissolution test, some knowledge or prediction of the permeability properties of the drug is beneficial. If, for example, the drug is absorbed from the upper intestine and is likely to be dosed in the fasted state, the most appropriate dissolution conditions may be a short test (~15–30 minutes) in a medium simulating gastric fluid in the fasted state (see Table 22.1). Alternatively, if it is advised that a drug should be administered with food and the drug is known to be well absorbed throughout the length of the gastrointestinal tract, a far longer dissolution test may be more appropriate. This could perhaps be several hours in duration with a range of media such as, initially, simulated gastric fluid to mimic the fed state, followed by simulated intestinal fluid to mimic both fed and fasted states.

The volumes of fluid in, and the degree of agitation of, the stomach and intestines vary enormously, particularly between the fed and the fasted states. Consequently it is difficult to choose a representative volume and degree of

agitation for an in vitro test. Guidance given to industry on the dissolution testing of immediate-release solid oral dosage forms suggests volumes of 500, 900 or 1000 mL and gentle agitation conditions.

Stability in physiological fluids

The stability of drugs in physiological fluids (in the case of orally administered drugs, the gastrointestinal fluids) depends on two factors:

- the chemical stability of the drug across the gastrointestinal pH range, i.e. the drug's pH stability profile between pH 1 and pH 8, and
- its susceptibility to enzymatic breakdown by the gastrointestinal fluids.

Means of assessing the chemical stability of a drug are discussed in Chapters 24 and 44. The stability of a drug in gastrointestinal fluids can be assessed by simulated gastric and intestinal media or by obtaining gastrointestinal fluids from humans or animals. The latter provides a harsher assessment of gastrointestinal stability but is more akin to the in vivo setting. In general, the drug is incubated with either real or simulated fluid at 37°C for a period of 3 hours and the drug content analysed. A loss of more than 5% of drug indicates potential instability. Many of the permeability methods described below can be used to identify whether gastrointestinal stability is an issue for a particular drug.

For drugs that will still be in the gastrointestinal lumen when they reach the colonic region, resistance to the bacterial enzymes present in this part of the intestine needs to be considered. The bacterial enzymes are capable of a whole host of reactions. There may be a significant portion of a poorly soluble drug still in the gastrointestinal tract by the time it reaches the colon. If the drug is

Table 22.2 Dissolution medium to simulate intestinal conditions in the fasted state (proposed by Dressman et al 1998)

Component	Concentration/amount
Potassium dihydrogen phosphate	0.029 M
Sodium hydroxide	qs to pH 6.8
Sodium taurocholate (bile salt)	5 mM
Lecithin	1.5 mM
Potassium chloride	0.22 M
Distilled water	qs to 1000 mL

pH = 6.8
Osmolarity = 280–310 mOsmol
Buffer capacity = 10 ± 2 mEq/L/pH

absorbed along the length of the gastrointestinal tract and is susceptible to degradation or metabolism by the bacterial enzymes within the tract, its absorption and hence its bioavailability are liable to be reduced. Similarly, for sustained- or controlled-release products that are designed to release their drug along the length of the gastrointestinal tract, the potential of degradation or metabolism by bacterial enzymes should be assessed. If the drug is metabolized to a metabolite which can be absorbed, the potential toxicity of this metabolite should be considered.

Permeability

There is a wealth of techniques available for either estimating or measuring the rate of permeation across membranes that are used to gain an assessment of oral absorption in humans. These range from computational (in silico) predictions to both physicochemical and biological methods. The biological methods can be further subdivided into in vitro, in situ and in vivo methods. In general, the more complex the technique, the more information that can be gained and the more accurate is the assessment of oral absorption in humans. The range of techniques is summarized in Table 22.4. Some of the more widely used ones are discussed below.

Partition coefficients

One of the first properties of a molecule that should be predicted or measured is its partition coefficient between an oil and a water phase (log P). This gives a measure of the lipophilicity of a molecule, which can be used as a prediction as to how well it will be able to cross a biological membrane. As discussed in Chapter 21,

Table 22.4 Some of the models available for predicting or measuring drug absorption

Model type	Model	Description
Computational	clog P	Commercial software that calculates octanol/water partition coefficient based on fragment analysis, known as the Leo–Hansch method
	mlog P	Method of calculating log P, known as the Moriguchi method (see text)
Physicochemical	Partition coefficient	Measure of lipophilicity of drug, usually measured between octanol and aqueous buffer via a shake-flask method
	Immobilized artificial membrane	Measures partition into more sophisticated lipidic phase on an HPLC column
Cell culture	Caco-2 monolayer	Measures transport across monolayers of differentiated human colon adenocarcinoma cells
	HT-29	Measures transport across polarized cell monolayer with mucin-producing cells
Excised tissues	Cells	Measures uptake into cell suspensions, e.g. erythrocytes
	Freshly isolated cells	Measures uptake into enterocytes; however, the cells are difficult to prepare and are short-lived
	Membrane vesicles	Measures uptake into brush border membrane vesicles prepared from intestinal scrapings or isolated enterocytes
	Everted sacs	Measures uptake into intestinal segments/sacs
	Everted intestinal rings	Studies the kinetics of uptake into the intestinal mucosa
	Isolated sheets	Measures the transport across sheets of intestine
In situ studies	In situ perfusion	Measures drug disappearance from either closed or open loop perfusate of segments of intestine of anaesthetized animals
	Vascularly perfused intestine	Measures drug disappearance from perfusate and its appearance in blood
In vivo studies	Intestinal loop	Measures drug disappearance from perfusate of loop of intestine in awake animal
Human data	Loc-I-Gut	Measures drug disappearance from perfusate of human intestine
	High-frequency capsule	Non-invasive method; measures drug in systemic circulation
	InteliSite capsule	Non-invasive method; measures drug in systemic circulation
	Bioavailability	Deconvolution of pharmacokinetic data

octanol is usually chosen as the solvent for the oil phase as it has similar properties to biological membranes. If the aqueous phase is at a particular pH, the distribution coefficient at that pH is measured (log *D*); this then accounts for the ionization of the molecule at that pH. In the case of a weakly acidic or a weakly basic drug, the log *D* measured at an intestinal pH (e.g. 6.8) is liable to give a better prediction of the drug's ability to cross the lipid gastrointestinal membrane than its partition coefficient, log *P*, which does not take the degree of ionization into account.

One of the most common ways of measuring partition coefficients is to use the shake flask method; this is discussed in Chapters 2 and 24. It relies on the equilibrium distribution of a drug between an oil and an aqueous phase. Prior to the experiment the aqueous phase should be saturated with the oil phase and vice versa. The experiment should be carried out at constant temperature. The drug should be added to the aqueous phase and the oil phase which, in the case of octanol, as it is less dense than water, will sit on top of the water. The system is mixed and then left to reach equilibrium (usually at least 24 hours). The two phases are separated and the concentration of drug is measured in each phase and a partition coefficient calculated (Fig. 22.2). As discussed in Chapter 21, within a homologous series, increasing lipophilicity (log *P* or log *D*) tends to result in greater absorption. A molecule is unlikely to cross a membrane (i.e. be absorbed via the transcellular passive route) if it has a log *P* less than 0.

Instead of determining log *P* experimentally, computational methods can be used to estimate it. There are a number of software packages available to do this. There is a reasonably good correlation between calculated and measured values. Log *P* can be estimated by breaking down the molecule into fragments and calculating the contribution of each fragment to overall lipophilicity (often called the *clog P*). Another way of estimating log *P* is the Moriguchi method, which uses 13 parameters for hydrophobic and hydrophilic atoms, proximity effects, unsaturated bonds, intramolecular bonds, ring structures, amphoteric properties and several specific functionalities

to obtain a value for the partition coefficient. This is often called the *m*log *P*. The advantages of these methods are in drug discovery, where an estimate of the lipophilicity of many molecules can be obtained before they are actually synthesized.

Another, more sophisticated physicochemical means of estimating how well a drug will partition into a lipophilic phase is by investigating how well the molecule can be retained on a high-performance liquid chromatography (HPLC) column. HPLC columns can be simply coated with octanol to mimic octanol-aqueous partition or, more elaborately, designed to mimic biological membranes. For example the immobilized artificial membrane (IAM) technique provides a measure of how well a solute (i.e. the drug) in the aqueous phase will partition into biological membranes (i.e. be retained on the column). Good correlations between these methods and biological in vitro methods of estimating transcellular passive drug absorption have been obtained.

Cell culture techniques

Cell culture techniques for measuring the intestinal absorption of molecules have been increasingly used over recent decades and are now a well-accepted model for absorption. The cell line that is most widely used is Caco-2.

Caco-2 cells are a human colon carcinoma cell line that was first proposed and characterized as a model for oral drug absorption by Hidalgo et al in 1989. In culture, Caco-2 cells spontaneously differentiate to form a monolayer of polarized enterocytes. These enterocytes resemble those in the small intestine, in that they contain microvilli and many of the transport systems present in the small intestine, for example those for sugars, amino acids, peptides and the P-glycoprotein efflux transporter. Adjacent Caco-2 cells adhere through tight junctions. However, the tightness of these junctions is more like those of the colon than those of the leakier small intestine.

There are many variations on growing and carrying out transport experiments with Caco-2 monolayers. In general, the cells are grown on porous supports, usually for a period of 15–21 days in typical cell culture medium, Dulbecco's Modified Eagle Medium supplemented with 20% fetal bovine serum, 1% non-essential amino acids and 2 mM L-glutamine. The cells are grown at 37°C in 10% carbon dioxide at a relative humidity of 95%. The culture medium is replaced at least twice each week. Transport experiments are carried out by replacing the culture medium with buffers, usually Hanks Balanced Salt Solution adjusted to pH 6.5 on the apical surface and Hanks Balanced Salt Solution adjusted to pH 7.4 on the basolateral surface (Fig. 22.3).

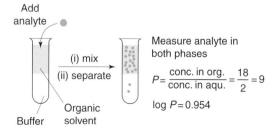

$$P = \frac{\text{conc. in org.}}{\text{conc. in aqu.}} = \frac{18}{2} = 9$$

$$\log P = 0.954$$

Fig. 22.2 Diagram of the shake-flask method for determining partition coefficient.

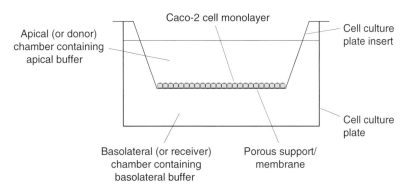

Fig. 22.3 Diagram of a Caco-2 cell culture system for determining apparent permeability.

After a short incubation period, usually about 30 minutes, when the cells are maintained at 37°C in a shaking water bath, the buffers are replaced with fresh buffers and a dilute solution of drug is introduced to the apical chamber. At regular intervals the concentration of the drug in the basolateral chamber is determined. The apparent permeability coefficient across cells can be calculated as follows:

$$P_{app} = dQ/dt(1/C_0 A) \qquad (22.1)$$

where P_{app} is the apparent permeability coefficient (cm/s), dQ/dt is the rate of drug transport (µg/s), C_0 is the initial donor concentration (mg/mL) and A is the surface area of the monolayer (cm²).

To check that the monolayer has maintained its integrity throughout the transport process, a marker for paracellular absorption, such as mannitol, which is often radiolabelled for ease of assay, is added to the apical surface. If less than 2% of this crosses the monolayer in an hour then the integrity of the monolayer has been maintained. Another way to check the integrity of the monolayer is by measuring the transepithelial resistance (TER).

To use the Caco-2 cells as an absorption model, a calibration curve needs to be generated. This is done for compounds for which the absorption in humans is known. Figure 22.4 shows the general shape of the curve of fraction absorbed in humans versus the apparent permeability coefficient in Caco-2 cells. As cells are biological systems and small changes in their source, method of culture and the way in which the transport experiment is performed will affect the apparent permeability of a drug, this curve can shift significantly to the right or left or alter in its steepness. Therefore, when carrying out Caco-2 experiments, it is important always to standardize the procedure within a particular laboratory and ensure that this procedure is regularly calibrated with a set of standard compounds.

Caco-2 monolayers can also be used to elucidate the mechanism of permeability. If the apparent permeability coefficient is found to increase linearly with increasing concentration of drug (i.e. the transport is not saturated), is the same whether the drug transport is measured from the apical to basolateral or the basolateral to apical direction, and is independent of pH, it can be concluded that the transport is a passive and not an active process. If the transport in the basolateral to apical direction is significantly greater than that in the apical to basolateral direction then it is likely that the drug is actively effluxed from the cells by a countermembrane transporter such as P-glycoprotein. If the transport of the drug is also inhibited by the presence of compounds that are known inhibitors of P-glycoprotein, such as verapamil, this gives a further indication that the drug is susceptible to P-glycoprotein efflux.

To help elucidate whether other membrane transporters are involved in the absorption of a particular drug, further competitive inhibition studies can be carried out with known inhibitors of the particular transporter. For example, the dipeptide glycosyl-sarcosine can be used to probe whether the dipeptide transporter is involved in the absorption of a particular drug.

To evaluate whether a compound is absorbed via the paracellular or the transcellular pathway, the tight junctions can be artificially opened with compounds such as

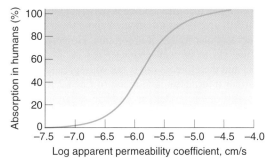

Fig. 22.4 The relationship between the fraction absorbed in humans and the apparent permeability coefficient in Caco cells.

EDTA, which chelates calcium. Calcium is involved in keeping the junctions together. If the apparent permeability of a compound is not affected by the opening of these junctions, which can be assessed by using a paracellular marker such as mannitol, one can assume the drug transport is via a transcellular pathway.

If the disappearance of drug on the apical side of the membrane is not mirrored by its appearance on the basolateral side, and/or the mass balance at the end of the transport experiment does not account for 100% of the drug, there may be a problem with binding to the membrane porous support. This will need investigation, or the drug may have a stability issue. The drug could be susceptible to enzymes secreted by the cells and/or to degradation by hydrolytic enzymes as it passes through the cells, or it may be susceptible to metabolism by cytochrome P450 within the cell. Thus the Caco-2 cells are not only capable of evaluating the permeability of drugs but have value in investigating whether two of the other potential barriers to absorption, stability and presystemic metabolism, are likely to affect the overall rate and extent of absorption.

Caco-2 cells are very useful tools for understanding the mechanism of absorption of drugs and have furthered significantly our knowledge of the absorption of a variety of drugs. Other advantages of Caco-2 cells are that they are a non-animal model, require only small amounts of compound for transport studies, can be used as a rapid screening tool to assess the permeability of large numbers of compounds in the discovery setting and can be used to evaluate the potential toxicity of compounds to cells.

The main disadvantages of Caco-2 monolayers as an absorption model are that, because of the tightness of the monolayer, they are more akin to the paracellular permeability of the colon rather than that of the small intestine and that they lack a mucus layer.

HT-29-A18C1, a subclone of a human intestinal adenocarcinoma cell line, can differentiate in culture to produce both absorptive cells containing a microvillus structure and mucus-secreting goblet cells. It also has a resistance similar to that of the small intestine and so it can be argued that this cell line is preferable to Caco-2 in that it will give better information about the transcellular and paracellular routes of absorption. However, this cell line has yet to be well characterized as an absorption model and therefore its use is not widespread.

Further information on the use of Caco-2 monolayers as an absorption model can be obtained from Artusson et al (1996).

Tissue techniques

A range of tissue techniques have been used as absorption models (Table 22.4). Two of the more popular ones

are the use of isolated sheets of intestinal mucosa and of everted intestinal rings. These are discussed in more detail below.

Isolated sheets of intestinal mucosa are prepared by cutting the intestine into strips. The musculature is then removed and the sheet mounted and clamped in a diffusion chamber or an Ussing chamber filled with appropriate biological buffers (Fig. 22.5). The transepithelial resistance is measured across the tissue to check its integrity. The system is maintained at 37°C and stirred so that the thickness of the unstirred water layer is controlled and oxygen provided to the tissue. The drug is added to the donor chamber and the amount accumulating in the receiver chamber is measured as a function of time. The permeability across the tissue can then be calculated.

Similar to cell monolayers, the two sides of the tissue can be sampled independently and thus fluxes from mucosal to serosal and from serosal to mucosal can be measured. Any pH dependence of transport can be determined by altering the pH of the buffers in the donor and/or receiver chambers. This system can also therefore be used to probe active transport.

One advantage of this technique over cell culture techniques is that permeability across different regions of the intestine can be assessed. It is particularly helpful to be able to compare permeabilities across intestinal and colonic tissue, especially when assessing whether a drug is suitable for a controlled-release delivery system. In addition, different animal tissues that permit an assessment of permeability in different preclinical models can

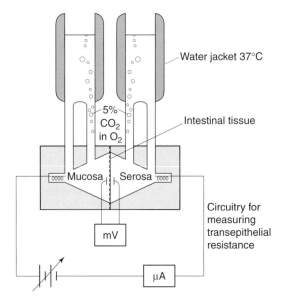

Fig. 22.5 Diagram of a diffusion chamber.

be used. The rat intestine is usually preferred for absorption studies as its permeability correlates well with that of human intestine. Human tissue and cell monolayers have also been used in this system.

Everted intestinal rings use whole intestinal segments rather than just sheets. The musculature is therefore intact. Intestinal segments are excised, again usually from rats. The segment is then tied at one end and carefully everted by placing it over a glass rod. It is cut into small sections or rings and these rings incubated in stirred oxygenated drug-containing buffer at 37°C. After a set period of time, drug uptake is quenched by quickly rinsing the ring with ice-cold buffer and carefully drying it. The ring is then assayed for drug content and the amount of drug taken up per gram of wet tissue over a specific period of time is calculated (mol g^{-1} time^{-1}). The advantage of using intestinal rings is that the test is relatively simple and quick to perform. A large number of rings can be prepared from each segment of intestine, which allows each animal to act as its own control. In addition, the conditions of the experiment can be manipulated and so provide an insight into the mechanisms of absorption.

The disadvantages of this system are that it is biological and that care must be taken to maintain the viability of the tissue for the duration of the experiment. As the drug is taken up into the ring, the tissue needs to be digested and the drug extracted from it before it is assayed. This results in lengthy sample preparation and complicates the assay procedure. In addition, as this is an uptake method, no polarity of absorption can be assessed.

Both these absorption models can be calibrated with a standard set of compounds similar to the Caco-2 model. A similarly shaped curve for the percentage of drug absorbed in humans versus apparent permeability or uptake (mole per weight of tissue) for the isolated sheet and everted ring methods, respectively, is obtained.

Perfusion studies

Many variations of intestinal perfusion methods have been used as absorption models over the years. Again, in general, because of its relative ease of use and similarity to the permeability of the human intestine, the rat model is preferred. In situ intestinal perfusion models have the advantage that the whole animal is used, with the nerve, lymphatic and blood supplies intact. Therefore there should be no problem with tissue viability and all the transport mechanisms present in a live animal should be functional.

The animal is anaesthetized and the intestine exposed. In the open loop method a dilute solution of drug is pumped slowly through the intestine and the difference in drug concentration between the inlet and outlet concentrations is calculated (Fig. 22.6). An absorption rate constant or effective permeability coefficient across the intestine can be calculated as follows:

$$P_{eff} = Q \ln(C_i - C_0)/2\pi rl \qquad (22.2)$$

where P_{eff} is the effective permeability coefficient (cm/s), Q is the flow rate in mL/s, C_i is the initial drug concentration, C_0 is the final drug concentration, r is the radius of the intestinal loop (cm), and, l is the length of intestinal loop (cm).

In the closed loop method a dilute solution of drug is added to a section of the intestine and the intestine closed. The intestine is then excised and drug content analysed immediately and after an appropriate time or time intervals, depending on the expected rate of absorption. Again, assuming a first-order rate process and hence an exponential loss of drug from the intestine, an absorption rate constant and effective permeability can be calculated. Like the intestinal ring method, the closed loop in situ perfusion model requires a lengthy digestion, extraction and assay procedure to analyse the drug remaining in the intestinal loop.

There is a lot of fluid moving in and out of the intestine and so the drug concentrations in both these in situ perfusion methods need to be corrected for fluid flux. This is normally done by gravimetric means or by using a non-absorbable marker to assess the effect of fluid flux on the drug concentration. As with other absorption models, correlations have been made with standard compounds where the fraction absorbed in humans is known; similar-shaped curves have been obtained (see Fig. 22.4). In these models the 'absorption rate' is calculated by

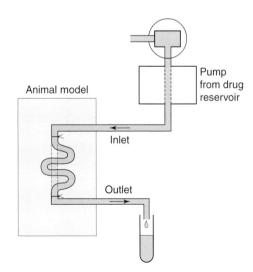

Fig. 22.6 Diagram of an in situ rat perfusion.

measuring the disappearance of the drug from the lumen and not its accumulation in the plasma. It is therefore important to check that the drug is not degraded in the lumen or intestinal wall as drug that has disappeared will be erroneously assumed to have been absorbed.

More sophisticated techniques are those involving vascular perfusion. In these techniques, either a pair of mesenteric vessels supplying an intestinal segment or the superior mesenteric artery and portal vein perfusing almost the entire intestine are cannulated. The intestinal lumen and sometimes the lymph duct are also cannulated for the collection of luminal fluid and lymph, respectively. This model, although complicated, is very versatile as drug can be administered into the luminal or the vascular perfusate. When administered to the intestinal lumen, drug absorption can be evaluated from both its disappearance from the lumen and its appearance in the portal vein. Using this method, both the rate and extent of absorption can be estimated, as well as carrier-mediated transport processes. Collection of the lymph allows the contribution of lymphatic absorption for very lipophilic compounds to be assessed. One of the other advantages of this system is the ability to determine whether any intestinal metabolism occurs before or after absorption.

A further extension of this model is to follow the passage of drugs from the intestine through the liver, and several adaptations of rat intestinal-liver perfusion systems have been investigated. Such a combined system gives the added advantage of assessing the first-pass or presystemic metabolism through the liver, and determining the relative importance of the intestine and liver in presystemic metabolism.

The disadvantage of these perfusion systems is that as they become more complex, a larger number of animals is required to establish suitable perfusion conditions and the reproducibility of the technique. However, in general, as the complexity increases so does the amount of information obtained.

Assessment of permeability in humans

Intestinal perfusion studies Until relatively recently, the most common way to evaluate the absorption of drugs in humans was by performing bioavailability studies and deconvoluting the data available to calculate an absorption rate constant. This rate constant, however, is dependent on the release of the drug from the dosage form and is affected by intestinal transit and presystemic metabolism. Therefore, very often it does not reflect the true intrinsic intestinal permeability of a drug.

Extensive studies have been carried out using a regional perfusion technique which has afforded a greater insight into human permeability (Loc-I-Gut). The Loc-I-Gut is a multichannel tube system with a proximal and a distal balloon (Fig. 22.7). These balloons are 100 mm apart and allow a segment of intestine 100 mm long to be isolated and perfused. Once the proximal balloon passes the ligament of Treitz, both balloons are filled with air, thereby preventing mixing of the luminal contents in the segment of interest with other luminal contents. A non-absorbable marker is used in the perfusion solution to check that the balloons work to occlude the region of interest. A tungsten weight is placed in front of the distal balloon to facilitate its passage down the gastrointestinal tract.

Drug absorption is calculated from the rate of disappearance of the drug from the perfused segment. This technique has afforded greater control in human intestinal perfusions, primarily because it isolates the luminal contents of interest, and has greatly facilitated the study of permeability mechanisms and the metabolism of drugs and nutrients in the human intestine (Knutson et al 1989, Lennernäs et al 1992).

Non-invasive approaches There is concern that the invasive nature of perfusion techniques can affect the function of the gastrointestinal tract, in particular the fluid content, owing to the intubation process altering the absorption and secretion balance. To overcome this problem, several engineering-based approaches have been developed to evaluate drug absorption in the gastrointestinal tract. These include high-frequency (HF) capsules (Fuhr et al 1994) and the InteliSite capsule (Wilding 1997).

The transit of the high-frequency capsule down the gastrointestinal tract is followed by X-ray fluoroscopy. Once the capsule reaches its desired release site, drug release is triggered by a high-frequency signal that leads to rupturing of a latex balloon that has been loaded with drug. Concerns about X-ray exposure and the difficulties of loading the drug into the balloon have limited the use of this technique.

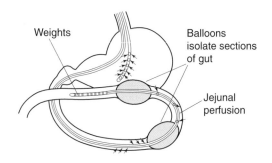

Fig. 22.7 Diagram of the Loc-I-Gut.

The InteliSite capsule is a more sophisticated system for measuring drug absorption. Either a liquid or a powder formulation can be filled into the capsule, the transit of which is followed by γ-scintigraphy (see later in this chapter). Once the capsule reaches its desired release site, it is activated by exposure to a radiomagnetic field that induces a small amount of heat in the capsule's electronic assembly. The heat causes the shape-memory alloys in the device to straighten. This rotates the inner sleeve of the capsule with respect to an outer sleeve and allows a series of slots in the two sleeves to become aligned and the enclosed drug to be released. For both these systems blood samples need to be taken to quantify drug absorption.

Presystemic metabolism

Presystemic metabolism is the metabolism that occurs before the drug reaches the systemic circulation. Therefore, for an orally administered drug, this includes the metabolism that occurs in the gut wall and the liver. As discussed above, perfusion models that involve both the intestines and the liver allow an evaluation of the presystemic metabolism in both organs. In other models it is sometimes possible to design mass balance experiments that will assess whether presystemic intestinal metabolism is likely to occur.

Intestinal cell fractions, such as brush border membrane preparations that contain an abundance of hydrolytic enzymes, and homogenized preparations of segments of rat intestine can also be used to determine intestinal presystemic metabolism. Drugs are incubated with either brush border membrane preparations or gut wall homogenate at 37°C and the drug content analysed.

Various liver preparations, for example subcellular fractions such as microsomes, isolated hepatocytes and liver slices, are used to determine hepatic metabolism in vitro. These are classified as phase I metabolism, which involves reduction or hydrolysis but mostly oxidation, and phase II metabolism, which follows phase I and involves conjugation reactions. Microsomes are prepared by high-speed centrifugation of liver homogenates (100 000 g) and are composed mainly of fragments of the endoplasmic reticulum. They lack cystolic enzymes and cofactors and are therefore only suitable to evaluate some of the metabolic processes (phase I metabolism) of which the liver is capable. Hepatocytes must be freshly and carefully prepared from livers and are only viable for a few hours. It is therefore difficult to obtain human hepatocytes. Hepatocytes are very useful for hepatic metabolism studies as it is possible to evaluate most of the metabolic reactions, i.e. both phase I and II metabolism. Whole liver slices again have the ability to evaluate

both phase I and II metabolism. Because they are tissue slices rather than cell suspensions, and because they do not require enzymatic treatment in their preparation, this may be why a higher degree of in vivo correlation can be achieved with liver slices than with hepatocytes and microsomes. The reader is referred to a review by Carlile et al (1997).

ASSESSMENT OF BIOAVAILABILITY

The measurement of bioavailability gives the net result of the effect of the release of drug into solution in the physiological fluids at the site of absorption, its stability in those physiological fluids, its permeability and its presystemic metabolism on the rate and extent of drug absorption by following the concentration–time profile of drug in a suitable physiological fluid. The concentration–time profile also gives information on other pharmacokinetic parameters, such as the distribution and elimination of the drug. The most commonly used method of assessing the bioavailability of a drug involves the construction of a blood plasma concentration–time curve, but urine drug concentrations can also be used and are discussed below.

Plasma concentration–time curves

When a single dose of a drug is administered orally to a patient, serial blood samples are withdrawn and the plasma assayed for drug concentration at specific periods of time after administration. This enables a plasma concentration–time curve to be constructed. Figure 22.8 shows a typical plasma concentration–time curve following the administration of an oral tablet.

At zero time, when the drug is first administered, the concentration of drug in the plasma will be zero. As the tablet passes into the stomach and/or intestine it disintegrates, the drug dissolves and absorption occurs. Initially the concentration of drug in the plasma rises as the rate of absorption exceeds the rate at which the drug is being removed by distribution and elimination. Concentrations continue to rise until a maximum (or peak) is attained. This represents the highest concentration of drug achieved in the plasma following the administration of a single dose, often termed the C_{pmax} (maximum plasma concentration). It is reached when the rate of appearance of drug in the plasma is equal to its rate of removal by distribution and elimination.

The ascending portion of the plasma concentration–time curve is sometimes called the *absorption phase*. Here the rate of absorption outweighs the rate of removal of drug by distribution and elimination. Drug absorption does not usually stop abruptly at the time of peak concentration but may continue for some time into

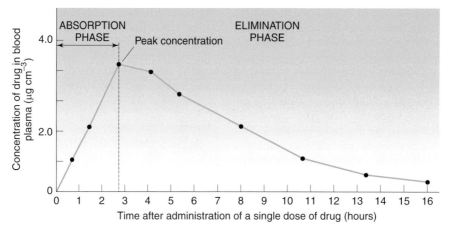

Fig. 22.8 A typical blood plasma concentration–time curve obtained following the peroral administration of a single dose of a drug in a tablet.

the descending portion of the curve. The early descending portion of the curve can thus reflect the net result of drug absorption, distribution, metabolism and elimination. In this phase the rate of drug removal from the blood exceeds the rate absorption and therefore the concentration of the drug in the plasma declines.

Eventually drug absorption ceases when the bioavailable dose has been absorbed, and the concentration of drug in the plasma is now controlled only by its rate of elimination by metabolism and/or excretion. This is sometimes called the *elimination phase* of the curve. It should be appreciated, however, that elimination of a drug begins as soon as it appears in the plasma.

Several parameters based on the plasma concentration–time curve that are important in bioavailability studies are shown in Figure 22.9, and are discussed below.

Minimum effective (or therapeutic) plasma concentration It is generally assumed that some minimum concentration of drug in the plasma must be reached before the desired therapeutic or pharmacological effect is achieved. This is called the *minimum effective* (or *minimum therapeutic*) *plasma concentration*. Its value not only varies from drug to drug but also from individual to individual and with the type and severity of the disease state. In Figure 22.9 the minimum effective concentration is indicated by the lower line.

Maximum safe concentration The concentration of drug in the plasma above which side-effects or toxic effects occur is known as the *maximum safe concentration*.

Therapeutic range or window A range of plasma drug concentrations is also assumed to exist over which the desired response is obtained yet toxic effects are avoided. This range is called the *therapeutic range* or

therapeutic window. The intention in clinical practice is to maintain plasma drug concentrations within this range.

Onset The *onset* may be defined as the time required to achieve the minimum effective plasma concentration following administration of the dosage form.

Duration The *duration* of the therapeutic effect of the drug is the period during which the concentration of drug in the plasma exceeds the minimum effective plasma concentration.

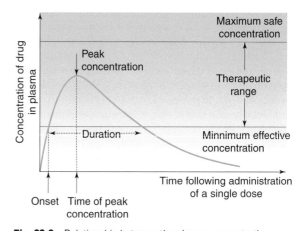

Fig. 22.9 Relationship between the plasma concentration–time curve obtained following a single extravascular dose of a drug and parameters associated with the therapeutic or pharmacological response.

Peak concentration The *peak concentration* represents the highest concentration of the drug achieved in the plasma, often referred to as the C_{pmax}.

Time of peak concentration This is the period of time required to achieve the peak plasma concentration of drug after the administration of a single dose. This parameter is related to the rate of absorption of the drug and can be used to assess that rate. It is often referred to as the T_{max}.

Area under the plasma concentration–time curve This is related to the total amount of drug absorbed into the systemic circulation following the administration of a single dose, and is often known as the AUC. However, changes in the area under the plasma concentration–time curve need not necessarily reflect changes in the total amount of drug absorbed but can reflect modifications in the kinetics of distribution, metabolism and excretion.

Use of plasma concentration–time curves in bioavailability studies

In order to illustrate the usefulness of plasma concentration–time curves in bioavailability studies in the assessment of the rate and extent of absorption, the administration of single equal doses of three different formulations, A, B and C, of the same drug to the same healthy individual by the same route of administration on three separate occasions can be considered. The assumption is made that sufficient time is allowed to elapse between the administration of each formulation such that the systemic circulation contained no residual concentration of drug and no residual effects from any previous administrations. It is also assumed that the kinetics and pattern of distribution of the drug, its binding phenomena, the kinetics of elimination and the experimental conditions under which each plasma concentration–time profile is obtained are the same on each occasion. The plasma concentration–time profiles for the three formulations are shown in Figure 22.10. The differences between the three curves are attributed solely to differences in the rate and/or extent of absorption of the drug from each formulation.

The three plasma profiles in Figure 22.10 show that each of the three formulations (A, B and C) of the same dose of the same drug results in a different peak plasma concentration. However, the areas under the curves for formulation A and B are similar, and this indicates that the drug is absorbed to a similar extent from these two formulations. Consideration of the times at which the peak plasma concentrations occur for formulations A and B shows that the drug is absorbed faster from A than from B. This means that formulation A shows a fast onset of therapeutic action but as its peak plasma concentration exceeds the maximum safe concentration, it is likely that

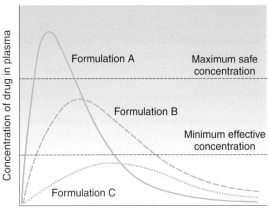

Fig. 22.10 Plasma concentration–time curves for three different formulations of the same drug administered in equal single doses by the same extravascular route.

this formulation will result in toxic side-effects. Formulation B, which has a slower rate of absorption than A, shows a slower therapeutic onset than A but its peak plasma concentration lies within the therapeutic range. In addition, the duration of action of the therapeutic effect obtained with formulation B is longer than that obtained with A. Hence formulation B appears to be superior to formulation A from a clinical viewpoint in that its peak plasma concentration lies within the therapeutic range of the drug and the duration of the therapeutic effect is longer.

Formulation C gives a much smaller area under the plasma concentration–time curve, indicating that a lower proportion of the dose has been absorbed. This, together with the slower rate of absorption from formulation C (the time of peak concentration is longer than for formulations A and B), results in the peak plasma concentration not reaching the minimum effective concentration. Thus formulation C does not produce a therapeutic effect and consequently is clinically ineffective as a single dose.

This simple hypothetical example illustrates how differences in bioavailability exhibited by a given drug from different formulations can result in a patient being either over-, under- or correctly medicated.

It is important to realize that the study of bioavailability based on drug concentration measurements in the plasma (or urine or saliva) is complicated by the fact that such concentration–time curves are affected by factors other than the biopharmaceutical factors of the drug product itself. Factors such as:

- body weight
- sex and age of the test subjects

- disease states
- genetic differences in drug metabolism
- excretion and distribution
- food and water intake
- concomitant administration of other drugs
- stress, and
- time of administration of the drug

are some of the variables that can complicate the interpretation of bioavailability studies. As far as possible, studies should be designed to control these factors.

Although plots such as those in Figure 22.10 can be used to compare the relative bioavailability of a given drug from different formulations, they cannot be used indiscriminately to compare different drugs. It is quite usual for different drugs to exhibit different rates of absorption, metabolism, excretion and distribution, different distribution patterns and differences in their binding phenomena. All of these will influence the concentration–time curve. Therefore it would be extremely difficult to attribute differences in the concentration–time curves obtained for different drugs presented in different formulations to differences in their bioavailabilities.

Cumulative urinary drug excretion curves

Measurement of the concentration of intact drug and/or its metabolite(s) in the plasma can also be used to assess bioavailability.

When a suitable specific assay method is not available for the intact drug in the urine or the specific assay method available for the parent drug is not sufficiently sensitive, it may be necessary to assay the principal metabolite or intact drug plus its metabolite(s) in the urine to obtain an index of bioavailability. Measurements involving metabolite levels in the urine are only valid when the drug in question is not subject to metabolism prior to reaching the systemic circulation. If an orally administered drug is subject to intestinal metabolism or first-pass liver metabolism, then measurement of the principal metabolite or of intact drug plus metabolites in the urine would give an overestimate of the systemic availability of that drug. It should be remembered that the definition of bioavailability is in terms of the extent and the rate at which intact drug appears in the systemic circulation after the administration of a known dose.

The assessment of bioavailability by urinary excretion is based on the assumption that the appearance of the drug and/or its metabolites in the urine is a function of the rate and extent of absorption. This assumption is only valid when a drug and/or its metabolites are extensively excreted in the urine, and where the rate of urinary excretion is proportional to the concentration of the

intact drug in the blood plasma. This proportionality does not hold if:

- the drug and/or its metabolites are excreted by an active transport process into the distal kidney tubule
- the intact drug and/or its metabolites are weakly acidic or weakly basic (i.e. their rate of excretion is dependent on urine pH)
- the excretion rate depends on the rate of urine flow.

The important parameters in urinary excretion studies are the cumulative amount of intact drug and/or metabolites excreted and the rate at which this excretion takes place. A cumulative urinary excretion curve is obtained by collecting urine samples (resulting from the total emptying of the bladder) at known intervals after a single dose of the drug has been administered. Urine samples must be collected until all drug and/or its metabolites have been excreted (this is indicated by the cumulative urinary excretion curve becoming parallel to the abscissa) if a comparison of the extent of absorption of a given drug from different formulations or dosage forms is to be made. A typical cumulative urinary excretion curve and the corresponding plasma concentration–time curve obtained following the administration of a single dose of a given drug by the oral route to a subject is shown in Figure 22.11.

The initial segments (X–Y) of the curves reflect the *absorption phase* (i.e. where absorption is the dominant process) and the slope of this segment of the urinary excretion curve is related to the rate of absorption of the

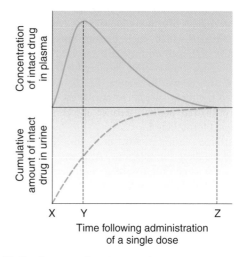

Fig. 22.11 Corresponding plots showing the plasma concentration–time curve (*upper curve*) and the cumulative urinary excretion curve (*lower curve*) obtained following the administration of a single dose of a drug by the peroral route.

drug into the blood. The total amount of intact drug (and/or its metabolite(s)) excreted in the urine at point Z corresponds to the time at which the plasma concentration of intact drug is zero and essentially all the drug has been eliminated from the body. The total amount of drug excreted at point Z may be quite different from the total amount of drug administered (i.e. the dose) either because of incomplete absorption or because of the drug being eliminated by processes other than urinary excretion.

Use of urinary drug excretion curves in bioavailability studies

In order to illustrate how cumulative urinary excretion curves can be used to compare the bioavailabilities of a given drug from different formulations, let us consider the urinary excretion data obtained following the administration of single equal doses of the three different formulations, A, B and C, of the same drug to the same healthy individual by the same extravascular route on three different occasions. Assume that these give the plasma concentration–time curves shown in Figure 22.10. The corresponding cumulative urinary excretion curves are shown in Figure 22.12.

The cumulative urinary excretion curves show that the rate at which drug appeared in the urine (i.e. the slope of the initial segment of each urinary excretion curve) from each formulation decreases in the order A > B > C. Because the slope of the initial segment of the urinary excretion curve is related to the rate of drug absorption, the cumulative urinary excretion curves indicate that the rates of absorption of drug from the three formulations decrease in the order A > B > C. Inspection of the corresponding plasma concentration–time curves in Figure 22.10 shows that this is the case, i.e. peak concentration

times (which are inversely related to the rate of drug absorption) for the three formulations increase in the order A > B > C. Although Figure 22.12 shows that the rate of appearance of drug in the urine from formulation A is faster than from B, the total amount of drug eventually excreted from these two formulations is the same, i.e. the cumulative urinary excretion curves for formulations A and B eventually meet and merge. As the total amount of intact drug excreted is assumed to be related to the total amount absorbed, the cumulative urinary excretion curves for formulations A and B indicate that the extent of drug absorption from these two formulations is the same. This is confirmed by the plasma concentration–time curves for formulations A and B in Figure 22.10 that exhibit similar areas under their curves.

Thus both the plasma concentration–time curves and the corresponding cumulative urinary excretion curves for formulations A and B show that the extent of absorption from these formulations is equal despite the drug being released at different rates from the respective formulations.

Consideration of the cumulative urinary excretion curve for C shows that this formulation not only results in a slower rate of appearance of intact drug in the urine but also that the total amount of drug eventually excreted is much less than from the other two formulations. Thus the cumulative urinary excretion curve suggests that both the rate and extent of drug absorption are reduced in the case of formulation C. This is confirmed by the plasma concentration–time curve shown in Figure 22.10 for formulation C. Formulation C exhibits a longer peak concentration time and a smaller area under the curve than do formulations A and B. Thus it can be concluded that cumulative urinary excretion curves may be used to compare the rate and extent of absorption of a given drug presented in different formulations provided that the conditions mentioned previously apply.

Absolute and relative bioavailability

Absolute bioavailability

The absolute bioavailability of a given drug from a dosage form is the fraction (or percentage) of the administered dose which is absorbed intact into the systemic circulation. Absolute bioavailability may be calculated by comparing the total amount of intact drug that reaches the systemic circulation after the administration of a known dose of the dosage form via a route of administration with the total amount that reaches the systemic circulation after the administration of an equivalent dose of the drug in the form of an intravenous bolus injection. An intravenous bolus injection is used as a reference to compare the systemic availability of the drug administered via different routes. This is because when a drug is

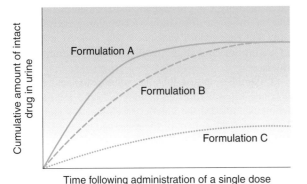

Fig. 22.12 Cumulative urinary excretion curves corresponding to the plasma concentration–time curves shown in Fig. 22.10 for three different formulations of the same drug administered in equal single doses by the same extravascular route.

delivered intravenously, the entire administered dose is introduced directly into the systemic circulation, i.e. it has no absorption barriers to cross, and is therefore considered to be totally bioavailable.

The absolute bioavailability of a given drug using plasma data may be calculated by comparing the total areas under the plasma concentration–time curves obtained following the administration of equivalent doses of the drug via an absorption site and via the intravenous route in the same subject on different occasions. Typical plasma concentration–time curves obtained by administering equivalent doses of the same drug by the intravenous route (bolus injection) and the gastrointestinal route are shown in Figure 22.13.

For equivalent doses of administered drug:

$$\text{absolute bioavailability} = \frac{(\text{AUC}_T)_{\text{abs}}}{(\text{AUC}_T)_{\text{iv}}} \quad (22.3)$$

where $(\text{AUC}_T)_{\text{abs}}$ is the total area under the plasma concentration–time curve following the administration of a single dose via an absorption site and $(\text{AUC}_T)_{\text{iv}}$ is the total area under the plasma concentration–time curve following administration by rapid intravenous injection.

If different doses of the drug are administered by both routes, a correction for the sizes of the doses can be made as follows:

$$\text{absolute bioavailability} = \frac{(\text{AUC}_T)_{\text{abs}}/D_{\text{abs}}}{(\text{AUC}_T)_{\text{iv}}/D_{\text{iv}}} \quad (22.4)$$

where D_{abs} is the size of the single dose of drug administered via the absorption site and D_{iv} is the size of the dose of the drug administered as an intravenous bolus injection.

tion. Sometimes it is necessary to use different dosages of drugs via different routes. Often the dose administered intravenously is lower to avoid toxic side-effects and for ease of formulation. Care should be taken when using different dosages to calculate bioavailability data as sometimes the pharmacokinetics of a drug are non-linear and different doses will then lead to an incorrect figure for the absolute bioavailability if calculated using a simple ratio, as in Eqn 22.4.

Absolute bioavailability using urinary excretion data may be determined by comparing the total cumulative amounts of unchanged drug ultimately excreted in the urine following administration of the drug via an absorption site and the intravenous route (bolus injection) on different occasions to the same subject.

For equivalent doses of administered drug:

$$\text{absolute bioavailability} = \frac{(X_u)_{\text{abs}}}{(X_u)_{\text{iv}}} \quad (22.5)$$

where $(X_u)_{\text{abs}}$ and $(X_u)_{\text{iv}}$ are the total cumulative amounts of unchanged drug ultimately excreted in the urine following administration of equivalent single doses of drug via an absorption site and as an intravenous bolus injection, respectively.

If different doses of drug are administered:

$$\text{absolute bioavailability} = \frac{(X_u)_{\text{abs}}/D_{\text{abs}}}{(X_u)_{\text{iv}}/D_{\text{iv}}} \quad (22.6)$$

The absolute bioavailability of a given drug from a particular type of dosage form may be expressed as a fraction or, more commonly, as a percentage.

Measurements of absolute bioavailability obtained by administering a given drug in the form of a simple aqueous solution (that does not precipitate on contact with or dilution by gastrointestinal fluids) by both the oral and the intravenous routes provide an insight into the effects that factors associated with the oral route may have on bioavailability, e.g. presystemic metabolism by the intestine or liver, the formation of complexes between the drug and endogenous substances (e.g. mucin) at the site of absorption and drug stability in the gastrointestinal fluids.

It should be noted that the value calculated for the absolute bioavailability will only be valid for the drug being examined if the kinetics of elimination and distribution are independent of the route and time of administration and also of the size of dose administered (if different doses are administered by the intravenous route and absorption site). If this is not the case, one cannot assume that the observed differences in the total areas under the plasma concentration–time curves or in the total cumulative amounts of unchanged drug ultimately excreted in the urine are due entirely to differences in bioavailability.

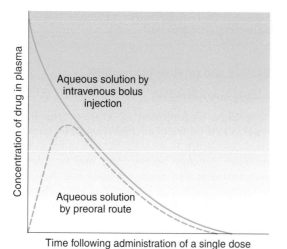

Fig. 22.13 Typical plasma concentration–time curves obtained by administering equivalent doses of the same drug by intravenous bolus injection and by the peroral route.

Relative bioavailability

In the case of drugs that cannot be administered by intravenous bolus injection, the relative (or comparative) bioavailability is determined rather than the absolute bioavailability. In this case the bioavailability of a given drug from a 'test' dosage form is compared to that of the same drug administered in a 'standard' dosage form. The latter is either an orally administered solution (from which the drug is known to be well absorbed) or an established commercial preparation of proven clinical effectiveness. Hence relative bioavailability is a measure of the fraction (or percentage) of a given drug that is absorbed intact into the systemic circulation from a dosage form relative to a recognized (i.e. clinically proven) standard dosage form of that drug.

The relative bioavailability of a given drug administered as equal doses of a test dosage form and a recognized standard dosage form, respectively, by the same route of administration to the same subject on different occasions may be calculated from the corresponding plasma concentration–time curves as follows:

$$\text{relative bioavailability} = \frac{(\text{AUC}_T)_{\text{test}}}{(\text{AUC}_T)_{\text{standard}}} \qquad (22.7)$$

where $(\text{AUC}_T)_{\text{test}}$ and $(\text{AUC}_T)_{\text{standard}}$ are the total areas under the plasma concentration–time curves following the administration of a single dose of the test dosage form and of the standard dosage form, respectively.

When different doses of the test and standard dosage forms are administered, a correction for the size of dose is made as follows:

$$\text{relative bioavailability} = \frac{(\text{AUC}_T)_{\text{abs}}/D_{\text{test}}}{(\text{AUC}_T)_{\text{standard}}/D_{\text{standard}}} \qquad (22.8)$$

where D_{test} and D_{standard} are the sizes of the single doses of the test and standard dosage forms, respectively.

Like absolute bioavailability, relative bioavailability may be expressed as a fraction or as a percentage. Urinary excretion data may also be used to measure relative bioavailability as follows:

$$\text{relative bioavailability} = \frac{(X_u)_{\text{test}}}{(X_u)_{\text{standard}}} \qquad (22.9)$$

where $(X_u)_{\text{test}}$ and $(X_u)_{\text{standard}}$ are the total cumulative amounts of unchanged drug ultimately excreted in the urine following the administration of single doses of the test dosage form and the standard dosage form, respectively. If different doses of the test and standard dosage forms are administered on separate occasions, the total amounts of unchanged drug ultimately excreted in the urine per unit dose of drug must be used in this equation.

It should be noted that measurements of relative and absolute bioavailability based on urinary excretion data may also be made in terms of either the total amounts of principal drug metabolite or of unchanged drug plus its metabolites ultimately excreted in the urine. However, the assessment of relative and absolute bioavailability in terms of urinary excretion data is based on the assumption that the total amount of unchanged drug (and/or its metabolites) ultimately excreted in the urine is a reflection of the total amount of intact drug entering the systemic circulation (as discussed in the earlier section on cumulative urinary excretion curves).

Relative bioavailability measurements are often used to determine the effects of dosage form differences on the systemic bioavailability of a given drug. Numerous dosage form factors can influence the bioavailability of a drug. These include the type of dosage form (e.g. tablet, solution, suspension, hard gelatin capsule), differences in the formulation of a particular type of dosage form, and manufacturing variables employed in the production of a particular type of dosage form. A more detailed account of the influence of these factors on bioavailability is given in Chapter 21.

Bioequivalence

An extension of the concept of relative bioavailability, which essentially involves comparing the total amounts of a particular drug that are absorbed intact into the systemic circulation from a test and a recognized standard dosage form, is that of determining whether test and standard dosage forms containing equal doses of the same drug are equivalent or not in terms of their systemic availabilities (i.e. rates and extents of absorption). This is called *bioequivalence*.

Two or more chemically equivalent products (i.e. products containing equal doses of the same therapeutically active ingredient(s) in identical types of dosage form which meet all the existing physicochemical standards in official compendia) are said to be bioequivalent if they do not differ *significantly* in their bioavailability characteristics when administered in the same dose under similar experimental conditions. Hence, in those cases where bioavailability is assessed in terms of plasma concentration–time curves, two or more chemically equivalent drug products may be considered bioequivalent if there is no significant difference between any of the following parameters: maximum plasma concentration (C_{max}), time to peak height concentration (T_{max}) and area under the plasma concentration–time curve (AUC).

In conducting a bioequivalence study, it is usual for one of the chemically equivalent drug products under test to be a clinically proven, therapeutically effective product that serves as a standard against which the other 'test' products may be compared. If a test product and the standard product are found to be bioequivalent then it is reasonable to expect that the test product will also be therapeutically effective, i.e. the test and the reference products are therapeutically equivalent. Bioequivalence studies are therefore important in determining whether chemically equivalent drug products manufactured by different companies are therapeutically equivalent, i.e. each will produce identical therapeutic responses in patients.

If two chemically equivalent drug products are absolutely bioequivalent, their plasma concentration–time and/or cumulative urinary excretion curves would be superimposable. In such a case there would be no problem in concluding that these products were bioequivalent. Nor would there be a problem in concluding bioinequivalence if the parameters associated with the plasma concentration–time and/or cumulative urinary excretion profiles for the test differed from the standard product by, for instance, 50%. However, a problem arises in deciding whether the test and standard drug products are bioequivalent when such products show relatively small differences in their plasma concentration–time curves and/or cumulative urinary excretion curves.

The problem is, how much of a difference can be allowed between two chemically equivalent drug products to still permit them to be considered bioequivalent? Should this be 10%, 20%, 30% or more? The magnitude of the difference that could be permitted will depend on the significance of such a difference on the safety and therapeutic efficacy of the particular drug. This will depend on such factors as the toxicity, the therapeutic range and the therapeutic use of the drug. In the case of a drug with a wide therapeutic range, the toxic effects of which occur only at relatively high plasma concentrations, chemically equivalent products giving quite different plasma concentration–time curves (Fig. 22.14) may still be considered satisfactory from a therapeutic point of view, although they are not strictly bioequivalent.

In the case of the hypothetical example shown in Figure 22.14, provided that the observed difference in the rates of absorption (as assessed by the times of peak plasma concentration), and hence in the times of onset, for formulations X and Y is not considered to be therapeutically significant, both formulations may be considered to be therapeutically satisfactory. However, if the drug in question was a hypnotic, in which case the time of onset for the therapeutic response is important, then the observed difference in the rates of absorption would become more important and the two formulations may be considered to be non-equivalent.

If the times of peak plasma concentration for formulations X and Y were 0.5 and 1.0 hour, respectively, it is likely that both formulations would still be deemed to be therapeutically satisfactory despite a 100% difference in their times of peak plasma concentration. However, if the

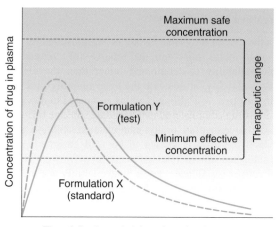

Fig. 22.14 Plasma concentration–time curves for two chemically equivalent drug products administered in equal single doses by the same extravascular route.

times of peak plasma concentration for formulations X and Y were 2 and 4 hours, respectively, these formulations might no longer be regarded as being therapeutically equivalent even though the percentage difference in their peak plasma concentration was the same.

It is difficult to quote a universally acceptable percentage difference that can be tolerated before two chemically equivalent drug products are regarded as being bioinequivalent and/or therapeutically inequivalent. In the case of chemically equivalent drug products containing a drug which exhibits a narrow range between its minimum effective plasma concentration and its maximum safe plasma concentration (e.g. digoxin), the concept of bioequivalence is fundamentally important, as in such cases small differences in the plasma concentration–time curves of chemically equivalent drug products may result in patients being overmedicated (i.e. exhibiting toxic responses) or undermedicated (i.e. experiencing therapeutic failure). These two therapeutically unsatisfactory conditions are illustrated in Figure 22.15a and b, respectively.

Despite the problems of putting a value on the magnitude of the difference that can be tolerated before two chemically equivalent drug products are deemed to be bioinequivalent, a value of 20% for the tolerated difference used to be regarded as a general criterion for determining bioequivalence. Thus if all the major parameters in either the plasma concentration–time or cumulative urinary excretion curves for two or more chemically equivalent drug products differ from each other by less than 20%, these products could be judged to be bioequivalent. However, if any one or more of these

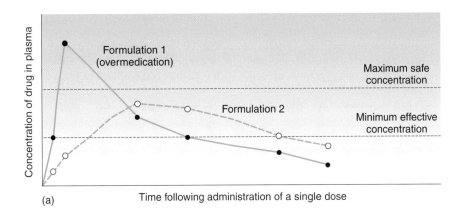

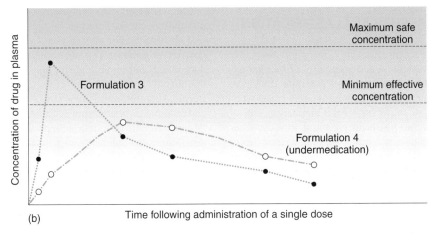

Fig. 22.15 Plasma concentration–time curves for chemically equivalent drug products administered in equal single doses by the same extravascular route, showing potential consequences of bioinequivalence for a drug having a narrow therapeutic range, i.e. (a) overmedication and (b) undermedication (after Chodos & Di Santo 1973).

parameters differ by more than 20% then there might be a problem with the bioequivalence of the test product(s) with respect to the standard product. However, recently some regulatory authorities have been adopting more stringent requirements for bioequivalence, involving statistical models and considerations of average, population and individual pharmacokinetics.

A further crucial factor in establishing bioequivalence, or in determining the influence that the type of dosage form, route of administration, etc., have on the bioavailability of a given drug, is the proper design, control and interpretation of such experimental studies.

ASSESSMENT OF SITE OF RELEASE IN VIVO

There are many benefits of being able to assess the fate of a dosage form in vivo and the site and release pattern of the

drug. Particularly for drugs that show poor oral bioavailability, or in the design and development of controlled- or sustained-release delivery systems, the ability to follow the transit of the dosage form and the release of drug from it is advantageous. The technique of γ-scintigraphy is now used extensively and enables a greater knowledge and understanding to be gained of the transit and fate of pharmaceuticals in the gastrointestinal tract.

γ-Scintigraphy is a versatile, non-invasive and ethically acceptable technique that is capable of obtaining information both quantitatively and continuously. The technique involves the radiolabelling of a dosage form with a γ-emitting isotope of appropriate half-life and activity. Technetium-99m is often the isotope of choice for pharmaceutical studies because of its short half-life (6 hours). The radiolabelled dosage form is administered to a subject who is positioned in front of a γ-camera. γ-Radiation emitted from the isotope is focused by a collimator and detected by a scintillation crystal and its associated circuitry. The signals are assembled by computer software to form a two-dimensional image of the dosage form in the gastrointestinal tract. The anatomy of the gastrointestinal tract can be clearly seen from liquid dosage forms, and the site of disintegration of solid dosage forms identified. The release of the radiolabel from the dosage form can be measured by following the intensity of the radiation. By coadministration of a radiolabelled marker and a drug in the same dosage form, and simultaneous imaging and taking of blood samples, the absorption site and release rate of a drug can be determined (for example with the InteliSite capsule described earlier in this chapter). When used in this way, the technique is often referred to as *pharmacoscintigraphy*.

BIOPHARMACEUTICAL CLASSIFICATION SCHEME

As a result of the plethora and variability of biopharmaceutical properties of existing and potential drugs, an attempt has been made to arrange drugs in a small number of groups. A scientific basis for a biopharmaceutical classification scheme has been proposed that classifies drugs into four classes according to their aqueous solubility across the gastrointestinal pH range and their permeability across the gastrointestinal mucosa (Amidon et al 1995). Two of the four potential barriers to absorption (see Fig. 22.1) are thus addressed by the scheme.

The scheme was originally proposed for the identification of immediate-release solid oral products for which in vivo bioequivalence tests may not be necessary. It is also useful to classify drugs and predict bioavailability issues that may arise during the various stages of the development process and is utilized by the regulatory authorities.

The four classes are defined in terms of high and low aqueous solubility and high and low permeability.

- Class I – high solubility/high permeability
- Class II – low solubility/high permeability
- Class III – high solubility/low permeability
- Class IV – low solubility/low permeability.

A drug is considered to be highly soluble where the highest dose strength is soluble in 250 mL or less of aqueous media over the pH range 1–8. The volume is derived from the minimum volume anticipated in the stomach when a dosage form is taken in the fasted state with a glass of water. If the volume of aqueous media needed to dissolve the drug in pH conditions ranging from 1 to 8 is greater than 250 mL then the drug is considered to have low solubility. The classification therefore takes into account the dose of the drug as well as its solubility.

A drug is considered to be highly permeable when the extent of absorption in humans is expected to be greater than 90% of the administered dose. Permeability can be assessed using one of the methods discussed earlier in this chapter that has been calibrated with known standard compounds or by pharmacokinetic studies.

Class I drugs Class I drugs will dissolve rapidly when presented in immediate-release dosage form, and are also rapidly transported across the gut wall. Therefore (unless they form insoluble complexes, are unstable in gastric fluids or undergo presystemic clearance) it is expected that such drugs will be rapidly absorbed and thus show good bioavailability. Examples of class I drugs are the β-blockers propranolol and metoprolol.

Class II drugs In contrast, for drugs in class II, the dissolution rate is liable to be the rate-limiting step in oral absorption. For class II drugs it should therefore be possible to generate a strong correlation between in vitro dissolution and in vivo absorption (discussed earlier in this chapter). Examples of class II drugs are the nonsteroidal antiinflammatory drug ketoprofen and the antiepileptic carbamazepine. This class of drug should be amenable to formulation approaches to improve the dissolution rate and hence oral bioavailability.

Class III drugs Class III drugs are those that dissolve rapidly but which are poorly permeable. Examples are the H_2-antagonist ranitidine and the β-blocker atenolol. It is important that dosage forms containing class III drugs release them rapidly in order to maximize the amount of time these drugs, which are slow to permeate the gastrointestinal epithelium, are in contact with it.

Class IV drugs Class IV drugs are those that are classed as poorly soluble and poorly permeable. These drugs are liable to have poor oral bioavailability or the oral absorption may be so low that they cannot be given by the oral route. The diuretics hydrochlorothiazide and frusemide are examples of class IV drugs. Forming prodrugs of class IV compounds or finding an alternative route of delivery are approaches that have to be adopted to significantly improve their absorption into the systemic circulation.

SUMMARY

This chapter discusses the range of current approaches to assessing the biopharmaceutical properties of drugs that are intended for oral administration. Methods of measuring and interpreting bioavailability data are described. The concepts of bioequivalence and the biopharmaceutical classification of drugs are introduced. It is imperative that the biopharmaceutical properties of drugs are fully understood, both in the selection of candidate drugs during the discovery process and in the design and development of efficacious immediate- and controlled-release dosage forms.

REFERENCES

Amidon, G.L., Lennernäs, H., Shah, V.P., Crison, J.R.A. (1995) Theoretical basis for a biopharmaceutic drug classification: the correlation of in vitro drug product dissolution and in vivo bioavailability. *Pharmaceutical Research*, **12**, 413-420.

Artusson, P., Palm, K., Luthman, K. (1996) Caco-2 monolayers in experimental and theoretical predictions of drug transport. *Advanced Drug Delivery Reviews,* **22**, 67-84.

Carlile, D.J., Zomorodi, K., Houston, J.B. (1997) Scaling factors to relate drug metabolic clearance in hepatic microsomes, isolated hepatocytes and the intact liver – studies with induced livers involving diazepam. *Drug Metabolism and Disposition,* **25**, 903-911.

Chodos, D.J., Di Santo, A.R. (1973) *Basis of Bioavailability*. Upjohn Company, Kalamazoo, Michigan.

Dressman, J.B., Amidon, G.L., Reppas, C., Shah, V.P. (1998) Dissolution testing as a prognostic tool for oral drug absorption: immediate release dosage forms. *Pharmaceutical Research*, **15**, 11-22.

Fuhr, U., Staib, A.N., Harder, S. et al. (1994) Absorption of ipsapirone along the human gastrointestinal. *British Journal of Clinical Pharmacology,* **38**, 83-86.

Hidalgo, I.J., Raub, T.J., Borchardt, R.T. (1989) Characterization of the human colon carcinoma cell line (Caco-2) as a model system for intestinal epithelium permeability. *Gastroenterology*, **96**, 736-749.

Knutson, L., Odlind, B., Hallgren, R. (1989) A new technique for segmental jejunal perfusion in man. *American Journal of Gastroenterology*, **84**, 1278-1284.

Lennernäs, H., Abrenstedt, O., Hallgren, R., Knutson, L., Ryde, M., Palzow, L.K. (1992) Regional jejunal perfusion, a new in vivo approach to study oral drug absorption in man. *Pharmaceutical Research*, **9**, 1243-1251.

Wilding, I. (1997) Non invasive techniques to study human drug absorption. *European Journal of Pharmaceutical Science*, **5**, 518-519.

23

Dosage regimens

J. H. Collett

DOSAGE REGIMENS: THEIR INFLUENCE ON THE CONCENTRATION–TIME PROFILE OF A DRUG IN THE BODY

The subject of dosage regimens is concerned with the dose, time of administration and drug plasma levels factors associated with *multiple* dosing of a drug. The influence that physiological factors, the physicochemical properties of a drug and dosage form factors can have in determining whether a therapeutically effective concentration of a drug is achieved in the plasma following peroral administration of a *single* dose of drug has been discussed previously in Chapters 20 and 21.

Some drugs such as hypnotics, analgesics and antiemetics may provide effective treatment following the administration of a single dose. However, the duration of most illnesses is longer than the therapeutic effect produced by the administration of a single dose of a drug in a conventional dosage form, i.e. a dosage form that is formulated to give rapid and complete drug release. In such cases, doses of the drug are usually administered on a repetitive basis over a period of time determined by the nature of the illness. For instance, one 250 mg ampicillin capsule may be administered every 6 hours for a period of 5 days to treat a bacterial infection. Such a dosing regimen, in which the total dose of drug (i.e. in this example 5 g) administered over 5 days is given in the form of multiple doses (i.e. each of 250 mg) at given intervals of time (i.e. every 6 hours), is known as a *multiple dosage regimen*.

The proper selection of both the dose size and the frequency of administration is an important factor which influences whether a satisfactory therapeutic plasma concentration is achieved and maintained over the prescribed course of drug treatment. Thus the design of a multiple dosage regimen is crucial to successful drug therapy.

ONE-COMPARTMENT OPEN MODEL OF DRUG DISPOSITION IN THE BODY

In order to understand how the design of a dosage regimen can influence the time course of a drug in the body, as measured by its plasma concentration–time curve, let us consider that the complex kinetic processes of drug input, output and distribution in the body may be represented by the pharmacokinetic model of drug disposition, the one-compartment open model, shown in Figure 23.1.

In the case of a one-compartment open model, the drug is considered to be distributed instantly throughout the whole body following its release and absorption from the dosage form. Thus the body behaves as a single compartment in which absorbed drug is distributed so rapidly that a concentration equilibrium exists at any given time between the plasma, other body fluids and the tissues into which the drug has become distributed.

To assume that the body behaves as a one-compartment open model does not necessarily mean that the drug concentrations in all body tissues at any given time are equal. The model does assume, however, that any changes that occur in the plasma reflect quantitatively changes occurring in the concentration of drug at the site(s) of action.

Rate of drug input versus rate of drug output

In a one-compartment open model, the overall kinetic processes of drug input and drug output are described by first-order kinetics. In the case of a perorally administered dosage form, the process of drug input into the body compartment involves drug release from the dosage form and passage of drug across the cellular membranes constituting the gastrointestinal barrier. The rate of drug input or absorption represents the net result of all these processes. The rate of drug input (absorption) at any given time is proportional to the concentration of drug, which is assumed to be in an absorbable form, in solution in the gastrointestinal fluids at the site(s) of absorption, i.e. the effective concentration, C_e, of drug at time, t.

Hence:

$$\text{rate of drug input at time } t \,\alpha\, C_e \qquad (23.1)$$

and

$$\text{rate of drug input at time } t = -k_a C_e \qquad (23.2)$$

where k_a is the apparent absorption rate constant.

The negative sign in Eqn 23.2 indicates that the effective concentration of drug at the absorption site(s) decreases with time. The apparent absorption rate constant gives the proportion (or fraction) of drug which enters the body compartment per unit time. Its units are time^{-1}, e.g. hours^{-1}.

Unlike the rate of drug input into the body compartment, the apparent absorption rate constant, k_a, is independent of the effective concentration of drug at the absorption site(s). Since the rate of drug input is proportional to the effective drug concentration, the rate of drug input will be maximal following administration of a dose of drug contained in a peroral dosage form which gives rapid and complete drug release. The rate of drug input will decrease gradually with time as a consequence of the effective drug concentration at the absorption site(s) decreasing progressively with time, chiefly as a result of absorption into the body compartment. Other processes, such as chemical degradation and movement of drug away from the absorption site(s), will also contribute to the gradual decrease in the effective drug concentration with time.

In the case of a one-compartment open model, the rate of drug output or elimination is a first-order process. Consequently, the magnitude of this parameter at any given time is dependent on the concentration of drug in the body compartment at that time. Immediately following administration of the first dose of peroral dosage form, the rate of drug output from the body will be low since little of the drug will have been absorbed into the body compartment. However, as absorption proceeds, initially at a higher rate than the rate of drug output, the net concentration of drug in the body will increase with time. Likewise, the rate of drug output from the body compartment will also increase with time. Since the rate of drug output is increasing with time whilst the rate of drug input into the body compartment is decreasing with

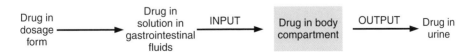

Fig. 23.1 One-compartment open model of drug disposition for a perorally administered drug.

time, the situation is eventually reached when the rate of drug output begins to exceed the rate of drug input. Consequently, the net concentration of drug in the body compartment will reach a peak value and then begin to fall with time. The ensuing decreases in the net concentration of drug in the body will also cause the rate of drug output to decrease with time.

These changes in the rates of drug input and output, relative to each other, with time are responsible for the characteristic shape of the concentration time course of a drug in the body shown in Figure 23.2 following peroral administration of a single dose of drug.

It is evident from the preceding discussion, and Figure 23.2, that the greater the rate of drug input relative to the rate of drug output from the body compartment over the net absorption phase, the higher will be the peak concentration achieved in the body or plasma following peroral administration of a single dose of drug. This explains why increases in dose size and formulation changes in dosage forms, which produce increases in the effective concentration of drug at the absorption site(s), result in higher peak plasma and body concentrations being obtained for a given drug. It should also be noted that any unexpected decrease in the rate of drug output relative to the rate of drug input, which may occur as the result of renal impairment, is also likely to result in higher plasma and body concentrations of drug than expected and the possibility of the patient exhibiting undesirable side-effects of the drug. The adjustment of dosage regimens in cases of patients having severe renal impairment is considered later in this chapter.

Elimination rate constant and biological half-life of a drug

In the case of a one-compartment open model, the rate of elimination or output of a drug from the body compartment follows first-order kinetics (see Chapter 7) and is related to the concentration of drug, C_t, remaining in the body compartment at time t, by the following equation:

$$\text{rate of elimination at time } t = -k_e C_t \quad (23.3)$$

where k_e is the apparent elimination rate constant. The negative sign in Eqn 23.3 indicates that elimination is removing drug *from* the body compartment.

The apparent elimination rate constant of a drug gives the proportion or fraction of that drug which is eliminated from the body per unit time. Its units are in terms of time^{-1}. The apparent elimination constant of a given drug thus provides a quantitative index of the persistence of that drug in the body.

An alternative parameter used is the biological or elimination half-life of the drug, $t_{1/2}$. The biological half-life of a given drug is the time required for the body to eliminate 50% of the drug which it contained. Thus, the larger the biological half-life exhibited by a drug, the slower will be its elimination from the body or plasma.

For a drug whose elimination follows first-order kinetics, the value of its biological half-life is independent of the concentration of drug remaining in the body or plasma. Hence, if a single dose of a drug having a biological half-life of 4 hours was administered

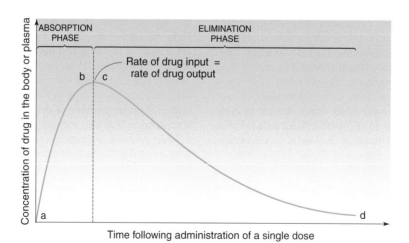

a–b rate of drug absorption > rate of drug elimination
c–d rate of drug elimination > rate of drug absorption

Fig. 23.2 Concentration–time course of a drug in the body following peroral administration of a single dose of drug which confers one-compartment open model characteristics on the body.

perorally, then after the peak plasma concentration had been reached, the plasma concentration of drug would fall by 50% every 4 hours until the entire drug had been eliminated or a further dose was administered. The relationship between the numbers of half-lives elapsed and the percentage of drug eliminated from the body following administration of a single dose is given in Table 23.1.

An appreciation of the relationship between the percentage of drug eliminated from the body and the number of biological half-lives elapsed is useful when considering how much drug is eliminated from the body over the time interval between successive doses in a multiple dosage regimen. The biological half-life of a drug varies from drug to drug and even, for a given drug, varies from patient to patient. Some biological half-lives for various drugs are given in Table 23.2.

For a drug whose elimination follows first-order kinetics, the biological half-life of the drug, $t_{1/2}$, is related to the apparent elimination rate constant, k_e, of that drug according to the following equation:

$$t_{1/2} = \frac{0.693}{k_e} \tag{23.4}$$

This equation indicates that the biological half-life of a drug will be influenced by any factor that influences the apparent elimination rate constant of the drug. This explains why factors such as genetic differences between individuals, age and type of disease can affect the biological half-life exhibited by a given drug. The biological half-life of a drug is an important factor which influences the plasma concentration–time curve obtained following peroral administration of a multiple dosage regimen.

Table 23.2   The biological half-life ranges for phenobarbitone, digoxin and theophylline

Drug	Biological half-life (hours)
Phenobarbitone	50–120
Digoxin	36–51
Theophylline	3–8

Concentration–time curve of a drug in the body following the peroral administration of equal doses of a drug at fixed intervals of time

In discussing how the design of multiple peroral dosage regimens can influence the concentration–time course of a drug in the body, the following assumptions have been made.

- The drug confers upon the body the characteristics of a one-compartment open model.
- The values of the apparent absorption rate and apparent elimination rate constants for a given drug do not change during the period for which the dosage regimen is administered to a patient.
- The fraction of each administered dose which is absorbed by the body compartment remains constant for a given drug.
- The aim of drug therapy is to achieve promptly and maintain a concentration of drug at the appropriate site(s) of action which is both clinically efficacious and safe for the desired duration of drug treatment. This aim is assumed to be achieved by the prompt attainment and maintenance of plasma concentrations of drug which lie within the therapeutic range of the drug.

If the time interval between each perorally administered dose is longer than the time required for complete elimination of the previous dose, then the plasma concentration time profile of a drug will exhibit a series of isolated single dose profiles as shown in Figure 23.3.

Consideration of the plasma concentration–time profile shown in Figure 23.3 in relation to the minimum effective and maximum safe plasma concentrations for the drug reveals that the design of this particular dosage regimen is unsatisfactory. The plasma concentration only lies within the therapeutic range of the drug for a relatively short period of time following the administration of each dose and the patient remains undermedicated for relatively long periods of time. If the dosing time interval is reduced such that it is now shorter than the time required for complete elimination of the previous dose,

Table 23.1   Relationship between the amount of drug eliminated and the number of half-lives elapsed

Number of half-lives elapsed	Percentage of drug eliminated
0.5	29.3
1.0	50.0
2.0	75.0
3.0	87.5
3.3	90.0
4.0	94.0
4.3	95.0
5.0	97.0
6.0	98.4
6.6	99.0
7.0	99.2

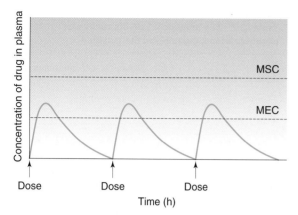

Fig. 23.3 Plasma concentration–time curve following peroral administration of equal doses of a drug at time intervals that allow complete elimination of the previous dose (MSC, maximum safe plasma concentration of the drug; MEC, minimum effective plasma concentration of the drug).

then the resulting plasma concentration–time curve exhibits the characteristic profile shown in Figure 23.4.

Figure 23.4 shows that at the start of this multiple dosage regimen, the maximum and minimum plasma concentrations of drug observed during each dosing time interval tend to increase with successive doses. This increase is a consequence of the time interval between successive doses being less than that required for complete elimination of the previous absorbed dose. Consequently the total amount of the drug remaining in the body compartment at any time after a dose is equal to

the sum of that remaining from all the previous doses. The accumulation of drug in the body and plasma with successively administered doses does not continue indefinitely. Providing drug elimination follows first-order kinetics, the rate of drug elimination will increase as the average concentration of drug in the body (and plasma) rises. If the amount of drug supplied to the body compartment per unit dosing time interval remains constant, then a situation is eventually reached when the overall rate of elimination of drug from the body over the dosing time interval, becomes equal to the overall rate at which drug is being supplied to the body compartment over the dosing time interval. The overall rate of elimination has effectively caught up with the overall rate of supply of drug to the body compartment over each dosing time interval. This is due to the elimination rate increasing as the residual concentration of drug in the plasma rises (since elimination is first order here).

When the overall rate of drug supply equals the overall rate of drug output from the body compartment, a *steady state* is reached with respect to the *average* concentration of drug remaining in the body over each dosing time interval. There is some variability of short time periods but overall the average drug concentration remains constant. At steady state, the amount of drug eliminated from the body over each dosing time interval is equal to the amount of drug that was absorbed into the body compartment following administration of the previous dose.

Figure 23.5 shows that the amount of drug in the body, as measured by the plasma concentration of drug, fluctuates between maximum and minimum values, which remain more or less constant from dose to dose. At steady state the average concentration of drug in the plasma, $C^{ss}_{average}$, over successive dosing time intervals remains constant.

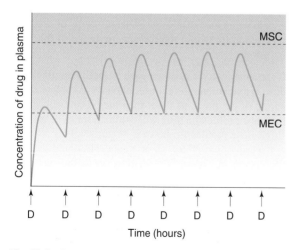

Fig. 23.4 Plasma concentration–time curve following peroral administration of equal doses, D, of a drug every 4 hours (MSC, maximum safe plasma concentration of the drug; MEC, minimum effective plasma concentration of the drug).

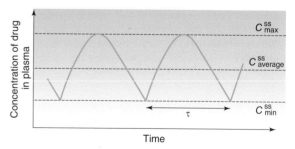

Fig. 23.5 Fluctuation of concentration of drug in the plasma at steady state resulting from repetitive peroral administration of equal doses, D, of drug at a fixed interval of time, t. C^{ss}_{max}, C^{ss}_{min} and $C^{ss}_{average}$ represent the maximum, minimum and average plasma concentrations of drug, respectively, achieved at steady state.

For a drug administered repetitively in equal doses and at equal time intervals, the time required for the average plasma concentration to attain the corresponding steady-state value is a function only of the biological half-life of the drug and is independent of both the size of the dose administered and the length of the dosing time interval. The time required for the average plasma concentration to reach 95% of the steady-state value corresponding to the particular multiple dosage regimen is 4.3 times the biological half-life of the drug. The corresponding figure for 99% is 6.6 times. Therefore, depending on the magnitude of the biological half-life of the drug being administered, the time taken to attain the average steady-state plasma concentration may range from a few hours to several days.

From a clinical viewpoint, the time required to reach steady state is important since for a properly designed multiple dosage regimen, the attainment of steady state corresponds to the achievement and maintenance of maximal clinical effectiveness of the drug in the patient.

It should be noted that for a drug such as phenytoin, whose elimination is not described by first-order kinetics, the peroral administration of equal doses at fixed intervals of time may not result in the attainment of steady-state plasma levels of the drug. If the concentration of such drug in the body rises sufficiently following repetitive administration, the pathway responsible for its elimination may become saturated with drug. If this occurs, the rate of elimination would become maximal and could not increase to cope with any further rises in the average concentration of drug in the body. Hence the overall rate of elimination would not become equal to the overall rate of supply of drug to the body over each dosing time interval, and the condition necessary for the attainment of steady state would not be achieved. If repetitive administration continued the same rate, the average concentration of drug in the body and plasma would tend to continue to accumulate, rather than reaching a plateau.

IMPORTANT FACTORS INFLUENCING STEADY-STATE PLASMA CONCENTRATIONS OF A DRUG

Dose size and frequency of administration

In designing a multiple dosage regimen which balances patient convenience with achievement and maintenance of maximal clinical effectiveness, only two parameters can be adjusted for a given drug: the size of dose and the frequency of administration. Let us consider how the maximum, minimum and average steady-state plasma concentrations of drug are influenced by these parameters.

Size of dose

Figure 23.6 illustrates the effects of changing the dose size on the concentration of drug in the plasma following repetitive administration of peroral doses at equal intervals of time. As the size of the administered dose is increased, the higher are the corresponding maximum, minimum and average plasma drug levels, C_{max}^{ss}, C_{min}^{ss} and $C_{average}^{ss}$ respectively, achieved at steady state. What may not be so well appreciated is that the larger the size of dose administered, the larger the fluctuation between C_{max}^{ss} and C_{min}^{ss} during each dosing time interval. Large fluctuations between C_{max}^{ss} and C_{min}^{ss} can be hazardous, particularly with a drug such as digoxin which has a narrow therapeutic range. In the case of such a drug, it is possible that C_{max}^{ss} could exceed the maximum safe plasma concentration of the drug. Figure 23.6 also illustrates that the time required to attain steady-state plasma concentrations of drug is independent of the size of the administered dose.

Interval of time between successive equal doses

Figure 23.7 illustrates the effects of constant doses administered at various dosing intervals which are multiples of the biological half-life of the drug $t_{1/2}$. The uppermost plasma concentration–time curve in Figure 23.7 shows

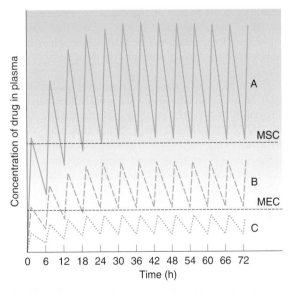

Fig. 23.6 Diagrammatic representation of the effect of dose size on the plasma concentration–time curve obtained following peroral administration of equal doses of a given fixed drug at fixed intervals of time equal to the biological half-life of the drug. Curve A, dose = 250 mg. Curve B, dose = 100 mg. Curve C, dose = 40 mg.

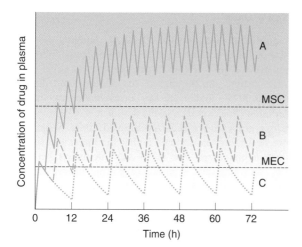

Fig. 23.7 Diagrammatic representation of the effect of changing the dosing time interval, t, on the plasma concentration–time curve obtained following repetitive peroral administration of equal size doses of a given drug. Curve A, dosing time interval = 3 hours ($0.5t_{1/2}$). Curve B, dosing time interval = 6 hours ($t_{1/2}$). Curve C, dosing time = 12 hours ($2t_{1/2}$).

that the repetitive administration of doses at a time interval which is less than the biological half-life of the drug results in higher steady-state plasma drug concentrations being obtained. The higher steady-state concentration is a consequence of the extent of elimination of the drug from the body over a dosing time interval equal to $0.5\ t_{1/2}$ being smaller than that which is eliminated when the dosing time interval is equal to $t_{1/2}$ (see Table 23.1).

Figure 23.7 also shows that repetitive administration of doses at time intervals greater than the biological half-life of the drug results in the lower steady-state plasma drug concentrations being obtained. This decrease is a consequence of a greater proportion of the drug being eliminated over a dosing time interval equal to $2t_{1/2}$ as compared to that which is eliminated when the dosing time interval is equal to $t_{1/2}$.

Summary of the effects of dose size and frequency of administration

Consideration of the effects of administered dose size and the dosage time interval on the amount of a given drug achieved in the body, as measured by the plasma concentration of drug, following repetitive peroral administration of equal doses of the drug has revealed the following relationships:

- The magnitude of the fluctuations between the maximum and minimum steady-state amounts of drug in the body is determined by the size of dose administered or, more accurately, by the amount of drug absorbed following each dose administered.
- The magnitude of the fluctuations between the maximum and minimum steady-state plasma concentrations of a drug is an important consideration for any drug which has a narrow therapeutic range, e.g. digoxin. The administration of smaller doses at more frequent intervals is a means of reducing the steady-state fluctuations without altering the average steady-state plasma concentration of the drug. For example, a 500 mg dose of drug given every 6 hours will provide the same $C_{average}^{ss}$ value as a 250 mg dose of the same drug given every 3 hours, whilst the C_{max} and C_{min} fluctuation for the latter dose will be decreased by a half.
- The average maximum and minimum amounts of drug achieved in the body at steady state are influenced by either the dose size, the dosage time interval in relation to the biological half-life of the drug, or both. The greater the dose size and the smaller the dosage time interval relative to the biological half-life of the drug, the greater are the average, maximum and minimum steady-state amounts of drug in the body.
- For a given drug, the time taken to achieve steady state is independent of dose size and the dosage time interval.
- If the maximum safe and minimum effective plasma drug concentrations are represented by the dashed lines shown in Figures 23.6 and 23.7, respectively, then it is evident that the proper selection of dose size and dosage time interval is important with respect to achieving and maintaining steady-state plasma concentrations which lie within the therapeutic range of the particular drug being administered.

It is evident from the preceding discussion that the proper selection of the dose size and the dosage time interval is crucial in ensuring that a multiple dosage regimen provides steady-state concentrations of drug in the body which are both clinically efficacious and safe.

Mathematical relationships which predict the values of the various steady-state parameters achieved in the body following repetitive administration of doses at constant intervals of time have been used to assist the design of clinically acceptable multiple dosage regimens. For example, a useful equation for predicting the average amount of drug achieved in the body at steady state, $D_{average}^{ss}$, following repetitive peroral administration of equal doses, D, at a fixed time interval, τ, is given by:

$$D^{ss}_{average} = \frac{FDt_{1/2} 1.44}{\tau} \qquad (23.5)$$

where F is the fraction of drug absorbed following administration of a dose, D, of drug (thus $F \cdot D$ is the bioavailable dose of drug) and $t_{1/2}$ is the biological half-life of the drug. The average amount of a given drug in the body at steady state, $D^{ss}_{average}$, is related to the corresponding average plasma concentration of the drug by the factor known as the *apparent volume of distribution* of the drug, i.e.:

$$D^{ss}_{average} = V_d C^{ss}_{average} \qquad (23.6)$$

where V_d is the apparent volume of distribution of the drug and $C^{ss}_{average}$ is the average steady-state plasma concentration of the drug. Eqn 23.5 can be rewritten in terms of the average steady-state plasma concentration of the drug as follows:

$$C^{ss}_{average} = \frac{FDt_{1/2} 1.44}{\tau V_d} \qquad (23.7)$$

If the value of the average body amount or the average plasma concentration of a given drug at steady state which gives a satisfactory therapeutic response in a patient is known, then Eqn 23.5 or Eqn 23.7, respectively, can be used to estimate either the size of dose which should be administered repetitively at a preselected constant dosage time interval or the dosage time interval that a preselected dose should be administered repetitively. In order to illustrate a dosage regimen calculation, based on the average steady-state plasma concentration of a drug, consider the following worked example.

An antibiotic is to be administered on a repetitive basis to a male patient weighing 76 kg. The antibiotic is commercially available in the form of tablets each containing 250 mg of the drug. The fraction of the drug which is absorbed following peroral administration of one 250 mg tablet is 0.9. The antibiotic has been found to exhibit a biological half-life of 3 hours and the patient has an apparent volume of distribution of 0.2 litre kg^{-1} of body weight. What dosage time interval should be selected to administer this drug on a repetitive basis in order that a therapeutic average steady-state plasma concentration of 16 mg L^{-1} will be achieved?

Using Eqn 23.7:

$$C^{ss}_{average} = \frac{FDt_{1/2} 1.44}{\tau V_d} \qquad (23.8)$$

where the average steady-state plasma concentration of drug, $C^{ss}_{average}$ = 16 mg L^{-1}, the fraction of each administered dose absorbed, F = 0.9, the size of administered dose, D = 250 mg, the biological half-life of the drug,

$t_{1/2}$ = 3 hours and the apparent volume of distribution, V_d = 0.2 litre kg^{-1} of patient's body weight.

Hence, for a patient weighing 76 kg, the value of:

$$V_d = 0.2 \times 76 \text{ litres}$$

$$= 15.2 \text{ litres}$$

To calculate the dosage time interval, τ, requires substitution of the above values into Eqn 23.7 which gives:

$$16 = \frac{0.9 \times 250 \times 3 \times 1.44}{\tau \times 15.2}$$

$$\tau = \frac{0.9 \times 250 \times 3 \times 1.44}{16 \times 15.2}$$

$$= \frac{972.0}{243.2} \text{ hours}$$

$$\approx 4 \text{ hours}$$

Thus one 250 mg tablet should be administered every 4 hours in order to achieve the required averaged average steady-state plasma concentration.

Mathematical equations which predict the maximum or minimum steady-state plasma concentrations of a drug achieved in the body followed by repetitive administration of equal doses at a fixed interval of time are also available for drugs whose time course in the body is described by the one-compartment open pharmacokinetic model.

Concept of 'loading doses'

As discussed earlier, the time required for a given drug to reach 95% of the average steady-state plasma concentration is 4.3 biological half-lives, when equal doses of the drug are administered repetitively at equal intervals of time. Thus, for a drug with a long half-life of 24 hours it would take more than 4 days for the average drug concentration in the plasma to reach 95% of its steady-state value. Since the attainment of steady-state plasma concentrations is normally associated with the attainment of maximal clinical effectiveness of the drug, it is conceivable that a number of days could elapse before a patient experienced the full therapeutic benefit of a drug having a long half-life. To reduce the time required for onset of the full therapeutic effect of a drug, a large single dose of the drug may be administered initially in order to achieve a peak plasma concentration which lies within the therapeutic range of the drug and is approximately equal to the value of C^{ss}_{max} required. This initial dose is known as the 'loading dose' or 'priming dose'.

Thereafter smaller, equal doses are administered repetitively at suitable fixed intervals of time in order to maintain the plasma concentrations of drug at the maximum, minimum and average state levels which provide the patient with the full therapeutic benefit of the drug. These smaller, equal doses are known as '*maintenance doses*'. As a general rule, the loading dose should be twice the size of the maintenance dose if the selected dosage time interval corresponds to the biological half-life of the drug.

Figure 23.8 illustrates how rapidly therapeutic steady-state plasma concentrations of drug are achieved when the dosage regimen consists of an initial loading dose followed by equal maintenance doses at fixed intervals of time in comparison to a 'simple' multiple dosage regimen consisting of doses that are equal in size and are administered at the same dosage time intervals as the maintenance doses.

Influence of changes in the apparent elimination rate constant of a drug: the problem of patients with renal impairment

Whilst the loading dose, maintenance dose and dosage time interval may be varied in order to design a clinically efficacious multiple dosage regimen, one factor cannot normally be adjusted. That factor is the apparent elimination rate constant exhibited by the particular drug being administered. However, the elimination rate constant of a given drug does vary from patient to patient and is influenced by whether the patient has normal or impaired renal function.

Figure 23.9 indicates the effects produced by changes in the apparent elimination rate constant on the plasma concentration–time curve obtained following repetitive, peroral administration of equal doses of a given drug at equal intervals of time. Any reduction in the apparent elimination rate constant of a drug will produce a proportional increase in the biological half-life exhibited by that drug. This reduction, in turn, will result in a greater degree of accumulation of the drug in the body following repetitive administration before steady-state drug levels are achieved. The greater degree of drug accumulation is a consequence of a smaller proportion of the drug being eliminated from the body over each fixed dosage time interval when the biological half-life of the drug is increased.

Patients who develop severe renal impairment normally exhibit smaller apparent elimination rate constants and consequently longer biological half-lives for drugs which are eliminated substantially by renal excretion than do patients with normal renal function. For instance, the average apparent elimination rate constant for digoxin may be reduced from 0.021 h^{-1} in patients with normal renal function to 0.007 h^{-1} in severe renal impairment. The average steady-state amount of drug in the body is only achieved and maintained when the overall rate of drug supply equals the overall rate of elimination of drug from the body over successive dosing time intervals. Any reduction in the overall rate of elimination of a drug as a result of renal disease without a corresponding compensatory reduction in the overall rate of drug supply will result in increased steady-state amounts in the body. This effect, in turn, may lead to side-effects and toxic effects if the

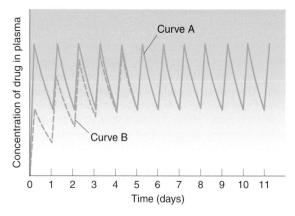

Fig. 23.8 Diagrammatic representation of how the initial administration of a loading dose followed by equal maintenance doses at fixed intervals of time ensures rapid attainment of steady-state plasma levels for a drug having a long biological half-life of 24 hours. Curve A represents the plasma concentration–time curve obtained following peroral administration of a loading dose of 500 mg followed by a maintenance dose of 250 mg every 24 hours. Curve B represents the plasma concentration–time curve obtained following peroral administration of a 250 mg dose every 24 hours.

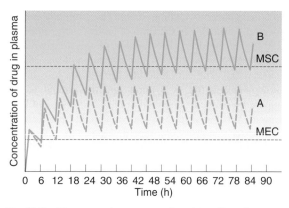

Fig. 23.9 Diagrammatic representation of the effect of changing the biological half-life of a given drug on the plasma concentration–time curve exhibited by the drug following peroral administration of one 250 mg dose every 6 hours. Curve A, biological half-life of drug = 6 hours. Curve B, biological half-life of drug = 12 hours.

increased steady-state levels of drug exceed the maximum safe concentration of the drug.

In order to illustrate this concept, let us consider that curves A and B in Figure 23.9 correspond to the plasma concentration–time curves obtained for a given drug in patients having normal renal function and severe renal impairment, respectively, and that the upper and lower dashed lines represent the maximum safe and minimum effective plasma concentrations, respectively. It is thus evident that administration of a drug according to a multiple dosage regimen which produces therapeutic steady-state plasma levels of drug in patients with normal renal function will give plasma drug concentrations which exceed the maximum safe plasma concentration of the drug in patients with severe renal impairment. Hence adjustment of multiple dosage regimens in terms of dose size, frequency of administration or both is necessary if patients suffering with renal disease are to avoid the possibility of overmedication.

Influence of the 'overnight no-dose period'

In our discussions so far, we have considered that multiple dosage regimens consist of doses being administered at uniform time intervals around the clock. In practice, it is unusual to administer doses under such conditions. If a multiple dosage regimen requires a dose to be administered 'four times a day' it is unlikely that a dose will be administered at exactly 6-hourly intervals around the clock. Instead, the four doses are likely to be administered during the 'waking' hours of each day according to

such time schedules as, say, 10 am–2 pm–6 pm–10 pm or 9 am–1 pm–5 pm–9 pm. The significant feature of both these dosing schedules is that the patient will experience an overnight no-dose period of 12 hours. Whilst overnight no-dose periods undoubtedly give patients periods of undisturbed sleep, such periods may also cause problems in maintaining therapeutic steady-state plasma concentrations of drug in the body.

It is conceivable that overnight no-dose periods of 8–12 hours could result in substantial decreases occurring in the amount of drug in the plasma and body, particularly for drugs having biological half-lives which are relatively short compared to the overnight no-dose period. For instance, in the case of a drug having a biological half-life of 4 hours, an overnight no-dose period of 12 hours would correspond to the elapse of three biological half-lives and consequently, a large reduction in the amount of drug in the body.

The potential problems of overnight no-dose periods with respect to maintaining therapeutic steady-state drug levels in patients are illustrated in Figure 23.10. This figure shows that for a drug having a biological half-life of 4 hours, a multiple dosage regimen comprising one 60 mg dose administered perorally four times each day according to a 9 am–1 pm–5 pm–9 pm timetable does not permit a true steady state to be attained. Thus the concentration of drug in the plasma does not fluctuate between constant maximum and minimum values over successive dosage time intervals as would occur if the doses were administered every 4 hours around the clock.

Furthermore, Figure 23.11 shows that even if a loading does of 120 mg were included in the dosage regimen in

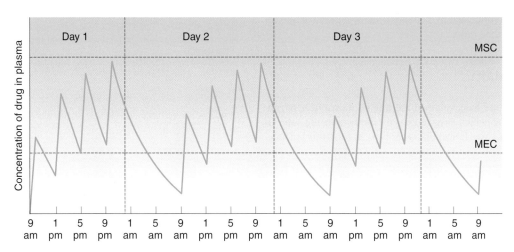

Fig. 23.10 Diagrammatic representation of the variation in the concentration of a drug in the plasma accompanying the peroral administration of a single dose of 60 mg four times a day according to the time schedule 9 am–1 pm–5 pm–9 pm. The biological half-life of the drug is 4 hours.

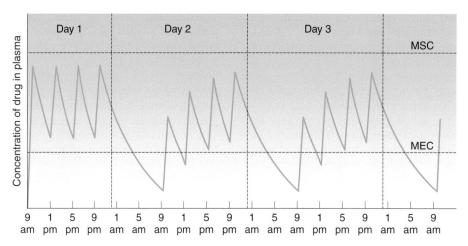

Fig. 23.11 Diagrammatic representation of the variation in the concentration of drug in the plasma accompanying the peroral administration of a loading dose of 120 mg followed by single maintenance doses of 60 mg four times a day according to the time schedule 9 am–1 pm–5 pm–9 pm. The biological half-life of the drug is 4 hours.

order to ensure that a true steady state was obtained before the first overnight no-dose period, the steady state would not be reestablished after the first overnight no-dose period. If the upper and lower dashed lines in Figures 23.10 and 23.11 represent the therapeutic range of the drug, then the patient would experience periods during which the level of drug in the plasma and body would fall below that necessary to elicit its therapeutic effect. Hence, unless the therapeutic range of the drug is sufficiently large to accommodate the fluctuations in drug concentration associated with overnight no-dose periods, problems could arise with regard to maintaining therapeutic drug levels in patients. The potential problems associated with overnight no-dose periods are even further complicated by patients who forget to take one of their daytime doses.

SUMMARY

This chapter has explained the interrelationship between the rate at which drug enters the body and the rate at which it leaves. It also discusses how, in turn, this balance influences the concentration of drug in the blood plasma at any given time. It is clearly important for pharmaceutical scientists to come to terms with this problem and then overcome it by finding ways of maintaining therapeutic drug levels appropriate to a particular disease state. This can be achieved by the careful design of the appropriate drug delivery system. This aspect of the design and formulation of modified-release drug delivery systems is discussed fully in the following chapter.

BIBLIOGRAPHY

Gibaldi, M. (1991) *Biopharmaceutics and Clinical Pharmacokinetics*, 4th edn. Lea and Febiger, Philadelphia.

Rowland, M., Tozer, T.N. (1995) *Clinical Pharmacokinetics: Concepts and Applications*, 3rd edn. Lea and Febiger, Philadelphia.

PART 5

DOSAGE FORM DESIGN AND MANUFACTURE

Pharmaceutical preformulation

J. I. Wells, M. E. Aulton

CONCEPT OF PREFORMULATION

Prior to the development of dosage forms, it is essential that certain *fundamental* physical and chemical properties of potential drug molecules and other *derived* properties of the drug powder are determined. This information dictates many of the subsequent events and approaches in formulation development. This first learning phase is known as *preformulation*. The meaning of the word is quite literal in that it defines the steps to be undertaken before formulation proper. It is normal for preformulation to be performed on potential active drugs (at this stage often referred to as new chemical entities (NCEs) or new drug candidates). In the case of the formulation of generic products of existing drugs, sufficient information is usually known prior to formulation.

Preformulation will give pointers to the feasibility of the various possible dosage forms and to any potential problems of instability and poor in vivo dissolution, and thus bioavailability. It should also give some guidance to the suitability of potential excipients to be used in subsequent formulation. This chapter covers the pertinent aspects of physicochemical preformulation. In parallel, pharmaceutical companies perform biopharmaceutical preformulation studies. These are referred to in Part 4 of this book.

Almost all new drugs are marketed as tablets, capsules or both (see Table 24.1). Only a few drugs are marketed as an injection. However, formulations for the intravenous route are always required during early toxicity, metabolic, bioavailability and clinical studies to provide a precise drug dosing. Other dosage forms may be required (Table 24.1) but these are drug specific and depend to a large extent on the successful development of tablets, capsules and injections.

A recommended list of information required in preformulation is shown in Table 24.2. It is assembled, recognizing their relative importance and probable existence of only limited quantities of new bulk drug (mg rather than g). Investigators must be pragmatic and generate data of immediate relevance, especially if likely dosage forms are known. At this stage care must be taken in interpretation of any data generated as the early samples may be impure and the presence of impurities may affect many measured properties. In some ways this is not a problem as long as the preformulation scientist is aware of this. Preformulation attempts to get 'ball park' figures on which to base future decisions. More precise data can be generated later once the new drug is available in larger quantities and in a more pure form.

It is worth mentioning at this point that all the analytical techniques discussed here are those commonly used in formulation itself. However, there is often a need to adapt these techniques to cope with the small amount of often precious NCE available to the preformulation team.

It is important therefore to gain as much information as possible from these small amounts of material. In this context, preformulation work is often prioritized to yield the key information early in these studies. Two fundamental properties are mandatory for a new compound

Table 24.1 Frequency distribution of dosage form types manufactured in the UK

Dosage form	Frequency (%)
Tablets	46
Liquid oral	16
Capsules	15
Injections	13
Suppositories and pessaries	3
Topicals	3
Eye preparations	2
Aerosols (inhalation)	1
Others	1

Table 24.2 Preformulation drug characterization

Test	Method/function/ characterization
1 Spectroscopy	Simple UV assay
2 Solubility	Phase solubility, purity
aqueous	Intrinsic solubility, pH effects
pK_a	Solubility control, salt formation
salts	Solubility, hygroscopicity, stability
solvents	Vehicles, extraction
partition coeff K_w^o	Lipophilicity, structure activity
dissolution	Biopharmaceutics
3 Melting point	DSC – polymorphism, hydrates, solvates
4 Assay development	UV, TLC, HPLC
5 Stability (in solution and solid state)	Thermal, hydrolysis, oxidation, photolysis, metal ions, pH
6 Microscopy	Morphology, particle size
7 Powder flow	Tablet and capsule formulation
bulk density	
angle of repose	
8 Compression properties	Excipient choice
9 Excipient compatibility	Excipient choice

and these should be determined first. This is the concept of *minimum preformulation*. These properties are

1. intrinsic solubility (C_o),
2. dissociation constant (pK_a).

Independent of this pharmaceutical profiling (Table 24.2), analysts will generate data (Table 24.3) to confirm structure and purity and this should be used to complement and confirm pharmaceutical data. Their greater training and knowledge in analysis will assist in the identification of suitable stability-indicating assays by, for example, high-performance liquid chromatography (HPLC).

SPECTROSCOPY

The first step in preformulation is to establish a simple quantitative analytical method. Most drugs absorb light in the ultraviolet wavelengths (190–390 nm) since they are generally aromatic and may contain double bonds. Using the UV spectrum of the drug, it is possible to choose an analytical wavelength (often the wavelength of maximum absorption, λ_{max}) suitable to quantify the amount of drug in a particular solution. Excitation of the molecule in solution causes a loss in light energy and the net change from the

intensity of the incident light (I_o) and the transmitted light (I) can be measured. The amount of light absorbed by a solution of drug is proportional to the concentration (C) and the path length of the solution (l) through which the light has passed. Equation 24.1 is the Beer–Lambert Law where e is the molar extinction coefficient.

$$\text{Absorbance } (A) = \log_{10}(I_o/I) = eCl \qquad (24.1)$$

In pharmaceutical science, it is usual to use the *specific absorption coefficient* $E_{1cm}^{1\%}$ (E_1^1) where the sample path length is 1 cm and the solution concentration is 1% w/v (10 mg mL^{-1}) since doses of drugs and concentrations are generally expressed in units of weights rather than molarity. The relationship between specific absorption coefficient, molar extinction coefficient and molecular weight is given by:

$$E_1^1 = 10e/MW \qquad (24.2)$$

UV analysis is a very simple and convenient quantitative technique that is suitable at this early stage of preformulation but it suffers from being non-indicating of the molecule absorbing the UV light. It must be replaced later in the process once more material becomes available for an assay (usually HPLC, see later in this chapter) that will give a precise indication of the molecule and its degradation products.

Table 24.3	Analytical preformulation
Attribute	**Test**
Identity	Nuclear magnetic resonance (NMR)
	Infrared spectroscopy (IR)
	Ultraviolet spectroscopy (UV)
	Thin-layer chromatography (TLC)
	Differential scanning calorimetry (DSC)
	Optical rotation, where applicable
Purity	Moisture (water and solvents)
	Inorganic elements
	Heavy metals
	Organic impurities
	Differential scanning calorimetry (DSC)
Assay	Titration
	Ultraviolet spectroscopy (UV)
	High-performance liquid chromatography (HPLC)
Quality	Appearance
	Odour
	Solution colour
	pH of slurry (saturated solution)
	Melting point

SOLUBILITY

Aqueous solubility

The availability of drug is always limited at this stage and the preformulation scientist may only have 50 mg with which to work. As the compound is new, the quality is invariably poor, so that a large number of unknown impurities may be present and often the first crystals crystallize out as a metastable polymorph. Accordingly, as a minimum, the approximate values of solubility and pK_a must be determined. Solubility dictates the ease with which formulations of aqueous solutions for oral gavage and intravenous injection are obtained for preclinical studies. A knowledge of the candidate's pK_a allows the informed use of pH to maintain solubility and to allow the informed choice of salts required to achieve good bioavailability from the solid state (Chapter 21), improve stability (Chapter 44) and improve powder properties (Chapters 12 and 13).

Kaplan (1972) suggested that unless a compound has an aqueous solubility in excess of 1% (10 mg mL^{-1}) over the pH range 1–7 at 37°C, potential bioabsorption problems may occur. Similarly, if the intrinsic dissolution rate is greater than 1 mg cm^{-2} min^{-1} then absorption will be unimpeded. Dissolution rates less than 0.1 mg cm^{-2} min^{-1}

were likely to give dissolution rate-limited absorption. This 10-fold difference in dissolution rate translates to a lower limit for solubility of 1 mg mL^{-1}. Under sink conditions, dissolution rate and solubilities can be assumed at the preformulation stage to be proportional for most drugs.

A solubility of less than 1 mg mL^{-1} indicates the need for a salt, particularly if the drug will be formulated as a tablet or capsule. In the range 1–10 mg mL^{-1} serious consideration should be given to salt formation. When the solubility of the drug cannot be manipulated in this way (neutral molecules, glycosides, steroids, alcohols or where the pK_a is less than 3 for an acid or greater than 10 for a base) then liquid filling in soft or hard gelatin capsules may be necessary. These would contain the drug in an oily or hydrophilic (but not aqueous) solvent (discussed more fully in Chapters 34 and 35).

Intrinsic solubility (C$_0$)

An increase in solubility in acidic aqueous solution compared with that in pure water suggests a weak base. An increase in solubility in alkaline solutions suggests a weakly acid drug. In both cases a dissociation constant (pK_a) can be measured and this will indicate whether the formation of suitable salts is possible. An increase in both acidic and alkaline solubility of the NCE suggests either amphoteric or zwitterion behaviour. In this case there will be two pK_as, one acidic and one basic. This can occur in large molecules composed of both acidic and basic functional groups.

No change in NCE solubility over a range of pHs suggests a non-ionizable, neutral molecule with no measurable pK_a. Solubility manipulation will require either alternative solvents or complexation.

When the purity of the drug sample can be assured, the solubility value obtained in acid for a weak acid or alkali for a weak base can be assumed to be the *intrinsic solubility* (C$_0$), i.e. the fundamental solubility of the NCE when completely unionized. The solubility should ideally be measured at two temperatures:

- 4°C to ensure physical and chemical stability on extended short-term storage until more definitive data are available. The maximum density of water occurs at 4°C and this leads to a minimum aqueous solubility
- 37°C to support biopharmaceutical evaluation.

However, since absolute purity is often in doubt with preformulation samples, the presence of impurities could either increase or decrease the NCE's apparent solubility (or alternatively have no effect). The problem for preformulation scientists at this early stage is that they will not

know which of these options is taking place. A reasonably accurate estimation of this crucial solubility can be made by use of a phase-solubility diagram (Fig. 24.1). The data are obtained from a series of experiments in which the ratio of the amount of drug to the amount of dissolving solvent is varied.

As an example, assume that the compound is a base and the estimate of its solubility in 0.1 M NaOH was 1 mg mL^{-1}. Four solutions of 3 mL can be set up containing, say, 3, 6, 12 and 24 mg of drug. Each of these will be saturated (as they equal or exceed the NCE's estimated solubility) and give the phase ratios shown in Figure 24.1. Three millilitres is the smallest volume which can be manipulated for either centrifugation or filtration and dilution of UV analysis. The vials should be agitated continuously overnight and then the concentration in solution determined.

Any deviation from the horizontal is indicative of the presence of impurities. A large amount of drug, with its inherent impurities, will either promote or suppress solubility. In the cases where the observed result changes with the amount of solvent, the line is extrapolated to zero phase ratio, where solubility will be independent of solvent level and the true intrinsic solubility of the drug. It would, of course, be impossible to measure this directly.

pK_a from solubility data

Seventy-five percent of all drugs are weak bases, 20% are weak acids and only 5% are non-ionic, amphoteric or alcohols. It is therefore appropriate to consider the Henderson–Hasselbalch equations for weak acids and bases. More detail on the derivation and usage of these equations is given in Chapter 3.

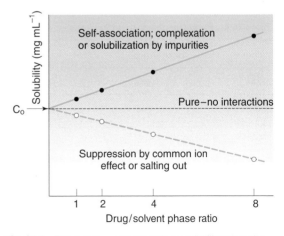

Fig. 24.1 Effect of drug: solvent ratio on solubility when the drug is impure.

For weak acids:

$$pH = pK_a + \log_{10}([A^-]/[HA]) \qquad (24.3)$$

and for weak bases:

$$pH = pK_a + \log_{10}([B]/[BH^+]) \qquad (24.4)$$

Equations 24.3 and 24.4 can be used to:

- determine pK_a by following changes in solubility
- predict solubility at any pH provided that the intrinsic solubility (C_o) and pK_a are known
- facilitate the selection of suitable salt-forming compounds and predict the solubility and pH properties of the salts.

Albert & Serjeant (1984) give a detailed account of how to obtain precise pK_a values by potentiometry, spectroscopy and conductivity.

Salts

A major improvement in solubility can be achieved by forming a salt. A salt is a chemical combination of two ionizable components – one acidic and one basic relative to the other. Either the acidic or the basic moiety may be the drug. If the pK_a (acid) and pK_a (base) are too close (<about 0.5 units), a stable salt may not form. Some molecules do not form salts, such as those that do not dissociate when dissolved in water; examples of such molecules are steroids and alcohols.

Some acceptable pharmaceutical salt counter-ions and their pK_as are shown in Table 24.4. As an example, the consequences of changing chlordiazepoxide to various salt forms, in terms of pK_a, pH of a saturated solution of salt and aqueous solubility, are shown in Table 24.5.

In some cases, salts prepared from strong acids (e.g. hydrochloride) or bases (e.g. sodium, potassium) are freely soluble but very hygroscopic. This does lead to instability in tablet or capsule formulations since some drug will partially dissolve in its own adsorbed films of moisture. It is often better to use a weaker acid or base to form the salt provided any solubility requirements are met. A less soluble salt will generally be less hygroscopic and form less acidic or basic solutions (see Table 24.5).

The future potential dosage form may also influence the choice of salt. Injections should ideally lie in the pH range 3–9 to prevent vessel or tissue damage and pain at the injection site. Oral syrups should not be too acidic to enhance palatability. Packaging may also be susceptible; for example, excessive alkalinity will attack glass.

From Table 24.5, it can be seen that not only does the intrinsic pH of the base solution fall significantly if salt forms are produced but, as a consequence, the solubility increases exponentially (Eqns 24.3 and 24.4). This has important implications in vivo. A weak base with an intrinsic solubility greater than 1 mg mL^{-1} will be freely soluble in the gastrointestinal tract, especially in the stomach. However, it is usually better to formulate with a salt since it will control the pH of the diffusion layer (the saturated solution immediately adjacent to the dissolving surface and known as the pH microenvironment, discussed further in Chapter 21). For example, although chlordiazepoxide base itself ($C_S = 2$ mg mL^{-1} at pH$_{sat}$ = 8.3) meets the requirements for satisfactory in vivo solubility (Kaplan 1972), commercial capsules contain the more water-soluble chlordiazepoxide hydrochloride ($C_S = 165$ mg mL^{-1} at pH$_{sat}$ = 2.53).

A weakly basic drug will have a high dissolution rate and high solubility in the stomach but as it moves down

Table 24.4 Potential pharmaceutical salts					
Basic drugs			**Acidic drugs**		
Anion	pKa	% Usage	Cation	pKa	% Usage
Hydrochloride	−6.10	43.0	Potassium	16.00	10.8
Sulfate	−3.00, +1.96	7.5	Sodium	14.77	62.0
Mesylate	−1.20	2.0	Lithium	13.82	1.6
Maleate	1.92, 6.23	3.0	Calcium	12.90	10.5
Phosphate	2.15, 7.20,	3.2	Magnesium	11.42	1.3
Salicylate	12.38	0.9	Diethanolamine	9.65	1.0
Tartrate	3.00	3.5	Zinc	8.96	3.0
Lactate	3.00	0.8	Choline	8.90	0.3
Citrate	3.10	3.0	Aluminium	5.00	0.7
Succinate	3.13, 4.76, 6.40	0.4	Others		8.8
Acetate	4.21, 5.64	1.3			
Others	4.76	31.4			

Table 24.5 Theoretical solubility and pH of salts of chlordiazepoxide

Salt	pKa	Salt pH	Solubility (mg mL^{-1})
Base	4.80	8.30	2.0
Hydrochloride	−6.10	2.53	<165*
Maleate	1.92	3.36	57.1
Tartrate	3.00	3.90	17.9
Benzoate	4.20	4.50	6.0
Acetate**	4.76	4.78	4.1

* Maximum solubility of chlordiazepoxide hydrochloride, achieved at pH 2.89, is governed by crystal lattice energy and common ions.
** Chlordiazepoxide acetate may not form as the pK_a of acetate is too high and too close to that of drug ion.

the gastrointestinal tract, the pH rises and dissolution rate and solubility fall. Conversely, a weak acid has minimal dissolution in the stomach but becomes more soluble and its dissolution rate increases down the gut. Paradoxically, as dissolution rate increases, so bioabsorption of the molecule falls because the drug is ionized. Thus a weakly basic drug is ideal for peroral administration since it will dissolve in its ionic form in the stomach and then be absorbed in its neutral form in the small intestine. It is therefore probably not a coincidence that 75% of all commercially available drugs are weak bases.

The dissolution rate of a particular salt is usually much greater than the parent drug. Sodium and potassium salts of weak acids dissolve much more rapidly than the parent acid and some comparative data are shown in Table 24.6. On the basis of bulk pH, these salts would be expected to have lower dissolution rates in the stomach. However, the pH of the diffusion layer

(discussed in Chapter 21 and determined by measuring the pH of a saturated bulk solution) is higher than the pH of gastric fluid (which is approximately pH 1.5) because of their buffering action. The pH is the saturated unbuffered aqueous solution (calculated pH in Table 24.6) and the dissolution rate is governed by this pH and not the bulk media pH.

In the intestine, the salt does not depress the pH, unlike the acid which is neutralized, and the diffusion layer pH is again raised to promote dissolution. Providing that the acid forming the salt is strong, the pH of the solution adjacent to the dissolving surface will be that of the salt, whereas for the dissolving free base, it will be the pH of the bulk dissolving media. With weak bases, their salts dissolve rapidly in the stomach but there is no absorption since the drug is ionized and absorption is delayed until the intestine. Any undissolved drug, as salt, rapidly dissolves since the higher diffusion layer pH compensates for the higher bulk pH which would be extremely unfavourable to the free base. Data for chlordiazepoxide are shown in Table 24.5. The maleate salt has a predicted solubility of 57 mg mL^{-1} but, more importantly, reduces the pH by 5 units. By controlling diffusion layer pH, the dissolution rate can increase many fold, independent of its position in the gastrointestinal tract. This is particularly important in the development of controlled-release products.

Different salts of a drug rarely change its basic pharmacology but only its physical properties. However, the salt form does change the physicochemical properties of the drug. Changes in dissolution rate and solubility affect the rate and extent of absorption (bioavailability). Such changes have been found to affect the intensity of drug response.

Consequently each new drug candidate has to be examined to choose the most suitable salt because each potential salt can behave very differently. Thus each

Table 24.6 Dissolution rates of weak acids and their sodium salts

Drug	pK_a	pH (at C$_s$)	Dissolution rate (mg cm^{-2} min^{-1}) × 10^2	
			Dissolution media	
			0.1M HCl (pH 1.5)	Phosphate (pH 6.8)
Salicylic acid	3.0	2.40	1.7	27
Sodium salicylate	–	8.78	1870	2500
Benzoic acid	4.2	2.88	2.1	14
Sodium benzoate	–	9.35	980	1770
Sulfathiazole	7.3	4.97	<0.1	0.5
Sodium sulfathiazole	–	10.75	550	810

requires separate preformulation screening. The regulatory authorities treat each salt as a different chemical entity, particularly in the context of their biopharmaceutics and toxicity testing.

Solvents

It is generally necessary for the pharmaceutical scientist to formulate an injection even if there is no intention to market one. This is because it will be needed for preclinical and early clinical testing. The first choice of solvent is obviously water. However, although the drug may be freely soluble, it may be unstable in aqueous solution. Chlordiazepoxide hydrochloride is such an example. Accordingly, water-miscible solvents can be used (a) as a solvent in formulations to improve solubility or stability and (b) in analysis to facilitate extraction and separation (e.g. chromatography).

Oils are used in emulsions, topicals (creams and ointments), intramuscular injections and liquid-fill oral preparations (soft and hard gelatin capsules) when aqueous pH and solvent solubility and stability are unattainable. Table 24.7 shows a range of solvents to fulfil these needs.

Aqueous methanol is widely used in HPLC and is the standard solvent in sample extraction during analysis and stability testing. It is often made slightly acidic or alkaline to increase solvent power and ensure consistent ionic conditions for UV analysis. Other pharmaceutical solvents are available but are generally only required in special cases. The most acceptable non-aqueous solvents pharmaceutically are glycerol, propylene glycol and ethanol. Generally, for a lipophilic drug (i.e. a partition coefficient (log P) >1; see next section), solubility doubles through this series.

Where the amount of available drug is limited and the aqueous solubility is inadequate, it is better to measure the solubility in aqueous solvent mixtures rather than in a pure organic solvent. Whereas solubilities at other levels and their mixtures can be predicted, the solubility in pure solvent is often inconsistent because of cosolvent effects. Furthermore, formulations rarely use pure non-aqueous solvent, particularly injections. For example, ethanol should only be used up to 10% in an injection to prevent haemolysis and pain at the injection site.

Partition coefficient (K_w^o) (log P)

The partition coefficient is the solvent:water quotient of drug distribution. In other words, it is a measure of the relative solubility of a drug in other solvents compared with its solubility in water. As an example, if the drug is twice as soluble in an oil than water under otherwise identical conditions, it will have a K_w^o of 2. K is used as the symbol for partition coefficient and the superscript and subscript indicate the solvents used (oil and water in this case). The determination and relevance of partition coefficient are discussed further in Chapter 2.

When these ratios are much larger, it is common practice to use the logarithmic ratio, log P (i.e. the log of partition coefficient, log P = log $[K_w^o]$). For example, a $[K_w^o]$ of 1000 is the same as a log P of 3. Thus the higher a drug's $[K_w^o]$ or log P, the greater its oil solubility compared with its aqueous solubility.

This has a number of applications which are relevant to preformulation.

- *Solubility* – both aqueous and in mixed solvents.
- *Drug absorption in vivo* – applied to a homologous series for structure–activity relationships (SAR).
- *Partition chromatography* – choice of column (in HPLC) or plate (in TLC) and choice of mobile phase (eluant).

Table 24.7   Recommended solvents for preformulation screening

Solvent	Dielectric constant (ε)	Solubility parameter (δ)	Application
Water	80	24.4	All
Methanol	32	14.7	Extraction, separation
0.1M HCl (pH 1.1)			Dissolution (gastric), acidic extraction
0.1M NaOH (pH 13.1)			Basic extraction
Buffer (pH 6–7)			Dissolution (intestinal)
Ethanol	24	12.7	Formulation
Propylene glycol	32	12.6	Formulation
Glycerol	43	16.5	Formulation
PEG 300 or 400	35		Formulation

Solvent solubility

The relative polarities of solvents can be scaled using dielectric constant (ε), solubility parameter (δ), interfacial tension (γ) and hydrophilic–lipophilic balance (HLB). The best solvent in any given application is the one whose polarity matches that of the solute; an ideal, fully compatible solution can be formed when $\delta_{solvent} = \delta_{solute}$. This can be ascertained by determining solubility maxima, using a substituent contribution approach or the dielectic requirement of the system.

The most useful scale of polarity for a solute is K_w^o (the oil:water partition coefficient described above) since the other approaches do not allow easy estimates for the behaviour of crystalline solids. For a wide range of drugs, it is possible to relate solvent solubility and the partition coefficient. Yalkowski & Roseman (1981) derived the following expression for 48 drugs in propylene glycol.

$$\log C_S = \log C_w + \int (0.89)\log P + 0.03 \quad (24.5)$$

Equation 24.5 can be applied more generally by introducing a factor ϕ to account for the relative solvent power of pharmaceutical solvents. Table 24.8 lists some examples (Yalkowski et al 1975).

Equation 24.5 now becomes, for a wide range of solvents:

$$\log C_S = \log C_o + \int (\log \phi + 0.89 \log P + 0.03) \quad (24.6)$$

Methodology and structure–activity prediction

Choice of non-aqueous solvent (oil) The oil:water partition is a measure of the relative lipophilicity (oil-loving) nature of a compound, usually in the unionized state (HA or B), between an immiscible lipophilic solvent or oil and an aqueous phase. Many different partition solvents have been used (Leo et al 1971) but the largest data base has been generated using n-octanol. The solubility parameter of octanol ($\delta = 10.24$) lies midway in the range for drugs (8–12) although some non-polar

($\delta < 7$) and polar drugs ($\delta > 13$) are encountered. This allows measurable results between equal volumes of oil and aqueous phases. Whilst n-octanol is a good model for the in vivo situation, some researchers argue that others are better. However, its previous widespread usage and corresponding extensive database have resulted in it becoming the standard 'oily solvent'.

In the *shake flask method* the drug, predissolved in one of the phases, is shaken with the other partitioning solvent for 30 minutes, allowed to stand for 5 minutes and then the majority of the lower aqueous phase (octanol has a density of 0.8258 g mL^{-1} and therefore rises to the top) is run off and centrifuged for 60 minutes at 2000 rpm. The aqueous phase is assayed before (ΣC) and after partitioning (C_w) (the aqueous concentration) to give $K_w^o = (\Sigma C - C_w)/C_w$.

If the transfer of solute to the oil phase is small, ΔC_w is small and any resulting analytical error increases error in the estimate of K_w^o. Indeed, to encourage greater movement of drug from the aqueous layer, a considerably more polar non-aqueous solvent, n-butanol, has been used. Where the partition coefficient is high, it is usual to reduce the ratio of the oil phase from 1:1 to 1:4 or 1:9 in order to increase the aqueous concentration (C_w) to a measurable level. For a 1:9 oil:water ratio, $K_w^o = (10 \, \Sigma C - C_w)/C_w$.

In general, polar solvents are advocated to correlate biological activity with physicochemical properties. Solvents that are less polar than octanol are termed *hyperdiscriminating* while more polar solvents, e.g. butanols and pentanols, are *hypodiscriminating*. This concept refers to the discriminating power of a partitioning solvent within a homologous series. With n-butanol, the values of log P tend to be close while with heptane and other inert hydrocarbons, the differences in solute lipophilicities are exaggerated. n-Octanol generally gives a range consistent with other physicochemical properties when compared to drug absorption in the GI tract. Hyperdiscriminating solvents reflect more closely the transport across the blood–brain barrier, while hypodiscriminating solvents give values consistent with buccal absorption (Fig. 24.2). A good correlation exists between the solvent water content at saturation and solvent lipophilicity of a range of solvents.

Certainly, it is imperative to standardize on methodology, especially the choice of solvent. Where solubility constraints allow, this should be n-octanol. Since the existing data bank and previous experience are so extensive, it aids the interpretation and usefulness of the data generated.

Structure–activity relationships Since the pioneering work of Meyer and Overton, numerous studies on correlating molecular structure and biological activity have been reported. These structure–activity relationships

Table 24.8 Solvent power (ϕ) of some pharmaceutical solvents	
Solvent	Relative solvent power (ϕ)
Glycerol	0.5
Propylene glycol	1
PEG 300 or 400	1
Ethanol	2
DNA, DMF	4

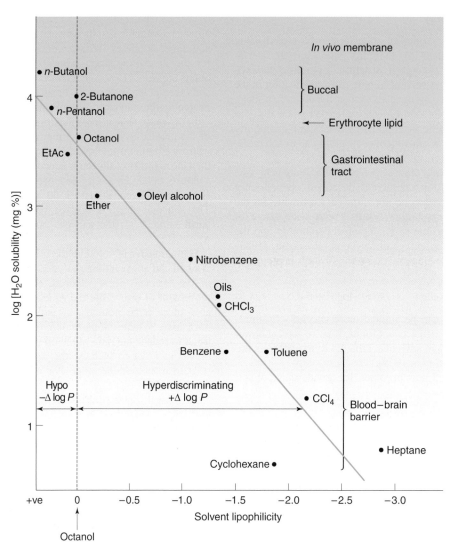

Fig. 24.2 Discriminating power of partitioning solvents as a function of their water capacity.

(SAR) can rationalize drug activity and, particularly in modern medicinal chemistry, facilitate a scientific approach to the design of more effective, elegant structural analogues.

The application of SAR depends on a sound knowledge of the physicochemical properties of each new drug candidate in a therapeutic class, and preformulation is an essential information source.

It is assumed in SAR that:

$$\log K_w^o = a \times \log K_w^{octanol} + b \qquad (24.7)$$

This relationship (in which a and b are constants for a series of similar molecules) holds for all polar and semipolar solvents. However, correlations are poor with non-polar solvents (hexane to *iso*-octane) and this seems to be related to water content. Given the importance of water, it is imperative that the octanol is saturated with the aqueous phase and the aqueous phase with octanol prior to any determination, otherwise the partitioning behaviour of the drug will be influenced by the mutual partitioning of the two solvents.

While the aqueous phase is most often water, it is better to measure log P under controlled pH. All drugs capable of ionization, and with a measurable pK_a, will have intrinsic buffer capacity affecting the aqueous pH. Depending on the degree of dissociation, this will lead to an apparent K_w^o rather than the true (absolute) value, when the drug is unionized.

Since the ionized species will have greater aqueous solubility and lower lipophilicity to HA or BOH then the measured K_w^o (apparent) will be inevitably lower. Accordingly, K_w^o (true) should be measured at >2 pH units away from the pK_a (pK_a −2 (acid); pK_a + 2 (base)) to ensure the drug is in its unionized form. The aqueous phase should contain a suitable buffer to ensure this. Given the importance of log P (log [*]) in SAR, comparative data generated in a therapeutic class ($R_n.X$, where X is the therapeutic nucleus and n is a number of substituents R) should also be determined at physiological pH 7.4.

Quantitative SAR (QSAR) is based on the premise that drug absorption is a multipartitioning process (repeated adsorption and desorption) across cellular membranes and is dependent on the lipophilicity of the drug, and the rate of penetration is proportional to the drug partition coefficient in vitro. Clearly, the ionic condition in vivo will affect any correlation and accordingly for dissociating drugs, the in vitro conditions should be similar. The widespread use of *n*-octanol in these studies (Hansch & Dunn 1972) and the existence of many excellent correlations in vivo are probably not fortuitous. *n*-Octanol exhibits hydrogen bonding acceptor and donor properties typical of many biological macromolecules. The partial polarity of *n*-octanol allows the inclusion of water, which is also a feature of biological lipid membranes and leads to a more complex partitioning behaviour than a less polar, essentially anhydrous solvent.

The effect of salt formation on the measured log P is shown in Table 24.9. Generally the log P differs from between 3 and 4 (K_w^o from 1000 to 10 000) when compared with the parent compound. Thus the lipophilicity falls by 3–4 orders of magnitude and this accounts for the significant increase in the aqueous solubility of the salts. The physicochemical model for biological activity assumes that activity of a compound is related to these factors associated with molecular structure:

- electronic (charge)
- steric (spatial size)
- hydrophobic effects (partitioning).

Account must also be taken of structural and theoretical aspects so that:

$$\text{Biological activity} = f\,[(\text{electronic}) + (\text{steric}) + (\text{hydrophobic}) + (\text{structural/theoretical})] \quad (24.8)$$

Steric effects occur when there is a direct interaction between the substituent and the parent nucleus and is related to substituent bulk. High positive values of the steric effect parameter, E_s, indicate significant steric effects with intra- and intermolecular hindrance to a reaction or finding at the active site.

The hydrophobic component is measured by the distribution between an aqueous phase and an immiscible lipid phase and parallels drug adsorption and distribution in vivo. A relationship has been demonstrated between partition coefficient within a series and the structure of the molecule and this, in turn, related to biological effect. This has led to the wider application of SAR which, by other modifications and calculations, has led to what is known as quantitative SAR (QSAR).

While all these calculations and estimations are useful, log P remains the most useful physical parameter and undoubtedly the most reliable data. Correlations still come from experimentally derived partition values for the analogues in a series.

Dissolution

The dissolution rate of a drug is only important where it is the rate-limiting step in the absorption process. Kaplan (1972) suggested that provided the solubility of a drug exceeded 10 mg mL^{-1} at pH <7 then no bioavailability- or dissolution-related problems were to be expected. Below 1 mg mL^{-1}, such problems were quite possible and salt formation could improve absorption and solubility by controlling the pH of the microenvironment independently of the drug and dosage form's position within the GI tract.

Intrinsic dissolution rate

When dissolution is solely controlled by diffusion (transport control), the rate of diffusion is directly proportional to the saturated concentration of the drug in solution (i.e. solubility). Under these conditions the rate constant k_1 is defined by:

$$k_1 = 0.62 D^{2/3} v^{1/6} \omega^{1/2} \quad (24.9)$$

where v is the kinematic viscosity and ω is the angular velocity of a rotating disc of drug. By maintaining the

Table 24.9 The effect of salt formation on the log P of some weakly basic drugs

Free base and hydrochloride salt	log P (free base)	log P (hydrochloride salt)	Δlog P
Chlorpromazine	5.35	1.51	3.84
Promazine	4.49	0.91	3.58
Trifluopromazine	5.19	1.78	4.28
Trifluoperazine	5.03	1.69	3.34
Diphenylhydramine	3.30	−0.12	3.42
Propranolol	3.18	−0.45	3.63
Phenylpropanolamine	1.83	−1.09	2.92

dissolution fluid viscosity and rotational speed of the sample constant, the dissolution rate (dC/dt) from a constant surface area (A) will be constant and related solely to solubility. Under sink conditions ($C_S \gg C$) the following equation applies.

$$dC/dt = \frac{A}{V} k_1 C_S \qquad (24.10)$$

Intrinsic dissolution rate (IDR) is given by:

$$IDR = k_1 C_S \text{ (mg cm}^2 \text{ min}^{-1}) \qquad (24.11)$$

This constant rate differs from the dissolution from conventional dosage forms, which is known as total dissolution (mg mL^{-1}), where the exposed surface area (A) is uncontrolled as disintegration, deaggregation and dissolution proceed (Wells 1988). Accordingly, the IDR is independent of formulation effects and measures the intrinsic properties of the drug and salts as a function of dissolution media, e.g. pH, ionic strength and counter-ions.

Measurement of intrinsic dissolution rate A compressed disc of material can be made by slow compression of 500 mg of drug in a 13 mm IR disc punch and die set to a high compaction pressure greater than 500 MPa (to ensure zero porosity) and a long dwell time (to improve compaction).

The metal surfaces in contact should be prelubricated with, for example, stearic acid (5% w/v in chloroform). The compressed disc is fixed to the holder of the rotating basket apparatus using a low melting paraffin wax and successively dipped so that the top and sides of the disc are coated. The lower circular face should be cleared of residual wax using a scalpel and carefully scraped to remove any stearic acid transferred from the punch face.

The coated disc is rotated at 100 rpm, 20 mm from the bottom of a 1 litre flat-bottomed dissolution flask containing 1 litre of fluid at 37°C. The amount of drug release is then monitored, usually by UV spectrometry, with time. The slope of the line divided by the exposed surface area gives the IDR (mg cm^2 min^{-1}).

Each candidate should be measured in 0.05 M HCl (gastric) and phosphate buffer pH 7 (intestinal) and distilled water, especially if sink conditions are not possible for a weak base at pH 7 or a weak acid in 0.05 M HCl. Sink conditions maintain the bulk concentration (C) at a low level, otherwise the rate of dissolution is progressively reduced and the plot of concentration against time becomes non-linear. It is recommended that C should not exceed $0.1 C_S$.

By comparing the IDR of a salt in water with that obtained in acidic and alkaline solutions, or the free base with its salts in the same medium, a measure of the salt's ability to control its immediate microenvironment will emerge.

The equation derived from a combination of Equation 24.11 and the appropriate Henderson–Hasselbalch equation (Chapter 3):

$$IDR = k_1 [C_0(1 + \text{antilog } [pK_a - pH])] \qquad (24.12)$$

shows that the rate of dissolution of a drug candidate is clearly a function of its intrinsic solution (C_0), its dissociation constant (pK_a) and either the pH of the bulk dissolution medium or microenvironment created by the dissolving salt. This is why, when minimum preformulation was discussed at the beginning of this chapter, these were regarded as the two most important characteristics on which to obtain data in the very early stages of preformulation. Using the measured rate of the free base at known bulk pH, expected rates in other media, using the experimental salts, can be calculated and compared with experimental values.

Measurement of IDR can be useful diagnostically. The importance of improvements in the IDR, due to microenvironmental pH control, lies in the improvement in vivo of a salt over the parent drug. Where no increase is found, there is likely to be no advantage in using that particular salt. Improvements are obviously more likely if the salt former is strong. For a weak base, the hydrochloride ($pK_a = -6.10$) offers the best advantage but this may prove, in some instances, disappointing due to the common ion effect in vivo with Cl$^-$ ions.

Common ion effect

An interaction often overlooked is the common ion effect. A common ion often reduces the solubility of a slightly soluble electrolyte significantly. 'Salting out' results from the removal of water molecules that can act as a solvent due to the competing hydration of other ions. The reverse process, 'salting in', arises with larger anions, e.g. benzoate, salicylate, which open the water structure. These hydrotropes increase the solubility of poorly water-soluble compounds, e.g. diazepam.

Hydrochloride salts often exhibit suboptimal solubility in gastric juice due to the abundance of Cl$^-$ ions there (Table 24.10). Other small inorganic counter-ions, other than Cl$^-$, such as nitrate, sulfate and phosphate, have also been implicated.

To identify a common ion interaction, the IDR of the hydrochloride (or inorganic) salt should be compared between (a) water, (b) water containing 1.2% w/v NaCl and (c) 0.05 M HCl and 0.9% w/v NaCl in 0.05 M HCl. Both saline media contain 0.2M Cl$^-$, which is typically encountered in fluids in vivo.

A common ion effect with Cl$^-$ will result in a significantly reduced IDR in the presence of sodium chloride. Other salt forms are then worth considering, e.g. tosylate, mesylate, etc., but the parent molecule will still remain

Table 24.10 Examples of weakly basic drugs which have decreased solubility in acidic and Cl⁻ solutions

Chlortetracycline
Demethylchlortetracycline
Methacycline
Demeclocycline
Phenazopyridine
Cyproheptadine
Bromhexine
Triamterine

sensitive to Cl⁻. Solubilities will be suppressed in the presence of saline, although not to the same extent since Cl⁻ is not involved in the dissolving microenvironment. Any improvement with the new salt can be assessed by again measuring the IDR with and without saline. Since some compounds are sensitive to other counter-ions, e.g. nitrate, sulfate and phosphate, this can be demonstrated by including the appropriate sodium salt in the dissolution medium. Phase solubility studies have indicated that basic amine drugs are more soluble in organic acids than inorganic. Where a hydrochloride salt exhibits suboptimal solubility then the next logical choice is probably a salt of toluene sulphonic acid (tosylate: $pK_a = -1.34$). Mesylate, napsylate, besylate and maleate salts offer progressively weaker acidic alternatives.

With low-solubility amine drugs, the salts of polyhydroxy acids, e.g. lactate, often give the greatest aqueous solubility due to their accessible hydroxy groupings.

MELTING POINT

The determination of melting point during preformulation studies is important since it is a simple test requiring only small amounts of material that can yield much valuable information regarding the thermal properties of the material. It can also assist at this stage in making predictions about the potential stability of the NCE. There is, for example, and possibly somewhat surprisingly, a link between melting point and solubility. This is discussed later in this section.

Techniques

The melting point of a drug can be measured using these techniques:

- capillary melting
- hot stage microscopy
- differential scanning calorimetry or thermal analysis.

Capillary melting

Capillary melting (the observation of melting in a capillary tube in a heated metal block) gives information about the melting range but it is difficult to assign an accurate melting point using this technique.

Hot stage microscopy

This is the visual observation of melting under a microscope equipped with a heated and lagged sample stage. The heating rate is controllable and other transitions can be observed and recorded. It is more precise since the phase transitions (first melt, 50% melt and completion) can be registered on a recorder as the melting proceeds and, by virtue of high magnification, the values are more accurate.

Differential scanning calorimetry and differential thermal analysis

Neither of the previous methods is as versatile as either differential thermal analysis (DTA) or differential scanning calorimetry (DSC). An additional advantage is that the sample size required for these is only 2–5 mg.

DTA measures the temperature difference between the sample and a reference as a function of temperature or time when heating at a constant rate. DSC is similar to DTA, except that the instrument measures the amount of energy required to keep the sample at the same temperature as the reference, i.e. it measures the enthalpy of transition.

When no physical or chemical change occurs within the sample then there is neither a temperature change nor input energy to maintain an isotherm. However, when phase changes occur then latent heat suppresses a temperature change and the isothermal energy required registers as an electrical signal generated by thermocouples. Crystalline transitions, fusion, evaporation and sublimation are changes in state which can be quantified (Fig. 24.3).

The major concern in preformulation is polymorphism and the measurement of melting point and other phase changes are the primary diagnostic tool. Later confirmation by IR spectroscopy and X-ray diffraction is advisable.

Polymorphism

A polymorph is a solid material with at least two different molecular arrangements which give distinct crystal species. These differences disappear in the liquid or vapour state. Polymorphism is discussed further in Chapter 8. Of concern here are the relative stabilities,

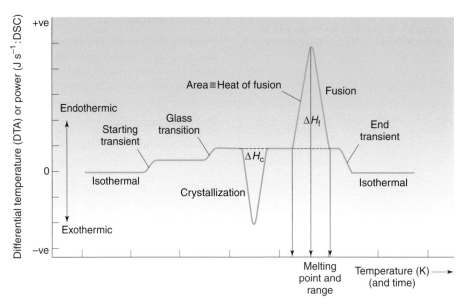

Fig. 24.3 Schematic differential scanning calorimeter thermogram.

dissolution rates and solubilities of potential or real polymorphs. The highest melting species is generally most stable and other polymorphs are metastable and can convert to the stable form. There are also potentially large differences in their physical properties so that they behave as distinct chemical entities. Solubility (particularly important in suspension dosage forms and biopharmaceutically), melting point, density, crystal shape, optical and electrical properties and vapour pressure are often very different for each polymorph.

Polymorphism is remarkably common, particularly within certain structural groups: 63% of barbiturates, 67% of steroids and 40% of sulfonamides exhibit polymorphism. The steroid progesterone has five polymorphs, while the sulfonamide sulfabenzamide has four polymorphs and three solvates. The biopharmaceutical importance of polymorphism is illustrated by the data for fluprednisolone (Fig. 24.4).

It is convention to number the polymorphs in order of stability at room temperature starting with Form I using Roman numerals; Form 1 and Form A are also used for the most stable polymorph. Conventionally, Form I usually has the highest melting point and lowest solubility; in suspension formulation it is essential to use the least soluble polymorph because of Ostwald ripening in which transition to a more stable, less soluble polymorph can result in crystal growth.

Accordingly, in preformulation the following should be considered:

- How many polymorphs exist?
- How stable is each of the forms?
- Is there an amorphous glass?
- Can the metastable forms be stabilized?
- What is the solubility of each form?
- Will a more soluble form survive processing and storage?

Examination of solvates

Prior to the examination of any true polymorphs of the NCE, the presence of solvates (sometimes incorrectly and confusingly called false polymorphs or

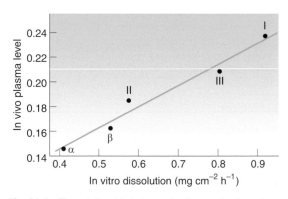

Fig. 24.4 The relationship between in vitro and in vivo release from fluprednisolone implants.

pseudopolymorphs) should be identified since different polymorphs are often obtained by changing the recrystallizing solvent. Trace levels of solvent are usual in early batches of new drug candidates (as residues from the final crystallization). These can become molecular additions within the crystal and change crystal habit.

The distinction between solvates and true polymorphs can be ascertained by observing the melting behaviour of the compound dispersed in silicone oil using hot stage microscopy. Hydrates and other solvates will evolve a gas (water or solvent vapour, respectively), causing bubbling of the oil. True polymorphs merely melt, forming a second globular phase. The temperature at which the solvent volatizes will be close to the boiling point of the solvent.

Examination of true polymorphism

After the study of the potential presence of hydrates or other solvates, the evaluation of true polymorphism can proceed. Most polymorphs are obtained by solvent manipulation. Typical solvents inducing polymorphic change are: water, methanol, ethanol, acetone, chloroform; *n*-propanol, isopropanol alcohol, *n*-butanol, *n*-pentanol; toluene and benzene. Polymorphs can also be produced without the presence of solvent by thermal techniques, notably sublimation and recrystallization from the melt. Supercooling of the melt is particularly useful in discovering unstable modifications.

The initial difficulty is to measure the melting point of the metastable form, and here heating rate is critical. Too rapid heating will obscure the endotherm, while too slow a heating rate may allow other transitions to occur or encourage decomposition. Often, therefore, comparison at two rates, e.g. $2°C$ and $20°C \text{ min}^{-1}$, is advisable.

The difference in melting point (ΔT_m) between the stable and metastable polymorphs is a measure of the stability of the metastable polymorph. Where $\Delta T_m < 1°C$ then neither is significantly more stable and either may be obtained upon conventional crystallization. If ΔT_m is 25–50°C then the lower melting species will be difficult to crystallize and will revert rapidly. The closer the two melting points ($\Delta T_m = 1$–25°C) then the unstable form(s) can normally be obtained easily before a solid–solid transformation occurs. This can be suppressed by using small samples since individual crystals of even highly unstable forms can be melted.

If it appears that polymorphism is occurring, or likely, then a cooperative study with the bulk chemists should determine the most stable (chemical and physical) form. Differences in solubility and melting point must also be assessed and then a decision made to determine which form to progress through to the next stage of formulation. Small differences in stability but higher solubility of a relatively metastable form may lead to a preferential choice of a polymorph other than Form I. A case in point is cimetidine where the commercial product does not contain the most stable polymorph as this is too insoluble. However, the polymorph used is 'stable enough' to fulfil all regulatory and shelf life requirements.

Crystal purity

Thermal analysis has been widely used as a method of purity determination. This is particularly pertinent at the preformulation stage since early samples of a new drug are inevitably 'dirty' while improvements in synthetic route are made. Thermal analysis is rapid and will discriminate 0.002 mole % of impurity.

Solubility

The most important reason for determining melting point during preformulation is crystalline solubility. Such studies are particularly important, because the scarcity of available drug powder often precludes accurate solubility determinations. Melting point and solubility are related via the latent heat of fusion which is the amount of heat generated during melting or fusion. A crystal with weak bonds has a low melting point and low heat of fusion. Conversely a strong crystal lattice leads to a high melting point and a high heat of fusion. Since solubility also requires the disruption of crystal structure to allow molecular dispersion in the solvent, it is also influenced by intermolecular forces.

Polymorphs differ in melting point and solubility. The existence of different crystal arrangements for the same compound inevitably leads to differences in crystal lattice energy since intermolecular distances will be different in the alternative forms. This effect is shown for riboflavine in Figure 24.5.

ASSAY DEVELOPMENT

The assumption that the drug is stable may not be valid since drugs are notoriously unstable, particularly as hydrolysis is often the predominant cause. In order to follow drug stability, both in solution and solid phase, it is mandatory to have suitable stability-indicating assays. In the early stages of preformulation, simple UV spectroscopy can be used but later, chromatography is required to separate the drug from its degradation products and any excipients. UV analysis is good for a quick quantitative determination in early preformulation studies but it is 'non-indicating'. This means that the UV absorption pattern will not indicate uniquely what is being assayed. Thus if any degradation products have

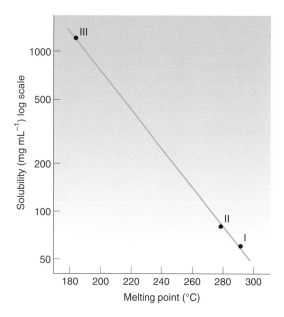

Fig. 24.5 The relationship between solubility and melting point for three polymorphs of riboflavine.

similar or identical UV absorption characteristics to the parent compound, they cannot be differentiated.

Thin-layer chromatography (TLC) is widely used in a semi-quantitative mode to estimate impurity levels, to establish the number of impurities and for collecting samples from the plate for subsequent HPLC (high performance (pressure) liquid chromatography). HPLC is now acknowledged as the most versatile and useful technique in pharmaceutical analysis and the method of choice in preformulation stability assessment.

UV spectroscopy

The principles of UV spectroscopy were enumerated earlier and will serve to quantify many of the subsequent physical constants and solubilities above. TLC and particularly HPLC have superseded UV spectroscopy as the basic analytical tools in stability assessment. However, certain UV techniques are worthy of discussion.

Molecular weight

To a first approximation, the molar extinction coefficient (e) of a chromophore (absorbing molecular group) is unaffected by distant substituent groups in a molecule. If, therefore, e of the chromophore is known from another related compound in the series, the molecular weight of the new derivative can be calculated from the absorbance of a solution of known concentration since molecular weight = $10 \, e/E_1^1$.

pK_a

pK_a measurement by spectroscopy is indicated when solubility is too low, or when the pK_a is particularly low (<2) or high (>11), for determination by potentiometry. The method depends upon determining the ratio of molecular species (neutral molecule at pH <pK_a−2 (acid), pH >pK_a+2 (base)) to the ionized species in a series of seven buffers (pH = ±1 of pK_a). An analytical wavelength (λ) is chosen where the greatest difference in absorbance exists between the molecular species and the pure ionized moiety at two pH units from the pK_a.

Thin-layer chromatography (TLC)

All chromatographic procedures emanate from the Russian botanist Tswett who in 1906 separated plant pigments by pipetting solutions on to the top of packed glass tubes. Tswett's work led to the development of column chromatography and to HPLC. Other workers used paper as a support and before the advent of HPLC, paper chromatography was used for simplicity and speed. TLC arose from a need to satisfactorily separate lipids which paper techniques could not achieve but it was soon realized that the technique was also considerably more flexible. Paper chromatography is limited by the cellulose support whereas the thin layer of material on a glass plate can be prepared from a slurry of a wide variety of different chemical types, e.g. silica gel, celite, alumina, cellulose (analogous to paper chromatography) and chemically modified celluloses. More recently, with the advent of reverse-phase chromatography, C_2, C_8 and C_{18} silanized and diphenyl silica have been used.

TLC separation times were found to be considerably shorter than paper chromatography, spots were more compact and resolution better. Additionally, submicrogram samples could be separated and recovered if necessary (by scraping away the spot using a fine spatula), reextracted and injected onto HPLC.

TLC is now generally regarded as a reliable and sensitive qualitative technique for the separation of complex mixtures in stability samples to go forward to further analysis. In a typical analysis, extracted samples are spotted 20 mm from the bottom of a square glass plate, 200 mm × 200 mm coated with a dry slurry of silica (250 μm thick) and placed in a closed tank, containing a 10 mm layer of eluting solvent, which has produced a saturated vapour phase. The sample is developed (separated) by the capillary movement of the solvent up the plate and, in this respect, is similar to HPLC. Consequently, TLC and HPLC are complementary. TLC will quantify the number of components (since they can be seen) and estimate their concentration by reference to standards run concurrently, while HPLC can quantify their level, confident that all have been separated. Observation of the most suitable developing solvent for TLC (particularly HPTLC (high performance TLC) and reverse-phase TLC) will be a useful guide to identifying the ideal mobile phase for HPLC.

High-performance liquid chromatography (HPLC)

High-performance (pressure) liquid chromatography (HPLC) is essentially liquid column chromatography performed by eluting under pressure. Much of the basic theory of TLC and HPLC is the same. By pumping the eluting solvent (mobile phase) under a pressure of up to 40 MPa and a flow rate of up to 3 mL min^{-1}, the column can be much smaller and use much smaller particle size packing material (stationary phase). This results in shorter retention times (solute time on column), high sensitivity (typically 1 ng) and the need for only a small sample volume (0–50 μL). Yet it is highly selective (has high separation power) for the resolution of complex mixtures.

HPLC methods can be divided into two distinct modes.

Normal-phase HPLC

Normal-phase HPLC is performed by eluting a silica-packed column, which is hydrophilic, with a non-polar mobile phase. The mobile phase is usually hexane to which is added one or more of the following, in increasing order of polarity: chloroform (CHCl$_3$), tetrahydrofuran (THF), acetonitrile (ACN), isopropyl alcohol (IPA) or methanol (MeOH). Separation is achieved by partition with successive differential adsorption and desorption of both the solute and solvents during passage down the column. Polar solutes are retained whereas more lipophilic molecules are not. By increasing the polarity of the mobile phase (e.g. by adding MeOH or IPA), polar solutes are eluted more quickly while non-polar solutes are better retained and their order of retention is changed. Decreasing solvent polarity increases polar solute retention and facilitates the elution of lipophilic molecules.

In general, normal-phase HPLC is used for moderately polar solutes (freely soluble in methanol). Non-polar hydrocarbon-soluble solutes are difficult to retain and very polar and water-soluble solutes are difficult to elute sufficiently.

Reverse-phase HPLC

When the solute is eluted by a polar (largely aqueous) mobile phase over a hydrophobic stationary phase, the chromatography is known as reverse phase. Solute behaviour is the reverse of that described for normal-phase HPLC which uses a hydrophilic silica stationary phase. Separation between the stationary phase and mobile phase is solvophobic, analogous to partitioning.

A degree of hydrophobicity of the stationary phase can be achieved by bonding a coating on to the silica support. The most common bonded phases are the alkyl silanes: octodecylsilane (ODS), octysilane (OS) and trimethysilane (TMS). The predominantly aqueous mobile phase usually contains methanol, ACN and/or THF to modify solvent polarity by matching the lipophilicity of the solutes in order to facilitate good chromatography. Ionization control can be achieved in the range pH 2–8. The inclusion of 1–2% acetic acid or diethylamine is used to suppress the ionization of weak acids and bases respectively. *Ion-suppression chromatography* is used to increase lipophilicity and improve retention of polar solutes.

In general, polar solutes have short retention times in reverse-phase HPLC while non-polar compounds are retained. Increasing the mobile phase polarity (by increasing the water concentration) shortens retention for polar solutes while retaining less polar compounds. Decreasing solvent polarity (by decreasing water concentration) helps retain polar compounds while more lipophilic solutes are eluted more rapidly. Non-aqueous reverse phase (NARP HPLC), where THF or methylene chloride replaces water in the mobile phase, is used to separate lipophilic solutes.

The great flexibility of choice in mobile phase (by using solvents ranging from water to hexane), the increasing number of available stationary phases (particularly bonded phases) and the inherent sensitivity of HPLC produce a powerful analytical technique. It is the method of choice in preformulation stability studies.

DRUG AND PRODUCT STABILITY

Wherever possible, commercial pharmaceutical products should have a shelf life of 3 years. The potency should not fall below an acceptable minimum. This is usually 95% under the recommended storage conditions without the generation of toxic degradation products. Additionally, the product should still look and perform as it did when first manufactured.

Drug and product stability are discussed in detail in Chapter 44. The following discussion covers those aspects that it is important to examine and understand at the preformulation stage. By investigating the intrinsic stability of the drug at this point of its development, it is possible for the preformulation scientist to advise on formulation approaches and indicate types of excipient, specific protective additives and packaging which are likely to improve the integrity of the drug and product. Typical stress conditions during a preformulation study are shown in Table 24.11.

Drug degradation occurs by four main processes:

- hydrolysis
- oxidation
- photolysis
- trace metal catalysis.

Hydrolysis and oxidation are the most common pathways and in general light and metal ions catalyse a subsequent oxidative process.

Temperature

Thermal effects are superimposed on all four chemical processes. Typically, a 10°C increase in temperature can produce a 2–5-fold increase in decay. Often the increase in reaction rate with temperature follows an Arrhenius-type relationship (see Chapter 7). A plot of the log of the reaction rate against the reciprocal of absolute temperature yields a straight line. The reaction rate can then be calculated at any temperature and the relationship allows a prediction of shelf life at room temperature by extrapolation. This assumption forms the basis of accelerated stability tests.

However, the mechanism or pathway of the chemical breakdown often changes with temperature. This will be indicated by a discontinuity or 'knee joint' in the Arrhenius plot. This is not easily detected and would inevitably lead to erroneous conclusions, if based on extrapolation of elevated temperature data to predict shelf lives at room temperature or under refrigeration. Reaction mechanisms often change about 50°C and this is a sensible ceiling.

Order of reaction

The time course of degradation depends on the number of reactants, whose concentration influences the rate. These are discussed in Chapter 7. Most pharmaceutical degradations occur by first-order kinetics (logarithmic) but some are zero order or pseudo zero order, e.g. aspirin in aqueous suspension, whilst a few are second order, e.g. chlorbutol hydrolysis.

It is often more convenient to express reaction rates in terms of time. The most common is the *half-life*, the time at which the concentration of the original compound has halved ($t_{1/2}$ or t_{50}). The shelf life of a product can be likewise expressed as t_{95} (i.e. the time for 5% loss), etc.

In the absence of a definitive value for the activation energy (E_a), which can be obtained from the slope of the Arrhenius plot, it is prudent to assume a low value (e.g. 40 kJ mol^{-1}), since this will lead to higher reaction rates and any prediction of shelf life will be conservative. Values for a wide range of drug degradation reactions are 40–400 kJ mol^{-1} but are usually in the range 60–250 kJ mol^{-1} with a mean of 83 kJ mol^{-1}.

Hydrolysis

The most likely cause of drug instability is hydrolysis. Water plays a dominant role and in many cases it is implicated passively as a solvent vector between two reacting species in solution. In the 'dry' state, water from the air may be adsorbed onto the surface of solid particles and any partial dissolution of the drug will result in a liquid layer that is a saturated solution. Consequently studies in dilute solution can be completely misleading and a poor predictor of so-called 'solid-state' stability (discussed later in this chapter).

Hydrolytic reactions involve nucleophilic attack of labile bonds, e.g. lactam > ester > amide > imide, by water on the drug in solution and are first order.

When attack is by a solvent other than water it is known as *solvolysis*.

A number of conditions catalyse the breakdown:

- presence of OH$^-$
- presence of H$_3$O$^+$
- presence of divalent metal ions
- ionic hydrolysis (protolysis) is quicker than molecular
- heat

Table 24.11 Stress conditions used in preformulation stability assessment

Test	Conditions
Solid	
Heat (°C)	4, 20, 30, 40, 40/75% RH, 50 and 75
Moisture uptake	30, 45, 60, 75 and 90% RH at RT*, **
Physical stress	Ball milling
Aqueous solution	
pH	1, 3, 5, 7, 9 and 11 at RT and 37°C Reflux in 1 M HCl and 1 M NaOH
Light+	UV (254 and 366 nm) and visible (south-facing window) at RT.
Oxidation+	Sparging with oxygen at RT; UV may accelerate breakdown

* RT is ambient room temperature. Can vary between 15° and 25°C.
** Saturated solutions of MgBr$_2$, KNO$_2$, NaBr, NaCl and KNO$_3$ respectively.
+ At pH of maximum stability in simple aqueous solution.

- light
- solution polarity and ionic strength
- high drug concentrations.

The influence of pH

The degradation of most drugs is catalysed by extremes of pH, i.e. high $[H_3O^+]$ or high $[OH^-]$, and most drugs have their maximum stability between pH 4 and 8. Where the maximum stability of a drug in a particular system dictates wider values in the dosage form, it is important for injection formulations that they have a low buffer capacity to prevent unnecessary challenge to the homeostatic pH (7.4) of blood.

Weakly acidic and basic drugs are most soluble when ionized and it is then that instability is most likely since they are charged. This leads to a problem since many potent drugs are extremely poorly soluble and pH ionization is the most obvious method to obtain a solution. In some cases, therefore, the inclusion of a water-miscible solvent in the formulation will increase stability by:

- suppressing ionization
- reducing the extreme of pH required to achieve solubility
- reducing the water activity by reducing the polarity of the solvent, e.g. 20% propylene glycol in a chlordiazepoxide hydrochloride injection.

Reactions in aqueous solution are usually catalysed by pH and this is monitored by measuring degradation rates against pH, keeping temperature, ionic strength and solvent concentration constant. Suitable buffers include acetate, citrate, lactate, phosphate and ascorbate (an intrinsic antioxidant).

Solvolysis

Where the reacting solvent is not water, then breakdown is termed *solvolysis*. Furthermore, the definition can be extended to include any change in solvent polarity (usually measured as dielectric constant) as a result of increased ionic strength. Phenobarbitone is considerably more stable in preparations containing water-miscible solvents whereas aspirin, which undergoes extensive hydrolysis, is degraded rapidly in aqueous solvents. Both effects are directly related to the dielectric constant (polarity) of the solvent. In general, if a compound produces degradation products which are more polar then the addition of a less polar solvent will stabilize the formulation. If the degradation products are less polar, then the vehicle should be more polar to improve stability. With the hydrolysis of neutral non-polar drugs, e.g. steroids, the transition state will be non-polar with no net charge. In this case solvents will not affect the rate of

decomposition and can be used with impunity to increase solubility.

Oxidation

The degree of oxidation is influenced by the environment, i.e. light, trace metals, oxygen and oxidizing agents. Reduction is a complementary reaction and there is a mutual exchange of electrons. Oxidation is a loss of electrons and an oxidizing agent must be able to take electrons. In organic molecules, oxidation is synonymous with dehydrogenation (the loss of hydrogen) and this is the mode of action of polyhydroxyphenol antioxidants, e.g. hydroquinone. However, most antioxidants function by providing electrons or labile H^+ that will be accepted by any free radical to terminate the chain reaction. A prerequisite for effective antioxidant activity in any particular preparation is that the antioxidant is more readily oxidized than the drug, i.e. it is sacrificial.

Chelating agents

Chelating agents are molecules that are capable of forming complexes with the drug involving more than one bond. For example, ethylene diamine is bidentate (two links), tripyridyl is tridentate (3) and ethylene diamine tetraacetic acid (EDTA) is hexadentate (6). The latter is particularly effective and widely used as a pharmaceutical chelating agent.

Photolysis

Oxidation, and to some extent hydrolysis, is often catalysed by light. The energy associated with this radiation increases as wavelength decreases, so that the energy of UV visible > IR and is independent of temperature (Table 24.12).

When molecules are exposed to electromagnetic radiation they absorb light (photons) at characteristic wavelengths which causes an increase in energy which can:

- cause decomposition
- be retained or transferred
- be converted to heat
- result in light emission at a new wavelength (fluorescence, phosphorescence).

Natural sunlight lies in the wavelength range 290–780 nm of which only the higher energy (UV) range (290–320 nm) causes photodegradation of drugs. Fluorescent lighting tubes emit visible light and potentially deleterious UV radiation in the range 320–380 nm, while conventional tungsten filament light bulbs are safe, emitting radiations > 390 nm.

Table 24.12 Relationship between wavelength and associated energy of various forms of light

Type of radiation	Wavelength (nm)	Energy
UV	50–400	287–72
Visible	400–750	72–36
IR	750–10 000	36–1

Thus photolysis is prevented by suitable packaging: such as amber glass bottles, cardboard outers and aluminium foil overwraps and blisters. Clear flint glass absorbs around 80% in the 290–320 nm range whereas amber glass absorbs more than 95%. Plastic containers, by comparison, absorb only 50%.

Solid-state stability

Many of the processes of composition apply generally, particularly when the drug is in solution. However, certain important distinctions arise with the stability of drugs in the solid state, e.g. in tablets and capsules. This is a difficult area to study, largely due to the complexities of formulated systems and the practical difficulties in obtaining quantitative data. The paucity of published data must not be interpreted to mean that this area is unimportant, especially given the popularity of tablets and capsules.

In all solid dosage formulations, there will be some free moisture (contributed by excipients as well as the drug). This will be present either as absorbed or adsorbed water. In the case of tablets, a significant percentage of water, typically 1–2% w/w, is required to facilitate good compression. This residual free water can act as a vector for chemical reactions between drug and excipients. The adsorbed moisture films are saturated with drug compared with the dilute solutions encountered in injectables. The ionic equilibria are quite different and comparison is quite meaningless. They should not be extrapolated glibly to the solid state.

Hygroscopicity

A substance which absorbs sufficient moisture from the atmosphere to dissolve itself is *deliquescent*. A substance which loses water to form a lower hydrate or becomes anhydrous is termed *efflorescent*. These are extreme cases and usually most pharmaceutical compounds either are impassive to the water available in the surrounding atmosphere or lose or gain some water from the atmosphere, depending on the relative humidity (RH). Materials unaffected by RH are termed *non-hygroscopic*

while those in a dynamic equilibrium with water in the atmosphere are *hygroscopic*.

Ambient RH (approximately 0% at the poles and deserts, 55% in temperate climates and 87% in the tropics) can vary widely and continually depending on the weather and air temperature and these cyclic changes lead to constant variations in the moisture content of unprotected bulk drug and excipients. The constant sinusoidal change in day and night temperatures is the major influence.

Pharmaceutical air conditioning is usually set below 50% RH and very hygroscopic products, e.g. effervescent tablets that are particularly moisture sensitive, are made and stored below 40% RH. Tablets and capsules must be hydrophilic to facilitate wetting, deaggregation and dissolution during drug delivery. As a paradox, they must have limited hygroscopicity to ensure good chemical and physical stability under all reasonable climatic conditions. Good packaging (see Chapter 42) will accommodate moisture challenge, e.g. glass bottles, foil blisters and desiccant. However, preformulation studies on the drug and potential excipient combinations should provide the basis for more robust formulations and a wider, more flexible and cheaper choice of pack, while still reducing significantly any hydrolytic instability due to absorbed free moisture. Drug salts should be chosen to be non-hygroscopic. As a working limit, this should mean that they take up less than 0.5% water up to 95% RH.

Stability assessment

The testing protocols used in preformulation to ascertain the stability of formulated products must be performed in solution and in the solid state since the same drug (or its salts) will be used in both an injection and a capsule, for example. These protocols are discussed for drugs and formulated products in Chapter 44 and a suggested scheme for preformulation samples has been shown in Table 24.11.

MICROSCOPY

The microscope has two major applications in pharmaceutical preformulation:

- basic crystallography, to determine crystal morphology (structure and habit), polymorphism and solvates
- particle size analysis.

Most pharmaceutical powders have crystals in the range 0.5–300 μm. However, the distributions are often smaller, typically 0.5–50 μm, to ensure good blend homogeneity and rapid dissolution.

A lamp-illuminated, mono-objective microscope fitted with polarizing filters above and below the stage is more than adequate. For most preformulation work, a 10× eyepiece and a 10× objective are ideal, although occasionally, with micronized powders and when following solid–solid and liquid–liquid transitions in polymorphs, 10 × 20 may be required.

Crystal morphology

Crystals are characterized by repetition of atoms or molecules in a regular three-dimensional structure which is absent in glasses and some polymers. There are six crystal systems (cubic, tetragonal, orthorhombic, monoclinic, triclinic and hexagonal) that have different internal structures and spatial arrangements.

Without changing the internal structure, which occurs with polymorphism, crystals can adopt different external structures. This is known as *crystal habit*, of which five types are recognized that occur in all six crystal systems:

- *tabular* – moderate expansion of two parallel faces
- *platy* – plates
- *prismatic* – columns
- *acicular* – needle-like
- *bladed* – flat acicular.

Conditions during crystallization will contribute to changes in crystal habit and may be encountered in early batches of a new drug substance until the synthetic route has been optimized. Crystal habit can be modified by:

- *excessive supersaturation*, which tends to transform a prism or isodiametric (granular) crystals to a needle shape
- *cooling rate and agitation*, which change habit since they change the degree of supersaturation. Naphthalene gives thin plates (platy) if rapidly recrystallized in cold ethanol or methanol whereas slow evaporation yields prisms
- *changing the crystallizing solvent*, which preferentially adsorbs on to certain faces, inhibiting their growth. Resorcinol produces needles from benzene and squat prisms from butyl acetate
- *the addition of cosolvents or other solutes and ions*, which change habit by poisoning crystal growth in one or more directions. Sodium chloride is usually cubic but the presence of urea produces an octahedral habit.

Particle size analysis

Small particles are particularly important in low-dose, high-potency drug candidates since large particle populations are necessary to ensure adequate blend homogeneity (coefficient of variation <1–2%), and for any drug whose aqueous solubility is poor (<1 mg mL^{-1}), since dissolution rate is directly proportional to surface area (inversely proportional to particle size).

There are numerous methods of particle sizing and these are discussed in Chapter 9. Sieving is usually unsuitable during preformulation due to the lack of bulk material. The simplest but unfortunately the most tedious method for small quantities is the microscope. The Coulter Counter (an electric stream sensing zone method of size analysis in which electrolyte displacement is measured by conductivity changes as the sample is drawn through a small hole) and laser light scattering are widely used for routine bulk analysis and research.

POWDER FLOW PROPERTIES

Of primary importance when handling a drug powder is its flow characteristics. When limited amounts of drug are available, these can be evaluated by measurements of bulk density and angle of repose. These are extremely useful derived parameters for assessing the impact of changes in drug powder properties as new batches become available. Standard powder technology techniques for measuring these properties (see Chapter 13) are used in preformulation but they need to be adapted for the small amounts of powder available (see below).

Changes in particle size and shape are generally very apparent on microscopic examination. An increase in crystal size or a more uniform shape will generally lead to better flow properties.

Bulk density

Carr and Neumann developed a simple test to evaluate flowability of a powder by comparing the poured (fluff) density (ρ_{Bmin}) and tapped density (ρ_{Bmax}) of a powder and the rate at which it packed down. A useful, empirical guide is given by the Carr's Compressibility Index.

$$\text{Carr's Index (\%)}$$
$$= \frac{\text{Tapped density} - \text{Poured density}}{\text{Tapped density}} \times 100 \quad (24.13)$$

It is a simple index that can be determined on small quantities of powder and may be interpreted as in Table 24.13.

A similar index has been defined by Hausner (1967):

$$\text{Hausner ratio}$$
$$= \frac{\text{Tapped density}\,(\rho_{Bmax})}{\text{Poured density}\,(\rho_{Bmin})} \quad (24.14)$$

Table 24.13 Carr's Index as an indication of powder flow

Carr's Index (%)	Type of flow
5–15	Excellent
12–16	Good
18–21	Fair to passable*
23–35	Poor*
33–38	Very poor
>40	Extremely poor

* May be improved by glidant, e.g. 0.2% Aerosil

A Hausner ratio of less than 1.25 (equivalent to 20% Carr) indicates good flow, while greater than 1.5 (equivalent to 33% Carr) indicates poor flow. A Hausner ratio between 1.25 and 1.5 added glidant normally improves flow.

Carr's Index and the Hausner ratio are one-point determinations and do not always reflect the ease or speed with which consolidation of the powder occurs. Indeed, some materials have high indices (suggesting poor flow) but they may consolidate rapidly, and vice versa. Rapid consolidation is essential for uniform filling on tablet machines when the powder flows at ρ_{Bmin} into the die and ideally consolidates to approaching ρ_{Bmax} prior to consolidation.

An empirical linear relationship exists between the change in bulk density and the log number of taps in a jolting volumeter. An example of a standard powder technology apparatus (shown in Fig. 13.13) adapted for smaller amounts of powder is shown in Figure 24.6. A small (10 mL) measuring cylinder is fixed into the neck of a standard cylinder in a standard jolting volumeter

and the apparatus used in exactly the same manner. The reduction in powder volume is plotted against the log of the number of taps. A common observation is that non-linearity occurs up to two taps and after 30 taps, when the bed consolidates more slowly. The slope of the linear region is a measure of the speed of consolidation and is useful for differentiating powders or blends with similar Carr's Index or Hausner ratio and to examine the benefit of glidants.

Angle of repose

When only gravity acts upon it, a static heap of powder will tend to form a conical mound. One limitation exists: the angle to the horizontal cannot exceed a certain value and this is known as the *angle of repose* (θ). If any particle temporarily lies outside this limiting angle, it will roll or slide down the adjacent surface under the influence of gravity, until the gravitational pull is balanced by the friction caused by interparticulate forces. Accordingly, there is an empirical relationship between angle of repose and the ability of the powder to flow. However, the exact value for angle of repose does depend on the method of measurement.

The angles of repose given in Table 24.14 may be used as a guide to flow. The interrelationship between angle of repose, Carr's Index and the expected powder flow is shown in Figure 24.7.

When only small quantities of powder are available, again a miniaturized version of a standard powder technology technique is used: the *angle of spatula*. This is achieved by picking up a quantity of powder on a spatula and estimating the angle of the triangular section of the powder heap viewed from the end of the spatula held horizontally. This is obviously crude but is useful during preformulation when only small quantities of drug are available.

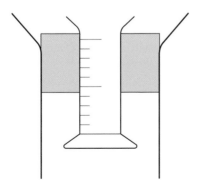

Fig. 24.6 Adaptation of the cylinder of a jolting volumeter for smaller quantities of powder.

Table 24.14 Angle of repose as an indication of powder flow properties

Angle of repose (degrees)	Type of flow
<20	Excellent
20–30	Good
30–34	Passable*
>40	Very poor

* May be improved by a glidant, e.g. 0.2% Aerosil

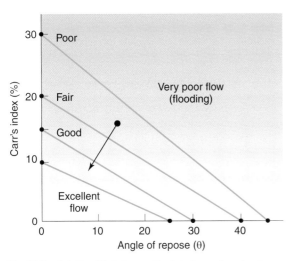

Fig. 24.7 Relationship between Carr's Index and angle of repose of a powder and its flow characteristics.

COMPRESSION PROPERTIES

The compression properties of most drug powders are generally poor and necessitate the addition of compression aids. When the dose is less than 50 mg, tablets can usually be prepared by direct compression with the addition of modern direct compression bases. At higher doses the preferred method would be wet massing.

Nonetheless, information on the compression properties of the pure drug is extremely useful. While it is true that the tableted material should be ductile, i.e. capable of permanent (plastic) deformation, it should also exhibit a degree of brittleness (fragmentation). Thus if the drug dose is high and it behaves plastically, the chosen excipients should fragment, e.g. lactose, calcium phosphate. If the drug is brittle or elastic, the excipients should be plastic, i.e. microcrystalline cellulose, or plastic binders should be used in wet massing. Obviously, as the dose is reduced, this becomes less important as the compactability of the formulation is then dictated by the excipients, in particular the diluent.

The compression properties (elasticity, plasticity, fragmentation and punch filming propensity) for small quantities of a new drug candidate can be established by the sequence outlined in Table 24.15. This provides a convenient method to elucidate as much information as possible about the compactability of the material using the minimum amount of material. An interpretation of the results follows.

Plastic material

When materials are ductile (i.e. they easily undergo plastic deformation) they deform by changing shape. Since there is no fracture, no new surfaces are generated during compression and a more intimate mix of magnesium stearate (as in Sample C) leads to poorer bonding. Since these materials bond after viscoelastic deformation, and this is time dependent, increasing the dwell time at compression (B) will increase bonding strength. Thus, a material exhibiting crushing strengths in order B > A > C would probably have plastic tendencies.

Fragmenting material

If a material is predominantly fragmenting, neither lubricant mixing time (C) nor dwell time (B) should affect tablet strength. Thus materials which show crushing strengths which are independent of the method of manufacture outlined in Table 24.15 are likely to exhibit fragmenting properties during compression and possess a high friability.

Elastic material

Some materials (paracetamol is an example) are hard and elastic and there is very little permanent change (either plastic flow or fragmentation) caused by compression; the material rebounds elastically when the compression load is released. If bonding is weak, the compact will self-destruct during ejection and the top of the compact will either detach (*capping*) or the whole cylinder will crack into horizontal layers (*lamination*). These phenomena are discussed more fully in Chapter 31.

Table 24.15 Scheme for the evaluation of drug compression properties			
	500 mg drug + 1% magnesium stearate		
Sample code	A	B	C
Blend in a tumbler mixer for	5 min	5 min	30 min
Compress 13 mm dia. compacts in an IR hydraulic press at for a dwell time of	75 MPa 2 s	75 MPa 30 s	75 MPa 2 s
Store tablets in a sealed container at room temperature to allow equilibration	24 h	24 h	24 h
Perform crushing strength on tablets and record load	A N	B N	C N

The following observations would be indicative of an elastic material.

- A will cap or laminate.
- B will probably maintain integrity but will be very weak.
- C will cap or laminate.

Elastic drug materials require a particularly plastic tableting diluent or wet massing to induce plasticity.

Punch filming (sticking)

Finally, the surface of the top and bottom punches should be examined for adhesion of drug. The punches can be dipped into a suitable extraction solvent, e.g. MeOH, and the drug level determined. This will probably be higher for A and B (Table 24.15) since magnesium stearate is an effective antiadherent and 30 minutes mixing (C) should produce a monolayer around each drug particle and suppress adhesion more effectively.

Sticking propensity is not always easy to detect in one-off compressions of this type, not even with a sophisticated compaction simulator. Punch sticking and the resultant tablet picking may often occur only after a long tableting run has resulted in a rise in temperature and led to adherence of successive layers of particles to the punch.

The performance of potentially sticky materials can be improved by:

- a change in salt form
- using high excipient ratios
- using abrasive inorganic excipients
- wet massing and/or
- the addition of magnesium stearate.

EXCIPIENT COMPATIBILITY

The successful formulation of stable and effective solid dosage forms depends on the careful selection of the excipients which are added to facilitate administration, promote the consistent release and bioavailability of the drug and protect it from degradation.

Thermal analysis can be used to investigate and predict any physicochemical interactions between components in a formulation and therefore can be applied to the selection of suitable chemically compatible excipients. Primary excipients recommended for initial screening for tablet and capsule formulations are shown in Table 24.16.

Method

The preformulation screening of drug:excipient interactions requires around 5 mg of drug, in a 50% mixture

Table 24.16 Suggested primary candidates as excipients for tablet and capsule formulations

Excipient	Function*
Lactose monohydrate	F
Dicalcium phosphate dihydrate	F
Dicalcium phosphate anhydrous	F
Microcrystalline cellulose	F
Maize starch	D
Modified starch	D
Polyvinylpyrrolidone	B
Sodium starch glycollate	D
Sodium croscarmellose	D
Magnesium stearate	L
Colloidal silica	G

* B, binder; D, disintegrant; F, filler/diluent; G, glidant; L, lubricant.

with the excipient, to maximize the likelihood of observing an interaction. Mixtures should be examined under nitrogen to eliminate oxidative effects at a standard heating rate (2, 5 or 10°C min^{-1}) in a DSC apparatus, over a temperature range which will encompass any thermal changes likely to occur in both the drug and excipient.

The melting range and any other transitions of the drug will be known from earlier investigations into purity, polymorphism and solvates. For all potential excipients (Table 24.16) it is sensible to retain, in a reference file, representative thermograms for comparison.

Interpretation

A scheme for interpreting DSC data from individual components and their mixtures is shown in Figure 24.8.

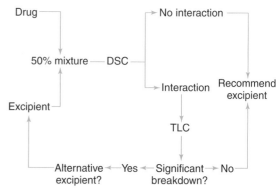

Fig. 24.8 Scheme to identify chemically compatible excipients using DSC with confirmatory TLC.

Where an interaction is suspected but the thermal changes are small, the incompatibility should be confirmed by TLC. Where such confirmation is required, samples (50:50 mixtures of drug and excipient) should be sealed in small neutral glass test tubes and stored for either 7 days at 50°C or 14 days at 37°C.

Basically, the thermal properties of a physical mixture are the sum of the individual components, and this thermogram can be compared with those of the drug and the excipient alone. An interaction on DSC will show as changes in melting point, peak shape and area and/or the appearance of a transition. However, there is invariably some change in transition temperature and peak shape and area by virtue of mixing two components and this is not due to any detrimental interaction. In general, provided that no new thermal events occur, no interaction can be assigned. Chemical interactions are indicated by the appearance of new peaks or where there is gross broadening or elongation of an exo- or endothermic change. Second-order transitions produce changes usually observed as steps in the baseline. Such observations may be indicative of the production of eutectic or solid solution type melts. The excipient is then probably chemically reactive and incompatible with the drug and should be avoided.

The advantages of DSC over more traditional, routine compatibility screens, typically TLC, are that no long-term storage of the mixture is required prior to evaluation nor is any inappropriate thermal stress (other than the DSC itself, which has drug and excipient controls)

required to accelerate the interactions. This, in itself, may be misleading if the mode of breakdown changes with temperature and elevated temperatures fail to reflect the degradation path occurring under normal (room temperature) storage.

It is important to view the results of such incompatibility testing with caution. For example, magnesium stearate is notoriously incompatible with a wide range of compounds when tested. Yet, since it is only used at low levels, typically 0.25–0.75%, such apparent incompatibility rarely produces a problem in practice on long-term storage and use.

SUMMARY

Preformulation studies have a significant part to play in anticipating formulation problems and identifying logical paths in both liquid and solid dosage form technology (Fig. 24.9). The need for adequate drug solubility cannot be overemphasized. The availability of good solubility data should allow the selection of the most appropriate salt for development. Stability studies in solution will indicate the feasibility of parenteral or other liquid dosage form and can identify methods of stabilization. In parallel, solid-state stability, as assessed by DSC, TLC and HPLC analysis of both drug alone and in the presence of tablet and capsule excipients, will indicate the most acceptable vehicles for solid dosage forms.

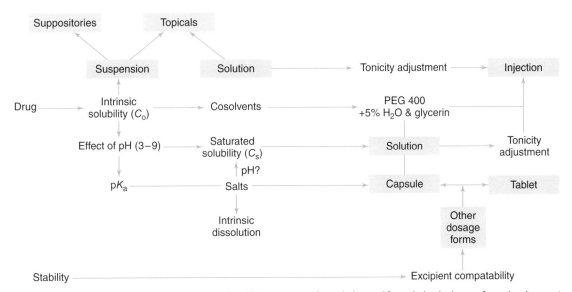

Fig. 24.9 A generic development pathway: the relationship between preformulation and formulation in dosage form development. The formulation stages are shown in boxes and the preformulation stages are unboxed.

By comparing the physicochemical properties of each drug candidate within a therapeutic group (using C_S, pK_a, melting point K_w°), the preformulation scientist can assist the synthetic chemist to identify the optimum molecule, provide the biologist with suitable vehicles to elicit pharmacological response and advise the bulk chemist about the selection and production of the best salt with appropriate particle size and morphology for subsequent processing.

REFERENCES

Albert, A.A., Serjeant, E.P. (1984) *Ionization Constants of Acids and Bases*. Wiley, New York.

Hausner, H.H. (1967) Friction Conditions In A Mass Of Metal Powder, International Journal of Powder Metallurgy, 3 (4), 7-13.

Kaplan, S.A. (1972) Relationships between aqueous solubility of drugs and their bioavailability, *Drug Metabolism Reviews*, **1**, 15-32.

Leo, A., Hansch, C., Elkins, D. (1971) Partition coefficients and their uses, Chemical Reviews, 71(6), 525-555.

Wells, J.I. (1988) *Pharmaceutical Preformulation – The Physicochemical Properties of Drug Substances*. Taylor and Francis, London.

Yalkowski, S.H., Amidon, G.L., Zografi, G., Flynn, G.L. (1975) Solubility of nonelectrolytes in polar solvents III: Alkyl p-aminobenzoates in polar and mixed solvents. *Journal of Pharmaceutical Science,* **64**, 48.

Yalkowski, S.H., Roseman, T. (1981) *Solubilisation of drugs by cosolvents*. Chapter 3 in *Techniques of Solubilization of Drugs*, 91-113, ed. S.H. Yalkowski, Marcel Dekker Inc, New York.

BIBLIOGRAPHY

Bastin, R.J., Bowker, M.J., Slater, B.J. (2000) Salt selection and optimisation procedures for pharmaceutical new chemical entities. *Organic Process Research and Development,* **4**(5), 427-435.

Colin, R.G. et al (2004) Applications of high throughput technologies to drug substance and drug product development. *Computers and Chemical Engineering*, **28**, 943-953.

Connors, K.A., Amidon, G.L., Kennon, L. (1979) *Chemical Stability of Pharmaceuticals*. Wiley, New York

Corrigan, O I. (2004) *Salt Forms: Pharmaceutical Aspects*. Encyclopedia of Pharmaceutical Technology, Marcel Dekker, New York.

The article is called *Salt Forms: Pharmaceutical Aspects* and is a monograph in *Encyclopedia of Pharmaceutical Technology* edited by J SwarbrickDavies, G. (2001) Changing the salt, changing the drug. *Pharmaceutical Journal*, **266**(7138), 322-323.

Forbes, R.T. (2005) *Preformulation polymorph screening*. 10th Arden House European Conference, Cambridge. Royal Pharmaceutical Society of Great Britain and AAPS, London.

Hansch, C., Leo, A.J. (1979) *Substituent Constants for Correlation Analysis in Chemistry and Biology*. Wiley, New York.

Hansch, C., Dann, W.J. (1972) Linear relationships between lipophilic character and biological activity of drugs, Journal of Pharmaceutical Sciences, 61(1), 1-19.

Jones, T.M. (1981) Pharmaceutical powder flow assessment. *International Journal of Pharmaceutical Technology and Product Manufacture*, **2**, 17.

Lipinski, C.A. (2002) Drug-like properties and the cause of poor solubility and poor permeability. *Journal of Pharmacological and Toxicological Methods*, **44**, 235.

McCrone, W.C., McCrone, L.B., Delly, J.G. (1978) *Polarized Light Microscopy*. Ann Arbor Science, Michigan.

Mendenhall, D.W. (2001) Trends in formulation science: building in developability. *AAPS Newsmagazine*, 13.

Morris, K.R. (1994) An integrated approach to the selection of optimal salt form for a new drug candidate. *International Journal of Pharmaceutics*, **105**, 209-217.

Perrin, D.D., Dempsey, B., Serjeant, E.P. (1981) *pK_a Predictions for Organic Acids and Bases*. Chapman and Hall. London.

Pryde, A., Gilbert, M.T. (1979) *Applications of High Performance Liquid Chromatography*. Chapman and Hall, London.

Rekker, R.F. (1977) *The Hydrophobic Fragmental Constant*. ed. W.T. Nauta and R.F. Rekker, Elsevier, Amsterdam.

Storey, R. (2005) *The use of high throughput screening as part of solid form selection*. 10th Arden House European Conference, Cambridge. Royal Pharmaceutical Society of Great Britain and AAPS, London.

25

Solutions

M. R. Billany

INTRODUCTION

An understanding of the properties of solutions, the factors that affect solubility and the process of dissolution is essential because of the importance of solutions in so many areas of pharmaceutical formulation. The fundamentals of solutions and their properties are covered in Chapters 2 and 3 and it is recommended that they be read in conjunction with this chapter for a full understanding of the principles involved in the formulation of solutions.

Ways of expressing solubility and definitions of terms are also explained in these earlier chapters but it is worth reiterating that a solution is a homogeneous one-phase system consisting of two or more components. The solvent, or mixture of solvents, is the phase in which the dispersion occurs, and the solute is the component which is dispersed as molecules or ions in the solvent.

In general, the solvent is present in the greater amount but there are several exceptions. For example, a common pharmaceutical syrup formulation contains 66.7% w/w of sucrose as the solute in 33.3% w/w of water as the solvent.

For most pharmaceutical solutions, the solvent system is likely to be liquid and the solute will be either a liquid or a solid, although solid dispersions, in which both solute and solvent are solids, can be prepared and are used for the improvement of the bioavailability of poorly soluble drugs. As the solute is present as a molecular dispersion, it will exhibit a fast rate of dissolution, owing to its very high specific surface area. In addition, the particles are already in a deaggregated and wetted state and so there is little air adsorbed on the particle surfaces to inhibit dissolution. There may even be a slight increase in actual solubility.

Solutions of gases in liquids are characteristic of pressurized aerosols, in which the propellant gas is dispersed or dissolved in the solvent under pressure. On activation of the valve mechanism, the propellant ejects the product from the container. The propellant immediately evaporates, leaving the active agent in the form of tiny droplets or particles or within a foam structure.

ADVANTAGES AND DISADVANTAGES OF SOLUTIONS AS AN ORAL DOSAGE FORM

Although tablets and capsules are more widely used than liquid preparations for oral administration, the latter possess several advantages.

- Liquids are easier to swallow than solids and are therefore particularly acceptable for paediatric and geriatric use.

- A drug must usually be in solution before it can be absorbed. If it is administered in the form of a solution, the drug is immediately available for absorption. Therefore, the therapeutic response is faster than if using a solid dosage form, which must first disintegrate in order to allow the drug to dissolve in the gastrointestinal fluid before absorption can begin. Even if the drug should precipitate from solution in the acid conditions of the stomach, it will be in a sufficiently wetted and finely divided state to allow rapid absorption to occur.

- A solution is an homogeneous system and therefore the drug will be uniformly distributed throughout the preparation. In suspension or emulsion formulations, dose variation can occur as a result of phase separation on storage.

- Some drugs, including aspirin and potassium chloride, can irritate and damage the gastric mucosa, particularly if localized in one area, as often occurs after the ingestion of a solid dosage form. Irritation is reduced by the administration of a solution of a drug because of its immediate dilution by the gastric contents.

There are, however, several problems associated with the manufacture, transport, stability and administration of solutions.

- Liquids are bulky and therefore inconvenient to transport and store. If the container should break, the whole of the product is immediately and irretrievably lost.

- The stability of ingredients in aqueous solution is often poorer than if formulated as a tablet or capsule, particularly if they are susceptible to hydrolysis. The shelf life of a liquid dosage form is often much shorter than that of the corresponding solid preparation. Not only is the stability of the drug important but also the stability of any excipients, such as surfactants, preservatives, flavours and colours. The chemical stability of some ingredients in solution, however, can be improved by the use of a mixed solvent system. The inclusion of a surfactant above its critical micelle concentration can also improve chemical stability because the hydrolytic degradation of a material may be reduced by its solubilization within the micelles.

- Solutions often provide suitable media for the growth of microorganisms and may therefore require the incorporation of a preservative.

- Most liquid preparations are designed so that the normal dosage of the drug is present in 5 mL, or a multiple of 5 mL, of product. Accurate dosage depends on the ability of the patient to use a 5 mL spoon or a volumetric dropper.

- The taste of a drug, which is often unpleasant, is always more pronounced when in solution than in a solid form. Solutions can, however, easily be sweetened and flavoured to make them more palatable.

CHOICE OF SOLVENT

Aqueous solutions

Water is the solvent most widely used as a vehicle for pharmaceutical products, because of its physiological compatibility and lack of toxicity. It possesses a high dielectric constant, which is essential for ensuring the dissolution of a wide range of ionizable materials. In some cases this property may be an advantage but the lack of selectivity can be responsible for aqueous solutions containing unwanted substances such as inorganic salts and organic impurities. This is one reason why water is rarely used for the extraction of active constituents from vegetable sources.

Types of pharmaceutical water

For many preparations potable water can be used. This is water freshly drawn from the mains system and which is suitable for drinking. If this type is unobtainable, then a suitable, though more expensive, alternative is pharmacopoeial purified water, which has been freshly boiled and cooled immediately before use to destroy any vegetative microorganisms that are likely to be present. Purified water must, however, be used on all occasions where the presence of salts, often dissolved in potable water, is undesirable. Purified water is normally prepared by the distillation or deionization of potable water or by the process of reverse osmosis.

Water for injections must be used for the formulation of parenteral solutions and is obtained by sterilizing pyrogen-free distilled water immediately after its collection. For the formulation of aqueous solutions of drugs, such as aminophylline which is sensitive to the presence of carbon dioxide, water for injections free from carbon dioxide must be used. Similarly, drugs which are liable to oxidation, such as chlorphenamine (chlorpheniramine) and metoclopramide, require water for injections free from dissolved air to be used. These are both obtained from apyrogenic distilled water in the same way as before but are then boiled for at least 10 minutes, cooled, sealed in their containers while excluding air, and then sterilized by autoclaving (see Chapter 18).

Approaches to the improvement of aqueous solubility

Although water is very widely used in pharmaceutical preparations, it may not be possible to ensure complete solution of all ingredients at all normal storage temperatures. Strongly ionized materials are likely to be freely soluble in water over a wide pH range and should cause no problems. Similarly, weak acids and weak bases should be adequately soluble at favourable pHs. Even if in solution, it is still important to ensure that the concentration of any material is not close to its limit of solubility, as precipitation may occur if the product is cooled or if any evaporation of the vehicle should occur. For unionized drugs or for weak electrolytes at a pH that is unfavourable for extensive ionization, one or more of the following methods should be used to improve aqueous solubility.

Cosolvency

The solubility of a weak electrolyte or non-polar compound in water can often be improved by altering the polarity of the solvent. This can be achieved by the addition of another solvent that is both miscible with water and in which the compound is also soluble. Vehicles used in combination to increase the solubility of a drug are called cosolvents, and often the solubility in this mixed system is greater than can be predicted from the material's solubility in each individual solvent.

Because it has been shown that the solubility of a given drug is maximal at a particular dielectric constant of any solvent system, it is possible to eliminate those solvent blends possessing other dielectric constants. In some cases, however, it has been shown that the chemical nature of the solvent system used may be of greater importance. A more detailed explanation of the effects of the molecular structure of the solute and the physicochemical properties of the solvent can be found in Chapter 2.

The choice of suitable cosolvents is somewhat limited for pharmaceutical use because of possible toxicity and irritancy, particularly if required for oral or parenteral use. Ideally, suitable blends should possess values of dielectric constant between 25 and 80. The most widely used system that will cover this range is a water/ethanol blend. Other suitable solvents for use with water include sorbitol, glycerol, propylene glycol and syrup. For example, a blend of propylene glycol and water is used to improve the solubility of co-trimoxazole in oral solutions, and paracetamol is formulated as an elixir by the use of alcohol, propylene glycol and syrup. For external application to the scalp, betamethasone valerate is available dissolved in a water/isopropyl alcohol mixture.

For further details covering the suitability of different cosolvents, see under their individual headings in this chapter.

pH control

A large number of drugs are either weak acids or weak bases, and therefore their solubilities in water can be influenced by the pH of the system. A quantitative application of the Henderson–Hasselbalch equation will enable the solubility of such a drug in water at a given pH to be determined, provided its pK_a and the solubility of its unionized species are known (see Chapter 3). The solubility of a weak base can be increased by lowering the pH of its solution, whereas the solubility of a weak acid is improved by an increase in pH. Some compounds will accept or donate more than one hydrogen ion per molecule, and will therefore possess more than one pK_a value and so exhibit a more complex solubility profile.

In controlling the solubility of a drug in this way, it must be ensured that the chosen pH does not conflict with other product requirements. For example, the chemical stability of a drug may also depend on pH, and in many cases the pH of optimum solubility will not coincide with the pH of optimum stability. This may also be true for other ingredients, especially colours, preservatives and flavours.

The pH of solutions for parenteral and ophthalmic use, for application to mucous membranes or for use on abraded skin must also be controlled, as extremes can cause pain, irritation and even tissue damage. This is particularly true for subcutaneous, intramuscular and intraspinal injections because the solutions will not be rapidly diluted after administration.

In some instances the bioavailability of drugs may be influenced by the pH of their solutions (see Chapter 21), and changes in pH can also affect a preservative's activity by altering the extent to which it is ionized. Often a compromise must be reached during formulation to ensure that the stability and solubility of all ingredients, physiological compatibility and bioavailability are all adequate for the product's intended purpose.

The values of molar solubilities and dissociation constants of drugs that are reported in the literature, or determined during preformulation studies, are usually for the drug alone in distilled water. These values may differ in the final formulation owing to the presence of other ingredients. For example, the inclusion of cosolvents such as alcohol or propylene glycol with water will lower the dielectric constant of the vehicle and therefore increase the solubility of the unionized form of the drug. This lowering of the polarity of the solvent system will also reduce the degree of dissociation of the drug and increase its pK_a. As this effect will increase the concen-

tration of the unionized (less soluble) species, an increase in the pH of the system may be necessary in order to maintain solubility.

It must be appreciated that maximum solubility may best be achieved by a judicious balance between pH control and concentration of cosolvent, and can be determined, as before, by the Henderson–Hasselbalch equation, substituting the new values both for pK_a and for the molar solubilities of the unionized species.

Suitable buffer systems for the control of pH are discussed later in this chapter but care must be taken because the solubilities of sparingly soluble electrolytes can be decreased still further by the addition of a soluble electrolyte, should they contain a common ion. The opposite can be true if they do not possess common ions.

As the solubilities of non-electrolytes are not significantly affected by pH, other methods of improving their solubilities must be found.

Solubilization

The solubility of a drug that is normally insoluble or poorly soluble in water can often be improved by the addition of a surface-active agent above its critical micelle concentration. Surfactant molecules form different types of micelles, ranging from simple spherical structures to more complex liposomes, niosomes and liquid crystals. Details of their formation and structure can be found in Chapter 6. This phenomenon of micellar solubilization has been widely used for the formulation of solutions of poorly soluble drugs. In aqueous systems, non-polar molecules will dissolve in the interior of the micelle, which consists of the lipophilic hydrocarbon moiety.

The amount of surfactant to be used for this purpose must be carefully controlled. A large excess is undesirable because of cost, possible toxicity and its effect on product aeration during manufacture. Excessive amounts may also reduce the bioavailability of a drug if it is strongly adsorbed within the micelle. An insufficient amount of surfactant, however, may not solubilize all the drug, or may lead to precipitation either due to temperature fluctuations on storage or on dilution of the product.

Reference to Figure 6.16 will show that hydrophilic surfactants possessing HLB values above 15 will be particularly valuable as solubilizing agents.

The surfactant chosen must be non-toxic and non-irritant, bearing in mind its intended route of administration. It must also be miscible with the solvent system, compatible with the other ingredients, free from disagreeable odour and taste and be non-volatile.

Examples include the solubilization of fat-soluble vitamins such as phytomenadione using polysorbates. This enables their inclusion with water-soluble vitamins in the same aqueous-based formulation. For parenteral administration of these vitamins, a mixture of glyco-cholic acid and lecithin provides a mixed micelle system.

The solubility of amiodarone hydrochloride can similarly be improved, although this drug can exhibit autosolubilization at high concentrations.

The solubilization of iodine to produce iodophores is achieved by the use of macrogol ethers. These products exhibit several advantages over simple iodine solutions, including an improved chemical stability, reduced loss of active agent due to sublimation, less corrosion of surgical instruments and, in some cases, enhanced activity.

Polyoxyethylated castor oil is used as a solubilizing agent for a number of intravenous injections, including the immunosuppressant ciclosporin and the anticancer drug paclitaxel, both formulated as intravenous infusions. Care must be taken with this surfactant, as anaphylactic reactions are known to occur after it is injected.

Other drugs that have been solubilized include antibiotics such as griseofulvin, which has been formulated with cetomacrogol. Poloxamers (polyoxyethylene/polyoxypropylene copolymers), some of which are also suitable for parenteral administration, are used to maintain the clarity of solutions for oral use (Garcia Sagredo et al 1994). Lanolin derivatives have also been used for the solubilization of volatile and essential oils.

The solubility of phenolic compounds such as chloroxylenol, which is normally soluble in water up to 0.03%, can be improved by solubilization with soaps. By combining the beneficial effects of solubilization and cosolvency in one formulation, a 5% chloroxylenol solution can be formulated. Potassium ricinoleate is the soap and is formed in situ by the reaction between potassium hydroxide and castor oil, while ethanol and terpineol are included as cosolvents.

To ensure that the optimum concentration of surfactant is chosen, a known weight or volume is added to each of a series of vials containing the solvent. Whilst ensuring adequate temperature control, varying amounts of solubilisate (the material to be solubilized) are added to each vial in ascending order of concentration. The maximum concentration of drug that will form a clear solution with a given concentration of surfactant can be determined visually or by optical density measurement (Fig. 25.1a), and is known as the maximum additive concentration (MAC). This method can be repeated for different amounts of surfactant to enable a graph to be constructed of MAC against surfactant concentration, from which the optimum amount of solubilizing agent can be chosen for any required amount of drug (Fig. 25.1b).

Alternatively, a ternary-phase diagram can be constructed (Fig. 25.2) that will present a more comprehensive picture of the effects of solubilisate, surfactant and solvent concentrations on the physical characteristics of the system.

The three axes form the three sides of an equilateral triangle, each axis representing 0–100% of one of the components. Point A thus represents a formulation consisting of 50% solubilisate, 20% surfactant and 30% water. A number corresponding to the physical state of each product made can be placed on the appropriate place on the graph (e.g. 1 = clear solution, 2 = emulsion, 3 = transparent gel, etc.) and by enclosing each of these product types within a boundary, a phase diagram can be constructed. The area designating suitable formulations, which will usually be clear solutions, becomes immediately apparent and the best can then be chosen, bearing in mind the properties required for this type of product.

It is also important to ensure that the formulation chosen does not lie too close to a phase boundary, as the true positions of these can vary depending on the actual storage temperature of the product. In general, the degree of

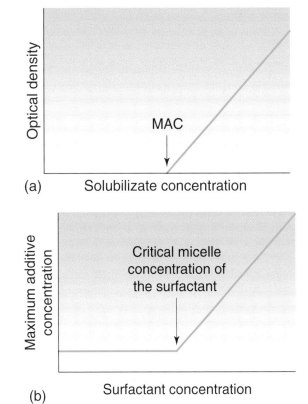

Fig. 25.1 (a) Graph of optical density of a solubilizate/surfactant/solvent system against solubilisate concentration showing the maximum additive concentration (MAC). (b) Determination of the MAC for a range of concentrations of a given surfactant will provide the data for this graph, enabling the optimum concentration of the surfactant to be chosen for the solubilization of a given concentration of active agent.

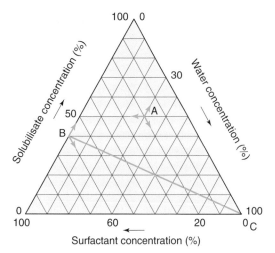

Fig. 25.2 Construction of a ternary-phase diagram.

solubilization of a drug increases as the temperature increases. From this type of phase diagram, the physical composition of diluted preparations can also be shown. Point B, for example, represents a product consisting of 40% solubilisate and 60% surfactant. The construction of a straight line from here to point C (100% water) represents the dilution of the product with increasing concentrations of water.

Should the concentration of drug to be included in the product be fixed, then the third axis can be used to represent varying concentrations of a third excipient such as a cosolvent. These values must, however, be plotted as percentage drug plus excipient to ensure a maximum value of 100%.

Alternatives to the use of surface-active agents as solubilizing agents include the cyclodextrins (Szejtli 1994). This range of compounds is based on a series of glucopyranose units that form cyclical structures resembling hollow cylinders (Fig. 25.3). As the inside surface of the ring is hydrophobic, owing to the presence of –CH$_2$– groups, drugs that are poorly soluble in water can be accommodated here. The outer part of the structure is hydrophilic and therefore freely soluble in water (Stella & Rajewski 1997).

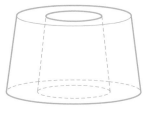

Fig. 25.3 Representation of the structure of cyclodextrins.

There are three natural cyclodextrins, the α, β and γ forms, the ring structures of which are composed of 6, 7 and 8 glucopyranose units respectively, as well as an expanding series of derivatives.

Poorly soluble drugs of appropriate size slot into the interior of these structures, forming soluble inclusion complexes, usually with one 'host' molecule per cyclodextrin molecule (Pagington 1987). Examples of marketed drugs formulated with cyclodextrins include a range of prostaglandins for parenteral infusion, an antiseptic gargle based on iodine and an oral liquid containing the antifungal drug itraconazole. There is also a number of eye drop formulations available containing cyclodextrins for enhanced delivery of corticosteroids.

Complexation

In some cases it may be possible to interact a poorly soluble drug with a soluble material to form a soluble intermolecular complex. As most complexes are macromolecular, however, they tend to be inactive, being unable to cross lipid membranes. It is therefore essential that complex formation is easily reversible, so that the free drug is released during, or before, contact with biological fluids.

It is not easy to predict whether a given drug will complex with a particular compound to improve solubility. Many complexes are not water soluble and may, in fact, be better suited for the prolonged release of the drug. Several well-known examples are in general use, however, and include the complexation of iodine with a 10–15% solution of polyvinylpyrrolidone to improve the aqueous solubility of the active agent. Similarly, the interaction of salicylates and benzoates with xanthines, such as theophylline or caffeine, is carried out for the same effect.

Chemical modification

As a last resort, chemical modification of a drug may be necessary in order to produce a water-soluble derivative. Examples include the synthesis of the sodium phosphate salts of hydrocortisone, prednisolone and betamethasone. The water-soluble chloramphenicol sodium succinate has no antibacterial activity of its own but is suitable for parenteral administration as a solution in order to obtain high blood levels, after which it is converted back to the less soluble active base. There are many examples of poorly soluble acids and bases being converted to a salt form to increase water solubility.

Particle size control

The size and shape of very small particles, if less than 1 micrometre diameter, can affect their solubilities. As particle size decreases, solubility will increase and molecular dispersions of drugs in solid/solid solutions can exhibit improved bioavailability owing to the increase in solubility of the dispersed drug. In practice, however, this phenomenon has little application in the formulation of solutions but is of particular relevance in suspension formulation.

Non-aqueous solutions

If it is not possible to ensure complete solution of the ingredients at all storage temperatures, or if the drug is unstable in aqueous systems, it may be necessary to use an alternative, non-aqueous solvent. The use of non-aqueous systems may also have other advantages. For example, the intramuscular injection of solutions of drugs in oils is often used for depot therapy, and some drugs are specifically synthesized to improve their oil solubilities. The propionate and benzoate esters of testosterone and oestradiol, respectively, are good examples of this. The oily solution remains as discrete globules within the muscle tissue, releasing the drug slowly into the surrounding tissue by partitioning. An aqueous solution containing water-soluble drugs would diffuse readily and, being miscible with tissue fluid, would cause the drug to be released immediately.

It is essential that, in choosing a suitable solvent, its toxicity, irritancy and sensitizing potential are taken into account, as well as its flammability, cost, stability and compatibility with other excipients. It will be obvious that there is a greater choice of solvents available for inclusion into products for external application than those for internal use, and that for parenteral products the choice is limited even further. A far wider range of solvents, however, is available for use as part of the manufacturing process of pharmaceutical products. In these instances the solvent is removed before packaging and is therefore not present in the final product. Examples include acetone, light petroleum and chloroform, although the latter is also used as a flavour and preservative in some extemporaneously prepared formulations. The following is a classification of some of the more widely used non-aqueous solvents in pharmaceutical preparations.

Fixed oils of vegetable origin

These are non-volatile oils that consist mainly of fatty acid esters of glycerol. Almond oil, for example, which consists of glycerides mainly of oleic acid, is used as a solvent for oily phenol injections, water being unsuitable because of the caustic nature of aqueous phenol solutions. Of similar chemical composition is arachis oil, which is used as the solvent in dimercaprol injection.

Olive oil, sesame oil, maize oil, cottonseed oil, soya oil and castor oil are all suitable for parenteral use, the latter also being used as the solvent in miconazole eye drops and in some formulations of triamcinolone ear drops.

Ethyl oleate, which is a useful solvent for both ergocalciferol injection and testosterone propionate injection, is less viscous than the oils described above and therefore more easily injected intramuscularly. Of similar viscosity is benzyl benzoate, which can be used as an alternative solvent for dimercaprol.

Veterinary formulations may also contain these solvents, arachis oil, for example, being used for hexachlorophene in the treatment of fascioliasis in ruminants.

Oils tend to be unpleasant to use externally, however, unless presented as an emulsion. Arachis oil is one of the few examples and is used as the solvent in methyl salicylate liniment.

Alcohols

Ethyl alcohol is the most widely used solvent in this class, particularly for external application, where its rapid evaporation after application to the skin imparts a cooling effect to such products as salicylic acid lotion. It is also particularly useful for the extraction of crude drugs, being more selective than water. At concentrations greater than 15%, ethanol exhibits antimicrobial activity but because of its toxicity, it is used orally or parenterally only at low concentrations, usually as a cosolvent with water.

If required for external use then industrial methylated spirit (IMS), which is free from excise duty, is usually included rather than the more expensive ethanol. Because IMS contains 5% methyl alcohol as a denaturant, it is rendered too toxic for internal use.

An alcohol possessing similar properties is isopropyl alcohol, which is used externally as a solvent for dicophane. Its main advantage is that it is less likely to be abused than ethanol and so denaturation is not necessary.

Polyhydric alcohols

Alcohols containing two hydroxyl groups per molecule are known as glycols but because of their toxicity, they are rarely used internally. One important exception to this is propylene glycol:

$$CH_3CH(OH)CH_2OH$$

which is often used in conjunction with water or glycerol as a cosolvent. It is used, for example, in the formulation of digoxin injection, phenobarbital injection and some formulations of diazepam injection, co-trimoxazole intravenous infusion and as the diluent for both chloramphenicol ear drops and some brands of hydrocortisone ear drops, and in many preparations for oral use.

The lower molecular weight polyethylene glycols (PEGs) or macrogols have the general formula:

$$HOCH_2(CH_2CH_2O)_nCH_2OH$$

and are available in a range of viscosity grades. PEG 400, for example, is used as a solvent in clotrimazole topical solution. They are also widely used as cosolvents with alcohol or water, although their main use is in the formulation of water-miscible ointment bases. There are also other glycols available which, although rarely included in products for human use, can be used for extraction processes or as solvents in the formulation of veterinary and horticultural solutions. Examples include dipropylene glycol, diethylene glycol, ethylene glycol and their monoethyl ethers. Glycerol, an alcohol possessing three hydroxyl groups per molecule, is also widely used, particularly as a cosolvent with water for oral use. At higher concentrations it is used in, for example, phenol and glycerol injection.

Dimethylsulfoxide

This is a highly polar compound and is thought to aid the penetration of drugs through the skin. Although used mainly as a solvent for veterinary drugs, it is used as a carrier for idoxuridine, an antiviral agent, for application to human skin.

Ethyl ether

This material is widely used for the extraction of crude drugs but because of its own therapeutic activity, it is not used for the preparation of formulations for internal use. It is, however, used as a cosolvent with alcohol in some collodions.

Liquid paraffin

The oily nature of this material makes it unpleasant to use externally, although it is often used as a solvent for the topical application of drugs in emulsion formulations. At one time light liquid paraffin was widely used as the base for oily nasal drops. (These are now rarely used because of the possibility of causing lipoidal pneumonia if they are inhaled into the lungs.) It has a minor use in veterinary formulation as a solvent in, for example, anthelminthic drenches containing carbon tetrachloride.

Miscellaneous solvents

Isopropyl myristate and isopropyl palmitate are used as solvents for external use, particularly in cosmetics, where their low viscosity and lack of greasiness make them pleasant to use. Dimethylformamide and dimethylacetamide have both been used as solvents in veterinary formulations but their toxicities render them unsuitable for human use. Kerosene is also limited in its application, being used mainly as a solvent for insecticides such as pyrethrum and piperonyl butoxide.

Xylene is present in some ear drops for human use to dissolve ear wax, and glycofurol is a useful solvent for parenteral products, particularly the intramuscular injection of antibiotics.

As with aqueous systems, it may be possible to improve the solubility of a drug in a particular vehicle by the addition of a cosolvent. For example, nitrocellulose is poorly soluble in both alcohol and ether but adequately soluble in a mixture of both. The formulation of digoxin injection, too, is best achieved by the inclusion of both ethyl alcohol and propylene glycol.

OTHER FORMULATION ADDITIVES

Buffers

These are materials which, when dissolved in a solvent, will enable the solution to resist any change in pH should an acid or an alkali be added. The choice of suitable buffer depends on the pH and buffering capacity required. It must be compatible with other excipients and have a low toxicity. Most pharmaceutically acceptable buffering systems are based on carbonates, citrates, gluconates, lactates, phosphates or tartrates. Borates can be used for external application but not to mucous membranes or to abraded skin.

Although solutions of drugs that are themselves weak electrolytes will act as buffers, their buffering capacities are not usually sufficiently robust and should be enhanced by one of the systems described above.

As the pH of most body fluids is 7.4, products such as injections, eye drops and nasal drops should, in theory, be buffered at this value to avoid irritation. Many body fluids themselves, however, have a buffering capacity and when formulating low-volume intravenous injections or eye drops, a wider pH range can be tolerated. This is potentially useful should a compromise be necessary when choosing a pH that is physiologically acceptable for a drug whose optimum stability, solubility and/or bioavailability may depend on different pHs. Further details on the use of buffers are given in Chapter 3.

Density modifiers

It is rarely necessary to control the density of solutions except when formulating spinal anaesthetics. Solutions of lower density than cerebrospinal fluid will tend to rise after injection and those of higher density will fall. Careful control of both the density of such injections and the position of the patient on the operating table will enable precise control of the area to be anaesthetized. The terms used to describe the density of injections in relation to that of spinal fluid are isobaric, hypobaric and hyperbaric, meaning of equal, lower and higher density, respectively. The most widely used material for density modification is dextrose.

Isotonicity modifiers

Solutions for injection, for application to mucous membranes and large-volume solutions for ophthalmic use must be made isoosmotic with tissue fluid to avoid pain and irritation.

The most widely used isotonicity modifiers are dextrose and sodium chloride. Isotonicity adjustments can only be made after the addition of all other ingredients, because each ingredient will contribute to the overall osmotic pressure of a solution.

Viscosity enhancement

It may be difficult for aqueous-based topical solutions to remain in place on the skin or in the eyes for any significant time because of their low viscosities. To counteract this effect, low concentrations of gelling agents can be used to increase the apparent viscosity of the product. Examples include povidone, hydroxyethylcellulose and carbomer.

Preservatives

When choosing a suitable preservative it must be ensured that:

- adsorption of the preservative from the product onto the container does not occur, and
- its efficiency is not impaired by the pH of the solution or by interactions with other ingredients.

For example, many of the widely used parahydroxybenzoic acid esters can be adsorbed into the micelles of some non-ionic surfactants and, although their presence can be detected by chemical analysis, they are in fact unable to exert their antimicrobial activities. It is only by full microbiological challenge testing that the efficiency of a preservative system can be properly assessed.

A more comprehensive discussion on the preservation of pharmaceuticals can be found in Chapter 43.

Reducing agents and antioxidants

The decomposition of pharmaceutical products by oxidation can be controlled by the addition of reducing agents such as sodium metabisulphite or antioxidants such as butylated hydroxyanisole or butylated hydroxytoluene. For unit-dose parenteral products, such as injections of nicotinamide and ascorbic acid, it is possible to use water for injections free from dissolved air and to replace the air in the headspace by nitrogen or another inert gas.

Sweetening agents

Low molecular weight carbohydrates, and in particular sucrose, are traditionally the most widely used sweetening agents. Sucrose has the advantage of being colourless, very soluble in water, stable over a pH range of about 4–8 and, by increasing the viscosity of fluid preparations, will impart to them a pleasant texture in the mouth. It will mask the tastes of both salty and bitter drugs and has a soothing effect on the membranes of the throat. For this reason, despite its cariogenic properties, sucrose is particularly useful as a vehicle for antitussive preparations.

Polyhydric alcohols such as sorbitol and mannitol also possess sweetening power and can be included in preparations for diabetic use, where sucrose is undesirable. Other less widely used bulk sweeteners include maltilol, lactilol, isomalt, fructose and xylitol. Treacle, honey and liquorice are now very rarely used, having only a minor application in some extemporaneously prepared formulations.

Artificial sweeteners can be used in conjunction with sugars and alcohols to enhance the degree of sweetness, or on their own in formulations for patients who must restrict their sugar intake. They are also termed intense sweeteners because, weight for weight, they are hundreds and even thousands of times sweeter than sucrose and are therefore rarely required at a concentration greater than about 0.2%.

Only six artificial sweeteners are permitted for oral use within the European Union, the most widely used being the sodium or calcium salts of saccharin (E954). Both salts exhibit high water solubility and are chemically and physically stable over a wide pH range. Less widely used are aspartame (E951), which is a compound of L-aspartic acid and L-phenylalanine, acesulfame potassium (E950), thaumatin (E957), sodium cyclamate (E952) and neohesperidine DC (E959). The main disadvantage of all artificial sweeteners is their tendency to impart a bitter or metallic aftertaste, and they are therefore often formulated with sugars to mask this.

Flavours and perfumes

The simple use of sweetening agents may not be sufficient to render palatable a product containing a drug with a particularly unpleasant taste. In many cases, therefore, a flavouring agent can be included. This is particularly useful in paediatric formulations to ensure patient compliance. The inclusion of flavours has the additional advantage of enabling the easy identification of liquid products.

Flavouring and perfuming agents can be obtained from either natural or synthetic sources. Natural products include fruit juices, aromatic oils such as peppermint and lemon, herbs and spices, and distilled fractions of these. They are available as concentrated extracts, alcoholic or aqueous solutions, syrups or spirits and are particularly widely used in the manufacture of products for extemporaneous use. Artificial perfumes and flavours are of purely synthetic or semi-synthetic origin, often having no natural counterpart. They tend to be cheaper, more readily available, less variable in chemical composition and more stable than natural products. They are usually available as alcoholic or aqueous solutions or as powders. Because of their limited solubilities, it is usual to include a cosolvent such as ethanol to ensure clarity.

The choice of a suitable flavour can only be made as a result of subjective assessment and, as consumer preferences vary considerably, this is not easy. Some guidance can, however, be gained by reference to Table 25.1, which shows that certain flavours are particularly useful for the masking of one or more of the basic taste sensations of saltiness, bitterness, sweetness and sourness. These tastes are detected by sensory receptors on various areas of the tongue, whereas the more subtle flavours are detected by the olfactory receptors.

In some cases there is a strong association between the use of a product and its flavour or perfume content. For example, products intended for the relief of indigestion are often mint flavoured. This is because for many years mint has been used in such products for its carminative effect but even in products containing other active agents, the odour and taste of mint are now firmly associated with antacid activity. Similarly, the odour of terpineol is often associated with antiseptic activity and, in a competitive market; it may therefore be unwise to alter these flavours or perfumes to any appreciable extent.

The fact that personal preferences for flavours and perfumes often vary with age can also aid the formulator. Children, in general, prefer fruity tastes and smells whereas adults choose flowery odours and acid flavours. Other suitable materials for the masking of unpleasant tastes include menthol, peppermint oil and chloroform. In addition to having their own particular tastes and odours, they also act as desensitizing agents by exerting a mild anaesthetic effect on the sensory taste receptors.

Flavour-enhancing agents such as citric acid for citrus fruits and glycine or monosodium glutamate for general use are now becoming more widely used.

Colours

Once a suitable flavour has been chosen, it is often useful to include a colour associated with that flavour in order to improve the attractiveness of the product. Another reason for the inclusion of colours is to enable easy product identification, particularly of poisonous materials, including weed killers and mineralized methylated spirit, and, for example, to differentiate between the many types of antiseptic solution used in hospitals for the disinfection of skin, instruments, syringes, etc.

The presence of a strongly coloured degradation product, which does not affect the use of the product, may occasionally be masked by the use of a suitable colour. It is, however, essential to ensure that any colour chosen is acceptable in the country in which the product is to be sold. A colour that is acceptable in one country may not be acceptable in another and as aspects of colour legislation can change quite frequently, it is necessary to ensure that only the latest regulations are consulted. The legal departments of most dye manufacturers are usually willing to supply up-to-date information.

The proliferation of nomenclature that exists for most colours can also cause confusion. For example, the water-soluble dye amaranth is also known as Bordeaux S, Cl Food Red 9 and Cl Acid Red 27. It has been allocated the Colour Index Number 16185 by the Society of Dyers and Colourists and the American Association of Textile Chemists and Colorists. Under the USA Food, Drug and Cosmetics Act it is known as FD and C Red Number 2, and a directive of the Council of European Communities has allocated it the reference number E123.

As with flavours and perfumes, there is a range of both natural and synthetic colours. The former, which tend to be more widely acceptable, can be classified into carotenoids, chlorophyll, anthocyanins and a miscellaneous group which includes riboflavines, melanoidins (caramel) and betanin, extracted from beetroot. They can, however, exhibit the usual problems associated with natural products, namely variations in availability and

Table 25.1 Suitable masking flavours for various product tastes	
Taste of product	Suitable masking flavour
Salty	Apricot, butterscotch, liquorice, peach, vanilla
Bitter	Anise, chocolate, mint, passion fruit, wild cherry
Sweet	Vanilla, fruits, berries
Sour	Citrus fruits, liquorice, raspberry

chemical composition, both of which may cause formulation difficulties.

Synthetic or 'coal tar' dyes tend to give bright colours and are generally more stable than natural materials. Most of those that are suitable for pharmaceutical use are the sodium salts of sulphonic acids, and therefore they may be incompatible with cationic drugs. Care must also be taken to ensure that any dye used is not adversely affected by pH or by ultraviolet radiation, or by the inclusion of oxidizing or reducing agents or surfactants.

TYPES OF LIQUID PREPARATIONS

The terminology used for the titles of different forms of liquid preparation for both oral and topical use can sometimes be confusing, with overlap between definitions and more than one definition being appropriate for one particular product. Furthermore, definitions can vary between different official compendia and may be at variance with definitions used within the pharmaceutical industry. This section attempts to give an overview of the types of pharmaceutical solution available.

Liquids for cutaneous application

Lotions and liniments

Lotions can be formulated as solutions and are designed to be applied to the unbroken skin without friction. They may contain humectants, so that moisture is retained on the skin after application of the product, or alcohol, which evaporates quickly, imparting a cooling effect and leaving the skin dry.

Liniments, in contrast, are intended for massage into the unbroken skin and can contain such ingredients as methyl salicylate or camphor as counterirritants.

Paints and collodions

Liquids for application to the skin or mucous membranes in small amounts are often termed paints, and are usually applied with a small brush. The solvent is normally alcohol, acetone or ether, which evaporates quickly leaving a film on the skin that contains the active agent. A viscosity modifier such as glycerol is often added to ensure prolonged contact with the skin.

Collodions are similar preparations which, after evaporation of the solvent, leave a tough, flexible film that will seal small cuts or hold a drug in intimate contact with the skin. The film former is usually pyroxylin (nitrocellulose) in an alcohol/ether or alcohol/acetone solvent blend. Often a plasticizer such as castor oil and an adherent such as colophony resin are included.

Ear preparations

Also known as otic or aural products, these are simple solutions of drugs in water, glycerol, propylene glycol or alcohol/water mixtures for local use, and include antibiotics, antiseptics, cleansing solutions and wax softeners. They are applied to the external auditory canal as drops, sprays or washes.

Eye preparations

These are small-volume sterile liquids designed to be instilled onto the eyeball or within the conjunctival sac for a local effect.

Irrigations

Irrigations are sterile, large-volume aqueous-based solutions for the cleansing of body cavities and wounds. They should be made isotonic with tissue fluid.

Nasal preparations

These are formulated as small-volume solutions in an aqueous vehicle, oils being no longer used for nasal administration. Because the buffering capacity of nasal mucus is low, formulation at a pH of 6.8 is necessary. Nasal drops should also be made isotonic with nasal secretions using sodium chloride, and viscosity can also be modified using cellulose derivatives if necessary. Active agents for administration by this route for local use include antibiotics, antiinflammatories and decongestants. The nasal route is also of major importance for specific types of drugs, and a full description of this method of drug delivery can be found in Chapter 37.

Oral liquids

This is a general term used to describe a solution, suspension or emulsion in which the active ingredient is dissolved or dispersed in a suitable liquid vehicle.

Elixirs

The terms 'mixture' and 'elixir' are often confused, although an elixir is strictly a solution of a potent or nauseous drug in a clear, sweetened solution. If the active agent is sensitive to moisture, it may be formulated as a flavoured powder or granulation by the pharmaceutical industry and then simply dissolved in water immediately prior to administration. The dosage is usually taken using a 5 mL medicine spoon, although smaller volumes can be given using a volumetric dropper.

Linctuses

A linctus is a viscous preparation, usually prescribed for the relief of cough. It normally consists of a simple solution of the active agent in a high concentration of sucrose, often with other sweetening agents. This type of product, which is also designed to be administered in multiples of 5 mL, should be sipped slowly and not be diluted beforehand. The syrup content has a demulcent action on the mucous membranes of the throat. For diabetic use, the sucrose is usually replaced by sorbitol and/or synthetic sweeteners.

Mixtures and draughts

Mixtures are usually aqueous preparations that can be in the form of either a solution or a suspension. Most preparations of this type are manufactured on a small scale as required, and are allocated a shelf life of a few weeks before dispensing. Doses are usually given in multiples of 5 mL using a metric medicine spoon. A draught is a mixture of which only one or two large doses of about 50 mL are given, although smaller doses are often necessary for children.

Oromucosal preparations

These are designed for application to the throat or oral cavity and can include solids and semi-solids as well as solutions.

Mouthwashes and gargles

These aqueous solutions are for the prevention and treatment of mouth and throat infections and can contain antiseptics, analgesics and/or astringents. They are usually diluted with warm water before use.

Gingival and sublingual preparations

These are in the form of sprays or drops for application to specific areas of the oral mucosa such as the gums for the prevention and treatment of periodontal disease or under the tongue to enable fast absorption of active agents into the systemic circulation.

Parenteral products

Sterile solutions for injection or infusion into the body are also available.

Rectal preparations

Aqueous or oily solutions, as well as emulsions and suspensions, are available for the rectal administration of medicaments for cleansing, diagnostic or therapeutic reasons, and are termed enemas.

Intermediate products

Aromatic waters and spirits

There are many pharmaceutical solutions that are designed for use during the manufacture of other preparations and which are rarely administered themselves. Aromatic waters, for example, are aqueous solutions of volatile materials and are used mainly for their flavouring properties. Examples include anise water, which also has carminative properties, and chloroform water, which also acts as a preservative.

They are usually manufactured as concentrated waters and are then diluted, traditionally 1:40, in the final preparation.

Spirits are also alcoholic solutions but of volatile materials, which are mainly used as flavouring agents.

Extracts, infusions and tinctures

Infusions, extracts and tinctures are terms used for concentrated solutions of active principles from animal or vegetable sources. Infusions are prepared by extracting the drug using 25% alcohol but without the application of heat. Traditionally these preparations are then diluted 1:10 in the final product. Extracts are similar products that are then concentrated by evaporation. Tinctures are alcoholic extracts of drugs but are relatively weak compared with extracts.

Syrups

Syrups are concentrated solutions of sucrose or other sugars to which medicaments or flavourings are often added. For example, tolu syrup is used as a cough expectorant and orange syrup contains dried bitter orange peel as a flavouring agent. Although syrups are used in the manufacture of other preparations, such as mixtures or elixirs, they can also be administered as products in their own right, the high concentrations of sugars imparting a sweetening effect.

As syrups can contain up to 85% of sugars, they are capable of resisting bacterial growth by virtue of their osmotic effect. Syrups can contain lower concentrations of sugars but will often include sufficient of a polyhydric alcohol such as sorbitol, glycerol or propylene glycol in order to maintain a high osmotic gradient. In addition, by acting as cosolvents they will help to prevent crystallization and to maintain solubility of all ingredients.

However, in a closed container, it is possible for surface dilution of a syrup to take place. This occurs as a result of solvent evaporation that condenses on the upper internal surfaces of the container and then flows back on to the surface of the product, thereby producing a diluted layer which provides an ideal medium for the growth of certain microorganisms. For this reason syrups often contain additional preservatives.

A further problem with the storage and use of syrups involves the crystallization of the sugar within the screw cap used to seal the containers, thereby preventing its release. This can be avoided by the addition of the polyhydric alcohols previously mentioned or by the inclusion of invert syrup, which is a mixture of glucose and fructose.

STABILITY OF SOLUTIONS

Both the chemical and the physical stability of solutions in their intended containers are important. A solution must retain its initial clarity, colour, odour, taste and viscosity over its allocated shelf life. Clarity can easily be assessed by visual examination or by a measurement of its optical density after agitation. Colour too may be assessed both visually and spectrophotometrically, and equipment suitable for the measurement of rheological properties of solutions has been covered earlier.

The stability of flavours and perfumes is perhaps more difficult to assess. Although chromatographic methods are used with varying success to quantify these properties, considerable reliance must be placed on the organoleptic powers of a panel of assessors, who must be screened to ensure that their powers of olfaction and gustation are sufficiently sensitive. If a suitable majority of the panel members is unable to detect a difference between a stored sample and a freshly prepared reference material, it may be assumed that the taste or odour of the sample has not changed significantly.

MANUFACTURE OF SOLUTIONS

For both small- and large-scale manufacture of solutions the only equipment necessary is suitable mixing vessels, a means of agitation and a filtration system to ensure clarity of the final solution. During manufacture, the solute is simply added to the solvent in a mixing vessel and stirring is continued until dissolution is complete. If the solute is more soluble at elevated temperatures, it may be advantageous to apply heat to the vessel, particularly if the dissolution rate is normally slow. Care must be taken, however, should any volatile or thermolabile materials be present. Size reduction of solid materials to increase their surface areas should also speed up the process of solution.

Solutes present in low concentrations, particularly dyes, are often predissolved in a small volume of the solvent and then added to the bulk. Volatile materials such as flavours and perfumes are, where possible, added at the end of a process and after any cooling, to reduce loss by evaporation. Finally, it must be ensured that significant amounts of any of the materials are not irreversibly adsorbed on to the filtration medium used for final clarification. For a discussion of suitable packaging materials and containers for solutions, see Chapter 42.

REFERENCES

Garcia Sagredo, F., Guzman, M., Molpereces, J., Aberturas, M.R. (1994) Pluronic copolymers – characteristics, properties and pharmaceutical applications. *Pharmaceutical Technology Europe*, **1**, 46-56; **2**, 38-44.

Pagington, I.S. (1987) β-cyclodextrin: the success of molecular inclusion. *Chemistry in Britain*, **23**, 455.

Stella, V.J., Rajewski, R.A. (1997) Cyclodextrins: their future in drug formulation and delivery. *Pharmaceutical Research*, **14**, 556-567.

Szejtli, J. (1994) Medicinal applications of cyclodextrins. *Medicinal Research Reviews*, **14**, 353-386.

BIBLIOGRAPHY

Florence, A.T., Attwood, D. (2006) *Physicochemical Principles of Pharmacy*, 4th edn. Pharmaceutical Press, London.

Martin, A. (1993) *Physical Pharmacy*, 4th edn. Lea and Febiger, Philadelphia.

Sweetman, S.C. (2004) *Martindale – The Complete Drug Reference*, 34th edn. Pharmaceutical Press, London.

26

Clarification

A. M. Twitchell

INTRODUCTION

Clarification is a term used to describe processes that involve the removal or separation of a solid from a fluid, or a fluid from another fluid. The term 'fluid' encompasses both liquids and gases. Clarification can be achieved using either filtration or centrifugation techniques, both of which are described in this chapter.

In pharmaceutical processing there are two main reasons for such processes:

- to remove unwanted solid particles from either a liquid product or from air
- to collect the solid as the product itself (e.g. following crystallization).

FILTRATION

Types of filtration

Solid/fluid filtration

Solid/fluid filtration can be defined as the separation of an insoluble solid from a fluid by means of a porous medium that retains the solid but allows the fluid to pass. It is the most common type of filtration encountered during the manufacture of pharmaceutical products. Solid/fluid filtration may be further subdivided into two types, namely solid/liquid filtration and solid/ gas filtration.

Solid/liquid filtration   There are numerous applications of solid/liquid filtration in pharmaceutical processing, some of which are listed below:

- Improvement of the appearance of solutions, mouthwashes, etc., to give them a 'sparkle' or 'brightness'; this is often referred to as 'clarifying' a product.
- Removal of potential irritants, e.g. from eye drop preparations or solutions applied to mucous membranes.

- Production of water of appropriate quality for pharmaceutical production.
- Recovery of desired solid material from a suspension or slurry, e.g. to obtain a drug or excipient after a crystallization process.
- Certain operations, such as the extraction of vegetable drugs with a solvent, may yield a turbid product with a small quantity of fine suspended colloidal matter. This can be removed by filtration.
- Sterilization of liquid or semi-solid products where processes involving heat (such as autoclaving) are not appropriate.
- Detection of microorganisms present in liquids. This can be achieved by analysing a suitable filter on which the bacteria are retained. This method can also be used to assess the efficiency of preservatives.

Solid/gas filtration There are two main applications of solid/gas filtration in pharmaceutical processing. One of particular importance in manufacturing is the removal of suspended solid material from air in order to supply air of the required standard for either processing equipment or manufacturing areas. This includes the provision of air for equipment such as fluidized-bed processors (see Chapters 29 and 30), film-coating machinery (Chapter 33) and bottle-cleaning equipment, so that product appearance and quality are maintained. The use of suitable filters also enables the particulate contamination of air in manufacturing areas to be at an appropriate level for the product being manufactured; for example, air free from microorganisms can be supplied to areas where sterile products are being manufactured.

It is also often necessary to remove particulate matter generated during a manufacturing operation from the process air in order to prevent the material being vented to the atmosphere. Examples of this include filtering of exhaust air from fluidized-bed and coating processes.

Fluid/fluid filtration

Flavouring oils are sometimes added to liquid preparations in the form of a spirit, i.e. dissolved in alcohol. When these spirits are added to aqueous-based formulations some of the oil may come out of solution, giving the product a degree of turbidity. Removal of the oil droplets by passing them through an appropriate filter (a liquid/liquid filtration process) is used to produce the desired product appearance.

Compressed air is used in a number of pharmaceutical processes, e.g. film-coating spray guns (Chapter 33), bottle-cleaning equipment and fluid energy mills (Chapter 10). Before use, the compressed air needs to be filtered to ensure that any entrained oil or water droplets are removed. This is an example of a liquid/gas filtration process.

Mechanisms of filtration

The mechanisms by which material may be retained by a filter medium (i.e. the surface on or in which material is deposited) are discussed below.

Straining/sieving

If the pores in the filter medium through which the fluid is flowing are smaller than the material that is required to be removed, the material will be retained. Filtration occurs on the surface of the filter in this case, and therefore the filter can be very thin (typically around 100 μm). Filter media of this type are referred to as membrane filters. Because filtration occurs on the surface there is a tendency for them to become blocked unless the filter is carefully designed (see later). Filters employing the straining mechanism are used where the contaminant level is low or small volumes need to be filtered.

Examples of the use of membrane filters include the removal of bacteria and fibres from parenteral preparations.

Impingement

As a flowing fluid approaches and passes an object, for example a filter fibre, the fluid flow pattern is disturbed, as shown in Figure 26.1. Suspended solids may, however, have sufficient momentum that they do not follow the fluid path but impinge on the filter fibre and are retained, owing to attractive forces between the particle and the fibre. Where the pores between filter fibres are larger than the material being removed, some particles may follow the fluid streamlines and miss the fibre, this being more likely if the particles are small (owing to their lower momentum) and as the distance from the centre of the fibre towards which they approach increases. To ensure the removal of all unwanted material, filter media using the impingement mechanism must be sufficiently thick so that material not

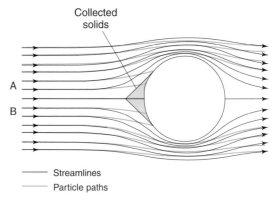

Fig. 26.1 Filtration by impingement.

trapped by the first fibre in its path is removed by a subsequent one. These types of filter are therefore referred to as depth filters. The fluid should flow through the filter medium in a streamlined manner to ensure the filter works effectively, as turbulent flow may carry the particles past the fibres. Depth filters are the main type of filter used for removing material from gases.

Attractive forces

Electrostatic and other surface forces may exert sufficient hold on the particles to attract and retain them on the filter medium (as occurs during the impingement mechanism).

Air can be freed from dust particles in an electrostatic precipitator by passing the air between highly charged surfaces, which attract the dust particles.

Autofiltration

Autofiltration is the term used to describe the situation when filtered material (termed the filter cake) acts as its own filter medium. This mechanism is used by the metafilter which is covered later in this chapter.

Factors affecting the rate of filtration

The filtration process chosen must remove the required 'contaminants' or product but must also do so at an acceptably fast rate to ensure that the manufacturing process can be carried out economically. The laboratory Buchner funnel and flask (Fig. 26.2) is a convenient filter that can be used to illustrate the factors that influence the rate at which a product can be filtered. This filter is used for solid/liquid filtration processes but the same basic principles are valid whatever filtration process is being evaluated.

The rate of filtration (volume of filtered material (V, m^3) obtained in unit time (t, s)) depends on the following factors:

- The area available for filtration (A, m^2), which in this case is the cross-sectional area of the funnel.
- The pressure difference (ΔP, Pa) across the filter bed (filter medium and any cake formed). With the Buchner funnel apparatus, this difference is due to the 'head' of unfiltered suspension and therefore it decreases as filtration proceeds and the level drops. Note that it is the pressure difference across the filtration medium that is important, and this can be increased by drawing a vacuum in the collection flask. The difference between atmospheric pressure and the lower pressure in the flask is added to the pressure due to the unfiltered product to give the total pressure difference.

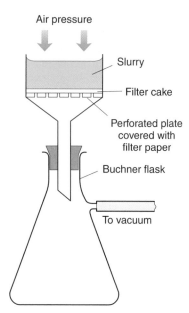

Fig. 26.2 Buchner funnel and vacuum flask.

- The viscosity of the fluid passing through the filter, i.e. the filtrate (μ, Pa s). A viscous fluid will filter more slowly than a mobile one owing to the greater resistance to movement offered by more viscous fluids (see Chapter 4).
- The thickness of the filter medium and any deposited cake (L, m). The cake will *increase* in thickness as filtration proceeds so if this is not removed, the rate of filtration will fall.

Darcy's equation

The above factors are combined in the Darcy equation:

$$\frac{V}{t} = \frac{KA\Delta P}{\mu L} \qquad (26.1)$$

In this equation the driving force for this particular 'rate process' is the pressure difference across the filter, and the resistance to the process is a function of the properties of the filter bed, its thickness and the viscosity of the filtrate. The contribution to resistance to filtration from the filter medium is usually small compared to that of the filter cake, and can often be neglected in calculations.

The proportionality constant K (m^2) expresses the permeability of the filter medium and cake and will increase as the porosity of the bed increases. It is clearly desirable that K should be large in order to maximize the filtration rate. If K is taken to represent the permeability of the cake, it can be shown that K is given by:

$$K = \frac{e^2}{5(1-e)^2 S^2} \qquad (26.2)$$

where e is the porosity of the cake and S is the surface area of the particles comprising the cake. If the solid material is one that forms an impermeable cake, the filtration rate may be improved by adding a filter aid (discussed later), which aids the formation of open porous cakes.

Methods used to increase filtration rate

Darcy's equation can be used to determine ways in which the filtration rate can be increased or controlled in practice. These are now discussed.

Increase the area available for filtration The total volume of filtrate flowing through the filter will be directly proportional to the area of the filter, and hence the rate of filtration can be increased by using either larger filters or a number of small units in parallel. Both of these approaches will also distribute the cake over a larger area and thus decrease the value of L, thereby further increasing the filtration rate.

Increase the pressure difference across the filter cake The simplest filters, e.g. a laboratory filter funnel, use the gravitational force of the liquid 'head' to provide the driving force for filtration. Often this driving force is too low for an acceptably fast filtration rate and there is a requirement to increase it. If a vacuum is 'pulled' on the far side of the filter medium (see Fig. 26.1) then the pressure difference can be increased up to atmospheric pressure, i.e. approximately 100 kPa or 1 bar. In practice, however, it will be less, as liquids will boil in the collecting vessel if the pressure is reduced to too low a value (discussed in Chapter 46). Despite the limited pressure difference generated, vacuum filtration is used in the laboratory where there are safety advantages in using glassware, because if the glassware is damaged it will implode rather than explode. One important industrial filter, the rotary vacuum filter, also utilizes a vacuum; this is described later in this chapter.

With industrial-scale liquid filtration, commonly used means of obtaining a high-pressure difference are either pumping the material to be filtered into the filter using a suitable pump, or using a pressurized vessel to drive the liquid through the filter. Most industrial filters have positive-pressure feed, the pressure used being limited only by the pump capacity and the ability of the filter to withstand the high-pressure stress. Pressures up to 1.5 MPa (15 bar) are commonly used.

Although increasing the ΔP value in the absence of any other changes will cause a proportional increase in filtration rate, care needs to be taken to ensure that a phenomenon known as cake compression does not occur. Too high an applied pressure may cause the particles making up the cake to deform and therefore decrease the voidage (bed porosity). It can be seen from Eqn 26.2 that small decreases in the value of the poros-ity (e) lead to large decreases in cake permeability (K), and therefore in the filtration rate. The effect of decreasing K greatly outweighs any increase in filtration rate arising from a thinner cake. There is also a danger of 'blinding' the filter medium at high pressures by forcing particles into it. This is most likely in the early stages before a continuous layer of cake has formed. As a general rule, filtration should start at moderate pressure, which can be increased as filtration proceeds and the cake thickness builds up.

Decrease the filtrate viscosity The flow through a filter cake can be considered as the total flow through a large number of capillaries formed by the voids between the particles of the cake. The rate of flow through each capillary is governed by Poiseuille's Law, which is a mathematical relationship that includes viscosity as a factor contributing to the resistance to flow. To increase the filtration rate, the viscosity of the filtrate can be reduced in most cases by heating the formulation to be filtered. Many industrial filters, e.g. the metafilter, can be fitted with a steam jacket which can control temperature and hence viscosity. Care needs to be taken with this approach, however, when filtering formulations containing volatile components, or if components are thermolabile. In such cases, dilution of the formulation with water may be an alternative means of reducing the viscosity providing that the increase in filtration rate exceeds the effect of increasing the total volume to be filtered.

Decrease the thickness of filter cake Darcy's equation (Eqn 26.1) shows that the filtration rate falls off as the cake increases in thickness. This effect is commonly observed when filtering in the laboratory using filter paper in a funnel. In some cases, if the cake is allowed to build up the process slows to an unacceptable rate, or may almost stop. In these situations it may be necessary to remove the cake periodically or maintain it at a constant thickness, as occurs for example with the rotary drum filter. As previously mentioned, the cake thickness can be kept lower by using a larger filter area.

Increase the permeability of the cake One way of increasing the permeability of the cake is to include filter aids. A filter aid is a material that, when included in the formulation to be filtered, forms a cake of a more open, porous nature and thus increases the K value in Darcy's equation. In addition, it may reduce the compressibility of the cake and/or prevent the filtered material blocking the filter medium. Filter aids that are used include diatomite (a form of diatomaceous earth) and perlite (a type of volcanic glass) which has been used in the filtration of, for example, penicillin and streptomycin. The use of filter aids is obviously not appropriate if the filtered material is the intended end product.

Filtration equipment

The filtration equipment described in this chapter is that used for filtering liquids. Equipment for filtering gases (mainly air) is also available.

Equipment selection

Ideally the equipment chosen should allow a fast filtration rate to minimize production costs, be cheap to buy and run, be easily cleaned and resistant to corrosion, and be capable of filtering large volumes of product before the filter needs stripping down for cleaning or replacing.

There are a number of product-related factors that should be considered when selecting a filter for a particular process. These include:

- the chemical nature of the product. Interactions with the filter medium may lead to leaching of the filter components, degradation or swelling of the filter medium or adsorption of components of the filtered product on the filter. All of these may influence the efficiency of the filtration process or the quality of the filtered product
- the volume to be filtered and the filtration rate required. These dictate the size and type of equipment and the amount of time needed for the filtration process
- the operating pressure needed. This is important in governing the filtration rate (Eqn 26.1) and influences whether a vacuum filter (where the pressure difference is limited to approximately 100 kPa) is appropriate. High operating pressures require that the equipment be of sufficient strength and that appropriate safe operating procedures be adopted
- the amount of material to be removed. This will influence the choice of filter, as a large 'load' may necessitate the use of prefilters or may require a filter where the cake can be continuously removed
- the degree of filtration required. This will dictate the pore size of membrane filters or the filter grade to be used. If sterility is required then the equipment should itself be capable of being sterilized and care must be taken to ensure that contamination does not occur after the product has passed the filter
- the product viscosity and filtration temperature. A high product viscosity may require elevated pressures to be used. The incoming formulation can be heated or steam-heated jackets can be fitted to the equipment. Care should be taken to ensure the equipment seals, etc., can operate at elevated temperatures.

Industrial filtration equipment

Filters for liquid products may be classified by the method used to drive the filtrate through the filter medium. Filters can be organized into three classes, namely gravity, vacuum and pressure filters.

Gravity filters   Filters that rely solely on gravity generate only low operating pressures and therefore use on a large scale is limited. Gravity filters are, however, simple and cheap, and are frequently used in laboratory filtration where volumes are small and a low filtration rate is relatively unimportant.

Vacuum filters

The rotary vacuum filter   In large-scale filtration, continuous operation is often desirable and this may be difficult to achieve when it is necessary to filter slurries containing a high proportion of solids. The rotary vacuum filter is continuous in operation and has a system for removing the cake so that it can be run for long periods handling concentrated slurries. A rotary drum filter is shown in section in Figure 26.3. It can be visualized as two concentric cylinders with the annular space between them divided into a number of septa by radial partitions. The outer cylinder is perforated and covered with a filter cloth. Each septum has a radial connection to a complicated rotating valve whose function is to perform the sequence of operations listed in Table 26.1.

The cylinder rotates slowly in the slurry, which is kept agitated, and a vacuum applied to the segments draws filtrate into the septa, depositing cake on the filter cloth. When the deposited cake leaves the slurry bath, vacuum is maintained to draw air through the cake, thus aiding liquid removal. This is followed by washing and then further drainage in the drying zone. The cake is removed by the scraper blade aided by compressed air forced into the septa. It is the function of the rotary valve to direct these services into each septum when it is required.

Rotary filters can be up to 2 m in diameter and 3.5 m in length, with a filtration area of around 20 m^2. Cake compression rollers are often fitted to improve the efficiency of washing and draining if the cake on the drum becomes cracked. Difficult solids, which tend to block the filter cloth, necessitate a preliminary precoat of a thickness of filter aid to be deposited on the cloth prior to filtration of the slurry. During the actual filtration, the scraper knife is set to move slowly inwards, removing the blocked outer layer of the filter aid and exposing fresh surface.

If removal of the cake presents problems, a string discharge filter may be employed. This is useful for filtration of the fermentation liquor in the manufacture of antibiotics, when a felt-like cake of mould mycelia must be removed. The filter cloth in this case has a number of bands passing round the drum and over two additional

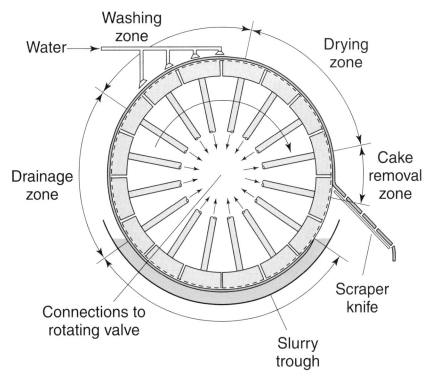

Fig. 26.3 Rotary drum filter.

Table 26.1 Rotary vacuum filter operation

Zone	Position	Service	Connected to
Pick-up	Slurry trough	Vacuum	Filtrate receiver
Drainage	–	Vacuum	Filtrate receiver
Washing	Wash sprays	Vacuum	Wash water receiver
Drying	–	Vacuum	Wash water receiver
Cake removal	Scraper knife	Compressed air	Filter cake conveyor

In some cases, for example when the solid is the required product, the same receiver may be used for filtrate and for wash water.

small rollers, as shown in Figure 26.4. In operation, the bands lift the cake off the filter medium. The cake is broken by the sharp bend over the rollers and collected, and the bands return to the drum.

The advantages of the industrial rotary vacuum filter can be summarized as follows:

- It is automatic and continuous in operation, so that labour costs are very low.
- The filter has a large capacity.
- Variation of the speed of rotation enables the cake thickness to be controlled, and for solids that form

an impenetrable cake the thickness may be limited to less than 5 mm. On the other hand, if the solids are coarse and form a porous cake, the thickness may be 100 mm or more.

Disadvantages of the rotary vacuum filter include the following:

- The rotary filter is a complex piece of equipment with many moving parts and is very expensive. In addition to the filter itself, ancillary equipment such as vacuum pumps,

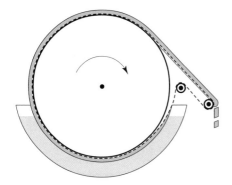

Fig. 26.4 String discharge rotary drum filter.

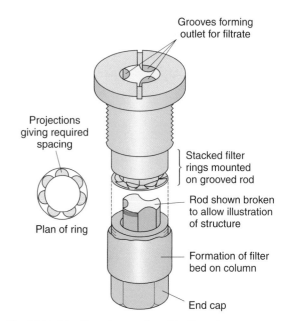

Fig. 26.5 Metafilter. Construction of the filter element.

vacuum receivers and traps, slurry pumps and agitators are required.

- The cake tends to crack because of the air drawn through by the vacuum system, so that washing and drying are not efficient.
- Being a vacuum filter, the pressure difference is limited to 100 kPa (1 bar). Yet some hot filtrates may boil due to the reduced pressure.
- The rotary filter is suitable only for straightforward slurries, being less satisfactory if the solids form an impermeable cake or will not separate cleanly from the cloth.

Small rotary vacuum filter units with a drum approximately 120 mm long and 75 mm diameter are also available (Steadfast Equipment). These are simpler in construction than the larger industrial-type units as they do not have a cake-washing facility. They have disposable filter drums and can filter batches from around 100 to 700 litres at a rate of 1–2 L/min.

The rotary filter is most suitable for continuous operation on large quantities of slurry, especially if the slurry contains considerable amounts of solids, that is, in the range 15–30%.

Examples of pharmaceutical applications include the collection of calcium carbonate, magnesium carbonate and starch, and the separation of the mycelia from the fermentation liquor in the manufacture of antibiotics.

Pressure filters   Pressure filters feed the product to the filter at a pressure greater than that which would arise from gravity alone. This is the most common type of filter used in the processing of pharmaceutical products.

The metafilter   In its simplest form, the metafilter consists of a grooved drainage rod on which is packed a series of metal rings. These rings, usually made of stainless steel, are about 15 mm inside diameter, 22 mm outside diameter and 0.8 mm in thickness, with a number of semicircular projections on one surface (Fig. 26.5). The height of the projections and the shape of the section of the ring are such that when the rings are packed together and tight-

ened on the drainage rod, channels are formed that taper from about 250 μm down to 25 μm. One or more of these packs is mounted in a vessel and the filter operated by pumping in the slurry under pressure.

In this form the metafilter can be used for separating coarse particles but for finer particles, a bed of a suitable material (such as a filter aid) is first built up over the rings by recirculating a filter aid suspension. The pack of rings, therefore, serves essentially as a base on which the true filter medium is supported.

The advantages of the metafilter can be summarized as follows:

- It possesses considerable strength and high pressures can be used with no danger of bursting the filter medium.
- As there is no filter medium as such, the running costs are low and it is very economical.
- The metafilter can be made from materials (such as stainless steel) that can provide excellent resistance to corrosion and avoid contamination of the product.
- By selecting a suitable grade of material to form the filter bed, it is possible to remove very fine particles. In fact, it is possible to sterilize a liquid using this filter.

The small surface area of the metafilter restricts the amount of solid that can be collected. This, together with the ability to separate very fine particles, means that the metafilter is used almost exclusively for clarifying liquids where the contaminant level is low. Furthermore, the strength of the metafilter permits the use of high pressures (up to 15 bar), making the method suitable for viscous liquids.

Specific examples of pharmaceutical uses include the clarification of syrups, injection solutions and intermediates such as insulin liquors.

Cartridge filters Cartridge filters are now commonly used in the preparation of pharmaceutical products, as they possess a very large filtration area in a small unit and are easy and relatively cheap to operate. In simple form, they consist of a cylindrical cartridge containing highly pleated material (e.g. PTFE or nylon) or 'string-wound' material (i.e. wound like a ball of string). This cartridge then fits in a metal supporting cylinder and the product is pumped under pressure into one end of the cylinder surrounding the filter cartridge. The filtrate is forced through the filter cartridge from the periphery to the inner hollow core, from where it exits through the other end of the support cylinder. The filter cartridges are often disposable and are good for applications where there is a low contaminant level, e.g. during the filtration of liquid products as they are filled into bottles.

Cross-flow microfiltration It is possible to form membrane filters within 'hollow fibres'. The membrane, which may consist of polysulphone, acrylonitrile or polyamide, is laid down within a fibre which forms a rigid porous outer support (Fig. 26.6). The lumen of each fibre is small, typically 1–2 μm. However, a large number of them can be contained in a surrounding shell to form a cartridge which may have an effective filtration area of over 2 m².

In use, the liquid to be treated is pumped through the cartridge in a circulatory system, so that it passes through many times. The filtrate, which in this technique is often called the 'permeate', flows radially through the membrane and porous support. The great advantage of this mode of operation is that the high fluid velocity and turbulence minimize blocking of the membranes. Fresh liquid enters the system from a reservoir as filtration proceeds. Because the fluid flow is across the surface, rather than at right angles, this technique is known as cross-flow microfiltration.

The method has been used for fractionation of biological products by first using a filter of pore size sufficient to let through all the molecules equal to or smaller in size than those required, and then passing the permeate through a second filter that will retain the required molecules while passing smaller unwanted molecules. Blood plasma can be processed to remove alcohol and water and prepare concentrated purified albumin. The process has also been used for the recovery of antibiotics from fermentation media.

CENTRIFUGATION

Centrifugal force can be used either to provide the driving force (ΔP) for the filtration process (refer to Darcy's equation above, Eqn 26.1) or to replace the gravitational force in sedimentation processes (refer to Stokes' Law, Chapter 4 and Chapter 6). Centrifuges are often used in the laboratory to separate solid material from a liquid, the solid typically forming a 'plug' at the bottom of the test tube at the end of the process.

Principles of centrifugation

If a particle (mass = m, kg) spins in a centrifuge (radius r, m) at a velocity (v, m s^{-1}) then the centrifugal force (F, N) acting on the particle equals mv^2/r. The same particle experiences gravitational force (G, N) = $m\,g$ (where g = the gravitational constant).

The centrifugal effect (C) is the ratio of these two forces, so $C = F/G$, i.e. C indicates how many times greater F is than G. Therefore, $C = v^2/g\,r$. If the rotational velocity is taken to be $\pi\,d\,n$, where n is rotation speed (s^{-1}) and d is the diameter of rotation (m), then $C = 2.01\,d\,n^2$.

In order to increase the centrifugal effect, it is therefore more efficient to increase the centrifuge speed than to use a larger diameter at the same speed. Larger centrifuges also generate greater pressures on the centrifuge wall for the same value of C, and are therefore more costly to make.

Industrial centrifuges

There are two main types of centrifuge used to achieve separation on an industrial scale: those using perforated baskets, which perform a filtration-type operation (work like a spin-dryer), and those with a solid-walled vessel, where particles sediment towards the wall under the influence of the centrifugal force.

Perforated-basket centrifuges (centrifugal filters)

A diagram of a perforated-basket centrifuge is shown in Figure 26.7. It consists of a stainless steel perforated

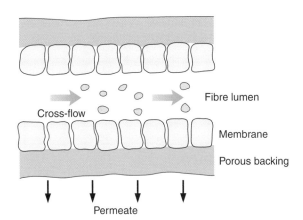

Cross-flow

Fibre lumen

Membrane

Porous backing

Permeate

Fig. 26.6 Cross-flow microfiltration through an individual fibre.

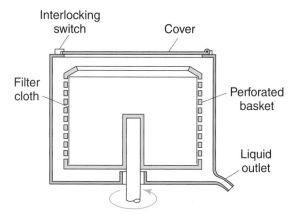

Fig. 26.7 Centrifugal dewatering filter.

basket (typically 1–2 m in diameter) lined with a filter cloth. The basket rotates at a speed which is typically < 25 s^{-1}, higher speeds tending to stress the basket excessively. The product enters centrally and is thrown outwards by centrifugal force and held against the filter cloth. The filtrate is forced through the cloth and removed via the liquid outlet; the solid material is retained on the cloth. The cake can be washed if required by spraying water into the centrifuge.

The centrifugal filter has been used for separating crystalline materials from the preparation liquor, e.g. in the preparation of drug crystals, and for removing precipitated proteins from, for example, insulin. It has the advantages of being compact and efficient, a 1 m diameter centrifuge being able to process about 200 kg in 10 minutes. It can also handle concentrated slurries which might block other filters. The spinning action gives a product with a low moisture content (typically around 2% w/w) which saves energy during subsequent drying.

The centrifuge described above is operated batchwise but continuous centrifuges are available for large-scale work. These have means for automatic discharge of the cake from a basket, which rotates around a horizontal axis in contrast to the vertical axis. Most of the energy required to run a centrifuge is used to bring it up to operating speed and little more is needed to maintain that speed. Continuous centrifuges are therefore cheaper to run but the initial cost is considerably more.

Tubular-bowl centrifuges (centrifugal sedimenters)

These consist of a cylindrical 'bowl', typically around 100 mm in diameter and 1 m long, that rotates at a high speed, 300–1000 s^{-1}. The product enters at the bottom and centrifugal force causes solids to be deposited on the wall as it passes up the bowl, the clear liquid overflowing from the top (Fig. 26.8). This type of centrifuge can also be

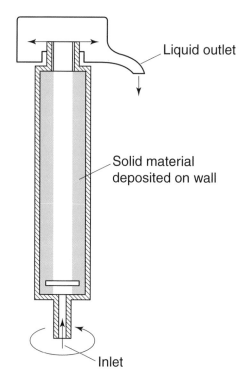

Fig. 26.8 Tubular-bowl centrifuge.

adapted to separate immiscible liquids. The inlet rate needs to be controlled so that there is sufficient time for sedimentation to occur before the product leaves the bowl.

The uses of centrifugal sedimenters include:

- liquid/liquid separation, e.g. during antibiotic manufacture and purification of oils from natural source
- the removal of very small particles
- the removal of solids that are compressible or 'slimy' and which easily block the filter medium
- the separation of blood plasma from whole blood (a C of approximately 3000 is required)
- the separation of different particle size fractions, and
- examining the stability of emulsions.

These centrifuges are compact, have a high separating efficiency and are good for separating 'difficult' solids. However, they have a limited capacity and are complicated to construct in order to achieve the required speed and minimize vibration.

BIBLIOGRAPHY

Meltser, T.H. (1987) *Filtration in the Pharmaceutical Industry.* Marcel Dekker, New York.
Rushdon, A. (2000) *Solid-liquid Filtration and Separation Technology.* Wiley, New York.

27

Suspensions and emulsions

M. R. Billany

INTRODUCTION

A coarse suspension is a dispersion of finely divided, insoluble solid particles (the disperse phase) in a fluid (the dispersion medium or continuous phase). Most pharmaceutical suspensions consist of an aqueous dispersion medium, although in a few instances it may be an organic or oily liquid. A disperse phase with a mean particle diameter of up to 1 μm is usually termed a colloidal dispersion and includes such examples as aluminium hydroxide and magnesium hydroxide suspensions. A solid in liquid dispersion, in which the particles are above colloidal size, is termed a coarse suspension.

An emulsion may be defined as two immiscible liquids, one of which is finely subdivided and uniformly distributed as droplets throughout the other. The system is stabilized by the presence of an emulsifying agent. The dispersed liquid or internal phase usually consists of globules of diameters down to 0.1 μm which are distributed within the external or continuous phase.

The physical properties of both colloidal and coarse suspensions and of emulsions are discussed in Chapter 6.

PHYSICAL PROPERTIES OF WELL-FORMULATED SUSPENSIONS AND EMULSIONS

The product must remain sufficiently homogeneous for at least the period between shaking the container and removing the required amount.

The sediment or creaming produced on storage, if any, must be easily resuspended by moderate agitation of the container.

The product may need to be thickened in order to reduce the settling rate of the particles or the creaming rate of oil globules. The resulting viscosity must not be so high that removal of the product from the container and transfer to the site of application are difficult.

Any suspended particles should be small and uniformly sized in order to give a smooth, elegant product, free from a gritty texture.

PHARMACEUTICAL APPLICATIONS OF SUSPENSIONS

Suspensions can be used as oral dosage forms, applied topically to the skin, eye or mucous membrane surfaces, or given parenterally by injection.

Suspensions as oral drug delivery systems

Many people have difficulty in swallowing solid dosage forms and therefore require the drug to be dispersed in a liquid.

Some materials are required to be present in the gastrointestinal tract in a finely divided form, and their formulation as suspensions will provide the desired high surface area. Solids such as kaolin, magnesium carbonate and magnesium trisilicate, for example, are used for the adsorption of toxins or to neutralize excess acidity. A dispersion of finely divided silica in dimethicone 1000 is used in veterinary practice for the treatment of 'frothy bloat'.

The taste of most drugs is more noticeable if it is in solution rather than in an insoluble form. Paracetamol is available both in solution as paediatric paracetamol oral solution and also as a suspension. The latter is more palatable and therefore particularly suitable for children. For the same reason, chloramphenicol mixtures can be formulated as suspensions containing the insoluble chloramphenicol palmitate.

Suspensions for topical administration

Suspensions of drugs can also be formulated for topical application (see Chapter 38). They can be fluid preparations, such as calamine lotion, which are designed to leave a light deposit of the active agent on the skin after quick evaporation of the dispersion medium. Some suspensions, such as pastes, are semi-solid in consistency and contain high concentrations of powders dispersed, usually, in a paraffin base. It may also be possible to suspend a powdered drug in an emulsion base, as in zinc cream.

Suspensions for parenteral use and inhalation therapy

Suspensions can also be formulated for parenteral administration in order to control the rate of absorption of the drug. By varying the size of the dispersed particles of active agent, the duration of activity can be controlled. The absorption rate of the drug into the blood stream will then depend simply on its rate of dissolution. If the drug is suspended in a fixed oil such as arachis or sesame, the product will remain after injection in the form of an oil globule, thereby presenting to the tissue fluid a minimal surface area from which the partitioning of drug can occur. The release of drug suspended in an aqueous vehicle will be faster, as some diffusion of the product will occur along muscle fibres and become miscible with tissue fluid. This will present a larger surface area from which the drug can be released.

Vaccines for the induction of immunity are often formulated as dispersions of killed microorganisms, as in cholera vaccine, the injectable version of which is now being replaced in many countries by orally delivered suspensions. Alternatively, the constituent toxoids can be adsorbed on to a substrate of aluminium hydroxide or phosphate, as in adsorbed diphtheria and tetanus vaccine. Thus a prolonged antigenic stimulus is provided, resulting in a high antibody titre.

Some X-ray contrast media are also formulated in this way. Barium sulfate, for the examination of the alimentary tract, is available as a suspension for either oral or rectal administration, and propyliodone is dispersed in either water or arachis oil for examination of the bronchial tract.

The adsorptive properties of fine powders are also used in the formulation of some inhalations. The volatile components of menthol and eucalyptus oil would be lost from solution very rapidly during use, whereas a more prolonged release is obtained if the two active agents are adsorbed on to light magnesium carbonate prior to the preparation of a suspension.

Chapter 36 describes some aspects of the formulation of aerosols, many of which are also available as suspensions of the active agent in a mixture of propellants.

Solubility and stability considerations

If the drug is insoluble or poorly soluble in a suitable solvent, then formulation as a suspension is usually required. Some eye drops, notably hydrocortisone acetate and neomycin eye drops, are formulated as suspensions because of the poor solubility of hydrocortisone in a suitable solvent.

The degradation of a drug in the presence of water may also preclude its use as an aqueous solution. In this case it may be possible to synthesize an insoluble derivative that can then be formulated as a suspension.

Prolonged contact between the solid drug particles and the dispersion medium can be considerably reduced by preparing the suspension immediately prior to issue to the patient. Amoxicillin, for example, is provided by the manufacturer as the trihydrate salt mixed with the other powdered or granulated ingredients. The pharmacist then makes the product up to volume with water immediately before issue to the patient, allocating a shelf life of either 7 or 14 days at a temperature below 25°C.

FORMULATION OF SUSPENSIONS

Particle size control

It is first necessary to ensure that the drug to be suspended is of a fine particle size prior to formulation. This is to ensure a slow rate of sedimentation of the suspended particles. Large particles, if greater than about 5 μm diameter, will also impart a gritty texture to the product and may cause irritation if injected or instilled into the eyes. The ease of administration of a parenteral suspension may depend upon particle size and shape, and it is quite possible to block a hypodermic needle with particles over about 25 μm diameter, particularly if they are acicular in shape rather than isodiametric. A particular particle size range may also be chosen in order to control the rate of dissolution of the drug and hence its bioavailability.

Even though the particle size of a drug may be small when the suspension is first manufactured, there is always a degree of crystal growth that occurs on storage, particularly if temperature fluctuations occur. This is because the solubility of the drug may increase as the temperature rises but on cooling, the drug will crystallize out. This is a particular problem with slightly soluble drugs such as paracetamol.

If the drug is polydispersed, then the very small crystals of less than 1 micrometre diameter will exhibit a greater solubility than the larger ones. Over a period of time the small crystals will become even smaller, whereas the diameters of the larger particles will increase. It is therefore advantageous to use a suspended drug of a narrow size range. The inclusion of surface-active agents or polymeric colloids, which adsorb on to the surface of each particle, may also help to prevent crystal growth.

Different polymorphic forms of a drug may exhibit different solubilities, the metastable state being the most soluble. Conversion of the metastable form, in solution, to the less soluble stable state, and its subsequent precipitation, will lead to changes in particle size.

Use of wetting agents

Some insoluble solids may be easily wetted by water and will disperse readily throughout the aqueous phase with only minimal agitation. Most, however, will exhibit varying degrees of hydrophobicity and will not be easily wetted. Some particles will form large porous clumps within the liquid, whereas others remain on the surface and become attached to the upper part of the container. The foam produced on shaking will be slow to subside because of the stabilizing effect of the small particles at the liquid/air interface.

To ensure adequate wetting, the interfacial tension between the solid and the liquid must be reduced so that the adsorbed air can be displaced from the solid surfaces by the liquid. The particles will then disperse readily throughout the liquid, particularly if an intense shearing action is used during mixing. If a series of suspensions is prepared, each containing one of a range of concentrations of wetting agent, then the concentration to choose will be the lowest that provides adequate wetting.

The following are the most widely used wetting agents for pharmaceutical products.

Surface-active agents

Figure 6.16 shows that surfactants possessing an HLB value between about 7 and 9 are suitable for use as wetting agents. The hydrocarbon chains would be adsorbed by the hydrophobic particle surfaces, whereas the polar groups project into the aqueous medium and become hydrated. Wetting of the solid occurs as a result of a fall in interfacial tension between both the solid and the liquid and, to a lesser extent, between the liquid and air.

Most surfactants are used at concentrations of up to about 0.1% as wetting agents and include, for oral use, the polysorbates (Tweens) and sorbitan esters (Spans).

For external application, sodium lauryl sulfate and sodium dioctylsulfosuccinate can also be used.

The choice of surfactant for parenteral administration is obviously more limited, the main ones used being the polysorbates, some of the poloxamers (polyoxyethylene/polyoxypropylene copolymers) and lecithin.

Disadvantages in the use of this type of wetting agent include excessive foaming and the possible formation of a deflocculated system, which may not be required.

Hydrophilic colloids

These materials include acacia, bentonite, tragacanth, alginates, xanthan gum and cellulose derivatives. They will behave as protective colloids by coating the solid hydrophobic particles with a multimolecular layer. This will impart a hydrophilic character to the solid and so promote wetting. These materials are also used as suspending agents and may, like surfactants, produce a deflocculated system, particularly if used at low concentrations.

Solvents

Materials such as alcohol, glycerol and glycols, which are water miscible, will reduce the liquid/air interfacial tension. The solvent will penetrate the loose agglomerates of powder, displacing the air from the pores of the individual particles, so enabling wetting to occur by the dispersion medium.

Flocculated and deflocculated systems

Having incorporated a suitable wetting agent, it is then necessary to determine whether the suspension is flocculated or deflocculated and to decide which state is preferable. Whether or not a suspension is flocculated or deflocculated depends on the relative magnitudes of the forces of repulsion and attraction between the particles. The effects of these particle–particle interactions have been adequately covered in Chapter 6.

In a deflocculated system, the dispersed particles remain as discrete units and, because the rate of sedimentation depends on the size of each unit, settling will be slow. The supernatant of a deflocculated system will continue to remain cloudy for an appreciable time after shaking, due to the very slow settling rate of the smallest particles in the product, even after the larger ones have sedimented. The repulsive forces between individual particles allow them to slip past each other as they sediment. The slow rate of settling prevents the entrapment of liquid within the sediment, which thus becomes compacted and can be very difficult to redisperse. This phenomenon is also called caking or claying and is the most serious of all the physical stability problems encountered in suspension formulation.

The aggregation of particles in a flocculated system will lead to a much more rapid rate of sedimentation or subsidence because each unit is composed of many individual particles and is therefore larger. The rate of settling will also depend on the porosity of the aggregate, because if it is porous the dispersion medium can flow through, as well as around, each aggregate or floccule as it sediments.

The nature of the sediment of a flocculated system is also quite different from that of a deflocculated one. The structure of each aggregate is retained after sedimentation, thus entrapping a large amount of the liquid phase. As explained in Chapter 6, aggregation in the primary minimum will produce compact floccules, whereas a secondary minimum effect will produce loose floccules of higher porosity. Whichever occurs, the volume of the final sediment will still be large and will easily be redispersed by moderate agitation.

In a flocculated system the supernatant quickly becomes clear, as the large flocs that settle rapidly are composed of particles of all sizes. Figure 27.1 illustrates the appearance of both flocculated and deflocculated suspensions at given times after shaking.

In summary, deflocculated systems have the advantage of a slow sedimentation rate, thereby enabling a uniform dose to be taken from the container, but when settling does occur, the sediment is compacted and difficult to redisperse. Flocculated systems form loose sediments which are easily redispersible but the sedimentation rate is fast and there is a danger of an inaccurate dose being administered; also, the product will look inelegant.

Controlled flocculation

A deflocculated system with a sufficiently high viscosity to prevent sedimentation would be an ideal formulation. It cannot be guaranteed, however, that the system would remain completely homogeneous during the entire shelf life of the product. Usually a compromise is reached in which the suspension is partially flocculated to enable easy redispersion, should it be necessary, and viscosity is controlled so that sedimentation rate is at a minimum.

So the next stage of the formulation process, after the addition of the wetting agent, is to ensure that the product exhibits the correct degree of flocculation. Underflocculation will give those undesirable properties that are associated with deflocculated systems. An overflocculated product will look inelegant and, to minimize settling, the viscosity of the product may have to be so high that any necessary redispersion would be difficult.

Controlled flocculation is usually achieved by a combination of particle size control, the use of electrolytes to

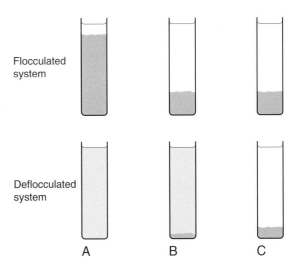

Fig. 27.1 The sedimentation behaviour of flocculated and deflocculated suspensions. Within a few minutes of manufacture (a), there is no apparent change within the deflocculated system compared to its initial appearance. Even after several hours (b), there is still little obvious change, except that the concentration of solids in the lower layers has increased at the expense of the upper layers owing to slow particle sedimentation. There is a small amount of compact sediment. After prolonged storage (c), depending on the physical stability of the system, the supernatant has cleared, leaving a compact sediment. In the flocculated system at (a) there is some clear supernatant with a distinct boundary between it and the sediment. At (b) there is a larger volume of clear supernatant with a relatively large volume of a porous sediment, which does not change further even after prolonged storage (c).

control zeta potential and the addition of polymers to enable crosslinking to occur between particles. Some polymers have the advantage of becoming ionized in an aqueous solution and can therefore act both electrostatically and sterically. These materials are also termed polyelectrolytes.

Flocculating agents

In many cases, after the incorporation of a non-ionic wetting agent a suspension will be found to be deflocculated, either because of the reduction in solid/liquid interfacial tension or because of the hydrated hydrophilic layer around each particle forming a mechanical barrier to aggregation. The use of an ionic surfactant to wet the solid could produce either a flocculated or a deflocculated system, depending on any charge already present on the particles. If particles are of opposite charge to that of the surfactant then neutralization will occur. If a high charge density is imparted to the suspended particles then deflocculation will be the result.

If it is necessary for the suspension to be converted from a deflocculated to a partially flocculated state, this may be achieved by the addition of electrolytes, surfactants and/or hydrophilic polymers.

Electrolytes The addition of an inorganic electrolyte to an aqueous suspension will alter the zeta potential of the dispersed particles and if this value is lowered sufficiently, flocculation may occur.

The Schultz–Hardy rule shows that the ability of an electrolyte to flocculate hydrophobic particles depends on the valency of its counter-ions. Although they are more efficient, trivalent ions are less widely used than mono- or divalent electrolytes because they are generally more toxic. If hydrophilic polymers, which are usually negatively charged, are included in the formulation they may be precipitated by the presence of trivalent ions.

The most widely used electrolytes include the sodium salts of acetates, phosphates and citrates. The concentration chosen will be that which produces the desired degree of flocculation. Care must be taken not to add excessive electrolyte or charge reversal may occur on each particle, so forming, once again, a deflocculated system.

Surfactants Ionic surface-active agents may also cause flocculation by neutralizing the charge on each particle, thus resulting in a deflocculated system. Non-ionic surfactants will, of course, have a negligible effect on the charge density of a particle but may, because of their linear configurations, adsorb onto more than one particle, thereby forming a loose flocculated structure.

Polymeric flocculating agents Starch, alginates, cellulose derivatives, tragacanth, carbomers and silicates are examples of polymers that can be used to control flocculation. Their linear branched-chain molecules form a gel-like network within the system and become adsorbed on to the surfaces of the dispersed particles, thus holding them in a flocculated state. Although some settling can occur, the sedimentation volume is large, and usually remains so for a considerable period.

Care must be taken to ensure that, during manufacture, blending is not excessive as this may inhibit the crosslinking between adjacent particles and result in the adsorption of each molecule of polymer on to one particle only. If this should occur then a deflocculated system may result because the formation of the hydrophilic barrier around each particle will inhibit aggregation. A high concentration of polymer may have a similar effect if the whole surface of each particle is coated. It is essential that areas on each suspended particle remain free from adsorbate, so that crosslinking can recur after the product is sheared. Further details of the use of polymers can be found in the next section.

RHEOLOGY OF SUSPENSIONS

An ideal pharmaceutical suspension would exhibit a high apparent viscosity at low rates of shear so that, on storage, the suspended particles would either settle only very slowly or, preferably, remain permanently suspended. At higher rates of shear, such as those caused by moderate shaking of the product, the apparent viscosity should fall sufficiently for the product to be poured easily from its container. The product, if for external use, will then spread easily without excessive dragging, but must not be so fluid that it runs off the skin surface. If intended for injection the product should pass easily through a hypodermic needle with only moderate pressure applied to the syringe plunger. It would then be important for the initial high apparent viscosity to be reformed after a short time to maintain adequate physical stability.

A flocculated system partially fulfils these criteria. In such a system pseudoplastic or plastic behaviour (see Chapter 4) is exhibited as the structure progressively breaks down under shear. The product then shows the time-dependent reversibility of this loss of structure, which is termed thixotropy.

A deflocculated system, however, would exhibit newtonian behaviour owing to the absence of such structures and may even, if high concentrations of disperse phase are present, exhibit dilatancy.

Although a flocculated system may exhibit some thixotropy and plasticity, unless a high concentration of disperse phase is present it may not be sufficient to prevent rapid settling, particularly if a surfactant or an electrolyte is present as a flocculating agent. In these cases suspending agents may be used to increase the apparent viscosity of the system.

Suitable materials are the hydrophilic polymers discussed above. These exert their effect by entrapping the solid dispersed particles within their gel-like network, so preventing sedimentation. At low concentrations, many suspending agents can be used to control flocculation and it must be realized that if large quantities are to be used to enhance viscosity, the degree of flocculation may also be altered.

VISCOSITY MODIFIERS

The following materials are those most widely used for the modification of suspension viscosity.

Polysaccharides

Acacia

This natural material is often used as a suspending agent for extemporaneously prepared suspensions. Acacia is not a good thickening agent and its value as a suspending agent is largely due to its action as a protective colloid. It is therefore useful for preparations containing tinctures of resinous materials that precipitate on addition to water. It is essential to ensure that any precipitated resin is well coated by the protective colloid before any electrolyte (which should be well diluted) is added. Acacia is not very effective for dense powders and for these it is often combined with other thickeners such as tragacanth, starch and sucrose in compound tragacanth powder.

Because of the stickiness of acacia it is rarely used in preparations for external use.

Tragacanth

This product will form viscous aqueous solutions. Its thixotropic and pseudoplastic properties make it a better thickening agent than acacia and it can be used for both internal and external products. Like acacia, it is mainly, though not exclusively, used for the extemporaneous preparation of suspensions with a short shelf life.

Tragacanth is stable over a pH range of 4–7.5 but takes several days to hydrate fully after dispersion in water. The maximum viscosity of its dispersions is not achieved, therefore, until after this time and can also be affected by heating. There are several grades of this material and only the best quality is suitable for use as a pharmaceutical suspending agent.

Alginates

Alginic acid, a polymer of D-mannuronic acid, is prepared from kelp. Its salts have suspending properties similar to those of tragacanth. Alginate mucilages must not be heated above 60°C as depolymerization occurs with a consequent loss in viscosity. They are most viscous immediately after preparation, after which there is a fall to a fairly constant value after about 24 hours. Alginates exhibit a maximum viscosity over a pH range of 5–9 and at low pH the acid is precipitated. Sodium alginate (Manucol) is the most widely used material in this class but it is, of course, anionic and will be incompatible with cationic materials and with heavy metals. The addition of calcium chloride to a sodium alginate dispersion will produce calcium alginate, which has a much higher viscosity. Several different viscosity grades are commercially available.

Starch

Starch is rarely used on its own as a suspending agent but is one of the constituents of compound tragacanth powder, and it can also be used with carmellose sodium.

Xanthan gum (Keltrol)

This is an anionic heteropolysaccharide produced by the action of *Xanthomonas campestris* on corn sugars. It is very soluble in cold water and is one of the most widely used thickening agents for the extemporaneous preparation of suspensions for oral use. It is used in concentrations up to about 2% and is stable over a wide pH range.

Water-soluble celluloses

Several cellulose derivatives are available that will disperse in water to produce viscous colloidal solutions suitable for use as suspending agents.

Methylcellulose (Celacol, Methocel)

This is a semi-synthetic polysaccharide of the general formula:

$$[C_6H_7O_2(OH_2)OCH_3]_n$$

Several grades are available, depending on their degree of methylation and on the chain length. The longer the chain, the more viscous is its solution. For example, a 2% solution of methylcellulose 20 exhibits an apparent viscosity of 20 millipascal seconds (mPas) and methylcellulose 4500 has value of 4500 mPas at 2% concentration. Because these products are more soluble in cold water than in hot, they are often dispersed in warm water and then, on cooling with constant stirring, a clear or opalescent viscous solution is produced. Methylcelluloses are non-ionic and therefore stable over a wide pH range and are compatible with many ionic additives.

Hydroxyethylcellulose (Natrosol)

This compound has hydroxyethyl instead of methyl groups attached to the cellulose chain and is also available in different viscosity grades. It has the advantage of being soluble in both hot and cold water and will not gel on heating. Otherwise it exhibits the same properties as methylcellulose.

Carmellose sodium (sodium carboxymethylcellulose)

The chemical structure of this material can be

represented by:

$$[C_6H_{10-x}O_5(CH_2COONa)_x]_n$$

where x represents the degree of substitution, usually about 0.7, which in turn affects its solubility. The viscosity of its solution depends on the value of n, which represents the degree of polymerization. The numerical suffix of a commercial product gives an indication of the viscosity of a 2% solution. For example, sodium carboxymethylcellulose 50 at a concentration of 2% will have a viscosity of 50 mPa s. It is widely used at concentrations of up to 1% in products for oral, parenteral or external use.

Microcrystalline cellulose (Avicel)

This material is partially hydrolysed cellulose and contains crystals of colloidal dimensions which disperse readily in water (but are not soluble) to produce thixotropic gels. It is a widely used suspending agent and the rheological properties of its dispersions can often be improved by the incorporation of additional hydrocolloid, in particular carboxymethylcellulose, methylcellulose or hydroxypropyl methylcellulose. These will aid dispersion and also stabilize the product against the flocculating effects of added electrolyte.

Hydrated silicates

There are three important materials within this classification, namely bentonite, magnesium aluminium silicate and hectorite. They belong to a group called the montmorillonite clays. They hydrate readily, absorbing up to 12 times their weight of water, particularly at elevated temperatures. As with most naturally occurring materials, they may be contaminated with spores and this must be borne in mind when considering a sterilization process and choosing a preservative system.

Bentonite

This has the general formula:

$$Al_2O_3.4SiO_2.H_2O$$

It is used at concentrations of up to 2–3% in preparations for external use, such as calamine lotion.

Magnesium aluminium silicate (Veegum)

Also known as attapulgite, this material disperses and swells readily in water by absorbing the aqueous phase into its crystal lattice. Several grades are available, differing in their particle size, their acid demand and the vis-

cosity of their dispersions. They can be used both internally and externally at concentrations of up to about 5% and are stable over a pH range of 3.5–11. Veegum/ water dispersions will exhibit thixotropy and plasticity with a high yield value but the presence of salts can alter these rheological properties because of the flocculating effect of their positively charged counter-ions. Some grades, however, have a higher resistance to flocculation than others.

This material is often combined with organic thickening agents such as sodium carboxymethylcellulose or xanthan gum to improve yield values and degree of thixotropy and to control flocculation (Ciullo 1981).

Hectorite

This material is similar to bentonite and can be used at concentrations of 1–2% for external use. It is also possible to obtain synthetic hectorites (Laponite) that do not exhibit the batch variability or level of microbial contamination associated with natural products and which can also be used internally.

As with other clays, it is often advantageous to include an organic gum to modify its rheological properties.

Carbomers (carboxypolymethylene)

This material is a totally synthetic copolymer of acrylic acid and allyl sucrose. It is used at concentrations of up to 0.5%, mainly for external application, although some grades can be taken internally. When dispersed in water it forms acidic, low-viscosity solutions which, when adjusted to a pH of between 6 and 11, become highly viscous.

Colloidal silicon dioxide (Aerosil)

When dispersed in water, this finely divided product will aggregate, forming a three-dimensional network. It can be used at concentrations of up to 4% for external use but has also been used for thickening non-aqueous suspensions.

TYPES OF EMULSION

Pharmaceutical emulsions usually consist of a mixture of an aqueous phase with various oils and/or waxes. If the oil droplets are dispersed throughout the aqueous phase, the emulsion is termed oil-in-water (o/w). A system in which the water is dispersed throughout the oil is a water-in-oil (w/o) emulsion. It is also possible to form multiple emulsions. For example, many small water droplets can be enclosed within larger oil droplets, which are themselves then dispersed in water. This gives a water-in-oil-in-water (w/o/w) emulsion. The alternative o/w/o emulsion is also possible.

If the dispersed globules are of colloidal dimensions (1 nm to 1 μm diameter) the preparation, which is quite often transparent or translucent, is called a microemulsion. This type has similar properties to a micellar system and will therefore exhibit the properties of hydrophobic colloids. As the size of the dispersed droplets increases, more of the characteristics of coarse dispersions will be exhibited (see Chapter 6).

Tests for identification of emulsion type

Several simple methods are available for distinguishing between o/w and w/o emulsions (Table 27.1). The most common of these involve:

- miscibility tests with oil or water – the emulsion will only be miscible with liquids that are miscible with its continuous phase
- conductivity measurements – systems with aqueous continuous phases will readily conduct electricity, whereas systems with oily continuous phases will not
- staining tests – either a water-soluble or an oil-soluble dye is blended with the emulsion. Microscopic examination will show whether the continuous phase or the dispersed droplets are coloured.

FORMULATION OF EMULSIONS

Because of the very wide range of emulsifying agents available, considerable experience is required to choose the best emulgent system for a particular product. The final choice will depend to a large extent on the properties

and use of the final product and the other materials required to be present.

Choice of emulsion type

The decision as to whether an o/w or a w/o emulsion is to be formulated will eliminate many unsuitable emulsifying systems.

Fats or oils for oral administration, either as medicaments in their own right or as vehicles for oil-soluble drugs, are invariably formulated as oil-in-water emulsions. In this form they are pleasant to take and the inclusion of a suitable flavour in the aqueous phase will mask any unpleasant taste.

Emulsions for intravenous administration must also be of the o/w type, although intramuscular injections can also be formulated as w/o products if a water-soluble drug is required for depot therapy.

Emulsions are most widely used for external application. Semi-solid emulsions are termed creams and more fluid preparations are called either lotions or, if intended for massage into the skin, liniments. Both o/w and w/o types are available.

Oil-in-water emulsions are used for the topical application of water-soluble drugs, mainly for local effect. They do not have the greasy texture associated with oily bases and are therefore pleasant to use and easily washed from skin surfaces.

Water-in-oil emulsions will have an occlusive effect by inhibiting the evaporation of eccrine secretions. This will hydrate the upper layers of the stratum corneum and so is particularly useful for dry skin conditions. This, in turn, may influence the absorption rates of drugs from these preparations. This type of emulsion is also useful for cleansing the skin of oil-soluble dirt, although

Table 27.1 Tests for identification of emulsion type

Oil-in-water emulsions	Water-in-oil emulsions
Miscibility tests Are miscible with water but immiscible with oil	Are miscible with oil but not with water

Staining tests by incorporation of an oil-soluble dye
Macroscopic examination
  Paler colour than a w/o emulsion
Microscopic examination
  Coloured globules on a colourless background
	
	More intense colouration than with an o/w emulsion
	
	Colourless globules against a coloured background

Conductivity tests Water, being the continous phase, will conduct electricity throughout the system. Two electrodes, when placed in such a preparation with a battery and suitable light source connected in series, will cause the lamp to glow	A preparation in which oil is the continuous phase will not conduct electricity. The lamp will not glow, or will only flicker spasmodically

its greasy texture is not always cosmetically acceptable. Oil-in-water emulsions are less efficient as cleansers but are usually more acceptable to the consumer, particularly for use on the hands. Similarly, moisturizing creams, designed to prevent moisture loss from the skin and thus inhibit drying of the stratum corneum, are more efficient if formulated as w/o emulsions, which produce a coherent, water-repellent film.

Choice of oil phase

In many instances the oil phase of an emulsion is the active agent and therefore its concentration in the product is predetermined. Liquid paraffin, castor oil, cod liver oil and arachis oil are all examples of medicaments which are formulated as emulsions for oral administration. Cottonseed oil, soya bean oil and safflower oil are used for their high calorific value in emulsions for intravenous feeding. Examples of externally applied oils that are formulated as emulsions include turpentine oil and benzyl benzoate.

Many emulsions for external use contain oils that are present as carriers for the active agent. It must be realized that the type of oil used may also have an effect on both the viscosity of the product and the transport of the drug into the skin (see Chapter 38). One of the most widely used oils for this type of preparation is liquid paraffin. This is one of a series of hydrocarbons that also includes hard paraffin, soft paraffin and light liquid paraffin. They can be used individually or in combination with each other to control emulsion consistency. This will ensure that the product can be spread easily but will be sufficiently viscous to form a coherent film over the skin. The film-forming capabilities of the emulsion can be further modified by the inclusion of various waxes, such as beeswax, carnauba wax or higher fatty alcohols. Continuous films can therefore be formed that are sufficiently tough and flexible to prevent contact between the skin and aqueous-based irritants. These preparations are called barrier creams and many are of the w/o variety. The inclusion of silicone oils, such as dimethicone at 10–20%, which have exceptional water-repellent properties, may also permit the formulation of o/w products that are equally effective.

A variety of fixed oils of vegetable origin is also available, the most widely used being arachis, sesame, cottonseed and maize. Those expressed from seeds or fruits are often protein rich and contain useful vitamins and minerals. They are often, therefore, formulated for oral administration as emulsions. Because of their lack of toxicity, they can be used both internally and externally as vehicles for other materials.

Emulsion consistency

The texture or 'feel' of a product intended for external use must also be considered. A w/o preparation will have a greasy texture and often exhibits a higher apparent viscosity than o/w emulsions. This fact is often used to convey a feeling of richness to many cosmetic formulations. Oil-in-water emulsions will, however, feel less greasy or sticky on application to the skin, will be absorbed more readily because of their lower oil content and can be more easily washed from the skin surface.

Ideally emulsions should exhibit the rheological properties of plasticity/pseudoplasticity and thixotropy (see Chapter 4). A high apparent viscosity at the very low rates of shear caused by movement of disperse-phase globules is necessary in order to retard this movement and maintain a physically stable emulsion. It is important, however, that these products should flow freely when shaken, poured from the container or injected through a hypodermic needle. Therefore, at these high rates of shear, a much lower apparent viscosity is required. This change in apparent viscosity must be reversible after a suitable time delay so as to retard creaming and coalescence.

For an externally applied product, a wide range of emulsion consistencies can be tolerated. Low-viscosity lotions and liniments can be formulated that are dispensed from a flexible plastic container via a nozzle. Only light shearing is then required to spread this type of product over the skin surface. This is particularly advantageous for painful or inflamed skin conditions.

The main disadvantage with low-viscosity emulsions is their tendency to cream easily, especially if formulated with a low oil concentration. It is rarely possible to formulate low-viscosity w/o products because of the consistency of the oil phase.

Emulsions of high apparent viscosity for external use are termed creams and are of a semi-solid consistency. They are usually packed into collapsible plastic or aluminium tubes, although large volumes or very high-viscosity products are often packed into glass or plastic jars.

It is important not to ignore the patient/consumer acceptability of topically applied preparations, particularly in a competitive market.

There are several methods by which the rheological properties of an emulsion can be controlled.

Volume concentration of the disperse phase

A qualitative application of the Einstein equation to the behaviour of emulsions shows that the viscosity of the product as a whole would be higher than the viscosity of the continuous phase on its own. So, as the concentration of disperse phase increases, so does the apparent viscosity of the product.

Care must be taken to ensure that the disperse-phase concentration does not increase above about 60% of the total, as phase inversion may occur.

Particle size of the disperse phase

It is possible, under certain conditions, to increase the apparent viscosity of an emulsion by a reduction in mean globule diameter. This can be achieved by homogenization. There are two postulated mechanisms for this occurrence:

1. A smaller mean globule size can cause increased flocculation. In a flocculated system a significant part of the continuous phase is trapped within aggregates of droplets, thus effectively increasing the apparent disperse-phase concentration. Emulsions consisting of polydispersed droplets will tend to exhibit a lower viscosity than a monodispersed system, due to differences in electrical double-layer size and thus in the energy of interaction curves. These variations in interaction between globules during shear may be reflected in their flow behaviour.
2. If a hydrophilic colloid is used to stabilize the emulsion it will form a multimolecular film round the dispersed globules. A reduction in mean globule size will increase the total surface area and therefore more colloid will be adsorbed onto the droplet surface. This will effectively increase the volume concentration of the dispersed phase.

The particle size of the disperse phase is therefore controlled mainly by the method and conditions of manufacture of the emulsion, and by the type of emulgent used and its concentration.

Viscosity of the continuous phase

It has been well documented that a direct relationship exists between the viscosity of an emulsion and the viscosity of its continuous phase. Syrup and glycerol, which are used in oral emulsions as sweetening agents, will increase the viscosity of the continuous phase. Their main disadvantage is in increasing the density difference between the two phases and thus possibly accelerating creaming.

Hydrocolloids, when used as emulsifying agents in o/w emulsions, will stabilize them not only by the formation of multimolecular layers around the dispersed globules but also by increasing the continuous-phase viscosity. They do not have the disadvantage of altering the density of this phase. If oil is the continuous phase, then the inclusion of soft or hard paraffin or certain waxes will increase its viscosity.

Nature and concentration of the emulsifying system

It has already been shown that hydrophilic colloids, as well as forming multimolecular films at the oil/water interface, will also increase the viscosity of the continuous phase of an o/w emulsion. Obviously, as the concentration of this type of emulgent increases so will the viscosity of the product.

Surface-active agents forming condensed monomolecular films will, by the nature of their chemical structure, influence the degree of flocculation in a similar way, by forming linkages between adjacent globules and creating a gel-like structure. A flocculated system will exhibit a greater apparent viscosity than its deflocculated counterpart and will depend on surfactant concentration.

Choice of emulsifying agent

Toxicity and irritancy considerations

The choice of emulgent to be used will depend not only on its emulsifying ability but also on its route of administration and, consequently, on its toxicity. Although there is no approved list of emulsifying agents for use in pharmaceutical products, there is an approved list of emulsifiers as food additives for use in the European Union. It can be assumed that emulsifiers contained in this list would be suitable for internally used pharmaceutical emulsions. The regulations mainly include naturally occurring materials and their semi-synthetic derivatives, such as the polysaccharides, as well as glycerol esters, cellulose ethers, sorbitan esters and polysorbates.

It will be noted that most of these are non-ionic. These have a tendency to be less irritant and less toxic than their anionic, and particularly their cationic, counterparts. The concentrations of ionic emulsifying agents necessary for emulsification will be irritant to the gastrointestinal tract and have a laxative effect. Thus they should not be used for oral emulsions.

When choosing an emulgent for parenteral use, it must be realized that only certain types of non-ionic material are suitable. These include lecithin, polysorbate 80, methylcellulose, gelatin and serum albumin.

Formulation by the HLB method

It has already been shown that physically stable emulsions are best achieved by the presence of a condensed layer of emulgent at the oil/water interface, and that the complex interfacial films formed by a blend of an oil-soluble emulsifying agent with a water-soluble one produce the most satisfactory emulsions.

A useful method has been devised for calculating the relative quantities of these emulgents necessary to produce the most physically stable emulsion for a particular oil/water combination. This is called the hydrophile-lipophile balance (HLB) method. Although originally applied to non-ionic surface-active agents, its use has been extended to ionic emulgents. Each surfactant is allocated an HLB number representing the relative proportions of the lipophilic and hydrophilic parts of the molecule. High numbers (up to a theoretical maximum of 20) therefore indicate a surfactant exhibiting mainly hydrophilic or polar properties, whereas low numbers represent lipophilic or non-polar characteristics. Table 27.2 gives HLB values for some commonly used emulsifying agents. The concept of HLB values is discussed more fully in Chapter 6.

Each type of oil used will require an emulgent of a particular HLB number in order to ensure a stable product. For an o/w emulsion, for example, the more polar the oil phase, the more polar must be the emulgent system.

Table 27.3 gives the required emulgent HLB value for particular oil phases for both types of emulsion.

Example calculations If a formulation contains a mixture of oils, fats or waxes the total HLB required can be calculated. The following example of an o/w emulsion will show this:

Liquid paraffin	35%
Wool fat	1%
Cetyl alcohol	1%
Emulsifier system	7%
Water	to 100%

Table 27.2 HLB values for some pharmaceutical surfactants	
Sorbitan trioleate (Span 85)	1.8
Oleic acid	4.3
Sorbitan monooleate (Span 80)	4.3
Sorbitan monostearate (Span 60)	4.7
Sorbitan monolaurate (Span 20)	8.6
Polysorbate 60 (polyoxyethylene sorbitan monostearate)	14.9
Polysorbate 80 (polyoxyethylene sorbitan monooleate) (Tween 80)	15.0
Polysorbate 20 (polyoxyethylene sorbitan monolaurate) (Tween 20)	16.7
Potassium oleate	20.0
Sodium dodecyl (lauryl) sulfate	40.0

Table 27.3 Required HLB values for a range of oils and waxes		
	For a w/o emulsion	For an o/w emulsion
Beeswax	5	12
Cetyl alcohol	–	15
Liquid paraffin	4	12
Soft paraffin	4	12
Wool fat	8	10

The total percentage of oil phase is 37 and the proportion of each is:

Liquid paraffin	$35/37 \times 100$ =	94.6%
Wool fat	$1/37 \times 100$ =	2.7%
Cetyl alcohol	$1/37 \times 100$ =	2.7%

The total required HLB number is obtained as follows:

Liquid paraffin (HLB 12)	$94.6/100 \times 12$ =	11.4
Wool fat (HLB 10)	$2.7/100 \times 10$ =	0.3
Cetyl alcohol (HLB 15)	$2.7/100 \times 15$ =	0.4
Total required HLB		= 12.1

From theoretical considerations, this particular formulation requires an emulgent blend of HLB 12.1 in order to produce the most stable emulsion. It must be realized, however, that the presence of other ingredients, particularly those that may partition into the oil phase, can also affect the required HLB value. It is therefore often necessary to prepare a series of emulsions using blends of a given pair of non-ionic emulsifying agents covering a wide range of HLB values. This is also important if the required HLB for an oil phase is not available. The HLB value of the emulgent blend giving the most stable emulsion is the required value for that oil phase.

Assuming that a blend of sorbitan monooleate (HLB 4.3) and polyoxyethylene sorbitan monooleate (HLB 15) is to be used as the emulsifying system, the proportions of each to be added to the emulsion to provide an HLB of 12.1 are calculated as follows.

Let A be the percentage concentration of the hydrophilic and B the percentage of the hydrophobic surfactants required to give a blend having an HLB value of x. Then:

$$A = \frac{100(x - \text{HLB of } B)}{(\text{HLB of } A - \text{HLB of } B)} \text{ and } B = 100 - A$$

In our example, therefore:

$$A = \frac{100(12.1 - 4.3)}{(15 - 4.3)} = 72.9$$

$$B = 100 - 72.9 = 27.1$$

The total concentration of emulgent needed for each formulation will depend on the physical characteristics required but a good starting point would be to add an amount approximately equal to 20% of the volume of the oil phase and then increase or decrease this amount as necessary. In this example the total percentage of emulgent blend in the formulation is 7 and so the percentage of each emulsifier will be:

Sorbitan monooleate	$7 \times 27.1/100 = 1.90$
Polyoxyethylene sorbitan monooleate	$7 - 1.90 = 5.10$

The series of trial emulsions can then be assessed for stability, based on the fact that the degree of creaming or separation is at a minimum at the optimal HLB value. Should several of the series show equally poor or equally good stability, resulting in an inability to choose a suitable HLB value, then the total emulgent concentration may be increased or reduced, respectively, and the manufacture of the series repeated.

Having determined the best HLB value for a given pair of emulgents, that value can now be used to assess the suitability of other emulgent blends that may give a better emulsion than the one containing the emulgent used for the initial trials.

It must be remembered that, in choosing an emulsifier blend, the effect of chemical structure on the type of interfacial film must be taken into account. Condensed films are produced by emulgents having long, saturated hydrocarbon groups, thus providing maximum cohesion between adjacent molecules. In most cases it has been found that the most stable emulsions are formed when both emulsifying agents are of the same hydrocarbon chain length.

Use of phase-inversion temperature

The use of the HLB system has several disadvantages, including the inability to take into account the effects of temperature, the presence of additives and the concentration of the emulsifier. It is possible to overcome some of these problems.

An o/w emulsion stabilized by non-ionic emulgents will, on heating, undergo phase inversion to form a w/o product. This is because, as the temperature increases, the HLB value of a non-ionic surfactant will decrease as it becomes more hydrophobic. At the temperature at which the emulgent has equal hydrophilic and hydrophobic tendencies (the phase-inversion temperature PIT), the emulsion will invert.

The stability of an emulsion has been related to the phase-inversion temperature of its emulsifying agent (see Chapter 6).

CLASSIFICATION OF EMULSIFYING AGENTS

The inclusion of an emulsifying agent or agents is necessary to facilitate actual emulsification during manufacture and also to ensure emulsion stability during the shelf life of the product.

The different methods by which emulsifying agents (also called emulsifiers or emulgents) exert their effects have been detailed in Chapter 6 but the one factor common to all of them is their ability to form an adsorbed film around the dispersed droplets between the two phases. There are many types of emulgent available but for convenience they can be divided into two main classifications:

- synthetic or semi-synthetic surface-active agents and
- naturally occurring materials and their derivatives.

These divisions are quite arbitrary and some materials may justifiably be placed in more than one category.

Synthetic and semi-synthetic surface-active agents

There are four main categories of these materials, depending on their ionization in aqueous solutions: anionic, cationic, non-ionic and amphoteric. The latter are not widely used as emulsifying agents although one example, lecithin, is used to stabilize intravenous fat emulsions.

In many instances these surfactants require the presence of an auxiliary non-ionic emulsifying agent in order to form a complex monomolecular film at the oil/water interface

Anionic surfactants

In aqueous solutions these compounds dissociate to form negatively charged anions that are responsible for their emulsifying ability. They are widely used because of their cheapness but because of their toxicity are only used for externally applied preparations.

Alkali metal and ammonium soaps Emulgents in this group consist mainly of the sodium, potassium or ammonium salts of long-chain fatty acids, such as:

$$\text{Sodium stearate } C_{17}H_{35}COO^- \text{ Na}^+$$

They produce stable o/w emulsions but because, in acidic conditions, these materials will precipitate out as the free fatty acids, they are most efficient in an alkaline medium.

This type of emulgent can also be formed in situ during the manufacture of the product by reacting an alkali such as potassium, sodium or ammonium hydroxide with a fatty acid. The latter may be a constituent of a vegetable oil. Oleic acid and ammonia, for example, are reacted together to form the soap responsible for stabilizing white liniment.

These emulgents are incompatible with polyvalent cations, often causing phase reversal, and it is therefore essential that deionized water is used in their preparation.

Soaps of divalent and trivalent metals Only the calcium salts are commonly used and are often formed in situ during preparation of the product by interacting the appropriate fatty acid with calcium hydroxide. For example, oleic acid is reacted with calcium hydroxide to produce calcium oleate, which is the emulsifying agent for both zinc cream BP and some formulations of oily calamine lotion.

These emulgents will only produce w/o emulsions.

Amine soaps A number of amines form salts with fatty acids. One of the most important of these is based on triethanolamine $N(CH_2CH_2OH)_3$ and is widely used in both pharmaceutical and cosmetic products. For example, triethanolamine stearate forms stable o/w emulsions and is usually made in situ by a reaction between triethanolamine and the appropriate fatty acid.

Sulfated and sulfonated compounds The alkyl sulfates have the general formula $ROSO_3^- M^+$, where R represents a hydrocarbon chain and M^+ is usually sodium or triethanolamine. An example is sodium lauryl sulfate, which is widely used to produce o/w emulsions. It is used with cetostearyl alcohol to produce emulsifying wax, which stabilizes such preparations as aqueous cream and benzyl benzoate application.

Sulfonated compounds are much less widely used as emulgents. Materials of this class include sodium dioctylsulfosuccinate, and are more often used as wetting agents or for their detergency.

Cationic surfactants

In aqueous solutions these materials dissociate to form positively charged cations that provide the emulsifying properties. The most important group of cationic emulgents consists of the quaternary ammonium compounds. Although these materials are widely used for their disinfectant and preservative properties, they are also useful o/w emulsifiers.

Because of the toxicity of cationic surfactants, they tend to be used only for the formulation of antiseptic creams, where the cationic nature of the emulgent is also responsible for the product's antiseptic properties.

Cetrimide (cetyl trimethylammonium bromide) is one of the most useful of these cationic emulgents and is used at a concentration of 0.5% with 5% cetostearyl alcohol for the formulation of cetrimide cream.

Non-ionic surfactants

These products range from oil-soluble compounds stabilizing w/o emulsions to water-soluble materials giving o/w products. Non-ionic emulgents are particularly useful because of their low toxicity and irritancy; some can therefore be used for orally and parenterally administered preparations. They also have a greater degree of compatibility with other materials than do anionic or cationic emulgents and are less sensitive to changes in pH or to the addition of electrolytes.

Being non-ionic, the dispersed globules may not possess a significant charge density. To reduce the tendency for coalescence to occur in an o/w emulsion, it is necessary that the polar groups be well hydrated and/or sufficiently large to prevent close approach of the dispersed droplets in order to compensate for the lack of charge.

Most non-ionic surfactants are based on:

- a fatty acid or alcohol (usually with 12–18 carbon atoms), the hydrocarbon chain of which provides the hydrophobic moiety
- an alcohol (-OH) and/or ethylene oxide grouping ($-OCH_2CH_2-$), which provide the hydrophilic part of the molecule.

By varying the relative proportions of the hydrophilic and hydrophobic groupings, many different products can be obtained.

Glycol and glycerol esters Glyceryl monostearate (a polyhydric alcohol fatty acid ester) is a strongly hydrophobic material that produces weak w/o emulsions. The addition of small amounts of sodium, potassium or triethanolamine salts of suitable fatty acids will produce a 'self-emulsifying' glyceryl monostearate, which is a useful o/w emulsifier. Self-emulsifying monostearin is glyceryl monostearate to which anionic soaps (usually oleate or stearate) have been added. This combination is used to stabilize hydrocortisone lotion.

Other polyhydric alcohol fatty acid esters are also available either in the pure form or in the 'self-emulsifying' form containing small proportions of a primary emulsifier, and include glyceryl monooleate, diethylene glycol monostearate and propylene glycol monooleate.

Sorbitan esters These are produced by the esterification of one or more of the hydroxyl groups of sorbitan with either lauric, oleic, palmitic or stearic acids. The structure of sorbitan stearate is shown below.

This range of surfactants exhibits lipophilic properties and tends to form w/o emulsions. They are, however, much more widely used with polysorbates to produce either o/w or w/o emulsions.

Polysorbates   Polyethylene glycol derivatives of the sorbitan esters give us polysorbates. These have the general formula:

where R represents a fatty acid chain. Variations in the type of fatty acid used and in the number of oxyethylene groups in the polyethylene glycol chains produce a range of products of differing oil and water solubilities. Polyoxyethylene 20 sorbitan monooleate, for example, contains 20 oxyethylene groups in the molecule. This number must not be confused with the one given as part of the official name (polysorbate 80) or in the trade name (Tween 80), which is included in order to identify the type of fatty acid in the molecule.

Polysorbates are generally used in conjunction with the corresponding sorbitan ester to form a complex condensed film at the oil/water interface (see Formulation by the HLB method, earlier).

Other non-ionic oil-soluble materials, such as glyceryl monostearate, cetyl or stearyl alcohol or propylene glycol monostearate, can be incorporated with polysorbates to produce 'self-emulsifying' preparations. For example,

Polawax contains cetyl alcohol with a polyoxyethylene sorbitan ester.

Fatty alcohol polyglycol ethers   These are condensation products of polyethylene glycol and fatty alcohols, usually cetyl or cetostearyl:

$$ROH + (CH_2CH_2O)_n \rightarrow RO(CH_2CH_2O)_nH$$

where R is a fatty alcohol chain.

Perhaps the most widely used is macrogol cetostearyl ether (22) or cetomacrogol 1000, which is polyethylene glycol monocetyl ether. This is a very useful water-soluble o/w emulgent but because of its high water solubility, it is necessary to include an oil-soluble auxiliary emulsifier when formulating emulsions. Cetomacrogol emulsifying ointment includes cetomacrogol 1000 and cetostearyl alcohol and is used to stabilize cetomacrogol creams.

They can also be produced with shorter polyoxyethylene groups as lipophilic w/o emulsifiers. Combinations of lipophilic and hydrophilic ethers can be used together to produce stable emulsions.

Fatty acid polyglycol esters   The stearate esters or polyoxyl stearates are the most widely used of this type of emulgent. Polyoxyethylene 40 stearate (in which 40 represents the number of oxyethylene units) is a water-soluble material often used with stearyl alcohol to give o/w emulsions.

Poloxalkols   Poloxalkols are polyoxyethylene/polyoxypropylene copolymers with the general formula:

$$OH(C_2H_4O)_a(C_3H_6O)_b(C_2H_4O)_a$$

and comprise a very large group of compounds, some of which are used as emulsifying agents for intravenous fat emulsions.

Higher fatty alcohols   The hexadecyl (cetyl) and octadecyl (stearyl) members of this series of saturated aliphatic monohydric alcohols are useful auxiliary emulsifying agents. Part of their stabilizing effect comes from their ability to increase the viscosity of the preparation, thereby retarding creaming. Cetostearyl alcohol will also form complex interfacial films with hydrophilic surface-active agents, such as sodium lauryl sulfate, cetrimide or cetomacrogol 1000, and so stabilize o/w emulsions.

Naturally occurring materials and their derivatives

Naturally occurring materials often suffer from two main disadvantages: they show considerable batch-to-batch variation in composition, and hence in emulsifying properties, and many are susceptible to bacterial or mould growth. For these reasons they are not widely used in manufactured products requiring a long shelf life but rather for extemporaneously prepared emulsions designed for use within a few days of manufacture.

Natural polysaccharides

The most important emulsifying agent in this group is acacia. This stabilizes o/w emulsions by forming a strong multimolecular film round each oil globule and so coalescence is retarded by the presence of a hydrophilic barrier between the oil and water phases.

Because of its low viscosity, creaming will occur readily and therefore a suspending agent such as tragacanth or sodium alginate can also be included. Because of its sticky nature, the use of acacia is limited to products for internal application.

Semi-synthetic polysaccharides

In order to reduce the problems associated with batch-to-batch variation, semi-synthetic derivatives are available as o/w emulgents or stabilizers.

Several grades of methylcellulose and carmellose sodium are available and exert their action in a similar way to that of acacia. Methylcellulose 20, for example, is used at a concentration of 2% to stabilize liquid paraffin oral emulsion.

Sterol-containing substances

Beeswax, wool fat and wool alcohols are all used in the formulation of emulsions. Beeswax is used mainly in cosmetic creams of both o/w and w/o type. Beeswax is used as a stabilizer for w/o creams.

Wool fat (anhydrous lanolin) consists chiefly of normal fatty alcohols with fatty acid esters of cholesterol and other sterols. It will form w/o emulsions of low disperse-phase concentration, and it can also be incorporated for its emollient properties. Some individuals exhibit sensitization to this material and, because of its characteristic odour and the need to incorporate antioxidants, it is not widely used. It is, however, to be found in low concentrations in many ointments, where its water-absorbing properties are of great value. It can be employed as an emulsion stabilizer with a primary emulsifying agent, for example with calcium oleate in oily calamine lotion, with beeswax in proflavine cream, and with cetostearyl alcohol in zinc and ichthammol cream.

Because wool fat has some ideal properties, attempts have been made to improve its less desirable characteristics by physical and chemical modification. It has been converted by a reaction with ethylene oxide to give a range of polyoxyethylene lanolin derivatives. These non-ionic products are mainly water soluble and are used as o/w emulgents possessing the properties of emollience.

The principal emulsifying agent in wool fat is wool alcohols, which consist mainly of cholesterol together with other alcohols. They are an effective w/o emulgent, being more powerful than wool fat, and are used in the formulation of hydrous ointment. They are also incorporated as wool alcohols ointment into other ointment bases which, although not emulsions, will readily mix with aqueous skin secretions and easily wash off the skin. Wool alcohols do not have the same strong odour as wool fat but do require the presence of an antioxidant.

Finely divided solids

Certain finely divided solids can be adsorbed at the oil/water interface to form a coherent film that physically prevents coalescence of the dispersed globules. If the particles are preferentially wetted by the aqueous phase then o/w products will result, whereas preferential wetting by the oil will produce w/o emulsions.

Montmorillonite clays (such as bentonite and aluminium magnesium silicate) and colloidal silicon dioxide are used mainly for external use. Aluminium and magnesium hydroxides are also used internally. For example, liquid paraffin and magnesium hydroxide oral emulsion is stabilized by the incorporation of the magnesium hydroxide.

Other formulation additives

Buffers

The inclusion of buffers (see Chapters 3 and 25) may be necessary to maintain chemical stability, control tonicity or ensure physiological compatibility. It must be remembered, however, that the addition of electrolytes may have profound effects on the physical stability of suspensions and emulsions.

Density modifiers

From a qualitative examination of Stokes' Law (see Chapters 4 and 6), it can be seen that if the disperse and continuous phases both have the same densities then sedimentation or creaming will not occur. Minor modifications to the aqueous phase of a suspension or emulsion by incorporating sucrose, dextrose, glycerol or propylene glycol can be achieved. However, because of the differing coefficients of expansion this can only be possible over a small temperature range.

Humectants

Glycerol, polyethylene glycol and propylene glycol are examples of suitable humectants that can be incorporated at concentrations of about 5% into aqueous suspensions for external application. They are used to prevent the product from drying out after application to the skin.

They can also be added to an emulsion formulation in order to reduce the evaporation of the water, either from the packaged product when the closure is removed or from the surface of the skin after application. High concentrations, if used topically, may actually remove moisture from the skin, thereby dehydrating it.

Antioxidants

Before including an antioxidant in emulsion formulations, it is essential to ensure that its use is not restricted in whichever country it is desired to sell the product. In Britain, butylated hydroxyanisole (BHA) is widely used for the protection of fixed oils and fats at concentrations of up to 0.02% and for some essential oils up to 0.1%. A similar antioxidant is butylated hydroxytoluene (BHT), which is recommended as an alternative to tocopherol at a concentration of 10 ppm to stabilize liquid paraffin. Other antioxidants widely used for emulsion formulation include the propyl, octyl and dodecyl esters of gallic acid, recommended for use at concentrations up to 0.001% for fixed oils and fats and up to 0.1% for essential oils.

The efficiency of an antioxidant in a product will depend on many factors, including its compatibility with other ingredients, its oil/water partition coefficient, the extent of its solubilization within micelles of the emulgent, and its sorption onto the container and its closure. It must be realized, therefore, that the choice of antioxidant and the concentration at which it is to be used can only be determined by testing its effectiveness in the final product and in the package in which the product is to be sold.

Flavours, colours and perfumes

The use of these ingredients is discussed in Chapter 25 and the information there will be directly applicable to suspension and emulsion formulation.

Adsorption of these materials on to the surfaces of the disperse phase of a suspension may occur, and because of the high surface area of the dispersed powders in this type of formulation, their effective concentrations in solution may be significantly reduced. The finer the degree of subdivision of the disperse phase, the paler may appear the colour of the product for a given concentration of dye.

It must also be realized that the inclusion of these adjuvants may alter the physical characteristics of both suspensions and emulsions. Either the presence of electrolytes or their effect on pH can influence the degree of flocculation.

Sweetening agents

Suitable sweeteners are discussed in Chapter 25. High concentrations of sucrose, sorbitol or glycerol, which will exhibit newtonian properties, may adversely affect the rheological properties of the suspension. Synthetic sweeteners may be salts and can affect the degree of flocculation.

PRESERVATION OF SUSPENSIONS AND EMULSIONS

It is essential that a suitable preservative be included as part of an emulsion or suspension formulation, particularly if naturally occurring materials are to be used. This is to prevent the growth of microorganisms that may be present in the raw material and/or introduced into the product during use. Some of the natural products, particularly if they are to be applied to broken skin, should be sterilized before use. Bentonite, for example, may contain *Clostridium tetani* but can be sterilized by heating the dry powder at 160°C for 1 hour or by autoclaving aqueous dispersions.

Care must be taken to ascertain the extent of inactivation, if any, of the preservative system caused by interaction with other excipients. Solubilization by wetting agents and emulgents, interaction with polymers or adsorption onto suspended solids or globules, particularly kaolin or magnesium trisilicate, may reduce the availability of preservatives.

Because of the complex systems involved and the many factors to be taken into consideration, it is necessary to test the efficiency of a new preservative in the finished product and container by suitable challenge testing procedures.

Chapter 43 provides a comprehensive coverage of the microbiological preservation of pharmaceuticals, including suspensions and emulsions.

PHYSICAL STABILITY OF SUSPENSIONS

The physical stability of a suspension is normally assessed by the measurement of its rate of sedimentation, the final volume or height of the sediment, and the ease of redispersion of the product.

The first two parameters can be assessed easily by a measurement of the total initial volume or height of the suspension (V_0) and the volume or height of the sediment (V_t), as shown in Figure 27.1. By plotting the value of V_t/V_0 against time for a series of trial formulations (all initial values will equal unity), it can be seen, by an assessment of the slope of each line, which suspension shows the slowest rate of sedimentation. When the value of V_t/V_0 becomes constant this indicates that sedimentation has ceased.

Alternatively, the term flocculation value can be used, which is a ratio of the final volume or height of the sediment and the volume or height of the fully sedimented cake of the same system which has been deflocculated.

Attempts have also been made to equate the zeta potential of the suspended particles with the physical stability, particularly the degree of flocculation, of the system using electrophoresis.

The ease of redispersion of the product can be assessed qualitatively by simply agitating the product in its container. The use of a mechanical shaker will eliminate variations in shaking ability.

PHYSICAL STABILITY OF EMULSIONS

A stable emulsion is one in which the dispersed globules retain their initial character and remain uniformly distributed throughout the continuous phase. Various types of deviation from this ideal behaviour can occur. Explanations for emulsion stability have been given in Chapter 6. This section will concentrate on methods of improving emulsion stability in practice.

Creaming and its avoidance

This is the separation of an emulsion into two regions, one of which is richer in the disperse phase than the other. An everyday example is the creaming of milk, when fat globules slowly rise to the top of the product. This is not a serious instability problem as a uniform dispersion can be reobtained simply by shaking the emulsion. Creaming is, however, undesirable pharmaceutically because of the increased likelihood of coalescence of the droplets, owing to their close proximity to each other. A creamed emulsion is also inelegant and, if the emulsion is not shaken adequately, there is a risk of the patient obtaining an incorrect dosage.

Consideration of the qualitative application of Stokes' Law (see Chapters 4 and 9) will show that the rate of creaming can be reduced by the following methods.

Production of an emulsion of small droplet size

This factor usually depends on the method of manufacture. An efficient emulsifying agent will not only stabilize

the emulsion but also facilitate the actual emulsification process to give a product of fine globule size.

Increase in the viscosity of the continuous phase

Many auxiliary emulsifying agents, in particular the hydrophilic colloids, are viscosity enhancers and this property is part of their emulsifying capability. For example, the inclusion of methylcellulose will reduce the mobility of the dispersed droplets in an o/w emulsion. The addition of soft paraffin will have the same effect on water droplets in a w/o emulsion.

Storage of the product at a low temperature (but above freezing point) will increase the viscosity of the continuous phase and also reduce the kinetic energy of the system. This will decrease the rate of migration of the globules of the disperse phase. It is unwise, however, to rely solely on this method of controlling creaming, as storage conditions after the product is sold are outside the control of the manufacturer.

Reduction in the density difference between the two phases

Creaming could be prevented altogether if the densities of the two phases were identical. In practice, this method is never used, as it could only be achieved over a very narrow temperature range owing to differences in the coefficients of expansion between different ingredients.

Control of disperse-phase concentration

It is not easy to stabilize an emulsion containing less than 20% disperse phase as creaming will readily occur. A higher disperse-phase concentration would result in a hindrance of movement of the droplets and hence in a reduction in rate of creaming. Although it is theoretically possible to include as much as 74% of an internal phase, it is usually found that at above about 60% concentration, phase inversion occurs.

Finally, it must be realized that some of the factors above are interrelated. For example, homogenization of the emulsion would decrease globule size and, by thus increasing their number, increase the viscosity of the product.

Flocculation prevention

Flocculation involves the aggregation of the dispersed globules into loose clusters within the emulsion. The individual droplets retain their identities but each cluster behaves physically as a single unit. This, as we have already seen, would increase the rate of creaming. As flocculation must precede coalescence, any factor preventing or retarding flocculation would therefore maintain the stability of the emulsion.

Flocculation in the secondary minimum (see Fig. 6.3) occurs readily and cannot be avoided. Redispersion can easily be achieved by shaking. Primary minimum flocculation, however, is more serious and redispersion is not so easy.

The presence of a high charge density on the dispersed droplets will ensure the presence of a high energy barrier, and thus reduce the incidence of flocculation in the primary minimum. Care must be taken to ensure that the effects of any ions in the product are taken into consideration very early in the formulation process. This is particularly important when formulating emulsions for parenteral nutrition which contain high levels of electrolytes (Washington 1990).

Coalescence (breaking, cracking)

The coalescence of oil globules in an o/w emulsion is resisted by the presence of a mechanically strong adsorbed layer of emulsifier around each globule. This is achieved by the presence of either a condensed mixed monolayer of lipophilic and hydrophilic emulgents or a multimolecular film of a hydrophilic material. Hydration of either of these types of film will hinder the drainage of water from between adjacent globules which is necessary prior to coalescence. As two globules approach each other, their close proximity causes their adjacent surfaces to flatten. As a change from a sphere to any other shape results in an increase in surface area and hence in total surface free energy, this globule distortion will be resisted and drainage of the film of continuous phase from between the two globules will be delayed.

The presence of long, cohesive hydrocarbon chains projecting into the oil phase will prevent coalescence in a w/o emulsion.

CHEMICAL INSTABILITY OF EMULSIONS

Although it is not possible to list every incompatibility, the following general points will illustrate the more common chemical problems that can cause the coalescence of an emulsion.

It is necessary to ensure that any emulgent system used is not only physically but also chemically compatible with the active agent and with the other emulsion ingredients. Ionic emulsifying agents, for example, are usually incompatible with materials of opposite charge. Anionic and cationic emulgents are thus mutually incompatible.

It has already been demonstrated that the presence of electrolyte can influence the stability of an emulsion by either:

- reducing the energy of interaction between adjacent globules, or
- a salting-out effect, by which high concentrations of electrolytes can strip emulsifying agents of their hydrated layers and so cause their precipitation.

In some cases phase inversion may occur rather than demulsification. If, for example, a sodium soap is used to stabilize an o/w emulsion, then the addition of a divalent electrolyte such as calcium chloride may form the calcium soap, which will stabilize a w/o emulsion.

Emulgents may also be precipitated by the addition of materials in which they are insoluble. It may be possible to precipitate hydrophilic colloids by the addition of alcohol. For this reason care must be taken if tinctures are to be included in emulsion formulations.

Changes in pH may also lead to the breaking of emulsions. Sodium soaps may react with acids to produce the free fatty acid and the sodium salt of the acid. Soap-stabilized emulsions are therefore usually formulated at an alkaline pH.

Oxidation

Many of the oils and fats used in emulsion formulation are of animal or vegetable origin and can be susceptible to oxidation by atmospheric oxygen or by the action of microorganisms. The resulting rancidity is manifested by the formation of degradation products of unpleasant odour and taste. These problems can also occur with certain emulsifying agents, such as wool fat or wool alcohols. Oxidation of microbiological origin is controlled by the use of antimicrobial preservatives, and atmospheric oxidation by the use of reducing agents or, more usually, antioxidants. Some examples are mentioned earlier in this chapter.

Microbiological contamination

The contamination of emulsions by microorganisms can adversely affect the physicochemical properties of the product, causing such problems as gas production, colour and odour changes, hydrolysis of fats and oils, pH changes in the aqueous phase, and breaking of the emulsion. Even without visible signs of contamination, an emulsion can contain many bacteria and, if these include pathogens, may constitute a serious health hazard. Most fungi and many bacteria will multiply readily in the aqueous phase of an emulsion at room temperature, and many moulds will also tolerate a wide pH range. Some of the hydrophilic colloids, which are widely used as emulsifying agents, may provide a suitable nutritive medium for use by bacteria and moulds. Species of the genus Pseudomonas can utilize polysorbates, aliphatic hydrocarbons and compounds. Some fixed oils, including arachis oil, can be used by some Aspergillus and Rhizopus species, and liquid paraffin by some species of Penicillium.

A few emulgents, particularly those from natural sources, may introduce heavy contamination into products in which they are used. Because bacteria can reproduce in resin beds, deionized water may be unsatisfactory and even distilled water, if incorrectly stored after collection, can be another source of contamination. Oil-in-water emulsions tend to be more susceptible to microbial spoilage than water-in-oil products. For example, the continuous oil phase acts as a barrier to the spread of microorganisms throughout the product and the less water there is present, the less growth there is likely to be.

It is therefore necessary to include an antimicrobial agent to prevent the growth of any microorganisms that might contaminate the product. Suitable candidates are discussed in Chapter 43.

Adverse storage conditions

Adverse storage conditions may also cause emulsion instability. It has already been explained that an increase in temperature will cause an increase in the rate of creaming, owing to a fall in apparent viscosity of the continuous phase. The temperature increase will also cause an increased kinetic motion, both of the dispersed droplets and of the emulsifying agent at the oil/water interface. This effect on the disperse phase will enable the energy barrier to be easily surmounted and thus the number of collisions between globules will increase. Increased motion of the emulgent will result in a more expanded monolayer, and so coalescence is more likely. Certain macromolecular emulsifying agents may also be coagulated by an increase in temperature.

At the other extreme, freezing of the aqueous phase will produce ice crystals that may exert unusual pressures on the dispersed globules and their adsorbed layer of emulgent. In addition, dissolved electrolyte may concentrate in the unfrozen water, thus affecting the charge density on the globules. Certain emulgents may also precipitate at low temperatures.

The growth of microorganisms within the emulsion can cause deterioration and it is therefore essential that these products are protected as far as possible from the ingress of microorganisms during manufacture, storage and use, and that they contain adequate preservatives.

STABILITY TESTING OF EMULSIONS

Methods of assessing stability

Macroscopic examination

The physical stability of an emulsion can be assessed by an examination of the degree of creaming or coalescence occurring over a period of time. This is carried out by calculating the ratio of the volume of the creamed or separated part of the emulsion and the total volume. These values can be compared for different products.

Globule size analysis

If the mean globule size increases with time (coupled with a decrease in globule numbers), it can be assumed that coalescence is the cause. It is therefore possible to compare the rates of coalescence for a variety of emulsion formulations by measuring changes in globule size and number. Microscopic examination, electronic particle counting devices (such as the Coulter counter) and laser diffraction sizing are most widely used (detailed in Chapter 9).

Viscosity changes

It has already been shown that many factors influence the viscosity of emulsions. Any variation in globule size or number, or in the orientation or migration of emulsifier over a period of time, may be detected by a change in apparent viscosity. Suitable methods and equipment are detailed in Chapter 4.

In order to compare the relative stabilities of a range of similar products, it is often necessary to speed up the processes of creaming and coalescence. This can be achieved in one of the following ways.

Accelerated stability tests

To assess the physical stability of suspensions and emulsions, macroscopic examination and measurement of apparent viscosity are of value. In addition, for emulsions, microscopic evaluation of globule size distribution and numbers will provide further evidence of changes in physical stability.

Storage at adverse temperatures An assessment of these parameters at elevated temperatures for emulsions and coarse suspensions would give a speedier indication of a rank order of degree of instability but it is essential to correlate these results with those taken from suspensions stored at ambient temperatures.

By exaggerating the temperature fluctuations to which any product is subjected under normal storage conditions, it may be possible to compare the physical stabilities of a series of suspensions or emulsions. Temperature cycles consisting of storage for several hours at about 40°C followed by refrigeration or freezing until instability becomes evident have been used successfully. The continual formation and melting of small ice crystals will disrupt the adsorbed layer of emulgent at the oil/water interface and any weakness in the structure of the film will quickly become apparent. Similarly, normal temperature fluctuations can be used but at increased frequencies of only a few minutes at each extreme. This method of accelerated stability testing is particularly useful for the assessment of crystal growth in suspensions. Measurement of particle size is usually carried out microscopically, by laser diffraction or by use of a Coulter counter. It is of course important to ensure that the suspension is deflocculated so that each individual particle is measured, rather than each floccule.

Centrifugation A qualitative examination of Stokes' Law (see Chapters 4, 6 and 9) would indicate that centrifugation is a suitable method for artificially increasing the rate of sedimentation of a suspension. Again, it is not always possible to predict accurately the behaviour of such a system when stored under normal conditions from data obtained after this type of accelerated testing. The process of centrifugation may destroy the structure of a flocculated system that would remain intact under normal storage conditions. The sediment formed would become tightly packed and difficult to redisperse, whether or not the initial suspension was flocculated or deflocculated. This method may, however, give a useful indication of the relative stabilities of a series of trial products, particularly if used at speeds no faster than 200–300 rpm.

Rheological assessment Although apparent viscosity measurements are also used as a tool to assess physical stability, the high shear rates involved may also destroy the structure of a suspension or emulsion. Very low rates of shear, using for example the Brookfield viscometer with Helipath stand, can give an indication of the change in the structure of the system after various storage times. For suspensions it may be possible to combine the results from sedimentation techniques with those from rheological assessments.

A measurement of the residual apparent viscosity after breaking down the structure of the suspension can be used as a routine quality control procedure after manufacture.

MANUFACTURE OF SUSPENSIONS

It is important to ensure initially that the powder to be suspended is in a suitably fine degree of subdivision in order to ensure adequate bioavailability, minimum sedimentation rate and impalpability. Suitable size reduction equipment and the relative merits of wet and dry milling are detailed in Chapter 10.

For the extemporaneous preparation of suspensions on a small scale, the powdered drug can be mixed with the suspending agent and some of the vehicle using a pestle and mortar. It may also be necessary, at this stage, to include a wetting agent to aid dispersion. Other soluble ingredients should then be dissolved in another portion of the vehicle, mixed with the concentrated suspension and then made up to volume.

It is often preferable, particularly on a larger scale, to make a concentrated dispersion of the suspending agent first. This is best accomplished by adding the material slowly to the vehicle while mixing. Suitable mixers are described under 'Manufacture of emulsions' and can include either an impeller type of blender or a turbine mixer. This stage is important as it is necessary to ensure that agglomerates of the suspending agent are fully broken up. If they are not, then the surface of each agglomerate may gel and cause the powder inside to remain non-wetted. Very intense shearing, however, can destroy the polymeric structure of the suspending agent and it may be better to use milder shearing and then allow the dispersion to stand until full hydration has been achieved. This may be instantaneous or may, as with tragacanth, take several hours. If the suspending agent is blended with one of the water-soluble ingredients, such as sucrose, this will also aid dispersion.

The drug to be suspended is then added in the same way, along with the wetting agent. For very hydrophobic drugs, wetting may be facilitated by mixing under reduced pressure. This has the additional advantage of de-aerating the product and thus improving its appearance. Other ingredients should now be added, preferably dissolved in a portion of the vehicle, and the whole made up to volume if necessary. Finally, homogenization (see under 'Manufacture of emulsions') is performed to ensure complete dispersion of the drug and the production of a smooth and elegant preparation.

It is also possible, though much less widely used, to suspend an insoluble drug by precipitating it from a solution. This can be accomplished either by double decomposition or, if it is a weak acid or a weak base, by altering the pH of its solution or by precipitating the drug from a water-miscible solvent on the addition of water. This method may be of use if the drug is required to be sterile but is degraded by heat or irradiation. A soluble form of the drug is dissolved in a suitable vehicle, sterilized by filtration and then precipitated to form a suspension.

In normal circumstances aqueous suspensions can be autoclaved, as long as the process does not adversely affect either physical or chemical stability.

MANUFACTURE OF EMULSIONS

It has already been explained that the smaller the globules of the disperse phase, the slower will be the rate of creaming in an emulsion. The size of these globules can also affect the viscosity of the product. In general it has been found that the best emulsions with respect to physical stability and texture possess a mean globule diameter of between 0.5 and 2.5 μm. The choice of suitable equipment for the emulsification process depends mainly on the intensity of shearing required to produce this optimum particle size. Other considerations, however, include the volume and viscosity of the emulsion and the interfacial tension between the oil and the water. The presence of surfactants, which will reduce interfacial tension, will aid the process of emulsification as well as promoting emulsion stability.

In many cases simple blending of the oil and water phases with a suitable emulgent system may be sufficient to produce satisfactory emulsions. Further processing using an homogenizer can also be carried out to reduce globule size still further. The initial blending may be accomplished on a small scale by the use of a pestle and mortar or by using a mixer fitted with an impeller type of agitator, the size and type of which will depend primarily on the volume and viscosity of the emulsified product.

A more intense rate of shearing can be achieved using a turbine mixer (see Chapter 12) such as the Silverson mixer-homogenizer. In this type of machine the short, vertical or angled rotor blades are enclosed within a stationary perforated ring and connected by a central rod to a motor. The liquids are therefore subjected to intense shearing, caused initially by the rotating blades and then by the forced discharge through the perforated ring. Different models are available for a variety of batch sizes up to several thousand litres and can include inline models.

The mixing vessel may also be fitted with baffles in order to modify the circulation of the liquid and may be jacketed so that heating or cooling can be applied.

Homogenizers are often used after initial mixing to enable smaller globule sizes to be produced. They all work on the principle of forced discharge of the emulsion under pressure through fine interstices, formed by closely packed metal surfaces, in order to provide an intense shearing action.

If two immiscible liquids are subjected to ultrasonic vibrations, alternate regions of compression and rarefaction are produced. Cavities are then formed in the regions of rarefaction, which then collapse with considerable force, causing emulsification. The required frequency of vibration is usually produced electrically but mechanical methods are also available. Unfortunately, this method of emulsification is limited to small-scale production.

Colloid mills are also suitable for the preparation of emulsions on a continuous basis. The intense shearing of the product between the rotor and the stator, which can be variably separated, will produce emulsions of very small globule size.

It is important to ensure that methods of manufacture developed on a laboratory scale can be easily extended to large-scale production, and without any change in the quality of the product.

During manufacture, it is usual to add the disperse phase to the continuous phase during the initial mixing. The other ingredients are dissolved, prior to mixing, in the phase in which they are soluble. This is particularly important when making w/o emulsions. Oil-in-water emulsions, however, are sometimes made by the phase-inversion technique, in which the aqueous phase is slowly added to the oil phase during mixing. Initially a w/o emulsion is formed but as further aqueous phase is added, the emulsion inverts to form the intended product. This method often produces emulsions of very low mean droplet size.

Should any of the oily ingredients be of solid or semisolid consistency, they must be melted before mixing. It is also essential that the aqueous phase be heated to the same temperature to avoid premature solidification of the oil phase by the colder water on mixing but before emulsification has taken place. This also has the advantage of reducing the viscosity of the system, so enabling shear forces to be transmitted through the product more easily. Because of the increased kinetic motion of the emulgent molecules at the oil/water interface, however, it is necessary to continue stirring during the cooling process to avoid demulsification.

Volatile ingredients, including flavours and perfumes, are usually added after the emulsion has cooled. It must, however, be sufficiently fluid when cooled to enable adequate blending. Ingredients that may influence the physical stability of the emulsion, such as alcoholic solutions or electrolytes, require to be diluted as much as possible before adding slowly and with constant mixing.

RELEASE OF DRUGS FROM SUSPENSION AND EMULSION FORMULATIONS

Drug release from suspensions

After the oral administration of a suspension the drug, which is already in a wetted state, is presented to the gastrointestinal fluids in a finely divided form. Dissolution therefore begins immediately. The rate of absorption of the drug into the blood stream is therefore usually faster than for the same drug in a solid dosage form, but not as fast as that from a solution. The rate of release of a drug from a suspension is also dependent upon the viscosity of the product. The more viscous the preparation, the slower is likely to be the release of the drug. Care must therefore be taken to ensure that the physical characteristics of the suspension do not change on addition to an acid medium, if this might affect the rate of release of the drug.

Because the rate of release of an active agent from a suspension is usually slower than the release from solution, drugs are often formulated as suspensions for intramuscular, intraarticular or subcutaneous injection in order to prolong drug release. This is often termed depot therapy. Methylprednisolone, for example, which is available as the water-soluble sodium succinate salt, can be synthesized as the insoluble acetate ester. After intramuscular injection as a suspension, the rate of release is sufficiently slowed to maintain adequate blood levels for up to 14 days.

Drug release will occur even more slowly if the drug is suspended in an oil that, after injection, will remain as a globule, so providing a minimal area of contact with tissue fluid.

Sustained-release preparations formulated as suspensions for oral use are less common but one example is the use of the Pennkinetic system. This involves the complexation of drugs such as hydrocortone and dextromethorphan with tiny ion exchange resin particles that are then coated with ethylcellulose (Chang 1992). After ingestion, the drug is slowly released by exchanging with ions present in the gastrointestinal tract. One of the main difficulties in the formulation of this type of product is to ensure that ions are not present in any of its ingredients.

Drug release from emulsions

The main commercial use of emulsions is for the oral, rectal and topical administration of oils and oil-soluble drugs. Lipid emulsions are also widely used for intravenous feeding, although the choice of emulgent is very limited and globule size must be kept below 4 micrometre diameter to avoid the formation of emboli. Quite often, however, the high surface area of dispersed oil globules will enhance the rate of absorption of lipophilic drugs.

The emulsion can also be used as a sustained-release dosage form. The intramuscular injection of certain water-soluble vaccines formulated as w/o emulsions can provide a slow release of the antigen and result in a greater antibody response and hence a longer-lasting immunity. Other drugs have also been shown to have this effect, the rate of release being dependent mainly upon the oil/water partition coefficient of the drug and its rate of diffusion across the oil phase.

It is also possible to formulate multiple emulsion systems in which an aqueous phase is dispersed in oil droplets, which in turn are dispersed throughout another aqueous external phase, producing a water-in-oil-in-water (w/o/w) emulsion. These products can also be used for the prolonged release of drugs that are incorporated into the internal aqueous phase. They have the advantage of exhibiting a lower viscosity than their w/o counterparts and hence are easier to inject.

Similarly, o/w/o emulsions can be formulated and are also under investigation as potential sustained-release bases. Multiple emulsions, however, tend to be stable only for a relatively short time, although the use of polymers as alternatives to the traditional emulsifying agents may improve their physical stability (Florence & Whitehill 1982).

REFERENCES

Chang, R.K. (1992) Formulation approaches for sustained release oral suspensions. *Pharmaceutical Technology,* **16**, 134-136.

Ciullo, P.A. (1981) Rheological properties of magnesium aluminium silicate/xanthan gum dispersions. *Journal of the. Society of Cosmetic Chemists*, **Sep/Oct**, 32.

Florence, A.T., Whitehill, D. (1982) Stabilisation of water/oil/water multiple emulsions by polymerisation of the aqueous phase. *Journal of Pharmacy and Pharmacology*, **34**, 687-691.

Washington, C. (1990) The stability of intravenous fat emulsions in parenteral nutrition mixtures. *International Journal of Pharmaceutics*, **66**, 1-21.

BIBLIOGRAPHY

Florence, A.T., Attwood, D. (2006) *Physicochemical Principles of Pharmacy*, 4th edn. Pharmaceutical Press, London.

28

Powders and granules

M. P. Summers

POWDERED AND GRANULATED PRODUCTS AS DOSAGE FORMS

The term 'powder', when used to describe a dosage form, describes a formulation in which a drug powder has normally been mixed with other powdered excipients to produce the final product. The function of the added excipients depends upon the intended use of the product. Colouring, flavouring and sweetening agents, for example, may be added to powders for oral use.

Conventionally, the title 'powder' should be restricted to powder mixes for internal use and alternative titles are used for other powdered formulations, e.g. dusting powders, which are for external use. The more descriptive title 'oral powder' to differentiate powders for internal use is recommended.

Granules which are used as a dosage form consist of powder particles that have been aggregated to form a larger particle, which is usually 2–4 mm in diameter, sufficiently resistant to withstand handling. This is much larger than granules prepared as an intermediate for tablet manufacture. The processes involved in forming granules from powders are discussed in Chapter 29.

Powdered and granulated products are traditionally dispensed as:

- bulk powders or granules for internal use
- divided powders or granules (i.e. single-dose preparations) for internal use
- dusting powders for external use.

Other preparations which are presented as powders or granules include:

- insufflations for administration to ear, nose or throat
- antibiotic syrups to be reconstituted before use
- powders for reconstitution into injections
- dry-powder inhalers.

The *British Pharmacopoeia* contains other categories of this type of product that are not currently used as dosage forms.

Advantages and disadvantages of powdered and granulated products

The advantages of this type of preparation are as follows:

- Solid preparations are more chemically stable than liquid ones. The shelf life of powders for antibiotic syrups, for example, is 2–3 years but once they are reconstituted with water, it is 1–2 weeks. The instability observed in liquid preparations is usually the primary reason for presenting some injections as powders to be reconstituted just prior to use.
- Powders and granules are a convenient form in which to dispense drugs with a large dose. The dose of compound magnesium trisilicate oral powder is 1–5 g and, although it is feasible to manufacture tablets to supply this dose, it is often more acceptable to the patient to disperse a powder in water and swallow it as a draught.
- Orally administered powders and granules of soluble medicaments have a faster dissolution rate than tablets or capsules, as these must first disintegrate before the drug dissolves. Drug absorption from such powdered or granulated preparations will therefore be faster than from the corresponding tablet or capsule, if the dissolution rate limits the rate of drug absorption.

The disadvantages of powders and granules are as follows:

- Bulk powders or granules are far less convenient for the patient to carry than a small container of tablets or capsules, and are as inconvenient as liquid preparations, such as mixtures. Modern packaging methods for divided preparations, such as heat-sealable laminated sachets, mean that individual doses can be conveniently carried.
- The masking of unpleasant tastes may be a problem with this type of preparation. A method of attempting this is by formulating the powder into a pleasantly tasting or taste-masked effervescent product, whereas tablets and capsules are a more common alternative for low-dose products.
- Bulk powders or granules are not suitable for administering potent drugs with a low dose. This is because individual doses are extracted from the bulk using a 5 mL spoon. This method is subject to such variables as variation in spoon fill (e.g. 'level' or 'heaped' spoonfuls) and variation in the bulk

density of different batches of a powder. It is therefore not an accurate method of measurement. Divided preparations have been used for more potent drugs, but tablets and capsules have largely replaced them for this purpose.
- Powders and granules are not a suitable method for the administration of drugs which are inactivated in, or cause damage to, the stomach; these should be presented as enteric-coated tablets, for example.

DISPENSED PREPARATIONS

Bulk powders

The mixed ingredients are packed into a suitable bulk container, such as a wide-mouthed glass jar. Because of the disadvantages of this type of preparation, the constituents are usually relatively non-toxic medicaments with a large dose, e.g. magnesium trisilicate and chalk, as present in compound magnesium trisilicate oral powder. Relatively few proprietary examples exist, although many dietary/food supplements are packed in this way.

They should be administered using a device suitable for measuring the dose.

Divided powders

Divided powders are similar formulations to bulk powders but individual doses are separately wrapped.

Traditionally, single doses were wrapped in paper. This was unsatisfactory for most products, particularly if the ingredients were hygroscopic, volatile or deliquescent. Modern packaging materials of foil and plastic laminates have replaced such paper wrappings because they offer superior protective qualities and are amenable to use on high-speed packing machines.

Effervescent powders can now be packed in individual dose units because of the protective qualities of laminates. Such powders contain, for example, sodium bicarbonate and citric acid, which react and effervesce when the patient adds the powder to water to produce a draught. It is important to protect the powder from the ingress of moisture during manufacture and on subsequent storage to prevent the reaction occurring prematurely.

All powders and granules should be stored in a dry place to prevent deterioration due to ingress of moisture. Even if hydrolytic decomposition of susceptible ingredients does not occur, the particles will adhere and cake, producing an inelegant, often unusable product.

Bulk granules

One disadvantage of bulk powders is that, because of particle size differences, the ingredients may segregate (see Chapter 12), either on storage in the final container or in the hoppers of packaging machines. If this happens the product will be non-uniform and the patient will not receive the same dose of the ingredients on each occasion. This can be prevented by granulating the mixed powders.

Bulk granules therefore contain similar medicaments to powders, i.e. those with low-toxicity, high-dose drugs. Methylcellulose granules, for example, are used as a bulk-forming laxative and have a dose of 1–4 g daily. Many proprietary preparations contain similar bulk-forming laxatives.

Divided granules

These are granulated products in which sufficient for one dose is individually wrapped. Effervescent granules can be formulated and presented in this manner. The comments on packaging materials discussed under 'Divided powders' above are equally pertinent to divided granules.

Dusting powders

Dusting powders contain ingredients used for therapeutic, prophylactic or lubricant purposes and are intended for external use.

Only sterile dusting powders should be applied to open wounds. Such preparations should be prepared using materials and methods designed to ensure sterility and to avoid the introduction of contaminants and the growth of microorganisms.

Dusting powders for lubricant purposes or superficial skin conditions need not be sterile but they should be free from pathogenic organisms. As minerals such as talc and kaolin may be contaminated at source with spores of organisms causing tetanus and gangrene, these should be sterilized before they are incorporated into the product. Talc dusting powder is a sterile cutaneous powder containing starch and purified talc in which the talc is sterilized before incorporation with the starch, or the final product is subject to a suitable terminal sterilization procedure.

Dusting powders are normally dispensed in glass or metal containers with a perforated lid. The powder must flow well from such a container, so that it can be dusted over the affected area. The active ingredients must therefore be diluted with materials having reasonably good flow properties, e.g. purified talc or maize starch.

Hexachlorophane dusting powder contains an antibacterial agent and talc dusting powder is used as a lubricant to prevent chafing. Proprietary products are available, usually for the treatment of bacterial or fungal infections, e.g. Canesten powder (clotrimazole) is used as an antifungal agent.

Insufflations

Insufflations are medicated powders which are blown into regions such as the ear, nose and throat using an insufflator. The use of traditional insufflations declined because they were not very acceptable, being more inelegant and less convenient to apply than other topical preparations. A second problem was that if the powder contained a drug that had systemic activity it was difficult, with the conventional insufflator, to ensure that the same dose was delivered on each occasion.

Some potent drugs are now presented in this way because they are rapidly absorbed when administered as a fine powder via the nose (see Chapter 37 for a detailed discussion of the nasal route of administration). To enhance convenience and ensure that a uniform dose is delivered on each occasion, devices have been developed to replace the traditional insufflator. Sufficient drug for one dose may be presented in a hard gelatin capsule diluted with an inert, soluble diluent such as lactose. The capsule is placed in the body of the insufflator and is broken when the device is assembled. The drug is inhaled by the patient as a fine powder.

Dry-powder inhalers

The use of dry-powder systems for pulmonary drug delivery is now extensive. This dosage form has developed into one of the most effective methods of delivering active ingredients to the lung for the treatment of asthma and chronic obstructive pulmonary disease. Its popularity is reflected in the number of commercial preparations available in a number of sophisticated and increasingly precise devices. Pulmonary delivery is discussed fully in Chapter 36, and the reader is referred there for further information.

PREPARATIONS REQUIRING FURTHER TREATMENT AT TIME OF DISPENSING

Oral antibiotic syrups

For patients who have difficulty taking capsules and tablets, e.g. young children, a liquid preparation of a drug offers a suitable alternative. However, many antibiotics are physically or chemically unstable when formulated as a solution or suspension. The method used to overcome this instability problem is to manufacture the dry ingredients of the intended liquid preparation in a suitable container in the form of a powder or granules. When the pharmacist dispenses the product, a given quantity of water is added to reconstitute the solution or suspension. This enables sufficient time for warehousing and distribution of the product and storage at the pharmacy without degradation. Once it is reconstituted, the patient is warned of the short shelf life. A shelf life of 1–2 weeks for the reconstituted syrup should not be a serious problem for the patient. Examples are Erythroped suspension and amoxicillin oral suspension.

Powders for injection

Injections of medicaments that are unstable in solution must be made immediately prior to use and are presented as sterile powders in ampoules. Sufficient diluent, e.g. sterile water for injections, is added from a second ampoule to produce the required drug concentration and the injection is used immediately. The powder may contain suitable excipients in addition to the drug, e.g. sufficient additive to produce an isotonic solution when the injection is reconstituted.

BIBLIOGRAPHY

British Pharmacopoeia (latest edition). Stationery Office, London.
Compendium of Data Sheets and Summaries of Product Characteristics (published annually). Datapharm Publications, London.
Monthly Index of Medical Specialties (MIMS). Haymarket Medical Publications, London.

Granulation

M. P. Summers, M. E. Aulton

INTRODUCTION

Granulation is the process in which *primary powder particles* are made to adhere to form larger multi-particle entities called *granules*. Pharmaceutical granules typically have a size range between 0.2 and 4.0 mm, depending on the subsequent use of the granules. In the majority of cases this will be undertaken during the production of tablets or capsules, when granules will be made as an intermediate product and have a typical size range between 0.2 and 0.5 mm, whereas larger granules are used as a dosage form in their own right (see Chapter 28).

Granulation normally commences after initial dry mixing of the necessary powdered ingredients so that a uniform distribution of each ingredient through the mix is achieved. After granulation, the granules will either be packed (when used as a dosage form) or they may be mixed with other excipients prior to tablet compaction or capsule filling.

Reasons for granulation

The reasons why granulation is often necessary are as follows:

To prevent segregation of the constituents of the powder mix

Segregation (or demixing, see Chapter 12) is primarily due to differences in the size or density of the components of the mix, the smaller particles and/or denser particles concentrating at the base of a container with the large particles and/or less dense above them. An ideal granulation will contain all the constituents of the mix in the correct proportion in each granule and segregation of the ingredients will not occur (Fig. 29.1).

It is also important to control the particle size distribution of the granules because, although the individual components may not segregate, if there is a wide size

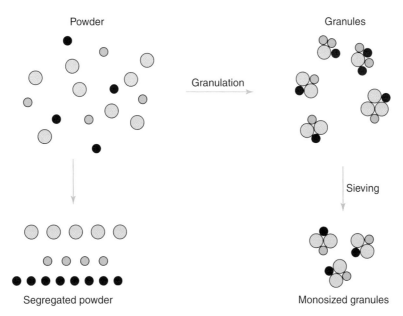

Fig. 29.1 Schematic diagram to illustrate how granulation can prevent powder segregation.

distribution, the granules themselves may segregate. If this occurs in the hoppers of sachet-filling machines, capsule-filling machines or tablet machines, products having large weight variations will result. This is because these machines fill by volume rather than weight and if different regions in the hopper contain granules of different sizes (and hence bulk density), a given volume in each region will contain a different weight of granules. This will lead to an unacceptable distribution of the drug content within the batch of finished product even though the drug is evenly distributed, weight per weight, through the granules.

To improve the flow properties of the mix

Many powders, because of their small size, irregular shape or surface characteristics, are cohesive and do not flow well. Poor flow will often result in a wide weight variation within the final product due to variable fill of tablet dies, etc. Granules produced from such a cohesive system will be larger and more isodiametric, both factors contributing to improved flow properties.

To improve the compaction characteristics of the mix

Some primary powder particles are difficult to compact even if a readily compactable adhesive is included in the blend, but granules of the same formulation are often more easily compacted and produce stronger tablets. This is associated with the distribution of the adhesive within the granule and is a function of the method employed to produce the granule. Often solute migration (see Chapter 30) occurring during the postgranulation drying stage results in a binder-rich outer layer to the granules. This in turn leads to direct binder–binder bonding which assists the consolidation of weakly bonding materials.

Other reasons

The above are the primary reasons for the granulation of pharmaceutical products but there are other reasons which may necessitate the granulation of powdered material:

- The granulation of toxic materials will reduce the hazard associated with the generation of toxic dust which may arise when handling powders. Suitable precautions must be taken to ensure that such dust is not a hazard during the granule drying process. Thus granules should be non-friable and have a suitable mechanical strength.
- Materials which are slightly hygroscopic may adhere and form a cake if stored as a powder. Granulation may reduce this hazard as the granules will be able to absorb some moisture and yet retain their flowability because of their size.
- Granules, being denser than the parent powder mix, occupy less volume per unit weight. They are therefore more convenient for storage or shipment.

Methods of granulation

Granulation methods can be divided into two types: *wet* methods which utilize a liquid in the process and *dry* methods in which no liquid is used.

In a suitable formulation a number of different excipients will be needed in addition to the drug. The common types used are diluents, to produce a unit dose weight of suitable size, and disintegrating agents which are added to aid the break-up of the granule when it reaches a liquid medium, e.g. on ingestion by the patient. Adhesives in the form of a dry powder may also be added, particularly if dry granulation is employed. These ingredients will be mixed before granulation.

Dry granulation

In the dry methods of granulation the primary powder particles are aggregated at high pressure. There are two main processes. Either a large tablet (known as a '*slug*') is produced in a heavy-duty tableting press (a process known as *slugging*) or the powder is squeezed between two rollers to produce a sheet of material (*roller compaction*). In both cases these intermediate products are broken using a suitable milling technique to produce granular material which is usually sieved to separate the desired size fraction. The unused fine material may be reworked to avoid waste. This dry method may be used for drugs which do not compress well after wet granulation or those which are sensitive to moisture.

Wet granulation (involving wet massing)

Wet granulation involves the massing of a mix of dry *primary powder particles* using a *granulating fluid*. The granulating fluid contains a solvent that must be volatile, so that it can be removed by drying, and non-toxic. Typical liquids include water, ethanol and isopropanol either alone or in combination. The granulation liquid may be used alone or, more usually, as a solvent containing a dissolved *adhesive* (also referred to as a *binder* or *binding agent*) which is used to ensure particle adhesion once the granule is dry.

Water is commonly used for economical and ecological reasons. The disadvantages of water as a solvent are that it may adversely affect drug stability, causing hydrolysis of susceptible products, and it needs a longer drying time than organic solvents. This long drying time increases the length of the process and again may affect stability because of the extended exposure to heat. The primary advantage of water is that it is non-flammable which means that expensive safety precautions such as the use of flame-proof equipment need not be taken. Organic solvents are used when water-sensitive drugs are processed, as an alternative to dry granulation or when a rapid drying time is required.

In the traditional wet granulation method, the wet mass is forced through a sieve to produce wet granules which are then dried. A subsequent screening stage breaks agglomerates of granules and removes the fine material which can be recycled. Variations of this traditional method are dependent upon the equipment used but the general principle of initial particle aggregation using a liquid remains in all of the processes.

Effect of granulation method on granule structure

The type and capacity of granulating mixers significantly influence the work input and time necessary to produce a cohesive mass, adequate liquid distribution and intragranular porosity of the granular mass. The method and conditions of granulation affect intergranular and intragranular pore structure by changing the degree of packing within the granules. It has been shown that precompacted granules, consisting of drug and binder particles, are held together by simple bonding formed during consolidation. Granules prepared by wet massing consist of intact drug particles held together in a sponge-like matrix of binder. Fluidized-bed granules are similar to granules prepared by the wet massing process but possess greater porosity, and the granule surface is covered by a film of binding agent. With spray-dried systems, the granules consist of spherical particles composed of an outer shell with an inner core of particles. Thus the properties of the granule are influenced by the manufacturing process.

GRANULATION MECHANISMS

Particle bonding mechanisms

To form granules, bonds must be formed between powder particles so that they adhere and these bonds must be sufficiently strong to prevent breakdown of the granule to powder in subsequent handling operations.

The five primary bonding mechanisms between particles are:

1. adhesion and cohesion forces in the immobile liquid films between individual primary powder particles
2. interfacial forces in mobile liquid films within the granules
3. the formation of solid bridges after solvent evaporation
4. attractive forces between solid particles
5. mechanical interlocking.

Different types of mechanism were identified in each group and the ones discussed below are those which are of relevance to pharmaceutical granulations.

Adhesion and cohesion forces in immobile films

If sufficient liquid is present in a powder to form a very thin, immobile layer, there will be an effective decrease in interparticulate distance and increase in contact area between the particles. The bond strength between the particles will be increased because of this, as the van der Waals forces of attraction are proportional to the particle diameter and inversely proportional to the square of the distance of separation.

This situation will arise with adsorbed moisture and accounts for the cohesion of slightly damp powders. Although such films may be present as residual liquid after granules prepared by wet granulation have been dried, it is unlikely that they contribute significantly to the final granule strength. In dry granulation, however, the pressures used will increase the contact area between the adsorption layers and decrease the interparticulate distance and this will contribute to the final granule strength.

Thin, immobile layers may also be formed by highly viscous solutions of adhesives and so the bond strength will be greater than that produced by the mobile films discussed below. The use of starch mucilage in pharmaceutical granulations may produce this type of film.

Interfacial forces in mobile liquid films

During wet granulation liquid is added to the powder mix and will be distributed as films around and between the particles. Sufficient liquid is usually added to exceed that necessary for an immobile layer and produce a mobile film. The three states of water distribution between particles are illustrated in Figure 29.2.

At low moisture levels, termed the *pendular state*, the particles are held together by lens-shaped rings of liquid. These cause adhesion because of the surface tension forces of the liquid–air interface and the hydrostatic suction pressure in the liquid bridge. When all the air has been displaced from between the particles, the *capillary state* is reached and the particles are held by capillary suction at the liquid–air interface which is now only at the granule surface. The *funicular state* represents an intermediate stage between the pendular and capillary states. Moist granule tensile strength increases about three times from the pendular to capillary state.

It may appear that the state of the powder bed is dependent upon the total moisture content of the wetted powders but the capillary state may also be reached by

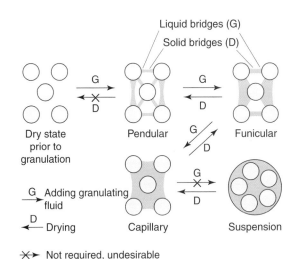

Fig. 29.2 Water distribution between particles of a granule during formation and drying.

decreasing the separation of the particles. In the massing process during wet granulation, continued kneading/mixing of material originally in the pendular state will densify the wet mass, decreasing the pore volume occupied by air and eventually producing the funicular or capillary state without further liquid addition.

In addition to these three states, a further state, the droplet, is illustrated in Figure 29.2. This will be important in the process of granulation by spray drying of a suspension. In this state, the strength of the droplet is dependent upon the surface tension of the liquid used.

These wet bridges are only temporary structures in wet granulation because the moist granules will be dried. They are, however, a prerequisite for the formation of solid bridges formed by adhesives present in the liquid or by materials which dissolve in the granulating liquid.

Solid bridges

These can be formed by:

- partial melting
- hardening binders and
- crystallization of dissolved substances.

Partial melting   Although not considered to be a predominant mechanism in pharmaceutical materials, it is possible that the pressures used in dry granulation methods may cause melting of low melting point materials where the particles touch and high pressures are developed. When the pressure is relieved, crystallization will take place, binding the particles together.

Hardening binders This is the common mechanism in pharmaceutical wet granulations when an adhesive is included in the granulating solvent. The liquid will form liquid bridges, as discussed above, and the adhesive will harden or crystallize on drying to form solid bridges to bind the particles. Adhesives such as polyvinylpyrrolidone, the cellulose derivatives (such as carboxymethylcellulose) and pregelatinized starch function in this way.

Crystallization of dissolved substances The solvent used to mass the powder during wet granulation may partially dissolve one of the powdered ingredients. When the granules are dried, crystallization of this material will take place and the dissolved substance then acts as a hardening binder. Any material soluble in the granulating liquid will function in this manner, e.g. lactose incorporated into powder blends granulated with water.

The size of the crystals produced in the bridge will be influenced by the rate of drying of the granules; the slower the drying time, the larger the particle size. It is therefore important that the drug does not dissolve in the granulating liquid and recrystallize because it may adversely affect the dissolution rate of the drug if crystals larger than that of the starting material are produced.

Attractive forces between solid particles

In the absence of liquids and solid bridges formed by binding agents, there are two types of attractive force which can operate between particles in pharmaceutical systems.

Electrostatic forces may be of importance in causing powder cohesion and the initial formation of agglomerates, e.g. during mixing. In general they do not contribute significantly to the final strength of the granule.

Van der Waals forces, however, are about four orders of magnitude greater than electrostatic forces and contribute significantly to the strength of granules produced by dry granulation. The magnitude of these forces will increase as the distance between adjacent surfaces decreases and in dry granulation this is achieved using pressure to force the particles together.

Mechanisms of granule formation

In the dry methods, adhesion of particles takes place because of applied pressure. A compact or sheet is produced which is larger than the granule size required and therefore the required size can be attained by milling and sieving.

In wet granulation methods, liquid added to dry powders has to be distributed through the powder by the mechanical agitation produced in the granulator. The particles adhere to each other because of liquid films and further agitation and/or liquid addition causes more

particles to adhere. The precise mechanism by which a dry powder is transformed into a bed of granules varies for each type of granulation equipment but the mechanism discussed below serves as a useful broad generalization of the process.

The proposed granulation mechanism can be divided into three stages.

Nucleation

Granulation starts with particle–particle contact and adhesion due to liquid bridges. A number of particles will join to form the pendular state illustrated in Figure 29.2. Further agitation densifies the pendular bodies to form the capillary state and these bodies act as nuclei for further granule growth.

Transition

Nuclei can grow by two possible mechanisms: either single particles can be added to the nuclei by pendular bridges or two or more nuclei may combine. The combined nuclei will be reshaped by the agitation of the bed.

This stage is characterized by the presence of a large number of small granules with a fairly wide size distribution. Providing that the size distribution is not excessively large, this point represents a suitable endpoint for granules used in capsule and tablet manufacture as relatively small granules will produce a uniform tablet die or capsule fill. Larger granules may give rise to problems in small-diameter dies due to bridging across the die and uneven fill.

Ball growth

Further granule growth produces large, spherical granules and the mean particle size of the granulating system will increase with time. If agitation is continued, granule coalescence will continue and produce an unusable, overmassed system, although this is dependent upon the amount of liquid added and the properties of the material being granulated.

Although ball growth produces granules which may be too large for pharmaceutical purposes, some degree of ball growth will occur in planetary mixers and it is an essential feature of some spheronizing equipment.

The four possible mechanisms of ball growth are illustrated in Figure 29.3.

Coalescence Two or more granules join to form a larger granule.

Breakage Granules break into fragments which adhere to other granules, forming a layer of material over the surviving granule.

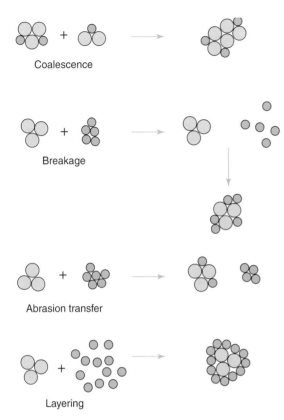

Fig. 29.3 Mechanisms of ball growth during granulation.

Abrasion transfer Agitation of the granule bed leads to attrition of material from granules. This abraded material adheres to other granules, increasing their size.

Layering When a second batch of powder mix is added to a bed of granules, the powder will adhere to the granules, forming a layer over the surface and thus increasing the granule size. This mechanism is only of relevance to the production of layered granules using spheronizing equipment.

There will be some degree of overlap between these stages and it will be very difficult to identify a given stage by inspection of the granulating system. For end-product uniformity, it is desirable to finish every batch of a formulation at the same stage and this may be a major problem in pharmaceutical production.

Using the slower processes such as the planetary mixer, there is usually a sufficient length of time to stop the process before overmassing. In faster granulation equipment, the duration of granulation can only be used as a control parameter when the formulation is such that granule growth is slow and takes place at a fairly uniform rate. In many cases, however, the transition from a non-granulated to an overmassed system is very rapid and monitoring equipment is necessary to stop the granulation at a predetermined point, known as granulation endpoint control.

PHARMACEUTICAL GRANULATION EQUIPMENT

Wet granulators

There are three main types of granulator used in the pharmaceutical industry for wet granulation.

Shear granulators

The older shear granulators have largely disappeared and have been replaced by the much more efficient high-speed mixer/granulators. In the traditional shear (or planetary) granulation process, dry-powder blending usually has to be performed as a separate initial operation using different powder-mixing equipment. The older process suffered from a number of major disadvantages: its long duration, the need for several pieces of equipment and the high material losses which can be incurred because of the transfer stages between the different equipment. The process served the industry well for many years but the advantages of modern mixer/granulators proved too attractive.

High-speed mixer/granulators

This type of granulator (e.g. Diosna) is used extensively for pharmaceutical granulation. They were developed from traditional planetary mixers in order to speed up the process and to reduce the number of pieces of equipment and separate process steps required. The machines have a stainless steel mixing bowl containing a three-bladed main impeller which revolves in the horizontal plane and a three-bladed auxiliary chopper (breaker blade) which revolves in either the vertical or horizontal plane (Fig. 29.4). The main blade is designed to rotate at about 150–300 rpm and the high-speed chopper rotates at about 1500 and 3000 rpm.

The unmixed dry powders are placed in the bowl and mixed by the rotating impeller for a few minutes. Granulating liquid is then added via a port in the lid of the granulator whilst the impeller is turning. The granulating fluid is mixed into the powders by the impeller. The chopper is usually switched on when the moist mass is formed as its function is to break up the wet mass to produce a bed of granular material. Once a satisfactory granule has been produced, the granular product is discharged, passing through a wire mesh, which breaks up

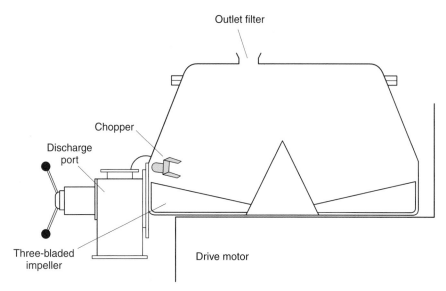

Fig. 29.4 High-speed mixer/granulator.

any large aggregates, into the bowl of a fluidized-bed drier.

Like most modern process equipment, high-speed mixer/granulators are available in a wide range of sizes. These are often designed to have similar geometric and powder movement characteristics in an attempt to minimize scale-up problems when a product moves from development to production. Bowl volumes between 1 L and 1250 L are available. The weight of powder that each one holds will depend on its bulk density and the optimum fill capacity (working volume) of each bowl. Bowls are manufactured from high-quality polished stainless steel.

The advantage of the process is that powder blending, wet massing and granulation are all performed in a few minutes in the same piece of equipment. The process needs to be controlled with care as the granulation progresses so rapidly that a usable granule can be transformed very quickly into an unusable, overmassed system. Thus it is often necessary to use a suitable monitoring system to indicate the end of the granulation process, i.e. when a granule of the desired properties has been attained. The process is also sensitive to variations in raw materials but this may be minimized by using a suitable endpoint monitor.

A variation of the Diosna type of design is the Collette UltimaGral mixer (GEA Collette, Vanguard) (Fig. 29.5). This is based on the bowl and overhead drive of the planetary mixer but the single paddle of a planetary mixer is replaced with two mixing shafts. One of these carries three blade arms which rotate in the horizontal plane at

the base of the bowl and the second carries smaller blades which act as the chopper and rotate rapidly in the upper regions of the granulating mass. Thus the operation principle is similar to that of the Diosna type described above.

This design is available in sizes ranging from 10 L to 200 L volume (capable of processing about 3 kg to 80 kg batches, respectively). The main mixing blade rotates at 450–600 rpm in the 10 L model and at 150–200 rpm in the 200 L model. This rotational speed variation is to attempt to maintain the same linear velocity of movement of the blades as this has been found to help scale-up. In all models the high-speed chopper rotates at 1500–3000 rpm.

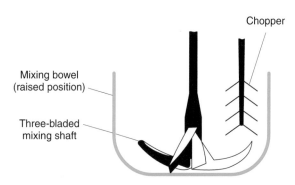

Fig. 29.5 Collette-Gral type of granulator: mixing shafts and bowl.

An attractive feature of high-speed granulators is the fact that the product is usually granular and a separate step to granulate the wet mass is avoided (the granules being produced by the action of the high-speed chopper). Occasionally this is not fully satisfactory and the moist mass then has to be transferred to a granulator such as an oscillating granulator (Fig. 29.6). The rotor bars of the granulator oscillate at an adjustable rate between 60 and 100 rpm and force the moist mass through the sieve screen, the size of which determines the granule size. The mass should be sufficiently moist to form discrete granules when sieved. If excess liquid is added at the wet massing stage, strings of material will be formed and if the mix is too dry, the mass will be sieved to powder and granules will not be formed.

This type of granulator can also deal with the size reduction of dry material. They are available in a range of sizes capable of dealing with 300–500 kg of wet mass per hour or 700–1200 kg/h of dry mass.

Fluidized-bed granulators

Fluidized-bed granulators (e.g. Aeromatic-Fielder, Glatt, Vanguard) have a similar design and operation to fluidized-bed driers, i.e. the powder particles are fluidized in a stream of air, but in addition granulation fluid is sprayed from a nozzle onto the bed of powders (Fig. 29.7).

Heated and filtered air is blown or sucked through the bed of unmixed powders to fluidize the particles and mix the powders; fluidization is actually a very efficient mixing process. Granulating fluid is pumped from a reservoir through a spray nozzle or multiple nozzles positioned over the bed of particles. A variety of spray nozzles is available to cope with a wide range of products. The granulating fluid causes the primary powder particles to adhere when the droplets and powders collide. Escape of material from the granulation chamber is prevented by exhaust filters which are periodically agitated to reintroduce the collected material into the fluidized bed. Sufficient liquid is sprayed to produce granules of the required size at which point the spray is turned off – but the fluidizing air continued. The wet granulates are then dried in the heated fluidizing air stream.

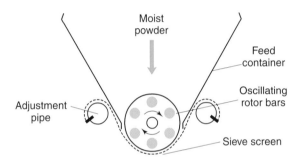

Fig. 29.6 Oscillating granulator.

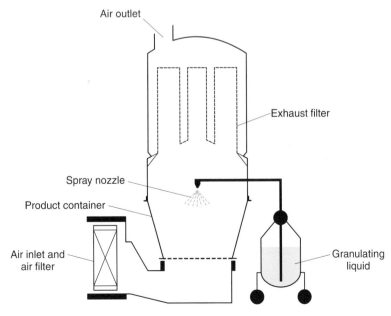

Fig. 29.7 Fluidized-bed granulator.

Commercial apparatus ranges from laboratory models that, by changing the bowl, have a volume between 0.2 and 2 L, giving a capacity of a few grams up to about 1 kg, up to production machines. A wide range is available to cope with the wide variety of production volumes encountered in the pharmaceutical industry. They can be obtained in sizes suitable for batches between 5 kg and a massive 1550 kg, these calculations being based on an optimum 70% bowl fill and a powder/granule bulk density of 0.5 kg/L.

Advantages of fluidized-bed granulation Fluidized-bed granulation has many advantages over conventional wet massing. All the granulation processes, which normally need separate equipment in the conventional method, are performed in one unit, saving labour costs, transfer losses and time. Another advantage of the process is that automation of the process can be achieved once the conditions affecting the granulation have been optimized.

Disadvantages of fluidized-bed granulation On the downside, the equipment is initially expensive and optimization of process (and product) parameters affecting granulation needs extensive development work, not only during initial formulation work but also during scale-up from development to production scale. Similar development work for the traditional process and that using high-speed granulators is not as extensive.

This long and very product-specific development process has proved to be a serious problem with fluidized-bed granulation in the pharmaceutical industry. There are numerous apparatus, process and product parameters which affect the quality of the final granule; these are listed in Table 29.1. The extent of this list, coupled with the fact that each formulation presents its own individual development problems, has led to fluidized-bed granulation not fulfilling its full potential in pharmaceutical production. This is exacerbated by the reality that most pharmaceutical companies have a wide range of products made at relatively small batch size, unlike other industries (fertilizers, herbicides, foodstuffs) where fluidized-bed granulation is used successfully and extensively. Intelligent computer control of the whole process is available but requires careful setting up to cope with this sensitivity to small changes in formulation and process variables.

Spray driers

These differ from the method discussed above in that a dry, granular product is made from a solution or a suspension rather than initially dry primary powder particles. The solution or suspension may be of drug alone, a single excipient or a complete formulation.

The process of spray drying is discussed more fully in Chapter 30. The resultant granules are free-flowing hollow spheres and the distribution of the binder in such granules (at the periphery following solute migration during drying) results in good compaction properties.

This process can be used to make tablet granules although it is probably economically justified for this purpose only when suitable granules cannot be produced by the other methods. Spray drying can convert hard elastic materials into more ductile materials. Spray-dried lactose is the classic example and its advantages over α-lactose monohydrate crystals when compacted are discussed in Chapter 31.

The primary advantages of the process are the short drying time and the minimal exposure of the product to heat due to the short residence time in the drying chamber. This means that little deterioration of heat-sensitive

Table 29.1 Apparatus, process and product variables influencing fluidized-bed granulation

Apparatus parameters	Process parameters	Product parameters
Air distribution place	Bed load	Type of binder
Shape of granulator body	Fluidizing air flow rate	Quantity of binder
Nozzle height	Fluidizing air temperature	Binder solvent
Positive or negative pressure operation	Fluidizing air humidity	Concentration of granulating solution
	Atomization	Temperature of granulating solution
	Nozzle type	Starting materials
	Spray angle	Fluidization
	Spraying regime	Powder hydrophobicity
	Liquid flow rate	
	Atomizing air flow rate	
	Atomizing air pressure	
	Droplet size	

materials takes place and it may be the only process suitable for this type of product.

Spheronizers/pelletizers

For some applications it may be desirable to have a dense, spherical pellet of the type difficult to produce with the equipment above. Such pellets are used for controlled drug release products following coating with a suitable polymer coat and filling into hard gelatin capsules. Capsule filling with a mixture of coated and non-coated drug-containing pellets would give some degree of programmed drug release after the capsule shell dissolves.

A commonly used process involves the separate processes of wet massing, followed by extrusion of this wet mass into rod-shaped granules and subsequent spheronization of these granules. Because this process is used so frequently to produce modified-release multiparticulates, this process will be discussed in some detail.

Extrusion/spheronization

Extrusion/spheronization is a multi-step process used to make uniformly sized spherical particles. It is primarily used as a method to produce multiparticulates for controlled drug release applications. The major advantage over other methods of producing drug-loaded spheres or pellets is the ability to incorporate high levels of active ingredients without producing excessively large particles (i.e. minimal excipients are necessary).

The main steps of the process are:

- *dry mixing of ingredients* to achieve a homogeneous powder dispersion
- *wet massing* to produce a sufficiently plastic wet mass
- *extrusion* to form rod-shaped particles of uniform diameter
- *spheronization* to round off these rods into spherical particles
- *drying* to achieve the desired final moisture content
- *screening* (optional) to achieve the desired narrow size distribution.

Applications of extrusion/spheronization

Potential applications are many but relate mainly to controlled drug release and improved processing.

Controlled drug release Both immediate-release and controlled-release pellets can be formed. In turn, these pellets can either be filled into hard gelatin capsule shells or compacted into tablets to form unit dosage forms. Pellets can contain two or more ingredients in the same individual unit or incompatible ingredients can be manufactured in separate pellets.

Pellets can be coated in sub-batches to give, say, rapid-, intermediate- and slow-release pellets in the same capsule shell. Dense multiparticulates disperse evenly within the GI tract and have less variable gastric emptying and intestinal transit times than single units, such as coated monolithic tablets.

Processing The process of extrusion/spheronization can be used to increase the bulk density, improve flow properties and reduce the problems of dust usually encountered with low-density, finely divided active and excipient powders.

Extrusion/spheronization is a more labour-intensive process than other forms of granulation and therefore should only be considered when other methods of granulation are either not satisfactory for that particular formulation or are inappropriate (i.e. when spheres are required).

Desirable properties of pellets

Uncoated pellets have:

- uniform spherical shape
- uniform size
- good flow properties
- reproducible packing (into hard gelatin capsules)
- high strength
- low friability
- low dust
- smooth surface
- ease of coating

and once coated:

- maintain all of the above properties, and
- have desired drug release characteristics.

Process

Dry mixing of ingredients This uses normal powder mixing equipment.

Wet massing This stage also employs normal equipment and processes as used in wet granulation. There are two major differences in the granulation step compared with granulation for compaction:

- amount of granulation fluid. and
- the importance of achieving a uniform dispersion of fluid.

The amount of fluid needed to achieve spheres of uniform size and sphericity is likely to be greater than that for a similar tablet granulation. Poor liquid dispersion will produce a poor-quality product.

Extrusion Extrusion produces rod-shaped particles of uniform diameter from the wet mass. The wet mass is forced through dies and shaped into small cylindrical particles with uniform diameter. The extrudate particles break at similar lengths under their own weight. Thus the extrudate must have enough plasticity to deform but not so much that the extruded particles adhere to other particles when collected or rolled in the spheronizer.

There are many designs of extruder but generally they can be divided into three classes, based on their feed mechanism:

- screw-feed extruders (axial or endplate, dome and radial)
- gravity-feed extruders (cylinder roll, gear roll, radial)
- piston-feed extruders (ram).

The first two categories (shown in Fig. 29.8) are used for both development and production but the latter is only used for experimental development work as it is easy to add instrumentation.

The primary extrusion process variables are:

- the feed rate of the wet mass
- the diameter of the die
- the length of the die
- water content of the wet mass. The properties of the extrudate, and thus the resulting spheres, are very dependent on the plasticity and cohesiveness of the wet mass. In general, an extrudable wet mass needs to be wetter than that appropriate for conventional granulation by wet massing.

Spheronization The function of the fourth step in the process (i.e. spheronization) is to round off the rods produced by extrusion into spherical particles.

This process is carried out in a relatively simple piece of apparatus (Fig. 29.9). The working part consists of a bowl having fixed side walls, with a rapidly rotating bottom plate or disc. The rounding of the extrudate into spheres is dependent on frictional forces generated by particle–particle and particle–equipment collisions.

The bottom disc has a grooved surface to increase these forces. Two geometric patterns are generally used:

- a cross-hatched pattern with grooves running at right angles to one another, and
- a radial pattern with grooves running radially from the centre of the disc.

The transition from rods to spheres during spheronization occurs in various stages. These are best described by examining the diagrams in Figure 29.10.

If the moist mass is too dry spheres will not be formed; the rods will only transform as far as dumbbells.

Drying A drying stage is required in order to achieve the desired moisture content. Drying is often the final step in the process. Drying of the pellets can be accomplished in any dryer that can be used for conventional wet granulations, including tray dryers and fluidized-bed dryers. Both are used successfully for extrusion/spheronization. If solute migration (see Chapter 30) occurs during drying of the wet spheres, this may result in:

- increased initial rate of dissolution
- stronger pellets, and
- modified surfaces which might reduce the adhesion of any added film coats.

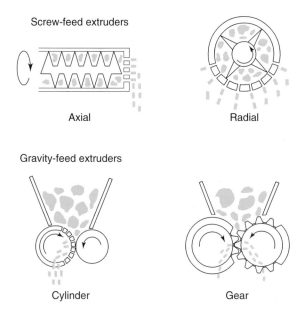

Screw-feed extruders

Axial   Radial

Gravity-feed extruders

Cylinder   Gear

Fig. 29.8 Schematic representation of production extruders.

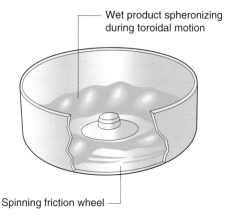

Wet product spheronizing during toroidal motion

Spinning friction wheel

Fig. 29.9 A spheronizer showing the characteristic toroidal (rope-like) movement of the forming pellets in the spheronizer bowl during operation.

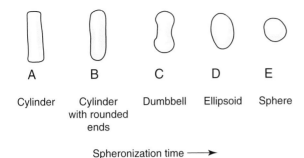

A	B	C	D	E
Cylinder	Cylinder with rounded ends	Dumbbell	Ellipsoid	Sphere

Spheronization time ⟶

Fig. 29.10 Representation of a mechanism of spheronization. The diagram shows a transition from cylindrical particles (a) into cylindrical particles with rounded edges (b), then dumbbells (c), to ellipsoids (d) and finally spheres (e).

Screening (optional) Screening may be necessary in order to achieve the desired narrow size distribution. Normal sieves are used. If all the previous stages are performed efficiently and with careful development of process and formulation conditions, this step may not be necessary.

Formulation variables

The composition of the wet mass is critical in determining the properties of the particles produced. During the granulation step a wet mass is produced which must be plastic, deform when extruded and break off to form uniformly sized cylindrical particles which are easily deformed into spherical particles. Thus the process has a complex set of requirements that are strongly influenced by the ingredients of the pellet formulation.

Summary

Extrusion/spheronization is a versatile process capable of producing spherical granules having very useful properties. Because it is more labour intensive than more common wet massing techniques, its use should be limited to those applications where a sphere is required and other granulation techniques are unsuitable.

The most common application of the process is to produce spherical pellets for controlled drug release.

Care must be taken to understand the required properties of the pellets and the manner in which the process and formulation influence the ability to achieve these aims.

Developments of the standard extrusion/spheronization process allow heated extrusion of formulations containing excipients which melt and bind the ingredients together. This is *melt granulation*. Low melting point waxes are used in the process.

Rotorgranulation

This process allows the direct manufacture of spheres suitable for controlled-release solid dosage forms from dry powder in one process. The powder mix is added to the bowl and wetted with granulating liquid from a spray or multiple sprays (Fig. 29.11). The base plate rotates at high speed and centrifugal force keeps the moist mass at the edges of the rotor. Here the velocity difference

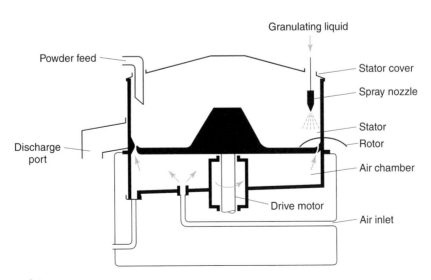

Granulating liquid

Powder feed — Stator cover

Spray nozzle

Discharge port — Stator

Rotor

Air chamber

Drive motor

Air inlet

Fig. 29.11 Rotorgranulator.

between the rotor and static walls, combined with the upward flow of air around the rotor plate, causes the mass to move in a toroidal motion, resulting in the formation of discrete spherical pellets. This is an almost identical motion to that occurring in spheronizers, as shown in Figure 29.10. The resulting spheres (actually, of course, wet granules) are dried by the heated inlet air from the air chamber which also acts as a positive-pressure seal during granulation.

Using this technique, it is possible to continue the process and coat the pellets by subsequently spraying coating solution on to the rotating dried pellets. Additionally, layered pellets can be produced by using uncoated pellets as nuclei in a second granulation with a powder mix of a second ingredient or ingredients.

Rotorgranulators (e.g. Freund, Vanguard) are manufactured in size ranges between 45 L and 450 L capacity. Again, the corresponding fill weights will depend upon the bulk density of the formulation and the optimum operating capacity of each bowl. This range requires corresponding bowl and rotor disc diameters between 300 and 1400 mm. Discs with different surface roughness patterns are available to cope with a wide range of materials. They also come with an adjustable air gap around the plate to assist in the manipulation of resulting granule size. Powder charging and discharging are made easy and there is precise powder feeding. Intelligent computer control of the whole process is available.

Dry granulators

Dry granulation converts primary powder particles into granules using the application of pressure without the intermediate use of a liquid. It therefore avoids heat/temperature combinations which may cause degradation of the product.

Two pieces of equipment are necessary for dry granulation: first, a machine for compressing the dry powders into compacts or flakes and second, a mill for breaking up these intermediate products into granules.

Slugging

The dry powders can be compacted using a conventional tablet machine or, more usually, a large heavy-duty rotary press can be used. This process is often known as 'slugging', the compacts made in the process (typically 25 mm diameter by about 10–15 mm thick) being termed 'slugs'. A hammer mill is suitable for breaking the compacts. This is an old process that is being replaced by the more modern roller compaction. Many pharmaceutical tableting materials suffer from a property known as *work hardening* which

results in poor recompaction of these already compacted granules.

Roller compaction

Roller compaction is an alternative gentler method, the powder mix being squeezed between two counterrotating rollers to form a compressed sheet (Fig. 29.12). The roller rotation speeds can be adjusted to allow variation in the compression time as the material passes between the rollers. Additionally, roller pressure can be adjusted and is maintained constant during a run by means of a hydraulic control system to yield resulting granules of constant crushing strength. Even rollers with different surface grooves are available if a particular product is troublesome.

The sheet so formed is normally weak and brittle and breaks immediately into flakes that can be somewhat similar to cornflakes in their geometry. These flakes need gentler treatment to break them into granules. An oscillating granulator of the type shown in Figure 29.6 can be

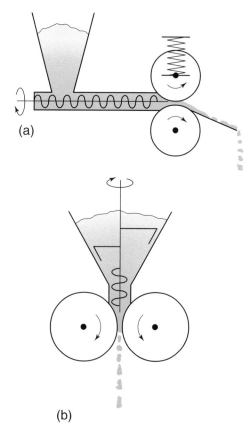

Fig. 29.12 Roller compaction: (a) Alexanderwerk and (b) Protec types.

used with care but often the conversion of these flakes to granules can be achieved by screening alone. Separation of fines (small powder particles) formed during the size reduction stage is often necessary. With suitable documentation, these may be recycled.

Advantages of the roller compaction process

- The process is economical as it dispenses with the intermediate stages of wet massing and drying, and thus the associated energy and other processing costs.
- It can cope with a wide range of materials, particle size, bulk density and flowability. However, experience has shown that not all materials respond to roller compaction as they do not possess suitable deformation or cohesion properties.
- There are relatively low investment costs compared with alternative granulation processes using multiple, and more expensive, equipment.
- The process is easily scaled up.
- The product has uniform properties with respect to its mechanical strength.
- Additionally, the more gentle 'squeeze' of roller compactors leaves the resulting granules capable of further compaction into tablets without the work-hardening problems encountered with slugging.

Again, like most modern pharmaceutical process machinery, a wide range of sizes is available capable of operating with a wide range of throughputs and compaction forces (e.g. Alexanderwerk, Powtec). In the case of roller compactors, this range is enormous, being available for throughputs between 10 and 2000 kg/h and compaction forces between 16 and 64 kN/cm of roller length. This is achieved by the choice of machines with roller diameters of between 100 mm and 450 mm and roller lengths of 30 mm to 115 mm This allows a wide range of APIs (active pharmaceutical ingredients, i.e. drugs) and excipients to be processed (or co-processed) and enables easy scale-up from a few hundred grams in development to very large-scale production of a successful product.

The Protec or Hutt type (Fig. 29.12b) has a vertical screw feeder in the hopper which produces an even flow of the material. Due to its design, it also has a precompacting and de-aerating effect on the powder charge. The speed of this screw, and that of the rollers, can be adjusted to provide control to the process.

BIBLIOGRAPHY

There are many published papers in the field of pharmaceutical granulation and only a very limited number is listed below.

Alvarez, L., Concheiro, A., Gomez-Amoza, J.L., Souto, C., Martinez-Pacheco R. (2002) Effect of microcrystalline cellulose grade and process variables on pellets prepared by extrusion-spheronisation. *Drug Development and Industrial Pharmacy,* **28**(4), 451-456.

Baert, L. (1992) Correlation of extrusion forces, raw materials and sphere characteristics. *Journal of Pharmacy and Pharmacology*, **44**, 676-678.

Das, S., Jarowski, C.I. (1979) Effect of granulating method on particle size distribution of granules and disintegrated tablets. *Drug Development and Industrial Pharmacy,* **5**, 479.

Erkoboni, D.F. (2003) Extrusion/spheronisation. *Drugs and the Pharmaceutical Sciences Series,* (eds) Ghebre-Sellassie I. and Martin C., Marcel Dekker, 2003. **133**, 277-322.

Farag Badawy, S.I. (2000) Effect of process parameters on compressibility of granulation manufactured in a higher-shear mixer. *International Journal of Pharmaceutics,* **198**(1), 51-61.

Faure, A., Grimsey, I.M., Rowe, R.C., York, P., Cliff, M.J. (1999) Applicability of a scale-up methodology for the wet granulation process in Collette Gral high shear mixer granulators. *European Journal of Pharmaceutical Sciences,* **8**, 85-93.

Gandhi, R., Kaul, C.L., Panchagnula, R. (1999) Extrusion and spheronization in the development of oral controlled-release dosage forms. *Pharmaceutical Science and Technology Today*, **2**(4), 160-181.

Gergely, G. (1981) Granulation – a new approach. *Manufacturing Chemist and Aerosol News,* **52**, 43.

Keleb, E.I., Vermeire, A., Vervaet, C., Jean Paul Remon (2004) Extrusion granulation and high shear granulation of lactose and highly dosed drugs: a comparative study. *Drug Development and Industrial Pharmacy,* **30**(6), 679-691.

Landin, M., York, P., Cliff, M.J., Rowe, R.C. (1999) Scale up of a pharmaceutical granulation in planetary mixers. *Pharmaceutical Development and Technology,* **4**(2), 145-150.

Law, M.F., Deasy, P.B., McLaughlin, J.P., Gabriel, S. (1997) Comparison of two commercial brands of microcrystalline cellulose for extrusion-spheronization. *Journal of Microencapsulation,* **14**(6), 713-723.

Lindberg, N.O., Leander, L. (1982) Instrumentation of a Kenwood major domestic-type mixer for studies of granulation. *Drug Development and Industrial Pharmacy,* **8**, 775.

Lodaya, M., Mollan, M., Ghebre-Sellassie I. et al (2003) Twin-screw wet granulation. *Drugs and the Pharmaceutical Sciences Series,* Eds. Ghebre-Sellassie I. and Martin C., Marcel Dekker, **133**, 323-343.

Maejima, T. et al (1998) Application of tumbling melt granulation (TMG) method to prepare controlled-release fine granules. *Chemical and Pharmaceutical Bulletin,* **46**(3), 534-536.

Nurnberg, E., Wunderlich, J. (1998) Manufacturing pellets by extrusion and spheronization (Part I). *Pharmaceutical Technology Europe,* **11**(2), 41-47; Part II **11**(3).

Ogaua, S., Kanijitra T., Miyanoto, Y., Miyajitra, M., Sato, H., Takayana, K., Nagai, T. (1994) A new attempt to solve the scale-up problem for granulation using response surface methodology. *Journal of Pharmaceutical Sciences,* **83**(3), 439-443.

Parikh, D.M. (1997) *Handbook of Pharmaceutical Granulation Technology.* Marcel Dekker, New York.

Rubino, O.R. (1999) Fluid-bed technology: overview and criteria for process selection. *Pharmaceutical Technology,* **6**, 104-113.

Shah, R.D., Mohan Kabadi, Pope, D.G., Aysburger, L.L. (1995) Physico-mechanical characterization of the extrusion-spheronization process. Part II: Rheological determinants for successful extrusion and spheronization. *Pharmaceutical Research,* **12**(4), 496-507.

Thoma, K., Ziegler, I. (1998) Investigations on the influence of the type of extruder for pelletization by extrusion-spheronization I. Extrusion behavior of formulations. *Drug Development and Industrial Pharmacy,* **24**(5), 401-411; II Sphere characteristics. *Drug Development and Industrial Pharmacy,* **24**(5), 413-422.

Vilhelmsen, T., Kristensen, J., Schaefer, T. et al (2004) Melt pelletization with polyethylene glycol in a rotary processor. *International Journal of Pharmaceutics,* **275**, 141-153.

Wørts, O. (1998) Wet granulation – fluidized bed and high shear techniques compared. *Pharmaceutical Technology Europe,* **10**(11), 27-30.

Zhang, F., McGinty, J.M. (1999) Properties of sustained-release tablets prepared by hot-melt etrusion. *Pharmaceutical Development and Technology,* **4**(2), 241-250.

30

Drying

M. E. Aulton

CHAPTER CONTENTS

INTRODUCTION

Drying is an important operation in primary pharmaceutical manufacture (i.e. the synthesis of drugs, also called active pharmaceutical ingredients (APIs)) since it is usually the last stage of manufacturing before packaging, often following a crystallization step. It is important that the residual moisture is rendered low enough to prevent product deterioration during storage and ensure free-flowing properties during use. It is equally important (and probably encountered more frequently) in secondary (dosage form) manufacture following the common operation of wet granulation (see Chapter 29) during the preparation of granules prior to tablet compaction. Hence, stability (see Chapter 44), flow properties (see Chapter 13) and compactability (see Chapter 31) are all influenced by residual moisture.

This chapter is concerned with drying to the 'dry' solid state starting with either a wet solid or a solution or suspension. The former is usually achieved by exposing the wet solid to moving, relatively dry air (elevated temperatures to accelerate the process are common). The latter is possible with equipment such as the spray dryer (see later in this chapter) that is capable of producing a dry product from solution or suspension in one operation.

Most pharmaceutical materials are not completely free from moisture (i.e. they are not 'bone dry') but contain some residual water, the amount of which may vary with the temperature and humidity of the ambient air to which they are exposed. This is discussed in more detail in this chapter.

For the purpose of this chapter, drying is defined as the removal of all or most of the liquid associated with a wet pharmaceutical product. All drying processes of relevance to pharmaceutical manufacturing involve evaporation or sublimation of the liquid phase and the removal of the subsequent vapour. The process must provide the latent heat for these processes without significant temperature rise. Naturally the latter will enhance the potential of thermal degradation of the product. In the majority of cases the 'liquid' will be water but more volatile organic solvents, such as isopropanol, may also need to be removed in a drying process. The physical principles of aqueous or organic solvent drying are similar regardless of the nature of the liquid though volatile solvents are normally recovered by condensation rather than being vented into the atmosphere. This is for environmental and economic reasons. Also, the toxicity and flammability of organic solvents pose additional safety and process considerations.

DRYING OF WET SOLIDS

Fundamental properties and interrelationships

An understanding of this operation requires some preliminary explanation of the following important terms. To avoid confusion and repetition, these terms will be defined and explained in the context of water (the most commonly used pharmaceutical solvent) but the explanations and concepts are equally applicable to other relevant liquids (e.g. ethanol, isopropanol, etc.).

Moisture content of wet solids

The moisture content of a wet solid is expressed as kg of moisture associated with 1 kg of the moisture-free or 'bone-dry' solid. Thus a moisture content of 0.4 means that 0.4 kg of water is present per kg of the 'bone-dry' solid that will remain after complete drying. It is sometimes calculated as percentage moisture content; thus this example would be quoted as 40% moisture content.

Total moisture content

This is the total amount of liquid associated with a wet solid. Some of this water can be easily removed by the simple evaporative processes employed by most pharmaceutical dryers and some cannot. The amount of easily removable water (*unbound water*) is known as the *free moisture content* and the moisture content of the water that is more difficult to remove in practice (*bound water*) is the *equilibrium moisture content*. Thus the total moisture content of a solid is equal to its free moisture content plus its equilibrium moisture content.

Unbound water   The unbound water associated with a wet solid exists as a liquid and it exerts its full vapour pressure. It can be removed readily by evaporation. During a drying process this unbound water is readily lost but the resulting solid will not be completely free from water molecules as it remains in contact with atmospheric air that inevitably contains water itself. Consequently the resulting solid is often known as *air dry*.

Equilibrium moisture content

As mentioned above, evaporative drying processes will not remove all the possible moisture present in a wet product because the drying solid equilibrates with the moisture that is naturally present in air. The moisture content of a solid under steady-state ambient conditions is termed the *equilibrium moisture content*. Its value will change with the temperature and humidity of the air, and with the nature of the solid (see later in this chapter).

Bound water Part of the moisture present in a wet solid may be adsorbed on surfaces of the solid or be absorbed within its structure to such an extent that it is prevented from developing its full vapour pressure and therefore from being easily removed by evaporation. Such moisture is described as 'bound water' and is more difficult to remove than unbound water. Adsorbed water is attached to the surface of the solid as individual water molecules which may form a mono-(or bi-) layer on the solid surface. Absorbed bound water exists as a liquid but is trapped in capillaries within the solid by surface tension. As such, it cannot exert its full vapour pressure and is not easily lost by evaporation.

Moisture content of air

An added complication to the drying process is that the drying air also contains moisture. Many pharmaceutical plants have air-conditioning systems to reduce the humidity of the incoming process air but removing water from air is a very expensive process and therefore not all the water will be removed. The moisture content of air is expressed as kg of water per kg of 'bone-dry' (water-free) dry air.

The moisture content of air is not altered by changes in its temperature alone, only by changes in the amount of moisture taken up by the air. The moisture content of air should be carefully distinguished from the relative humidity.

Relative humidity (RH) of air

Ambient air is a simple solution of water in a mixture of gases and as such follows the rules of most solutions – such as increased water solubility with increasing temperature, a maximum solubility at a particular temperature (saturation) and precipitation of the solute on cooling (condensation, rain!). Incidentally, this is exactly why rain is sometimes called precipitation.

At a given temperature air is capable of 'taking up' (i.e. dissolving) water vapour until it is saturated (at 100% RH). Lower relative humidities can be quantified in terms of *percentage relative humidity*, which is given by:

$$\frac{\text{Vapour pressure of water vapour in the air}}{\substack{\text{Vapour pressure of water vapour in air} \\ \text{saturated at the same temperature}}} \times 100 \quad (30.1)$$

This is *approximately* equal to the *percentage saturation*, which is:

$$\frac{\text{Mass of water vapour present per kg of dry air}}{\substack{\text{Mass of water vapour required to saturate} \\ \text{1 kg of dry air at the same temperature}}} \times 100 \quad (30.2)$$

Percentage saturation is the more fundamental measure but the expression 'relative humidity' is most commonly used. The two differ only very slightly in practice and only because water vapour does not behave exactly like an ideal gas.

These relationships show that the relative humidity of air is dependent not only on the amount of moisture in the air but also on its temperature. This is because the amount of water required to saturate air is itself dependent on temperature. As mentioned before, in ambient air water is in solution in the air gases and in this case its solubility increases with increasing temperature. If the temperature of the air is raised whilst its moisture content remains constant, the air will theoretically be capable of taking up more moisture and therefore its *relative* humidity falls. A reexamination of Equations 30.1 and 30.2 will show this.

It is important to understand the difference between moisture content and relative humidity of air. This is important in many contexts (powder properties, granulation, drying, compaction, storage conditions) but these terms are often confused.

An additional complication to be taken into account is that *during* a drying process both the temperature and moisture content of the drying air (and therefore its relative humidity) could change significantly. This arises from two separate factors:

- uptake into the drying air of evaporated water vapour from the drying solid. If evaporation is high and vapour removal inefficient, the drying efficiency will rapidly fall
- the cooling of the supply air (and consequently the product) as the air transfers latent heat to the wet solid. This phenomenon is known as *evaporative cooling*. If the cooling is excessive the temperature of the air may fall to a value known as the *dew point*. Here the solubility of water in the cooler air is reduced to such a point that it is exceeded and liquid water will condense and be deposited.

Relationship between equilibrium moisture content, relative humidity and the nature of the solid

The equilibrium moisture content of a solid exposed to moist air varies with the relative humidity and with the nature of the solid, as shown in some typical plots (Fig. 30.1). If we assume that the atmospheric conditions are of the order of 20°C and 70–75% relative humidity, a mineral such as kaolin will contain about 1% bound moisture, while a starch-based product may have as much as 30% or more.

Loss of water from wet solids

As explained above, unbound water is easily lost by evaporation until the equilibrium moisture content of the

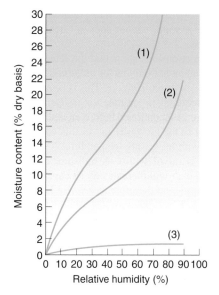

Fig. 30.1 Typical equilibrium moisture contents at 20°C.
(1) Starch-based materials. (2) Textiles and fibrous materials.
(3) Inorganic substance, such as kaolin.

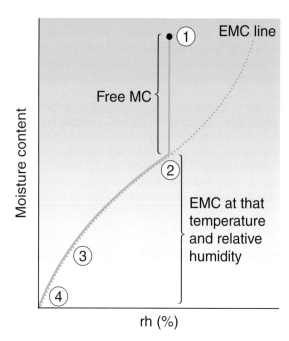

Fig. 30.2 Loss of water from a drying solid. The wet solid prior to drying is at condition (1). It can lose water by evaporation to position (2), its equilibrium moisture content at that RH. The only way the solid can lose more water is to reduce the RH of the atmosphere, to (3) with silica gel or to (4) with phosphorus pentoxide.

solid is reached. This is shown in Figure 30.2. Once the solid reaches its equilibrium moisture content, extending the time of drying will not change the moisture content since an equilibrium situation has been reached. The only way to reduce the moisture content of the solid shown in Figure 30.2 is to reduce the relative humidity of the ambient air. This can be achieved on a large scale with an air-conditioning system. On a laboratory scale, desiccators are used. Silica gel (a common laboratory and packaging desiccant) does not directly take water from a solid; instead it acts by removing the water from the air, thereby reducing its relative humidity to around 5–10%. This in turn causes the equilibrium to move along the drying curve in Figure 30.2 to the left, thus reducing the moisture content of the solids. Phosphorus pentoxide works in an identical manner but it has an even greater affinity for the water in the storage air.

If dried materials are exposed to humid ambient conditions they will quickly regain moisture from the atmosphere since this relationship is an equilibrium. Figure 30.1 shows this. Thus it is unnecessary to 'overdry' a product and there is no advantage in drying to a moisture content lower than that which the material will have under the normal conditions of use.

If low residual moisture content is necessary due to a hydrolytic instability in the material, the dried product must be efficiently sealed during or immediately after the drying process to prevent ingress of moisture. It also worthy of note that some solid pharmaceutical materials perform better when they contain a small amount of

residual water. Powders will flow better; the flow of very dry powders is inhibited by static charge. Tablet granules have superior compaction properties with a small amount (1–2 %) of residual moisture.

TYPES OF DRYING METHOD

Choice of drying method

When considering how to dry a material, the following points should be considered:

- heat sensitivity of the material being dried
- physical characteristics of the material
- nature of the liquid to be removed
- the scale of the operation
- the necessity for asepsis
- available sources of heat (steam, electrical).

The general principles for efficient drying can be summarized as:

- large surface area for heat transfer
- efficient heat transfer per unit area (to provide sufficient latent heat of vaporization or heat of sublimation in the case of freeze drying)

- efficient mass transfer of evaporated water through any surrounding boundary layers, i.e. sufficient turbulence to minimize boundary layer thickness
- efficient vapour removal, i.e. low relative humidity air moving at adequate velocity.

Dryers in the pharmaceutical industry

The types and variety of drying equipment have reduced in recent years as pharmaceutical companies strive for standardization and globalization of manufacturing. The types of dryers that have proved the most successful have become commonplace and less efficient (or more damaging) drying processes have largely disappeared. An additional trend is the manufacture of 'mini' versions of manufacturing equipment to be used in formulation and process development. Previously, sometimes very distinctly different dryers were used in laboratories but this resulted in numerous problems during scale-up. The use of the miniaturized production equipment (processing just a few hundred grams) will minimize later problems during the scaling to manufacturing batches (typically a few hundred kilograms).

Types of pharmaceutical dryers

A variety of pharmaceutical dryers are still used and it is convenient to categorize these according to the heat transfer method that they employ, i.e. convection, conduction or radiation.

CONVECTIVE DRYING OF WET SOLIDS

Dynamic convective dryers

Fluidized-bed dryer

An excellent method of obtaining good contact between the warm drying air and wet particles is found in the *fluidized-bed dryer*. The general principles of the technique of *fluidization* will be summarized before discussing its application to drying.

Consider the situation in which particulate matter is contained in a vessel, the base of which is perforated, enabling a fluid to pass through the bed of solids from below. The fluid can be liquid or gas but air will be assumed for the purposes of this description, as it is directly relevant to the drying process.

If the air velocity through the bed is increased gradually and the pressure drop through the bed is measured, a graph of the operation shows several distinct regions, as indicated in Figure 30.3. At first, when the air velocity is low, the region A to B, flow takes place between the particles without causing disturbance but as the velocity is

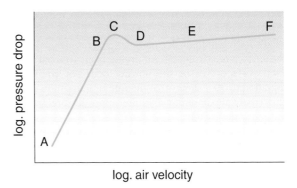

Fig. 30.3 Effect of air velocity on pressure drop through a fluidized bed.

increased a point is reached, C, when the pressure drop has attained a value where the frictional drag on the particle is equal to the force of gravity on the particle. Rearrangement of the particles occurs to offer least resistance, D, and eventually they are suspended in the air and can move. The pressure drop through the bed decreases slightly because of the greater porosity at D. Further increase in the air velocity causes the particles to separate and move freely and the bed is *fully fluidized,* region D to E. Any additional increase in velocity separates the particles further, that is, the bed expands, without appreciable change in the pressure drop. In the region E to F, fluidization is irregular, much of the air flowing through in bubbles; the term *boiling bed* is used to describe this. At a very high air flow rate, F, the air velocity is sufficient to entrain the solid particles and transport them out of the top of the bed in a process known as *pneumatic transport*.

The important factor is that fluidization produces conditions of great turbulence, the particles mixing with good contact between air and particles. Hence, if hot air is used, the turbulent conditions lead to high heat and mass transfer rates, the fluidized-bed technique therefore offering a means of rapid drying.

The fluidized-bed dryer was developed to make use of this process of fluidization to improve the efficiency of heat transfer and vapour removal compared with the older static tray dryers that it replaced. A reason for this is the more efficient transfer of the required latent heat of evaporation from the air to the drying solid. The rate of heat transfer in convective drying may be written as:

$$\text{Rate of heat transfer } (dH/dt) = h_c\, A\, \Delta T \qquad (30.3)$$

where h_c is a heat transfer coefficient (see Chapter 46) for convective heat transfer, A is the surface area available for heat transfer, and ΔT is the difference in temperature between the drying air and the solid to be dried. The heat transfer coefficient is high in a fluidized bed as the vigorous motion of the particles reduces the thickness of the boundary layer. Also, the process fluidizes individual powder particles or granules and thus the surface area available for drying is maximized to the total surface area of the powder bed. An equivalent equation to 30.3 shows that the rate of mass transfer (in this case vapour removal in the opposite direction) is similarly improved.

Heat and mass transfer are therefore relatively efficient and the process, even for a large manufacturing batch, takes between about 20 and 40 minutes.

The arrangement of a typical fluidized-bed dryer is shown in Figure 30.4. Sizes are available with capacities ranging from about 400 g to 1200 kg. These are now manufactured so that dryers throughout the range have similar geometric and hydrodynamic features to aid manufacturing scale-up from laboratory experiments.

Advantages of fluidized-bed drying

1. Efficient heat and mass transfer give high drying rates, so that drying times are short. Apart from obvious economic advantages, the heat challenge to thermolabile materials is minimized.
2. The fluidized state of the bed ensures that drying occurs from the surface of all the individual particles. Hence, most of the drying will occur at a constant rate.
3. The temperature of a fluidized bed is uniform throughout (as a result of the turbulence) and can be controlled precisely.

4. The turbulence in a fluidized bed causes some attrition to the surface of the granule. This produces a more spherical free-flowing product.
5. The free movement of individual particles reduces the risk of soluble materials migrating during drying (see later in this chapter).
6. Keeping the granules separate during drying also reduces the problems of aggregation and reduces the need for a sieving stage after drying.
7. The fluidization containers can be mobile, making handling and movement around the production area simple, thus reducing labour costs.
8. Short drying times mean that the unit has a high product output from a small floor space.

Disadvantages of fluidized-bed drying

1. The turbulence of the fluidized state may cause excessive attrition of some materials, with damage to some granules and the production of too much dust.
2. Fine particles may become entrained in the fluidizing air and must be collected by bag filters, with care to avoid segregation and loss of fines.
3. The vigorous movement of particles in hot dry air can lead to the generation of charges of static electricity, and suitable precautions must be taken. A mixture of air with a fine dust of organic materials such as starch and lactose can explode violently if ignited by sparking caused by static

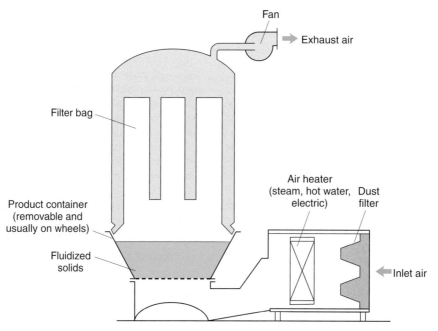

Fig. 30.4 Fluidized bed dryer.

charges. The danger is increased if the fluidized material contains a volatile solvent. Adequate electrical earthing is essential and, naturally, is fitted as standard on all modern dryers.

CONDUCTIVE DRYING OF WET SOLIDS

In this process the wet solid is in thermal contact with a hot surface and the bulk of heat transfer occurs by conduction.

Vacuum oven

This equipment is a good example of a conduction dryer though it is not used so extensively as it was formerly. The vacuum oven (Fig. 30.5) consists of a jacketed vessel sufficiently strong in construction to withstand a vacuum within the oven and possibly steam pressure in the jacket. In addition, the supports for the shelves form part of the jacket, giving a larger area for conduction heat transfer. The oven should be closed by a door that can be locked tightly to give an airtight seal. The oven is connected through a condenser and liquid receiver to a vacuum pump, although if the liquid to be removed is water and the pump is of the ejector type that can handle water vapour, the pump can be connected directly to the oven.

Operating pressure can be as low as 0.03–0.06 bar, at which water boils at 25–35°C. Some ovens may be large (for example, about 1.5 m cube and with 20 shelves).

The main advantage of a vacuum oven is that drying takes place at a low temperature and since there is little air present, there is minimum risk of oxidation. The temperature of the drying solid can rise to the steam or heating water temperature at the end of the drying but this is not usually harmful.

Vacuum ovens are rarely used nowadays for production but are still worthy of mention as they may be the only method available to dry particularly thermolabile or oxygen-sensitive materials. Additionally, small-scale ones are frequently found in development laboratories where they are commonly used for the drying of small development samples, particularly when the heat stability of the drug or formulation is uncertain.

RADIATION DRYING OF WET SOLIDS

Radiant heat transmission

Heat transmission by radiation differs from heat transfer by conduction or convection in that no transfer medium (solid, liquid or gaseous) needs be present. Heat energy in the form of radiation can cross empty space or travel through the atmosphere virtually without loss. If it falls on a body capable of absorbing it then it appears as heat, although a proportion may be reflected or transmitted.

Use of microwave radiation

Microwave radiation in the wavelength range 10 mm to 1 m has been found to be an efficient heating and drying method. Microwave dryers are used in the pharmaceutical industry.

Generation and action of microwaves

Microwaves are produced by an electronic device known as a magnetron. Microwave energy can be reflected down a rectangular duct (termed a waveguide) or simply beamed through a transparent polypropylene window into the drying chamber. To avoid interference with radio and television, it is permitted to operate only at certain frequencies which are normally 960 and 2450 MHz.

The penetration of microwaves into the wet product is so good that heat is generated uniformly within the solid.

When microwaves fall on substances of suitable electronic structure (small polar molecules, such as water), the electrons in the molecule attempt to resonate in sympathy with the radiation. The resulting molecular 'friction' results in the generation of heat. The large molecules of the solids do not resonate as well as, say, water molecules, so further heating may be avoided once the water is removed. This is indicated clearly by the 'loss factors' listed in Table 30.1. The loss factor is the ratio of the microwave energy absorbed by individual molecules to the microwave energy provided. Thus the higher the number, the greater the absorption of microwave energy. Table 30.1 lists these values for some common solvents and excipients. Clearly, the absorption of the microwave energy is far greater for small polar molecules than larger and less polar molecules.

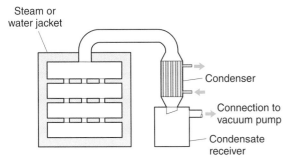

Fig. 30.5 Vacuum oven (schematic).

Steam or water jacket

Condenser

Connection to vacuum pump

Condensate receiver

Table 30.1 Microwave energy loss factors for some pharmaceutical solvents and excipients

Material	Loss factor
Methanol	13.6
Ethanol	8.6
Water	6.1
Isopropanol	2.9
Acetone	1.25
Maize starch	0.41
Magnesium carbonate	0.08
Lactose	0.02

A microwave dryer for granulates

Figure 30.6 is a sketch of a microwave dryer used for drying granulates. It is designed to operate under a slight vacuum. That, in itself, is not essential for the use of microwaves but the air flow through the chamber facilitates the continuous removal of evaporated solvent. The radiation is generated by multiple magnetrons each producing 0.75 kW at 2450 MHz. The radiation passes through the polypropylene window into the drying chamber where it is absorbed by the liquid in the wet granules contained on a tray. The heat generated in the mass drives off the moisture.

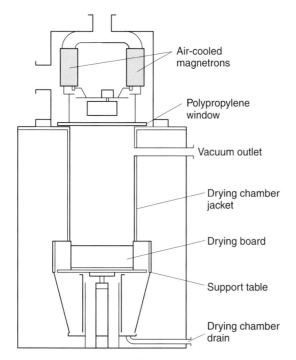

Fig. 30.6 Microwave dryer (courtesy of T K Fielder).

Labels: Air-cooled magnetrons; Polypropylene window; Vacuum outlet; Drying chamber jacket; Drying board; Support table; Drying chamber drain

The evolved vapour is drawn away in the air flow as it is formed. When drying is nearly complete, the radiation field intensity within the chamber will rise since the dry solids do not absorb as readily as water. This rise is detected and the magnetrons are progressively turned down automatically to give an accurate control of the final moisture content and minimize the danger of overheating.

Advantages of microwave drying

The following advantages are claimed for microwave drying:

1. It provides rapid drying at fairly low temperatures.
2. The thermal efficiency is high since the dryer casing and the air remain cool. Most of the microwave energy is absorbed by the liquid in the wet material.
3. The bed is stationary, avoiding problems of dust and attrition.
4. Solute migration is reduced as there is uniform heating of the wet mass.
5. Equipment is highly efficient and refined. All the requirements of product and operator safety have been incorporated into machines without detracting from GMP considerations.
6. Granulation endpoint is possible by measuring the residual microwave energy (as this rises sharply within the dryer when there is little solvent left to evaporate).

Disadvantages of microwave drying

1. The batch size of commercial production microwave dryers is smaller than the batch sizes available for fluidized-bed drying.
2. Care must be taken to shield operators from the microwave radiation, which can cause damage to organs such as the eyes and testes. This is ensured by 'fail-safe' devices preventing generation of microwaves until the drying chamber is sealed.

DRYERS FOR SOLUTIONS AND SUSPENSIONS

The objective of these dryers is to generate a large surface area in the liquid for heat and mass transfer and to provide an effective means of collecting the dry solid. The most useful type disperses the liquid to a spray of small droplets – the spray dryer.

Spray dryer

The spray dryer provides a large surface area for heat and mass transfer by atomizing the liquid to small droplets.

These are sprayed into a stream of hot air, so that each droplet dries to an individual solid particle. Thus particle formation and drying occur in the one process.

There are many forms of spray dryer (e.g. GEA Niro) and Figure 30.7 shows a typical design in which the drying chamber resembles a cyclone. This ensures good circulation of air, facilitates heat and mass transfer and encourages the separation of dried particles from the moving air by the centrifugal action.

Atomizer

The character of the particles is controlled by the droplet size so the type of atomizer is important. Early simple jet atomizers tended to block easily as a result of rapid evaporation and deposition of solid on the nozzle. This caused the flow rate to vary and this had a detrimental effect on the uniformity and predictability of droplet size.

This was resolved by the use of rotary types of atomizer, one form of which is shown in Figure 30.8. Liquid is fed on to the disc that is rotated at high speed (10 000–30 000 revolution/min). A film is formed and spreads from the small disc to a larger, inverted hemispherical bowl, becoming thinner, and eventually being dispersed from the edge in a fine spray of uniform droplet size. In addition, the rotary atomizer has the advantage of being equally effective with

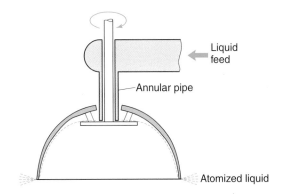

Fig. 30.8 Rotary atomizer.

either solutions or suspensions of solids and it can operate efficiently at various feed rates.

Modern two-fluid nozzles have overcome the problems of earlier jet atomizers and have proved successful. In this context, the two fluids are the liquid product and the atomizing air. Two-fluid nozzles can handle feed rates between 30 and 80 L/h. They can be positioned either to spray their droplets co-currently into the air stream from the top of the dryer, or to spray from the base of the dryer in what is known as 'fountain mode'. The two-fluid nozzles produce a narrow droplet size range with the mean size being affected by nozzle position. In general, a nozzle used co-currently will produce smaller droplets than one used in fountain mode. Rotary atomizers produce droplets in the mid-range. To illustrate this, data from one experiment performed under similar conditions showed that the mean droplet size from a co-current two-fluid nozzle was 2 μm, from a rotary atomizer was 50 μm and from a two-fluid nozzle used in fountain mode was 100 μm.

Chamber

The air enters the chamber tangentially and rotates the drying droplets around the chamber to increase their residence time and therefore time for drying. For pharmaceutical purposes, it is usual to filter the air and to heat it indirectly by means of a heat exchanger. Dust carried over in the air outlet stream may be recovered by a cyclone separator or filter bag. It is also possible to recycle up to 60% of the exhaust air to the air inlet of the dryer. This greatly improves the efficiency of the process.

A range of sizes of spray dryer is available, from a laboratory model with a volume of 100–200 mL capable of producing just a few grams of experimental material from aqueous or organic solution, through a pilot-scale model with a chamber diameter of 800 mm and a height of 3 m capable of evaporating 7 kg of water per hour, to a production-scale model that could have a chamber diameter of 3.5 m and be 6 m high (or even larger) with

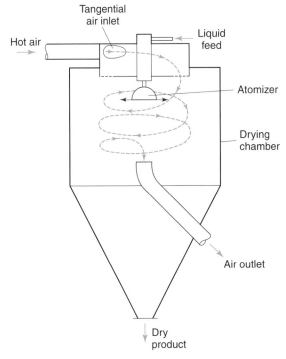

Fig. 30.7 Spray dryer.

an evaporative capacity of about 50–100 kg water per hour. Larger spray dryers, with a capacity of up to 4000 kg/h, are used in other industries, notably in food production. Typically, modern spray dryers have a 60° cone at the base of the hollow cylinder.

Product

Spray-dried products are easily recognizable, being uniform in their appearance. The particles have a characteristic shape, in the form of hollow spheres sometimes with a small hole. This arises from the drying process, since the droplet enters the hot air stream and dries on the outside to form an outer crust with liquid still in the centre. This liquid then vaporizes and the internal vapour escapes by blowing a hole in the sphere. Figure 30.9 shows the mechanism of formation of the spherical product.

Intelligent computer control is available to control process parameters as these, in turn, can affect particle size, bulk density, moisture content, dissolution rate and dispersibility of the resulting product.

Advantages of the spray-drying process

1. There are millions of small droplets which give a large surface area for heat and mass transfer, so that evaporation is very rapid. The actual drying time of a droplet is only a fraction of a second, and the overall time in the dryer only a few seconds.
2. Because evaporation is very rapid, the droplets do not attain a high temperature. Most of the heat is used as latent heat of vaporization and the temperature of the particles is kept low by evaporative cooling.
3. The characteristic particle form allows efficient particle packing and thus gives the product a high bulk density. It also leads to rapid dissolution because of the large surface area.
4. Provided that a suitable atomizer is used, the resulting powder will have a uniform and controllable particle size.
5. The product is free-flowing, with almost spherical particles, and is especially convenient for tablet manufacture as it has excellent flow and compaction properties.
6. In many cases spray drying will increase the dissolution rate and bioavailability of poorly water-soluble drugs (APIs).
7. Labour costs are low, the process yielding a dry, free-flowing powder from a dilute solution, in a single operation with no handling.
8. It can be used as a continuous process if required.

Disadvantages of the spray-drying process

1. The equipment is very bulky and, with the ancillary equipment, is expensive.
2. The overall thermal efficiency is rather low since the air must still be hot enough when it leaves the dryer to avoid condensation of moisture. Also, large volumes of heated air pass through the chamber without contacting a particle and thus not contributing directly to the drying process.

Uses of the spray-drying process

The spray dryer can be used for drying almost any substance, in solution or in suspension. It is most useful for thermolabile materials, and particularly if handled continuously and in reasonably large quantities.

Examples of both soluble and insoluble substances that are spray dried include citric acid, sodium phosphate, gelatin, starch, barium sulfate and calcium phosphate. The process is also used for some powdered antibiotic formulations where the spray-dried powder is packaged and distributed. This is then reconstituted as a syrup at the time of dispensing. The dry product is spray dried from a formulation containing all the necessary ingredients, including colours and flavours. Since only water is removed in the spray-drying process, these products must be reconstituted with pure water only.

Spray drying is also capable of producing spherical particles in the respirable range of 1–7 μm that are necessary for the delivery of drugs from dry powder inhalers (see Chapter 36).

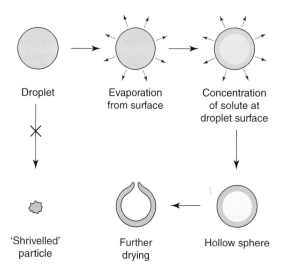

Droplet

Evaporation from surface

Concentration of solute at droplet surface

'Shrivelled' particle

Further drying

Hollow sphere

Fig. 30.9 Formation of product in spray drying.

It is possible to operate spray dryers aseptically using heated filtered air to dry products such as serum hydrolysate. Also, some spray dryers operate in a closed circuit mode with an inert gas to minimize oxidation of the product. Volatile solvents can be recovered from such systems.

Pharmaceutical spray drying has been reviewed by Wendel & Çelik (1997) and the reader is referred to this article if additional information is required.

Fluidizing spray dryer

A development of the spray dryer is the fluidized spray dryer (Niro). This has a small fluidized bed mounted in the base of the cone at the point where the product is collected. The moving air created in the fluidized bed overcomes any cohesion of spray-dried particles after they fall into the collection chamber. This allows spheres with a higher moisture content to be handled and also ones made from stickier and more cohesive substances than were previously possible to process.

FREEZE DRYING

Freeze drying is a process used to dry extremely heat-sensitive materials. It can allow the drying, without excessive damage, of proteins, blood products and even microorganisms which retain a small but significant viability.

In this process, the initial liquid solution or suspension is frozen, the pressure above the frozen state is reduced and the water removed by sublimation. Thus an overall liquid-to-vapour transition takes place, as with all the previous dryers discussed, but all three states of matter are involved: liquid to solid, then solid to vapour.

The theory and practice of freeze drying are based on an understanding and application of the phase diagram for the water system.

The phase diagram for water

The phase diagram for the water system is shown in Figure 30.10. It consists of three separate areas. Each area represents a single phase of water – vapour, liquid or solid. Two phases can coexist along a line under the conditions of temperature and pressure defined by any point on the line. The point O is the one unique point where all three phases can coexist and is known as the *triple point*. Its coordinates for pure water are a pressure of 610 Pa (as a comparison, atmospheric pressure is approximately 10^5 Pa) and a temperature of 0.0075°C.

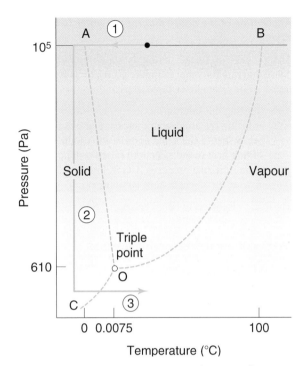

Fig. 30.10 The phase diagram for water (not to scale) with freeze-drying process superimposed (see text for explanation).

The lines on the phase diagram represent the interphase equilibrium lines which show:

- the boiling point of water as it is lowered by reduction of the external pressure above the water (BO in Fig. 30.10)
- the variation of the melting point of ice on reduction of the external pressure above it. There is a very slight rise in the melting point (AO)
- the reduction of the vapour pressure exerted by ice as the temperature is reduced (CO).

On heating ice at *atmospheric* pressure, it will melt when the temperature rises to 0°C, i.e. at this temperature the ice will change to liquid water. Continued heating at atmospheric pressure will raise the temperature of the water to 100°C. If heating is continued, the liquid water will be converted into water vapour at 100°C.

If, however, solid ice is maintained at a pressure below the triple point then on heating, the ice will sublime and pass directly to water vapour without passing through the liquid phase. This sublimation, and therefore drying, will only occur at a temperature below that of the triple point. Thus it will only happen if the pressure is prevented from rising above the triple point pressure during the process. To ensure that this is so, the vapour evolved must be removed as fast as it is formed.

Application of the phase diagram of water to freeze drying

The process of freeze drying is superimposed on the phase diagram for water in Figure 30.10. In its basic form freeze drying comprises three steps:

1. freezing the solution
2. reducing the atmospheric pressure above the ice to below that of the triple point of the product
3. adding heat to the system to raise the temperature to the sublimation curve (CO in Fig. 30.10) to provide the latent heat of sublimation.

These are discussed in detail below.

Stages of the freeze-drying process

Freezing stage

The liquid material is frozen before the application of vacuum to avoid frothing. The depression of the freezing point caused by the presence of dissolved solutes means that the solution must be cooled to well below the normal freezing temperature for pure water and it is usual to work in the range −10 to −30°C, typically below −18°C. The presence of dissolved solutes will shift the pure-water phase diagram. Since the subsequent stage of sublimation is slow, several methods are used at this stage to produce a large frozen surface to speed up that later stage.

Shell freezing This is employed for fairly large volumes such as blood products. The bottles are rotated slowly and almost horizontally in a refrigerated bath. The liquid freezes in a thin shell around the inner circumference of the bottle. Freezing is slow and large ice crystals form which is a drawback of this method as they may damage blood cells and reduce the viability of microbial cultures.

In vertical spin freezing, the bottles are spun individually in a vertical position so that centrifugal force forms a circumferential layer of solution which is cooled by a blast of cold air. The solution supercools and freezes rapidly with the formation of small ice crystals.

Centrifugal evaporative freezing This is a similar method where the solution is spun in small containers within a centrifuge. This prevents foaming when a vacuum is applied. The vacuum causes boiling at room temperature and this removes so much latent heat that the solution cools quickly and snap freezes. About 20% of the water is removed prior to freeze drying and there is no need for separate refrigeration. Ampoules are usually frozen in this way, a number being spun in a angled position (approximately 30° to the horizontal) in a special centrifuge head so that the liquid is thrown outwards and freezes as a wedge with a larger surface area.

Vacuum application stage

The containers and the frozen material must be connected to a source of vacuum sufficient to drop the pressure below the triple point and remove the large volumes of low-pressure vapour formed during drying. Again, an excess vacuum is normal in practice to ensure that the product in question is below the triple point of the formulation.

Commonly a number of bottles or vials are attached to individual outlets of a manifold which is connected to vacuum.

Sublimation stage

Heat of sublimation must be supplied. It may be thought that, as the process takes place at a low temperature, the additional heat needed to sublime the ice will be small. In fact, the latent heat of sublimation of ice is 2900 kJ kg^{-1}, appreciably larger than the latent heat of evaporation of water at atmospheric pressure. This heat must be supplied for the process to take place.

Sublimation can only occur at the frozen surface. It is a slow process (approximately 1 mm thickness of ice per hour) and is surface area dependent. This step must therefore be considered at the freezing stage (as discussed above). The procedures discussed earlier not only increase the surface area, but also reduce the thickness of ice to be sublimated.

Primary drying Under those conditions the ice sublimes, leaving a porous solid which still contains about 0.5% moisture after primary drying. Further reduction can be effected by secondary drying. During the primary drying, the latent heat of sublimation must be provided and the vapour removed.

Heat transfer Heat transfer is critical; insufficient heat input prolongs the process, which is already slow, and excess heat will cause melting.

Small ampoules may be left on the centrifuge head or may be placed on a manifold; in either case heat from the atmosphere is sufficient. Large volumes, bottles of blood for example, are placed in individually heated cylinders or are connected to a manifold when heat can be taken from the surrounding environment that must be replaced by some form of input heat.

In all cases, heat transfer must be controlled since only about 5 W m^{-2} K^{-1} is needed and overheating will lead to melting. It is important to appreciate that, although a significant amount of heat is required, there should be no significant increase in temperature; the added heat should be sufficient to provide the latent heat of sublimation only and little sensible heat.

Vapour removal The vapour formed must be removed continually to prevent the pressure within the container rising above the triple point pressure and thus preventing sublimation. To reduce the pressure sufficiently, it is necessary to use efficient vacuum pumps, usually two-stage rotary pumps on the small scale and ejector pumps on the large scale. On the small scale, vapour is absorbed by a desiccant such as phosphorus pentoxide or is cooled in a small condenser with solid carbon dioxide. Mechanically refrigerated condensers are used on the large scale.

For vapour flow to occur, the vapour pressure at the condenser must be less than that at the frozen surface and a low condenser temperature is necessary. On the large scale, vapour is commonly removed by pumping but the pumps must be of large capacity and must not be affected by moisture. The extent of the necessary pumping capacity will be realized from the fact that, under the pressure conditions used during primary drying, 1 g of ice will form 1000 litres of water vapour. Ejector pumps are most satisfactory for this purpose.

Rate of drying   The rate of drying in freeze drying is very slow, the ice being sublimated at a rate of about only 1 mm thickness per hour. The drying rate curve illustrated in Figure 30.11 shows a similar shape to a normal drying curve, the drying being at constant rate during most of the time.

Computer control enables the drying cycle to be monitored. There is an optimum vapour pressure for a maximum sublimation rate and the heat input and other variables are adjusted to maintain this value. Continuous freeze drying is possible in modern equipment where the vacuum chamber is fitted with a belt conveyor and vacuum locks. Despite these advances, the overall drying rate is still slow.

Secondary drying

The removal of the final amounts of residual moisture at the end of primary drying is performed by raising the

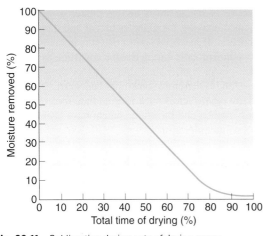

Fig. 30.11   Sublimation drying: rate of drying curve.

temperature of the solid to as high as 50 or 60°C. A high temperature is permissible for many materials because the small amount of moisture remaining at the end of primary drying is not sufficient to cause spoilage.

Packaging

Attention must be paid to packaging freeze-dried products to ensure protection from moisture during storage. Containers should be closed without contacting the atmosphere, if possible, and ampoules, for example, are sealed on the manifold while still under vacuum. Otherwise, the closing must be carried out under controlled atmospheric conditions. The dry material often needs to be sterile.

Advantages of freeze drying

Freeze drying, as a result of the character of the process, has certain special advantages:

1. Drying takes place at very low temperatures, so that enzyme action is inhibited and chemical decomposition, particularly hydrolysis, is minimized.
2. The solution is frozen such that the final dry product is a network of solid occupying the same volume as the original solution. Thus the product is light and porous.
3. The porous form of the product gives ready solubility of the freeze-dried product.
4. There is no concentration of the solution prior to drying. Hence, salts do not concentrate in the wet state and denature proteins, as occurs with other drying methods.
5. Since the process takes place under high vacuum, there is little contact with air and oxidation is minimized.

Disadvantages of freeze drying

There are two main disadvantages of freeze drying:

1. The porosity, ready solubility and complete dryness of the product result in one with a very hygroscopic nature. Unless dried in the final container and sealed in situ, packaging requires special consideration.
2. The process is very slow and uses complicated plant that is very expensive. It is not a general method of drying, therefore, but is limited to certain types of valuable products that, because of their heat sensitivity, cannot be dried by any other means.

Uses of freeze drying

The method is used for those products which could not be dried by any other heat method. These include biological products; for example, some antibiotics, blood products, vaccines (such as BCG, yellow fever, smallpox), enzyme preparations (such as hyaluronidase) and microbiological cultures. The latter enables specific microbiological species and strains to be stored for long periods with viability of about 10% on reconstitution.

SOLUTE MIGRATION DURING DRYING

Solute migration is the phenomenon that can occur during drying which results from the movement of a solution within a wet system. The solvent moves towards the surface of a solid (from where it evaporates), taking any dissolved solute with it. Many drugs and binding agents are soluble in granulating fluid and during the drying of granulates these solutes can move towards the surface of the drying bed or granule and be deposited there when the solvent evaporates. Solute migration during drying can lead to localized variability in the concentration of soluble drugs and excipients within the dried product.

Migration associated with drying granules can be of two types: intergranular migration (between granules) and intragranular migration (within individual granules).

Intergranular migration

Intergranular migration, where the solutes move from granule to granule, may result in gross maldistribution of active drug. It can occur during the drying of static beds of granules (e.g. tray drying) since the solvent and accompanying solute(s) move from granule to granule towards the top surface of the bed where evaporation takes place. When the granules are compressed, the tablets may have a deficiency or an excess of drug. For example, experimentation found that only 12% of tablets made from a tray-dried warfarin granulate were within the USP limits for drug content.

Intragranular migration

Drying methods based on fluidization and vacuum tumbling keep the granules separate during drying and so prevent the intergranular migration that may occur in fixed beds. However, intragranular migration, where the solutes move towards the periphery of each granule, may take place.

Consequences of solute migration

Solute migration of either type can result in a number of problems and occasional benefits.

Loss of active drug

The periphery of each granule may become enriched, with the interior suffering depletion. This will be of no consequence unless the enriched outer layer is abraded and lost, as may happen during fluidized-bed drying when the fine drug-rich dust will be eluted in the air and carried to the filter bag or lost. The granules suffer a net loss of drug and as a result will be below specification with respect to quantity of active ingredient.

Mottling of coloured tablets

Coloured tablets can be made by adding soluble colour during wet granulation. Intragranular migration of the colour may give rise to dry granules with a highly coloured outer zone and a colourless interior (Fig. 30.12). During compaction granule fracture takes place and the colourless interior is exposed. The eye then sees the coloured fragments against a colourless background and the tablets appear mottled.

Migration may be reduced by using the insoluble aluminium 'lake' of the colouring material (in which the soluble dye is adsorbed strongly onto insoluble alumina particles) in preference to the soluble dye itself. Studies have indicated that the production of small granules, which do not fracture so readily, are preferable to larger ones if mottling is troublesome.

Migration of soluble binders

Intragranular migration may deposit a soluble binder at the periphery of the granules and so confer a 'hoop stress' resistance, making the granules harder and more resistant to abrasion. It has been shown that this migration can aid the bonding process during tablet compaction as a result of binder–binder (rather than drug–drug or drug–excipient) contact and is therefore sometimes beneficial.

Many other factors such as granulate formulation and drying method and moisture content have been shown to affect solute migration.

Influence of formulation factors on solute migration

Nature of substrate

The principles governing solute migration are similar to those of thin-layer chromatography. Thus, if the granule substrate has an affinity for the solute then migration will

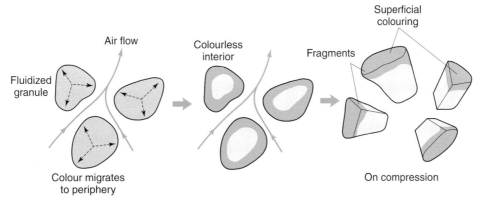

Fig. 30.12 Diagram of mottling caused by intragranular migration.

be impeded. Luckily, many of the common tablet excipients possess this affinity. The presence of absorbent materials, such as starch and microcrystalline cellulose, will minimize tablet solute migration.

The use of water-insoluble aluminium lakes (pigments) reduces mottling compared with water-soluble dyes. This effect has also been seen with film-coat colours.

Viscosity of granulating fluid

The popular granulating fluids are solutions of polymers whose viscosity is appreciably greater than water alone. This viscosity impedes the movement of moisture by increasing the fluid friction. Increasing the concentration and therefore the viscosity of PVP solution has been shown to slow the migration of drugs in fixed beds of wet granules. Solution of methylcellulose with comparable viscosities gave similar migration rates showing that the effect is due to viscosity alone and not to any specific action of either of the binders.

Influence of process factors on solute migration

Drying method

Intergranular migration in fixed beds of granules will occur whenever a particular method of drying creates a temperature gradient. This results in greater evaporation from the hotter zones.

In slow convective drying (e.g. during static tray drying), the maximum concentration of migrated solute will normally occur in the surface of the drying bed since the process of drying is slow enough to maintain a capillary flow of solvent/solute to the surface over a long period of time.

Drying by microwave radiation results in the uniform heating that is a characteristic of this technique which in turn minimizes solute migration.

Drying methods which keep the granules in motion will abolish the problem of intergranular migration but intragranular migration can still occur. This is marked in fluidized granules.

Initial moisture content

The initial moisture content of the granulate will also influence the extent of migration. The greater the moisture content, the greater will be the moisture movement before the pendular state is reached at which migration cannot continue as there is no longer a continuous layer of mobile liquid water within the wet solid (see Fig. 29.2).

Some practical means of minimizing solute migration

It may be useful to list the measures that can be taken to minimize migration:

- Use the minimum quantity of granulating fluid and ensure that it is well distributed. High-speed mixer/granulators give better moisture distribution than earlier equipment and granulates prepared in this way show less migration.
- Prepare the smallest granules that will flow easily and are generally satisfactory if mottling is troublesome.
- Avoid tray drying unless there is no alternative.
- If tray drying is unavoidable, then the dry granules should be remixed before compression. This will ensure that a random mix of enriched and depleted

granules will be fed to the tablet machines. This remixing will be more effective if the granule size is small since there will be a greater number of granules per die fill.

- If intragranular migration is likely to be troublesome, consider vacuum or microwave drying as an alternative to fluidized-bed drying.

REFERENCE

Wendel, S., Çelik, M. (1997) An overview of spray-drying applications. *Pharmaceutical Technology*, **10**, 124-144.

BIBLIOGRAPHY

Armstrong, N.A., March, G.A. (1974) Quantitative assessment of surface mottling of colored tablets. *Journal of Pharmaceutical Sciences*, **63**(1), 126-129.

Armstrong, N.A., March, G.A. (1976) Quantitative assessment of factors contributing to mottling of colored tablets I. manufacturing variables. *Journal of Pharmaceutical Sciences*, **65**(2), 198-200.

Armstrong, N.A., March, G.A. (1976) Quantitative assessment of factors contributing to mottling of colored tablets II. formulation variables. *Journal of Pharmaceutical Sciences*, **65**(2), 200-204.

Armstrong, N.A., March, G.A., De Blaey, C.J., Polderman, J. (1973) The use of adsorbents to prevent mottling in coloured tablets. *Journal of Pharmacy and Pharmacology*, **25** (suppl), 163-164.

Broadhead, J., Rouan, S.K., Hau, I., Rhodes, C.T. (1994) The effect of process and formulation variables on the properties of spray-dried beta-galactosidase. *Journal of Pharmacy and Pharmacology*, **46**(6), 458-467.

Chaudry, I.A., King, R.E. (1972) Migration of potent drugs in wet granulations. *Journal of Pharmaceutical Science*, **6**, 1121.

Masters, K. (1991) *Spray Drying Handbook*, 5th edn. Longman Scientific and Technical, Harlow, Essex.

Nielson, F. (1983) Spray drying of pharmaceuticals. *Manufacturing Chemist and Aerosol News*, **53**(7), 38-41.

Norhebel, G., Moss, A.A.H. (1971) *Drying of Solids in the Chemical Industry*. Butterworth and Co. (Publishers) Ltd, Sevenoaks, Kent.

Powell, M. (1983) Developments in freeze drying. *Manufacturing Chemist and Aerosol News,* **53**(7), 47-50.

Seager, H., Burt, I., Ryder, J. et al (1979) The effect of granule structure on the mechanical properties of tablets. *International Journal of Pharmaceutical Technology and Product Manufacture*, **1**, 36.

Travers, D.N. (1983) Problems with solute migration. *Manufacturing Chemist and Aerosol News*, **53**(3), 67-71.

Wan, L.S., Heng, P.W., Chia, C.G. (1991) Preparation of coated particles using a spray drying process with an aqueous system. *International Journal of Pharmacy*, **77**, 183-191.

Tablets and compaction

G. Alderborn

INTRODUCTION

The oral route is the most common way of administering drugs and among the oral dosage forms, tablets of various kinds are the most common type of solid dosage form in contemporary use. The term 'tablet' (from Latin *tabuletta*) is associated with the appearance of the dosage form, i.e. tablets are small disc-like or cylindrical specimens. The Latin name of the dosage form tablet in the *European Pharmacopoeia* is *compressi* which reflects the fact that the dominating process of tablet fabrication is powder compression in a confined space. Alternative preparation procedures are also in use, such as mouldings and freeze drying. Tablet-like preparations prepared by freeze drying are sometimes referred to as oral lyophilisates. Moulding, i.e. the shaping and hardening of a semi-solid mixture of active substances and excipients, and freeze drying will not be further described in this chapter.

The idea of forming a solid dosage form by powder compression is not new. In 1843 the first patent for a hand-operated device used to form a tablet was granted. The use of tablets as dosage forms became of interest to the growing pharmaceutical industry but within pharmacies, the pill (a dosage form for oral administration formed by hand into spherical particles about 4–6 mm in diameter) remained the most popular solid dosage form for a long time.

A tablet consists of one or more drugs (active ingredients) as well as a series of other substances used in the formulation of a complete preparation. In the *European Pharmacopoeia* (5th edition, 2005), tablets are defined as: 'solid preparations each containing a single dose of one or more active ingredients and usually obtained by compressing uniform volumes of particles'. Tablets are intended for oral administration. Some are swallowed whole, some after being chewed, some are dissolved or dispersed in water before being administered and some are retained in the mouth, where the active ingredient is released.

Thus, a variety of tablets exists and the type of excipients and also the way in which they are incorporated in the tablet vary between the different types. There are also other dosage forms that can be prepared in a similar way but which are administered by other routes, such as suppositories.

Tablets are used mainly for systemic drug delivery but also for local drug action. For systemic use, the drug must be released from the tablet, i.e. normally dissolved in the fluids of the mouth, stomach or intestine, and thereafter be absorbed into the systemic circulation, by which it reaches its site of action. Alternatively, tablets can be formulated for local delivery of drugs in the mouth or gastrointestinal tract, or can be used to increase temporarily the pH of the stomach.

Tablets are popular for several reasons:

- The oral route represents a convenient and safe way of drug administration.
- Compared to liquid dosage forms, tablets have general advantages in terms of the chemical and physical stability of the dosage form.
- The preparation procedure enables accurate dosing of the drug.
- Tablets are convenient to handle and can be prepared in a versatile way with respect to their use and the delivery of the drug.
- Finally, tablets can be relatively cheaply mass produced, with robust and quality-controlled production procedures giving an elegant preparation of consistent quality.

The main disadvantage of tablets as a dosage form concerns the bioavailability of poorly water-soluble or poorly absorbable drugs. In addition, some drugs may cause local irritant effects or otherwise cause harm to the gastrointestinal mucosa.

QUALITY ATTRIBUTES OF TABLETS

Like all other dosage forms, tablets should fulfil a number of specifications regarding their chemical, physical and biological properties. Quality issues relating to the final product are worth considering early in the development process (and thus early in this chapter) as they give an indication of the goal to be achieved during the development and manufacture of tablets.

Tests and specifications for some of these properties are given in pharmacopoeias. The most important of these are dose content and dose uniformity, the release of the drug in terms of tablet disintegration and drug dissolution, and the microbial quality of the preparation. In addition, the authorities and manufacturers define a set of other specifications. One such important property is the resistance of the tablet to attrition and fracture.

The quality attributes a tablet must fulfil can be summarized as follows:

1. The tablet should include the correct dose of the drug.
2. The appearance of the tablet should be elegant and its weight, size and appearance should be consistent.
3. The drug should be released from the tablet in a controlled and reproducible way.
4. The tablet should be biocompatible, i.e. not include excipients, contaminants and microorganisms that could cause harm to patients.

5. The tablet should be of sufficient mechanical strength to withstand fracture and erosion during handling at all stages of its lifetime.
6. The tablet should be chemically, physically and microbiologically stable during the lifetime of the product.
7. The tablet should be formulated into a product acceptable to the patient.
8. The tablet should be packed in a safe manner.

TABLET MANUFACTURING

Stages in tablet formation

Tablets are prepared by forcing particles into close proximity to each other by powder compression, which enables the particles to cohere into a porous, solid specimen of defined geometry. The compression takes place in a die by the action of two punches, the lower and the upper, by which the compressive force is applied. *Powder compression* is defined as the reduction in volume of a powder owing to the application of a force. Because of the increased proximity of particle surfaces accomplished during compression, bonds are formed between particles which provide coherence to the powder, i.e. a compact is formed. *Compaction* is defined as the formation of a solid specimen of defined geometry by powder compression.

The process of tableting can be divided into three stages (sometimes known as the compaction cycle) (Fig. 31.1).

Die filling

This is normally accomplished by gravitational flow of the powder from a hopper via the die table into the die (although presses based on centrifugal die filling are also used). The die is closed at its lower end by the lower punch.

Tablet formation

The upper punch descends and enters the die and the powder is compressed until a tablet is formed. During the compression phase, the lower punch can be stationary or can move upwards in the die. After maximum applied force is reached, the upper punch leaves the powder, i.e. the decompression phase.

Tablet ejection

During this phase the lower punch rises until its tip reaches the level of the top of the die. The tablet is

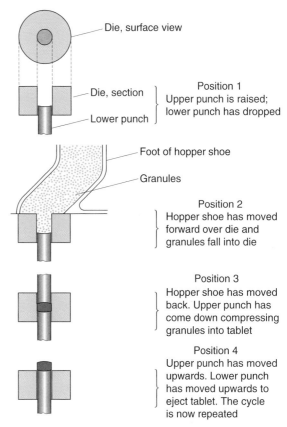

Fig. 31.1 The sequence of events involved in the formation of tablets.

subsequently removed from the die and die table by a pushing device.

Tablet presses

There are two types of press in common use during tablet production: the single-punch press and the rotary press. In addition, hydraulic presses are used in research and development work for the initial evaluation of the tableting properties of powders and the prediction of the effect of scale-up on the properties of the formed tablets (scale-up refers to the change to a larger apparatus for performing a certain operation on a larger scale).

Single-punch press (eccentric press)

A single-punch press possesses one die and one pair of punches (Fig. 31.2), i.e. a set of tableting tools. The powder is held in a hopper which is connected to a hopper shoe located at the die table. The hopper shoe moves to and fro over the die, by either a rotational or a

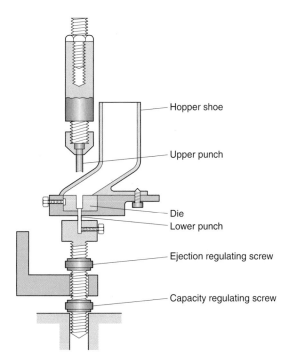

Fig. 31.2 A single-punch tablet press.

translational movement. When the hopper shoe is located over the die, the powder is fed into the die by gravitational powder flow. The amount of powder filled into the die is controlled by the position of the lower punch. When the hopper shoe is located beside the die, the upper punch descends and the powder is compressed. The lower punch is stationary during compression and the pressure is thus applied by the upper punch and controlled by the upper punch displacement. After ejection, the tablet is pushed away by the hopper shoe as it moves back to the die for the next tablet.

The output of tablets from a single-punch press is up to about 200 tablets per minute. A single-punch press thus has its primary use in the production of small batches of tablets, such as during formulation development and during the production of tablets for clinical trials.

Rotary press

The rotary press (also referred to as a multistation press) was developed to increase the output of tablets. The primary use of this machine is thus during scale-up in the latter part of the formulation work and during large-scale production. Outputs of over 10 000 tablets per minute can be achieved by rotary presses.

A rotary press operates with a number of dies and sets of punches, which can vary considerably from three for small rotary presses up to 60 or more for large presses. The dies are mounted in a circle in the die table and both the die table and the punches rotate together during operation of the machine, so that one die is always associated with one pair of punches (Figs 31.3 and 31.4). The vertical movement of the punches is controlled by tracks that pass over cams and rolls used to control the volume of powder fed into the die and the pressure applied during compression.

The powder is held in a hopper whose lower opening is located just above the die table. The powder flows by gravity onto the die table and is fed into the die by a feed frame. The reproducibility of the die feeding can be improved by a rotating device, referred to as a force-feeding device. During powder compression both punches operate by vertical movement. After tablet ejection, the tablet is knocked away as the die passes the feed frame.

Computerized hydraulic press

For computerized hydraulic presses the movement of the punches can be controlled and varied considerably. Thus, tablets can be prepared under controlled conditions with respect to the loading pattern and loading rate. Possible applications are the investigation of the sensitivity of a drug to such variations, or to mimic the loading pattern of production presses to predict scale-up problems. Because of this latter application, this type of press is also referred to as a 'compaction simulator'.

Instrumentation of tablet presses

Significant research on the process of tablet preparation was initiated in the 1950s and 1960s, i.e. about 100 years after the introduction of tablets as a dosage form. An

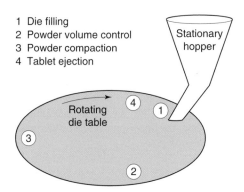

Fig. 31.3 Schematic illustration of the events involved in the formation of tablets with a rotary press.

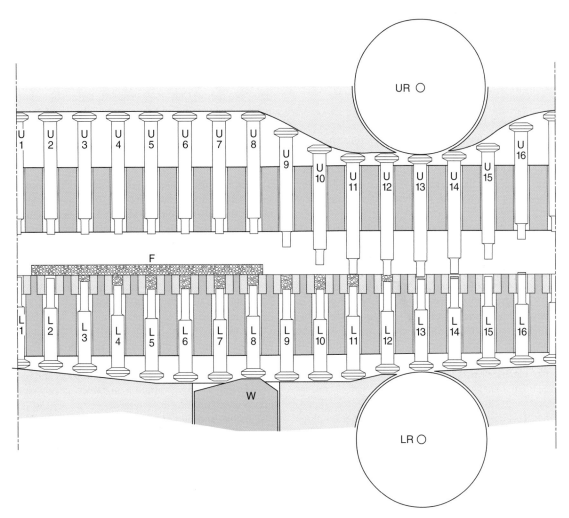

Fig. 31.4 Diagram of punch tracks of a rotary tablet press. UR, upper roller; LR, lower roller; W, powder volume adjuster; F, feed frame with granules. U1 to U8, upper punches in raised position; L1, lower punch at top position, tablet ejected; L2 to L7, lower punches dropping to lowest position and filling die with granules to an overfill at L7; L8, lower punch raised to expel excess granules giving correct volume; U9 to U12, upper punches lowering to enter die at U12; L13 and U13, upper and lower punches pass between rollers and granules are compacted to a tablet; U14 to U16, upper punch rising to top position; L14 to L16, lower punch rising to eject tablet.

important step in the development of such fundamental research was the introduction of instrumented tablet machines. By this instrumentation, the forces involved in the compaction process, i.e. the press forces from the upper and lower punches and the force transmitted to the die and the displacement of the upper and lower punch during the compression and decompression phases, could be recorded.

Instrumented presses are used in research, in development and in the production of tablets. In research and development, instrumented machines are used to provide fundamental information on the mechanical and compaction properties of powders that should be used in tablet formulations. With this application, the work is normally carried out by instrumented single-punch presses or instrumented hydraulic presses (compaction simulators). The two main applications for an instrumented press in research and development are:

1. to prepare tablets under defined conditions, e.g. in terms of applied force during compaction. These tablets are thereafter characterized by different procedures, such as imaging, surface area and tensile strength analysis
2. to describe and analyse the compression properties of materials by studying punch forces

and punch displacements during the compression and decompression phases. A series of different procedures exists, involving, for example, the assessment of deformation behaviour of particles during compression and friction properties during ejection. Some of these are described below.

In production, instrumented production machines, i.e. rotary presses, are used to control the tableting operation and to ensure that tablets of consistent quality are produced. Normally, only force signals are used on production machines and the variation in force signal during compression is monitored as it reflects variations in tablet weight.

Force transducers commonly used in the instrumentation of tablet machines are of two types. The most common type is called a *strain gauge*, which consists of wires through which an electric current is passed. The strain gauge is bonded to a punch or punch holder. During powder compression, a force is applied to the punches and they will temporarily deform. The magnitude of this deformation is dependent on the elastic modulus of the punches and the force applied. When the punch is deformed, the wire of the strain gauge is also deformed and the electrical resistance of the strain gauge will change. This change in electrical resistance can be recorded and calibrated in terms of a force signal. Another, less common type of force transducer employs piezoelectric crystals. These are devices which emit an electrical charge when loaded, the magnitude of which is proportional to the applied force.

Displacement transducers measure the distance which the punches travel during the compression and decompression processes. The most common type of displacement transducer delivers an analogue signal. It consists of a rod and some inductive elements mounted in a tube. When the rod moves within the tube, a signal is obtained which directly reflects the position of the rod. The movable rod is connected to the punch so that they move in parallel, i.e. the signal from the displacement transducer reflects the position of the punch. Digital displacement transducers are also used in instrumented tablet machines. Such transducers are based on differences in signal level depending on the position of an indicator.

Displacement transducers are necessarily mounted some distance from the punch tip. There is therefore a difference in the position given by the transducer and the real position of the punch tip owing to deformation of the punch along the distance between its tip and the connection point of the transducer. This deviation must be determined by a calibration procedure, e.g. by compressing the punch tips against each other, and a correction for this error must be made before the displacement data can be used.

The signals from the force and displacement transducers are normally amplified and sampled into a computer. After conversion into digital form, the signals are transformed into physically relevant units, i.e. N, Pa, mm, etc., and organized as a function of time. To obtain reliable data, the calibration of the signals, the resolution of the measuring systems and the reproducibility of the values must be carefully considered.

Tablet tooling

Tablets are formed in a variety of shapes. The most common tablet shapes are circular, oval and oblong but tablets may also have other shapes, such as triangular and diamond. From a side-view, tablets may be flat or convex and with or without bevelled edges. Tablets may also bear break marks or symbols and other markings. Break marks (or breaklines) are used to facilitate breaking of tablets in a controlled way to ensure reproducible doses. Markings are used to facilitate identification of a preparation and are of two types: embossed and debossed. Debossed markings are indented into the tablet and embossed markings are raised on the tablet surface. The size, shape and appearance of a tablet formed by powder compaction are controlled by the set of tools and by tooling design; a large variation in tablet size, shape and appearance can thus be obtained.

Punches and dies for rotary presses are designed in a standardized way and different standard configurations and terminology are in use. The terminology used in describing the punches includes head, neck, barrel, stem and tip and in describing the die includes face, chamfer and bore. The tools are normally fabricated in steel and different steels may be used. Due to the high forces applied to the powder bed, tools may be damaged and under normal use they become worn. The toughness, wear resistance and corrosiveness vary between different types of steels and the choice of steel grade depends on factors such as the tooling configuration, the formulation to be compacted and the cost. In addition, the surface of punches and dies may be coated with a thin layer of another metal, such as chrome, to modify its surface properties, such as hardness and corrosiveness.

Punches and dies are precision tools and they should thus be handled and stored with care. Manufacturing problems may be related to the quality of the compression tooling. Tooling inspection programmes should thus be used in the development and production of tablets.

Technical problems during tableting

A number of technical problems can arise during the tableting procedure, among which the most important are:

- high weight and dose variation of the tablets
- low mechanical strength of the tablets
- capping and lamination of the tablets
- adhesion or sticking of powder material to punch tips
- high friction during tablet ejection.

Such problems are related to the properties of the powder intended to be formed into tablets and also to the design and conditions of the press and the tooling. They should therefore be avoided by ensuring that the powder possesses adequate technical properties and also that a suitable, well-conditioned tablet press is used, e.g. in terms of the use of forced-feed devices and polished and smooth dies and punches.

Important technical properties of a powder that must be controlled to ensure the success of a tableting operation are:

- homogeneity and segregation tendency
- flowability
- compression properties and compactability
- friction and adhesion properties.

The technical properties of the powder are controlled by the ingredients of the formulation (i.e. the drug and excipients) and by the way in which the ingredients are combined into a powder during precompaction processing. The precompaction processing often consists of a series of unit operations in sequence. The starting point is normally the drug in a pure, most often crystalline form; the subsequent treatment of the drug particles is sometimes referred to as *downstream processing*. The unit operations used during this precompaction treatment are mainly particle size reduction, powder mixing, particle size enlargement and powder drying. For further details of these procedures see Chapters 10, 12, 29 and 30, respectively. Granulation of a fine powder is a common means used to preserve the fineness of the drug within larger particles that are suitable for tableting (see below) and granulation procedures are traditionally in common use in preparing a powder for tableting. To save time and energy, precompaction processing without a particle size enlargement operation is chosen if possible. This procedure is called tablet production by direct compression, or direct compaction.

Tablet production via granulation

Rationale for granulating powders prior to tableting

Because both granulation and tableting involve the formation of aggregates, tablet production by granulation is based on the combination of two size enlarge-

ment processes in sequence. The main rationales for granulating the powder (drug and filler mixture) before tableting are to:

- increase the bulk density of the powder mixture and thus ensure that the required volume of powder can be filled into the die
- improve the flowability of the powder in order to ensure that tablets with a low and acceptable tablet weight variation can be prepared
- improve mixing homogeneity and reduce segregation by mixing small particles which subsequently adhere to each other
- improve the compactability of the powder by adding a solution binder, which is effectively distributed on the particle surfaces
- ensure a homogeneous colour in a tablet by adding the colour in a manner that ensures its effective distribution over the particle surfaces
- affect the dissolution process for hydrophobic, poorly soluble particles by using a fine particulate drug which is thoroughly mixed with a hydrophilic filler and a hydrophilic binder.

Before granulation the drug might be processed separately in order to obtain a suitable quality in terms of solid-state and particulate properties, such as spray drying and milling. Normally, the drug exists in dry particulate form before granulation. However, it might be suspended or dissolved in a liquid and be added to the filler as a part of the agglomeration liquid.

Different procedures may be used to prepare a granulation, among which the most important are the use of convective mixers, fluidized-bed driers, spray driers and compaction machines. Chapter 29 discusses granulation in some detail but the process is summarized here in the context of tableting.

Granulation by convective mixing

Agitation of a powder by convection in the presence of a liquid, followed by drying, is the main procedure for the preparation of a pharmaceutical granulation. This is often considered to be the most effective means in terms of production time and cost to prepare good-quality granulations. The process is often referred to as *wet granulation*.

The ingredients to be granulated in a convective mixer are first dry mixed. The objective is to achieve a good homogeneity. As the components are often cohesive powders, a convective mixer operating at high intensity is normally used (a high-shear mixer). The mixture often consists of the drug and a filler. A disintegrant may also be included (i.e. an intragranular disintegrant) but it is also common to add the disintegrant to the dry granulation (i.e.

an extragranular disintegrant). After wet mixing, the wet mass is dried in a separate drier (usually a fluidized-bed dryer; see Chapter 30). Because granulation in a convective mixer is not a very well-controlled operation, large granules (above 1 mm) are often formed which must be broken down into smaller units. This is normally done by milling in a hammer mill or by pressing the granulation through a screen in an oscillating granulator. Granules ranging in size from about 100 to 800 µm are thus obtained.

The prepared granulation is finally dry-mixed with the other ingredients, for example in a double-cone mixer, before tableting. Common excipients added in this final mixing operation are disintegrants, lubricants, glidants and colourants. Figure 31.5 summarizes the sequence of unit operations used in the production of tablets with precompaction treatment by granulation.

Alternative granulation procedures

A series of alternative granulation procedures can be preferable in certain situations. Granulation in a fluidized-bed apparatus is less common than the use of convective mixers as it is considered to be more time-consuming. However, granulations of high quality in terms of homogeneity, flowability and compactability can be prepared by this operation.

By spray drying a suspension of drug particles in a liquid, which can contain a dissolved binder, relatively small spherical granules with uniform size can be prepared. The process is of limited use except for the prepa-ration of fillers or diluents for direct compaction. The granulation can show a good compactability and presents a possibility to granulate a drug suspension without a separate drying step for the drug substance.

The formation of granules by compacting the powder into large compacts which are subsequently comminuted into smaller granules is an alternative approach to granulation. The approach can be employed as a means to avoid exposure of the powder to moisture and heat and is also referred to as *dry granulation*. In addition, for powders of very low bulk density, compaction can be an effective means to increase markedly their bulk density. The formation of the compacts can be accomplished by powder compression in a die (slugging), giving relatively large tablet-like compacts, or by powder compression between rotating rollers (roller compaction), giving weak compacts with a flake or ribbon-like appearance. Roller compaction is a suitable operation for continuous granulation.

Tablet production by direct compaction

An obvious way to reduce production time and hence cost is to minimize the number of operations involved in the pretreatment of the powder mixture before tableting. Tablet production by direct compaction involves only two operations in sequence: powder mixing and tableting (Fig. 31.6). The advantage with direct compaction is primarily a reduced production cost. However, in a direct compactable formulation, specially designed fillers and dry binders are normally required, which usually are more expensive than the traditional ones. They may also require a larger number of quality tests before processing. As heat and water are not involved, product stability can be improved. Finally, drug dissolution might be faster from a tablet prepared by direct compaction owing to fast tablet disintegration into primary drug particles.

The disadvantages of direct compaction are mainly technological. In order to handle a powder of acceptable flowability and bulk density, relatively large particles

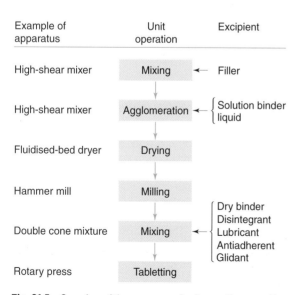

Fig. 31.5 Overview of the sequence of unit operations used in the production of tablets with precompaction treatment by granulation.

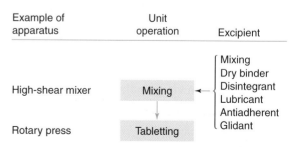

Fig. 31.6 Overview of the sequence of unit operations used in the production of tablets by direct compaction.

must be used which may be difficult to mix to a high homogeneity and be prone to segregation. Moreover, a powder consisting mainly of drug will be difficult to form into tablets if the drug itself has poor compactability. Finally, an even colouring of tablets can be difficult to achieve with a colourant in dry particulate form.

Direct compaction has been used mainly for two types of drug: firstly, relatively soluble drugs which can be processed as coarse particles (to ensure good flowability) and, secondly, relatively potent drugs which are present in a few milligrams in each tablet and can be mixed with relatively coarse excipient particles (in this latter case the flow and compaction properties of the formulation are controlled mainly by the excipients).

TABLET EXCIPIENTS

In addition to the active ingredient(s), a series of excipients are normally included in a tablet; their role is to ensure that the tableting operation can run satisfactorily and that tablets of specified quality are prepared. Depending on the intended main function, excipients to be used in tablets are subcategorized into different groups. However, one excipient can affect the properties of a powder or the tablet in a series of ways and many substances used in tablet formulations can thus be described as multifunctional. The functions of the most common types of excipients used in tablets are described below. Examples of substances used as excipients in tablets are given in Table 31.1.

Filler (or diluent)

In order to form tablets of a size suitable for handling, a lower limit in terms of powder volume and weight is required. Tablets weigh normally at least 50 mg. Therefore, a low dose of a potent drug requires the incorporation of a substance into the formulation to increase the bulk volume of the powder and hence the size of the tablet. This excipient, known as the filler or the diluent, is not necessary if the dose of the drug per tablet is high.

The ideal filler should fulfil a series of requirements, such as:

- be chemically inert
- be non-hygroscopic
- be biocompatible
- possess good biopharmaceutical properties (e.g. water soluble or hydrophilic)
- possess good technical properties (such as compactability and dilution capacity)
- have an acceptable taste
- be cheap.

Table 31.1 Examples of substances used as excipients in tablet formulation

Type of excipient	Example of substances
Filler	Lactose Sucrose Glucose Mannitol Sorbitol Calcium phosphate Calcium carbonate Cellulose
Disintegrant	Starch Cellulose Crosslinked polyvinyl pyrrolidone Sodium starch glycolate Sodium carboxymethyl cellulose
Solution binder	Gelatin Polyvinyl pyrrolidone Cellulose derivatives (e.g. hydroxypropylmethyl cellulose) Polyethylene glycol Sucrose Starch
Dry binder	Cellulose Methyl cellulose Polyvinyl pyrrolidone Polyethylene glycol
Glidant	Silica Magnesium stearate Talc
Lubricant	Magnesium stearate Stearic acid Polyethylene glycol Sodium lauryl sulfate Sodium stearyl fumarate Liquid paraffin
Antiadherent	Magnesium stearate Talc Starch Cellulose

As all these requirements cannot be fulfilled by a single substance, different substances have gained use as fillers in tablets, mainly carbohydrates but also some inorganic salts.

Lactose is the most common filler in tablets. It possesses a series of good filler properties, e.g. dissolves readily in water, has a pleasant taste, is non-hygroscopic, is fairly non-reactive and shows good compactability. Its main limitation is that some people have intolerance to lactose.

Lactose exists in both crystalline and amorphous forms. Crystalline lactose is formed by precipitation and, depending on the crystallization conditions, α-monohydrate or β-lactose (an anhydrous form) can be formed. By thermal treatment of the monohydrate form, crystalline α-anhydrous particles can be prepared. Depending on the crystallization conditions and the use of subsequent size reduction by milling, lactose of different particle sizes is obtained.

Amorphous lactose can be prepared by spray drying a lactose solution (giving nearly completely amorphous particles) or a suspension of crystalline lactose particles in a lactose solution (giving aggregates of crystalline and amorphous lactose). Amorphous lactose dissolves more rapidly than crystalline and shows better compactability. Its main use is therefore in the production of tablets by direct compaction. The amorphous lactose is, however, hygroscopic and physically unstable, i.e. it will spontaneously crystallize if crystallization conditions are met as a result of elevated temperature or high relative humidity (see Chapter 8 for more details).

Other sugars or sugar alcohols, such as glucose, sucrose, sorbitol and mannitol, have been used as alternative fillers to lactose, primarily in lozenges or chewable tablets because of their pleasant taste. Mannitol has a negative heat of solution and imparts a cooling sensation when sucked or chewed.

Apart from the sugars, perhaps the most widely used fillers are powdered celluloses of different types. Celluloses are biocompatible, chemically inert and have good tablet-forming and disintegrating properties. They are therefore used also as dry binders and disintegrants in tablets. They are compatible with many drugs but, owing to their hygroscopicity, may be incompatible with drugs prone to chemical degradation in the solid state.

The most common type of cellulose powder used in tablet formulation is microcrystalline cellulose. The name indicates that the particles have both crystalline and amorphous regions, depending on the relative position of the cellulose chains within the solid. The degree of crystallinity might vary depending on the source of the cellulose and the preparation procedure. The degree of crystallinity will affect the physical and technical properties of the particles, e.g. in terms of hygroscopicity and powder compactability.

Microcrystalline cellulose is prepared by hydrolysis of cellulose followed by spray drying. The particles thus formed are aggregates of smaller cellulose fibres. Depending on the preparation conditions, aggregates of different particle size can be prepared which have different flowabilities.

A final important example of a common filler is an inorganic substance, dicalcium phosphate dihydrate. This is insoluble in water and non-hygroscopic but is hydrophilic, i.e. easily wetted by water. The substance can be obtained in both a fine particulate form, mainly used in granulation, and an aggregated form. The latter possesses good flowability and is used in tablet production by direct compaction. Calcium phosphate is slightly alkaline and may thus be incompatible with drugs sensitive to alkaline conditions.

Disintegrant

A disintegrant is included in the formulation to ensure that the tablet, when in contact with a liquid, breaks up into small fragments, which promotes rapid drug dissolution. Ideally, the tablet should break up into individual drug particles in order to obtain the largest possible effective surface area during dissolution.

The disintegration process for a tablet occurs in two steps. First, the liquid wets the solid and penetrates the pores of the tablet. Thereafter, the tablet breaks into smaller fragments. The actual fragmentation of the tablet can also occur in steps, i.e. the tablet disintegrates into aggregates of primary particles which subsequently deaggregate into their primary drug particles. A deaggregation directly into primary powder particles will set up conditions for the fastest possible dissolution of the drug. A scheme for the release of the drug from a disintegrating tablet is shown in Figure 31.7.

Several mechanisms of action of disintegrants have been suggested, such as swelling of particles, exothermic wetting reaction, particle repulsion and particle deformation recovery. However, as two main processes are involved in the disintegration event, disintegrants to be used in plain tablets are here classified into two types:

1. *Disintegrants that facilitate water uptake.* These disintegrants act by facilitating the transport of liquids into the pores of the tablet, with the consequence that the tablet may break into fragments. One obvious type of substance that can promote liquid penetration is surface-active agents. Such substances are used to make the drug particle surfaces more hydrophilic and thus promote the wetting of the solid and the penetration of the liquid into the pores of the tablet. It has also been suggested that other substances can promote the liquid penetration, using capillary forces to suck water into the pores of the tablet.
2. *Disintegrants that will rupture the tablet.* Rupturing of tablets can be caused by swelling of the disintegrant particles during sorption of water.

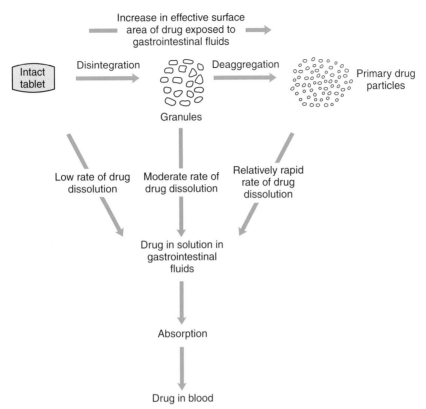

Fig. 31.7 Mechanistic representation of the drug release process from a tablet by disintegration and dissolution. (From Wells, J.I., Rubinstein, M.W. (1976) *Pharm. J.*, **217**, 629.)

However, it has also been suggested that non-swelling disintegrants can break the tablet and different mechanisms have been suggested. One such concerns a repulsion of particles in contact with water and another the recovery of deformed particles to their original shape in contact with water, i.e. particles which have been deformed during compaction.

The most traditional disintegrant in conventional tablets is starch, among which potato, maize and corn starches are the most common types used. The typical concentration range of starch in a tablet formulation is up to 10%. Starch particles swell in contact with water and this swelling can subsequently disrupt the tablet. However, it has also been suggested that starch particles may facilitate disintegration by particle–particle repulsion.

The most common and effective disintegrants act via a swelling mechanism and a series of effective swelling disintegrants has been developed which can swell dra-matically during water uptake and thus quickly and effectively break the tablet. These are normally modified starch or modified cellulose. High-swelling disintegrants are included in the formulation at relatively low concentrations, typically 1–5% by weight.

Disintegrants can be mixed with other ingredients prior to granulation and thus be incorporated within the granules (intragranular addition). It is also common for the disintegrant to be mixed with the dry granules before the complete powder mix is compacted (extragranular addition). The latter procedure will contribute to an effective disintegration of the tablet into smaller fragments. Disintegrants may also be incorporated as both an intragranular and an extragranular portion.

A third group of disintegrants functions by producing gas, normally carbon dioxide, in contact with water. Such disintegrants are used in effervescent tablets and normally not in tablets that should be swallowed as a solid. The liberation of carbon dioxide is obtained by the decomposition of bicarbonate or carbonate salts in contact with acidic water. The acidic pH is accomplished by the incorporation of a weak acid in the formulation, such as citric acid and tartaric acid.

Binder

A binder (also sometimes called adhesive) is added to a drug-filler mixture to ensure that granules and tablets can be formed with the required mechanical strength. Binders can be added to a powder in different ways:

- As a dry powder which is mixed with the other ingredients before wet agglomeration. During the agglomeration procedure, the binder might thus dissolve partly or completely in the agglomeration liquid.
- As a solution which is used as agglomeration liquid during wet agglomeration. The binder is here often referred to as a *solution binder*.
- As a dry powder which is mixed with the other ingredients before compaction (slugging or tableting). The binder is here often referred to as a *dry binder*.

Both solution binders and dry binders are included in the formulation at relatively low concentrations, typically 2–10% by weight. Common traditional solution binders are starch, sucrose and gelatin. More commonly used binders today, with improved adhesive properties, are polymers such as polyvinylpyrrolidone and cellulose derivatives (in particular hydroxypropyl methylcellulose). Important examples of dry binders are microcrystalline cellulose and crosslinked polyvinylpyrrolidone.

Solution binders are generally considered the most effective and this is therefore the most common way of incorporating a binder into granules; the granules thus formed are often referred to as binder–substrate granules. It is not uncommon, however, for a dry binder to be added to the dry binder–substrate granules before tableting in order to further improve the compactability of the granulation.

Glidant

The role of the glidant is to improve the flowability of the powder. Glidants are used in formulations for direct compaction but are often also added to a granulation before tableting to ensure that sufficient flowability of the tablet mass is achieved for high production speeds.

Traditionally, talc has been used as a glidant in tablet formulations, in concentrations of about 1–2% by weight. Today, the most commonly used glidant is probably colloidal silica, added in very low proportions (about 0.2% by weight). Because the silica particles are very small they adhere to the particle surfaces of the other ingredients (i.e. an ordered or structured mixture is

formed; see Chapter 12) and improve flow by reducing interparticulate friction. Magnesium stearate, normally used as a lubricant, can also promote powder flow at low concentrations (<1% by weight).

Lubricant

The function of the lubricant is to ensure that tablet formation and ejection can occur with low friction between the solid and the die wall. High friction during tableting can cause a series of problems, including inadequate tablet quality (capping or even fragmentation of tablets during ejection and vertical scratches on tablet edges) and may even stop production. Lubricants are thus included in almost all tablet formulations.

Lubrication is achieved by mainly two mechanisms: *fluid lubrication* and *boundary lubrication* (Fig. 31.8). In fluid lubrication a layer of fluid is located between and separates the moving surfaces of the solids from each other and thus reduces the friction. Fluid lubricants are seldom used in tablet formulations. However, liquid paraffin has been used, such as in formulations for effervescent tablets.

Boundary lubrication is considered as a surface phenomenon, as here the sliding surfaces are separated by only a very thin film of lubricant. The nature of the solid surfaces will therefore affect friction. In boundary lubrication, the friction coefficient and wear of the solids are higher than with fluid lubrication. All substances that can affect interaction between sliding surfaces can be described as boundary lubricants, including adsorbed gases. The lubricants used in tablet formulations acting by boundary lubrication are fine particulate solids.

A number of mechanisms have been discussed for these boundary lubricants, including that lubricants are

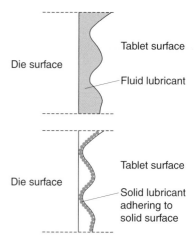

Fig. 31.8 Schematic illustration of lubrication mechanisms by fluid and boundary lubrication.

substances that show a low resistance towards shearing. The most effective of the boundary lubricants are stearic acid or stearic acid salts, primarily magnesium stearate. Magnesium stearate has become the most widely used lubricant owing to its superior lubrication properties. The stearic acid salts are normally used at low concentrations (<1% by weight).

Besides reducing friction, lubricants may cause undesirable changes in the properties of the tablet. The presence of a lubricant in a powder is thought to interfere in a deleterious way with the bonding between the particles during compaction, thus reducing tablet strength (Fig. 31.9). Because many lubricants are hydrophobic, tablet disintegration and dissolution are often retarded by the addition of a lubricant. These negative effects are strongly related to the amount of lubricant present and a minimum amount is normally used in a formulation, i.e. concentrations of 1% or below, often 0.25–0.5%. In addition, the way in which the lubricant is mixed with the other ingredients should also be considered. It can, for example, be important if the excipients are added sequentially to a granulation rather than simultaneously. The total mixing time and the mixing intensity are also important in this context.

The commonly observed retardation of disintegration and dissolution of tablets is related to the hydrophobic character of the most commonly used lubricants. In order to avoid these negative effects, more hydrophilic substances have been suggested as alternatives to the hydrophobic lubricants. Examples are surface-active agents and polyethylene glycol. A combination of hydrophobic and hydrophilic substances might also be used.

The lubricant's effect on friction and on the changes in tablet properties are related to the tendency of lubricants to adhere to the surface of drugs and fillers during dry mixing. Lubricants are often fine particulate substances which thus are prone to adhere to larger particles. In addition, studies on the mixing behaviour of magnesium stearate have indicated that this substance has the ability to form a film which can cover a fraction of the surface area of the drug or filler particles (the substrate particles). This film can be described as being continuous rather than particulate. A number of factors have been suggested to affect the development of such a lubricant film during mixing and hence also affect friction and changes in tablet properties, such as the shape and surface roughness of the substrate particles; the surface area of the lubricant particles; mixing time and intensity; and the type and size of mixer.

Concerning the tablet strength-reducing effect of a lubricant, apart from the degree of surface coverage of the lubricant film obtained during mixing, the compression behaviour of the substrate particles will also be important. Drugs and fillers can thus be evaluated in terms of their lubricant sensitivity, i.e. the reduction in tablet strength due to the addition of a lubricant compared to a tablet

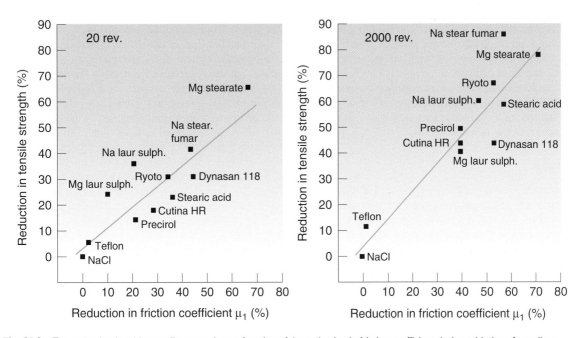

Fig. 31.9 The reduction in tablet tensile strength as a function of the reduction in friction coefficient during tableting of a sodium chloride powder mixed with 0.1% by weight of a series of lubricants admixed at two different mixing intensities. (From Hölzer & Sjögren 1981, with permission.)

formed from a powder without a lubricant. An important property for this lubricant sensitivity seems to be the degree of fragmentation the substrate particles undergo during compression (see below). It is thus assumed that, during compression, particle surfaces which are not covered with a lubricant film are formed during particle fragmentation and that these clean surfaces will bond differently from the lubricant-covered particle surfaces.

To explain the effect of lubricant film formation on the tensile strength of tablets, a coherent matrix model has been developed. This suggests that when a continuous matrix of lubricant-covered particle surfaces exists in a tablet, along which a fracture plane can be formed, the tablet strength is considerably lower than that of tablets formed from unlubricated powder. However, if the mixing and compression processes do not result in such a coherent lubricant matrix within the tablet, for example due to irregular substrate particles or particle fragmentation, the lubricant sensitivity appears to be lower.

Antiadherent

The function of an antiadherent is to reduce adhesion between the powder and the punch faces and thus prevent particles sticking to the punches. Many powders are prone to adhere to the punches, a phenomenon (known in the industry as *sticking or picking*) which is affected by the moisture content of the powder. Such adherence is especially prone to happen if the tablet punches have markings or symbols. Adherence can lead to a build-up of a thin layer of powder on the punches, which in turn will lead to an uneven and matt tablet surface with unclear markings or symbols.

Many lubricants, such as magnesium stearate, have also antiadherent properties. However, other substances with limited ability to reduce friction can also act as antiadherents, such as talc and starch.

Sorbent

Sorbents are substances that are capable of sorbing some quantities of fluids in an apparently dry state. Thus, oils or oil–drug solutions can be incorporated into a powder mixture which is granulated and compacted into tablets. Microcrystalline cellulose and silica are examples of sorbing substances used in tablets.

Flavour

Flavouring agents are incorporated into a formulation to give the tablet a more pleasant taste or to mask an unpleasant one. The latter can also be achieved by coating the tablet or the drug particles.

Flavouring agents are often thermolabile and so cannot be added prior to an operation involving heat. They are often mixed with the granules as an alcohol solution.

Colourant

Colourants are added to tablets to aid identification and patient compliance. Colouring is often accomplished during coating (see Chapter 33 for further information) but a colourant can also be included in the formulation prior to compaction. In the latter case, the colourant can be added as an insoluble powder or dissolved in the granulation liquid. The latter procedure may lead to a colour variation in the tablet caused by migration of the soluble dye during the drying stage (see Chapter 30 for more information on the phenomenon of solute migration).

TABLET TYPES

Classification of tablets

Several categories of tablets may be distinguished and the denomination and definitions of different types of tablets can be found in pharmacopoeias. The tablet dosage forms described in the *European Pharmacopoeia* (5th edn) appear in the monographs on tablets and on oromucosal preparations (solid oromucosal preparations are tablet preparations for use in the mouth where the active ingredient should be released for local action or for systemic uptake via the oral mucosa).

A possible means of classifying tablets is based on the drug release pattern from the tablets, i.e. immediate release, prolonged release and delayed release. The latter two types are also referred to as modified-release tablets. For immediate-release tablets, the drug is intended to be released rapidly after administration, or the tablet is dissolved and administered as a solution. This is the most common type of tablet and includes disintegrating, chewable, effervescent, sublingual and buccal tablets.

Modified-release tablets should normally be swallowed intact. The formulation and thus also the type of excipients used in such tablets might be quite different from those of immediate-release tablets. The drug is released from a prolonged-release tablet slowly at a nearly constant rate or alternatively as a series of pulses, i.e. pulsatile release. If the rate of release is constant during a substantial period of time, a zero-order type of release is obtained, i.e. $M = kt$ (where M is the cumulative amount of drug released and t is the release time). This is sometimes described as an ideal type of prolonged-release preparation.

For delayed-release tablets the drug is liberated from the tablet some time after administration. After this period has elapsed, the release is normally rapid. The most common type of delayed-release tablet is an enteric tablet, for which the drug is released in the upper part of the small intestine after the preparation has passed the stomach. However, a delayed release can also be combined with a slow drug release, e.g. for local treatment in the lower part of the intestine or in the colon.

The type of release obtained from immediate-, prolonged- and delayed-release tablets is illustrated in Figure 31.10. In the following sections, the most common types of tablets are described.

Disintegrating tablets

The most common type of tablet is intended to be swallowed and to release the drug in a relatively short time thereafter by disintegration and dissolution, i.e. the goal of the formulation is fast and complete drug release in vivo. Such tablets are often referred to as conventional or plain tablets. A disintegrating tablet includes normally at least the following type of excipients: filler (if the dose of the drug is low), disintegrant, binder, glidant, lubricant and antiadherent.

As discussed above, the drug is released from a disintegrating tablet in a sequence of processes, including tablet disintegration, drug dissolution and drug absorption (see Fig. 31.7). All these processes will affect, and can be rate-limiting steps for, the rate of drug bioavailability. The rate of the processes is affected by both formulation factors and production conditions.

The disintegration time of the tablet can be markedly affected by the choice of excipients, especially disintegrant (Fig. 31.11). The type of filler and lubricant can also be of significant importance for tablet disintegration.

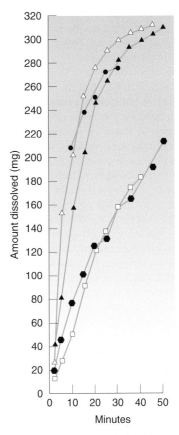

Fig. 31.11 The dissolution rate of salicylic acid, as assessed by an in vitro dissolution method based on agitated baskets, from tablets formed from mixtures of salicylic acid (325 mg) and a series of different types of starches as disintegrant. □ potato starch, ◆ arrowroot starch, ▲ rice starch, ● corn starch, △ compressible starch. (From Underwood, T.W., Cadwallader, D.E. (1972) *J. Pharm. Sci.*, **61**, 239.)

Tablet disintegration may also be affected by production conditions during manufacture. Important examples are the design of the granulation procedure (which will affect the physical properties of the granules), mixing conditions during the addition of lubricants and antiadherents, and the applied punch force during tableting and the punch force–time relationship. It has been reported that an increased compaction pressure can either increase or decrease disintegration time, or give complex relationships with maximum or minimum disintegration times.

For poorly water-soluble drugs, the dissolution rate is often the rate-limiting step for bioavailability. The dissolution rate is a function of the solubility and the surface area of the drug (see Chapter 2). Thus, dissolution rate will increase if the solubility of the drug is increased, e.g. by the use of a salt of the drug. It is also possible to speed up the dissolution process by incorporating into the

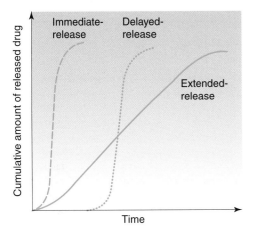

Fig. 31.10 Schematic representation of the cumulative amount of drug released from immediate-, extended- and delayed-release tablets.

formulation a substance that forms a salt with the drug during dissolution. This has been a common means to increase the dissolution rate of aspirin by using magnesium oxide in the formulation.

The drug dissolution rate will also increase with an increase in the surface area of the drug. Thus, control of drug particle size is important to control drug dissolution. However, a reduced particle size will make a powder more cohesive. A reduction in drug particle size might thus give aggregates of particles which are difficult to break up, with the consequence that the drug dissolution rate from the tablet will be reduced. It is thus important to ensure that the tablet is formulated in such a way that it will disintegrate and the aggregates thus formed break up into small drug particles so that a large surface area of the drug is exposed to the dissolution medium.

For drugs with poor absorption properties, the absorption can be affected (see Chapter 21) by modifying the drug's lipophilicity, e.g. by esterification of the drug. The use of substances in the formulation that affect the permeability of the gastrointestinal cell membranes, often referred to as absorption enhancers, is also a possible means of increasing the drug absorption rate and degree.

Single disintegrating tablets can also be prepared in the form of multilayers, i.e. the tablet consists of concentric or parallel layers cohered to each other. Multilayer tablets are prepared by repeated compression of powders and are made primarily to separate incompatible drugs from each other, i.e. incompatible drugs can be incorporated into the same tablet. Although intimate contact exists at the surface between the layers, the reaction between the incompatible drugs is limited. The use of parallel layered tablets where the layers are differently coloured represents an approach to preparing easily identifiable tablets.

Another variation of the disintegrating tablet is coated tablets which are intended to disintegrate and release the drug quickly (in contrast to coated tablets intended for modified release). The rationale for using coated tablets and detailed descriptions of the procedures used for tablet coating are given in Chapter 33.

Chewable tablets

Chewable tablets are chewed and thus mechanically disintegrated in the mouth. The drug is, however, normally not dissolved in the mouth but swallowed and dissolves in the stomach or intestine. Thus, chewable tablets are used primarily to accomplish a quick and complete disintegration of the tablet – and hence obtain a rapid drug effect – or to facilitate the administration of the tablet. A common example of the former is antacid tablets. In the latter case, the elderly and children in particular have difficulty in swallowing tablets and so chewable tablets are attractive forms of medication. Important examples are

vitamin tablets. Another general advantage of a chewable tablet is that this type of medication can be taken when water is not available.

Chewable tablets are similar in composition to conventional tablets except that a disintegrant is normally not included in the composition. Flavouring and colouring agents are common and sorbitol and mannitol are common examples of fillers.

Effervescent tablets

Effervescent tablets are dropped into a glass of water before administration, during which carbon dioxide is liberated. This facilitates tablet disintegration and drug dissolution; the dissolution of the tablet should be complete within a few minutes. As mentioned above, the effervescent carbon dioxide is created by a reaction in water between a carbonate or bicarbonate and a weak acid such as citric or tartaric.

Effervescent tablets are used to obtain rapid drug action, for example for analgesic drugs (Fig. 31.12), or to facilitate the intake of the drug, for example for vitamins.

The amount of sodium bicarbonate in an effervescent tablet is often quite high (about 1 g). After dissolution of such a tablet, a buffered water solution will be obtained which normally temporarily increases the pH of the stomach. The result is a rapid emptying of the stomach and the residence time of the drug in the stomach will thus be short. As drugs are absorbed more effectively in the small intestine than in the stomach, effervescent tablets can thus show a fast drug bioavailability, which can be advantageous, for example, for analgesic drugs. Another aspect of the short drug residence time in the

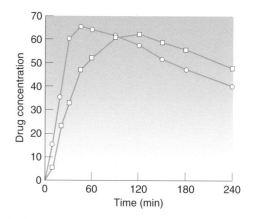

Fig. 31.12 Concentration of salicylates in plasma after administration of acetylsalicylic acid tablets (1 g). Circles, effervescent tablet; squares, conventional tablet. (From Ekenved, G., Elofsson, R., Sölvell, L. (1975) *Acta Pharm. Suec.*, **12**, 323.)

stomach is that drug-induced gastric irritation can be avoided, e.g. for aspirin tablets, as the absorption of aspirin in the stomach can cause irritation.

Effervescent tablets also often include a flavour and a colourant. A water-soluble lubricant is preferable in order to avoid a film of a hydrophobic lubricant on the surface of the water after tablet dissolution. A binder is normally not included in the composition.

Effervescent tablets are prepared by both direct compaction and by compaction via granulation. In the latter case, traditional wet granulation is seldom used; instead, granules are formed by the fusion of particles as a result of their partial dissolution during wet massing of a moistened powder.

Effervescent tablets should be packaged in such a way that they are protected against moisture. This is accomplished with waterproof containers, often including a dessicant, or with blister packs or aluminium foils.

Compressed lozenges

Compressed lozenges are tablets that dissolve slowly in the mouth and so release the drug dissolved in the saliva. Lozenges are used for systemic drug uptake or for local medication in the mouth or throat, e.g. with local anaesthesia, antiseptic and antibiotic drugs. The latter type of tablets can thus be described as slow-release tablets for local drug treatment.

Disintegrants are not used in the formulation but otherwise such tablets are similar in composition to conventional tablets. In addition, lozenges are often coloured and include a flavour. The choice of filler and binder is of particular importance in the formulation of lozenges, as these excipients should contribute to a pleasant taste or feeling during tablet dissolution. The filler and binder should therefore be water soluble and have a good taste. Common examples of fillers are glucose, sorbitol and mannitol. A common binder in lozenges is gelatin.

Lozenges are normally prepared by compaction at high applied pressures in order to obtain a tablet of high mechanical strength and low porosity which can dissolve slowly in the mouth.

Sublingual tablets and buccal tablets

Sublingual tablets and buccal tablets are used for drug release in the mouth followed by systemic uptake of the drug. A rapid systemic drug effect can thus be obtained without first-pass liver metabolism. Sublingual tablets are placed under the tongue and buccal tablets are placed in the side of the cheek.

Sublingual and buccal tablets are often small and porous, the latter facilitating fast disintegration and drug release.

Prolonged-release tablets

Classification of prolonged-release tablets

In recent years there has been great interest in the development and use of tablets which should be swallowed and thereafter slowly release the drug in the gastrointestinal tract. Such tablets are denominated in various ways, such as slow release, extended release, sustained release and prolonged release. They are often also referred to as controlled-release preparations. This latter term is somewhat misleading, as all tablets, irrespective of their formulation and use, should release the drug in a controlled and reproducible way. (The nomenclature for prolonged-release preparations is subject to some debate and no worldwide acceptable system exists. The reader is referred to Chapter 32 for further discussion on this subject.)

After release from the tablet, the drug should normally be absorbed into the systemic circulation. The aim is normally to increase the time period during which a therapeutic drug concentration level in the blood is maintained. However, the aim can also be to increase the release time for drugs that can cause local irritation in the stomach or intestine if they are released quickly. Examples of the latter are potassium chloride and iron salts. In addition, drugs for local treatment of diseases in the large intestine are sometimes formulated as prolonged-release tablets.

A prolonged-release tablet contains one dose of the drug which is released for a period of about 12–24 hours. The release pattern can vary, from being nearly continuous to two or more pulses. In the latter case, the pulses can correspond to a rapid release of the drug or can be a combination of a rapid release of one portion of drug followed by a slow release of a second portion.

A prolonged-release preparation can also be categorized as a single-unit or a multiple-unit dosage form. In the first case, the drug dose is incorporated into a single-release unit and in the latter is divided into a large number of small release units. A multiple-unit dosage form is often considered to give a more reproducible drug action.

There is a series of rationales behind the increased interest in administering drugs orally for systemic uptake in the form of prolonged-release tablets. However, the drug must fulfil certain criteria in order to render itself suitable for sustained-release medication, otherwise another type of tablet is a more feasible alternative. These rationales and criteria, as well as the pharmacokinetic aspects of prolonged-release drug administration, are described elsewhere in this book (see Chapters 23 and 32). In Chapter 32 the formulation principles used to achieve prolonged drug release are described.

Prolonged-release tablets are often categorized according to the mechanism of drug release. The following are the most common means used to achieve a slow, controlled release of the drug from tablets:

- drug transport control by diffusion
- dissolution control
- erosion control
- drug transport control by convective flow (accomplished by, for example, osmotic pumping)
- ion exchange control.

Diffusion-controlled release systems

In diffusion-controlled prolonged-release systems, the transport by diffusion of dissolved drugs in pores filled with gastric or intestinal juice or in a solid (normally polymer) phase is the release-controlling process. Depending on the part of the release unit in which the drug diffusion takes place, diffusion-controlled release systems are divided into matrix systems (also referred to as monolithic systems) and reservoir systems. The release unit can be a tablet or a nearly spherical particle of about 1 mm in diameter (a granule or a millisphere). In both cases the release unit should stay more or less intact during the course of the release process. In matrix systems, diffusion occurs in pores located within the bulk of the release unit and in reservoir systems, diffusion takes place in a thin water-insoluble film or membrane, often about 5–20 μm thick, which surrounds the release unit. Diffusion through the membrane can occur in pores filled with fluid or in the solid phase that forms the membrane.

Drug is released from a diffusion-controlled release unit in two steps:

1. The liquid that surrounds the dosage form penetrates the release unit and dissolves the drug. A concentration gradient of dissolved drug is thus established between the interior and the exterior of the release unit.
2. The dissolved drug will diffuse in the pores of the release unit or the surrounding membrane and thus be released or, alternatively, the dissolved drug will partition into the membrane surrounding the dose unit and diffuse in the membrane.

A dissolution step is thus normally involved in the release process but the diffusion step is the rate-controlling step. The rate at which diffusion will occur depends on three variables: the concentration gradient over the diffusion distance; the area and distance over which diffusion occurs; and the diffusion coefficient of the drug in the diffusion medium. Some of these variables are used to modulate the release rate in the formulation.

Reservoir systems In a reservoir system the diffusion occurs in a thin film surrounding the release unit (Fig. 31.13). This film is normally formed from a high molecular weight polymer. The diffusion distance will be constant during the course of the release and, as long as a constant drug concentration gradient is maintained, the release rate will be constant, i.e. a zero-order release ($M = kt$).

One possible process for the release of the drug from a reservoir system involves partition of the drug dissolved inside the release unit to the solid membrane, followed by transport by diffusion of the drug within the membrane. Finally, the drug will partition to the solution surrounding the release unit. The driving force for the release is the concentration gradient of dissolved drug over the membrane. The release rate can be described in a simplified way by the following equation, which also summarizes the formulation factors by which the release rate can be controlled, i.e.:

$$M/t = C\,A\,K\,D/l \qquad (31.1)$$

where C is the solubility of the drug in the liquid, A and l are the area and thickness of the membrane, D is the diffusion coefficient of the drug in the membrane, and K the partition coefficient for the drug between the membrane and the liquid at equilibrium.

In practice, the membrane surrounding the release unit often includes a water-soluble component. This can be small particles of a soluble substance, such as sucrose, or a water-soluble polymer, such as a water-soluble cellulose derivative (e.g. hydroxypropyl methylcellulose). In the latter case the polymer is used together with a water-insoluble polymer as the film-forming materials that constitute the coating. In such a membrane the water-soluble component will dissolve and form pores filled with liquid in which the drug can thereafter diffuse. The area and length of these pores will thus constitute the diffusion area and distance. These factors can be estimated from the porosity of the membrane (e) and the tortuosity (τ) of the pores (the tortuosity refers to the ratio between the actual transport distance in the pores between two positions and the transport distance

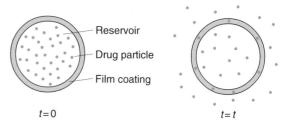

$t=0$ $t=t$

Fig. 31.13 Schematic illustration of the mechanism of drug release from a diffusion-based reservoir tablet (t = time).

in a solution). The release rate can thus be described in a simplified way as follows:

$$M/t = C \, A \, e \, D/l \, \tau \qquad (31.2)$$

The membrane porosity and pore tortuosity can be affected by the addition of water-soluble components to the membrane.

For oral preparations, the film surrounding the release units is normally based on high molecular weight, water-insoluble polymers, such as certain cellulose derivatives (e.g. ethyl cellulose) and acrylates. The film often also includes a plasticizer. In the case of drug release through liquid-filled pores, a small amount of a water-soluble compound is also added, as described above. Reservoir systems today are normally designed as multiple-unit systems rather than single units.

Matrix systems   In a matrix system the drug is dispersed as solid particles within a porous matrix formed of a water-insoluble polymer, such as polyvinyl chloride (Fig. 31.14). Initially, drug particles located at the surface of the release unit will be dissolved and the drug released rapidly. Thereafter, drug particles at successively increasing distances from the surface of the release unit will be dissolved and released by diffusion in the pores to the exterior of the release unit. Thus, the diffusion distance of dissolved drug will increase as the release process proceeds. The drug release, in terms of the cumulative amount of drug (*M*) released from a matrix in which drug particles are suspended, is considered to be proportional to the square root of time, i.e. $M = kt^{1/2}$.

The main formulation factors by which the release rate from a matrix system can be controlled are the amount of drug in the matrix, the porosity of the release unit, the length of the pores in the release unit (dependent on the size of the release unit and the pore tortuosity) and the solubility of the drug (which regulates the concentration gradient). The characteristics of the pore system can be affected by, for example, the addition of

soluble excipients and by the compaction pressure during tableting.

Matrix systems are traditionally designed as single-unit systems, normally tablets, prepared by tableting. However, alternative preparation procedures are also used, especially for release units that are smaller than tablets. Examples of such techniques are extrusion, spray congealing and casting.

Dissolution-controlled release systems

In dissolution-controlled prolonged-release systems, the rate of dissolution of the drug or another ingredient in the gastrointestinal juices is the release-controlling process. It is obvious that a sparingly water-soluble drug can form a preparation of a dissolution-controlled prolonged-release type. Reduced drug solubility can be accomplished by preparing poorly soluble salts or derivatives of the drug. An alternative means of achieving prolonged release based on the dissolution control principle is to incorporate the drug in a slowly dissolving carrier or by covering drug particles with a slowly dissolving coating. In the latter case, the release of the drug from such units occurs in two steps:

1. The liquid that surrounds the release unit dissolves the coating (rate-limiting dissolution step).
2. The solid drug is exposed to the liquid and subsequently dissolves.

In order to obtain a prolonged release based on dissolution of a coating, the tablet is formulated to release the drug in a series of consecutive pulses, i.e. a pulsatile release. This can be accomplished by dividing the drug dose into a number of smaller release units, often nearly spherical granules of about 1 mm in diameter, which are coated in such a way that the dissolution time of the coatings will vary (Fig. 31.15). A variation in dissolution time of the coating can be accomplished by varying its thickness or its solubility. Release units with different

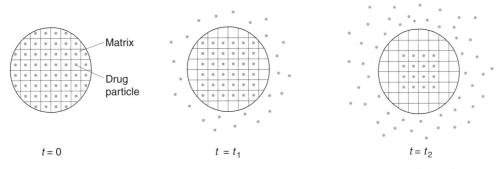

$t = 0$ $t = t_1$ $t = t_2$

Fig. 31.14   Schematic illustration of the mechanism of drug release from a diffusion–based matrix tablet (*t* = time).

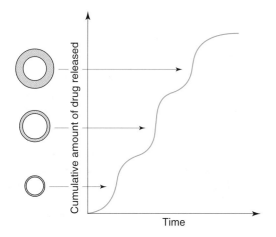

Fig. 31.15 Schematic representation of the cumulative amount of drug released from a dissolution-based (due to differences in coating thickness) pulsatile-release preparation.

release times will be mixed and formed into a disintegrating tablet.

Delayed-release tablets are also normally formulated as dissolution-controlled preparations. In the case of gastroresistant tablets, the dissolution is inhibited until the preparation reaches the higher pH of the small intestine, where the drug is released in a relatively short time.

Erosion-controlled release systems

In erosion-controlled prolonged-release systems, the rate of drug release is controlled by the erosion of a matrix in which the drug is dispersed. The matrix is normally formed by a tableting operation and the system can thus be described as a single-unit system. The erosion in its simplest form can be described as a continuous liberation of matrix material (both drug and excipient) from the surface of the tablet, i.e. surface erosion. The consequence will be a continuous reduction in tablet weight during the course of the release process (Fig. 31.16). Drug release from an erosion system can thus be described in two steps:

1. Matrix material, in which the drug is dissolved or dispersed, is liberated from the surface of the tablet.
2. The drug is subsequently exposed to the gastrointestinal fluids and mixed with (if the drug is dissolved in the matrix) or dissolved in (if the drug is suspended in the matrix) the fluid.

This release scheme is in practice a simplification, as erosion systems may combine different mechanisms for drug release. For example, the drug may be released both by erosion and by diffusion within the matrix. Thus, a mathematical description of drug release from an erosion system is complex. However, drug release can often approximate zero order for a significant part of the total release time.

The eroding matrix can be formed from different substances. One example is lipids or waxes, in which the drug is dispersed. Another example is polymers that gel in contact with water (e.g. hydroxyethyl cellulose). The gel will subsequently erode and release the drug dissolved or dispersed in the gel. Diffusion of the drug in the gel may occur in parallel.

Osmosis-controlled release systems

In osmosis-controlled prolonged-release systems, the flow of liquid into the release unit, driven by a difference in osmotic pressure between the inside and the outside of the release unit, is used as the release-controlling process. Osmosis can be defined as the flow of a solvent from a compartment with a low concentration of solute to a compartment with a high concentration. The two compartments are separated by a semi-permeable membrane, which allows flow of solvent but not of solute.

In the most simple type of osmosis-controlled drug release, the following sequence of steps is involved in the release process:

1. Osmotic transport of liquid into the release unit.
2. Dissolution of drug within the release unit.
3. Convective transport of a saturated drug solution by pumping of the solution through a single orifice or through pores in the semi-permeable membrane.

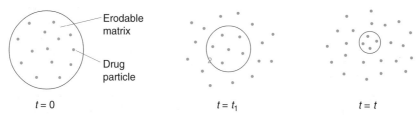

Fig. 31.16 Schematic illustration of the mechanism of drug release from an erosion tablet.

The pumping of the drug solution can be accomplished in different ways. One example is a tablet which includes an expansion layer, i.e. a layer of a substance that swells in contact with water, the expansion of which will press out the drug solution from the release unit. Alternatively, the increased volume of fluid inside the release unit will increase the internal pressure and the drug solution will thus be pumped out.

If the flow rate of incoming liquid to the release unit is the rate-controlling process, the drug release rate can be described as:

$$M/t = C\ V/t \qquad (31.3)$$

where V is the volume of incoming liquid. The flow rate of incoming liquid under steady-state conditions is a zero-order process and the release rate of the drug will therefore also be a zero-order process. The water flow is not affected by the flow and pH of the dissolution medium. However, the water flow rate and hence drug release rate can be affected by a number of formulation factors, such as the osmotic pressure of the drug solution within the release unit, the drug solubility, and the permeability and mechanical properties of the membrane.

Osmosis-controlled release systems can be designed as single-unit or multiple-unit tablets. In the first case, the drug solution can be forced out from the tablet through a single orifice (Fig. 31.17) formed in the membrane by boring with a laser beam. Alternatively, the drug solution can flow through a number of pores formed during the uptake of water. Such pores can be formed by the dissolution of water-soluble substances in the membrane or by straining of the membrane owing to the increased internal pressure in the release unit. In the case of multiple-unit release tablets, the transport occurs in formed pores.

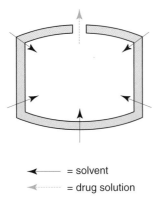

= solvent

= drug solution

Fig. 31.17 Schematic illustration of the mechanism of drug release from an osmosis-controlled release system designed as a single-unit tablet with a single release orifice.

TABLET TESTING

Test methods

In tablet formulation development and during manufacturing of tablets, a number of procedures are used to assess the quality of the tablets. Some test methods are described in pharmacopoeias and these tests are traditionally concerned with the content and the in vitro release of the active ingredient. Test methods not described in pharmacopoeias are sometimes referred to as non-compendial and concern a variety of quality attributes that need to be evaluated, such as the porosity of tablets. Below, some of the tests used in the quality evaluation of tablets are briefly described.

Uniformity of content of active ingredient

A fundamental quality attribute for all pharmaceutical preparations is the requirement for a constant dose of drug between individual tablets. In practice, small variations between individual preparations are accepted and the limits for this variation appear as standards in pharmacopoeias. Traditionally, uniformity of dose or dose variation between tablets is tested in two separate tests: uniformity of weight (mass) and uniformity of active ingredient.

The test for uniformity of weight is carried out by collecting a sample of tablets from a batch and determining their individual weights. The average weight of the tablets is then calculated. The sample complies with the standard if the individual weights do not deviate from the mean more than is permitted in terms of percentage.

If the drug substance forms the greater part of the tablet mass, any weight variation obviously indicates a variation in the content of active ingredient. Compliance with the standard thus helps to ensure that uniformity of dosage is achieved. However, in the case of potent drugs which are administered in low doses, the excipients form the greater part of the tablet weight and the correlation between tablet weight and amount of active ingredient can be poor (Fig. 31.18). Thus, the test for weight variation must be combined with a test for variation in content of the drug substance. Nevertheless, the test for uniformity of weight is a simple way to assess variation in drug dose, which makes the test useful as a quality control procedure during tablet production.

The test for uniformity of drug content is carried out by collecting a sample of tablets followed by a determination of the amount of drug in each. The average drug content is calculated and the content of the individual tablets should fall within specified limits in terms of percentage deviation from the mean.

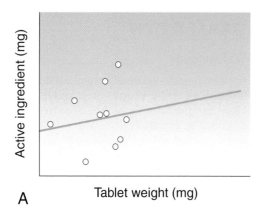

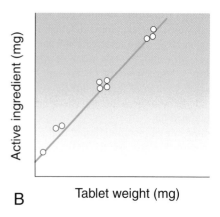

A Tablet weight (mg)

B Tablet weight (mg)

Fig. 31.18 Correlation between amount of active ingredient and tablet weight for (a) a low-dose (drug content 23% of tablet weight) and (b) a high-dose (drug content 90% of tablet weight) tablet. (From Airth, J.M., Bray, D.F., Radecka, C. (1967) *J. Pharm. Sci.*, **56**, 233–235.)

Disintegration

As discussed above, the drug release process from tablets often includes a step at which the tablet disintegrates into smaller fragments. In order to assess this, disintegration test methods have been developed and examples of such can be found in pharmacopoeias.

The test is carried out by agitating a given number of tablets in an aqueous medium at a defined temperature and the time to reach the endpoint of the test is recorded. The preparation complies with the test if the time to reach this endpoint is below a given limit. The endpoint of the test is the point at which all visible parts of the tablets have been eliminated from a set of tubes in which the tablets have been held during agitation. The tubes are closed at the lower end by a screen and the tablet fragments formed during the disintegration are eliminated from the tubes by passing the screen openings, i.e. disintegration is considered to be achieved when no tablet fragments remain on the screen (fragments of coating may remain).

A disintegration instrument (Fig. 31.19) consists normally of six chambers, i.e. tubes open at the upper end and closed by a screen at the lower. Before disintegration testing, one tablet is placed in each tube and normally a plastic disc is placed over the tablet. The tubes are placed in a water bath and raised and lowered at a constant frequency in the water in such a way that at the highest position of the tubes, the screen (and thus the tablet held down by the plastic disc) remains below the surface of the water.

Tests for disintegration do not normally seek to establish a correlation with in vivo behaviour. Thus, compliance with the specification is no guarantee of an

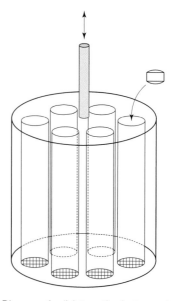

Fig. 31.19 Diagram of a disintegration instrument for the testing of tablet disintegration time.

acceptable release and uptake of the drug in vivo and hence an acceptable clinical effect. However, it is reasonable to assume that a preparation which fails to comply with the test is unlikely to be efficacious. Disintegration tests are, however, useful for assessing the potential importance of formulation and process variables on the biopharmaceutical properties of the tablet and as a control procedure to evaluate the quality reproducibility of the tablet during production.

Dissolution

Dissolution testing is the most important way to study, under in vitro conditions, the release of a drug from a solid dosage form and thus represents an important tool to assess factors that affect the bioavailability of a drug from a solid preparation. During a dissolution test, the cumulative amount of drug that passes into solution is measured as a function of time. The test thus describes the overall rate of all the processes involved in the release of the drug into a bioavailable form.

Dissolution studies are carried out for several reasons:

- To evaluate the potential effect of formulation and process variables on the bioavailability of a drug.
- To ensure that preparations comply with product specifications.
- To indicate the performance of the preparation under in vivo conditions.

This last point requires that in vitro dissolution data correlate with the in vivo performance of the dosage form, which must be experimentally verified. The term in vitro/in vivo correlation in this context is related to the correlation between in vitro dissolution and the release or uptake of the drug in vivo. The establishment of such a correlation is one of the most important aspects of a dissolution test for a preparation under formulation development and is discussed further in Chapter 22.

Dissolution is accomplished by locating the tablet in a chamber containing a flowing dissolution medium. So that the method is reproducible, all factors that can affect the dissolution process must be standardized. This includes factors that affect the solubility of the substance (i.e. the composition and temperature of the dissolution medium) and others that affect the dissolution process (such as the concentration of dissolved substance in, and the flow conditions of, the fluid in the dissolution chamber). Normally, the concentration of the drug substance in the bulk of the dissolution medium shall not exceed 10% of the solubility of the drug, i.e. sink conditions. Under sink conditions, the concentration gradient between the diffusion layer surrounding the solid phase and the concentration in the bulk of the dissolution medium is often assumed to be constant.

A number of compendial and non-compendial methods exist for dissolution testing, which can be applied to both drug substances and formulated preparations. With respect to preparations, the main test methods are based on forced convection of the dissolution medium and can be classified into two groups: stirred-vessel methods and continuous-flow methods.

Stirred-vessel methods

The most important stirred-vessel methods are the paddle method (Fig. 31.20) and the rotating-basket method (Fig. 31.21). Details of these can be found, for example, in monographs in the European or US pharmacopoeias. Both use the same type of vessel, which is filled with a dissolution medium of controlled volume and temperature. In the paddle method, the tablet is placed in the vessel and the dissolution medium is agitated by a rotating paddle. In the rotating-basket method, the tablet is placed in a small basket formed from a screen. This is then immersed in the dissolution medium and rotated at a given speed.

Continuous-flow methods

In the continuous-flow method, the preparation is held within a flow cell, through which the dissolution medium is pumped at a controlled rate from a large reservoir. The liquid which has passed the flow cell is collected for analysis of drug content. The continuous-flow cell method may have advantages over stirred-vessel methods, e.g. it maintains sink conditions throughout the experiment and avoids floating of the preparation.

The amount of drug dissolved is normally analysed more or less continuously as the concentration in the vessel as a function of time. However, sometimes a single measurement can be performed if required in the pharmacopoeial or product specification, i.e. the amount of drug dissolved within a certain time period is determined.

The composition of the dissolution medium might vary between different test situations. Pure water may be used but in many cases a medium that shows a closer resemblance to some physiological fluid is used. In such media the pH and ionic strength can be controlled and surface-active agents might be added to affect the surface tension of the liquid and the solubility of the drug. Such fluids are often referred to as simulated gastric or intestinal fluids. Also, other dissolution media might be used, such as solvent mixtures, if the solubility of the drug is very low.

Mechanical strength

The mechanical strength of a tablet is associated with the resistance of the solid specimen to fracturing and attrition. An acceptable tablet must remain intact during handling at all stages, i.e. during production, packaging, warehousing, distribution, dispensing and administration by the patient. Thus, an integrated part of the formulation and production of tablets is the determination of their mechanical strength. Such testing is carried out for several reasons, such as to:

- assess the importance of formulation and production variables for the resistance of a tablet to fracturing and attrition during formulation work, process design and scaling up
- control the quality of tablets during production (in-process and batch control)

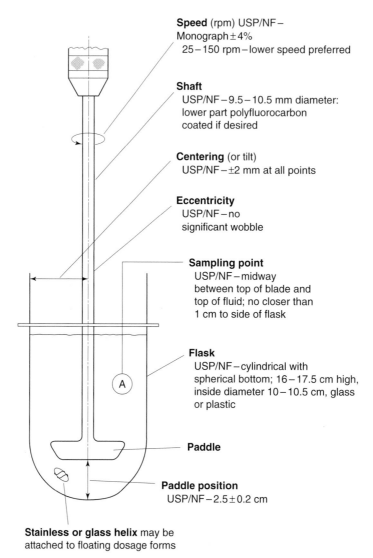

Speed (rpm) USP/NF –
Monograph ±4%
25–150 rpm – lower speed preferred

Shaft
USP/NF – 9.5–10.5 mm diameter:
lower part polyfluorocarbon
coated if desired

Centering (or tilt)
USP/NF – ±2 mm at all points

Eccentricity
USP/NF – no
significant wobble

Sampling point
USP/NF – midway
between top of blade and
top of fluid; no closer than
1 cm to side of flask

Flask
USP/NF – cylindrical with
spherical bottom; 16–17.5 cm high,
inside diameter 10–10.5 cm, glass
or plastic

Paddle

Paddle position
USP/NF – 2.5 ± 0.2 cm

Stainless or glass helix may be
attached to floating dosage forms

Fig. 31.20 Diagram of a dissolution instrument based on the rotating paddle method for the testing of tablet dissolution rate. (From Banakar 1992.)

• characterize the fundamental mechanical properties of materials used in tablet formulation.

A number of methods is available for measuring mechanical strength and they give different results. Also, the hardness of a tablet is sometimes measured by indentation test. The hardness of a specimen is associated with its resistance to local permanent deformation and is thus not a measure of the resistance of the tablet to fracturing.

The most commonly used methods for strength testing can be subcategorized into two main groups: attrition resistance methods (friability tests) and fracture resistance methods.

Attrition resistance methods

The idea behind attrition resistance methods is to mimic the kind of forces to which a tablet is subjected during handling between its production and its administration. These are also referred to as friability tests: a friable tablet is one that is liable to erode mechanically during handling. During handling, tablets are subjected to stresses from collisions and tablets sliding towards one another and other solid surfaces, which can result in the removal of small fragments and particles from the tablet surface. The result will be a progressive reduction in tablet weight and a change in its appearance. Such

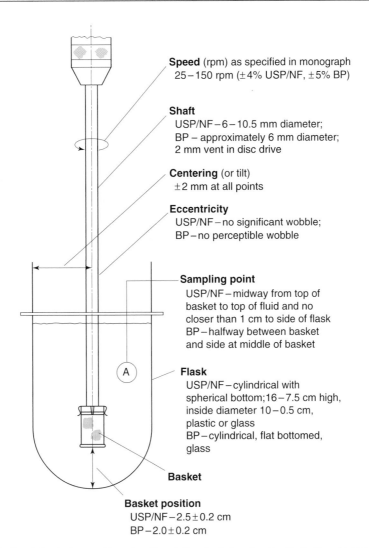

Speed (rpm) as specified in monograph
25–150 rpm (±4% USP/NF, ±5% BP)

Shaft
USP/NF–6–10.5 mm diameter;
BP – approximately 6 mm diameter;
2 mm vent in disc drive

Centering (or tilt)
±2 mm at all points

Eccentricity
USP/NF–no significant wobble;
BP–no perceptible wobble

Sampling point
USP/NF–midway from top of
basket to top of fluid and no
closer than 1 cm to side of flask
BP–halfway between basket
and side at middle of basket

Flask
USP/NF–cylindrical with
spherical bottom;16–7.5 cm high,
inside diameter 10–0.5 cm,
plastic or glass
BP–cylindrical, flat bottomed,
glass

Basket

Basket position
USP/NF–2.5±0.2 cm
BP–2.0±0.2 cm

Fig. 31.21 Diagram of a dissolution instrument based on the rotating-basket method for the testing of tablet dissolution rate. (From Banakar 1992.)

attrition can occur even though the stresses are not high enough to break or fracture the tablet into smaller pieces. Thus, an important property of a tablet is its ability to resist attrition so as to ensure that the correct amount of drug is administered and that the appearance of the tablet does not change during handling. Another application of a friability method is to detect incipient capping, as tablets with no visible defects can cap or laminate when stressed by an attrition method, e.g. a rotating cylinder.

The most common experimental procedure for determining attrition resistance involves the rotation of tablets in a cylinder followed by the determination of weight loss after a given number of rotations. Another approach is to shake tablets intensively in a jar of similar dimensions to a pack-jar. Normally, weight loss of less than 1% during a friability test is required. In addition, the tablets should not show capping or cracking during such testing.

Fracture resistance methods

Analysis of the fracture resistance of tablets involves the application of a load on the tablet and the determination of the force needed to fracture or break the specimen along its diameter. This has particular relevance in ensuring that the tablet remains intact during its removal from a blister pack.

In order to obtain a controlled loading during the test, care must be taken to ensure that the load is applied under defined and reproducible conditions in terms of the type of load applied (compression, pulling, twisting, etc.) and the loading rate.

For compressive loading of tablets, the test is simple and reproducible under controlled conditions and the diametric compression test has therefore a broad use during formulation development and tablet production. In such compression testing, the tablet is placed against a platen and the load is applied along its diameter by a movable platen. The tablet fails ideally along its diameter, i.e. parallel to the compression load, in a single fracture into two pieces of similar size (Fig. 31.22) and the fracture force is recorded. This mode of failure is actually a tensile failure even though it is accomplished here by compressive loading. The force needed to fracture the tablet by diametral compression is often somewhat unfortunately referred to as the crushing strength of the tablet. The term 'hardness' is also used in the literature to denote the failure force, which is in this context incorrect as hardness is a deformation property of a solid.

The force needed to fracture a tablet depends on the tablet's dimensions. An ideal test, however, should allow comparison between tablets of different sizes or even shapes. This can be accomplished by assessing the strength of the tablet, i.e. the force needed to fracture the tablet per unit fracture area. A strength test requires that the fracture mode (i.e. the method by which the crack is formed) can be controlled and that the stress state along the fracture plane can be estimated. The simplest and most common tensile strength test is the indirect diametral compression test described above. For a cylindrical flat-faced tablet, the tensile strength (σ_T) can be calculated by Eqn 31.4, provided that the tablet fails in a tensile fracture mode characterized by a single linear fracture across the diameter of the cylindrical specimen.

$$\sigma_T = 2F/\pi D h \qquad (31.4)$$

where F is the force needed to fracture the tablet and D and h are the diameter and the height of the cylindrical flat-faced tablet, respectively.

In practice, more complicated failure characteristics than tensile failure are often obtained during diametral compression (Fig. 31.23), which will prevent the strict application of the calculation procedure. It should be pointed out that the tensile strength of convex-faced tablets can also be calculated by using other equations.

Alternative procedures to measure the tensile strength of a tablet include breaking the tablet in a bending test or directly pulling the tablet apart until it fractures. The latter may be used to detect weaknesses in the compact in the axial direction, which is an indication of capping or lamination tendencies in the tablet.

FUNDAMENTAL ASPECTS OF THE COMPRESSION OF POWDERS

Mechanisms of compression of particles

The compressibility of a powder is defined as its propensity, when held within a confined space, to reduce in volume while loaded. The compression of a powder bed is normally described as a sequence of processes. Initially, the particles in the die are rearranged, resulting in a closer packing structure and reduced porosity. At a certain load the reduced space and the increased interparticulate friction will prevent any further interparticulate movement. The subsequent reduction of the tablet volume is therefore associated with changes in the dimensions of the particles.

Particles, either whole or a part, can change their shape temporarily by elastic deformation and permanently by plastic deformation (Fig. 31.24). Particles can also fracture into a number of smaller, discrete particles,

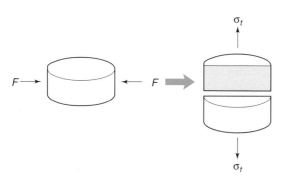

Fig. 31.22 Illustration of the tensile failure of a tablet during diametral compression.

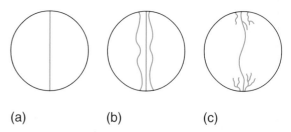

(a) (b) (c)

Fig. 31.23 Examples of different types of failure induced by diametral compression. (a) Simple tensile failure. (b) Triple cleft failure. (c) Failure due to shear at platen edges. (From Davies, P.N., Newton, J.M. (1996) Mechanical strength. In: Alderborn, G., Nyström, C. (eds) *Pharmaceutical Powder Compaction Technology*. Marcel Dekker, New York.)

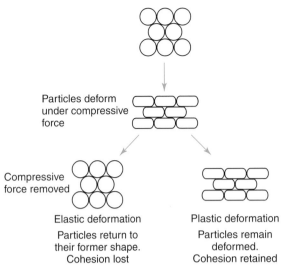

Particles deform under compressive force

Compressive force removed

Elastic deformation

Particles return to their former shape. Cohesion lost

Plastic deformation

Particles remain deformed. Cohesion retained

Fig. 31.24 Schematic illustration of particle deformation, elastic and plastic, during compression. (From Armstrong 1982.)

i.e. particle fragmentation. The particle fragments can then find new positions, which will further decrease the volume of the powder bed. When the applied pressure is further increased, the smaller particles formed could again undergo deformation. Thus, one single particle may undergo this cycle of events several times during one compression. As a consequence of compression, particle surfaces are brought into close proximity to each other and particle–particle bonds can be formed.

Elastic and plastic deformations of particles are time-independent processes, i.e. the degree of deformation is related to the applied stress and not the time of loading. However, deformation can also be time dependent, i.e. the degree of deformation is related to the applied stress and the time of loading. This deformation behaviour is referred to as viscoelastic and viscous deformation of a material. The consequence is that the compression behaviour of a material might depend on the loading conditions during the formation of a tablet in terms of the punch displacement–time relationship. Many pharmaceutical substances seem to have a viscous character, i.e. be strain rate sensitive, and the properties of the tablet are thus dependent on the punch displacement–time relationship for the compression process.

Elastic deformation can be described as a densification of the particle due to a small movement of the cluster of molecules or ions that forms the particle, e.g. a crystal lattice or a cluster of disordered molecules. Plastic deformation is considered to occur by the sliding of molecules along slip planes within the particles. For real crystals, such slip planes are formed at defects in the crystal lattice, especially dislocations.

The majority of powders handled in pharmaceutical production consist not of non-porous primary particles but rather of granules, i.e. porous secondary particles formed from small dense primary particles. For granules, a larger number of processes is involved in their compression. These can be classified into two groups:

- physical changes in the granules, i.e. the secondary particles
- physical changes in the primary particles from which the granules are formed.

The latter concern changes in the dimensions of the primary particles due to elastic and plastic deformation and fragmentation. Such processes may be significant for the strength of tablets. It is, for example, common for a capping-prone substance, when compacted as dense particles, to also be prone to cap or laminate during compaction in the form of granules, such as substrate–binder granules. However, in terms of the evolution of the tablet structure, the physical changes in the granules that occur during compression are of primary importance.

At low compression forces, the reduction in volume of the bed of granules can occur by a rearrangement within the die. However, granules are normally fairly coarse, which means that they spontaneously form a powder bed of relatively low voidage (i.e. the porosity of the intergranular spaces). Therefore, this initial rearrangement phase is probably of limited importance with respect to the total change in bed volume of the mass. With increased loading, a further reduction in bed volume therefore requires changes in the structure of the granules. The granules can deform, both elastically and permanently, but also densify, i.e. reduce their intragranular porosity. By these processes granules can still be described as coherent units but their shape and porosity will change.

Granules can also be broken down into smaller units by different mechanisms:

- Primary particles might be removed from the surface of granules when they slide against each other or against the die wall. This can be described as erosion or attrition, rather than fracturing. This mechanism occurs primarily for granules with a rough surface texture.
- Granules can fracture into a number of smaller ones, i.e. granule fragmentation.

Studies on the compression properties of granules formed from pharmaceutical substances have indicated that granules are not prone to fracture into smaller units during compression over a normal range of applied pressures. Thus, permanent deformation and densification dominate the compression event. However, for irregular, rough granules some attrition might occur. Deformation and densification of granules have been suggested to occur by the repositioning of primary particles within the granules, i.e. these processes involve an internal flow of primary particles. In this context, the terms 'degree' and 'mode' of deformation have been used to describe granule deformation. Degree of deformation refers to some quantitative change in the shape of the granules, whereas mode of deformation refers to the type of shape change, such as a flattening of the granule or a more complicated shape change towards irregular granules.

The dominating compression mechanisms for dense particles and granules are summarized in Table 31.2. The relative occurrence of fragmentation and deformation of solid particles during compression is related to the fundamental mechanical characteristics of the substance, such as their elasticity and plasticity. For granules, both the mechanical properties of the primary particles from which the granules are formed and the physical structure of the granule, such as their porosity and shape, will affect the relative occurrence of each compression mechanism.

Evaluation of compression behaviour

Procedures

The procedures used in research and development work to evaluate the compression behaviour of particles and the mechanisms of compression involved in the volume reduction process are of two types:

- characterization of ejected tablets
- characterization of the compression and decompression events.

Concerning the characterization of ejected tablets, the most important procedures used are inspection and the determination of the pore structure of the tablet, in terms of a mean pore size, pore size distribution and specific surface area. A less common approach is to calculate ratios between the mechanical strengths of tablets measured in different directions.

Concerning characterization of the compression and decompression events, these procedures are based on relationships between parameters that can be derived from the compaction process (Table 31.3). Some of the most common approaches used in this context are described below.

Inspection of tablets

The inspection of tablets, e.g. by scanning electron microscopy and by profilometry, is an important means of studying changes in the physical properties of particles during compression. Such changes include fragmentation into smaller particles, permanent shape changes due to deformation and finally, the formation of cracks within the particles. Such inspection will also give information about the relative positions of particles within the tablet and hence the interparticulate pore structure. The fracture path during strength testing, i.e. failure around or across the particles, can also be estimated from inspection of the tablet fracture surface.

In addition to the inspection of intact tablets, studies of the fragmentation of particles during compression can be obtained by analysing the size and size distribution of particles obtained by deaggregation of a tablet. Such deaggregation can occur spontaneously by disintegration of the tablet in a liquid or be created mechanically. Studies on such deaggregated tablets have indicated that powder compression can effectively reduce the size of particles and result in a wider particle size distribution of the cohered particles within a tablet.

Pore structure and specific surface area of tablets

One of the most important ways to study the evolution of tablet structure during compression is to measure some

---

Table 31.2 Dominating compression mechanisms for dense particles and granules (porous particles)

Dense particles	Granules
Repositioning of particles	Repositioning of granules
Particle deformation	Granule deformation
elastic	(permanent)
plastic	Granule densification
viscous/viscoelastic	Granule fragmentation/attrition
Particle fragmentation	Deformation of primary particles

Table 31.3 Parameters used in procedures to describe compression and decompression events

Upper punch force/pressure versus compression time[*]
Lower punch force/pressure versus compression time[†]
Upper punch force/pressure versus lower punch force/pressure
Upper punch force versus die wall force
Punch force versus punch displacement (mainly upper punch)
Tablet relative volume versus upper punch pressure/force
Tablet porosity versus upper punch pressure/force

[*]Used both during ordinary compression and also as prolonged loading after maximum applied force/pressure has been reached (referred to as stress relaxation measurements).
[†]Used primarily to describe the ejection phase.

characteristic of the pore structure of the tablet. Information on pore size distribution can be obtained by mercury intrusion measurements and by gas adsorption-desorption. However, the most common way to evaluate the pore system of a tablet has been to measure the surface area of the tablet by air permeability or gas adsorption. The former has also been used to derive an indication of the mean pore size in a tablet.

Fragmentation is a size reduction process and so can be assessed by measuring the specific surface area of a particulate solid before and after compaction, or measuring changes in tablet surface area with compaction pressure. The surface area of tablets can be determined by several procedures, including gas adsorption and mercury intrusion. Both these methods can provide useful information on particle fragmentation. However, by these methods it is difficult to differentiate between inter- and intraparticulate pores and the procedure might thus not reflect particle fragmentation only but also the formation or closure of cracks or intraparticulate pores.

A method which measures the external surface area is thus advantageous in this context. Air permeametry is one such method which also has the advantage of being simple and fast. The procedure involves the formation of tablets at a series of applied pressures, followed by the measurement of the tablet's specific surface area. The slope of the relationship between tablet surface area and applied pressure represents the degree of fragmentation and can be used to classify materials with respect to their fragmentation propensity (Fig. 31.25). It should be pointed out that the calculation of tablet surface area from air permeability measurements may give erroneous values as a result of the assumptions made in the derivation of the calculation procedure. In spite of this, the method has been shown to give useful data in terms of describing the fragmentation propensity of a substance.

The relationship between tablet surface area and applied pressure is, however, strongly dependent on the original surface area of the powder, i.e. the tablet surface area increases more markedly with applied pressure when the original particle size was smaller. Attempts have been made in the literature to derive an expression similar to those describing the size reduction of particles during milling (see Chapter 10), by which a measure of the propensity of particles to fragment independent of the original powder surface area can be calculated.

It is generally assumed that a change in the size of a particle affects the mechanics of particle deformation, i.e. how a particle responds to an applied load. Such a size-related change in the mechanics of particles can, for example, be attributed to a reduced probability of the presence of flaws in the crystal structure at which a catastrophic failure is initiated. It seems possible, therefore, that at a limiting particle size, fragmentation

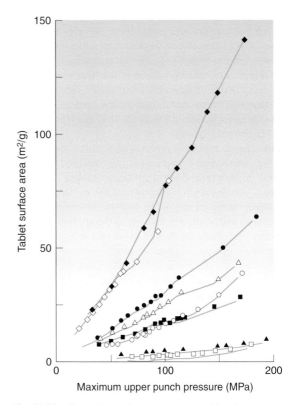

Fig. 31.25   The tablet surface area, measured by air permeametry, as a function of compaction pressure for a series of pharmaceutical substances. □ sodium chloride, ▲ sodium bicarbonate, ○ saccharose, ■ sodium citrate, △ ascorbic acid, ● lactose, ◇ paracetamol, ◆ Emcompress. (From Alderborn et al 1985.)

might cease. Examples of such transitions from a brittle to a plastic behaviour have been reported and the particle size at which this transition takes place is referred to as the critical particle size. This critical size has been suggested to vary markedly between different substances.

The use of surface area data to estimate particle fragmentation from gas adsorption and permeability measurements can only be applied to powders consisting of solid particles and not to those consisting of porous particles, such as granules. The problem for the latter type is related to the internal surface area and the intraparticulate porosity of the granules.

As granules are porous particles, there are two types of pore structure in a bed of granules, i.e. there will be pores both within and between the granules. The compression process will dramatically affect the pore structure and for tablets prepared from granules, it is in practice difficult to distinguish between inter- and intragranular pores.

It seems, though, that granules tend to keep their integrity during compaction and hence there are also these two types of pore structure in the resulting tablet. It has been shown that the porosity of the intragranular pore space constitutes a significant portion of the total porosity of a tablet formed from granules. As granules densify during compression, measures of their porosity before compression are not sufficient compensation for the intragranular part of the pore system.

In order to avoid the problem of defining the porosity of the intergranular pore space, a simplified approach based on air permeability measurements has been used instead to characterize the compression behaviour of granules. In this case, a tablet permeability coefficient is measured and studied in relation to the applied pressure. By this procedure, the change in intergranular tablet pore structure with applied pressure can be assessed, which is suggested to reflect the deformation and densification behaviour of granules during tableting.

Force–displacement profiles

The relationship between upper punch force and upper punch displacement during compression, often referred to as the force–displacement profile, has been used as a means to derive information on the compression behaviour of a powder and to make predictions on its tablet-forming ability. The area under a force–displacement curve represents the work or energy involved in the compression process. Different procedures have been used to analyse the curves.

One suggested approach is based on the division of the force–displacement curve into different regions (denoted E1, E2 and E3 in Fig. 31.26). It has been suggested that the areas of E1 and E3 should be as small as possible for a powder to perform well in a tableting operation and give tablets of a high mechanical strength. An alternative proposed approach is based on mathematical analysis of the force–displacement curve from the compression phase, e.g. in terms of a hyperbolic function.

Force–displacement curves have some use in pharmaceutical development as an indicator of the tablet-forming ability of powders, including the assessment of the elastic properties of materials from the decompression curve. They can also be used as a means to monitor the compression behaviour of a substance in order to document and evaluate reproducibility between batches. However, the interpretation of the force–displacement relationship in terms of mechanisms of particle compression, or compression mechanics, is not clarified, which limits the use of force–displacement curves in fundamental compression studies.

Force–displacement measurements have also been used in fundamental studies on the energy changes

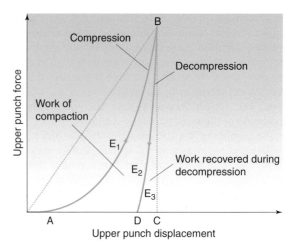

Fig. 31.26 The relationship between upper punch force and upper punch displacement during compression and decompression of a powder. (From Ragnarsson, G. (1996) Force–displacement and network measurements. In: Alderborn, G., Nyström, C. (eds) *Pharmaceutical Powder Compaction Technology.* Marcel Dekker, New York.)

during compaction of powders, i.e. a thermodynamic analysis of the process of compact formation. The energy applied to the powder can be calculated from the area under the force–displacement curve. This compaction energy is used to overcome friction between particles, to deform particles both permanently and reversibly and to create new particle surfaces by fragmentation. The thermal energy released during compaction can be assessed by calorimetry, i.e. the die is constructed as a calorimeter. The heat released during compression is the result of particle deformation, i.e. energy is consumed during deformation and thereafter partly released when the deformation is completed, and the result of the formation of interparticulate bonds.

Data have been reported indicating that the net effect of a compaction process is exothermal, i.e. more thermal energy is released during compaction than is applied to the powder in terms of mechanical energy. The main explanation for this is released bonding energy in the form of heat due to the formation of bonds between particles.

Tablet volume–applied pressure profiles

In both engineering and pharmaceutical sciences, the relationship between volume and applied pressure during compression is the main approach to deriving a mathematical representation of the compression process. A large number of tablet volume–applied pressure relationships exist. In addition to tablet volume and applied pressure parameters, such expressions include some constants which often are defined in physical terms. However, only for a few equations has the physical significance of the constants been generally accepted. Among these, the most recognized expression in pharmaceutical science is the tablet porosity–applied pressure function according to Heckel.

Heckel equation Tablet porosity can be measured either on an ejected tablet or on a powder column under load, i.e. in die. The latter approach is more common as it can be performed rapidly with a limited amount of powder. A problem might be that the compression time is different at each pressure, which could affect the profile for materials having pronounced time-dependent compression behaviour.

The compression of a powder can be described in terms of a first-order reaction where the pores are the reactant and the densification the product. Based on this assumption, the following expression was derived:

$$\ln(1/e) = KP + A \qquad (31.5)$$

where e is the tablet porosity, P the applied pressure, A a constant suggested to reflect particle rearrangement and fragmentation, and K the slope of the linear part of the relationship which is suggested to reflect the deformation of particles during compression. The reciprocal of the slope value K is often calculated and considered to represent the yield stress or yield pressure (P_y) for the particles, i.e.:

$$\ln(1/e) = (P/P_y) + A \qquad (31.6)$$

The yield stress is defined as the stress at which plastic deformation of a particle is initiated. To be able to use the Heckel yield pressure parameter to compare different substances, it is important to standardize the experimental conditions, such as tablet dimensions and speed of compaction.

Figure 31.27 shows a typical Heckel profile. The profile often shows an initial curvature (region I) which is associated with particle fragmentation and repositioning. Thereafter, the relationship is often linear over a substantial range of applied pressures (region II) and thus obeys the expression. The linear part is considered to reflect a situation where particle deformation controls the compression process and from the gradient of this linear part, the yield pressure can be calculated. Finally, the profile again deviates from the linear relationship (region III) and this curvature is considered to reflect elastic deformation of the whole tablet.

Strain rate sensitivity Another proposed use of yield pressure values from Heckel profiles is to assess the time-dependent deformation properties of particles during compression by comparing yield pressure values derived under compression at different punch velocities. A term denoted the *strain rate sensitivity* (SRS) has been proposed (Roberts & Rowe 1985) as a characteristic of the time dependency of a powder:

$$SRS = (P_y' - P_y'')/P_y'' \qquad (31.7)$$

where P_y' is the yield pressure derived at a high punch velocity and P_y'' is that derived at a low punch velocity. P_y' is normally higher than P_y'' and the SRS is thus a positive value.

The discussion on the use of Heckel profiles to derive a measure of the compression yield pressure is applicable to the compression of powders consisting of solid particles. It should be emphasized that the interpretation of $1/K$ in terms of a mean yield stress for the particles is under debate. Nevertheless, support has been presented that such an interpretation is valid for solid (non-porous) particles. For porous particles, i.e. granules and pellets, the Heckel procedure is inadequate for the derivation of a measure of deformability or granule strength. The problem of applying the Heckel approach to the compression of porous particles is related to the need to assess the porosity of the reactant pore system. The pore space of interest in relation to the Heckel equation is intergranular and the problem of quantifying this is discussed above.

Kawakita equation A promising means of assessing the compression mechanics of granules is to calculate a compression shear strength from the Kawakita equation. This was derived from the assumption that, during powder compression in a confined space, the system is in equilibrium at all stages, so that the product of a pressure term and a volume term is constant. The equation can be written in the following linear form:

$$P/C = (1/a\,b) + (P/a) \qquad (31.8)$$

where P is applied pressure, C the degree of volume reduction and a and b are constants. The degree of volume reduction relates the initial height of the powder

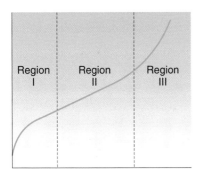

Fig. 31.27 A typical example of a Heckel profile indicating the three regions of powder compression. (From Sun, C., Grant, D.J.W. (2001) *Pharm. Dev. Technol.*, **6**, 193.)

column (h_o) to the height of the powder column (the compact) at an applied pressure P (h_p) as follows:

$$C = (h_o - h_p)/h_o \qquad (31.9)$$

The equation has been applied primarily to powders of solid particles. However, it has been suggested (Adams et al 1994) that the compression parameter $1/b$ corresponds to the strength of granules in terms of their compression strength. The procedure thus represents a possible means to characterize the mechanical property of granules from a compression experiment.

Evaluation of die wall friction during compression

Friction is a serious problem during tableting. Consequently, a series of procedures has been developed with the aim of assessing the friction between the powder or tablet and the die wall during compression and ejection, which can be used during tablet formulation to evaluate lubricants and formulations. These methods are based mainly on the use of force signals during powder compression or tablet ejection. The type of compression situation most commonly used in this context is a single-punch press with a movable upper punch and a stationary lower punch. In such a rig the force is applied by the upper punch and transmitted axially to the lower punch and also laterally to the die. The ejection of the tablet involves the application of an ejection force by the lower punch. Typical force profiles during compression in a single-punch press with a stationary lower punch are given in Figure 31.28.

When the descending upper punch establishes contact with the powder bed in the die, the force increases with compression time. The applied force rises to a maximum value and thereafter decreases during the decompression phase to zero. Parallel with the force trace from the upper punch, force traces from the lower punch and the die will be obtained. These can be described as transmitted forces and the force values are thus generally lower than the applied force. The force transmitted from the upper punch to the lower is considered to depend on a number of factors, including the friction between the powder and the die wall. These factors can be summarized in the following expression:

$$F_a = F_b\, e^{KL/D} \qquad (31.10)$$

where F_a and F_b are applied and transmitted forces, L and D are the length and diameter of the powder column within the cylindrical die (Fig. 31.29) and K is a constant. The constant K is a function of the friction coefficient between particles and the die wall. Thus, the transmission of force from the upper to the lower punch depends on the friction between the powder and the die wall. Both the difference in transmitted force, i.e. upper punch force–lower punch force, and the ratio between the upper and lower punch force, i.e. lower punch force/upper punch force (often denoted the R value), are used as measures of die wall friction during compression. For a well-lubricated powder, the force transmission corresponds to $R > 0.9$.

In addition to studies on transmitted forces during uniaxial compression of a powder, studies have been performed with the intention of describing the distribution of the compression pressure within the powder column in a more detailed way. A complex pressure pattern will be developed during the compression, an example of which is given in Figure 31.30. This distribution in pressure will probably be associated with local variations in porosity, pore size and strength within the tablet, caused by, for example, pressure-related variations in the degree of particle deformation within the tablet.

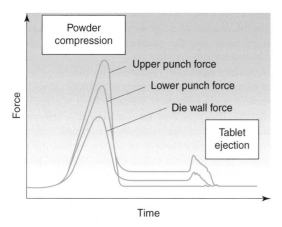

Fig. 31.28 Force–time signals (from punches and die) during uniaxial powder compression.

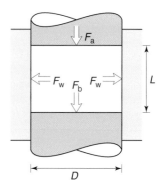

Fig. 31.29 Schematic illustration of punch and die wall forces involved during uniaxial powder compression in a cylindrical die.

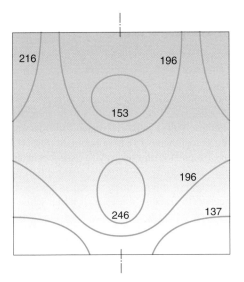

Fig. 31.30 The distribution of compression pressure (in MPa) during uniaxial powder compression. (From Train, D. (1957) *Trans. Inst. Chem. Engrs,* **35**, 258.)

After the upper punch has lost contact with the tablet and its force has consequently decreased to zero, the tablet will be positioned in the die in contact with the lower punch and the die wall. In this situation, the tablet will apply a force to both the lower punch and the die wall. The magnitude of these forces is dependent on the mechanical character of the particles formed into the tablet but also by the friction conditions at the interface between tablet and die wall.

The ejection of the tablet will result in an increased force signal from the lower punch, referred to as the ejection force. This is a function of the lateral die wall force but also of the friction condition at the interface between tablet and die wall. The maximum ejection force is thus also used as a measure of friction between tablet and die wall. One approach to assess friction during ejection is to calculate the dimensionless friction coefficient (μ) as the ratio between the ejection force (F_e) and the die wall force (F_w) at the beginning of the ejection phase, i.e.:

$$\mu = F_e/F_w \qquad (31.11)$$

To summarize, the following procedures are mainly used to derive measures of friction between powder or tablet and the die wall from force signals during tableting in a single-punch press:

- force difference between upper and lower punch
- force ratio between lower and upper punch
- maximum ejection force
- friction coefficient during ejection.

FUNDAMENTAL ASPECTS OF THE COMPACTION OF POWDERS

Bonding in tablets

The transformation of a powder into a tablet is fundamentally an interparticulate bonding process, i.e. the increased strength of the assembly of particles is the result of the formation of bonds between them. The nature of these bonds is traditionally subdivided into five types, known as the Rumpf classification:

1. Solid bridges
2. Bonding by liquids (capillary and surface tension forces)
3. Binder bridges (viscous binders and adsorption layers)
4. Intermolecular and electrostatic forces
5. Mechanical interlocking

In the case of compaction of dry powders, two of the suggested types of bond are often considered to dominate the process of interparticulate bond formation, i.e. bonding due to intermolecular forces and bonding due to the formation of solid bridges. Mechanical interlocking between particles is also considered as a possible but less significant bond type in tablets.

Bonding by intermolecular forces is sometimes also known as *adsorption bonding*, i.e. the bonds are formed when two solid surfaces are brought into intimate contact and subsequently adsorb to each other. Among the intermolecular forces, dispersion forces are considered to represent the most important bonding mechanism. This force operates in vacuum and in a gaseous or liquid environment up to a separation distance between the surfaces of approximately 10–100 nm.

The formation of solid bridges, also referred to as the *diffusion theory of bonding*, occurs when two solids are mixed at their interface and accordingly form a continuous solid phase. Such a mixing process requires that molecules in the solid state are movable, at least temporarily, during compression. An increased molecular mobility can occur due to melting or as a result of a glass–rubber transition of an amorphous solid phase.

Mechanical interlocking is the term used to describe a situation where strength is provided by interparticulate hooking. This phenomenon usually requires that the particles have an atypical shape, such as needle-shaped, or highly irregular and rough particles.

For tablets of a porosity in the range 5–30%, it is normally assumed that bonding by adsorption is the dominant bond type between particles. In tablets formed from amorphous substances or from substances with low melting points, it is possible that solid bridges can be formed across the particle–particle interface. It is also reasonable that if tablets of a very low porosity, i.e. close to zero, are formed, particles can fuse together to a significant degree.

Often granules, i.e. secondary particles formed by the agglomeration of primary particles, are handled in a tableting operation. When granules are compacted, bonds will be formed between adjacent granule surfaces. For granules that do not include a binder, the fusion of adjacent surfaces during compaction is probably not a significant bonding mechanism. Thus, intermolecular bonding forces acting between intergranular surfaces in intimate contact will probably be the dominant bond type in such tablets.

Granules often include a binder. When such binder–substrate granules are compacted it is reasonable to assume that the binder also plays an important role in the formation of intergranular bonds. The binder may fuse together locally and form binder bridges between granule surfaces which cohere the granules to each other. Such bridges may be the result of a softening or melting of binder layers during the compression phase. However, different types of adsorption bonds may be active between granule surfaces. These may be subdivided into three types: binder–binder, binder–substrate and substrate–substrate bonds.

For adsorption bonds between granules in a tablet, the location of the failure during fracturing of the tablet can vary. Fractures occurring predominantly through binder bridges between substrate particles, as well as predominantly at the interface between the binder and the substrate particle, may occur. The location of the failure has been attributed to the relative strength of the cohesive (binder bridge) and adhesive (binder–substrate interface) forces acting within the granules, which can be affected by, for example, the surface geometry of the substrate particles.

The main bond types in tablets formed from dense particles (interparticulate bonds) and from granules (intergranular bonds) are summarized in Table 31.4.

Table 31.4 Suggested predominant bond types in tablets formed from dense particles (interparticulate bonds) and from granules (intergranular bonds)

Interparticulate bonds	Intergranular bonds
Adsorption bonds (intermolecular forces)	Adsorption bonds of three types: binder–binder binder–substrate substrate–substrate
Solid bridges	Solid binder bridges

Compactability of powders and the strength of tablets

The compactability of a powder refers to its propensity to form a coherent tablet and thus represents a critical powder property in successful tableting operations. The ability of a powder to cohere is understood in this context in a broad sense, i.e. a powder with a high compactability forms tablets with a high resistance towards fracturing and without tendencies to cap or laminate (Fig. 31.31). In practice, the most common way to assess powder compactability is to study the effect of compaction pressure on the strength of the resulting tablet, as assessed by the force needed to fracture the formed tablet while loaded diametrically, or the tensile strength of the tablet. Such relationships are often nearly linear (Fig. 31.32) above a lower pressure threshold needed to form a tablet and up to a pressure corresponding to a tablet of a few percent porosity. At low porosities the relationship between

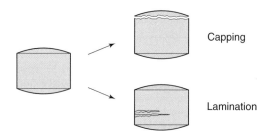

Fig. 31.31 Illustration of tablet defects referred to as capping and lamination.

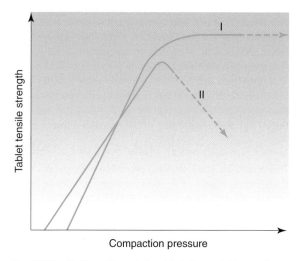

Fig. 31.32 Outline of the relationship between tablet tensile strength and compaction pressure for tablets showing no lamination (I) and for tablets showing lamination or capping (II).

tablet strength and compaction pressure will often level out. This relationship can thus be described simply in terms of a three-region relationship characterized by lower and upper tablet strength thresholds and an intermediate region in which the tablet strength is pressure dependent in an almost linear way.

Compactability profiles are sometimes also described by sigmoidal curves that can be divided principally into the three regions described above. At low pressures, the tensile strength of tablets increases as a power function with applied pressure, followed by a nearly linear region that finally levels off.

If cracks are formed in the tablet during tableting, e.g. during the ejection phase, this will often affect the assessed strength. Cracking and capping can often be induced at relatively high compaction pressures. This may be reflected as a drop in the tablet strength–compaction pressure profile.

A series of approaches to quantitatively describe or to model the compactability profile of a powder can be found in the literature. Some modelling approaches aim at describing the microstructure of a tablet in terms of an interparticulate bond structure and are based on the view that bond formation during compaction is significant for the development of coherence, i.e. it is postulated that the tensile strength of a tablet has some proportionality to the interparticulate bonds that act over the fracture area. Such models can thus be described as bond summation approaches and implicit is that all bonds are separated simultaneously during strength assessment. Since this is not consistent with the real mode of failure of a solid, the models are not fundamental approaches to understanding the strength of a tablet (see below).

Examples of such equations describing compactability profiles have been given by Leuenberger (1982) and Alderborn and co-workers (Alderborn 2003). In both cases the bond structure is modelled and related to an endpoint representing the maximum tensile strength (T_{max}) that can be obtained for tablets of a specific powder. Leuenberger's approach is based on the concept of effective numbers of interparticulate bonds in a cross-section of the tablet. It is assumed that over a cross-section of a tablet, a number of bonding and non-bonding sites exists. This number depends on the applied pressure during compression (P) and the tablet relative density (r, which is equivalent to 1 minus the tablet porosity, e). In the derivation of the expression, the term *compression susceptibility* (γ) was introduced, which described the compressibility of the powder and has the unit 1/pressure. The equation takes the following form:

$$T = T_{max} \left(1 - e^{[\gamma P \rho]}\right) \qquad (31.12)$$

The compactability profile as described by the expression stems from the origin of the tensile strength–

compaction pressure axes and the tensile strength will initially increase with compaction pressure and finally level off (compare discussion of compactability profiles above).

Alternatives to tablet strength–compaction pressure relationships for representing the compactability of powders are also used, such as the relationship between tablet strength and tablet porosity and the relationship between tablet strength and the work done by the punches during tablet formation.

Compaction is fundamentally a bonding process, i.e. strength is provided by bonds formed at the interparticulate junctions or contact sites during the compression process. Studies on the structure of fractured tablets indicate that a tablet generally fails by the breakage of interparticulate bonds, i.e. an interparticulate fracture process. However, especially for tablets of low porosity, the tablet can also fracture by breakage of the particles that form the tablet, i.e. a combination of an inter- and an intraparticulate fracture process. In general terms it seems, though, that the interparticulate contacts in a tablet represent the preferred failure path during fracturing. This conclusion is applicable to both tablets formed from solid particles and tablets formed from porous secondary particles (granules and pellets). Consequently, factors that affect the microstructure at the interparticulate junctions have been considered significant for the compactability of a powder.

Our understanding of the mechanical strength of a solid is based on the resistance of a solid body to fracture while loaded. It might seem reasonable that the sum of the bonding forces that cohere the molecules forming the solid will represent the strength of that solid. However, solids fail by a process of crack propagation, i.e. the fracture is initiated at a certain point within the solid and is thereafter propagated across a plane, thereby causing the solid to break. The consequence in terms of the strength of the solid is that the sum of the bonding forces acting over the fracture surface will be higher than the stress required to cause failure. It is known, for example, that for crystalline solids the theoretical strength due to the summation of intermolecular bonds is much higher than the measured strength of the solid.

In order to understand the strength of solids, the process of fracture has attracted considerable interest in different scientific areas. In this context important factors associated with the fracturing process and the strength of a specimen are the size of the flaw at which the crack is initiated and the resistance of the solid towards fracturing. The latter property can be described by the critical stress intensity factor, which is an indication of the stress needed to propagate a crack. Another fracture mechanics parameter, which is related to the critical stress intensity factor, is the strain energy release rate, which is a measure of the energy released during crack propagation.

By using the critical stress intensity factor, the tensile strength of the solid (T) is considered to relate to the flaw size (c) and the critical stress intensity factor (K_{IC}) in the following way:

$$T = f(K_{IC}/c^{1/2}) \qquad (31.13)$$

The critical stress intensity factor varies with tablet porosity. It has therefore been suggested that for compacts, such as tablets, factors such as the size of the particles within the tablet and the surface energy of the material will affect the critical stress intensity factor (Kendall 1988). These factors are also considered to control the interparticulate bond structure in a tablet.

Procedures to determine the critical stress intensity factor for a particulate solid have been described. Such a procedure involves normally the formation of a beam-shaped compact in which a notch is formed. When the compact is loaded, the fracture is initiated at the notch. The force needed to fracture the compact is determined and the critical stress intensity factor thereafter calculated. In order to assess a material characteristic, compacts of a series of porosities are formed and the series of values for the critical stress intensity factor subsequently determined is plotted as a function of the compact porosity (Fig. 31.33). The relationship is thereafter sometimes extrapolated to zero porosity and the value thus derived is sometimes considered a fundamental material characteristic.

In addition to the evaluation of compactability profiles and fracture mechanics studies, indices and expressions have been derived within pharmaceutical science which can be described as indicators of the compactability of a powder. There are several applications of such indicators during pharmaceutical development, such as:

- the evaluation of the compactability of small amounts of particles
- the selection of drug candidates during preformulation based on technical performance
- the detection of batch variations of drugs and excipients
- the selection of excipients and the evaluation of the compactability of formulations.

Examples of such indicators which have found industrial use are the indices of tableting performance derived by Hiestand and co-workers (Hiestand 1996). Hiestand derived three indices of tableting performance, among which the *bonding index* (BI) and the *brittle fracture index* (BFI) are suggested to reflect the compactability of the powder. These indices are dimensionless ratios between mechanical properties of compacts formed at some porosity. The BI is proposed to reflect the ability of particles to form a tablet of high tensile strength, whereas the BFI is proposed to reflect the ability of a tablet to resist fracturing and lamination during handling. These indices are defined as follows:

$$BI = T/H \qquad (31.14)$$

and

$$BFI = (T/T_o - 1)/2 \qquad (31.15)$$

where T is the tensile strength of a normal compact, T_o is the tensile strength of a compact with a small hole and H is the hardness of the compact.

Postcompaction tablet strength changes

The compactability of a powder is normally understood in terms of the ability of particles to cohere during the compression process and hence to form a porous specimen of defined shape. However, the mechanical strength of tablets can change, increase or decrease, during storage without the application of any external mechanical force. The underlying mechanisms for such changes are often a complex function of the combination of ingredients in the tablet and the storage conditions, such as relative humidity and temperature. In order to describe mechanisms responsible for postcompaction changes in tablet strength, studies on simple, one-component powders have been conducted (Table 31.5). The suggested mechanisms are probably active also in tablets formed from complete formulations of several components.

During storage at a fairly high relative humidity, tablets can be softer and their tensile strength reduced.

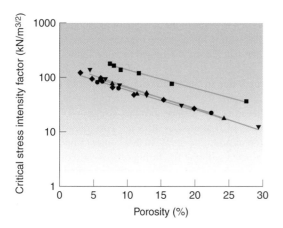

Fig. 31.33 A log-linear relationship between the critical stress intensity factor and the compact porosity for beams formed from polyethylene glycols of different molecular weight. (From Al-Nasassrah et al 1998.)

Table 31.5   Proposed mechanisms for postcompaction changes (increase or decrease) in the mechanical strength of tablets

Decreased tablet strength
Reduced bonding (intermolecular forces) due to condensation of water in tablet pores
Change in tablet microstructure due to dissolution of material in condensed water
Softening of amorphous material due to water absorption

Increased tablet strength
Formation of bonds due to crystallization of material dissolved in condensed water
Formation of bonds due to crystallization of amorphous material in rubbery state
Change in tablet microstructure due to viscous particle deformation
Change in tablet microstructure due to rearrangement of solid material in the amorphous state
Change in tablet microstructure due to polymorphic transformations

With increased relative humidity, the state of water adsorbed at the solid surface can change from an adsorbed gas to a liquid, i.e. water condenses in the tablet pores. Furthermore, if the solid material is freely soluble in water, it can dissolve. Both the presence of condensed water in the pores and the dissolution of a substance in the condensed water can drastically decrease tablet strength and eventually lead to the collapse of the whole tablet. However, the dissolution of a freely soluble substance in condensed pore water can also give an increase in tablet strength if the water is allowed to evaporate owing to a change in temperature or relative humidity. The result of this evaporation can be a crystallization of solid material, with the subsequent formation of solid bridges between particles in the tablet and increased tablet strength.

In addition to the mechanisms involving the presence of condensed pore water, several other mechanisms have been proposed to cause an increase in tablet strength during storage at a relative humidity at which condensation of water is unlikely to occur. One such mechanism is a continuing viscous deformation of particles after the compaction process is completed. This phenomenon is referred to as *stress relaxation* of tablets. The increase in tablet strength can be significant with no or minor detectable changes in its physical structure. However, viscous deformation of small parts of particles might change the microstructure of the tablet in terms of the relative orientation of particle surfaces and the geometry

of the interparticle voids and thus affect the resistance to fracturing of a tablet. A characteristic feature for stress relaxation changes is that the tablet strength changes occur for a limited time in connection with the compaction phase.

Explanations for observed changes in tablet strength due to the presence of amorphous material in tablets have been presented. If the amorphous substance absorbs or desorbs moisture, the mechanical strength of the tablet can change. This is probably related to an effect of absorbed moisture on the mechanical properties of the amorphous material. If the uptake of moisture allows the amorphous material to change from a glassy to a rubbery state, the amorphous phase may crystallize. Such crystallization can subsequently affect (normally increase) tablet strength.

Another mechanistic explanation for a storage-related increase in tablet strength which involves amorphous material is a process described as a restructuring of parts of the pore system due to a rearrangement of solid material. It has been reported, for example, that a marked increase in tablet strength during storage occurred in parallel with a change to a more open pore structure. Moreover, these changes do not necessarily occur immediately after compaction but can be initiated by exposure of the tablet to humid air for a certain period after compaction (Fig. 31.34). The restructuring of the pore system might be due to a diffusion-like transport of molecules or ions at the surface of particles, followed by a localization of material in zones where particle surfaces are close to each other. Such a mobility of molecules in the solid state has been shown by an amorphous phase.

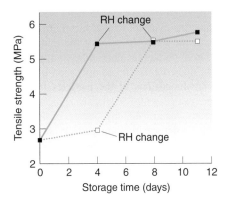

Fig. 31.34 The tensile strength of sodium chloride tablets as a function of storage time for tablets stored at different relative humidities. Open symbols: tablets stored 4 days at low, 4 days at high and 3 days at low relative humidity. Closed symbols: tablets stored 4 days at high, 4 days at low and 3 days at high relative humidity. (From Eriksson & Alderborn 1994.)

Finally, an increase in tablet strength during storage has also been explained by a change in the crystal structure of particles, from a less to a more stable crystal form, i.e. a polymorphic transformation.

RELATIONSHIPS BETWEEN MATERIAL PROPERTIES AND TABLET STRENGTH

Factors of importance for powder compactability

A number of empirical studies exist in the pharmaceutical literature with the aim of mapping factors that affect the structure of a tablet and its mechanical strength, i.e. tensile strength, resistance towards attrition and capping tendencies. These factors can be classified into three groups: material and formulation factors; processing factors (choice of tablet machine and operation conditions); and environmental factors (relative humidity, etc.).

Of special importance from a formulation perspective are the physical and mechanical properties of the particles used in the formulation and how these particles are combined in granulation and mixing steps. Relationships for powders consisting of one component, of two components, such as a filler and a lubricant or a dry binder, or of several components have been discussed in this context.

Compaction of solid particles

As discussed above, it is often assumed that the evolution of the interparticulate structure of a tablet, in terms of bonds between particles and the pores between the particles, will be significant for the mechanical strength of the tablet. Thus, the material-related factors that control the evolution of the microstructure of the tablet have been discussed as important factors for the compactability of a powder. In this context, the compression behaviour and the original dimensions of the particles have received special interest.

As already mentioned, the degree of fragmentation and permanent deformation that particles undergo during compression are significant for tablet structure and strength. It has been suggested that both fragmentation and deformation are strength-producing compression mechanisms. The significance of particle fragmentation has been considered to be related to the formation of small particles which constitute the tablet, with the consequence that a large number of contact sites between particles at which bonds can be formed will be developed and the voids between the particles will be reduced in size. The significance of permanent deformation has

been explained in terms of an effect on the area of contact of the interparticulate contact sites, with a subsequent increased bonding force. The relative importance of these mechanisms for the bonding between particles in a tablet and the resistance of a tablet towards fracturing has not, however, been fully clarified. Concerning elastic deformation, which is recoverable, this is considered as a disruptive rather than a bond-forming mechanism. Poor compactability, in terms of low tablet strength and capping/lamination, has been attributed to elastic properties of the solid. A summary of proposed advantages and disadvantages of the different particle compression mechanisms for the ability of the particles to form tablets is given in Table 31.6.

It is sometimes considered that one of the most important properties of particles for the mechanical strength of a tablet is their size before compaction. A number of empirical relationships between particle dimensions before compaction and the mechanical strength of the resultant tablet can thus be found in the literature. As a rule, it is normally assumed that a smaller original particle size increases tablet strength. However, it is also suggested that the effect of original particle size is in relative terms limited for powder compactability, with the possible exception of very small (i.e. micronized) particles. Reported data show, however, that different and sometimes complex relationships between particle size and tablet strength can be obtained, with maximum or minimum tablet strength values. Complex relationships might be associated with a change in the shape, structure (such as the formation of aggregates) or degree of disorder of the particles with particle size. It seems also that increased compaction pressure stresses the relationship between original particle size and tablet strength in absolute terms.

Expressions quantifying the relationship between tablet strength and original particle size have been presented in the literature, such as the following:

$$F = K \, d^{-a} \qquad (31.16)$$

where F is the force (N) needed to break the compact, d is the diameter (m) of the particle, and K and a are constants. The expression thus describes the general assumption that tablet strength increases with a reduced original particle size. The compactability of sodium chloride and hexamine is described by this equation (Fig. 31.35).

Some studies have specifically reported on the effect of original particle shape on tablet strength. The results indicate that, for particles that fragment to a limited degree during compression, an increased particle irregularity improved their compactability. However, for particles that fragmented markedly during compression, the original shape of the particles did not affect tablet

Table 31.6 Proposed advantages and disadvantages of the different compression mechanisms in relation to the tablet-forming ability of the powder

Compression mechanism	Advantages	Disadvantages	Others
Fragmentation	No effect of particle shape Low sensitivity to additives Strain-rate insensitive	May cause fracturing of tablets (capping, etc.)	Bond-forming ability (and tablet strength) dependent on degree of particle fragmentation
Plastic deformation	Resistant towards fracturing of tablets (capping, etc.) Strain-rate insensitive	Sensitive to additives and variations in original particle shape	Bond-forming ability (and tablet strength) dependent on degree of particle deformation
Elastic deformation	–	May cause fracturing of tablets (capping, etc.)	–
Time-dependent deformation	–	Strain rate sensitive Prone to change tablet strength after compaction due to stress relaxation	–

strength. Moreover, an increased compaction pressure increased the absolute difference in strength of compacts of different original particle shape. Thus, the shape characteristics of particles that fragment markedly during compression seem not to affect the microstructure and

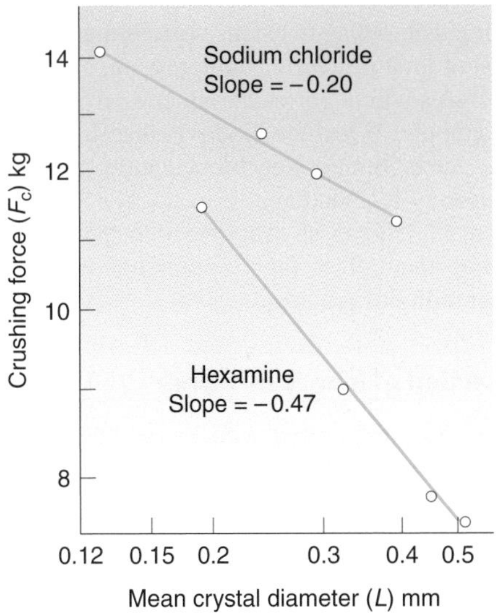

Fig. 31.35 The relationship (log–log scales) between the force needed to break the tablet and the original diameter of the particles of sodium chloride and hexamine. (From Shotton, E., Ganderton, D. J. (1961) *Pharm. Pharmacol. Suppl.*, **13**, 144T.)

the tensile strength of tablets but the converse applies for particles that showed limited fragmentation.

Compaction of granules

The rationales for granulating a powder mixture before tableting have been discussed above, one reason being to ensure good tableting behaviour, including the compactability. When granules are compacted, the mechanical characteristics of the primary particles and the properties of other excipients will affect the tableting behaviour of the powder. For example, it is a common experience that capping-prone material will show capping tendencies in the granulated form of the substance also. However, the design of the granulation process, such as the method of granulation, will control the physical properties of the granules formed, e.g. in terms of granule porosity and strength, which subsequently will affect the evolution in the microstructure of the tablets during compaction. Thus, the evolution of the intergranular tablet microstructure during compression as well as the evolution in tablet strength are related to the following factors:

- the composition of the granules (e.g. choice of filler and binder)
- the physical properties of the granules (e.g. porosity and mechanical strength).

During compression of granules, the granules tend to keep their integrity and the formed tablet can in physical terms be described as granules bonded together. When subjected to a load, tablets formed from granules often fail because of breakage of these bonds. Hence, the bonding force of the intergranular bonds and the structure of the intergranular pores will be significant for the tensile strength of the tablets.

In terms of the physical properties of granules, porosity, compression shear strength and shape are significant properties that influence compactability. In general terms, increased porosity, decreased compression shear strength and increased irregularity (Fig. 31.36) will increase the compactability of the granules. As discussed above, pharmaceutical granules seem to fragment to only a limited degree during compression. The importance of these granule properties for compactability has thus been discussed in terms of a sequential relationship between the original physical character of the granules, the degree of deformation they undergo during compression and the area of contact and the geometry of the intergranular pores of the formed tablet. The formation of large intergranular areas of contact and a closed pore system promote a high tablet strength.

Traditionally, the most important means of controlling the compactability of granules has been to add a binder to the powder to be granulated. This is normally done by adding the binder in a dissolved form, thereby creating binder–substrate granules. An increased amount of binder can correspond to an increased compactability but this is not a general rule. The importance of the presence of a binder for the compactability of such granules can be explained in two ways. First, it has been suggested that intergranular bonds that involve binder-coated granule surfaces can be described as comparatively strong, i.e. difficult to break. Second, binders are often comparatively deformable substances, which can reduce the compression shear strength of the whole granule and thus facilitate the deformation of the granules during compression. An increased degree of granule deformation is sometimes proposed to increase the compactability of the granules. Thus, the binder might have a double role in the compactability of granules, i.e. increase granule deformation and increase bond strength. Except for the presence of a binder in the granules, the combination of fillers in terms of the hardness and dimensions of the particles can affect the compression shear strength and hence the deformation properties of the granules during compression.

In the preparation of binder–substrate granules, the intention is normally to spread out the binder homogenously within the granules, i.e. all substrate particles are more or less covered with a layer of binder. However, it is possible that the binder will be concentrated at different regions within the granules, e.g. due to solute migration during drying. The question of the importance of a relatively homogeneous distribution versus a peripheral localization of the binder, i.e. concentration at the granule surface, has been addressed in the literature. It has been argued that a peripheral localization of the binder in the granules before compression should be advantageous, as the binder can thereby be used most effectively for the formation of intergranular bonds. However, the opposite has also been suggested, i.e. a homogeneous binder distribution is advantageous for the compactability of granules. This observation was explained by assuming that, owing to extensive deformation and some attrition of granules during compression, new extragranular surfaces will be formed originating from the interior of the granule. When the binder is distributed homogeneously, such compression-formed surfaces will show a high capacity for bonding.

Figure 31.37 gives an overview of the physical granule properties that affect the compression behaviour and compactability of granules.

Compaction of binary mixtures

Most of the fundamental work on powder compaction has been carried out on one-component powders. It is, however, of obvious interest to derive knowledge that enables the prediction of the tableting behaviour of mixtures of powders from information on the behaviour of the individual components. In this context, powder mixtures of two components, i.e. binary mixtures, have often been the system of choice in pharmaceutical studies. Binary mixtures can be of two types: simple physical mixtures, i.e. nearly randomized mixtures of

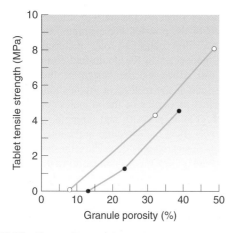

Fig. 31.36 The tensile strength of tablets formed from granules of a series of porosities and of two different shapes. Open symbol: irregular granules. Closed symbol: nearly spherical granules. (From Johansson, B., Alderborn, G. Unpublished data.)

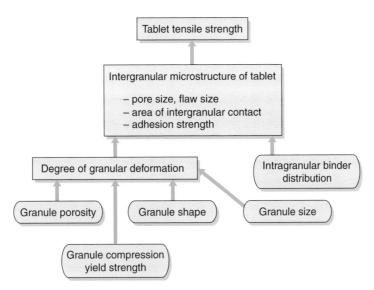

Fig. 31.37 Overview of proposed physical granule properties of importance for the compactability of granules.

particles, and interactive (ordered) mixtures. Most of the studies in this context are empirical, although models for the compaction of binary powder mixtures have been derived.

Concerning simple binary mixtures, the importance of the relative proportions of the ingredients has been studied in relation to the compactability of or compression parameters for the respective single component. The mixture can show a linear dependence of the properties of the single powders but deviations from such a simple linear relationship, both positively and negatively, have also been reported. Such non-linear behaviour has been explained in terms of differences between the components in their mechanical and adhesive properties.

Interactive mixtures, especially their compactability after the admixture of lubricants and dry binders, have been the subject of study. Concerning the tablet strength-reducing effect of a lubricant mixed with solid particles, it depends on the surface coverage of the lubricant film obtained during mixing, on the compaction properties of the lubricant per se and on the compression behaviour of the substrate particles. Lubricant sensitivity, also referred to as dilution capacity, seems to be strongly related to the fragmentation propensity of the substrate particles, as discussed earlier.

Concerning the tablet strength-increasing effect of a dry binder mixed with solid particles, similar factors seem to control the compactability of the dry binder mixture as for the lubricant mixture, i.e. the degree of surface coverage of the substrate particle, the binding capacity and deformability of the dry binder and the fragmentation propensity of the substrate particles (Fig. 31.38).

The dilution capacity of interactive mixtures between granules and lubricants or dry binders seems to be related to the degree of deformation the granules undergo during compression, i.e. a high degree of deformation will give a lower sensitivity to a lubricant but also a less positive effect of a dry binder.

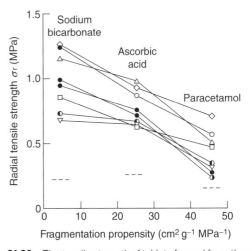

Fig. 31.38 The tensile strength of tablets formed from three substrate substances of different fragmentation propensities in binary mixtures with some fine particulate dry binders, i.e. microcrystalline cellulose, methylcellulose and polyvinylpyrrolidone of different particle size. The dotted lines represent the tensile strength of tablets formed from the single substrate substances. (From Nyström & Glazer 1985.)

REFERENCES

Adams, M.J., Mullier, M.A., Seville, J.P.K. (1994) Agglomerate strength measurement using a uniaxial confined compression test. *Powder Technology*, **78**, 5.

Alderborn, G. (2003) A novel approach to derive a compression parameter indicating effective particle deformability. *Pharmaceutical Development and Technology*, **8**, 367.

Al-Nasassrah, M.A., Podczeck, F., Newton, J.M. (1998) The effect of an increase in chain length on the mechanical properties of polyethylene glycols. *European Journal of Pharmaceutics and Biopharmaceutics*, **46**, 31.

Banakar, U.V. (1992) *Pharmaceutical Dissolution Testing*. Marcel Dekker, New York.

Eriksson, M., Alderborn, G. (1994) Mechanisms of post-compaction changes in tensile strength of sodium chloride compacts prepared from particles of different dimensions. *International Journal of Pharmaceutics*, **109**, 59.

Hiestand, E.N. (1996) Rationale for and the measurement of tableting indices. In: Alderborn, G., Nyström, C. (eds) *Pharmaceutical Powder Compaction Technology*. Marcel Dekker, New York.

Hölzer, A.H., Sjögren, J. (1981) Evaluation of some lubricants by the comparison of friction coefficients and tablet properties. *Acta Pharmaceutica Suecica*, **18**, 139.

Kendall, K. (1988) Agglomerate strength. *Powder Metallurgy*, **31**, 28.

Leuenberger, H. (1982) The compressibility and compactability of powder systems. *International Journal of Pharmaceutics*, **12**, 41.

Nyström, C., Glazer, M. (1985) Studies on direct compression of tablets. XIII. The effect of some dry binders on the tablet strength of compounds with different fragmentation propensity. *International Journal of Pharmaceutics*, **23**, 255.

Roberts, R., Rowe, R. (1985) The effect of punch velocity on the compaction of a variety of materials. *Journal of Pharmacy and Pharmacology*, **37**, 377.

BIBLIOGRAPHY

Alderborn, G., Nyström, C. (eds) (1996) *Pharmaceutical Powder Compaction Technology*. Marcel Dekker, New York.

Alderborn, G., Pasanen, K., Nyström, C. (1985) Studies on direct compression of tablets. XI. Characterization of particle fragmentation during compaction by permeametry measurements of tablets. *International Journal of Pharmaceutics*, **23**, 79.

Armstrong, N.A. (1982) Causes of tablet compression problems. *Manufacturing Chemist*, **October**, 62.

Chien, Y.W. (1992) *Novel Drug Delivery Systems*, 2nd edition. Marcel Dekker, New York.

Chulia, D., Deleuil, M., Pourcelot, Y. (1991) *Powder Technology and Pharmaceutical Processes*. Elsevier, Amsterdam.

Duberg, M., Nyström, C. (1986) Studies on direct compression of tablets. XVII. Porosity-pressure curves for the characterization of volume reduction mechanisms in powder compression. *Powder Technology*, **46**, 67.

European Pharmacopoeia, 5th edition (2005) Council of Europe, Strasbourg.

Lieberman, H.A., Lachman, L., Schwartz, J.B. (1989) *Pharmaceutical Dosage Forms: Tablets*, 2nd edition, vols 1–3. Marcel Dekker, New York.

Podczeck, F. (1998) *Particle-particle Adhesion in Pharmaceutical Powder Handling*. Imperial College Press, London.

Sandell, E. (1993) *Industrial Aspects of Pharmaceutics*. Swedish Pharmaceutical Press, Stockholm.

Stanley-Wood, N.G. (1983) *Enlargement and Compaction of Particulate Solids*. Butterworths, London.

Modified-release peroral dosage forms

J. H. Collett, R. C. Moreton

CHAPTER CONTENTS

MAINTENANCE OF THERAPEUTIC DRUG CONCENTRATIONS BY MODIFIED-RELEASE PERORAL DOSAGE FORMS

For many disease states the ideal dosage regimen is that by which an acceptable therapeutic concentration of drug at the site(s) of action is attained immediately and is then maintained constant for the desired duration of the treatment. It is evident from Chapter 23 that, provided dose size and frequency of administration are correct, therapeutic 'steady-state' plasma concentrations of a drug can be achieved promptly and maintained by the repetitive administration of conventional peroral dosage forms. However, there are a number of potential limitations associated with this. In the context of this discussion a 'conventional' peroral oral dosage form is assumed to be one that is designed to release rapidly the complete dose of drug contained therein immediately following administration. In addition, the released drug is assumed to be in a form which is therapeutically active and immediately available for absorption into the systemic circulation.

These limitations are as follows.

- The concentration of drug in the plasma and hence at the site(s) of action of the drug fluctuates over successive dosing intervals, even when the so-called 'steady-state' condition is achieved. Hence it is not possible to maintain a therapeutic concentration of drug which remains constant at the site(s) of action for the duration of treatment. At best, the mean value of the maximum and minimum plasma concentrations associated with each successive dose remains constant for the period of drug treatment.
- The inevitable fluctuations of steady-state concentrations of drug in the plasma, and hence at the site(s) of action, can lead to a patient being over- or undermedicated for periods of time if the values of C_{max}^{ss} and C_{min}^{ss} (Chapter 23) rise or fall, respectively, beyond the therapeutic range of the drug.
- For drugs with short biological half-lives, frequent doses are required to maintain steady-state plasma concentrations within the therapeutic range. For such drugs the maintenance of therapeutic plasma concentrations is particularly susceptible to the consequence of forgotten doses and the overnight no-dose period. Lack of patient compliance, which is more likely in the case of regimens requiring frequent administration of conventional dosage forms, is often an important reason for therapeutic inefficiency or failure. Clearly, not even a peroral dosage regimen which has been designed to

perfection can achieve and maintain clinically efficacious concentrations of a drug at its site(s) of action if the patient does not comply with it.

These limitations and requirements led pharmaceutical scientists to consider presenting therapeutically active molecules in 'extended-release' preparations. In reality, the scientists were attempting to take the control of medication away from the patient, and to some extent the physician, and to place it in the drug delivery system.

Over the years an enormous amount of work has been put into designing drug delivery systems that can eliminate or reduce the cyclical plasma concentrations seen after conventional drug delivery systems are administered to a patient according to a specified dosage regimen.

One of the first commercially available products to provide sustained release of a drug was Dexedrine Spansules® made by Smith Kline & French. After this many more sustained-release products came to the market, some successful, others potentially lethal. Each delivery system was aimed at eliminating the cyclical changes in plasma drug concentration seen after the administration of a conventional delivery system. A variety of terms was used to describe these systems:

- *Delayed release* indicates that the drug is not being released immediately following administration but at a later time, e.g. enteric-coated tablets, pulsatile-release capsules.
- *Repeat action* indicates that an individual dose is released fairly soon after administration, and second or third doses are subsequently released at intermittent intervals.
- *Prolonged release* indicates that the drug is provided for absorption over a longer period of time than from a conventional dosage form. However, there is an implication that onset is delayed because of an overall slower release rate from the dosage form.
- *Sustained release* (SR) indicates an initial release of drug sufficient to provide a therapeutic dose soon after administration, and then a gradual release over an extended period.
- *Extended release* (ER) dosage forms release drug slowly, so that plasma concentrations are maintained at a therapeutic level for a prolonged period of time (usually between 8 and 12 hours).
- *Controlled-release* (CR) dosage forms release drug at a constant rate and provide plasma concentrations that remain invariant with time.
- *Modified-release* (MR) dosage forms are defined by the USP as those whose drug release characteristics of time course and/or location are chosen to accomplish therapeutic or convenience objectives not offered by conventional forms, whereas an

extended-release (ER) dosage form allows a twofold reduction in dosing frequency or increase in patient compliance or therapeutic performance. It is interesting to note that the USP considers that the terms controlled release, prolonged release and sustained release are interchangeable with extended release. From a biopharmaceutical perspective this is not strictly a concern.

Repeat-action versus sustained-action drug therapy

A repeat-action tablet or hard gelatin capsule may be distinguished from its sustained-released counterpart by the fact that the repeat-action product does not release the drug in a slow, controlled manner and consequently does not give a plasma concentration–time curve which resembles that of a sustained-release product. A repeat-action tablet usually contains two doses of drug, the first being released immediately following peroral administration in order to provide a rapid onset of the therapeutic response. The release of the second dose is delayed, usually by means of an enteric coat. Consequently, when the enteric coat surrounding the second dose is breached by the intestinal fluids, the second dose is released immediately. Figure 32.1 shows that the plasma concentration–time curve obtained following the administration of one repeat-action preparation exhibits the 'peak and valley' profile associated with the intermittent administration of conventional dosage forms. The primary advantage provided by a repeat-action tablet over a conventional one is that two

(or occasionally three) doses are administered without the need to take more than one tablet.

Modified release

The term 'modified release (MR)' will be used in this chapter to describe peroral dosage forms that continuously release drugs at rates which are sufficiently controlled to provide periods of prolonged therapeutic action following each administration of a 'single dose'. Although all MR products could be described literally as controlled-release systems, the term 'controlled release' will only be used in this chapter to describe a peroral sustained-release product which is able to maintain a constant therapeutic steady-state concentration of drug in the plasma, the tissues or at the site of action. This use of the term is in accordance with the proposals of Chien (1995).

The degree of precision of control over the rate of drug release from an MR dosage form varies according to the particular formulation technique employed. Consequently, depending on the degree of control over release (and consequently over drug absorption) that is achieved, peroral MR products are generally designed to provide either:

- the prompt achievement of a plasma concentration of drug that remains essentially constant at a value within the therapeutic range of the drug for a satisfactorily prolonged period of time, or
- the prompt achievement of a plasma concentration of drug which, although not remaining constant, declines at such a slow rate that the plasma concentration remains within the therapeutic range for a satisfactorily prolonged period of time.

Typical drug plasma concentration–time profiles corresponding to the above criteria for modified-release products are shown in Figure 32.2.

Kinetic pattern of drug release required for the ideal modified controlled-release peroral dosage form

If it is assumed that the drug to be incorporated into the ideal MR dosage form confers upon the body the characteristics of a one-compartment open model, then the basic kinetic design of such a product may be represented diagrammatically as shown in Figure 32.3.

To achieve a therapeutic concentration promptly in the body and then to maintain that concentration for a given period of time requires that the total drug in the dosage form consist of two portions: one that provides the initial priming/loading dose, D_i, and one that provides the maintenance or sustained dose, D_m.

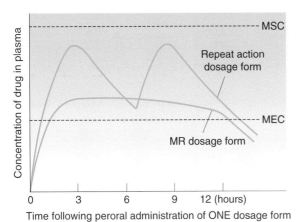

Fig. 32.1 Plasma concentration–time curves obtained following peroral administration of (a) one repeat-action dosage form containing two doses, and (b) one MR dosage form containing the same drug. MSC = maximum safe concentration, MEC = minimum effective concentration (see Chapter 23).

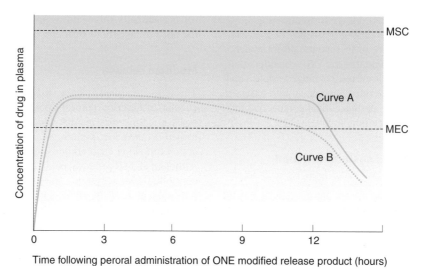

Fig. 32.2 Typical plasma concentration–time profiles for MR peroral products which, following rapid attainment of a therapeutic plasma concentration of drug, provide a period of prolonged therapeutic action by either (a) maintaining a constant therapeutic plasma concentration (curve A) or (b) ensuring that the plasma concentration of drug remains within the therapeutic range for a satisfactorily prolonged period of time (curve B).

The initial priming dose of drug D_i is released rapidly into the gastrointestinal fluids immediately following administration of the MR dosage form (see step 1 in Fig. 32.3). The released dose is required to be absorbed into the body compartment rapidly following a first-order kinetic process that is characterized by the apparent absorption rate constant, k_a^1 (see step 2 in Fig. 32.3). The aim of this initial rapid release and subsequent absorption of the initial priming dose is the rapid attainment of a therapeutic concentration of drug in the body. This priming dose provides a rapid onset of the desired therapeutic response in the patient.

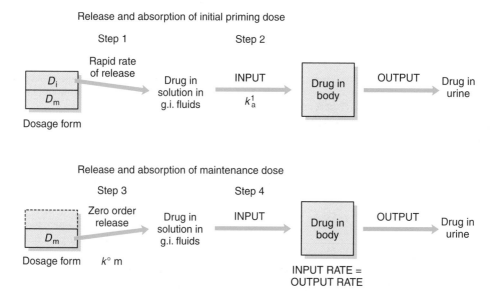

Fig. 32.3 A one-compartment open model of drug disposition in which the source of drug input is an ideal MR peroral drug product. D_i is the initial priming dose of drug in the dosage form; D_m is the maintenance dose of drug in the dosage form; k_a^1 is the first-order apparent absorption rate constant of drug from the priming dose; k_m^o is the zero-order release rate constant of drug from the maintenance dose.

Following this period of rapid drug release, the portion D_m of drug remaining in the dosage form is released at a slow but defined rate (see step 3 in Fig. 32.3). In order to maintain a constant plasma level of drug, the maintenance dose, D_m, must be released by the dosage form according to zero-order kinetics. It thus follows that the rate of drug release will remain constant and be independent of the amount of the maintenance dose remaining in the dosage form at any given time. The rate of release of the maintenance dose may be characterized by the zero-order rate constant k_m^o.

Two further conditions must be fulfilled in order to ensure that the therapeutic concentration of drug in the body remains constant:

1. The zero-order rate of drug release from the maintenance dose must be rate determining with respect to the rate at which the released drug is subsequently absorbed into the body. The kinetics of absorption of the maintenance dose will thus be characterized by the same zero-order release rate constant, k_m^o (step 3 in Fig. 32.3).
2. The rate at which the maintenance dose is released from the dosage form, and hence the rate of absorption (input) of drug into the body, must be equal to the rate of drug output from the body when the concentration of drug in the body is at the required therapeutic value (see step 4 in Fig. 32.3).

In practice, it is difficult to design an ideal modified- or controlled-release product that is capable of releasing the maintenance dose at a precise controlled rate which is in mass balance with the rate of drug elimination corresponding to the required therapeutic concentration of drug in the plasma. There are problems in achieving and maintaining zero-order release and absorption of the maintenance dose of drug in the presence of all the variable physiological conditions associated with the gastrointestinal tract (see Chapter 20). In addition, the apparent elimination rate constant of a given drug varies from patient to patient, depending on such factors as genetic differences, age differences and differences in the severity of disease. Consequently it is likely that most peroral MR products in current use will not fall into the category of ideal MR/controlled-release peroral dosage forms. However, such products may be referred to simply as MR products and may be differentiated from their ideal counterparts by the following definition. A modified-release product/dosage form is a system in which a portion (the initial priming dose) of the drug is released immediately in order to achieve the desired therapeutic response promptly. The remaining dose of drug (the 'maintenance' dose) is then released slowly, thereby resulting in a therapeutic drug/tissue drug concentration which is prolonged but not maintained constant.

Formulation methods of achieving modified drug release

It is evident from the preceding discussion that formulation techniques that permit rapid release of the priming dose, followed by slow release of the maintenance dose, are required in order to design peroral MR products. All MR formulations use a chemical or physical 'barrier' to provide slow release of the maintenance dose. Many formulation techniques have been used to 'build' the barrier into the peroral dosage form. These include the use of coatings, embedding of the drug in a wax or plastic matrix, microencapsulation, chemical binding to ion exchange resins and incorporation in an osmotic pump. The initial rapidly releasing priming dose may be provided by incorporating that portion of the drug in a separate, rapidly releasing form, for instance as uncoated, rapidly releasing granules or pellets in a tablet or hard gelatin capsule. Alternatively, immediate and rapid release of the priming dose has been achieved by that portion of the drug being positioned at the surface of a porous wax or plastic matrix.

Potential advantages of modified-release dosage forms over conventional dosage forms

1. Improved control over the maintenance of therapeutic plasma drug concentration of drugs permits:
   - improved treatment of many chronic illnesses where symptom breakthrough occurs if the plasma concentration of drug drops below the minimum effective concentration, e.g. asthma, depressive illnesses
   - maintenance of the therapeutic action of a drug during overnight no-dose periods, e.g. overnight management of pain in terminally ill patients permits improved sleep
   - a reduction in the incidence and severity of untoward systemic side-effects related to high peak plasma drug concentrations
   - a reduction in the total amount of drug administered over the period of treatment. This contributes to the reduced incidence of systemic and local side-effects observed in the cases of many drugs administered in MR formulations.
2. Improved patient compliance, resulting from the reduction in the number and frequency of doses required to maintain the desired therapeutic response, e.g. one peroral MR product every 12 hours contributes to the improved control of

therapeutic drug concentration achieved with such products.

3. There is a reduction in the incidence and severity of localized gastrointestinal side-effects produced by 'dose dumping' of irritant drugs from conventional dosage forms, e.g. potassium chloride. The more controlled, slower release of potassium chloride from its peroral MR formulations minimizes the build-up of localized irritant concentrations in the gastrointestinal tract. Consequently, potassium chloride is now administered perorally almost exclusively in MR form.

4. It is claimed that cost savings are made from the better disease management that can be achieved with MR products.

Potential limitations of peroral modified-release dosage forms

1. Variable physiological factors, such as gastrointestinal pH, enzyme activities, gastric and intestinal transit rates, food and severity of disease, which often influence drug bioavailability from conventional peroral dosage forms, may also interfere with the precision of control of release and absorption of drugs from peroral MR dosage forms. The achievement and maintenance of prolonged drug action depend on such control.

2. The rate of transit of MR peroral products along the gastrointestinal tract limits the maximum period for which a therapeutic response can be maintained following administration of a 'single dose' to approximately 12 hours, plus the length of time that absorbed drug continues to exert its therapeutic activity.

3. MR products, which tend to remain intact, may become lodged at some site along the gastrointestinal tract. If this occurs, slow release of the drug may produce a high localized concentration that causes local irritation to the gastrointestinal mucosa. MR products which are formulated to disperse in the gastrointestinal fluids are less likely to cause such problems.

4. There are constraints on the types of drugs that are suitable candidates for incorporation into peroral MR formulations. For instance, drugs having biological half-lives of 1 hour or less are difficult to formulate for modified release. The high rates of elimination of such drugs from the body mean that an extremely large maintenance dose would be required to provide 8–12 hours of continuous therapy following a single administration. Apart from the potential hazards of administering such a large dose, the physical

size of the MR dosage form could make it difficult to swallow. Drugs having biological half-lives between 4 and 6 hours make good candidates for inclusion in MR formulations. Factors other than the biological half-life can also preclude a drug from being formulated as an MR product. Drugs that have specific requirements for their absorption from the gastrointestinal tract are poor candidates. In order to provide a satisfactory period of prolonged drug therapy, a drug is required to be well absorbed from all regions as the dosage form passes along the gastrointestinal tract.

5. MR products normally contain a larger total amount of drug than the single dose normally administered in a conventional dosage form. There is the possibility of unsafe overdosage if an MR product is improperly made and the total drug contained therein is released at one time or over too short a time interval. Consequently, it may be unwise to include very potent drugs in such formulations.

6. As a general rule, MR formulations cost more per unit dose than conventional dosage forms containing the same drug. However, fewer 'unit doses' of an MR formulation should be required.

DESIGN OF PERORAL MODIFIED-RELEASE DRUG DELIVERY SYSTEMS

Factors influencing design strategy

Having made the decision that a drug is to be included in a modified-release delivery system intended for oral administration, it is necessary to take account of the physiology of the gastrointestinal tract, the physico-chemical properties of the drug, the design of the dosage form, the drug release mechanism, the particular disease factors, and the biological properties of the drug. All of these can influence or interact with one another.

Physiology of the gastrointestinal tract and drug absorption

The influence of gastrointestinal physiology on drug delivery is discussed in detail in Chapter 20. It should also be noted that the residence time of a dosage form in the gastrointestinal tract is influenced by both stomach emptying time and intestinal transit time. It has been reported that:

- solution and pellets (<2 mm) leave the stomach rapidly

- single dose units (>7 mm) can stay in the stomach for up to 10 hours if the delivery system is taken with a heavy meal
- the transit time through the small intestine is approximately 3 hours.

Physicochemical properties of the drug

Several physicochemical properties of the active drug can influence the choice of dosage form. This is discussed fully in Chapter 21. These properties include aqueous solubility and stability, pK_a, partition coefficient (or, more appropriately, permeability values) and salt form.

The aqueous solubility and intestinal permeability of drug compounds are of paramount importance. A classification has been made (Amidon et al 1995) whereby drugs can be considered to belong to one of four categories:

- high solubility and high permeability (best case)
- high solubility and low permeability
- low solubility and high permeability
- low solubility and low permeability (worst case).

This is codified as the Biopharmaceutical Classification System (explained and discussed in Chapter 22).

Consider first the influence of solubility. A drug that is highly soluble at intestinal pH and absorbed by passive diffusion (i.e. not site-specific absorption) would probably present the ideal properties for inclusion in an MR dosage form. However, there may be some problems associated with the choice of actual formulation. At the other end of the scale, compounds that have a low aqueous solubility (<1 mg mL^{-1}) may already posses inherent sustained-release potential as a result of their low rate of dissolution. The innate advantages of low aqueous solubility in relation to modified release would be negated if the drug also had low membrane permeability.

Having achieved dissolution of the drug in the gastrointestinal tract then permeability considerations become important. An indication of drug permeability values can be obtained using Caco-2 tissue culture models (discussed in Chapter 22). More than 90% absorption in vivo may be expected for compounds with permeability, P, values $> 4 \times 10^{-6}$ mm s^{-1}, whereas less than 20% absorption is expected when P is $<0.5 \times 10^{-6}$ mm s^{-1} (Bailey et al 1996). Drug candidates with a permeability $< 0.5 \times 10^{-6}$ mm s^{-1} are likely to be unsuitable for presentation as MR preparations.

Drug compounds that satisfy the solubility and permeability requirements should also ideally have:

- a biological half-life of between 4 and 6 hours so that accumulation in the body does not occur

- a lack of capability to form pharmacologically inactive metabolites by, for example, first-pass metabolism. Modified release is actually used for drugs which undergo first-pass metabolism but this should not be to such an extent that only inactive metabolites are left after the first pass
- a dosage not exceeding 325 mg in order to limit the size of the delivery system. There are a few examples where this dose is exceeded, e.g. Brufen Retard.

Choice of the dosage form

The first decision to be made is whether to formulate the active ingredient as a single or a multiple unit system. Single-unit dosage forms include tablets, coated tablets, matrix tablets and some capsules. A multiple-unit dosage form includes granules, beads, capsules and microcapsules.

Modified-release dosage forms include inert insoluble matrices, hydrophilic matrices, ion exchange resins, osmotically controlled formulations and reservoir systems.

The selection of the appropriate dosage form will need to take account of an acceptable level of variability of performance, the influence of GI tract structure and function on the delivery system, and the release mechanism and release profile of the dosage form.

Drug release mechanisms

The two basic mechanisms controlling drug release are *dissolution* of the active drug component and the *diffusion* of dissolved or solubilized species. Within the context of these mechanisms applied to MR dosage forms, there are four processes operating:

- Hydrating of the device (swelling of the hydrocolloid or dissolution of the channelling agent)
- Diffusion of water into the device
- Dissolution of the drug
- Diffusion of the dissolved (or solubilized) drug out of the device.

These mechanisms may operate independently, together or consecutively.

Drug delivery systems can be designed to have either continuous release, a delayed gastrointestinal transit while continuously releasing or delayed release. Drug release may be constant, declining or bimodal.

Constant release The general belief has been that the ideal MR system should provide and maintain constant drug plasma concentrations. This led to considerable effort being put into developing systems that release drugs at a constant rate. In general, these systems rely on diffusion of the drug or, occasionally, osmosis. However, with the advent of chronotherapy, i.e. drug delivered at both the appropriate time *and* rate, zero-order release may not be such a desirable goal in the future.

Declining release Drug release from these systems is commonly a function of the square root of time or it follows first-order kinetics. These systems cannot maintain a constant plasma drug concentration but can provide sustained release.

Bimodal release Although constant drug release may be ideal, this may not always be the case. If the gastrointestinal tract behaves as a one-compartment model (see Chapter 23), i.e. the different segments are homogeneous, then the situation is ideal. However, we know from Chapter 20 that absorption rate is not invariant along the gastrointestinal tract. So, whatever happens, the rate of release from the dosage form must regulate drug absorption; in other words, release rate must always be slower than absorption rate. This situation may not be easy to achieve; a release rate suited to absorption from the intestine may be far too great for that required in the stomach or colon. One possible solution to this problem is to prepare a dosage form that provides a rapid initial delivery of drug followed by a slower rate of delivery and then an increased rate at a later time.

FORMULATION OF MODIFIED-RELEASE DOSAGE FORMS

For convenience of description, oral modified-release delivery systems can be considered under the following headings:

- monolithic or matrix systems
- reservoir or membrane-controlled systems
- osmotic pump systems.

These are the main classes of delivery system and they are considered in turn below. However, there are other systems and the above is not an exhaustive list.

There is a basic principle that governs all these systems. In a solution, drug diffusion will occur from a region of high concentration to a region of low concentration. This concentration difference is the driving force for drug diffusion out of a system. Water diffuses into the system in an analogous manner. There is an abundance of water in the surrounding medium and the system should allow water penetration. The inside of the system normally has a lower water content initially than the surrounding medium.

Components of a modified-release delivery system

The components of a modified-release delivery system include:

- active drug
- release-controlling agent(s): matrix formers, membrane formers
- matrix or membrane modifier, such as channelling agents for wax (hydrophobic) matrices and solubilizers, and wicking agents for hydrophilic matrices
- solubilizer and/or pH modifier
- lubricant and flow aid, such as magnesium stearate, stearic acid, hydrogenated vegetable oil, sodium stearyl fumarate, talc or colloidal silicon dioxide
- supplementary coatings to extend lag time, further reduce drug release, etc.
- density modifiers (if required).

These types of components are virtually the same for all oral solid MR dosage forms. The differences are in the excipients, how they are incorporated into the formulation and what role they play.

The delivery systems may also be classified as inert, lipid or hydrophilic, depending on the nature of the excipients used. Suitable excipients for modified-release dosage systems are listed in Table 32.1.

Table 32.1 Suitable excipients for modified-release dosage forms categorized as inert, lipid or hydrophilic

Inert excipients
Dibasic calcium phosphate
Ethylcellulose
Methacrylate copolymer
Polyamide
Polyethylene
Polyvinyl acetate
Lipid excipients
Carnauba wax
Cetyl alcohol
Hydrogenated vegetable oils
Microcrystalline waxes
Mono- and triglycerides
PEG monostearate
Hydrophilic excipients
Alginates
Carbopol
Gelatin
Hydroxypropyl cellulose
Hydroxypropyl methylcellulose
Methylcellulose
Xanthan gum
Polyethylene oxide

Monolithic matrix delivery systems

These systems can be considered as two groups:

- those with drug particles dispersed in a soluble matrix, with drug becoming available as the matrix dissolves or swells and dissolves (*hydrophilic colloid matrices*)
- those with drug particles dispersed in an insoluble matrix, with drug becoming available as a solvent enters the matrix and dissolves the particles (*lipid matrices* and *insoluble polymer matrices*).

Drugs dispersed in a soluble matrix rely on a slow dissolution of the matrix to provide sustained release. Excipients used to provide a soluble matrix often are those used to make soluble film coatings. Alternatively, slowly dissolving fats and waxes can be used. Synthetic polymers, such as polyorthoesters and polyanhydrides, have been used. These undergo surface erosion with little or no bulk erosion. If the matrix is presented with a conventional tablet geometry, then on contact with dissolution media the surface area of the matrix decreases with time, with a concomitant decrease of drug release.

Drug particles may be incorporated into an insoluble matrix. Penetration of fluid into the device must precede drug release from these matrices. Fluid penetration is followed by dissolution of the drug particles and diffusion through fluid-filled pores. This type of delivery system would not be suitable for the release of compounds that are insoluble or which have a low aqueous solubility.

Excipients used in the preparation of insoluble matrices include hydrophobic polymers, such as polyvinyl acetate, ethylcellulose and some waxes.

It is useful to consider each of the matrix systems mentioned above separately.

Lipid matrix systems

Principle of design Wax matrices are a simple concept. They are easy to manufacture using standard direct compression, roller compaction or hot melt granulation.

The matrix compacts are prepared from blends of powdered components. The active compound is contained in a hydrophobic matrix that remains intact during drug release. Release depends on an aqueous medium dissolving the channelling agent, which leaches out of the compact, so forming a porous matrix of tortuous capillaries. The active agent dissolves in the aqueous medium and, by way of the water-filled capillaries, diffuses out of the matrix.

Wax matrices are a simple unsophisticated delivery system with a fairly coarse control of rate and extent of drug release. The release is generally not zero order and there are few opportunities to modify it.

These matrices are not now in common usage but the concept is worth considering. A typical formulation consists of:

- active drug
- wax matrix former
- channelling agent
- solubilizer and pH modifier
- antiadherent/glidant
- lubricant.

Matrix formers Hydrophobic materials that are solid at room temperature and do not melt at body temperature are used as matrix formers. These include hydrogenated vegetable oils, hydrogenated cottonseed oil, hydrogenated soya oil, microcrystalline wax and carnauba wax. In general, such waxes form 20–40% of the formulation. If too little matrix former is used, the formulation may break up during passage down the gastrointestinal tract and this, in turn, may lead to premature release of a large portion of the content of the tablet or capsule ('dose dumping'). If too much matrix former is added there is a risk that some of the drug will be completely encapsulated and not released from the device.

Channelling agents Channelling agents are chosen to be soluble in the gastrointestinal tract and to leach from the formulation. This leaves tortuous capillaries through which the dissolved drug may diffuse in order to be released. The drug itself can be a channelling agent but a water-soluble pharmaceutically acceptable solid material is more likely to be used. Typical examples include sodium chloride, sugars and polyols. The choice will depend on the drug and the desired release characteristics. These agents can be 20–30% of the formulation.

Solubilizers and pH modifiers It is often necessary to enhance the dissolution of the drug. This may be achieved by the inclusion of solubilizing agents, such as some of the polyethylene glycols (PEGs), polyols or surfactants. If the drug is ionizable then the inclusion of buffers or counter-ions may be appropriate. On occasion, the dissolution enhancer may also be the channelling agent.

Antiadherent/glidant Heat generated during compaction of the matrix can cause melting of the wax matrix-forming material and sticking to the punches. Something is needed to cope with the sticking; suitable antiadherents include talc and colloidal silicon dioxide.

These materials also act as glidants and improve the flow of formulations on the tablet machine. The typical amounts used will depend on the antiadherent used, for example 1–2% for colloidal silicon dioxide and 5–10% for talc.

This type of formulation usually does not need a lubricant per se, as the fats are themselves liquid-film lubricants, i.e. they melt during compaction. Magnesium stearate, if added, can also act as an antiadherent.

Insoluble polymer matrix systems

An inert matrix system is one in which a drug is embedded in an inert polymer which is not soluble in the gastrointestinal fluids. Drug release from inert matrices has been compared to the leaching from a sponge. The release rate depends on drug molecules in aqueous solution diffusing through a network of capillaries formed between compacted polymer particles. The concept of using inert matrices as drug delivery systems was considered in the late 1950s and led to the development of Duretter (Astra Hassle) and Gradumet (Abbott) technologies, and products such as Ferro-Gradumet (Abbott). There have been concerns that residual catalysts and initiators used in the preparation of the polymer(s) of the matrix could be leached along with active drug. The matrices remain intact during gastrointestinal transit and this has led to concerns that impaction may occur in the large intestine and that patients may be concerned to see the matrix 'ghosts' in stools. More recently there has been renewed interest in this type of matrix, and polymers such as ethylcellulose are finding favour.

The release rate of a drug from an inert matrix can be modified by changes in the porosity and tortuosity of the matrix, i.e. its pore structure. The addition of pore-forming hydrophilic salts or solutes will have a major influence, as can the manipulation of processing variables. Compression force controls the porosity of the matrix, which in turn controls drug release. Generally, a more rigid and less porous matrix will release drug more slowly than a less consolidated matrix.

The addition of excipients, such as lubricants, fillers, etc., is a necessary part of the formulation process. However, the presence of excipients is likely to influence drug release. It may be anticipated that water-soluble excipients will enhance the wetting of the matrix or increase its tortuosity and porosity on dissolution. Insoluble excipients can decrease the wettability of the matrix and reduce the penetration of the dissolving medium.

The particle size of the insoluble matrix components influences release rate, larger particles leading to an increase in release rate. This is attributed to these coarser particles producing matrices with a more open pore structure.

An increase in drug loading tends to enhance release rate but the relationship between the two is not clearly defined. One possible explanation may be a decrease in the tortuosity of the matrix. As may be expected, release rate can be related to drug solubility.

Drug release from insoluble matrices The release of drugs from insoluble matrices has been investigated and four types of drug matrix system can be considered:

- drug molecularly dissolved in the matrix and drug diffusion occurs by a solution-diffusion mechanism
- drug dispersed in the matrix and then, after dissolution of the drug, diffusion occurs via a solution-diffusion mechanism
- drug dissolved in the matrix and diffusion occurs through water-filled pores in the matrix
- drug dispersed in the matrix and then, after dissolution, diffusion occurs through water-filled pores.

The amount of drug released from matrix dosage forms is normally proportional to the square root of the time of exposure to the dissolution medium:

$$M_t = Kt^{0.5} \tag{32.1}$$

where M_t is the amount of drug released with time t, and K is a constant.

The amount of drug released decreases with time of exposure to the dissolution medium. The reason for this is that the drug is released initially from the surface region and there is then only a short diffusion pathway. As the period of dissolution progresses, the area of drug exposed to dissolution medium decreases. Also, an ever-increasing 'zone of depletion' is formed within the matrix as the drug dissolves and so the diffusion pathway increases in length.

A simple exponential relationship has been used to characterize drug release from non-swelling delivery systems:

$$\frac{M_t}{M_\infty} = Kt^n \tag{32.2}$$

where M_t/M_∞ is the fractional solute release, K is a constant and n is the diffusional exponent.

The numerical value of the diffusional exponent is indicative of the release mechanism and is influenced by the matrix aspect ratio (i.e. diameter:length ratio). If the matrix is presented as a thin film, a value of $n = 0.5$ would be indicative of Fickian diffusion, whereas values of n not equal to 0.5 are indicative of anomalous or non-Fickian process. Zero-order release is considered to be happening if $n = 1.0$. In other words, the rate of surface erosion is controlling the rate of drug release and not its rate of diffusion within the matrix.

Hydrophilic colloid matrix systems

These delivery systems are also called swellable-soluble matrices. In general, they comprise a compressed mixture of drug and water-swellable hydrophilic polymer. The systems are capable of swelling, followed by gel formation, erosion and dissolution in aqueous media. Their behaviour is in contrast to a true hydrogel, which swells on hydration but does not dissolve.

Principle of design of hydrophilic matrices The system comprises a mixture of drug, hydrophilic colloid, any release modifiers and lubricant/glidant. On contact with water, the hydrophilic colloid components swell to form a hydrated matrix layer. This then controls the further diffusion of water into the matrix. Diffusion of the drug through the hydrated matrix layer controls its rate of release. The outer hydrated matrix layer will erode as it becomes more dilute. The rate of erosion depends on the nature of the colloid.

Hydrophilic colloid gels can be regarded as a network of polymer fibrils that interlink in some way. There is also a continuous phase in the interstices between the fibrils through which the drug diffuses. These interstices connect together and are analogous to the tortuous capillaries seen in wax matrices.

The tortuosity of the diffusion path and the 'microviscosity' and interactions within the interstitial continuum govern the diffusion of the drug through the hydrated gel layer and hence the release of the drug.

Types of hydrophilic matrix

True gels These systems interact in the presence of water to form a crosslinked polymeric structure with a continuous phase trapped in the interstices of the gel network. The crosslinks are more than just random hydrogen bonds between adjacent polymer chains (e.g. alginic acid in the presence of di- or trivalent cations, gelatin). Here they limit the mobility of the polymer chains and give a structure to the gel (Fig. 32.4). The crosslinks can be chemical bonds or physical bonds, e.g. triple helix formations in gelatin gels which are based on hydrogen bonds. The portions of the polymer chains between crosslinks can move but the crosslinks restrict the overall movement of the chains.

Viscous or 'viscolized' matrices Not all matrix systems form 'true' gels. In reality, some are more properly described as very viscous solutions. In the presence of water, these systems form a matrix in which the increased viscosity occurs as a result of simple entanglement of adjacent polymer chains but without proper crosslinking (Fig. 32.5). It is a dynamic structure. The chains are able to move relative to one another and the drug diffuses through the interstitial continuum but the pathway is not fixed. Examples are hydroxypropyl methylcellulose and sodium alginate in water.

Comparison of different types of hydrocolloid matrix The differences between the various different types of hydrocolloid matrix are summarized in Table 32.2. It should be appreciated that these are simplifications. In general, bulk viscosity is not a good test for the functionality of either system. It may be satisfactory as a quality control test for the matrix-forming materials.

Advantages of hydrophilic matrix systems

- Comparatively simple concept.
- Excipients are generally cheap and are usually GRAS (generally regarded as safe).
- Capable of sustaining high drug loadings.
- Erodible, so reducing the possibility of 'ghost' matrices.

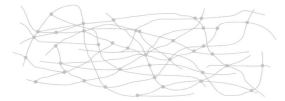

Fig. 32.4 Representation of a 'true' gel matrix.

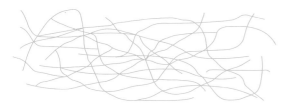

Fig. 32.5 Representation of a 'viscolized' matrix.

Table 32.2 Comparison of different types of hydrocolloid matrix

True gels	Viscous matrices
The diffusion pathway is via the continuous phase in the interstices of the gel	The diffusion pathway is via the continuous phase trapped between the adjacent polymeric chains
The crosslinks are more or less 'fixed' after the gel has formed	There are no 'fixed' crosslinks
The bulk viscosity of the gel is derived from the structure of the crosslinked polymeric chains with a contribution from the continuous phase	The bulk viscosity is related to the entanglement of adjacent polymer chains which are free to move within the continuous phase
Bulk viscosity generally does not correlate well with diffusion	Bulk viscosity may correlate with diffusion
Diffusion in the gel correlates with 'microviscosity'	

- Easy to manufacture using commonly available equipment by direct compression, wet granulation or roller compaction.
- Well-established technology.
- Possible to obtain different types of release profile: zero order, first order, biomodal, etc.

Disadvantages of hydrophilic matrix delivery systems

- Release of the drug is dependent on two diffusion processes: penetration of the water through the hydrated matrix into the non-hydrated core, and diffusion of the dissolved drug through the hydrated matrix.
- If the outer layer of the hydrated matrix erodes, this can complicate the release profile.
- Requires batch-to-batch consistency in the matrix-forming materials, other components and process parameters.
- Scale-up of manufacture can be a problem.
- Need optimal rate-controlling polymers for different actives.

These matrices are comparatively simple in concept. However, the events following hydration can be quite complex. The key is that there are two diffusion processes (water in and then drug out). The drug will only diffuse through a hydrated gel layer. This really only applies to drugs that are solid at room temperature. Liquid drugs may diffuse in the non-hydrated state and would not be suitable for some types of system.

Components of hydrophilic matrix delivery systems

- Active drug
- Hydrophilic colloid(s)
- (Matrix modifier)
- (Solubilizer and/or pH modifier)
- Compression aid
- Lubricant
- (Glidant).

Those components listed in parentheses are optional and not always necessary.

Matrix-forming agents for hydrophilic matrices Hydrophilic colloids, which on contact with water form a hydrated gel that remains 'sufficiently intact' during passage through the gastrointestinal tract, are suitable matrix-forming agents for hydrophilic matrices. Examples of hydrophilic colloids include:

- hydroxypropyl methylcellulose (high-viscosity grades)
- hydroxypropyl cellulose
- sodium carboxymethyl cellulose
- alginates
- xanthan gum

- xanthan gum/locust bean gum combinations
- carbopol
- polyethylene oxide.

These agents generally occupy 20–80% of the mass; the actual amount will depend on the drug and the desired release characteristics.

Hydration and swelling are the key factors in the functioning of a hydrophilic matrix, as has already been stated.

Gel modifiers for hydrophilic matrix delivery systems These are materials that are incorporated into the matrix to modify the diffusional characteristics of the gel layer, very often to enhance drug diffusion and hence release of the drug. Examples include sugars, polyols and soluble salts.

The type of modifier will depend very much on the chemical nature of the hydrocolloid(s) used. They may also modify the rate and extent of hydration of the hydrophilic matrix material.

Gel modifiers can have a number of other functions. For example, they may act to:

- allow more complete, more uniform hydration of the gel matrix
- allow more rapid hydration of the gel matrix
- associate with the matrix molecules and thus influence the interactions at a molecular level, e.g. crosslinking
- modify the environment in the interstices of the gel, either to speed up or slow down diffusion
- suppress or promote the ionization of ionizable polymers.

Few materials will have only a single action. It is more likely that they will work in several ways.

Solubilizers and pH modifiers for drugs in hydrophilic matrices Many drugs will not dissolve sufficiently in gastrointestinal fluids to allow them to be released from a hydrophilic colloid matrix. Dissolution can be improved by the inclusion of solubilizing agents (e.g. PEGs, polyols, surfactants, etc.). The only restriction is that the formulation can be formed into a tablet and that the material is acceptable. Many drugs are ionizable. The inclusion of appropriate counter-ions can facilitate release from the system. Some materials can act as both dissolution enhancer and matrix modifier; the amount of excipient needed will be determined by the amount of drug.

The above relates to the drug molecule rather than the matrix material. It is necessary for any drug to be in solution for diffusion to occur. For insoluble drugs, solubilization is therefore an important consideration.

With some gel materials the use of certain ions causes changes in the nature of the gel matrix.

The solubilizers and pH modifiers might also influence the release process through a direct effect on the matrix.

Different materials could augment crosslinking whereas others might perhaps weaken the crosslinks.

Lubricants for hydrophilic delivery systems   As with any tablet compacted on a tablet machine, a lubricant is necessary. Lubricants can have four functions:

- reduce interparticulate friction during compression and compaction
- reduce die wall friction
- prevent sticking to the punches
- improve flow of the formulation on to the machine and into the die.

The requirements for lubricants used in hydrophilic matrix tablets are no different from those for any other compressed tablet and are thus analogous to those for conventional immediate-release tablets and capsules. Generally the choice is not governed by the same constraints as in immediate release. For example, overblending or excess magnesium stearate may not be a major problem here.

It is not essential that the lubricant is soluble. Such lubricants are available but are generally not very effective and tend to be reserved for effervescent products.

Suitable lubricants and recommended concentrations to be included in the formulation are listed in Table 32.3.

Drug release from hydrophilic colloid matrices   The classic description of the events following immersion of a matrix in aqueous media is as follows:

- Surface drug (if water soluble) dissolves and gives a 'burst effect'.
- The hydrophilic polymer hydrates and an outer gel layer forms.

Table 32.3   Concentration of lubricants used in hydrophilic matrix systems

Lubricant	%
Hydrophobic lubricants	
Magnesium stearate	0.25–2
Calcium stearate	0.25–2
Stearic acid	1–4
Hydrogenated vegetable oil	1–4
Hydrophilic lubricants (the latter two examples are only partially soluble in water)	
Glyceryl palmitostearate	0.5–5
Glyceryl behenate	2–5
Sodium stearyl fumarate	0.25–2
Inorganic lubricants	
Colloidal silicon dioxide	0.05–0.25 as glidant
	0.2–1.0 as antiadherent
Talc	1–4 as antiadherent

- The gel layer becomes a barrier to uptake of further water and to the transfer of drug.
- Drug (if soluble) release occurs by diffusion through the gel layer; insoluble drug is released by erosion followed by dissolution.
- Following erosion, the new surface becomes hydrated and forms a new gel layer.

It may be anticipated that the relative importance of each release mechanism will depend on the physicochemical properties of the gel layer, the aqueous solubility of the drug and the mechanical attrition of the matrix in the aqueous environment.

When a drug/glassy polymer matrix is placed in an aqueous environment, the water penetrates the polymer network. As the amount of water increases, a transition from a glassy to a rubbery state occurs as the glass transition temperature is decreased by the presence of water to the temperature of the medium. The intake of solvent (water) induces stresses within the matrix polymer. Eventually the matrix polymer relaxes and this manifests itself as swelling. It is possible to differentiate three 'fronts' during hydration: eroding, diffusing and swelling.

The actual drug release mechanism depends on the relative contributions of swelling and dissolution. Drug release from swellable, soluble matrices is constant when swelling and eroding fronts synchronize but is non-linear when this is not the case. The release of sodium diclofenac from PVA and from HPMC matrices has been investigated. It was noted that if the fronts synchronized then the gel layer thickness was constant and zero-order release was observed. When synchronization did not take place, the gel layer tended to increase in thickness and there was a decrease in the amount released, providing non-linear kinetics.

MEMBRANE-CONTROLLED DRUG DELIVERY SYSTEMS

Membrane-controlled delivery systems function as follows. The rate-controlling part of the system is a membrane through which the drug must diffuse. To allow the drug to diffuse out, the membrane has to become permeable, e.g. through hydration by water normally present in the gastrointestinal tract or by the drug being soluble in a membrane component, such as the plasticizer. Unlike hydrophilic matrix systems, the membrane polymer does not swell on hydration to form a hydrocolloid matrix, and does not erode.

In membrane-controlled delivery systems, a drug reservoir, e.g. a tablet or multiparticulate pellet, is coated with a membrane. The drug should not diffuse in the solid state, although loading of the membrane might be an advantage if an initial release on contact with dissolution medium is desired. Aqueous medium diffusing into the system and forming a continuous phase through the membrane initiates drug diffusion and release.

The essential difference between a membrane and a matrix system is that in the former the polymer membrane is only at the surface of the system, whereas in the latter the polymer is throughout the whole system. In both cases the hydration of the polymer is the step that allows the drug to diffuse. With the classic membrane system there are the two diffusion processes: 'water in' followed by 'drug out'.

The delivery systems may be presented as either single or multiple units.

Components of a membrane-controlled system

The individual components of a typical membrane-controlled system can be listed in terms of core and coating as follows.

Core

- Active drug
- Filler or substrate
- (Solubilizer)
- Lubricant/glidant.

The exact composition of the core formulation will depend on the formulation approach adopted.

Coating

- Membrane polymer
- Plasticizer
- (Membrane modifier)
- (Colour/opacifier).

Single-unit systems

These are essentially tablet formulations. They differ from conventional dosage forms in that modified-release tablet cores should not disintegrate but dissolve. Also a formulation is required that allows water to penetrate and the drug to dissolve so that diffusion can occur.

Core formulation for single-unit systems

Generally, water-insoluble materials that compact by brittle fracture are not suitable if used alone. Suitable fillers include lactose, microcrystalline cellulose, dextrose, sucrose and polyols (mannitol, sorbitol, xylitol, etc.).

Care is needed in the choice of soluble fillers to minimize osmotic effects. An inappropriate choice will result in increased internal osmotic pressure followed by rup-

ture of the release-controlling membrane. The choice of solubilizer (if required) will be governed by the solubility characteristics of the drug. Materials that have been used include buffers, surfactants, polyols and PEGs.

Because single-unit cores are most often compressed tablets, a satisfactory lubricant system will also be required. Again, this is the same as for any tablet except that soluble lubricants may not be necessary. Suitable lubricants are listed in Table 32.3.

Multiple-unit systems

As the name implies, this type of dosage unit comprises more than one discrete unit. Typically, such systems comprise coated spheroids (pellets approximately 1 mm in diameter) filled into a hard gelatin capsule shell or, less commonly, compressed into a tablet.

There are two main approaches that can be adapted to the manufacture of drug-containing multiple units:

- the use of inert sugar spheres ('non-pareils') coated first with drug and then with the release-controlling membrane
- the formulation of small spheroids containing the drug using an extrusion/spheronization process (described in Chapter 29). This approach is better if a high drug loading is required.

Typical formulations comprise drug with combinations of lactose and microcrystalline cellulose. Other materials can be used. A typical formulation for a wet mass for extrusion/spheronization might comprise:

Ingredients	Parts by weight
Active drug	1–20
Lactose	60
Microcrystalline cellulose	40
Binder	2–4
Water	40

After spheronization the material is dried prior to coating (see Chapter 33).

Release-controlling membrane

The membrane is a critical part of the formulation as it controls the release of the drug. The requirement is that the polymer remains intact for the period of release, i.e. there should be no swelling or subsequent erosion, as seen in hydrophilic matrices. Typical polymers used include ethylcellulose, acrylic copolymers, e.g. Eudragit RL and RS grades, shellac and zein. Shellac and zein are natural products and their quality can vary; consequently they are used less frequently.

The release-controlling polymer is film-coated on to the system. For the coating to be successful, the coating droplets must coalesce. The plasticizer is used to lower the glass transition temperature (T_g) of the film (see Chapter 33). The choice of plasticizer will depend on the polymer used, the active drug and the desired release characteristics. In addition, the plasticizer may modify the diffusional characteristics of the membrane with respect to the drug. The final choice of plasticizer will probably be a compromise of all these different requirements.

Examples of suitable plasticizers for ethylcellulose films include dibutyl phthalate, diethyl phthalate, dibutyl sebecate and citric acid esters. These are water-insoluble materials; a water-soluble plasticizer might increase the permeability of the membrane excessively. The amount of plasticizer required will depend on the several factors mentioned above but is typically 10–25% of the polymer dry weight.

The smallest amount of plasticizer is used that will produce the most consistent result, i.e. complete coalescence of the droplets to form the film without making it too elastic, plastic, soft or permeable. The plasticizer is not present only for processing but is added to have an effect on the mechanical properties of the resulting film, i.e. film flexibility should be induced and maintained. Plasticizers should be permanent to avoid stability problems.

It may be necessary to add components to the coating formulation to modify the release characteristics of the film, particularly to increase the rate of release. Typically this will be a less hydrophobic, water-soluble component. Examples of such materials include polyethylene glycols, propylene glycol, glycerol, other polyols and water-soluble polymers. Some of these may also act as plasticizers. It is important to recognize that many materials can have different functions in a formulation and also to understand what the implications of these different functionalities are for the finished product.

Advantages of membrane-controlled systems

- For multiple-unit systems, the gastrointestinal transit of small particulates is more consistent than that of a larger single-unit system.
- Multiple-unit systems are also less likely to suffer from the problems associated with total dose dumping due to overall catastrophic failure of a film around a monolith (tablet), which would then release the whole dosage.
- In addition, multiple-unit systems allow the release mechanism to be optimized for individual drugs in a system delivering two or more active components.

Disadvantages of membrane-controlled systems

- Dose dumping can occur from single-unit systems as a result of film failure.
- Multiple-unit systems can be difficult to retain in the higher gastrointestinal tract.
- The control of the membrane characteristics in film-coated membranes can be difficult.
- Filling of the multiunit spheroids into capsules can be a problem owing to build-up of static charge.

Osmotic pump systems

In one sense osmotic pump systems are another form of membrane-controlled release drug delivery system and work in the following way. A drug is included in a tablet core which is water soluble, and which will solubilize (or suspend) the drug in the presence of water. The tablet core is coated with a semi-permeable membrane which will allow water to pass through into the core, which then dissolves. As the core dissolves, a hydrostatic pressure builds up and forces (pumps) drug solution (or suspension) through a hole drilled in the coating. The rate at which water is able to pass in through the membrane and how quickly the drug solution (or suspension) can pass out of the hole govern the rate of release.

The rate at which the drug solution/suspension is forced out can be modified by changes in the viscosity of the solution formed inside the system. The essential difference between an osmotic pump system and a 'classic' membrane-controlled system is that for the osmotic pump, only one diffusion process is required (in this case 'water in'). As mentioned above, in the 'classic' system two processes are key: water in, drug out.

Components of osmotic pump systems

Osmotic pump systems consist of a core and a coat. The core consists of the active drug, a filler or substrate, (viscosity modifier), (solubilizer) and lubricant/glidant. Coatings contain a membrane polymer, a plasticizer, (membrane modifier) and (colour/opacifier).

This is the same list of components as for matrix-controlled systems and the types of excipient used are essentially similar. However, it is important to remember that the diffusing species is only water. An agent must be included in the core which is soluble enough to generate the osmotic pressure. Also there must be a hole through which the drug solution/suspension can be pumped out. Otherwise, the same considerations apply for the formulation of the core as with other membrane-controlled systems. The film coating must also be fully coalesced and be free from unintentional pinholes and it should act as a semi-permeable membrane.

Advantages of osmotic pump systems

- They are well characterized and understood.
- The diffusing species is water.
- Modification of the rate of water diffusion is more straightforward than for many systems.
- The release mechanism is not dependent on the drug.
- They are suitable for a wide range of drugs.
- The coating technology is straightforward.
- They typically give a zero-order release profile after an initial lag.

Disadvantages of osmotic pump systems

- Size of hole is critical.
- Laser drilling is capital intensive.
- Integrity and consistency of the coating are essential. If the coating process is not well controlled there is a risk of film defects, which could result in dose dumping. The film droplets or particles must be induced to coalesce into a film with consistent properties.

Delivery systems for targeting to specific sites in the gastrointestinal tract

Systems that target specific sites in the gastrointestinal tract are a form of modified-release delivery system and are considered briefly here. Targeting of drugs in the gastrointestinal tract is considered useful as a means of taking advantage of and/or overcoming efflux systems (see Chapter 20), intestinal cell metabolism, specific carrier mechanisms and cell recognition sites. This can be achieved by careful design of gastric retentive delivery systems and by colonic drug delivery systems. These two systems are discussed below.

Gastric retentive systems

The advantages of using these drug delivery systems include reduced variability of drug release, local drug delivery and action, and enhanced bioavailability for those drugs with a restricted absorption window in the gastrointestinal tract.

Methods of achieving gastric retention include:

- the addition of passage-delaying agents, such as food material, for example triethanolamine myristate, or drugs, for example propantheline
- the use of high-density materials – high-density particles (>2.5 g/cm^3) have prolonged gastric residence times. Densification can be achieved by the addition of materials such as barium sulfate

- modification of the size/shape of delivery system by the use of unfolding polymer sheets, swelling hydrogel balloons or polymer units that are too large to pass through the pyloric sphincter
- bioadhesive systems – systems have been used which will adhere to surfaces such as the mucosa. When these systems are used for gastrointestinal delivery, problems are that high local concentrations of drug may result and there is a turnover of mucosa, leading to detachment of the delivery system
- the use of floating dosage forms – these systems resist gastric emptying by floating on the stomach contents. They should not alter the intrinsic emptying rate of the stomach and their specific gravity should be less than that of the stomach contents. Floating delivery systems that are used are (a) hydrodynamically balanced systems, (b) carbon dioxide-generating systems or (c) freeze-dried systems.

Colonic delivery systems

Applications for colonic delivery systems systems include local delivery for the treatment of inflammatory diseases, infections and diarrhoea, and also systemic delivery.

Design principles for these delivery systems make use of:

- the specific pH of the colon – pH-sensitive polymers are used in their manufacture, e.g. combinations of Eudragit 100-55 (which is soluble only above about pH 5.5) with Eudragit S (ditto pH 7.0). The principle is that drug is released at a specific pH environment
- small intestine transit times – these depend on timed release of the active drug
- colonic bacteria – the principle here is to coat the drug/delivery system with a polymer that is sensitive to bacteria in the colon. Degradation of the polymer permits release of the active drug. Polymers used include glassy amylase (mixed with ethylcellulose) or pectin as a thick compression coat, crosslinked with calcium, with different degrees of methoxylation or amidation, or mixed with ethylcellulose.

ACKNOWLEDGEMENTS

The authors wish to thank Dr L.G. Martini and Dr P.B. Geraghty (Glaxo SmithKline Pharmaceuticals, Harlow, UK) for their assistance and advice in the preparation of this chapter.

REFERENCES

Amidon, G.L., Lennernas, H., Shah, V.P., Crison, J.R. (1995). A theoretical basis for a biopharmaceutic drug classification: the correlation of in vitro drug product dissolution and in vivo bioavailability *Pharmaceutical Research*, **10**, 413.

Bailey, C.A., Bryla, P., Malick, A.W. (1996). The use of the intestinal epithelial cell culture model Cac-2 in pharmaceutical development. *Advanced Drug Delivery Reviews,* **22**, 85.

Chien Y.W. (1995) *Novel Drug Delivery Systems*. Marcel Dekker, New York.

33

Coating of tablets and multiparticulates

S. C. Porter

INTRODUCTION

Coatings may be applied to a wide range of oral solid dosage forms, including tablets, capsules, multiparticulates and drug crystals. Tablets, however, represent the class of dosage form that is most commonly coated, although coated multiparticulates have gained increasing popularity.

Definition of coating

Coating is a process by which an essentially dry, outer layer of coating material is applied to the surface of a dosage form in order to confer specific benefits that broadly range from facilitating product identification to modifying drug release from the dosage form.

Reasons for coating

The reasons for coating pharmaceutical oral solid dosage forms are quite varied. The more common reasons include the following (no order of importance implied):

1. Providing a means of protecting the drug substance (API) from the environment, particularly light and moisture, and thus potentially improving product stability.
2. Masking the taste of drug substances that may be bitter or otherwise unpleasant.
3. Improving the ease of swallowing large dosage forms, especially tablets. Tablets that are coated are considered by patients to be somewhat easier to swallow than uncoated tablets.
4. Masking any batch differences in the appearance of raw materials and hence allaying patient concern over products that would otherwise appear different each time a prescription is dispensed or product purchased, in the case of over-the-counter products.
5. Providing a means of improving product appearance and aiding in brand identification.
6. Facilitating the rapid identification of product by the manufacturer, the dispensing pharmacist and the patient. In this case, the coatings would almost certainly be coloured. It is important here to emphasize that efficient labelling and associated procedures are the only sure way of identifying a product. However, colour is a useful subliminal check.
7. Enabling the coated product (especially tablets) to be more easily handled on high-speed automatic filling and packaging equipment. In this respect,

the coating often improves product flow, increases the mechanical strength of the product and reduces the risk of cross-contamination by minimizing 'dusting' problems.
8. Imparting modified-release characteristics that allow the drug to be delivered in a more effective manner.

Types of coating process

Three main types are used in the pharmaceutical industry today:

- film coating
- sugar coating
- compression coating.

Film coating is the most popular technique and virtually all new coated products introduced to the market are film coated. Film coating involves the deposition, usually by a spraying method, of a thin film of a polymer formulation surrounding a tablet, capsule or multiparticulate core.

Sugar coating is a more traditional process closely resembling that used for coating confectionery products. It has been used in the pharmaceutical industry since the late 19th century. It involves the successive application of sucrose-based coating formulations, usually to tablet cores, in suitable coating equipment. The water evaporates from the syrup, leaving a thick sugar layer around each tablet. Sugar coats are often shiny and highly coloured.

Compression coating, although traditionally a less popular process, has gained increased interest in recent years as a means of creating specialized modified-release products. It involves the compaction of granular material around a preformed tablet core using specially designed tableting equipment. Compression coating is essentially a dry process.

Each of these processes will now be considered in turn and an overview of relevant coating processes and materials will be given.

FILM COATING

Film coating is the more contemporary and thus commonly used process for coating oral solid dosage forms. As mentioned above, it involves the deposition, usually by a spraying method, of a thin film of a polymer formulation to the surface of a tablet, capsule or multiparticulate core. Now all newly launched coated products are film coated rather than sugar coated, often for many of the reasons given in Table 33.1.

Table 33.1 Major differences between sugar and film coating

Features	Sugar coating	Film coating
Tablets		
Appearance	Rounded with high degree of polish	Retains contour of original core Usually not as shiny as sugar coat types
Weight increase due to coating materials	30–50%	2–3%
Logo or 'break' lines	Not possible	Possible
Other solid dosage forms	Coating possible but little industrial importance	Coating of multiparticulates very important in modified-release forms
Process		
Stages	Multistage process	Usually single stage
Typical batch coating time	8 hours, but easily longer	1.5–2 hours
Functional coatings	Not usually possible apart from enteric coating	Easily adaptable for controlled release

Types of film coatings

Film coatings may be classified in a number of ways but it is common practice to do so in terms of the intended effect of the applied coating on drug release characteristics. Hence film coatings may be designated as either:

- *immediate-release film coatings* – these are also known as 'non-functional' coatings but this is something of a misnomer. It is used to imply that the coating has no effect on biopharmaceutical properties but a coating, as explained, has many other properties and functions
- *modified-release film coatings* (also known as 'functional' coatings), which may be further categorized as either delayed-release (or enteric) or extended-release coatings.

Immediate-release coatings are usually readily soluble in water, while enteric coatings are only soluble in water at pH values in excess of 5–6 and are intended to either protect the drug while the dosage form is in the stomach (in the case of acid-labile drugs) or prevent release of the drug in the stomach (in the case of drugs that are gastric irritants). More recently, enteric coatings have been employed as an integral part of colonic drug delivery systems (Alvarez-Fuentes et al 2004). For the most part, extended-release coatings are insoluble in water. They are designed to ensure that the drug is released in a consistent manner over a relatively long period of time (typically 6–12 hours) and thus reduce the number of dosages that a patient needs to consume in each 24-hour period. Additionally, extended-release film coatings are used to modify drug release in such a way that desired

therapeutic benefits can more easily be achieved and thus drug efficacy improved.

Description of the film-coating process

Film coating involves the deposition, usually by a spray method, of a thin film of a polymer formulation around each tablet core. It is possible to use conventional panning equipment but more usually specialized equipment is employed to take advantage of the fast coating times and high degree of automation possible.

The coating liquid (solution or suspension) contains a polymer in a suitable liquid medium together with other ingredients such as pigments and plasticizers. This solution is sprayed on to a rotating, mixed tablet bed or fluidized bed. The drying conditions result in the removal of the solvent, leaving a thin deposit of coating material around each tablet core.

Process equipment

The vast majority of film-coated tablets are produced by a process which involves the atomization (spraying) of the coating solution or suspension on to a bed of tablets.

Modern pan-coating equipment is of the side-vented type (as shown in Fig. 33.1) and some typical examples include:

- Accela Cota – Manesty Machines, Liverpool, UK
- Hi-Coater – Freund Company, Japan
- Driacoater – Driam Metallprodukt GmbH, Germany
- HTF/150 – GS, Italy
- IDA – Dumoulin, France.

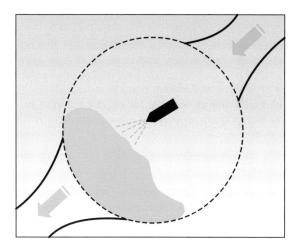

Fig. 33.1 Schematic of side-vented coating pan.

Examples of units that operate on a fluidized-bed principle include:

- GEA (Aeromatic-Fielder), Switzerland and UK
- Glatt AG, Switzerland and Germany.

Depending on the particular film-coating application involved, fluidized-bed equipment may be further divided into one of the three operating principles shown in Figure 33.2.

The coating formulation is invariably added as a solution or suspension via a spray gun. The design and operation of film-coating spray guns are similar in both perforated-pan and fluidized-bed coaters, although differences in performance of spray guns provided by dif-

ferent vendors, especially in perforated-pan processes, have been noted (Macleod & Fell 2002). A typical example of spray coating in a pan coater is shown in Figure 33.3.

Basic process requirements for film coating

The fundamental requirements of a film-coating process are more or less independent of the actual type of equipment being used and include:

- adequate means of atomizing the spray liquid for application to the tablet cores
- adequate mixing and agitation of the tablet bed. Spray coating relies upon each core passing

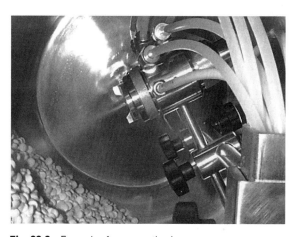

Fig. 33.3 Example of spray coating in a pan coater.

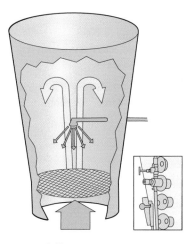 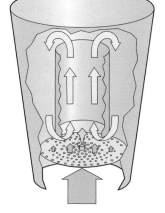 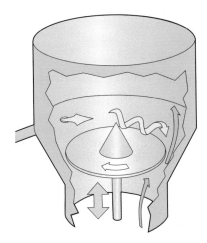

1. Top spray   2. Bottom spray   3. Tangential

Fig. 33.2 Schematics of fluid-bed coating equipment.

through the area of spraying. This is distinct from sugar coating, where each application of syrup is spread from tablet to tablet prior to drying (discussed later in this chapter)
- sufficient energy input in the form of heated drying air to evaporate the solvent. This is particularly important when applying aqueous-based coatings
- good exhaust facilities to remove dust- and solvent-laden air.

Film-coating formulations

Currently, the majority of film-coating processes involves the application of a coating liquid where a significant proportion of a major component (the solvent/vehicle) is removed by means of a drying process that is concurrent with the application of that coating liquid. Film-coating formulations typically comprise:

- polymer
- plasticizer
- colourants
- solvent/vehicle.

There are certain types of coating process that differ from this common approach. For example, some processes involve the application of hot-melt coatings that congeal on cooling (Jozwiakowski et al 1990), while others take advantage of recent developments in powder application technologies (Porter 1999).

It should be mentioned that all ingredients used in film-coating formulations must comply with the relevant regulatory and pharmacopoeial requirements current in the intended marketing area.

Film-coating polymers

The ideal characteristics of a film-coating polymer are discussed below.

Solubility

Polymer solubility is important for two reasons:

- It determines the behaviour of the coated product in the gastrointestinal tract (that is, the rate at which the drug will be released, and whether there will be any delay in the onset of drug release).
- It determines the solubility of the coating in a chosen solvent system (a factor that can have great influence on functional properties of the final coating).

Film coatings that are used on immediate-release products should utilize polymers that have good solubility in aqueous fluids to facilitate the rapid dissolution of the active ingredient from the finished dosage form follow-

ing ingestion. Such coatings are usually applied as solutions in an appropriate solvent system (with a strong preference being shown for water). However, film coatings used to modify the rate or onset of drug release from the dosage form tend to have limited or no solubility in aqueous media; such coatings are usually applied either as polymer solutions in organic solvents or as aqueous polymer dispersions (discussion later in this chapter).

Viscosity

Viscosity is very much a limiting factor with regard to the ease with which a film coating can be applied. High viscosity (typically that exceeding about 500 mPa s) complicates transfer of the coating liquid from the storage vessel to the spray guns, and subsequent atomization of that coating liquid. Ideally, therefore, polymers applied as solutions in a selected solvent should exhibit relatively low viscosities at the preferred concentration. This will help to facilitate easy, trouble-free spray application of the coating solution in industrial film-coating equipment.

Permeability

Appropriate permeability (to which the chosen polymer makes a significant contribution) is a key attribute when considering the various functional properties that film coatings are expected to possess. For example, coating permeability is of significant importance when the film coating is intended to:

- mask the unpleasant taste of the active ingredient in the dosage form
- improve stability of the dosage form by limiting exposure to atmospheric vapours and gases, particularly water vapour and oxygen
- modify the rate at which the active ingredient will be released from the dosage form.

These properties vary widely between the various polymers that might be considered for film-coating formulations.

Mechanical properties

In order to perform effectively for the purpose intended, a film coating must exist as a discrete, continuous coating around the surface of the product to be coated, and must be free from defects typically caused by the stresses to which the coating is likely to be exposed during the coating process.

Consequently, film-coating polymers should possess suitable characteristics with respect to:

- film strength, which greatly affects the ability of the coating to resist the mechanical stresses to which it will be exposed during the coating process and during subsequent handling of the coated product
- film flexibility, which imparts similar benefits to film strength and minimizes film cracking during handing or subsequent storage
- film adhesion, which is necessary to ensure that the coating remains adherent to the surface of the dosage form right up to the point of being consumed by the patient.

The generation and minimization of film-coating defects are discussed more fully later in this chapter.

Types of film-coating polymer: immediate-release coatings

Cellulose derivatives

Most cellulosic polymers used in film-coating formulations are substituted ethers of cellulose.

Hydroxypropyl methylcellulose (HPMC) is the most widely used of the cellulosic polymers. Its molecular structure is shown in Figure 33.4. It is readily soluble in aqueous media and forms films that have suitable mechanical properties and coatings that are relatively easy to apply. Coatings that utilize this polymer may be clear or coloured with permitted pigments. The polymer is the subject of monographs in the major international pharmacopoeia.

Other cellulosic derivatives used in film coatings, which have similar properties to HPMC, include *methylcellulose* (MC) and *hydroxypropyl cellulose* (HPC).

Vinyl derivatives

The most commonly used vinyl polymer in pharmaceutical applications is *polyvinyl pyrrolidone* (PVP). Unfortunately, this polymer has limited use in film-coating formulations because of its inherent tackiness.

A copolymer of vinyl pyrrolidone and vinyl acetate is considered a better film former than PVP. A more useful vinyl polymer is *polyvinyl alcohol* (PVA), a partial hydrolysate of polyvinyl acetate, which can be used to produce film coatings that have suitable mechanical properties and are highly adherent to pharmaceutical tablets. In addition, PVA exhibits good barrier properties to environmental gases (Okhamafe & York 1983) and water vapour (Jordan et al 1995).

Film coatings that use PVA as the primary polymer have mainly been exploited as special barrier coatings, helping to improve the stability of drug substances that are either sensitive to moisture (especially in countries that have humid climates) or are readily oxidized when exposed to atmospheric oxygen.

Recently, film coatings based on a copolymer of vinyl alcohol and ethylene glycol (Ziegler & Koller 2003) have become available. These coatings are less tacky than traditional PVA coatings and have the additional benefit of being extremely flexible, thus improving film robustness and allowing greater expansion capabilities should the tablet cores expand slightly during the coating process

Aminoalkyl methacrylate copolymers

These acrylic copolymers are readily soluble in aqueous media at low pH only, and thus are of prime importance in coating dosage forms where the need to achieve effective taste masking is a critical attribute (Dittgen et al 1997). These polymers are typically applied as solutions in organic solvents, although special forms may also be used to prepare aqueous polymer dispersions. An example of the molecular structure of this type of acrylic polymer is shown in Figure 33.5.

Types of film-coating polymer: modified-release coatings

Cellulose derivatives

As is the case with cellulosic polymers used in immediate-release applications, cellulosic polymers used for

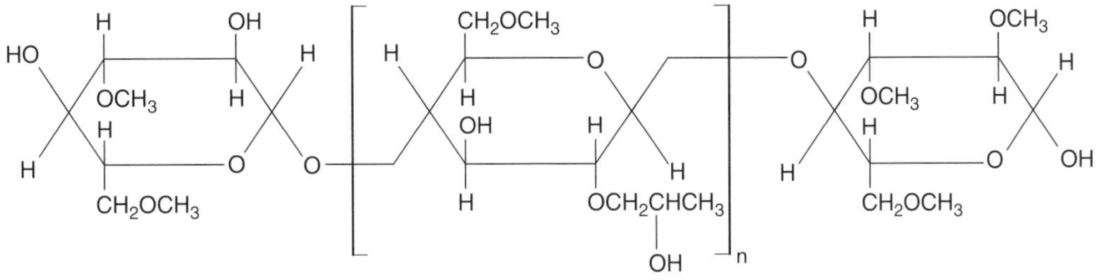

Fig. 33.4 Hydroxypropyl methylcellulose.

$$[- CH_2 - C(R_1)(R_2) - CH_2 - C(R_1)(R_3) - CH_2 - C(R_1)(R_4) - CH_2 - C(R_1)(R_4) -]_n$$

$$\text{Where: } R_1 = CH_3 \quad R_2 = COOC_4H_9 \quad R_3 = COOCH_3$$
$$R_4 = COOCH_2 - CH_2 - N(C_2H_2)_2$$

Fig. 33.5 Aminoalkyl methacrylate copolymer.

modified-release purposes are typically substituted ethers of cellulose. However, the level of substitution in this case is usually much higher, thus rendering the polymer insoluble in water. A typical example of such a cellulosic polymer is *ethyl cellulose* (EC), which is preferred for many extended-release applications (Porter 1989). Historically, ethyl cellulose has been applied as solutions in organic solvents, although aqueous polymer dispersions are commercially available.

Other cellulose derivatives used for modified-release applications include cellulose esters such as *cellulose acetate* (CA).

Methylmethacrylate copolymers

Acrylic ester polymers are typically insoluble in water but can be prepared with varying degrees of permeability to render them suitable for a variety of extended-release applications (Dittgen et al 1997). Originally intended for use as solutions in organic solvents, these polymers are commonly used today as aqueous polymer dispersions.

Methacrylic acid copolymers

The special functionality conferred by the presence of carboxylic acid groups enables this class of polymer to function as enteric coatings (Dittgen et al 1997). This is because the polymer is insoluble in water at the low pH that typifies conditions in the stomach but gradually becomes soluble as the pH rises towards neutrality, a condition that is more typical of the upper part of the small intestine. Currently, methacrylic acid copolymers are also commonly used as aqueous polymer dispersions. An example of the molecular structure of this type of acrylic polymer is shown in Figure 33.6.

$$[- CH_2 - C(CH_3)(COOH) - CH_2 - C(CH_3)(COOH_3) -]_n$$

Fig. 33.6 Methacrylic acid copolymer.

Phthalate esters

In terms of functionality, phthalate ester polymers exhibit similar properties to methacrylic acid copolymers (Chang 1990), in that they are most suited to delayed-release applications. Chemically, they are formed by the substitution of phthalic acid (or similar) groups into polymers that have been commonly used in other film-coating applications. Thus common examples of phthalate ester polymers are *hydroxypropylmethylcellulose phthalate* (HPMCP), *cellulose acetate phthalate* (CAP), and *polyvinyl acetate phthalate* (PVAP). Phthalate ester polymers may be applied as solutions in organic solvents or as aqueous polymer dispersions.

Plasticizers

Plasticizers are generally added to film-coating formulations to modify physical properties of the polymer. This is necessary because most acceptable film-coating polymers are brittle in nature. It is generally accepted that the mechanism by which plasticizers exert their effect is for plasticizer molecules to interpose themselves between the polymer molecules, thus increasing free volume and facilitating increased polymer chain motion within the structure of the coating. The positive benefits of this interaction include:

- increased film flexibility
- reduced residual stresses within the coating as it shrinks around the core during drying.

Examples of commonly used plasticizers are:

- polyols, such as polyethylene glycols and propylene glycol
- organic esters, such as diethyl phthalate and triethyl citrate
- oils/glycerides, such as fractionated coconut oil.

For a given application, it is often desirable to use plasticizers that are soluble in the solvent system being used.

Colourants

Pharmaceutically acceptable colourants are available in both water-soluble form (known as dyes) and water-insoluble form (known as pigments). The insoluble form is preferred in film-coating formulations, based on the fact that pigments tend to be more chemically stable towards light, provide better opacity and covering power, and provide a means of optimizing the permeability properties of the applied film coating. In addition, water-insoluble pigments will not suffer from the disadvantageous phenomenon of mottling (caused by solute migration, as discussed in Chapter 30) that can be observed with water-soluble dyes.

Examples of colourants are:

- iron oxide pigments
- titanium dioxide
- aluminium lakes (a pigment formed by bonding water-soluble colourants to approved substrata, such as fine alumina hydrate particles).

While the selection of a colourant is typically based on the need to achieve a certain visual effect and, to a lesser extent, the potential influence on film mechanical properties, an underlying selection criterion is that of regulatory acceptance. While there are many colourants that can be used, few have the fully global regulatory acceptance required to facilitate the world-wide use of the same formulation.

Solvents

Initially, film-coating processes were very much dependent on the use of organic solvents (such as *methanol/ dichloromethane* combinations or *acetone*) in order to achieve the rapid drying characteristics demanded by the process. Unfortunately, organic solvents possess many disadvantages (Hogan 1982) that are related to the following factors:

1. *Environmental issues* – the venting of untreated organic solvent vapour into the atmosphere is ecologically unacceptable, while efficient solvent vapour removal from gaseous effluent of coating processes is expensive.
2. *Safety issues* – organic solvents may be flammable (and thus explosive hazards) or expose plant operators to toxic hazards.
3. *Financial issues* – potentially unacceptable cost factors associated with the use of organic solvents are related to the need to build explosion-proof processing areas and provide suitable storage areas for hazardous materials. In addition, the relative expense of organic solvents as a raw material has also to be considered.
4. *Solvent residue issues* – for a given process, the amount of organic solvent retained in the film coat must be investigated, especially since there is increasing regulatory pressure to quantify and limit the residue levels.

Such disadvantages have provided the momentum for the current utilization of aqueous coating formulations as the preferred option. However, as a result of improved efficiency and decreased costs associated with solvent recovery, there has been an upsurge in interest in solvent coating but almost exclusively in modified-release coating applications.

Aqueous polymer dispersions

Essentially, all polymers used in modified-release film-coating applications are, in order to achieve their intended functionality, generally insoluble in water. Hence, they have been applied as solutions in organic solvents. The growing demand for aqueous formulations in modern film-coating processes thus initially caused a dilemma for pharmaceutical formulators, a dilemma that has ultimately been resolved by creating aqueous polymer dispersions of many of these polymers. The term 'aqueous polymer dispersion' is broadly used to describe polymer systems that are supplied as lattices, as well as those that have been formed into aqueous suspensions, and their use has been comprehensively reviewed by McGinity (1997).

Ideal characteristics of film-coated products

A film-coated product *and* its associated manufacturing process should be designed and controlled to ensure that the following characteristics are evident:

- Display even coverage and colour of the coating across the surface of each dosage unit within a batch, and from batch to batch.
- Show absence of defects that detract from finished product appearance or which affect dosage form functionality and stability.
- Be compliant with finished product specifications and any relevant compendial requirements.

Film-coating defects

Film coating is not a perfect process. Defects and imperfections in the coat can occur if the formulation of the coat and the core, or the coating process, is not adequately designed and controlled. The defects that are commonly attributed to film coating are usually:

- visual defects (usually seen with film-coated tablets), or
- defects that affect functional properties (such as those influencing drug release, and thus are usually associated with modified-release products).

By far the most common defects are those in the former category and these have been described in detail by Rowe

(1992), with suggestions for their resolution. Visual defects can be categorized as those relating to:

- *processing issues* – these are typically associated with an imbalance between the rate of delivery of the coating liquid and the rate of evaporation during the drying process. This imbalance results in either overwetting (where tablets or multiparticulates might become stuck together) or overdrying, when surface erosion of the tablets, as well as chipping of the tablet edges, may result.
- *formulation issues* – these are usually associated with some deficiency in the core (tablet or multiparticulate) or the coating. Core formulation issues often result in mechanical defects so that the core is not able to withstand the attritional effects of the coating process, leading to tablet breakage and erosion. Coating formulation issues often result in inadequate film mechanical strength, leading to film cracking and chipping, or inadequate film adhesion, resulting in film peeling and logo bridging.

SUGAR COATING

Sugar coating has long been the traditional method for coating pharmaceutical products (usually tablets). It involves the successive application of sucrose-based coating formulations to tablet cores in suitable coating equipment. Conventional panning equipment with manual application of syrup has been extensively used, although more specialized equipment and automated methods are now making an impact on the process. A comparison between sugar coating and film coating is tabulated in Table 33.1 and illustrated in Figure 33.7.

Types of sugar coatings

Sugar coatings are composed of ingredients that are readily soluble, or disintegrate rapidly, in water. Although it is technically feasible to apply sugar coatings to a wide range of pharmaceutical core materials, it is almost exclusively reserved for coating tablets. In general, sugar-coated tablets are intended to exhibit immediate-release attributes. However, one of the stages of the sugar-coating process, the sealing step (discussed below), involves the deposition of a polymer-based coating to the fresh surface of the tablets. At this stage, it is possible to use some of the speciality polymers (described earlier under film coating) that are either partially or completely insoluble in water, thus enabling the sugar-coated product to exhibit delayed (enteric)-release or extended-release characteristics.

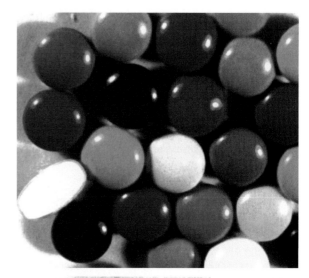

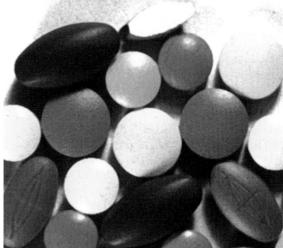

Fig. 33.7 Sugar- and film-coated tablets.

Ideal characteristics of sugar-coated tablets

Sugar-coated tablets should possess a smooth, rounded contour, with even colour coverage and a glossy finish. Those tablets that have been imprinted should exhibit high print quality (clear distinct print with no smudging or missing print). As is the case with film-coated tablets, sugar-coated tablets must be compliant with finished product specifications and any relevant compendial requirements.

Process equipment

Typically, tablets are sugar coated by a panning technique, using a traditional rotating sugar-coating pan with a supply of drying air (preferably being capable of being

- drying by directing air of the desired temperature onto the surface of the rolling mass of tablets.

Each of these substeps is now discussed in turn.

Sealing

Sugar coatings are aqueous formulations that are, quite literally, poured directly onto the tumbling tablets. Hence, water has an opportunity to penetrate directly into the tablet cores, potentially affecting product stability and possibly causing premature tablet disintegration. To prevent these problems, the cores are usually sealed initially with a water-proofing or sealing coat. Traditionally, alcoholic solutions of *shellac* were used for this purpose although the use of synthetic polymers, such as *cellulose acetate phthalate* or *polyvinyl acetate phthalate,* is now favoured. Unless a modified-release feature needs to be introduced, the amount of sealing coat applied has to be carefully calculated so that there is no negative influence on drug release characteristics for what should otherwise be an immediate-release product.

Subcoating

Sugar coatings are usually applied in quite substantial quantities to the tablet core (typically increasing the weight by as much as 50–100%) in order to round off the tablet edges. Much of this material build-up occurs during the subcoating stage and is achieved by adding bulking agents such as *calcium carbonate* to the sucrose solutions. In addition, antiadherents such as *talc* may be used to prevent tablets sticking together, and polysaccharide gums, such as *gum acacia*, may also be added as a binder in order to reduce brittleness.

Smoothing

The subcoating stage is notorious for producing a surface finish that is somewhat rough. To facilitate the application of the colouring layer (which requires a smooth surface), subcoated tablets are usually smoothed out by applying a sucrose coating that is often coloured with titanium dioxide to achieve the desired level of whiteness.

Colouring

Nearly all sugar-coated tablets are coloured, since visual elegance is usually considered to be of great importance with this type of coated dosage form. Colour coatings usually consist of sucrose syrups containing the requisite

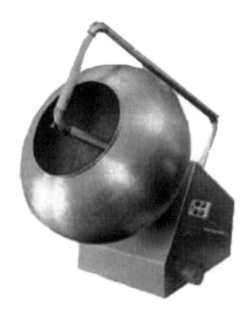

Fig. 33.8 Traditional sugar-coating pan.

thermostatically controlled) and an extraction system to remove dust- and moisture-laden air (illustrated in Fig. 33.8).

Traditional sugar-coating processes involve manual application techniques, whereby the coating liquid is ladled directly onto the surface of the cascading bed of tablets. In efforts to improve control and to speed up the sugar-coating process, many of the process equipment improvements discussed under film coating are used. Automated dosing techniques and control procedures can also now be employed to great effect.

Description of the sugar-coating process

Sugar coating is a multistage process and can be divided into the following steps:

1. Sealing of the tablet cores
2. Subcoating
3. Smoothing
4. Colouring
5. Polishing
6. Printing

At each stage of the coating process, multiple applications of the specified coating formulation are made using a sequential approach that involves:

- applying a predetermined amount of coating liquid
- allowing the coating liquid to be distributed throughout the tablet mass as the tablets tumble in the rotating pan

colouring materials. As with film coatings, colourants may be subdivided into either water-soluble dyes or water-insoluble pigments. Traditionally, water-soluble dyes have been used but in order to speed up the coating process and minimize colour migration problems, dyes have gradually been replaced with pigments. The actual colourants used must comply with regulations promulgated by the national legislation of the country where the products are to be marketed.

Polishing

Once the colour coating layers have been applied and dried, the tablet surface tends to be smooth but somewhat dull in appearance. To achieve the glossy finish that typifies sugar-coated products, a final stage involving the application of waxes is employed. Suitable waxes include *beeswax*, *carnauba wax* or *candelila wax*, applied as finely ground powders or as suspensions/solutions in an appropriate organic solvent.

Printing

It is common practice to identify all oral solid dosage forms with a manufacturer's logo, product name, dosage strength or other appropriate code. For sugar-coated products such identification can only be achieved by means of a printing process, which is typically an offset gravure process using special edible inks. However, alternative printing processes, such as inkjet and pad-printing processes, have also gained acceptance.

Sugar-coating defects

Sugar coating is technically and practically a difficult process that requires a great deal of skill and experience. Defects in the coating can occur without adequate process control. Although they may well have drug release or stability implications, defects associated with sugar-coated tablets are likely to be visual in nature. Common sugar-coat defects include:

- tablets that are rough in appearance (in which case the surface may also exhibit a marbled appearance as surface pits can become filled with wax during the polishing stage)
- tablets that are smooth but dull in appearance
- tablets that have pieces of debris (usually from broken tablets from the same batch) stuck to the surface
- tablets exhibiting poor colour uniformity
- tablets that split on storage as a result of inadequate drying (causing the tablets to swell).

COMPRESSION COATING

Compression coating differs radically from film coating and sugar coating. The process involves the compaction of granular material around preformed tablet cores (Fig. 33.9) using specially designed tableting equipment. Compression coating is essentially a dry process (although the coating formulation may have been produced by a wet-granulation process).

Description of the compression-coating process

Compression coating is based on a modification of the traditional tableting process. Tablet cores are first prepared and then mechanically transferred, on the same machine, to another, slightly larger die that has partially been filled with the coating powder. The tablet core is positioned centrally into this partially filled die, more coating powder is filled on top of the core and the whole composite mass undergoes a second compaction event. A detailed description of the compression-coating process has been given by Gunsel & Dusel (1990).

Traditionally, it has been used to separate incompatible materials (one contained in the tablet core and the second in the coating). With the traditional compression-coating process, there is still an interface layer (between the two layers) that may potentially compromise product stability. Thus it is also possible to apply two coating layers where the first coating layer is an inert, placebo formulation that effectively separates the core and the final coating layer, each of which contains a drug substance that is incompatible with the other.

Compression coating is a mechanically complex process that requires careful formulation and processing of the coating layer. Large or irregularly shaped granules will cause the core to tilt in the second die used for compression of the coating, increasing the likelihood of compressing an uneven or incomplete coating, with the core occasionally being visible at the tablet surface.

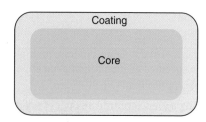

Fig. 33.9 Diagram of compression-coated tablet.

Types of compression coatings

Compression coatings are generally made from powdered ingredients that either dissolve, or readily disintegrate, in aqueous media and thus have commonly been used for immediate-release tablet products. There has been increased use of compression coatings for the purpose of creating modified-release products (Chopra 2003, Waterman & Fergione 2003).

COATING OF TABLETS

Overview of coating of tablets

Tablets are by far the most common type of oral solid dosage form that is coated. They may be coated with both immediate-release and modified-release coatings. Of the techniques available for applying coatings to tablets, the following are the most likely to be used:

- *Sugar coating* – while traditional pan-coating methods are often utilized, there is growing preference for automated techniques involving the application of thinner coatings so that batches can be completed within 1 work day (rather than the more traditional 3–5 days).
- *Film coating* – typically, pan-coating processes are preferred, although limited interest in using fluidized-bed processes for small tablets is also evident.
- *Compression coating* – more often used today for novel drug delivery applications, especially when partial coatings (for example, those applied only to the upper and lower faces of the tablets) are required.

Standards for coated tablets

In general, pharmacopoeias have similar requirements for coated and uncoated tablets, the differences being that:

- film-coated tablets must comply with the uniformity of mass test unless otherwise justified and authorized
- film-coated tablets must comply with the disintegration test for uncoated tablets except that the apparatus is operated for 30 minutes. The requirement for coated tablets other than those that are film coated is modified to include a 60-minute operating time. Furthermore, the test may be repeated using 0.1 N HCl in the event that any tablets fail to disintegrate in the presence of water.

COATING OF MULTIPARTICULATES

Coated multiparticulates, often referred to as 'pellets' or 'beads', commonly form the basis for a wide range of modified-release dosage forms (as described by Tang et al 2005). Typically used for extended-release products, interest has grown in this type of dosage form for delayed-release (enteric) applications as well. Coated multiparticulates possess many benefits compared to conventional non-disintegrating tablets (coated or otherwise) for a broad range of modified-release applications. These benefits are discussed more fully in Chapters 20 and 32 but are summarized here:

1. *Capitalizing on small size (typically 0.5–2.0 mm)* – gastrointestinal transit times can be somewhat erratic for non-disintegrating tablets (especially as a result of food effects); particles smaller than about 2.0 mm can pass through the constricted pyloric sphincter even during the gastric phase of the digestion process and distribute themselves more readily throughout the distal part of the gastrointestinal tract.
2. *Minimizing irritant effects* – whole, non-disintegrating tablets can potentially lodge in restrictions within the gastrointestinal tract, causing the release of drug to be localized and thus cause mucosal damage should the drug possess irritant effects. This potentially harmful effect can be minimized with multiparticulates since their small size reduces the likelihood of such entrapment, while the drug concentration is spread out over a larger number of discrete particles.
3. *Reducing the consequences of imperfect coatings* – film coatings, deposited using a spray technique, can potentially possess imperfections (such as pores) that could compromise the performance of modified-release dosage forms. Traditional coated tablets can be problematic in this regard since the whole dose could potentially be released quite rapidly if such imperfections (in the coating) exist. With multiparticulates, such a risk is greatly reduced since an imperfect coating on one or two pellets (out of 50–200 that constitute a single dosage unit) is likely to have little effect in terms of lack of benefit, or even harm, to the patient.
4. *Reducing the impact of poor coating uniformity* – film-coating processes are incapable of ensuring that every entity (tablet, pellet, etc.) within a batch of product will receive exactly the same amount of coating. With a tablet, the complete dose of drug is contained in that dosage unit, so any

tablet-to-tablet variation in the amount of coating applied can result in variable drug release from dosage unit to dosage unit. The types of process used for coating multiparticulates are renowned for achieving better uniformity of distribution of the coating material. A further advantage relates to the possible problem of 'dose dumping' resulting from a defect in a film coat. With multiparticulates, because the total dosage unit is made up of a large number of discretely coated particles, a defect in one pellet will only 'dump' a small fraction, say 1/200th, of the total unit dosage. This is likely to have no pharmacological consequences. In contrast, a defect in a coated monolithic tablet could release 24 hours worth of drug into a patient in just a few minutes.

Coated multiparticulates are traditionally filled into two-piece, hard gelatin capsules to form the final dosage unit, although they may also be compacted (as long as appropriate formulation and processing strategies are used to avoid rupturing of the coating) into tablets.

Types of multiparticulate

A number of different types of multiparticulates are illustrated in Figure 33.10. They are commonly film coated in order to create modified-release products.

Drug crystals

Drug crystals, as long as they are of the appropriate size and shape (elongated or acicular crystals should be avoided), can be directly coated with a modified-release film coating.

Irregular granules

Granulates, such as those regularly used to prepare tablets, can be film coated but variation in particle size distribution (from batch to batch), as well as the angular nature of such particles, can make it difficult to achieve uniform coating thickness around each particle.

Spheronized granules

Spheroidal particles simplify the coating process. The production of the spheroidal cores is detailed in Chapter 29.

Drug-loaded non-pareils

Another process for producing spheroidal particles involves the application of drug to the surface of 'non-pareils'. These are preformed spherical particles about 1 mm in diameter consisting primarily of sucrose and starch. Application of the drug uses either:

- a powder-dosing technique involving alternate dosing of powder (containing the drug substance) and binder liquid onto the surface of the non-pareils until the required dose of drug has been achieved, or
- spray application of drug, either suspended or dissolved in a suitable solvent (usually water) containing also a polymer binder (such as hydroxypropylmethylcellulose or polyvinyl pyrrolidone) onto the surface of the non-pareils.

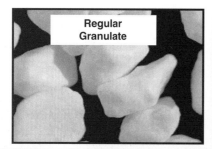
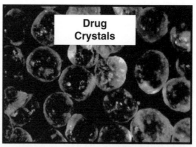
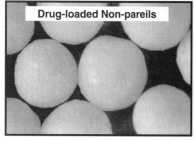
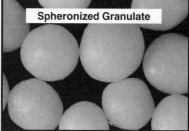
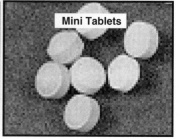

Fig. 33.10 Examples of film-coated multiparticulates.

Mini tablets

Many of the other types of multiparticulates described so far suffer from two potential batchwise drawbacks, namely:

- variation in particle size distribution
- variation in particle shape and surface roughness.

Such variability can result in variable coating thickness and thus product performance. This problem can be overcome by using mini compressed tablets (typically in the size range of 1–2 mm) produced using a modification of traditional tableting processes.

Mechanisms of drug release from multiparticulates

There are many factors that influence drug release from coated multiparticulates, some of which are related to the formulations used and others to the various manufacturing processes employed. Irrespective of the actual number of factors involved, it is generally accepted that the mechanisms of drug release (Ozturk et al 1990, Zhang et al 1991) can generally be ascribed to specific conditions.

Diffusion

Diffusion is primarily a process whereby drug will partition into the film coat membrane and permeate through it. The rate at which the drug is released by this mechanism is primarily influenced by the drug concentration gradient across the membrane, the thickness of the membrane, the solubility of the drug in the membrane and the permeability coefficient governing passage of the drug through the membrane.

Osmosis

Once water has passed through the film coating, dissolution of soluble components (excipients and drug) within the core can allow an osmotic pressure to be generated inside the coated particle that will influence the rate at which the drug will be pushed out through pores or a preformed aperture in the membrane.

Dialysis

Dialytic effects describe conditions where water-filled channels are formed in a microporous membrane (often created by the imperfections common to many applied film coatings) through which drug in solution can pass. The key factors influencing drug release by this mechanism include the length and tortuosity of these channels, as well as the solubility of the drug in water.

Erosion

Some coatings are designed to erode gradually with time, thereby releasing the drug contained within the pellet in a controlled manner. Examples of these types of coating are usually those that consist of natural materials such as shellac (the solubility of which in water increases with increasing pH) or waxes and fats that become soft enough to facilitate erosion as the coated multiparticulates are subjected to intense agitation as they pass through the gastrointestinal tract.

Processes for coating multiparticulates

Traditionally, multiparticulates were coated using pan-coating processes, often employing techniques very similar to those used in sugar coating. As coating processes evolved, spray application techniques became more prevalent and today, fluidized-bed processes are now preferred because of their ability to:

- enable discrete coatings to be applied to small particles while minimizing the risk of agglomeration
- ensure that coatings are uniformly deposited on the surface of each multiparticulate in the batch.

All the polymeric film-coating procedures described above can be used for the coating of multiparticulates. The fluidized bed is used in preference to the perforated pan. Another coating technique that is finding favour for the coating of modified-release pellets is hot-melt coating.

Hot-melt coating

Hot-melt coatings are usually applied to multiparticulates in order to mask taste and modify drug release. They consist of waxy materials (such as beeswax, synthetic spermaceti and other synthetic mono/diglycerides) that have melting points in the range of 55–65°C and exhibit melt viscosities that are typically less than 100 mPa s (in order to allow the formation of smooth coatings on the surfaces of particles). Hot-melt coatings are preferably applied to multiparticulates using fluidized-bed coating processes, as described by Kennedy & Niebergall (1996).

REFERENCES

Alvarez-Fuentes, J., Fernandez-Arevalo, M., Gonzalez-Rodriguez, M.L., Cirri, M., Mura, P. (2004) Development of enteric-coated timed-release matrix tablets for colon targeting. *Journal of Drug Targeting,* **12**(9-10), 607.

Chang, R-K. (1990) A comparison of rheological and enteric properties among organic solutions, ammonium salt aqueous solutions, and latex systems of some enteric polymers. *Pharmaceutical Technology,* **14**(10), 62.

Chopra, S.K. (2003) Procise: drug delivery systems based on geometric configuration. In: Rathbone, M.J., Hadgraft, J., Roberts, M.S. (eds) *Modified-Release Drug Delivery Technology (Drugs and the Pharmaceutical Sciences).* Marcel Dekker, New York.

Dittgen, M., Durrani, M., Lehmann, K. (1997) Acrylic polymers: a review of pharmaceutical applications. *S.T.P. Pharma Sciences,* **7**(6), 403.

Gunsel, W.C., Dusel, R.G. (1990) Compression-coated and layer tablets. In: Lieberman, H.A., Lachman, L., Schwartz, J.B. (eds) *Pharmaceutical Dosage Forms: Tablets*, vol 1, 2nd edn. Marcel Dekker, New York.

Hogan, J.E. (1982) Solvent versus aqueous film coating. *International Journal of Pharmaceutical Technology and Product Manufacture,* **3**, 7.

Jordan, M.P., Easterbrook, M.G., Hogan, J.E. (1995) Investigations into the moisture barrier properties of polyvinyl alcohol (PVA) tablet film coatings. *Proceedings of 1st World Meeting, APGI.APV,* Budapest, May 9-11.

Jozwiakowski, M.J., Jones, D.M., Franz, R.M. (1990) Characterization of a holt-melt fluid bed coating process for fine granules. *Pharmaceutical Research,* **7** (11), 1119.

Kennedy, J.P., Niebergall, P.J. (1996) Development and optimization of a solid dispersion hot-melt fluid bed coating method. *Pharmaceutical Development and* Technology, **1**(1), 51.

Macleod, G.S., Fell, J.T. (2002) Comparison of atomization conditions between different spray guns used in pharmaceutical film coating. *Pharmaceutical Technology Europe,* November Issue.

McGinity, J.W. (ed.) (1997) *Aqueous Polymeric Coatings For Pharmaceutical Dosage Forms*, 2nd edn (*Drugs and the Pharmaceutical Sciences* 79). Marcel Dekker, New York.

Okhamafe, A.O., York, P. (1983) Analysis of the permeation and mechanical properties of some aqueous-based film coating systems. *Journal of Pharmacy and Pharmacology,* **35**, 409.

Ozturk, A.G., Ozturk, S.S., Palsson, B.O., Wheatley, T.A., Dressman, J.B. (1990) Mechanism of release from pellets coated with an ethylcellulose-based film. *Journal of Controlled Release,* **14**, 203.

Porter, S.C. (1989) Controlled-release film coatings based on ethylcellulose *Drug Development and Industrial Pharmacy,* **15**(10), 1495.

Porter, S.C. (1999) A review of trends in film-coating technology. *American Pharmaceutical Review,* **2**(1), 32.

Rowe, R.C. (1992) Defects in film-coated tablets: aetiology and solutions. In: *Advances in Pharmaceutical Sciences*. Academic Press, London.

Tang, E.S.K., Chan, L.W., Heng, P.W.S. (2005) Coating of multiparticulates for sustained release. *American Journal of Drug Delivery,* **3**(1) 17.

Waterman, K.C., Fergione, M.B. (2003) Press-coating of immediate-release powders onto coated controlled-release tablets with adhesives. *Journal of Controlled Release*, **89**, 387.

Zhang, G., Schwartz, J.B., Schnaare, R.L. (1991) Bead coating. I. Change in release kinetics (and mechanism) due to coating levels. *Pharmaceutical Research,* **8**(3), 331.

Ziegler, R., Koller, J. (2003) Protection of light-sensitive active ingredients by instant-release coatings based on Kollicoat IR. Poster presented at AAPS Annual Meeting and Exposition, Salt Lake City, Utah, USA, October 26-30.

BIBLIOGRAPHY

Delporte, J.P. (1980) Some physical properties of two low viscosity hydroxypropyl methylcelluloses used for aqueous coating of pharmaceutical forms. *Journal de Pharmacie de Belgique,* **35**(6), 417.

Hard gelatin capsules

B. E. Jones

INTRODUCTION

The word 'capsule' is derived from the Latin *capsula*, meaning a small box. In current English usage it is applied to many different objects, ranging from flowers to spacecraft. In pharmacy, the word is used to describe an edible package made from gelatin or other suitable material which is filled with medicines to produce a unit dosage, mainly for oral use. There are two types of capsule, 'hard' and 'soft'; better adjectives would be 'two-piece' instead of 'hard' and 'one-piece' instead of 'soft'. The hard capsule consists of two pieces in the form of cylinders closed at one end; the shorter piece, called the 'cap', fits over the open end of the longer piece, called the 'body'.

RAW MATERIALS

Similar raw materials have been used in the manufacture of both types of capsule. Traditionally both contain gelatin, water, colourants and optional materials such as process aids and preservatives; in addition, soft capsules contain various plasticizers, such as glycerin and sorbitol. The major pharmacopoeias (European, Japanese and US) permit the use of gelatin or other suitable material. In recent years hard capsules have been manufactured from hypromellose in order to produce a shell with low moisture content (Ogura & Matsuura 1998) and soft capsules have been made from modified starch.

Gelatin

Gelatin is still the major component used for capsules and replacement polymer systems need to have the same basic properties. Gelatin possesses five basic properties that make it suitable for the manufacture of capsules:

1. It is non-toxic, widely used in foodstuffs, and acceptable for use worldwide.

2. It is readily soluble in biological fluids at body temperature.
3. It is a good film-forming material, producing a strong flexible film. The wall thickness of a hard gelatin capsule is about 100 μm.
4. Solutions of high concentration, 40% w/v, are mobile at 50°C. Other biological polymers, such as agar, are not.
5. A solution in water or in a water–plasticizer blend undergoes a reversible change from a sol to a gel at temperatures only a few degrees above ambient. This is in contrast to other films formed on dosage forms, where either volatile solvents or large quantities of heat are required to cause this change of state, e.g. tablet film coating. These types of film are formed by spraying and have a structure that could be described as formed of overlapping plates, whereas the gelatin films are homogeneous in structure, which gives them their strength.

Gelatin is a substance of natural origin that does not occur as such in nature. It is prepared by the hydrolysis of collagen, which is the main protein constituent of connective tissues (Jones R.T. 2004). Animal skins and bones are the raw materials used for the manufacture. There are two main types of gelatin: type A, which is produced by acid hydrolysis, and type B, which is produced by basic hydrolysis. The acid process takes about 7–10 days and is used mainly for porcine skins, because they require less pretreatment than bones. The basic process takes about 10 times as long and is used mainly for bovine bones. The bones must first be decalcified by washing in acid to give a soft sponge-like material, called ossein, and calcium phosphates are produced as a byproduct. The ossein is then soaked in lime pits for several weeks.

After hydrolysis, the gelatin is extracted from the treated material using hot water. The first extracts contain the gelatin with the highest physical properties and as the temperature is raised, the quality falls. The resulting weak solution of gelatin is concentrated in a series of evaporators and then chilled to form a gel. This gel is then extruded to form strands, which are then dried in a fluidized-bed system. The dried material is graded and then blended to meet the various specifications required.

The properties of gelatin that are most important to the capsule manufacturers are the Bloom strength and the viscosity. The Bloom strength is a measure of gel rigidity. It is determined by preparing a standard gel (6.66% w/v) and maturing it at 10°C. It is defined as the load in grams required to push a standard plunger 4 mm into the gel. The gelatin used in hard capsule manufacture is of a higher Bloom strength (200–250 g) than that used for soft capsules (150 g) because a more rigid film is required for the manufacturing process.

Many materials used in the manufacture of pharmaceuticals are manufactured from raw materials of bovine origin, e.g. stearates and gelatin. The outbreak of BSE, which started in the UK, has led to strict rules being introduced by the EU to minimize the risk of transmitting animal spongiform encephalopathy agents (TSE). The *European Pharmacopoeia* has included a general chapter on minimizing the risk of transmitting TSE agents via medicinal products and guidance on products at risk. Manufacturers of affected materials have to submit data to the European Department of the Quality of Medicines (EDQM) who will review it and issue a certificate of suitability for their product. This must then be submitted to the national regulatory authorities for medicinal products that contain these materials. The Scientific Steering Committee of the EU has collected data from many countries and has assigned to each a Geographical BSE Risk (GBR). There are four categories ranging from GBR I, which is a country in which BSE has never been detected and has in place a surveillance programme, e.g. New Zealand, to GBR IV which is a country in which the disease is prevalent, e.g. the UK. Currently gelatin for use in pharmaceuticals in the EU is sourced from bovine bones obtained from GBR I countries.

Colourants

The colourants that can be used are of two types: water-soluble dyes or insoluble pigments. To make a range of colours, dyes and pigments are mixed together as solutions or suspensions. The dyes used are mostly synthetic in origin and can be subdivided into the azo dyes (those that have an −N=N− linkage) and the non-azo dyes, which come from a variety of chemical classes. Most dyes used currently are of the non-azo class and the three most widely used are erythrosine (E127), indigo carmine (E132) and quinoline yellow (E104). Two types of pigment are used: iron oxides (E172), black, red and yellow, and titanium dioxide (E171), which is white and used to make the capsule opaque. The colourants that can be used to colour medicines are governed by legislation, which varies from country to country despite the fact that it is based on toxicological testing (Jones 1993). In the last 20 years there has been a move away from soluble dyes to pigments, particularly the iron oxides, because they are not absorbed on ingestion.

Process aids

The USNF describes the use of gelatin containing not more than 0.15% w/w of sodium lauryl sulfate for use in hard gelatin capsule manufacture. This functions as a wetting agent, to ensure that the lubricated metal moulds are uniformly covered when dipped into the gelatin solution.

Preservatives were formerly added to hard capsules as an in-process aid in order to prevent microbiological contamination during manufacture. Manufacturers operating their plants to GMP guidelines no longer use them. In the finished capsules, the moisture levels, 13–16% w/v, are such that the water activity will not support bacterial growth because the moisture is too strongly bonded to the gelatin molecule.

MANUFACTURE

The process in use today is the same as that described in the original patent of 1846 (Jones B.E. 2004). Metal moulds at room temperature are dipped into a hot gelatin solution which gels to form a film. This is dried, cut to length, removed from the moulds and the two parts are joined together. The difference today is that the operation is now fully automated, carried out as a continuous process on large machines housed in air-conditioned buildings. There is a limited number of specialist companies that manufacture empty capsule shells for supply to the pharmaceutical and health food industries, who fill them with their own products.

The first step in the process is the preparation of the raw materials. A concentrated solution of gelatin, 35–40%, is prepared using demineralized hot water, 60–70°C, in jacketed pressure vessels. This is stirred until the gelatin has dissolved and then a vacuum is applied to remove any entrapped air bubbles. Aliquots of this solution are then dispensed into suitable containers and the required amounts of dye solutions and pigment suspensions added. The viscosity is measured and adjusted to a target value by the addition of hot water. This latter parameter is used to control the thickness of capsule shells during production: the higher the viscosity, the thicker the shell wall produced. The prepared mixes are then transferred to a heated holding hopper on the manufacturing machine. Hypromellose solutions are prepared in a similar way but with the addition of a gelling agent, such as carrageenan, and a co-gelling agent, such as potassium chloride, to convert them into a gelling system.

The manufacturing machines are approximately 10 m long, 2 m wide and 3 m high. They consist of two parts,

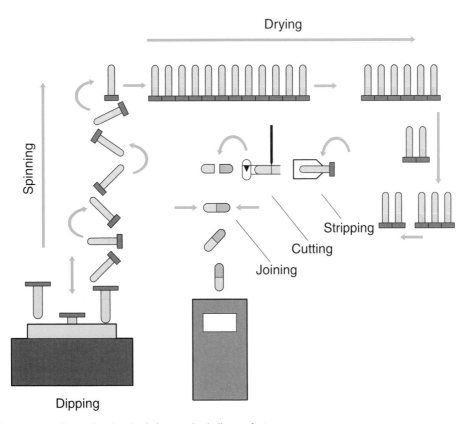

Fig. 34.1 The sequence of two-piece hard gelatin capsule shell manufacture.

which are mirror images of each other: on one half the capsule cap is made and on the other the capsule body. The machines are also divided into two levels, an upper and a lower. The moulds, commonly referred to as 'pins', are made of stainless steel and are mounted in sets on metal strips, called 'bars'. There are approximately 50 000 mould pins per machine. The machines are housed in large rooms where the humidity and temperature are closely controlled.

The sequence of events in the manufacturing process is shown in Figure 34.1. At the front end of the machine is a hopper, called a 'dip pan' or 'pot'. This holds a fixed quantity of gelatin at a constant temperature, between 45 and 55°C. The level of solution is maintained automatically by a feed from the holding hopper. Capsules are formed by dipping sets of moulds, which are at room temperature, 22°C, into this solution. A film is formed on the surface of each mould by gelling. The moulds are slowly withdrawn from the solution and then rotated during their transfer to the upper level of the machine, in order to form a film of uniform thickness. Groups of 'pin bars' are then passed through a series of drying kilns, in which large volumes of controlled humidity air are blown over them. When they reach the rear of the machine, the bars are transferred back to the lower level and pass through further drying kilns until they reach the front of the machine. Here the dried films are removed from the moulds, cut to the correct length, the two parts joined together and the complete capsule delivered from the machine. The mould pins are then cleaned and lubricated for the start of the next cycle. Hypromellose solutions behave in a similar way to gelatin except that the speed of gelling is slower than gelatin and thus the machine output is reduced.

The machines are normally operated on a 24-hour basis 7 days per week, stopping only for maintenance. The output per machine is over 1 million capsules per day, depending upon the size: the smaller the capsule, the higher the output.

The assembled capsules are not fully closed at this stage and are in a 'prelocked' position, which prevents them falling apart before they reach the filling machine. The capsules now pass through a series of sorting and checking processes, which can be either mechanical or electronic, to remove as many defective ones as possible. The quality levels are checked through the process using standard statistical sampling plans based on the Military Inspection Standards. If required, capsules can be printed at this stage. This is done using an offset gravure roll printing process using an edible ink based on shellac. The information printed is typically either the product name or strength, a company name or logo, or an identification code. The capsules are finally packed for shipment in moisture-proof liners, preferably heat-sealed aluminium foil bags, in cardboard cartons. In these containers they can be stored for long periods without deterioration in quality, provided they are not subjected to localized heating or sudden temperature changes that will affect their moisture content and dimensions.

Empty capsule properties

Empty capsules contain a significant amount of water that acts as a plasticizer for the gelatin film and is essential for their function (Jones R.T. 2004). During industrial filling and packaging operations, they are subjected to mechanical handling and because the gelatin walls can flex, these forces can be absorbed without any adverse effect. The standard moisture content specification for hard gelatin capsules is between 13% and 16% w/w. This value can vary depending upon the conditions to which they are exposed: at low humidities they will lose moisture and become brittle, and at high humidities they will gain moisture and soften. The moisture content can be maintained within the correct specification by storing them in sealed containers at an even temperature.

Capsules are readily soluble in water at 37°C. Their rate of solubility decreases when the temperature falls below this. Below about 30°C they are insoluble and simply absorb water, swell and distort. This is an important factor to take into account during disintegration and dissolution testing. Because of this most pharmacopoeias have set a limit of 37°C ± 1 for the media for carrying out these tests. Capsules made from hypromellose have a different solubility profile, being soluble at temperatures as low as 10°C (Chiwele et al 2000).

Capsule filling

Capsule sizes

Hard gelatin capsules are made in a range of fixed sizes; the standard industrial sizes in use today for human medicines are from 0 to 4 (Table 34.1). To estimate the fill weight for a powder, the simplest way is to multiply the body volume by its tapped bulk density (Jones 1998).

Table 34.1 Capsule size and body fill volumes	
Capsule size	Body volume (mL)
0	0.69
1	0.50
2	0.37
3	0.28
4	0.20

The fill weight for liquids is calculated by multiplying the specific gravity of the liquid by the capsule body volume multiplied by 0.9.

To accommodate special needs some intermediate sizes are produced, termed 'elongated sizes', that typically have an extra 10% of fill volume compared to the standard sizes, e.g. for 500 mg doses of antibiotics, elongated size 0 capsules are commonly used. The shape of the capsule has remained virtually unchanged since its invention over 150 years ago, except for the development of the self-locking capsule during the 1960s, when automatic filling and packaging machines were introduced. Filled capsules were subjected to vibration during this process, causing some to come apart and spill their contents. To overcome this, modern capsule shells have a series of indentations on the inside of the cap and on the external surface of the body which, when the capsule is closed after filling, form an interference fit sufficiently strong to hold them together during mechanical handling. The manufacturer of the empty shells can be identified from the types of indent, which are specific to each one.

Capsule shell filling

Hard capsules can be filled with a large variety of materials of different physicochemical properties. The limitations in the types of material that can be filled are shown in Table 34.2. Gelatin is a relatively inert material. The substances to be avoided are those which are known to react with gelatin, e.g. formaldehyde, which causes a crosslinking reaction that makes the capsule insoluble, or those that interfere with the integrity of the shell, e.g. substances containing free water, which can be absorbed by the gelatin, causing it to soften and distort. There is also a limitation on the size of capsule that can be easily swallowed and thus large doses of low-density formulations cannot be used.

The materials that have been filled into hard capsules are given in Table 34.3. The reason why such a range of materials can be handled is the nature of the capsule-filling process. Empty hard capsules are supplied in bulk containers. First, it is necessary for the filling machine to

Table 34.2 Limitations in properties of materials for filling into capsules

Must not react with gelatin
Must not contain a high level of 'free' moisture
The volume of the unit dose must not exceed the sizes of capsule available

Table 34.3 Types of material for filling into hard gelatin capsules

Dry solids
Powders
Pellets
Granules
Tablets
Semi-solids
Thermosoftening mixtures
Thixotropic mixtures
Pastes
Liquids
Non-aqueous liquids

orientate them so that they are all pointing in the same direction, i.e. body first. To do this, they are loaded into a hopper and from there pass down through tubes to a rectification section. Here the capsules are held in tight-fitting slots. Metal fingers strike them in the middle and because the bodies have the smaller diameter, they rotate away from the direction of impact. Next the capsules are sucked into pairs of bushings that trap the caps in the upper one, because of their greater diameter, thus separating them from the bodies. The bodies are then passed under the dosing mechanism and filled with material. Thus, providing a substance can be measured and dosed, it can be filled into capsules. The caps are then repositioned over the bodies and metal fingers push the bodies up into them to rejoin the two parts.

Capsule-filling machines

The same set of basic operations is carried out whether capsules are being filled on the bench for extemporaneous dispensing or on high-speed automatic machines for industrial products. The major difference between the many methods available is the way in which the dose of material is measured into the capsule body.

Filling of powder formulations

Bench-scale filling

There is a requirement for filling small quantities of capsules, from 50 to 10 000, in hospital pharmacies or in industry for special prescriptions or trials. There are several simple pieces of equipment available for doing this, e.g. the 'Feton' from Belgium or the 'Labocaps' from Denmark. These consist of sets of plastic plates which have predrilled holes to take from 30 to 100 capsules of a specific size. Empty capsules are fed into the holes, either manually or with a simple loading device.

The bodies are locked in their plate by means of a screw and the caps in their plate are removed. Powder is placed onto the surface of the body plate and is spread with a spatula so that it fills the bodies. The uniformity of fill weight is very dependent upon good flow properties of the powder. The cap plate is then repositioned over the body plate and the capsules are rejoined using manual pressure. Stainless steel versions of these devices are now available, e.g. Torpac Inc, USA, that can be cleaned and autoclaved to comply with GMP requirements.

Industrial-scale filling

The machines for the industrial-scale filling of hard gelatin capsules come in great variety of shapes and sizes, varying from semi- to fully automatic and ranging in output from 5000 to 150 000 per hour. Automatic machines can be either continuous in motion, like a rotary tablet press, or intermittent, where the machine stops to perform a function and then indexes round to the next position to repeat the operation on a further set of capsules.

The dosing systems can be divided into two groups:

- *Dependent* – dosing systems that use the capsule body directly to measure the powder. Uniformity of fill weight can only be achieved if the capsule is completely filled.
- *Independent* – dosing systems where the powder is measured independently of the body in a special measuring device. Weight uniformity is not dependent on filling the body completely. With this system the capsule can be part filled.

Dependent dosing systems

The auger Empty capsules are fed into a pair of ring holders (Fig. 34.2), the caps being retained in one half and the bodies in the other. The body holder is placed on a variable-speed revolving turntable; the powder hopper is pulled over the top of this plate, which revolves underneath it. In the hopper, a revolving auger forces powder down into the capsule bodies. The weight of powder filled into the body is dependent mainly upon the time the body is underneath the hopper during the revolution of the plate holder.

These machines are semi-automatic in operation, requiring an operator to transfer the capsule holders from one position to the next. They were first developed for large-scale use during the first half of the 20th century and are still widely used in many countries. The contact parts of these machines were originally made from cast iron but are now made from stainless steel to comply with GMP requirements. The machines are manufactured by many different makers but are all based on the original Colton Model No. 8 design. Their output varies between 15 000 and 25 000 per hour and is dependent upon the skill of the operator.

Independent dosing systems Most industrial machines in use in Europe and the USA are fully automatic and use dosing mechanisms that form a 'plug' of powder. This is a soft compact formed at low compression forces, between 10 and 100 N, which are significantly less than those used in tableting (10–100 kN). The reason the plug is soft is because it is not the final dosage form, unlike the tablet, as the material will be contained inside a capsule shell. There are two types of plug-forming machine: those that use a 'dosator' system and those that use a 'tamping finger and dosing disc' system.

Dosators This consists of a dosing tube inside which there is a movable spring-loaded piston, thus forming a variable-volume chamber in the bottom of the cylinder (Fig. 34.3). The tube is lowered open end first into a bed of powder, which enters the tube to fill the chamber and form a plug. This can be further consolidated by applying a compression force with the piston. The assembly is then raised from the powder bed and positioned over the capsule body. The piston is lowered, ejecting the powder plug into the capsule body. The weight of powder filled can be adjusted by altering the position of the piston inside the tube, i.e. increasing or decreasing the volume, and by changing the depth of the powder bed.

This system is probably the most widely used in the world and is the one that is described the most in the literature. Examples of machines that use this system are:

- *intermittent motion* – Zanasi (IMA), Pedini, Macophar and Bonapace. Their outputs range from 5000 to 60 000 per hour
- *continuous motion* – MG2, Matic (IMA). Their outputs range from 30 000 to 150 000 per hour.

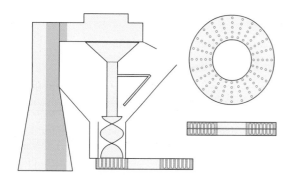

Fig. 34.2 An auger filling machine using the ring system, Model No. 8 (reproduced from Jones 2001, with permission).

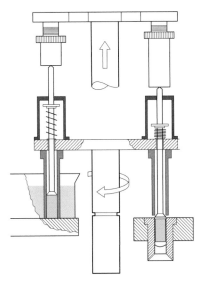

Fig. 34.3 A dosing tube or dosator-type machine, Zanasi RM63 (reproduced from Jones 2001, with permission).

Tamping finger and dosing disc The dosing disc forms the bottom of a revolving powder hopper (Fig. 34.4). This disc has in it a series of sets of accurately drilled holes in which powder plugs are formed by several sets of tamping fingers – stainless steel rods that are lowered into them through the bed of powder. At each position the fingers compress the material in the holes, building up a plug before they index on to the next position. As the disc rotates, material flows into the

holes. At the last position, the finger pushes the plug through the disc into a capsule body. The powder fill weight can be varied by the amount of insertion of the fingers into the disc, by changing the thickness of the dosing disc, and by adjusting the amount of powder in the hopper.

The machines that use this system are all intermittent in motion. Examples are manufactured by Robert Bosch, Harro Höfliger, PAM machinery, and Qualicaps.

Instrumented capsule-filling machines and simulators

Unlike tablet machines, few workers have instrumented capsule-filling machines. This is for a variety of reasons. Capsules are used only in the pharmaceutical and health food industries, as opposed to tablets, which are widely used by many other industries and for which there is therefore more incentive to do fundamental research. The tablet press is simple to quantify: there are two punches and a die that holds a specific volume of material. On a capsule-filling machine there are a variety of moving parts involved in dosing, which occurs in an unconfined bed of powder. The forces involved are small. As a result of this, comparatively few papers have been published on the topic. Machines that use the dosator system have been studied the most (Armstrong 2004). Strain gauges have been fixed to the piston that have enabled the compression forces (10–250 N) and ejection forces (1–20 N) in lubricated products to be measured. Distance transducers have been used to measure the relative movements of the piston and dosator. Simulators have also been built to overcome the problem of the machine parts moving but to date, these have had limited application (Armstrong 2004).

Pellet filling

Preparations formulated to give modified-release patterns are often produced as granules or coated pellets. They are filled on an industrial scale using machines adapted from powder use (Podczeck 2004). All have a dosing system based on a chamber with a volume that can easily be changed. Pellets are not compressed in the process and may have to be held inside the measuring devices by mechanical means, e.g. either by inverting the dosator or by applying suction to the dosing tube. In calculating the weight of particles that can be filled into a capsule, it is necessary to make an allowance for their size. Unlike powders, which have a much smaller size, they cannot fill all the available space within the capsule because of packing restrictions. The degree of this effect will be greater the smaller the capsule size and the larger the particle diameter.

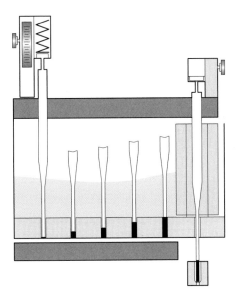

Fig. 34.4 A dosing disc and tamping finger machine, Höfliger & Karg (from Jones 2001, with permission).

Tablet filling

Tablets are placed in hoppers and allowed to fall down tubes, at the bottom of which is a gate device that will allow a set number of tablets to pass. These fall by gravity into the capsule bodies as they pass underneath the hopper. Most machines have a mechanical probe that is inserted into the capsule to check that the correct number of tablets has been transferred. Tablets for capsule filling are normally film coated to prevent dust generation, and are sized so that they can fall freely into the capsule body but without turning on their sides.

Semi-solid and liquid filling

Liquids can easily be dosed into capsules using volumetric pumps (Rowley 2004). The problem after filling is to stop leakage from the closed capsule. This can be done in one of two ways, either by formulation or by sealing of the capsule. Semi-solid mixtures are formulations that are solid at ambient temperatures and can be liquefied for filling by either heating (thermosoftening mixtures) or by stirring (thixotropic mixtures). After filling, they cool and solidify or revert to their resting state in the capsule to form a solid plug. Both types of formulations are filled as liquids using volumetric pumps. These formulations are similar to those that are filled into soft gelatin capsules but differ in one important respect: they can have melting points higher than 35°C, which is the maximum for soft capsules because this is the temperature used by the sealing rollers during their manufacture. Non-aqueous liquids, which are mobile at ambient temperatures, require the capsules to be sealed after filling. The industrially accepted method for this is to seal the cap and body together by applying a gelatin solution around the centre of the capsule after it has been filled. When this has been dried it forms a hermetic seal that prevents liquid leakage, contains odours inside the shell and significantly reduces oxygen permeation into the contents, protecting them from oxidation. An example of such equipment is the Qualicaps Hicapseal machine, which has outputs ranging from 40 000 to 100 000 per hour.

FORMULATION

All formulations for filling into capsules have to meet the same basic requirements:

1. They must be capable of being filled uniformly to give a stable product.
2. They must release their active contents in a form that is available for absorption by the patient.

3. They must comply with the requirements of the pharmacopoeial and regulatory authorities, e.g. dissolution tests.

In order to formulate rationally, it is necessary to take into account the mechanics of the filling machines and how each type of product is handled.

Powder formulation

The majority of products for filling into capsules are formulated as powders. These are typically mixtures of the active ingredient together with a combination of different types of excipients (Jones 1995; Table 34.4). The ones selected depend upon several factors:

- the properties of the active drug: its dose, solubility, particle size and shape
- the filling machine to be used
- the size of capsule to be used.

The latter factor defines the free space inside the capsule that is available to the formulator (Jones 1998). The easier active compounds to formulate are low-dose potent ones, which in the final formulation occupy only a small percentage of the total volume (< 20%) and so the properties of the mixture will be governed by the excipients chosen. Those compounds with a high unit dose, e.g. 500 mg of an antibiotic, leave little free space within the capsule and the excipients chosen must exert their effect at low concentrations (< 5%) and the properties of the mixture will be governed by that of the active ingredient.

Formulation for filling properties

There are three main factors in powder formulation:

- good flow (using free-flowing diluent and glidant)
- no adhesion (using lubricant)
- cohesion (plug-forming diluent).

The factor that contributes most to the uniform filling of capsules is good powder flow. This is because the powder bed, from which the dose is measured, needs to be homogeneous and packed reproducibly in order to achieve

---

Table 34.4 Types of excipient used in powder-filled capsules

Diluents, which give plug-forming properties
Lubricants, which reduce powder-to-metal adhesion
Glidants, which improve powder flow
Wetting agents, which improve water penetration
Disintegrants, which produce disruption of the powder mass
Stabilizers, which improve product stability

uniform fill weights. Packing is assisted by mechanical devices or suction pads on the filling machines. Low-dose actives can be made to flow well by mixing them with free-flowing diluents, e.g. lactose. The diluent is chosen also for its plug-forming properties: those most frequently used are lactose, maize starch and microcrystalline cellulose. When space is limited then either glidants, which are materials that reduce interparticulate friction, such as colloidal silicon dioxide, or lubricants, which are materials that reduce powder-to-metal adhesion, e.g. magnesium stearate, are added, enabling the dosing devices to function efficiently. Both these types of material exert their effect by coating the surfaces of the other ingredients, and thus the mixing of these into the bulk powder has a significant effect on their functioning.

Formulation for release of active ingredients

The first stage in active ingredient release is disintegration of the capsule shell. When capsules are placed in a suitable liquid at body temperature, 37°C, the gelatin starts to dissolve and within 1 minute the shell will split, usually at the ends. With a properly formulated product, the contents will start to empty out before all the gelatin has dissolved. The official tests for disintegration and dissolution were originally designed for tablets. Capsules have very different physical properties and after the contents have emptied out, the gelatin pieces remaining will adhere strongly to metal surfaces and may confuse the endpoint of the test.

The literature shows that the rate-controlling step in capsule disintegration and product release is the formulation of the contents, which ideally should be hydrophilic and dispersible (Jones 1987). The factors that can be modified to make the active ingredients readily available depend upon their properties and those of any excipients being used. The active ingredients have a fixed set of physicochemical properties which, except for the particle size, are out of the control of the formulator.

It has been shown that the particle size influences the rate of absorption for several compounds. For sulfisoxazole (Fig. 34.5), three different particle sizes were filled into capsules and administered to dogs; the smallest particle gave the highest peak blood level. This can be explained simply by the fact that the solution rate is directly proportional to the surface area of the particles: the smaller the particle, the greater the relative surface area. However, this is not a panacea for formulation problems because small particles tend to aggregate together and the effect is lost. It has been shown that the important factor with particle size is the 'effective surface area', which is the area of the active available to the dissolution fluid. This is related to the packing of particles and is a measure of how well the fluid can penetrate into the mass (Newton 2004).

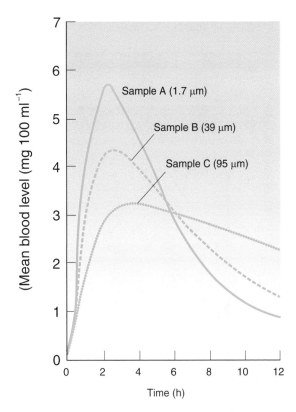

Fig. 34.5 Effect of particle size on bioavailability (after Fincher et al 1965, with permission).

Diluents are the excipients that are usually present in the greatest concentration in a formulation. They were classically defined as inert materials added to a mixture to increase its bulk to a more manageable quantity. Although they are relatively inert chemically, they do play a role in release. The case that first demonstrated this happened in Australia in the late 1960s. A capsule was reformulated that contained diphenylhydantoin, which is used for the treatment of epilepsy and is taken chronically. The diluent used was changed from calcium sulfate to lactose. In the months following this change, there was an upsurge in reports of side-effects similar to overdosing of product. It was demonstrated that the change had had a significant effect on the bioavailability of the active (Fig. 34.6). The change to lactose gave much higher blood levels of the drug, which was probably due to the fact that it is readily soluble whereas calcium sulfate is not.

Since this occurrence, the phenomenon has been shown to occur with other actives. The diluent used should be chosen in relationship to the solubility of the active. If a soluble diluent such as lactose is added to a poorly or insoluble compound, it will make the powder mass more hydrophilic, enabling it to break up more readily on

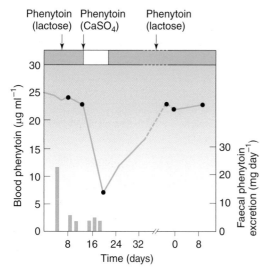

Fig. 34.6 Effect of diluent on bioavailability (after Tyrer et al 1970, with permission).

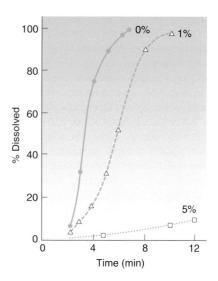

Fig. 34.7 Effect of lubricant on release of active ingredient (after Simmons et al 1972, with permission).

capsule shell disintegration. The converse is also true: actives that are readily soluble are best mixed with insoluble diluents such as starch or microcrystalline cellulose, because they help the powder mass to break up without interfering with their solubility in the medium.

Some excipients, such as lubricants and glidants, are added to formulations to improve their filling properties and these can sometimes have an effect on release. The important thing to avoid in formulations is materials that tend to make the mass more hydrophobic. The most commonly used lubricant for both encapsulation and tableting is magnesium stearate. Simmons et al (1972) studied the dissolution rate of chlordiazepoxide formulations with three levels of magnesium stearate: 0%, 1% and 5% (Fig. 34.7). They found that the dissolution rate was greatly reduced at the highest level of magnesium stearate, which they explained was due to the poor wetting of the powder mass. However, hydrophobic additives are not always deleterious because they reduce the cohesiveness of the powder mass. This was first demonstrated by Nakagawa et al (1980), who were studying the dissolution of different particle sizes of rifampicin with and without magnesium stearate (Fig. 34.8). They found that, for the larger particles (180–355 μm), the addition of magnesium stearate reduced the rate but for the smaller particles (<75 μm), it increased the rate. This is because magnesium stearate reduces the cohesiveness of the small particles so that they spread more rapidly through the dissolution medium than the unlubricated material. Augsburger (1988) studied the system hydrochlorthiazide, microcrystalline cellulose and various levels of magnesium stearate (Fig. 34.9). They filled capsules on

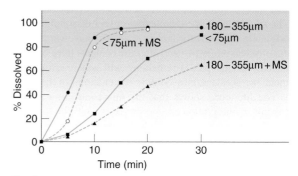

Fig. 34.8 Effect of lubricant on in vitro release of rifampicin (after Nakagawa et al 1980, with permission).

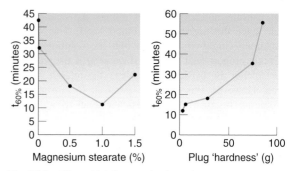

Fig. 34.9 Effect of lubricant on in vitro release of hydrochlorthiazide (after Mehta & Augsburger 1981, with permission).

an instrumented machine using the same compression force and found that as the concentration of magnesium stearate increased, the dissolution rate improved to a maximum value at about 1% w/v, after which it fell. They correlated this to the hardness of the powder plug, which followed a similar pattern, becoming softer, i.e. easier to break apart, as the concentration of lubricant increased. Above 1%, the plug becomes too hydrophobic for the increase in 'softness' to compensate for this.

The increase in the use of dissolution testing for control purposes has led to products being formulated for this factor. This has been achieved in two ways: by the addition of either surfactants or disintegrants. The addition of a wetting agent, sodium lauryl sulfate, has been studied by several workers. For poorly soluble drugs, the use of a soluble diluent together with 1% sodium lauryl sulfate gave the best results. Disintegrants were formerly never added to capsule formulations because starch, which was the most widely used tableting disintegrant, does not function well in this context. This is because the powder plug is much more porous than a tablet and the starch swells insufficiently to disrupt it. In more recent times 'superdisintegrants' have been introduced that either swell many-fold on absorbing water, e.g. sodium starch glycolate, or that act as wicks, attracting water into the plug, e.g. croscarmellose and crospovidone. These actions are sufficient to help break up the capsule plug. The choice of disintegrant is dependent upon the solubility of the active and the diluent, which governs whether either swelling or wicking, is the main disruptive force required (Mehta & Augsburger 1981).

Formulation optimization

The formulator has to produce a product that complies with the three formulation goals. Sometimes these are contradictory: for example, extra hydrophobic lubricant is required for filling machine performance, which could interfere with release. Therefore, in the development stage the formulation needs to be optimized so that it can meet the product specification. This can be done by using various statistical tools based on analysis of variance experiments that can identify the contribution of each excipient and process operation to the product performance, e.g. uniformity of fill weight and content, dissolution rate, disintegration, yield, etc. (Armstrong & James 1996).

The latest computer-based systems to aid the formulator are 'expert systems', which are based on neural networks coupled to a knowledge base (Lai et al 1996). The systems are set up using rules that have been established through experience and research. They enable a formulator to enter into the system the characteristics of the active ingredient and the type of product they would like to produce. The system then produces suggested formulations to try. This can significantly reduce the development time for a new product.

To summarize, the main factors in powder formulation release are:

- active ingredient, optimum particle size
- hydrophilic mass, relating solubility of active to excipients
- dissolution aids, wetting agent, superdisintegrant
- optimum formulation for filling and release.

Formulation for position of release

Many products are formulated to release their contents in the stomach. However, this may not always be the best place for the absorption of the active ingredient, and capsule formulation can be readily manipulated so that contents are released at various positions along the gastrointestinal tract (Jones 1991).

A common problem with oral dosage forms is making them easy to swallow. Certain people have great difficulty with this because the process is not a reflex and is controlled by the central nervous system. The capsule is a good shape for swallowing because the tongue will automatically align it with its long axis pointing towards the throat. Many tablets are now made this shape – called a 'caplet' – in order to facilitate swallowing. Patients who have difficulty swallowing should be instructed to do it either standing or sitting, in order to make full use of gravity, and to take a drink of water to lubricate the throat. They should drink a little water and hold it in the mouth. The capsule should be placed in the mouth and the head tilted forward. The capsule will now float on the water towards the back of the mouth and when the head is lifted the bolus of water and the capsule will go straight down the throat to the stomach.

In the stomach, the release of the active ingredient can be modified in a number of ways. It has been suggested that for some compounds, the best way to improve their absorption is for the dosage form to be retained in the stomach so that it will dissolve slowly, releasing a continuous flow of solution into the intestines. 'Floating capsules' have been made which contain various hydrophilic polymers, such as hypromellose, that swell on contact with water and form a mass that can float on the gastric liquids. Some compounds are destroyed at acid pHs and an enteric product can be made by either coating the filled capsule with an enteric film in a similar manner to a tablet or, more usually, by formulating the contents as pellets and coating them with an enteric polymer.

Much has been written in the literature about the advantages or disadvantages of making prolonged-release dosage forms as monolithic or as multiparticulate systems. The current consensus is that multiparticulates are better because they will be released in a stream from the stomach when the capsule shell disintegrates and will not be retained for variable periods of time, as would a monolithic product. They improve safety by avoiding the risk of the dose being dumped at one point, which could cause problems of local gastric irritation.

Certain compounds are absorbed only at specific locations along the intestines. If this window of absorption is known then a formulation can be made to release its contents in that region. There is currently an interest in targeting compounds to the distal parts of the intestines. This has been achieved in two ways. Products can be formulated to give a prolonged release and filled into a capsule that is enteric coated, e.g. Colpermin (Pharmacia Upjohn), an enteric-coated capsule filled with a prolonged-release formulation of peppermint oil. The capsule disintegrates in the duodenum and the contents slowly release the peppermint oil, which acts as a smooth muscle relaxant as it passes through the remainder of the tract. Products have also been prepared that have been coated with polymers that are enteric and are soluble only at higher pHs, 6–7. This pH is not reached until further along the small intestine, and so the contents are delivered to the more distal parts. Currently many new chemical entities are proteins or polypeptides and to make an oral dosage form, it is necessary to deliver them to the colon, thereby avoiding the proteolytic enzymes in the stomach and small intestine. The release mechanisms for these capsules are based on specific colonic conditions, e.g. coatings that are disrupted by colon-specific enzymes or by pressure (Nagata & Jones 2001).

Not all capsules administered by the oral route are intended for the gastrointestinal tract. Capsules have been used successfully for many years for products for inhalation. The active ingredient, which is micronized, is filled into the capsule either 'as is' or dispersed on a carrier particle. The weight filled into a capsule is much lower than for other types of product, typically less than 25 mg. These formulations are filled on automatic machines that have microdosing devices, and the product is administered by using a special inhaler. A capsule is placed in the device and the powder is released either by the halves of the capsule being forced apart or by the capsule wall being punctured by sharp pins or blades. The device is breath actuated. When the patient breathes in, the powder empties from the inhaler and the turbulent airflow dislodges the carrier particles (if present) and the active powder is inhaled into the lungs. The system has an added advantage over an aerosol device in that the patient can see how many doses they have taken by counting the number of capsules remaining.

REFERENCES

Armstrong, N.A. (2004) Instrumented capsule-filling machines and simulators. In: Podczeck, F., Jones, B.E. (eds) *Pharmaceutical Capsules*. Pharmaceutical Press, London.

Armstrong, N.A., James, K.C. (1996) *Pharmaceutical Experimental Design and Interpretation*. Taylor and Francis, London.

Augsburger, L.L. (1988) Instrumented capsule filling machines: methodology and application to product development. *S.T.P. Pharma*, **4**, 116-122.

Chiwele, I., Jones, B.E., Podczeck, F. (2000) The shell dissolution of various empty hard capsules. *Chemical and Pharmaceutical Bulletin*, **48**, 951-956.

Fincher, J.H., Adams, H.M., Beal, H.M. (1965) Effect of particle size on gastrointestinal absorption of sulfisoxazole in dogs. *Journal of Pharmaceutical Science*, **54**, 704-708.

Jones, B.E. (1987) Factors affecting drug release from powder formulations in hard gelatin capsules. *S.T.P. Pharma Sciences*, **3**, 777-783.

Jones, B.E. (1991) The two-piece gelatin capsule and the gastrointestinal tract. *S.T.P. Pharma Sciences*, **2**, 128-134.

Jones, B.E. (1993) Colours for pharmaceutical products. *Pharmaceutical Technology International*, **5**(4), 14-20.

Jones, B.E. (1995) Two piece capsules: excipients for powder products. European practice. *Pharmaceutical Technology Europe*, **7**(10), 25, 28-30, 34.

Jones, B.E. (1998) New thoughts on capsule filling. *S.T.P. Pharma Sciences*, **8**(5), 277-283.

Jones, B.E. (2001) Hard capsules. In: Swarbrick, J., Boylan, J.C. (eds) *Encyclopedia of Pharmaceutical Technology*, vol 1, 2nd edn. Marcel Dekker, New York.

Jones, B.E. (2004) The history of the medicinal capsule. In: Podczeck, F., Jones, B.E. (eds) *Pharmaceutical Capsules*. Pharmaceutical Press, London.

Jones, R.T. (2004) Gelatin: manufacture and physico-chemical properties. In: Podczeck, F., Jones, B.E. (eds) *Pharmaceutical Capsules*. Pharmaceutical Press, London.

Lai, S., Podczeck, F., Newton, J.M., Daumesnil, R. (1996) An expert system to aid the development of capsule formulations. *Pharmaceutical Technology Europe*, **8**(9), 60, 62, 64, 66, 68.

Mehta, A.M., Augsburger, L.L. (1981) A preliminary study of the effect of slug hardnes of drug dissolution from hard gelatin capsules filled on an automatic capsule-filling machine. *International Journal of Pharmaceutics*, **7**, 327-334.

Nagata, S., Jones, B.E. (2001) Hard two-piece capsules and the control of drug delivery. *European Pharmaceutical Review*, **5**(2), 41-46.

Nakagawa, H., Mohri, K., Nakashima, K., Sugimoto, I. (1980) Effects of particle size of rifampicin and addition of magnesium stearate on release of rifampicin from hard gelatin capsules. *Yakugaku Zasshi*, **100**, 1111-1117.

Newton, J.M. (2004) Drug release from capsules. In: Podczeck, F., Jones, B.E. (eds) *Pharmaceutical Capsules*. Pharmaceutical Press, London.

Ogura, T., Matsuura, S. (1998) HPMC capsules: an alternative to gelatin. *Pharmaceutical Technology Europe*, **10**(11), 32, 34, 36, 40, 42.

Podczeck, F. (2004) Dry filling of hard capsules. In: Podczeck, F., Jones, B.E. (eds) *Pharmaceutical Capsules*. Pharmaceutical Press, London.

Rowley, G. (2004) Filling of liquids and semi-solids into hard two-piece capsules. In: Podczeck, F., Jones, B.E. (eds) *Pharmaceutical Capsules*. Pharmaceutical Press, London.

Simmons, D.L., Frechette, M., Ranz, R.J., Chen, W.S., Patel, N.K. (1972) A rotating compartmentalized disk for dissolution rate determinations. *Canadian Journal of Pharmaceutical Science*, **7**, 62-65.

Tyrer, J.M., Eadie, M.J., Sutherland, J.M., Hopper, W.D. (1970) Outbreak of anticonvulsant intoxication in an Australian city. *British Medical Journal*, **IV**, 271-273.

35

Soft gelatin capsules

K. G. Hutchison, J. Ferdinando

CHAPTER CONTENTS

INTRODUCTION

The name 'soft gelatin capsules' is commonly abbreviated to 'softgels' and although the terms are interchangeable, 'softgels' will be used throughout this chapter for the sake of convenience and consistency.

When pharmaceutical formulation scientists are faced with the challenge of designing a solid oral dosage form for drug compounds, they have a number of choices. Over recent years, new drug molecules have tended to be more hydrophobic and therefore less soluble in aqueous systems. In the case of drugs for oral administration, it is becoming more difficult to formulate poorly water-soluble drugs into products from which the drug is fully released and well absorbed. One of the best methods to overcome this problem is to make a liquid formulation containing the drug. In order to convert this liquid formula into a solid dosage form, it may be encapsulated into soft gelatin capsules.

This chapter explains:

- why soft gelatin capsules are selected for formulation development
- how they are formulated, and
- how they are manufactured.

DESCRIPTION OF THE SOFT GELATIN CAPSULE DOSAGE FORM

Softgels consist of a liquid or a semi-solid matrix inside a one-piece outer gelatin shell (Fig. 35.1). Ingredients that are solid at room temperature can also be encapsulated into softgels providing they are at least semi-solid below approximately 45°C. The drug compound itself may be either in solution or in suspension in the capsule-fill matrix. The characteristics of the fill matrix may be hydrophilic (for example, polyethylene glycols) or lipophilic (such as triglyceride vegetable oils). Indeed, in

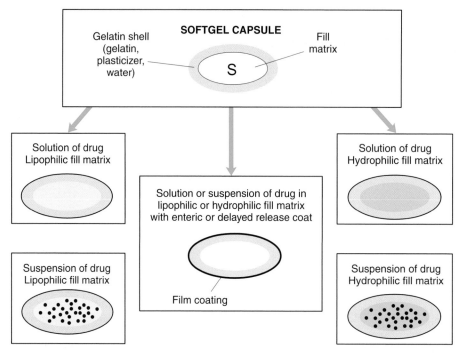

Fig. 35.1 Schematic diagram of different softgel formulations.

many formulations, the matrix may be a mixture of both the hydrophilic and lipophilic ingredients.

Significant advances have been made in recent years in the formulation of softgel fill matrices (see also Fig. 35.1). These include microemulsions and nanoemulsions encapsulated as preconcentrates in softgels. The term 'preconcentrate' means that the softgel fill matrix is a combination of lipophilic and hydrophilic liquids as well as surfactant components which, after oral administration, disperse to form, for example, a microemulsion. If the dispersion results in even smaller droplets in the nanoparticle range, then the dispersion is known as a nanoemulsion.

The softgel capsule shell consists of gelatin, water and a plasticizer. The shell may be transparent or opaque and can be coloured and flavoured if desired. Preservatives are not required owing to the low water activity in the finished product. The softgel can be coated with enteric-resistant or delayed-release coating material. Although virtually any shape of softgel can be made, oval or oblong shapes are usually selected for oral administration.

Softgels can be formulated and manufactured to produce a number of different drug delivery systems:

- Orally administered softgels containing solutions or suspensions that release their contents in the stomach in an easy-to-swallow, convenient unit dose form (Fig. 35.2). This is the most common type of softgel, already described above.
- Chewable softgels, where a highly flavoured shell is chewed to release the drug liquid fill matrix. The drug(s) may be present in both the shell and fill matrix.
- Suckable softgels, which consist of a gelatin shell containing the flavoured medicament to be sucked and a liquid matrix or just air inside the capsule.
- Twist-off softgels, which are designed with a tag to be twisted or snipped off, thereby allowing access to the fill material. This type of softgel can be very useful for unit dosing of topical medication, inhalations or indeed for oral dosing of a paediatric product (Fig. 35.3).
- Meltable softgels designed for use as 'patient-friendly' pessaries or suppositories.

RATIONALE FOR THE SELECTION OF SOFTGELS AS A DOSAGE FORM

There are a number of reasons why softgels may be selected as the most suitable dosage form. These are summarized in Table 35.1. In the majority of cases,

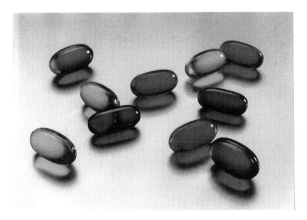

Fig. 35.2 Swallowable softgel capsules.

improved drug absorption is the primary reason for developing a softgel formulation (Ferdinando 2000). However, the other features listed should also be remembered because, either individually or collectively, they are important factors that determine the selection of this drug delivery system.

Improved drug absorption

Increased rate of absorption

Major advances have been made in the area of developing softgel formulations to address particular drug absorption issues. One of the best methods is presentation of the drug to the gastrointestinal tract in the form of a solution from which the drug can be rapidly absorbed. This can be achieved using a drug-solution matrix in a softgel formulation whereby absorption is significantly

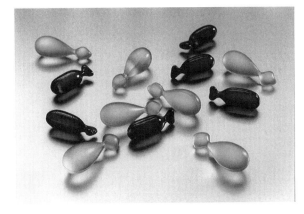

Fig. 35.3 Twist-off softgel capsules.

Table 35.1 Summary of the key features and advantages of the softgel dose form	
Features	**Advantages**
Improved drug absorption	Improved rate and extent of absorption and/or reduced variability, mainly for poorly water-soluble drugs
Patient compliance and consumer preference	Easy to swallow. Absence of poor taste or other sensory problem. Convenient administration of a liquid-drug dosage form
Safety – potent and cytotoxic drugs	Avoids dust-handling problems during dosage form manufacture; better operator safety and environmental controls
Oils and low melting point drugs	Overcomes problems with manufacture as compressed tablet or hard-shell capsules
Dose uniformity for low-dose drugs	Liquid flow during dosage form manufacture is more precise than powder flow. Drug solutions provide better homogeneity than powder or granule mixtures
Product stability	Drugs are protected against oxidative degradation by lipid vehicles and softgel capsule shells

faster than from other solid oral dosage forms, such as compressed tablets. This is because absorption of a poorly soluble drug from a tablet formulation is rate limited by the need for disintegration into granules, then drug dissolution into gastrointestinal fluid. With the solution-softgel approach, the shell ruptures within minutes to release the drug solution which is usually in a hydrophilic or highly dispersing vehicle that aids the rate of drug absorption. This may be a valuable attribute (a) for therapeutic reasons, such as the treatment of migraine or acute pain, or (b) where there is a limited absorptive region or 'absorption window' in the gastrointestinal tract. Figure 35.4 shows the faster absorption that can be achieved using a solution-softgel formulation compared to a tablet.

Increased bioavailability

As well as increasing the rate of absorption, softgels may also improve the extent of absorption. This can be

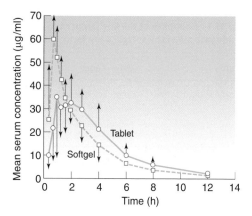

Fig. 35.4 Pharmacokinetic evaluation of softgels and tablets containing 400 mg ibuprofen (in 12 volunteers) (reproduced from Saano et al 1991).

particularly effective for hydrophobic drugs with relatively high molecular weight. An example of such a product is the protease inhibitor saquinavir, which has been formulated as a solution-softgel product (Perry & Noble 1988). The solution-softgel formulation provided around three times the bioavailability of saquinavir as measured by the area under the plasma–time curve (AUC) compared to a hard-shell capsule formulation.

In some cases a drug may be solubilized in vehicles that are capable of spontaneously dispersing into an emulsion on contact with gastrointestinal fluid. This is known as a *self-emulsifying system*. In other cases, a drug may be dissolved in an oil/surfactant vehicle that produces a microemulsion or a nanoemulsion on contact with gastrointestinal fluids. A nanoemulsion of progesterone has

been developed that provides a good example of this type of formulation. The vehicle consists of oils and surfactants in appropriate proportions. On contact with aqueous fluids, it produces an emulsion with an average droplet size less than 100 nm. The solubility of the drug is maintained as long as possible, delivering solubilized drug directly to the enterocyte membrane. This produces increased bioavailability compared to formulations in which the drug is dosed in the solid state. Figure 35.5 shows the plasma concentration–time profile for progesterone absorbed from the nanoemulsion formulation.

Softgel formulations may contain excipients – for example, one or more surfactants that can aid stability, wettability or even permeability of the drug (Aungst 2000).

Decreased plasma variability

High variability in drug plasma levels is a common characteristic of drugs with limited bioavailability. By dosing drug optimally in solution, the plasma level variability of such drugs can be significantly reduced. The cyclic polypeptide drug ciclosporin (Sandimmune Neoral®) benefits from such an approach by using a microemulsion preconcentrate in a softgel (Drewe et al 1992, Meinzer 1993).

Patient compliance and consumer preference

A number of self-medicating consumer preference studies have been carried out in an attempt to gauge the relative perception of softgels when compared to hard-shell capsules and tablets. The results of the studies showed consistently that softgels were perceived to be appealing dosage

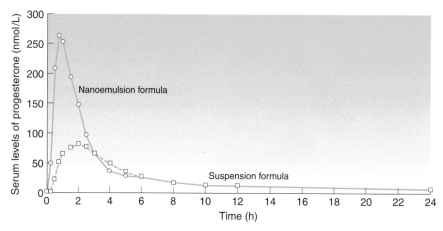

Fig. 35.5 Pharmacokinetic evaluation of progesterone comparing a softgel nanoemulsion solution of progesterone with a softgel containing a suspension of the drug in an oil following single dose administration in 12 healthy human volunteers (reproduced from Ferdinando 2000).

forms by most consumers and outperformed all other dosage forms in answering patient needs. The consumers expressed their preference for softgels in terms of (a) ease of swallowing, (b) absence of taste and (c) convenience.

One further aspect of improved compliance is that, if by using a drug solution in a softgel delivery system the bioavailability is enhanced, it may be possible to reduce the dose administered to achieve therapeutic effectiveness. In this way, it may also be possible to reduce the capsule size which will further improve patient compliance.

Safety for potent and cytotoxic drugs

The mixing, granulation and compression/filling processes used in preparing tablets and hard-shell capsules can generate a significant quantity of airborne powders. This can be of great concern for highly potent or cytotoxic compounds in terms of the operator and environmental protection required for satisfactorily safe product manufacture.

By preparing a solution or suspension of drug, where the active component is essentially protected from the environment by the liquid, such safety concerns can be significantly reduced.

Oils and low melting point drugs

When the pharmaceutical active is an oily liquid, has a melting point less than about 75°C or proves difficult to compress, liquid filling of softgels is an obvious approach to presenting a solid oral dosage form. If the drug is an oily liquid, then it can be encapsulated directly into a softgel without adding a further diluent excipient. Other low melting point drugs may be formulated with a diluent oil in order to ensure satisfactory liquid flow and dosing into softgels.

Dose uniformity of low-dose drugs

In pharmaceutical manufacture, liquid dosing avoids the difficulties of poor powder flow and therefore poor content uniformity. This is an important benefit for formulations containing low drug doses in the microgram region. Attempts to produce adequate mixtures of small quantities of a low-dose drug in larger quantities of powdered excipients for tableting or hard-shell filling are often unsuccessful. In contrast, improved homogeneity is achieved by dissolving the drug in a liquid, then encapsulating the liquid matrix in a softgel.

Product stability

If a drug is subject to oxidative or hydrolytic degradation, the preparation of a liquid-filled softgel may prove bene-

ficial. The liquid is prepared and encapsulated in a protective nitrogen atmosphere and the subsequent dried shell has very low oxygen permeability. By formulating in a lipophilic vehicle and packaging in well-designed blister packs using materials of low moisture transmission, the drug can be protected from moisture. Conversely, it is well accepted that by preparing a solution, the drug may be more reactive compared to the dry state and therefore potentially the drug may be less stable. The appropriate choice of excipients, an understanding of the drug degradation pathways and appropriate preformulation studies are vital to achieving a stable product.

MANUFACTURE OF SOFTGELS

Softgel capsules were used in the 19th century as a means of administering bitter-tasting or liquid medicines. These were manufactured individually by preparing a small sack of gelatin and allowing it to set. Each sack, or gelatin shell, was then filled with the medication and heat sealed. This method of manufacture was improved using a process that involved sealing two sheets of gelatin film between a pair of matching flat brass dies. Each die contained pockets into which the gelatin sheet was pressed and into which the medication was filled. The pressure between the two plates enabled individual capsules to be cut out from the die mould and these capsules were subsequently dried.

However, it was not until the invention of the rotary die encapsulation machine by Robert Pauli Scherer in 1933 that liquid fill capsules could be manufactured on a production scale. The rotary die process involves continuous formation of a heat seal between two ribbons of gelatin simultaneous with dosing of the fill liquid into each capsule. Although the speed and efficiency of the manufacturing process have improved greatly in recent years, the basic manufacturing principle remains essentially unchanged. The overall layout of a soft gelatin encapsulation machine is shown in Figure 35.6.

Before the encapsulation process takes place, two subprocesses are often carried out simultaneously, yielding the two components of a softgel. These are (a) the gel mass which will provide the softgel shell and (b) the fill matrix for the softgel contents.

The gel mass is prepared by dissolving the gelatin in water at approximately 80°C and under vacuum followed by the addition of the plasticizer, for example, glycerol. Once the gelatin is fully dissolved then other components such as colours, opacifier, flavours and preservatives may be added. The hot gel mass is then supplied to the encapsulation machine through heated transfer pipes by a casting method that forms two separate gelatin ribbons each

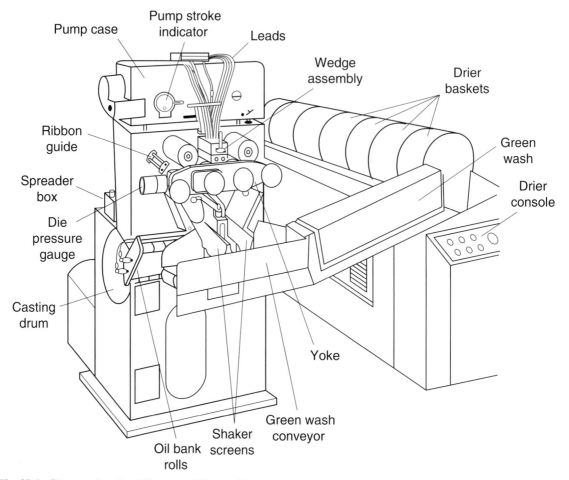

Fig. 35.6 Diagram of a soft gelatin encapsulation machine.

with a width of approximately 150 mm. During the casting process, the gelatin passes through the sol-gel transition and the thickness of each gel ribbon is controlled to ±0.1 mm in the range 0.5–1.5 mm. The thickness of the gel ribbons is checked regularly during the manufacturing process.

The two gel ribbons are then carried through rollers (at which a small quantity of vegetable oil lubricant is applied) and onwards to the rotary die encapsulation tooling (shown in Fig. 35.7). Each gel ribbon provides one half of the softgel. It is possible to make bicoloured softgels using gel ribbons of two different colours.

The liquid fill matrix containing the active drug substance is manufactured separately from preparation of the molten gel. Manufacture of the active fill matrix involves dispersing or dissolving the drug substance in the non-aqueous liquid vehicle using conventional mixer-homogenizers.

A number of different parameters are controlled during preparation of the active fill matrix, depending on the properties of the drug substance. For example, oxygen-sensitive drugs are protected by mixing under vacuum and/or inert gas; in some cases an antioxidant component may be added to the formulation. Also, if the drug substance is present as a suspension in the liquid fill matrix then it is important to ensure that particle size of the drug does not exceed approximately 200 μm. By doing this, it is possible to ensure that drug particles do not become entrapped within the capsule seal, potentially leading to loss of integrity of the softgel.

In the rotary die encapsulation process, the gel ribbon and the unit dose of liquid fill matrix are combined to form the softgel. The process involves careful control of three parameters:

- Temperature – this controls the heat available for capsule seal formation.

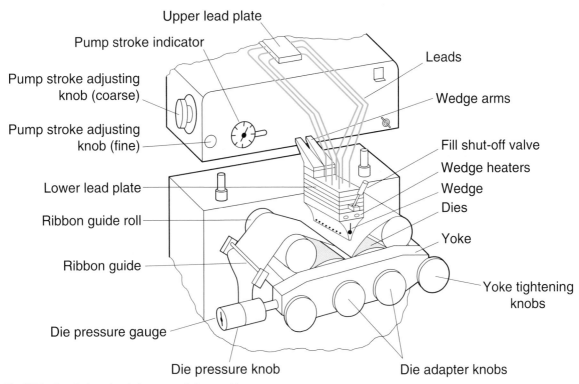

Fig. 35.7 Detail of a soft gelatin encapsulation machine.

- Timing – the timing of the dosing of unit quantities of fill matrix into the softgel during its formation is critical.
- Pressure – the pressure exerted between the two rotary dies controls the softgel shape and the final cut-out from the gel ribbon.

Figure 35.8 is a simplified diagram representing the mechanism of softgel formation using contrarotating dies and the wedge-shaped fill matrix injection system.

Accurately metered volumes of the liquid fill matrix are injected from the wedge device into the space between the gelatin ribbons as they pass between the die rolls. The wedge-shaped injection system is itself heated to approximately 40°C. The injection of liquid between the gel ribbons forces the gel to expand into the pockets of the dies, which govern the size and shape of the softgels. The ribbon continues to flow past the heated wedge injection system and is then pressed between the die rolls. Here the two softgel capsule halves are sealed together by the application of heat and pressure. The softgel capsules are cut automatically from the gel ribbon by raised rims around each die on the rollers.

After manufacture, the capsules are passed through a tumble dryer and then, to complete the drying process, they are spread onto trays and stacked in a tunnel dryer that supplies air at 20% relative humidity. The tunnel drying process may take 2–3 days or possibly as long as 2 weeks, depending on the specific softgel formulation. Finally, the softgels are inspected and packed into bulk containers in order to prevent further drying and for storage.

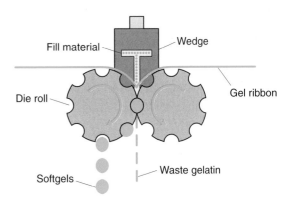

Fig. 35.8 Softgel formation mechanism.

FORMULATION OF SOFTGELS

Gelatin shell formulation

Typical softgel shells are made up of gelatin, plasticizer and materials that impart the desired appearance (colourants and/or opacifiers) and sometimes flavours. The following sections describe each of these materials, their functions, types and amounts most often used in manufacturing softgel shells.

Gelatin

A large number of different gelatin shell formulations are available depending on the nature of the liquid fill matrix. Most commonly, the gelatin is alkali-(or base-) processed (type B) gelatin and it normally constitutes 40% of the wet molten gel mass. Type A acid-processed gelatin can also be used.

Plasticizers

Plasticizers are used to make the softgel shell elastic and pliable. They usually account for 20–30% of the wet gel formulation. The most common plasticizer used in softgels is glycerol, although sorbitol and propylene glycol are also frequently used, often in combination with glycerol. The amount and choice of the plasticizer contribute to the hardness of the final product and may even affect the final product's dissolution or disintegration characteristics as well as physical and chemical stability. Plasticizers are selected on the basis of their compatibility with the fill formulation, ease of processing and desired properties of the final softgels, including hardness, appearance, handling characteristics and physical stability.

One of the most important aspects of softgel formulation is to ensure that there is minimum interaction or migration between the liquid fill matrix and the softgel shell. The choice of plasticizer type and concentration is important in ensuring optimum compatibility of the shell with the liquid fill matrix.

Water

The other essential component of the softgel shell is water. Water usually accounts for 30–40% of the wet gel formulation and its presence is important to ensure proper processing during gel preparation and softgel encapsulation. Following encapsulation, excess water is removed from the softgels through controlled drying. In dry softgels, the equilibrium water content is typically in the range 5–8% w/w which represents the proportion of water that is bound to the gelatin in the softgel shell. This level of water is important for good physical stability of softgels because in harsh storage conditions, softgels will become either too soft and fuse together or too hard and embrittled.

Colourants/opacifiers

Colourants (soluble dyes or insoluble pigments or lakes) and opacifiers are typically used at low concentrations in the wet gel formulation. Colourants can be either synthetic or natural and are used to impart desired shell colour for product identification. An opacifier, usually titanium dioxide, may be added to produce an opaque shell when the fill formulation is a suspension or to prevent photodegradation of light-sensitive fill ingredients. Titanium dioxide can either be used alone to produce a white opaque shell or in combination with pigments to produce a coloured opaque shell.

Properties of soft gelatin shells

Oxygen permeability

The gelatin shell of a soft gelatin capsule provides a good barrier against the diffusion of oxygen into the contents of the product. The quantity of oxygen (q) that passes through the gelatin is governed by the permeability coefficient (P), the area (A), thickness (h) of the shell particle, the pressure difference $(p_1 - p_2)$ and the time of diffusion (t) by the following equation:

$$q = \frac{PAt(p_1 - p_2)}{h} \qquad (35.1)$$

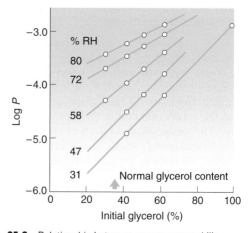

Fig. 35.9 Relationship between oxygen permeability coefficient and the glycerol concentration in the shell of softgels at room temperature and a range of relative humidity values (reproduced from Hom et al 1975).

The permeability coefficient (*P*) is related to the diffusion coefficient (*D*) and the solubility coefficient (*S*) by the equation $P = DS$. This relationship, described by Henry's Law, assumes no interaction between the gas and the polymeric film but *P* is clearly affected by the formulation of the gelatin shell as shown in Figure 35.9.

Figure 35.9 shows the relationship between oxygen permeability coefficient and the glycerol concentration in the gelatin shell of softgels at room temperature and relative humidity values from 31% to 80%. The oxygen permeability decreases with the % RH and the glycerol content in the gelatin shell formulation (Hom et al 1975). For maximum protection against the ingress of oxygen, the gelatin shell should be dry and formulated to contain about 30–40% glycerol.

Residual water content

Softgels contain littleF residual water and compounds which are susceptible to hydrolysis are protected if dissolved or dispersed in an oily liquid fill material and encapsulated as a soft gelatin capsule. Figure 35.10 shows the relationship between the equilibrium water content and the concentration of glycerol in the gelatin shell of a softgel capsule, stored at room temperature and environmental relative humidities of between 31% and 80%. The data show, for example, that the minimum water values are found at glycerol levels in the shell of between 30% and 40%. Such a formulation dried at 31% RH has a water content in the shell of about 7% (Hom et al 1975) and a water content in the fill in equilibrium with the atmosphere. The residual water content of most

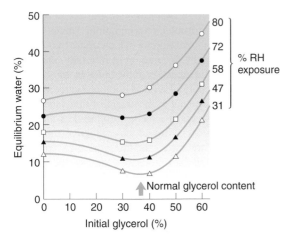

Fig. 35.10 The relationship between equilibrium water content and the concentration of glycerol in the shell of soft gelatin capsules at room temperature and a range of relative humidity values (reproduced from Hom et al 1975).

pharmaceutical compounds stored at 20% RH (the drying condition for softgels) is low and the water levels in the fills of softgels therefore are very small.

Formulation of softgel fill materials

In terms of formulation requirements, the softgel should be considered as a biphasic dosage form: a solid-phase capsule shell and a liquid-phase capsule fill matrix. Although it is possible to incorporate a drug in the shell of a softgel, the overwhelming majority of products have the active ingredient(s) within the fill matrix. The liquid-phase fill matrix is selected from components with a wide range of different physicochemical properties. The choice of components is made according to one or more of a number of criteria, including the following:

- capacity to dissolve the drug
- rate of dispersion in the gastrointestinal tract after the softgel shell ruptures and releases the fill matrix
- capacity to retain the drug in solution in the gastrointestinal fluid
- compatibility with the softgel shell
- ability to optimize the rate, extent and consistency of drug absorbed.

Types of softgel fill matrices

Lipophilic liquids/oils Trigylceride oils, such as soya bean oil, are commonly used in softgels. When used alone, however, their capacity to dissolve drugs is limited. Nevertheless, active ingredients such as hydroxycholecalciferol and other vitamin D analogues, plus steroids such as oestradiol, can be formulated into simple oily solutions for encapsulation in softgels.

Hydrophilic liquids Polar liquids with a sufficiently high molecular weight are commonly used. Polyethylene glycol (PEG) is the most frequently used, for example PEG 400 which has an average molecular weight of approximately 400 Da. Smaller hydrophilic molecules, such as ethanol or indeed water, can be incorporated in the softgel fill matrix in low levels, typically below 10% by weight.

Self-emulsifying oils A combination of a pharmaceutical oil and a non-ionic surfactant such as polyoxyethylene sorbitan monooleate can provide an oily formulation which disperses rapidly in the gastrointestinal fluid. The resulting oil/surfactant droplets enable rapid transfer of the drug to the absorbing mucosa and subsequent drug absorption.

Microemulsion and nanoemulsion systems A microemulsion of a lipid surfactant–polar liquid system is characterized by its translucent single-phase appearance. The droplet size is in the submicron range and light scattering by these droplets results in a faint blue coloration known as the Tyndall effect.

A nanoemulsion describes a similar system but containing emulsion droplets in the 100 nm size range. Microemulsion and nanoemulsion systems have the advantage of a high capacity to solubilize drug compounds and to retain the drug in solution even after dilution in gastrointestinal fluids.

In order to produce a microemulsion or nanoemulsion in the gastrointestinal tract, a 'preconcentrate' is formulated in the softgel fill matrix. In other words, the preconcentrate fill matrix contains a lipid component and one or more surfactants, which spontaneously form a microemulsion or a nanoemulsion on dilution in an aqueous environment such as in gastrointestinal fluid (Fig. 35.11). The resulting microemulsion or nanoemulsion is often stable for prolonged periods of time.

Suspensions Drugs that are insoluble in softgel fill matrices are formulated as suspensions. The continuous phase may be any of the vehicles described above. Suspension formulations provide significant advantages for certain low-solubility drugs which are very poorly absorbed after oral administration. With the appropriate choice of excipients, softgel suspensions can have improved bioavailability compared to compressed tablets or hard-shell capsules or even dilute aqueous solutions.

Lipolysis systems The advantage of the microemulsion approach lies in the high surface area presented by the microemulsion particles, which are essentially surfactant micelles swollen with solubilized oil and drug. This high surface area facilitates the rapid diffusion of drug from the dispersed oil phase into the aqueous intestinal fluids, until an equilibrium distribution is established. Thereafter, as drug is removed from the intestinal

fluids via enterocyte absorption, it is quickly replenished by the flow of fresh material from the microemulsion particles.

Formulation using the lipolysis systems

In addition to promoting the solubility of drug compounds, lipid formulations can also facilitate dissolution by taking advantage of lipolysis. This is because the lipid components of a softgel fill matrix, which comprise triglycerides or a partial (mono-/di-) glyceride, are often subject to intestinal fat digestion or lipolysis. Lipolysis is the term used to describe the action of the enzyme pancreatic lipase on triglycerides and partial glycerides, to form 2-monoglycerides and fatty acids. These 2-monoglycerides and fatty acids, known as lipolytic products, then interact with bile salts to form small droplets or vesicles. These vesicles are broken down into smaller and smaller vesicles, ultimately resulting in the formation of mixed micelles that are approximately 3–10 nm in size.

If a drug compound possesses higher solubility in lipolytic products than in triglyceride oils, then it is advantageous for lipolysis in the intestinal lumen to occur. In this way, the process of lipolysis promotes the formation of an excellent dissolution medium for the drug, namely lipolytic products. On the other hand, the absorption of a drug compound may be adversely affected by the presence of bile salt and in such a case, it may be advantageous for lipolysis to be reduced or blocked completely. It has been found that certain hydrophilic and lipophilic surfactants have the ability to block or promote lipolysis respectively (MacGregor et al 1997). These hydrophilic and lipophilic surfactants are often used in softgel fill matrix formulations.

It is possible to measure the rate and extent of lipolysis for a softgel fill matrix formulation. This is done by an in vitro pH stat measurement technique. In this, lipolysis is quantified by the amount of free fatty acids liberated by enzymatic digestion of the lipids in the softgel fill matrix. The quantity of a 1.0 M sodium hydroxide titrant is directly proportional to the extent of lipolysis.

The mixed intestinal micelles produced as a result of this lipolysis process are of physiological importance because these structures can transport high concentrations of hydrophobic molecules across the aqueous boundary layer which separates the absorptive membrane from the intestinal lumen. Thus, lipolytic products (i.e. fatty acids and monoglycerides), and hydrophobic drug, if present, reside in the hydrophobic core regions of mixed intestinal micelles. In contrast, the surface of the micelles remains hydrophilic and this facilitates rapid micellar diffusion across the aqueous boundary layer to the intestinal membrane. In the microclimate adjacent to the intestinal membrane, the pH is lower than in the

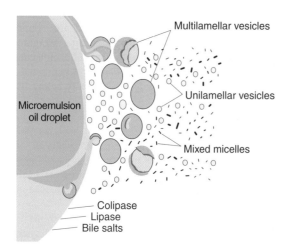

Fig. 35.11 Diagram of proposed nano/microemulsion dissolution mechanism.

intestinal lumen. This promotes demicellization, leading to the formation of a supersaturated solution of lipolytic products (and hydrophobic drug, if present) in close proximity to the enterocyte surface. These materials are then readily absorbed across the cell membrane by passive diffusion.

Mixed intestinal micelles comprising bile salts and lipolytic products can enhance the bioavailability of hydrophobic drugs whose absorption is normally dissolution rate limited. This is because mixed intestinal micelles can be very potent solubilizing agents for a wide range of hydrophobic drugs, much more so than simple bile salt micelles formed in the absence of lipolytic products. For example, under simulated physiological conditions, the aqueous solubility of cinnarizine in simple bile salt micelles is 4 µg/mL, compared to 0.5 µg/mL in aqueous buffer. However, in the presence of mixed micelles, the solubility of cinnarizine is further enhanced to approximately 44 µg/mL (Embleton et al 1995).

Taking cinnarizine as an example, it would be advantageous to formulate a softgel fill matrix that allows lipolysis to occur in the intestinal lumen because of the high drug solubility in lipolytic products. If the inhibition by a hydrophobic surfactant were allowed to occur, then it is highly likely that cinnarizine absorption would be impaired because of the reduced flow of drug into mixed micelles. However, if certain lipophilic surfactants, with an HLB less than 10, are added to the formulation, then the inhibitory effects of hydrophilic surfactants on lipolysis can be reduced or eliminated.

Two formulations containing cinnarizine, a hydrophobic drug whose absorption is normally dissolution rate limited, have been compared (Embleton et al 1995). Formulation [A] was prepared as a lipolysing formulation and [B] as a non-lipolysing formulation, as demonstrated by the in vitro model. Formulation [A] was composed of a digestible triglyceride oil, a hydrophilic surfactant and a lipophilic surfactant which was chosen on the basis of its ability to overcome the inhibitory effects of the hydrophilic surfactant on the in vitro triglyceride lipolysis. In vitro, this formulation exhibited 79% lipolysis after 60 minutes compared to the digestible oil alone. In contrast, the non-lipolysing formulation contained a lipophilic surfactant that did not overcome the inhibitory effects of the hydrophilic surfactant on the lipolysis of the triglyceride oil and was shown to lipolyse to an extent of only 3%. It is proposed that the oil in Formulation [A], which forms a fine oil-in-water emulsion on aqueous dilution, is rapidly digested, forming mixed intestinal micelles with endogenous bile. These micelles transport the drug to the intestinal membrane where the pH of the microclimate promotes micellar breakdown, facilitating enterocyte transport to the systemic circulation. In contrast, on dilution with aqueous

fluids, Formulation [B] forms a translucent microemulsion (as indicated by a blue tinge resulting from the Tyndall effect). As a result of this formulation failing to lipolyse and thereby remaining unaffected by enzymic activity, the drug is maintained within the oil phase, inhibiting the production of mixed intestinal micelles, hence restricting absorption of the drug.

The significance of the lipolysis process in enhancing the bioavailability of hydrophobic drugs was investigated further with an in vivo study. This study compared the bioavailability of cinnarizine (30 mg) orally administered as the lipolysing formulation [A] and non-lipolysing formulation [B] with a commercially available tablet, Formulation [C], to six beagle dogs. The $AUC_{(0-24h)}$ for Formulation [A] was significantly increased by 64% ($p < 0.01$) compared to the tablet preparation and by 48% ($p < 0.001$) compared to Formulation [B]. The C_{max} of Formulation [A] was approximately 75% higher than both Formulations [B] ($p < 0.001$) and [C] ($p < 0.01$) (see Fig. 35.12).

The results of this study have given a valuable insight into the effect of the microemulsion formulation on absorption of a hydrophobic drug in the gastrointestinal tract, and new information as to how the lipolysis process may influence bioavailability (Lacy et al 2000).

PRODUCT QUALITY CONSIDERATIONS

Ingredient specifications

All the ingredients of a softgel are controlled and tested to ensure compliance with pharmacopoeial specifications. However, additional specification tests may be added for certain excipients in order to ensure manufacture of a high-quality softgel product. For example, it is important to limit certain trace impurities such as aldehydes and peroxides that may be present in polyethylene glycol. The presence of high levels of these impurities gives rise to crosslinking of the gelatin polymer, leading to insolubilization through further polymerization. On prolonged storage, this can lead to slow dissolution of the capsule shell and subsequent retarded drug release.

The ingredient requiring the most careful control is gelatin itself. Once a particular grade of gelatin is used in the softgel formulation, the quality is controlled using parameters such as viscosity of a hot solution and Bloom strength of the gel. The Bloom strength is a measure of gel rigidity (see also Chapter 34).

In-process testing

During the encapsulation process the four most important tests are:

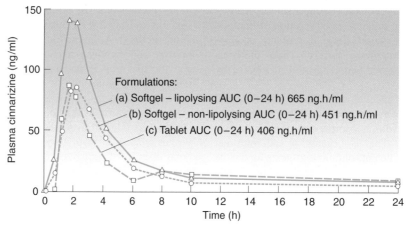

Fig. 35.12 Plasma concentration versus time curves for three formulations of cinnarizine in the dog (*n* = 6) (reproduced from Embleton et al 1995).

- the gel ribbon thickness
- softgel seal thickness at the time of encapsulation
- fill matrix weight and capsule shell weight
- softgel shell moisture level and softgel hardness at the end of the drying stage.

Appropriate control levels for these parameters are established during process development for each softgel product and are applied in routine production-scale manufacture.

Finished product testing

Finished softgels are subjected to a number of tests in accordance with compendial requirements for unit dose capsule products. These normally include capsule appearance, active ingredient assay and related substances assay as well as fill weight, content uniformity and microbiological testing.

REFERENCES

Aungst, B.J. (2000) Mini review: intestinal permeation enhancers. *Journal of Pharmaceutical Sciences*, **89**(4), 429-442.

Drewe, J., Meier, R., Vonderscherer, J. et al. (1992) Enhancement of the oral absorption of cyclosporin in man. *British Journal of Clinical Pharmacology*, **34**, 60-64.

Embleton, J., Hutchison, K.G., Lacy, J. et al. (1995) The effect of in-vivo lipolysis in improving the bioavailability of orally administered cinnarizine in self-emulsifying oily vehicles. American Association of Pharmaceutical Sciences Conference, Miami Beach.

Ferdinando, J.C. (2000) Formulation solutions – softgels. *Pharmaceutical Manufacturing and Packaging* Source Spring Issue, 69-73.

Hom, F.S., Veresh, S.A., Ebert, W.R. (1975) Soft gelatin capsules II: Oxygen permeability study of capsule shells *Journal of Pharmaceutical Sciences*, **64**(5), 851-857.

Lacy, J.E., Embleton, J.K., Perry, E.A. (2000) Delivery systems for hydrophobic drugs. US Patent 6,096,338.

MacGregor, K.J., Embleton, J.K., Lacy, J.E. et al. (1997) Influence of lipolysis on drug absorption from the gastrointestinal tract. *Advanced Drug Delivery Reviews*, **25**, 33-46.

Meinzer, A. (1993) Sandimmun® Neoral® Soft Gelatin Capsules. International Industrial Pharmaceutical Research Conference, Wisconsin, USA.

Perry, C.M., Noble, S. (1988) Saquinavir softgel capsule formulation. *Drugs*, **55**, 3.

Saano, V., Paronen, P., Peura, P. et al. (1991) Relative pharmacokinetics of three oral 400 mg ibuprofen dosage forms in healthy volunteers. *International Journal of Clinical Pharmacology, Therapy and Toxicology*, **29**(10), 381-385.

36

Pulmonary drug delivery

K. M. G. Taylor

INHALED DRUG DELIVERY

Drugs are generally delivered to the respiratory tract for the treatment or prophylaxis of airways diseases, such as bronchial asthma and cystic fibrosis. The administration of a drug at its site of action can result in a rapid onset of activity, which may be highly desirable, for instance when delivering bronchodilating drugs for the treatment of asthma. Additionally, smaller doses can be administered locally compared to delivery by the oral or parenteral routes, thereby reducing the potential incidence of adverse systemic effects and reducing drug costs. The pulmonary route is also useful where a drug is poorly absorbed orally, e.g. sodium cromoglicate, or where it is rapidly metabolized orally, e.g. isoprenaline. The avoidance of first-pass metabolism in the liver may also be advantageous, although the lung itself has some metabolic capability.

The lung may be used as a route for delivering drugs having systemic activity, because of its large surface area, the abundance of capillaries and the thinness of the air–blood barrier. This has been exploited in the treatment of migraine with ergotamine, and studies have demonstrated the potential for delivering proteins and peptides such as insulin and growth hormone via the airways.

Lung anatomy

The lung is the organ of external respiration, in which oxygen and carbon dioxide are exchanged between blood and inhaled air. The structure of the airways also prevents the entry of and promotes efficient removal of airborne foreign particles, including microorganisms.

The respiratory tract can be considered as comprising conducting (central) regions (trachea, bronchi, bronchioles, terminal and respiratory bronchioles) and respiratory (peripheral) regions (respiratory bronchioles and alveolar regions), although there is no clear demarcation between them (Fig. 36.1). The upper respiratory tract comprises the nose, throat, pharynx and larynx; the lower tract comprises the trachea, bronchi, bronchioles and the alveolar regions. Simplistically, the airways can be described by a symmetrical model in which each airway divides into two equivalent branches or generations. In fact, the trachea (generation 0) branches into two main bronchi (generation 1), of which the right bronchus is wider and leaves the trachea at a smaller angle than the left, and hence is more likely to receive inhaled material. Further branching of the airways ultimately results in terminal bronchioles. These divide to produce respiratory bronchioles, which connect with alveolar ducts leading to the alveolar sacs (generation 23). These contain

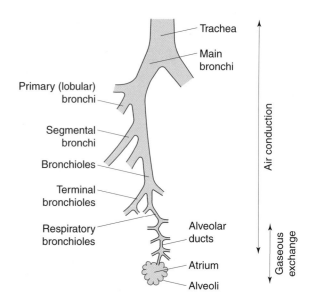

Fig. 36.1 Schematic representation of the human airways (reproduced with permission from Wilson & Washington 1989).

approximately $2-6 \times 10^8$ alveoli, producing a surface area of about 70–80 m^2 in an adult male.

The conducting airways are lined with ciliated epithelial cells. Insoluble particles deposited on the airways walls in this region are trapped by the mucus, swept upwards from the lungs by the beating cilia and swallowed.

Inhalation aerosols and the importance of size distribution

To deliver a drug into the airways, it must be presented as an aerosol (with the exception of medical gases). In pharmacy, an aerosol is defined as a two-phase system of solid particles or liquid droplets dispersed in air or other gaseous phase, having sufficiently small size to display considerable stability as a suspension.

The deposition of a drug/aerosol in the airways is dependent on four factors: the physicochemical properties of the drug, the formulation, the delivery/liberating device, and the patient (breathing patterns and clinical status).

The most fundamentally important physical property of an aerosol for inhalation is its size. The particle size of an aerosol is usually standardized by calculation of its aerodynamic diameter, d_a, which is the physical diameter of a unit density sphere which settles through air with a velocity equal to the particle in question. Therapeutic aerosols are heterodispersed (polydispersed) and the distribution of sizes is generally represented by the geometric standard deviation (GSD or σ_g), when size is log-normally distributed.

For approximately spherical particles:

$$d_a = d_p (\rho/\rho_0)^{1/2} \qquad (36.1)$$

where d_p is physical diameter, ρ is particle density and ρ_0 is unit density, i.e. 1 g/cm³.

When d_p is the mass median diameter (MMD), d_a is termed the mass median aerodynamic diameter (MMAD).

Influence of environmental humidity on particle size

As a particle enters the respiratory tract, the change from ambient to high relative humidity (approximately 99%) results in condensation of water on to the particle surface, which continues until the vapour pressure of the water equals that of the surrounding atmosphere. For water-insoluble materials, this results in a negligibly thin film of water; however, with water-soluble materials a solution is formed on the particle surface. As the vapour pressure of the solution is lower than that of pure solvent at the same temperature, water will continue to condense until equilibrium between vapour pressures is reached, i.e. the particle will increase in size. The final equilibrium diameter is constrained by the Kelvin effect, i.e. the vapour pressure of a droplet solution is higher than that for a planar surface and is a function of the particle's original diameter. Hygroscopic growth will affect the deposition of particles, resulting in deposition higher in the respiratory tract than would have been predicted from measurements of their initial size.

Particle deposition in the airways

The efficacy of a clinical aerosol is dependent on its ability to penetrate the respiratory tract. To penetrate to the peripheral (respirable) regions, aerosols require a size less than about 5 or 6 μm, with less than 2 μm being preferable for alveolar deposition. Literature values for 'respirable' size vary and must be considered alongside the environmental changes in size described above and the heterodispersed nature of inhalation aerosol size distributions. Larger particles or droplets are deposited in the upper respiratory tract and are rapidly cleared from the lung by the mucociliary action, with the effect that drug becomes available for systemic absorption and may potentially cause adverse effects. Steroid aerosols of sufficiently large size may deposit in the mouth and throat, with the potential to cause oral candidiasis. The size of aerosolized drug may be especially important in the treatment of certain conditions where penetration to the peripheral airways is particularly desirable, for instance

the treatment and prophylaxis of the alveolar infection *Pneumocystis carinii* pneumonia.

There are three main mechanisms responsible for particulate deposition in the lung: gravitational sedimentation, impaction and diffusion.

Gravitational sedimentation

From Stokes' Law, particles settling under gravity will attain a constant terminal settling velocity, V_t:

$$V_t = \frac{\rho g d^2}{18\eta} \qquad (36.2)$$

where ρ is particle density, g is the gravitational constant, d is particle diameter and η is air viscosity.

Thus, gravitational sedimentation of an inhaled particle is dependent on its size and density, in addition to its residence time in the airways. Sedimentation is an important deposition mechanism for particles in the size range 0.5–3 μm, in the small airways and alveoli, for particles that have escaped deposition by impaction.

Inertial impaction

Where a bifurcation occurs in the respiratory tract, the air stream changes direction and particles within the air stream, having sufficiently high momentum, will impact on the airways' walls rather than following the changing air stream. This deposition mechanism is particularly important for large particles having a diameter greater than 5 μm, and particularly greater than 10 μm, and is common in the upper airways, being the principal mechanism for deposition in the nose, mouth, pharynx and larynx and the large conducting airways. With the continuous branching of the conducting airways, the velocity of the air stream decreases and impaction becomes a less important mechanism for deposition.

The probability of impaction is proportional to:

$$\frac{V_t V \sin\theta}{gr} \qquad (36.3)$$

where θ is the change in airways direction, V is air-stream velocity and r is the airway's radius.

Brownian diffusion

Collision and bombardment of small particles by molecules in the respiratory tract produce Brownian motion. The resultant movement of particles from high to low concentrations causes them to move from the aerosol cloud to the airways' walls. The rate of diffusion is inversely proportional to the particle size, and thus diffusion is the predominant mechanism for particles smaller than 0.5 μm.

Other mechanisms of deposition

Although impaction, sedimentation and diffusion are the most important mechanisms for drug deposition in the respiratory tract, other mechanisms may occur. These include interception, whereby particles having extreme shapes, such as fibres, physically catch on to the airways' walls as they pass through the respiratory tract, and electrostatic attraction, whereby an electrostatic charge on a particle induces an opposing charge on the walls of the respiratory tract, resulting in attraction between particle and walls.

Effect of particle size on deposition mechanism

Different deposition mechanisms are important for different sized particles. Those greater than 5 µm will deposit predominantly by inertial impaction in the upper airways. Particles sized between 1 and 5 µm deposit predominantly by gravitational sedimentation in the lower airways, especially during slow, deep breathing, and particles less than 1 µm deposit by Brownian diffusion in the stagnant air of the lower airways. Particles of approximately 0.5 µm are inefficiently deposited, being too large for effective deposition by Brownian diffusion and too small for effective impaction or sedimentation, and they are often immediately exhaled. This size of minimum deposition should thus be considered during formulation, although for the reasons of environmental humidity discussed previously, the equilibrium diameter in the airways may be significantly larger than the original particle size in the formulation.

Breathing patterns

Patient-dependent factors, such as breathing patterns and lung physiology, also affect particle deposition. For instance, the larger the inhaled volume, the greater the peripheral distribution of particles in the lung, whereas increasing inhalation flow rate enhances deposition in the larger airways by inertial impaction. Breath-holding after inhalation enhances the deposition of particles by sedimentation and diffusion. Optimal aerosol deposition occurs with slow, deep inhalations to total lung capacity, followed by breath-holding prior to exhalation. It should be noted that changes in the airways resulting from disease states, for instance airways' obstruction, may affect the deposition profile of an inhaled aerosol.

Clearance of inhaled particles and drug absorption

Particles deposited in the ciliated conducting airways are cleared by mucociliary clearance within 24 hours and are ultimately swallowed. Insoluble particles penetrating to the alveolar regions, and which are not solubilized in situ, are removed more slowly. Alveolar macrophages engulf such particles and may then migrate to the bottom of the mucociliary escalator, or alternatively particles may be removed via the lymphatics.

Hydrophobic compounds are usually absorbed at a rate dependent on their oil/water partition coefficients, whereas hydrophilic materials are poorly absorbed through membrane pores at rates inversely proportional to molecular size. Thus, the airways' membrane, like the gastrointestinal tract, is preferably permeable to the unionized form of a drug. Some drugs, such as sodium cromoglicate, are partly absorbed by a saturable active transport mechanism, whilst large macromolecules may be absorbed by transcytosis. The rate of drug absorption, and consequently drug action, can be influenced by the formulation. Rapid drug action can generally be achieved using solutions or powders of aqueous soluble salts, whereas slower or prolonged absorption may be achieved using suspension formulations, powders of less soluble salts or novel drug delivery systems such as liposomes and microspheres.

FORMULATING AND DELIVERING THERAPEUTIC INHALATION AEROSOLS

There are currently three main types of aerosol-generating device for use in inhaled drug therapy: pressurized metered-dose inhalers, dry powder inhalers and nebulizers.

Pressurized metered-dose inhalers

Pressurized metered-dose inhalers (pMDIs) also referred to as metered-dose inhalers (MDIs), introduced in the mid-1950s, are the most commonly used inhalation drug delivery devices. In pMDIs, drug is either dissolved or suspended in liquid propellant(s) together with other excipients, including surfactants, and presented in a pressurized canister fitted with a metering valve (Fig. 36.2). A predetermined dose is released as a spray on actuation of the metering valve. When released from the canister, the formulation undergoes volume expansion in the passage within the valve and forms a mixture of gas and liquid before discharge from the orifice. The high-speed gas flow helps to break up the liquid into a fine spray of droplets.

Containers

Pharmaceutical aerosols may be packaged in tin-plated steel, plastic-coated glass or aluminium containers. In practice, pMDIs are generally presented in aluminium canisters, produced by extrusion to give seamless containers with a capacity of 10–30 mL. Aluminium is relatively inert and may be used uncoated where there is no chemical instability between container and contents.

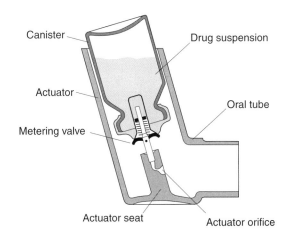

Fig. 36.2 The pressurized metered-dose inhaler (reproduced with permission from Morén 1981).

Alternatively, aluminium containers with an internal coating of a chemically resistant organic material, such as an epoxy resin or polytetrafluorine (PTFE), can be used.

Propellants

The propellants used in pMDI formulations are liquefied gases, traditionally chlorofluorocarbons (CFCs) and increasingly hydrofluoroalkanes (HFAs). At room temperature and pressure, these are gases but they are readily liquefied by decreasing temperature or increasing pressure. The head space of the aerosol canister is filled with propellant vapour, producing the saturation vapour pressure at that temperature. On spraying, medicament and propellant are expelled and the head volume increases. To reestablish the equilibrium, more propellant evaporates and so a constant pressure system with consistent spray characteristics is produced. The CFCs currently employed in pMDI formulations are trichlorofluoromethane (CFC-11), dichlorodifluoromethane (CFC-12) and dichlorotetrafluoroethane (CFC-114). Formulations generally comprise blends of CFC-11 and CFC-12 or CFC-11, CFC-12 and CFC-114 (Table 36.1),

together with a surfactant such as a sorbitan ester, oleic acid or lecithin, which acts as a suspending agent and lubricates the valve.

CFCs and HFAs are numbered using a universal system. The first digit is the number of carbon atoms minus 1 (omitted if zero), the second is the number of hydrogen atoms plus 1, and the third is the number of fluorine atoms. Chlorine fills any remaining valencies, given the total number of atoms required to saturate the compound. If asymmetry is possible, this is designated by a letter. The symmetrical isomer is assigned the number described above; of the asymmetrical isomers, that designated the letter *a* is the most symmetrical, *b* the next most symmetrical, and so on. The CFCs are perfectly miscible with each other and suitable blends give a useful intermediate vapour pressure, usually about 450 kPa. The vapour pressure of the mixture of propellants is given by Raoult's Law, i.e. the vapour pressure of a mixed system is equal to the sum of the mole fraction of each component multiplied by its vapour pressure:

$$P = p_a + p_b \tag{36.4}$$

where P is the total vapour pressure of the system and p_a and p_b are the partial vapour pressures of the components, *a* and *b*:

$$p_a = x_a p_a^o \tag{36.5}$$

$$p_b = x_b p_b^o \tag{36.6}$$

where x_a and x_b are the mole fractions and p_a^o and p_b^o are the partial vapour pressures of components *a* and *b*, respectively.

The reaction of CFCs with the ozone in the earth's stratosphere, which absorbs ultraviolet radiation at 300 nm, and their contribution to global warming are major environmental concerns. CFCs pass to the stratosphere, where in the presence of UV they liberate chlorine, which reacts with ozone. The depletion of stratospheric ozone results in increased exposure to the UV-B part of the UV spectrum, resulting in a number of adverse effects, in particular an increased incidence of skin cancer. The Montreal Protocol of 1987 was a global ban on

Table 36.1 Formulae and physicochemical properties of chlorofluorocarbons (CFCs) and hydrofluoroalkanes (HFAs) used in pMDI formulations

Number	Formula	Boiling point (°C)	Vapour pressure (kPa at 20°C)	Density (g/mL at 20°C)
11	CCl_3F	23.7	89 (0.89 bar)	1.49
12	CCl_2F_2	−29.8	568 (5.68 bar)	1.33
114	$C_2Cl_2F_4$	3.6	183 (1.83 bar)	1.47
134a	$C_2F_4H_2$	−26.5	660 (6.6 bar)	1.23
227	C_3F_7H	−17.3	398 (3.98 bar)	1.41

the production of the five worst ozone-depleting CFCs by the year 2000. This was amended in 1992, so that production of CFCs in developed countries was phased out by January 1996. In the European Union, all ozone-depleting CFCs were banned by the end of 1995. Pharmaceutical aerosols are currently exempted but this exemption is reviewed annually. In household and cosmetic aerosols, CFCs have been replaced by hydrocarbons such as propane and butane. Alternatively, compressed gases such as nitrogen dioxide, nitrogen and carbon dioxide may be used, for instance in food products. However, compressed gases do not maintain a constant pressure within the canister throughout its use, as the internal pressure is inversely proportionate to the head volume, and so product performance changes with age. For reasons of toxicity and inflammability, hydrocarbons are not considered appropriate alternatives to CFCs for inhalation products and so non-ozone depleting alternatives to CFCs have been developed.

Propellants HFA-134a (trifluoromonofluoroethane) and HFA-227 (heptafluoropropane) are non-ozone depleting, non-flammable HFAs, also called hydrofluorocarbons (HFCs), which have been widely investigated as alternatives to CFC-12 (see Table 36.1). However, these gases contribute to global warming and further replacements may be required in the future.

HFA-134a and HFA-227 have some physical properties, including density, which are similar to those of CFC-12 and, to a lesser extent, CFC-114. However, they present major formulation problems; in particular, they are poor solvents for the surfactants commonly used in MDI formulation and no alternative to CFC-11 is currently available. Ethanol is approved for use in formulations containing HFAs to allow dissolution of surfactants, and is included in marketed non-CFC MDI products. However, ethanol has low volatility and may consequently increase the droplet size of the emitted aerosols.

Metering valve

The metering valve of a pMDI permits the reproducible delivery of small volumes (25–100 µL) of product. Unlike the non-metering continuous-spray valve of conventional pressurized aerosols, the metering valve in pMDIs is used in the inverted position (Fig. 36.3). Depression of the valve stem allows the contents of the metering chamber to be discharged through the orifice in the valve stem and made available to the patient. After actuation, the metering chamber refills with liquid from the bulk and is ready to dispense the next dose. A corollary of this is that the pMDI needs to be primed, i.e. the metering chamber filled, prior to the first use by a patient. pMDI valves are complex in design and must protect the product from the environment, while also protecting

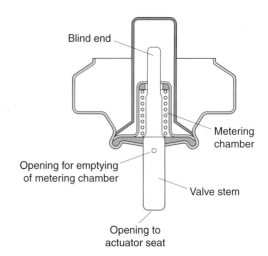

Fig. 36.3 The metering valve (reproduced with permission from Morén 1981).

against product loss during repeated use. The introduction of HFA propellants with different solvent properties has necessitated the development of new valve elastomers. The valve stem fits into the actuator, which is made of polyethylene or polypropylene. The dimensions of the orifice in the actuator play a crucial role, along with the propellant vapour pressure, in determining the shape and speed of the emitted aerosol plume.

Formulating metered-dose inhalers

Pressurized aerosols may be formulated as either solutions or suspensions of drug in the liquefied propellant. Solution preparations are two-phase systems. However, the propellants are poor solvents for most drugs. Cosolvents such as ethanol or isopropanol may be used, although their low volatility retards propellant evaporation. In practice, pressurized inhaler formulations have, until recently, been almost exclusively suspensions. These three-phase systems are harder to formulate and all the problems of conventional suspension formulation, such as caking, agglomeration, particle growth, etc., must be considered. Careful consideration must be given to the particle size of the solid (usually micronized to between 2 and 5 µm), valve clogging, moisture content, the solubility of active compound in propellant (a salt may be desirable), the relative density of propellant and drug, and the use of surfactants as suspending agents, e.g. lecithin, oleic acid and sorbitan trioleate (usually included at concentrations between 0.1 and 2.0% w/w). These surfactants are very poorly soluble (<<0.02% w/w) in HFAs and so ethanol is usually employed as a cosolvent, though alternative surfactants are being developed. Solution formulations of beclometasone dipropionate are now available. Evaporation of HFA propellant following actuation of these formulations results in smaller particle sizes than with conventional suspension formulations of the same drug, with consequent changes in its pulmonary distribution and bioavailability. The dose may be adjusted accordingly or the volatility of the product modified by the addition of a less volatile component, such as glycerol.

Filling metered-dose inhaler canisters

Canisters are filled by liquefying the propellant at reduced temperature or elevated pressure.

In cold filling, active compound, excipients and propellant are chilled and filled at about −60°C. Additional propellant is then added at the same temperature and the canister sealed with the valve. In pressure filling, a drug/propellant (CFC-11) concentrate is produced and filled at effectively room temperature and pressure (in fact, usually slightly chilled to below 20°C). The valve is crimped on to the canister and additional propellant (e.g. CFC-12) is filled at elevated pressure through the valve, in a process known as gassing. Pressure filling is most frequently employed for inhalation aerosols. However, no HFAs have the properties (high boiling point: 23.7°C) of CFC-11 so a single-stage pressure filling process has been developed for HFA-based formulations whereby a concentrated solution or suspension of drug in propellant, under pressure, is filled into canisters through the valve, followed by addition of further propellant.

Once filled, the canisters are leak tested by placing them in a water bath at elevated temperature, usually 50–60°C. Following storage to allow equilibration of the formulation and valve components, the containers are weighed to check for further leakage, prior to spray testing and insertion into actuators.

Advantages and disadvantages of metered-dose inhalers

The major advantages of pMDIs are their portability, low cost and disposability. Many doses (up to 200) are stored in the small canister and dose delivery is reproducible. The inert conditions created by the propellant vapour, together with the hermetically sealed container, protect drugs from oxidative degradation and microbiological contamination. However, pMDIs have disadvantages. They are inefficient at drug delivery. On actuation, the first propellant droplets exit at a high velocity, which may exceed 30 m/s. Consequently, much of the drug is lost through impaction of these droplets in the oropharyngeal areas. The mean emitted droplet size typically exceeds 40 μm, and propellants may not evaporate sufficiently rapidly for their size to decrease to that suitable for deep lung

deposition. Vaporization of the droplets is hindered by the low volatility of CFC-11, which is present in concentrations of at least 25% in most CFC-based formulations. Evaporation, such that the aerodynamic diameter of the particles is close to that of the original micronized drug, may not occur until 5 seconds after actuation.

An additional problem with pMDIs, which is beyond the control of the formulator and manufacturer, is their incorrect use by patients. Reported problems include:

- failure to remove the protective cap covering the mouthpiece
- the inhaler being used inverted
- failure to shake the canister
- failure to inhale slowly and deeply
- inadequate breath-holding
- poor inhalation/actuation synchronization.

Correct use by patients is vital for effective drug deposition and action. Ideally, the pMDI should be actuated during the course of slow, deep inhalation, followed by a period of breath-holding. Many patients find this difficult, especially children and the elderly. The misuse of pMDIs through poor inhalation/actuation coordination can be significantly reduced with appropriate instruction and counselling. However, it should be noted that even using the correct inhalation technique, only 10–20% of the stated emitted dose may be delivered to the site of action.

Spacers and breath-actuated metered-dose inhalers

Some of the disadvantages of pMDIs, namely inhalation/actuation coordination and the premature deposition of large propellant droplets high in the airways, can be overcome by using extension devices or 'spacers' positioned between the pMDI and the patient (Fig. 36.4), and thus these are frequently employed, with a pMDI, for administering aerosol medications to young children. The dose from a pMDI is discharged directly into the reservoir prior to inhalation. This reduces the initial droplet velocity, permits efficient propellant evaporation and removes

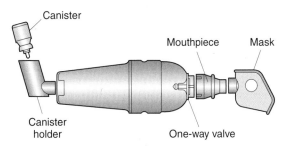

Fig. 36.4 The Nebuhaler® spacer device, fitted with a facemask for use by a child (courtesy of AstraZeneca).

the need for actuation/inhalation coordination. The disadvantage of traditional spacers is that they may be cumbersome because of their large volume, e.g. Nebuhaler® (AstraZeneca), though smaller, medium-volume spacers are now available, e.g. AeroChamber Plus® (Glaxo SmithKline). Alternatively, extension tubes may be built into the design of the pMDI itself as an extended mouthpiece, e.g. Syncroner® (Rhône-Poulenc Rorer) and Spacer Inhalers® (AstraZeneca). Breath-actuated pMDIs do not release drug until inspiration occurs. In the Autohaler® (3M), an inspiratory demand valve triggers a spring mechanism to release drug, whilst in the Easi-breathe® (Ivax), a vacuum in the device is released on inspiration to trigger actuation. Breath-actuated devices overcome the coordination problems of conventional pMDIs and are easy to use without adding bulk to the device.

Dry powder inhalers

In dry powder inhaler (DPI) systems, drug is inhaled as a cloud of fine particles. The drug is either preloaded in an inhalation device or filled into hard gelatin capsules or foil blister discs which are loaded into a device prior to use.

DPIs have several advantages over pMDIs. DPI formulations are propellant free and do not contain any excipient, other than a carrier (see below), which is usually lactose. They are breath-actuated, avoiding the problems of inhalation/actuation coordination encountered with pMDIs. DPIs can also deliver larger drug doses than pMDIs, which are limited by the volume of the metering valve and the maximum suspension concentration that can be employed without causing valve clogging. However, DPIs have several disadvantages. Liberation of powders from the device and the deaggregation of particles are limited by the patient's ability to inhale, which in the case of respiratory disease may be impaired. An increase in turbulent air flow created by an increase in inhaled air velocity increases the deaggregation of the emerging particles but also increases the potential for inertial impaction in the upper airways and throat, and so a compromise has to be found. Further, DPIs are exposed to ambient atmospheric conditions, which may reduce formulation stability. For instance, elevated humidity may cause powders to clump. Finally, DPIs are generally less efficient at drug delivery than pMDIs, such that twice the dose is often required for delivery from a DPI compared to the equivalent pMDI.

Formulating dry powder inhalers

To produce particles of a suitable size (preferably less than 5 μm), drug powders for use in inhalation systems are usually micronized. Alternatives are spray drying and supercritical fluid technology. The high-energy powders produced have poor flow properties because of their static, cohesive and adhesive nature. The flowability of a powder is affected by physical properties, including particle size and shape, density, surface roughness, hardness, moisture content and bulk density.

To improve their flow properties, poorly flowing drug particles are generally mixed with larger 'carrier' particles (usually 30–60 μm) of an inert excipient, usually lactose. Drug and carrier particles are mixed to produce an ordered mix in which the small drug particles attach to the surface of the larger carrier particles. This not only improves liberation of the drug from the inhalation device by improving powder flow, but also improves the uniformity of capsule or device filling. Once liberated from the device, the turbulent air flow generated within the inhalation device should be sufficient for the deaggregation of the drug/carrier aggregates. The larger carrier particles impact in the throat, whereas smaller drug particles are carried in the inhaled air deeper into the respiratory tract.

The success of DPI formulations depends on the adhesion of drug and carrier during mixing and filling of devices or hard gelatin capsules, followed by the ability of the drug to desorb from the carrier during inhalation such that free drug is available to penetrate to the peripheral airways. Adhesion and desorption will depend on the morphology of the particle surfaces and surface energies, which may be influenced by the chemical nature of the materials involved and the nature of powder processing. The performance of DPI systems is thus strongly dependent on formulation factors, and also on the construction of the delivery device and a patient's inhalation technique.

Unit-dose devices with drug in hard gelatin capsules

The first DPI device developed was the Spinhaler® (Rhône-Poulenc Rorer) for the delivery of sodium cromoglicate (Fig. 36.5). Each dose, contained in a hard gelatin capsule, is loaded individually into the device. The capsule, placed in a loose-fitting rotor, is pierced by two metal needles on either side of the capsule. Inhaled air flow though the device causes a turbovibratory air pattern as the rotor rotates rapidly, resulting in the powder being dispersed to the capsule walls and out through the perforations into the air. A minimum air flow rate of 35–40 L/min through the device is required to produce adequate vibrations by the rotor. The occurrence of lactose intolerance and local irritation, coughing and bronchoconstriction caused by the inhalation of large amounts of lactose has led to the development of an aggregated, carrier-free sodium cromoglicate capsule formulation for use in the Spinhaler. Other hard gelatin capsule-based devices,

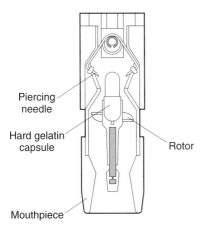

Piercing needle

Hard gelatin capsule

Rotor

Mouthpiece

Fig. 36.5 The Spinhaler® (reprinted from Bell et al 1971, with permission of Wiley-Liss Inc., a subsidiary of John Wiley and Sons, Inc.).

working on similar principles, have been marketed since, and some are still available, e.g. the Cyclohaler® (Du Pont).

Multidose devices with drug in foil blisters

The main disadvantage of hard gelatin capsule-based devices, namely the individual loading of each dose, has been overcome with the development of the Diskhaler® (GlaxoSmithKline). In this system, drug is mixed with a coarse lactose carrier and filled into an aluminium foil blister disc which is loaded, by the patient, into the device on a support wheel (Fig. 36.6). Each disc contains four or eight doses of drug and the blisters are pierced with a needle as a result of mechanical leverage of the

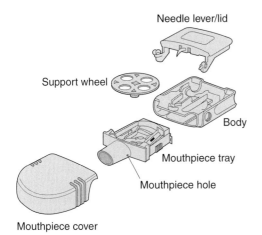

Needle lever/lid

Support wheel

Body

Mouthpiece tray

Mouthpiece hole

Mouthpiece cover

Fig. 36.6 The Diskhaler® (reproduced with permission from Sumby et al 1993).

lid. Air flow through the blister causes the powder to disperse as the patient inhales through the mouthpiece. The foil blisters are numbered, so that the patient knows the number of doses remaining.

Multidose devices with drug preloaded in inhaler

The evolution of the Diskhaler led to the production of the Accuhaler® or Diskus® Inhaler (GlaxoSmithKline), in which drug/carrier mix is preloaded into the device in foil-covered blister pockets containing 60 doses (Fig. 36.7). The foil lid is peeled off the drug-containing pockets as each dose is advanced, with the blisters and lids being wound up separately within the device, which is discarded at the end of operation. As each dose is packaged separately and only momentarily exposed to ambient conditions prior to inhalation, the Diskhaler and Accuhaler are relatively insensitive to humidity compared to hard gelatin capsule-based systems.

An alternative approach is a reservoir type of device, in which a dose is accurately measured and delivered from a drug reservoir. In the Clickhaler® DPI (Innovata Biomed), a drug–lactose blend is stored in a reservoir. Metering cups are filled by gravity from this reservoir and delivered to an inhalation passage, from which the dose is inhaled. The device is shaken before use. The device is capable of holding up to 200 doses and incorporates a dose counter which indicates the number of metered doses and informs patients when the device, which is discarded after use, is nearly empty. After the final dose has been dispensed, the push button locks to prevent further use.

The Turbohaler® (AstraZeneca) has overcome the need for both a carrier and the loading of individual doses (Fig. 36.8). The device contains a large number of doses (up to 200) of undiluted, loosely aggregated micronized drug, which is stored in a reservoir from which it flows on to a rotating disc in the dosing unit. The fine holes in the disc are filled and the excess drug is removed by scrapers. As the rotating disc is turned, by moving a turning grip back and forth, one metered dose is presented to the inhalation channel and this is inhaled by the patient, with the turbulent air flow created within the device breaking up any drug aggregates. A dose indicator is incorporated. The Turbohaler requires a higher inspiratory effort than the Diskhaler, owing to its higher internal resistance, and is more sensitive to humidity if not closed quickly after each use.

Future developments

Many devices are currently under development which reduce or eliminate the reliance on the patient's inspiratory effort to disperse the drug. This is advantageous as

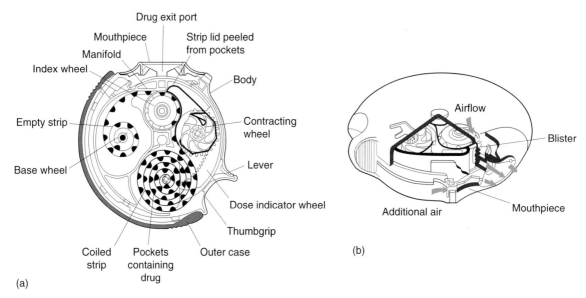

Fig. 36.7 The Accuhaler/Diskus® Inhaler, showing (a) a schematic diagram and (b) a cross-sectional representation of the device (reproduced with permission from Prime et al 1996).

inspiratory effort may be affected by the patient's age and/or clinical condition. For instance, Nektar Therapeutics have produced a device for the delivery of insulin as a fine powder, in which compressed air is used to disperse drug from a unit-dose package into a large holding chamber, from which it is inhaled by the patient. Another novel device, the Spiros® DPI (Dura) (Fig. 36.9), is a breath-actuated, effort-assisted device which uses a battery-powered impeller to deaggregate and aerosolize the drug powder, which is held in a rotating cassette. The device functions relatively independently of the patient's inspiratory flow rate and can be used with those patients who can only achieve low inspiratory flow rates.

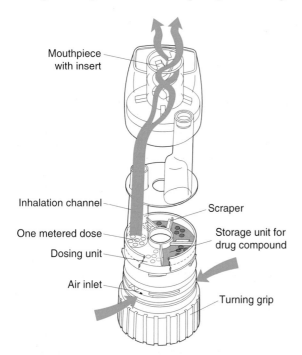

Fig. 36.8 The Turbohaler® (reproduced with permission from Wetterlin 1987).

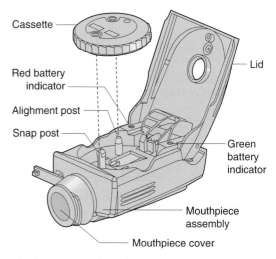

Fig 36.9 The Spiros® DPI (reproduced with permission from Nelson et al 1999).

Nebulizers

Nebulizers deliver relatively large volumes of drug solutions and suspensions and are frequently used for drugs that cannot be conveniently formulated into pMDIs or DPIs, or where the therapeutic dose is too large for delivery with these alternative systems. Nebulizers also have the advantage over metered-dose and dry powder systems in that drug may be inhaled during normal tidal breathing through a mouthpiece or facemask, and thus they are useful for patients such as children, the elderly and patients with arthritis, who experience difficulties with pMDIs.

There are three categories of commercially available nebulizer: jet, ultrasonic and vibrating-mesh.

Jet nebulizers

Jet nebulizers (also called air-jet or air-blast nebulizers) use compressed gas (air or oxygen) from a compressed gas cylinder, hospital air-line or electrical compressor to convert a liquid (usually an aqueous solution) into a spray. The jet of high-velocity gas is passed either tangentially or coaxially through a narrow Venturi nozzle, typically 0.3–0.7mm in diameter. An area of negative pressure, where the air jet emerges, causes liquid to be drawn up a feed tube from a fluid reservoir by the Bernoulli effect (Fig. 36.10). Liquid emerges as fine filaments, which collapse into droplets owing to surface tension. A proportion of the resultant (primary) aerosol leaves the nebulizer directly; the remaining large, non-respirable droplets impact on baffles or the walls of the nebulizer chamber and are recycled into the reservoir fluid.

Nebulizers are operated continuously and because the inspiratory phase of breathing constitutes approximately one-third of the breathing cycle, a large proportion of the emitted aerosol is not inhaled but is released into the environment. Open-vent nebulizers, incorporating inhalation and exhalation valves, e.g. the Pari LC® nebulizer (Pari), have been developed in which the patient's own breath boosts nebulizer performance, with aerosol production matching the patient's tidal volume and greatly enhancing drug delivery. On exhalation, the aerosol being produced is generated only from the compressor gas source, thereby minimizing drug wastage.

The rate of gas flow driving atomization is the major determinant of the aerosol droplet size and rate of drug delivery for jet nebulizers; for instance, there may be up to a 50% reduction in the mass median aerodynamic diameter when the flow rate is increased from 4 to 8 L/min, with a linear increase in the proportion of droplets less than 5 μm.

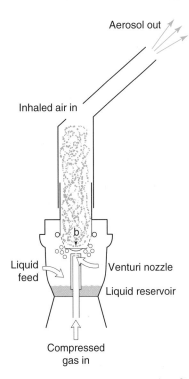

Fig. 36.10 Schematic diagram of a jet nebulizer. Compressed gas passes through a Venturi nozzle, where an area of negative pressure is created. Liquid is drawn up a feed tube and is fragmented into droplets. Large droplets impact on baffles (b), and small droplets are carried away in the inhaled air stream (reproduced with permission from Newman 1989).

Ultrasonic nebulizers

In ultrasonic nebulizers the energy necessary to atomize liquids comes from a piezoelectric crystal vibrating at high frequency. At sufficiently high ultrasonic intensities, a fountain of liquid is formed in the nebulizer chamber. Large droplets are emitted from the apex and a 'fog' of small droplets is emitted from the lower part (Fig. 36.11). Some models have a fan to blow the respirable droplets out of the device, whereas in others the aerosol only becomes available to the patient during inhalation.

Vibrating-mesh nebulizers

Recently, vibrating-mesh nebulizers have come commercially available, in which aerosols are generated by passing liquids through a vibrating mesh or plate with multiple apertures. The energy of vibration comes from a vibrating piezoelectric crystal attached to a horn transducer which transmits vibrations to a perforated plate with up to 6000 tapered holes (Fig. 36.12) or from an aerosol generator comprising a domed aperture plate,

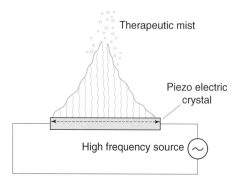

Fig. 36.11 Schematic diagram of an ultrasonic nebulizer (reproduced with permission from Atkins et al 1992).

with up to 10 000 tapered holes and a vibrational element which contracts and expands to generate the aerosol. These devices generate aerosols with a high fine particle fraction, deliver fluids very rapidly and have very small residual volumes (see below) compared to jet and ultrasonic nebulizers.

Formulating nebulizer fluids

Nebulizer fluids are formulated in water, occasionally with the addition of cosolvents such as ethanol or propylene glycol, and with the addition of surfactants for suspension formulations. Because hypoosmotic and hyperosmotic solutions may cause bronchoconstriction,

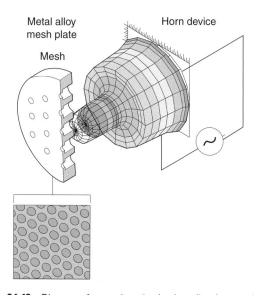

Fig. 36.12 Diagram of aerosol production in a vibrating-mesh nebulizer (courtesy of Omron Health Care).

as may high hydrogen ion concentrations, isoosmotic solutions of pH greater than 5 are usually employed. Stabilizers such as antioxidants and preservatives may also be included, although these may also cause bronchospasm and for this reason sulfites in particular are generally avoided as antioxidants in such formulations. Although chemically preserved multidose preparations are commercially available, nebulizer formulations are generally presented as sterile, isotonic unit doses (usually 1–2.5 mL) without a preservative.

Whilst most nebulizer formulations are solutions, suspensions of micronized drug are also available for delivery from nebulizers. In general, suspensions are poorly delivered from ultrasonic nebulizers, whereas with jet nebulizers the efficiency of drug delivery increases as the size of suspended drug is decreased, with little or no release of particles when they exceed the droplet size of the nebulized aerosol.

As the formulation of fluids for delivery by nebulizers is relatively simple, these devices are frequently the first to be employed when investigating the delivery of new entities to the human lung. Recently, they have been used for the delivery of peptides and liposomes. In general, ultrasonic nebulizers have not been successful for delivering either peptides or liposomes, because of denaturation resulting from the elevated temperatures produced. Consequently, ultrasonic nebulizers are expressly excluded for the delivery of recombinant human deoxyribonuclease in the management of cystic fibrosis. Jet nebulizers have been successfully used to deliver some peptide and liposome formulations, although the shearing forces that occur in the nebulizer may produce time-dependent damage to some materials.

Physicochemical properties of nebulizer fluids

The viscosity and surface tension of a liquid being nebulized may affect the output of nebulizers, as energy is required to overcome viscous forces and to create a new surface. However, the size selectivity of the nebulizer design and dimensions, with more than 99% of the primary aerosol mass being recycled into the reservoir liquid, means that changes in the size distribution of the primary aerosol resulting from changes in the properties of the solution being atomized may not always be reflected in the size distribution of the emitted aerosol. In general, the size of aerosol droplets is inversely proportional to viscosity for jet nebulizers and directly proportional to viscosity for ultrasonic nebulizers, with more viscous solutions requiring longer to nebulize to dryness and leaving larger residual volumes in the nebulizer following atomization. Surface tension effects are more complex but usually a decrease in surface tension is associated with a reduction in mean aerosol size.

Temperature effects during nebulization

The aerosol output from a jet nebulizer comprises drug solution and solvent vapour, which saturates the outgoing air. This causes solute concentration to increase with time and results in a rapid decrease in the temperature of the liquid being nebulized by approximately 10–15°C. This temperature decrease may be important clinically, as some asthma sufferers experience bronchoconstriction on inhalation of cold solutions. Further, the cooling effect within the reservoir fluid will reduce drug solubility and result in increased liquid surface tension and viscosity. Precipitation is uncommon with bronchodilators, which have high aqueous solubility, but problems may arise with less soluble drugs. In such instances the use of an ultrasonic nebulizer may be appropriate, as the operation of such devices may increase solution temperature by up to 10–15°C. As indicated, this temperature increase may have detrimental effects on heat-sensitive materials intended for nebulization. Vibrating-mesh nebulizers are reported to have a negligible effect on fluid temperature.

Duration of nebulization and residual volume

Clinically, liquids may be nebulized for a specified period of time or, more commonly, they may be nebulized to 'dryness', which may be interpreted as *sputtering time*, which is the time when air is drawn up the feed tube and nebulization becomes erratic, although agitation of the nebulizer permits treatment to be continued; *clinical time*, which is the time at which therapy is ceased following sputtering; or *total time*, which is the time at which the production of aerosol ceases.

Regardless of the duration of nebulization, not all the fluid in the nebulizer can be atomized. Some liquid, usually about 1 mL for jet and ultrasonic nebulizers, remains as the 'dead' or 'residual' volume, associated with the baffles, internal structures and walls of the nebulizer. Vibrating-mesh nebulizers have a much smaller residual volume. The proportion of drug retained as residual volume is more marked for smaller fill volumes; hence for a 2 mL fill volume, approximately 50% of fluid will remain associated with the nebulizer and be unavailable for delivery to the patient. This reduces to approximately 25% with a 4 mL fill volume, although there is a commensurate increase in the time necessary to nebulize to dryness. For this reason small-volume nebulizer fluids may be diluted to a larger volume by addition of a suitable diluent, usually sterile 0.9% sodium chloride solution.

Variability between nebulizers

Many different models of nebulizer and compressor are commercially available, and the size of aerosols produced and the dose delivered can vary enormously. For instance, in a study of 18 different commercially available jet nebulizers, operated according to the manufacturers' guidelines, aerosols were produced with MMADs ranging from 0.9 to 7.2 μm (Waldrep et al 1994). Variability may not only exist between different nebulizers but also between individual nebulizers of the same type, and repeated use of a single nebulizer may cause variability due to baffle wear and non-uniformity of assembly. Nebulizers, unlike the DPI and pMDI devices, are not manufactured by the producers of nebulizer solutions and suspension. The choice of nebulizer employed for their delivery is thus usually beyond the influence of the pharmaceutical manufacturer.

Novel delivery devices

A number of new inhalation devices are currently being developed, which do not fit neatly into the traditional categories of pMDI, DPI and nebulizers, since they operate on alternative principles. Two metered-dose liquid inhalers are the Respimat® (Boehringer Ingelheim, Fig. 36.13) and the AERx Pulmonary Delivery System® (Aradigm, Fig. 36.14). The Respimat Soft Mist® Inhaler is a handheld device with a multidose reservoir releasing a cloud of duration 1.5 seconds. This is much slower than for

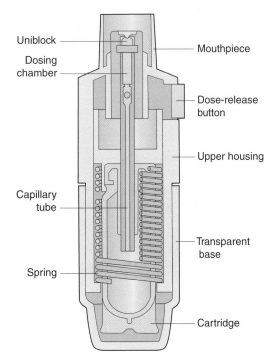

Fig. 36.13 The Respimat Soft Mist® Inhaler (©Boehringer Ingelheim International GmbH 2003–2004).

Airways and
mouthpiece assembly

Flow rate valve

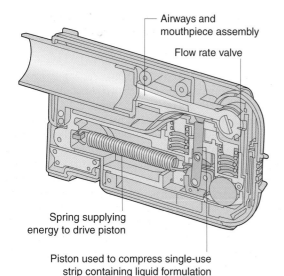

Spring supplying
energy to drive piston

Piston used to compress single-use
strip containing liquid formulation
which generates aerosol droplets

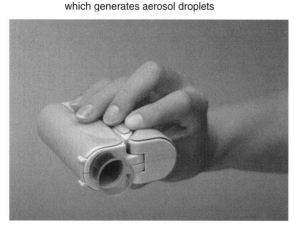

Fig. 36.14 The AERx® Pulmonary Delivery System (courtesy of Aradigm).

conventional pMDIs, allowing more time for coordination between actuation and inhalation. The device is mechanically actuated without employing a propellant. The aerosol generated by the device has lower velocity and smaller particle size than that generated with a conventional pMDI, resulting in superior peripheral lung deposition. The AERx Pulmonary Delivery System® has drug contained in unit-dose blister packs. Drug delivery is computer controlled and involves extrusion of liquid through a single-use nozzle containing numerous spherical holes, with exits approximately 1 μm in diameter. This produces very fine aerosols, suitable for delivery of peptides and proteins, such as insulin, to the peripheral airways. The device electronically monitors the patient's inspiratory flow rate with time, and releases drug at the inspiratory flow rate determined to be optimal for drug delivery.

METHODS OF AEROSOL SIZE ANALYSIS

The regional distribution of aerosols in the airways can be measured directly using γ-scintigraphy, by radiolabelling droplets or particles, usually with the short half-life γ-emitter technetium-99m (99mTc). However, more commonly, in vitro measurements of aerosol size are used to predict clinical performance. The principal methods that have been employed for size characterization of aerosols are microscopy, laser diffraction and cascade impaction.

Optical methods of measuring the physical size of deposited aerosols using microscopy are laborious and do not give an indication of their likely deposition within the humid airways while being carried in an air stream. With methods of analysis based on laser diffraction, aerosolized droplets or particles are sized as they traverse a laser beam to give a volume median diameter. Again, the aerodynamic properties of an aerosol are not being measured. In addition, spraying droplets into a beam exposes them to ambient conditions of temperature and humidity, which may result in solvent evaporation.

Cascade impactors and impingers

Cascade impactors comprise a series of progressively finer jets and collection plates, allowing fractionation of aerosols according to their MMAD as the aerosol is drawn through the device at a known flow rate. Traditional cascade impactors are constructed from metal. The most commonly used (Andersen type) comprises eight stages, with metal collection plates followed by a terminal filter. Multistage liquid impingers, working on the same principle, are constructed from glass or glass and metal and have three, four or five stages, with wet sintered glass collection plates followed by a terminal filter. Large, dense particles will deposit higher in the impactor, whereas smaller, less dense particles will follow the air flow and only deposit when they have been given sufficient momentum as they are accelerated through the finer jets lower in the impactor (Fig. 36.15). The first stage of the impactor is usually preceded by a 90° bend of metal or glass to mimic the human throat. The cut-off diameters for each stage at a particular air-flow rate can be determined using monodisperse aerosols or calculated using calibration curves. When determining the size of an aerosol, cumulative percentage undersize plots of deposited aerosol on each stage are plotted against the cut-off diameter for that stage to allow calculation of the MMAD. Such devices are used for aerodynamic assessment of fine particles in pMDIs and DPIs (USP and EP).

The five-stage liquid impinger (multistage liquid impinger, MSLI) (Fig. 36.16), with an appropriate induction port and mouthpiece adapter, is used to determine

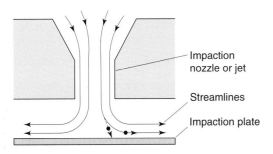

Fig. 36.15 Illustration of aerodynamic particle size separation by an impactor stage (reproduced with permission from Jaegfeldt et al 1987).

the aerodynamic size of DPIs (USP and EP) and pMDIs (EP). The MSLI may be operated at a flow rate between 30 and 100 L/min. At 60 L/min (i.e. 1 L/s), the effective cut-off diameters of stages 1, 2, 3 and 4 are 13.0, 6.8, 3.1 and 1.7 μm, respectively. The fifth stage comprises an integral filter which captures particles smaller than 1.7 μm. When testing DPIs to USP requirements, an air-flow rate (Q) calculated to produce a pressure drop of 4.0 kPa over the inhaler is employed. If this exceeds 100 L/min,

then 100 L/min is used. The cut-off diameters of each stage at flow rate (Q) can be calculated from:

$$D_{50'Q} = D_{50'Qn}(Q_n/Q)^{1/2} \qquad (36.7)$$

where $D_{50'Q}$ is the cut-off diameter at the flow rate Q and $D_{50'Qn}$ refers to the nominal cut-off values determined when Q_n is 60 L/min (values given above).

The use of cascade impaction methods to determine the size of aerosols has a number of disadvantages. The high flow rates employed (typically 28.3–60 L/min) result in rapid solvent evaporation and droplets may be re-entrained in the air stream whereas particles may 'bounce off' metal collection plates, although this latter effect may be reduced by coating the collection surface, for instance, with a silicone fluid or glycerol. These effects can result in a significant decrease in the measured aerosol size. Also, these measuring devices are operated at a constant air-flow rate. However, the dispersion of dry powder formulations and the deposition profile of inhaled aerosols will vary considerably with flow rate. To overcome the limitations of measurement at a single flow rate, an electronic lung has been developed, which uses a computer-controlled piston to draw air through the inhaler and into an impaction sizer, following a predetermined inhalation profile (Brindley et al 1994).

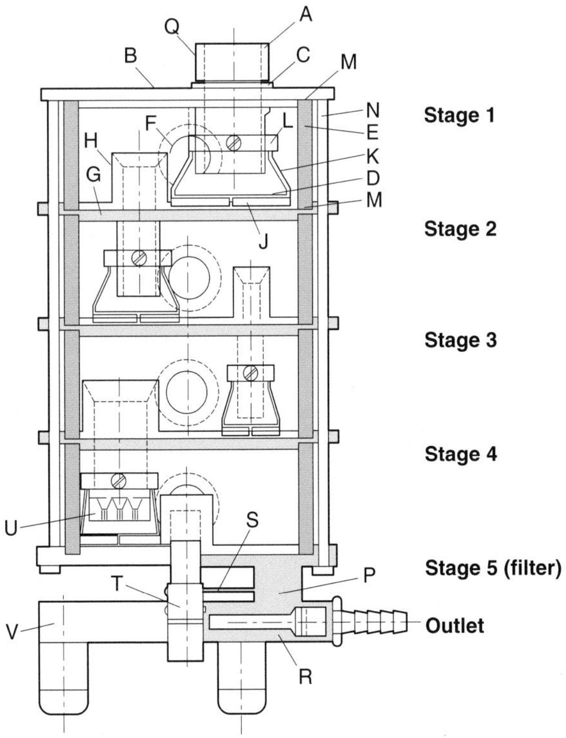

Fig. 36.16 The multistage liquid impinger (courtesy of AstraZeneca).

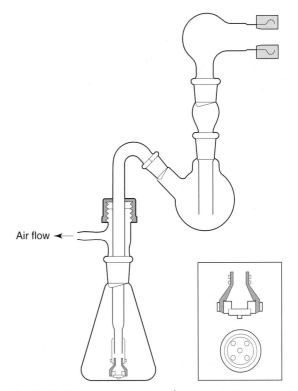

Fig. 36.17 The two-stage impinger (reproduced with permission from Hallworth & Westmoreland 1987).

Cascade impactor methods are invasive, laborious and time-consuming but necessary to derive information about median aerosol size and the polydispersity of the aerosol. To ensure that inhalation products are likely to be clinically effective, quality control measurements usually involve measurement of the emitted dose and the 'fine particle fraction' (that fraction of the emitted dose less than a stated size, usually 5 μm or sometimes 6.4 μm), which are combined to give a 'therapeutically useful' or 'respirable' dose or mass. For routine analysis, a simplified two-stage (twin) impinger is frequently employed (Fig. 36.17). Aerosol collected in the throat and the upper stage (stage 1) is considered 'non-respirable', whereas that collected in the lower stage (stage 2) is considered 'respirable'. For this glass device, the cut-off diameter for stage 2 is 6.4 μm, i.e. aerosols collected in this stage have an aerodynamic diameter less than 6.4 μm and for this measurement technique constitute the fine particle fraction. This two-stage impinger may be used for fine particle assessment of aerosols generated from pMDIs, DPIs and nebulizers (EP).

REFERENCES

Atkins, P.J, Barker, N.P., Mathisen, D. (1992) The design and development of inhalation drug delivery systems. In: Hickey, A.S.J. (ed.) *Pharmaceutical Inhalation Aerosol Technology*. Marcel Dekker, New York.

Bell, J.H., Hartley, P.S., Cox, J.S.G. (1971) Dry powder aerosols I: a new powder inhalation device. *Journal of Pharmaceutical Sciences*, **60**, 1559-1564.

Brindley, A., Sumby, B.S., Smith, I.J. (1994) The characterisation of inhalation devices by an inhalation simulator: the electronic lung. *Journal of Aerosol Medicine*, **7**, 197-200.

Hallworth, G.W., Westmoreland, D.G. (1987) The twin impinger: a simple device for assessing the delivery of drugs from metered dose pressurised aerosol inhalers. *Journal of Pharmacy and Pharmacology*, **39**, 966-972.

Jaegfeldt, H., Andersson, J.A.R., Trofast, E., Wetterlin, K.I.L. (1987) Particle size distribution from different modifications of Turbohaler. In: Newman, S.P., Morén, F., Crompton, G.K. (eds) *A New Concept In Inhalation Therapy*. Medicom Europe, Bussum.

Morén, F. (1981) Pressurised aerosols for oral inhalation. *International Journal of Pharmaceutics*, **8**, 1-10.

Nelson, H., Kemp, J.P., Bieler, S., Vaughan, L.M., Hill, M.R. (1999) Comparative efficacy and safety of albutarol sulfate Spiros inhaler and albuterol metered-dose inhaler. *Chest*, **115**, 329-335.

Newman, S.P. (1989) *Nebuliser Therapy: Scientific and Technical Aspects*. AB Draco, Lund.

Prime, D., Slater, A.L., Haywood, P.A., Smith, I.J. (1996) Assessing dose delivery from the Flixotide Diskus Inhaler – a multidose powder inhaler. *Pharmaceutical Technology Europe*, **8**(3), 23-34.

Sumby, B.S., Churcher, K.M., Smith, I.J. et al. (1993) Dose reliability of the Serevent Diskhaler system. *Pharmaceutical Technology International*, **6**(5), 20-27.

Waldrep, J.C., Keyhani, K., Black, M., Knight, V. (1994) Operating characteristics of 18 different continuous flow jet nebulizers with beclomethasone dipropionate liposome aerosol. *Chest*, **105**, 106-110.

Wetterlin, K.I.L. (1987) Design and function of Turbohaler. In: Newman, S.P., Morén, F., Crompton, G.K. (eds) *A New Concept In Inhalation Therapy*. Medicom Europe, Bussum.

Wilson, C.G., Washington, N. (1989) *Physiological Pharmaceutics: Biological Barriers to Drug Absorption*. Ellis Horwood, Chichester.

BIBLIOGRAPHY

Campen, L.V., Venthoye, G. (2002) Inhalation, dry powder. In: Swarbrick, J., Boylan, J.C. (eds) *Encyclopedia of Pharmaceutical Technology*, 2nd edn. Marcel Dekker, New York.

Hickey, A.S.J. (ed.) (2003) *Pharmaceutical Inhalation Aerosol Technology*, 2nd edn. Marcel Dekker, New York.

Munro, S.J.M., Cripps, A.L. (2002) Metered dose inhalers. In: Swarbrick, J., Boylan, J.C. (eds) *Encyclopedia of Pharmaceutical Technology*, 2nd edn. Marcel Dekker, New York.

Placke, M.E., Ding, J., Zimlich, W.C. (2002) Inhalation, liquids. In: Swarbrick, J., Boylan, J.C. (eds) *Encyclopedia of Pharmaceutical Technology*, 2nd edn. Marcel Dekker, New York.

Taylor, G., Kellaway, I. (2001) Pulmonary drug delivery. In: Hillery, A.M., Lloyd, A.W., Swarbrick, J. (eds) *Drug Delivery and Targeting for Pharmaceutical Scientists*. Taylor and Francis, London.

Taylor, K.M.G., McCallion, O.N.M. (2002 Ultrasonic nebulizers. In: Swarbrick, J., Boylan, J.C. (eds) *Encyclopedia of Pharmaceutical Technology*, 2nd edn. Marcel Dekker, New York.

Nasal drug delivery

P. M. Taylor

CHAPTER CONTENTS

INTRODUCTION

The nasal cavity has been considered as a route of drug administration for many decades, often for topical therapies such as decongestants. Recently, however, there has been a great deal of research investigating the nose as a route for systemic therapies, especially for peptides and proteins. Tables 37.1 and 37.2 show examples of topical nasal preparations, systemic preparations on the market and systemic preparations under investigation. The European market for drug delivery systems, with a value of $17.3 billion in 2003, represents about a quarter of the global market and of that European market, transnasal delivery is the second largest sector (after oral products) with a value of $3.87 billion (Datamonitor 2004).

There are many potential benefits to nasal administration:

- it is convenient
- there is a useful area for absorbing drugs, and
- there is a good systemic blood supply.

As with many other routes of delivery, there are also factors working against efficient drug absorption.

The aim of this chapter is to review the relevant features of nasal anatomy and physiology, outline the various factors that influence drug absorption and, finally, discuss the various formulation strategies and delivery systems that can be used for nasal drug delivery.

ANATOMY AND PHYSIOLOGY OF THE NOSE

The outermost part of the nose is the nasal vestibule, which runs for about 15 mm from the nostrils to the nasal valve (Fig. 37.1). The nasal cavity is behind the nasal valve and is about 60 mm long and has a volume of 20 mL and passes into the nasopharynx. The nasal cavity is divided vertically for most of its length by the nasal

Table 37.1 Examples of topical nasal preparations (taken from the BNF 50 2005)

Drug	Drug class	Use	Delivery system
Levocabastine	Antihistamine	Allergic rhinitis	Aqueous spray (pump)
Beclometasone dipropionate	Corticosteroid	Allergic and vasomotor rhinitis	Metered spray (pressurized) of aqueous suspension
Sodium cromoglycate	Cromoglycate	Allergic rhinitis	Aqueous spray (pump)
Ephedrine HCl	Sympathomimetic	Decongestant	Drops
Chlorhexidine HCl	Antimicrobial	*Staph.* infections (nostrils)	Cream

Table 37.2 Examples of marketed systemic nasal preparations (taken from the BNF 50 2005 and Behl et al 1998a)

Drug	Drug class	Use	Delivery system
Desmopressin	Pituitary hormone	Diabetes insipidus	Metered spray
Buserelin	Gonadorelin analogue	Prostate cancer, endometriosis	Metered spray (pump) and others
Nafarelin	Gonadorelin analogue	Prostate cancer, endometriosis	Metered spray and others
Sumatriptin	Serotonin agonist	Migraine	Unit-dose spray
Dihydroergotamine mesylate	Ergot alkaloid	Migraine	4-application spray
Nicotine	–	Cessation of smoking	Metered spray
Salmon calcitonin	Calcium regulator	Postmenopausal osteoporosis	Metered spray

septum, and the outer wall of each cavity contains three folds or indentations known as the nasal turbinates (or conchae). This folding means that the nasal cavity has a relatively large surface area for its volume – approximately 160 cm^2 (Chien 1992, Lee & Baldwin 1992, Mygind & Dahl 1998).

The normal functioning of the nose is closely related to its anatomy. The nose is a sensory organ that also conditions inspired air by warming and humidifying it before it reaches the lungs. Inspired air passes through the constriction of the nasal valve with a high linear velocity but the sharp change in direction of the flow into the nasal cavity and the presence of the turbinates (see Fig. 37.1) cause turbulent flow, bringing the air into close contact with the nasal lining. The large surface area of the nasal cavity and the rich underlying vasculature cause rapid heat and moisture transfer to the air. These are also factors that make the nasal cavity a good site for drug absorption.

Nasal mucosa and mucociliary clearance

The anterior part of the nose, from the nasal vestibule to the turbinates, is lined with squamous epithelium. The upper part of the cavity, accounting for about 5% of the total area, is lined with olfactory membrane. The latter contains the sensory olfactory cells as well as serous and mucosal cells; it is so placed because a large proportion of inspired air passes over this region. Most of the nasal

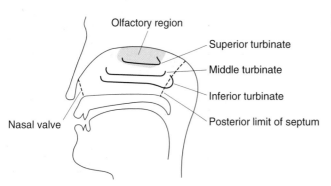

Fig. 37.1 Cross-section of human nasal cavity, showing major structures relevant to nasal drug administration.

cavity, however, is lined with mucous membrane containing a mixture of columnar cells, goblet cells and basal cells. The columnar cells in the forward third of the epithelium are non-ciliated; the remainder are covered with cilia. Cilia are hair-like projections on the exposed surface of epithelial cells. Each cell has about 300 cilia, measuring between 5 and 10 mm in length and 0.1–0.3 mm in diameter. The cilia beat in regular waves with a frequency of 10 Hz. Their role is to facilitate the movement of mucus from the nasal cavity to the nasopharynx and ultimately to the GI tract. The combined effect is known as mucociliary clearance (Marttin et al 1998, Schipper et al 1991).

Mucociliary clearance is a non-specific defensive function which also presents a barrier to drug absorption. The mucous layer is normally 5–20 μm thick and consists mostly of water, containing glycoproteins, ions and various other proteins such as enzymes and immunoglobulins. Glycoproteins give the mucus its viscous character, which causes foreign particles to become trapped, cleared to the GI tract and ultimately eliminated from the body. The mucus is actually divided into two layers, that closest to the cell surface being a less viscous, watery substance. This aids clearance by lubricating the passage of the mucus over the cell surfaces and easing the action of cilia. The cilia work in a ratchet-like way by engaging the viscous outer gel layer of the mucus, moving it towards the nasopharynx and then disengaging and returning to their starting position through the serous inner layer. The turnover time for mucus is variously quoted as approximately 10–15 minutes in total (Lee & Baldwin 1992) and 20 minutes for the half-life of mucociliary clearance (Schipper et al 1991).

Mucus presents a diffusional barrier to drug absorption. Any formulation must be able to overcome this, as well as remain in the region long enough to allow drug release and absorption. Various strategies for achieving these goals are given later in this chapter but it is important that any interruption to mucociliary clearance, whether from drug or excipient, should be minimal and temporary.

Nasal metabolism

The nasal route of administration avoids hepatic first-pass metabolism (see Chapter 20) but nasal mucosa does possess enzymatic activity as a protective mechanism against exogenous chemicals. Although not widely investigated yet, there is sufficient evidence to suggest that nasal first-pass metabolism may be a significant factor in the absorption of some drugs (Sarkar 1992). For example, there is a high content of cytochrome P450 enzymes; P450 monooxygenases can oxidize many nasally administered drugs, such as nasal decongestants and anaesthetics. Progesterone and testosterone have been found to be metabolized extensively in vitro,

although in vivo they have nasal bioavailabilities approaching 100% (relative to i.v. administration). Uneven distribution of enzymes is thought to be the reason for this apparent anomaly, greater activity being found in the olfactory mucosa used in the in vitro studies, whereas in vivo the steroids were probably absorbed rapidly by the less active respiratory mucosa.

There are many other types of enzyme in the nasal mucosa which can act on conventional drugs. Examples include dehydrogenases, hydroxylases, carboxylesterases, carbonic anhydrase and various phase II conjugative enzymes. Although these enzymes have usually been investigated for toxicological reasons, they may interfere with the efficient absorption of drugs. This is especially true for peptide- and protein-based drugs, as various enzymes, such as aminopeptidases, can significantly decrease the drug's bioavailability. It is now recognized that proteins and peptides are faced with substantial enzymatic, as well as physical, barriers to absorption across mucosal surfaces (Lee & Baldwin 1992).

The development of new nasal dosage forms should therefore include some consideration of the nature, extent and location of the drug's metabolism in the nose. Not all metabolism is undesirable, however, and certain enzymes, such as esterases, open the possibility of using prodrugs as a means of improving nasal drug delivery.

PHYSICOCHEMICAL FACTORS INFLUENCING DRUG ABSORPTION IN THE NASAL CAVITY

Investigation of how the physicochemical properties of various drugs influence their nasal absorption has provided some insight into the various mechanisms and routes of drug absorption. The most important properties are probably the size of the drug molecule, its charge or polarity, and its degree of hydrophilicity (or lipophilicity).

Molecular size and weight

McMartin et al (1987) compiled literature data for over 20 compounds ranging in molecular weight from 160 to 34 000 Da. Wherever possible, comparisons were made between absorption of the same compound after delivery by the nasal route in humans and rats and oral administration in humans. All three models showed similar effects: the absorption of small compounds (approx. 100 Da) was high, at around 80%, but this decreased markedly as molecular weight increased. Nasal absorption of a drug with a given molecular weight was slightly higher in rats than in humans but the greatest difference was seen between oral absorption and nasal absorption in humans. Drug absorption after nasal administration was very much higher than after oral delivery of a particular compound. Also, the molecular weight cut-off, beyond which absorption was negligible, was about two orders of magnitude better for nasal administration (about 20 000 Da compared to around 200 Da for peroral delivery).

Even though they relate to a small group of compounds, these data show the utility of the nasal route, and they led to the proposal that the drugs (which tended to be hydrophilic) were absorbed by non-specific diffusion through aqueous channels between the cells (the paracellular route), although other routes were a possibility. The molecular weight cut-off occurs because only molecules that are smaller than the channels can diffuse through them. The hypothesis that transport can occur through aqueous channels has received support in other studies using homologous series of hydrophilic compounds, such as polyethylene glycols (Donovan et al 1990) and labelled dextrans with molecular weights between 1260 and 45 500 Da (Fisher et al 1992).

Effect of pH and partition coefficient

Although molecular size is undoubtedly an important factor in influencing nasal absorption, the evidence in the preceding section tends to be based upon water-soluble compounds. More lipophilic compounds are likely to travel through one of the alternative routes, probably by partitioning across the mucosal cell membranes and diffusing through the cells (the transcellular route) at a slower rate than through the paracellular route. Most drugs can be ionized, and their partition coefficients are dependent upon environmental pH (unionized compounds will have a higher oil/water partition coefficient than ionized ones).

The pH at the surface of the mucosal cells has been reported to be 7.39 (Hirai et al 1981a) and the mucus layer itself is slightly acidic, at pH 5.5–6.5 (Chien 1992). It should be remembered that the local pH can be modified by a nasal formulation. Hirai et al (1981a) studied absorption in a perfused rat model of two model drug compounds at various pHs: a base (aminopyrine) and an acid (salicylic acid). The rate of absorption for both drugs increased as they became less ionized. Aminopyrine is absorbed more quickly at higher pHs, and the curve of absorption rate versus pH closely followed the degree of ionization versus pH curve. This suggests that the more lipophilic, unionized form of the drug is absorbed by passive diffusion through the mucosal cells. The salicylic acid was also absorbed more quickly in its unionized form (at low pH). The rate of absorption did not correspond with the degree of ionization; instead, it was higher than predicted. In this case it was suggested that there was another mechanism working alongside the slower diffusion through the cells, possibly the salicylic acid enhancing its own absorption. It is worth noting that despite both

of the model compounds being relatively small, there was no suggestion in this study of a fast absorption through intercellular channels.

Other mechanisms of drug absorption are also present in the nose. The absorption of benzoic acid decreases as pH increases but there was still appreciable absorption at pHs where the acid is completely ionised (Huang et al 1985), suggesting the existence of two methods of absorption. It is possible that low pHs can have a direct action on the nasal mucosa: the absorption of secretin was greater at low pHs, and histological examination of the epithelial cells found changes in their structure at pH 3 (Ohwaki et al 1987).

The effect of pH on peptide drugs is more complex than on conventional drugs, as peptides have a large number of ionizable groups of either charge. Peptides are characterized by their isoelectric point, the pH at which they have no net charge and where their solubility is often lowest. The nasal absorption of insulin (isoelectric point at pH 5.4), as measured by the reduction in blood sugar in dogs, was greatest at a solution pH of 3.1 (where there is a net positive charge on insulin) and lowest at pH 6.1 (near its isoelectric point). The absorption mechanisms of peptides are, however, complex, owing to their size and structure, and it is unlikely that the effect of pH on insulin absorption is due to a more favourable partitioning of the protein. Indeed, there could well have been direct effects on the epithelial cells at pH 3.1.

The role of the partition coefficient so far has largely been inferred from the relative proportions of the ionized to the unionized forms of the drug, but this relationship is not pronounced. The absorption of a series of barbiturates was studied at pH 6.0, when they would be largely unionized, and only a fourfold variation in absorption was found despite a nearly 50-fold range in the chloroform/water partition coefficient (Huang et al 1985). An investigation into the dependence of the absorption of a series of progesterone derivatives on their octanol/water partition coefficients gave a similar finding: absorption increased with partition coefficient, but to a markedly lower extent (Corbo et al 1989). The latter workers determined partition coefficients in a nasal mucosa-buffer system and found a much better correlation with absorption than the conventional oil/water models give. It is clear from these findings that an appropriate measure of partitioning must be used in order to determine the role of partitioning in nasal absorption but in general, it appears that partitioning is rarely the only factor controlling absorption.

Other physicochemical factors affecting nasal absorption

The solubility of the drug and its dissolution rate are important, especially if it is presented as a solid dosage form (e.g. a powder), as it must be able to cross the mucous layer before it can be absorbed by the epithelial cells. In addition, powder morphology and particle size influence the deposition of the drug inside the nasal cavity. All these factors must be considered in the design of formulations and will be addressed later in this chapter.

Physicochemical properties and mechanisms of absorption – a summary

The above discussion has shown that the influence of various properties on the absorption of drugs can provide valuable indicators about the mechanisms of drug absorption. It is also clear that the nasal absorption of drugs is a complicated affair, and there is rarely a single way in which a drug can be absorbed. Chien (1992) has written about the various absorption mechanisms; the summary given below is a broad generalization.

Aqueous channels between the cells provide a relatively good route for water-soluble compounds, with absorption being limited mostly by molecular size. Other drugs are absorbed by passive diffusion, possibly using a transcellular route, and there is evidence for active transport of some amino acids. Whatever the mechanism, combined literature data suggest that molecules with a molecular weight up to about 1000 Da should have a relatively good systemic bioavailability without the need for absorption promoters. Absorption promoters could increase this molecular weight limit to about 6000 Da but beyond this weight it is unlikely that large molecules could be absorbed without causing unacceptable damage to the nasal cavity.

STRATEGIES FOR IMPROVING DRUG AVAILABILITY IN NASAL ADMINISTRATION

There are three main ways to maximize the systemic bioavailability of drugs administered nasally:

- improve nasal residence time
- enhance nasal absorption
- modify drug structure to change physicochemical properties.

Increasing nasal residence time

Mucociliary clearance acts to remove foreign bodies and substances from the nasal mucosa as quickly as possible. One way of delaying clearance is to apply the drug to the anterior part of the nasal cavity, an effect which is largely determined by the type of dosage form used. The preparation could also be formulated with polymers such as methylcellulose, hydroxypropyl methylcellulose or poly-

acrylic acid (Carbopol), which increase the viscosity of the formulation and act as bioadhesives with the mucus (Schipper et al 1991). Increasing the residence time does not necessarily lead to increased absorption. This can be illustrated by considering insulin solutions with similar viscosities containing carboxymethylcellulose or Carbopol. The carboxymethylcellulose solutions do not enhance the absorption of insulin (Duchene et al 1988), whereas Carbopol solutions do (Morimoto et al 1985). Increasing the viscosity of solutions will decrease the rate of diffusion of molecules through them (hence the apparent lack of effect of carboxymethylcellulose) but the polymer may have other enhancing actions, such as opening the intercellular junctions, as has been suggested for Carbopol (Junginger 1990).

An interesting formulation development for lengthening residence time is the use of microspheres (Pereswetoff-Morath 1998). The absorption of insulin is increased by degradable starch microspheres which, although insoluble, swell in water and form a viscous, bioadhesive mass (Illum et al 1987). Subsequent studies indicate a more direct action of the microspheres on epithelial cells, whereby the swelling of the microspheres causes a temporary dehydration and shrinkage of the cells followed by opening of the tight intercellular junctions (Edman et al 1992). This makes the paracellular route more attractive.

Enhancing nasal absorption

Absorption enhancers work by increasing the rate at which drugs pass through the nasal mucosa. Many act by altering the structure of the epithelial cells in some way, but they should accomplish this while causing no damage or permanent change. General requirements of an ideal absorption enhancer at its concentration in use are as follows:

- It should give an effective increase in the absorption of the drug.
- It should not cause permanent damage or alteration to the tissues.
- It should not otherwise be irritant or toxic, either to the local tissues or to the rest of the body.
- It should be effective in small quantities.
- The enhancing effect should occur when absorption is required (i.e. there should not be a lag in its effect).
- The effect should be temporary and reversible.
- The enhancer should fulfil all other expectations of formulation excipients (e.g. stability and compatibility).

The major reason for developing and testing enhancers is to increase the absorption of peptides and proteins, because their size leads to a relatively poor bioavailability.

There is a large body of work investigating enhancers for nasal delivery. Much of this is focused on peptide delivery and the interested reader is directed to reviews written by Behl et al (1998b), Chien (1992) and Hinchcliffe & Illum (1999) for more detail on the various classes of enhancer.

Surfactants and bile salts have received considerable attention. Hirai et al (1981b) investigated surfactants of many types, including non-ionic ethers and esters, and anionic surfactants, for their effect on insulin absorption and found them to be particularly effective enhancers. Unfortunately, the enhancement usually correlates with mucosal damage, as the surfactants associate with cellular components such as membrane lipids and proteins. In some cases the association is so severe as to cause extraction of lipids or proteins and loss of epithelial cells. Surfactants are therefore unsuitable for therapeutic use as enhancers, although Hinchcliffe & Illum (1999) suggest they are experimentally useful as reference compounds guaranteed to cause enhancement.

Bile salts have greater potential as they appear to possess much of the enhancing activity but less of the damage potential of surfactants (bile salts possess some surface activity and can form micelles). Commonly studied bile salts include sodium cholate, sodium deoxycholate, sodium glycocholate and glycodeoxycholate, sodium taurocholate and taurodeoxycholate, all of which can cause enhancement at concentrations of 10–20 mM (Behl et al 1998b).

Several mechanisms have been proposed for the enhancing action of bile salts:

- Increasing cell membrane permeability by forming temporary channels through the lipid structure.
- Forming intercellular aqueous pores by opening the tight junctions between cells.
- Increasing the lipophilicity of charged drugs by forming ion pairs.
- Inhibition of proteolytic enzymes.

The most likely of these mechanisms for increasing the absorption of peptides is the opening of intercellular channels, rather than increasing cell permeability. The latter would probably require massive disruption of the cell before substantial quantities of peptide could pass. Although bile salts are claimed to be safer than surfactants, they can still cause damage to epithelial cells. Again there is a positive correlation between their enhancing activity and the damage caused.

Merkus et al (1993) have documented the damage potential of a number of bile salts and surfactants, using an index of morphological damage and a measurement of toxicity on the cilia (specifically the ciliary beat frequency, CBF). Decreases in CBF correspond to cellular damage, and measurement of CBF has the advantage of providing a relatively easy quantitative measure of toxicity which can be used to show the change in toxicity with time, including any reversal. Ciliotoxicity can also furnish another explanation for increased absorption, because a lower CBF tends to increase nasal residence time.

Sodium tauro-24,25-dihydrofusidate (STDHF) is an enhancer with a structure similar to bile salts that has been widely studied as an enhancer for proteins. It has good aqueous stability and solubility (>10% w/v) and is surface active, forming micelles at a critical micelle concentration of 2.5 mM. One study has found an approximately 10-fold increase in the bioavailability of human insulin and increases in the bioavailability of labelled dextrans ranging from about fourfold (40 000 Da dextran) up to 72 times (4000 Da) (Lee & Baldwin 1992). The degree of penetration enhancement depends on the concentration of the STDHF, reaching a maximum at around 0.3%. As this is over the critical micelle concentration, any further increase in STDHF concentration will see a rise in the number of micelles, not individual enhancer monomers. It can be concluded that the monomer concentration is more important for producing the enhancing effect than the number of micelles. The same authors claim that STDHF produces only a temporary increase in absorption and causes relatively little cell damage, although Merkus et al (1993) show that STDHF is ciliotoxic at its optimum enhancing concentration. It should be noted, however, that the ciliotoxicity depends on the model used, with a much lower degree of toxicity in human tissue than in the animal model used (chicken trachea).

Another group of surface-active materials is the phosphatidylcholines, for example lysophosphatidylcholine. These are similar to compounds that occur naturally as part of cell membranes and, as might be expected, one mechanism of action of phosphatidylcholines is to disrupt the cell membrane and increase its permeability. They may also inhibit proteolytic enzymes, and lysophosphatidylcholine is mucolytic. They are effective enhancers of protein absorption and, despite their proposed mechanism of action, do not cause the expected damage to the nasal lining. Dodecanoyl-l-α-phosphatidylcholine (DPPC) is one derivative which has been developed with a high activity and low toxicity profile. It is undergoing development as an enhancer for insulin. Early studies showed that DPPC increases the absorption of insulin in humans with little or no irritation to the nose, although more recent work suggests that the amount of insulin absorbed by this route may not be therapeutically useful (Hinchcliffe & Illum 1999).

Cyclodextrins (CD) are hollow cylindrical molecules made up of glucose units in a cyclic arrangement: α-CD has six glucose units, β-CD has seven and γ-CD has eight. These compounds have found a wide range of pharmaceutical uses, from solubility enhancement to taste masking, because of their ability to form 'inclusion complexes'. Here, part or all of a drug molecule inserts in the hollow central cavity of the cyclodextrin molecule. The complexed drug molecule takes on some of the physico-chemical properties of the cylcodextrin molecule. Derivatives of the cyclodextrins can be used to modify these properties. Cyclodextrins have polar outer surfaces and less polar interiors, so they tend to be water soluble but have the ability to accommodate hydrophobic molecules as part of the inclusion complex. This results in an increased aqueous solubility for the included species.

Cyclodextrins increase the bioavailability of lipophilic compounds by increasing their aqueous solubility, and hence their availability, at the surface of the nasal epithelium (Merkus et al 1999). As an example, dimethyl-β-cyclodextrin (DMβCD) gives an absolute bioavailability for oestradiol of 95% in rats and 67% in rabbits, a three-to fivefold increase compared with a control preparation. This has been supported by clinical data in humans showing that nasally administered oestradiol is effective as an oestrogen-replacement therapy in ovariectomized postmenopausal women.

Data are available to show the enhancement of absorption of other lipophilic compounds and even hydrophilic drugs. Hydrophilic drugs which have an enhanced absorption include peptides (e.g. buserelin) and proteins (e.g. calcitonin). The bioavailability of insulin is not increased to a therapeutic level. Insulin is one of the major goals for therapeutic administration via the nose but this has yet to be achieved at sufficient levels even with the use of enhancers. The mechanism of enhancement of hydrophilic drug absorption by cyclodextrins has yet to be fully elucidated, but it is probably the result of a direct action on the nasal epithelium rather than a modification of the drug's physicochemical properties.

One of the main benefits of using cyclodextrins, according to Merkus et al (1999), is their lack of toxicity, expressed as direct damage to the nasal cells, ciliotoxicity or more systemic effects. Particularly useful are the methylated-β-cyclodextrins, which exhibit a combination of high activity and low toxicity.

The enhancers reported so far all act directly on the nasal epithelium, with a consequent risk of irritation and cellular damage. Alternative molecules, such as chitosan (a polysaccharide derived from the shells of crustacea), that have different mechanisms of delivery have been studied (Illum 1998).

It is unlikely that there will be a single universal absorption enhancer and currently many of the most effective enhancers also cause damage to the nose. However, the volume of research and development work that has been conducted on these enhancers will make the nasal delivery of many drugs feasible.

Modifying drug structure

Structural modifications to the drug molecule are usually made in order to bestow more favourable physicochemical properties to the drug, for example increasing its aqueous solubility or improving its partitioning characteristics. Cyclodextrins can perform some of these functions, although they do not actually change the drug's structure. Some structural changes will be permanent, either by altering substituent groups on the molecule or by using different salt forms. However, they run the risk of changing the drug's therapeutic and toxicological profile and thus require regulatory approval, with its associated costs and lengthy studies.

An alternative is to use prodrugs, whereby the prodrug has favourable properties for absorption but is changed to the active drug on passing through the nasal epithelium. An example is the use of an ester (thereby increasing the drug's lipophilicity) that can be metabolized to the active drug by the esterases present in the nasal mucosa. Peptide and protein drugs especially may benefit from the formation of prodrugs (Krishnamoorthy & Mitra 1998).

NASAL DRUG DELIVERY SYSTEMS AND THEIR FORMULATION

General formulation issues

Nasal dosage forms must fulfil the functions of any other type of formulation. They must:

- be effective
- have an acceptable safety and stability, both chemical and microbiological
- be acceptable to the patient to ensure compliance.

If the formulation is a liquid it may commonly contain:

- antimicrobial preservatives (e.g. benzalkonium chloride)
- antioxidants (e.g. butylated hydroxytoluene)
- solubilizing agents or cosolvents (e.g. glycol derivatives)
- salts for adjusting pH and tonicity
- humectants, to minimize irritation to the nose (e.g. glycerol)
- viscosity-increasing agents (e.g. methylcellulose), and
- absorption enhancers.

Types of nasal dosage form and delivery system

The final dosage form used for nasal drug delivery is chosen after consideration of a wide range of issues, covering patient convenience, efficiency of drug delivery and formulation issues (Bommer 2000). The specifics of the dosage form or delivery system play a major role in the absorption of the drug by influencing its deposition. For example, as mentioned above, drugs deposited in the anterior part of the nasal cavity will be better absorbed than those applied further back.

Deposition mechanisms

There are three main ways of depositing inhaled particles on the nasal lining: impaction, sedimentation and diffusion (Kublik & Vidgren 1998).

Impaction Impaction occurs when there is a change in direction of the airflow – as happens when inspired air passes through the nasal valve – and the inertia of large or fast-moving particles carries them in their original direction. This is usually the main way of depositing particles in the turbulence caused by fast flow rates or with particles larger than 0.5–1 mm. Varying the flow rate from the device or the aerodynamic particle size are the means by which the formulator can influence this type of deposition.

Sedimentation Sedimentation happens when the air is moving slowly and the particles settle slowly under the force of gravity. This mode of deposition is described by Stokes' equation. The only control the formulator can have over this practically is by ensuring a slow flow rate and by modifying the drug particle size or formulation droplet size.

Diffusion The final method of deposition, diffusion, occurs by Brownian motion and is thus limited to very small particles ($< 0.5 \mu m$). Normally diffusion is not important, as the inspired particles are too large.

Nasal dosage forms

Nasal dosage forms will usually contain the drug in a liquid or powder formulation delivered by a pressurized or pump system. Several studies have looked at the influence of dosage form and delivery system on the deposition and absorption of drugs, and useful summaries are given by Kublik & Vidgren (1998) and Su (1991).

Liquid formulation Liquid formulations are usually aqueous solutions of the drug and thus have the general benefits and drawbacks of pharmaceutical solutions. They are relatively simple to develop and manufacture compared to solid dosage forms but often have a lower microbiological and chemical stability, requiring the use of various preservatives.

The liquid form can be soothing to the nasal lining but this may be countered by the excipients, such as the antimicrobial preservatives, which can cause irritation or ciliotoxicity. The simplest way to give a liquid is by nose drops but their cheapness and convenience are usually outweighed by the inaccuracy of dosing volume and the likelihood of too-rapid clearance by the liquid running straight into the oesophagus. Dosing accuracy can be improved by using unit-dose packs containing a predetermined volume but accurate placing of the drops still requires some skill and dexterity on the part of the user.

Squeezed bottles Squeezed bottles are often used for nasal decongestants and work by spraying a partially atomized jet of liquid into the nasal cavity. They give a better absorption of drug by directing the formulation into the anterior part of the cavity and covering a large part of the nasal mucosa. Deposition and volume are still subject to the technique of the user – whether the patient squeezes the bottle smoothly or in a series of vigorous squirts, for example. This type of delivery system, where the formulation is expelled through a plain orifice without any type of valve system, is subject to contamination by 'suck-back', as external material can be drawn back into the container as the pressure on it is released.

Metered-dose pump systems Metered-dose pump systems offer greater control over dosing than any of the previous systems. They can deliver solutions, suspensions or emulsions, with a predetermined volume between 25 and 200 μL, thus offering deposition over a large area. The formulation scientist is able to incorporate a high degree of control over the size and localization of the dose by changing various factors, such as the rheological and surface tension characteristics of the formulation and the design and geometry of the pump.

The interactions between these factors are complex but one example will show the type of control that is available. The angle at which the spray leaves the nozzle (the cone angle) will affect where the formulation is deposited. A small cone angle (about 35°) tends to be deposited towards the back of the nasal cavity and larger angles (tending towards 90°) will deposit further forward.

Metered-dose systems are also available as pressurized products. These permit the delivery of solid particulate preparations and present special formulation challenges because of the requirement to form a stable dispersion of the drug in the propellant system. Pressurized metered-dose systems give a good distribution of the formulation in the nasal cavity but there is evidence that it is not as even as the distribution from metered-dose pumps.

Particle size and dose volume are two important factors for controlling delivery from metered-dose systems. The optimum particle size for deposition in the nasal cavity is 10 μm (mass median diameter; Su 1991). In addition, particulate formulations tend to have a longer residence time in the nasal cavity than liquids, because they are removed more slowly by mucociliary clearance.

The volume of formulation that can be delivered is obviously limited by the size of the nasal cavity, and larger volumes tend to be cleared faster despite covering a larger area. Better absorption is often achieved by administering two doses, one in each nostril, rather than a single large dose (e.g. two 80 μL doses rather than one 140 μL; Kublik & Vidgren 1998).

SUMMARY

The nasal route is one of many which is receiving a large amount of attention as a way of delivering drugs into the systemic circulation. Much of the attention is focused on peptide and protein drugs, several of which have reached the market, and there is even the prospect of being able to use the nasal route to deliver vaccines (Illum 2003). The delivery systems for these drugs and vaccines are often complex formulations, as they are likely to incorporate absorption enhancers or technology to increase the time that the drug is in contact with the nasal lining.

The nasal route of administration is already a valuable way of delivering drugs to the body, and recent advances uphold the promise of the nasal route as a convenient way to administer a wider range of complex drugs.

REFERENCES

Behl, C.R., Pimplaskar, H.K., Sileno, A.P., de Meireles, J., Romeo, V.D. (1998a) Effects of physicochemical properties and other factors on systemic nasal drug delivery. *Advanced Drug Delivery Reviews*, **29**, 89-116.

Behl, C.R., Pimplaskar, H.K., Sileno, A.P. et al. (1998b) Optimization of systemic nasal drug delivery with pharmaceutical excipients. *Advanced Drug Delivery Reviews*, **29**, 117-133.

Bommer, R. (2000) Nasal drug delivery devices and packaging. *Pharmaceutical Technology*, **24**, 46-53.

British National Formulary 50 (2005) British Medical Association and Royal Pharmaceutical Society of Great Britain, London.

Chien, Y. (1992) Nasal drug delivery. In: Chien, Y. (ed.) *Novel Drug Delivery Systems*, 2nd edn. Marcel Dekker, New York.

Corbo, D.C., Huang, Y.C., Chien, Y.W. (1989) Nasal delivery of progestational steroids in ovariectomised rabbits 2. Effect of penetrant hydrophilicity. *International Journal of Pharmaceutics*, **50**, 253-260.

Datamonitor (2004) *Drug Delivery in Europe: Industry Profile*. Datamonitor Europe, London.

Donovan, M., Flynn, G., Amidon, G. (1990) Absorption of polyethylene glycols 600 through 2000: the molecular weight dependence of gastrointestinal and nasal absorption. *Pharmaceutical Research*, **7**, 863-868.

Duchene, D., Touchard, F., Peppas, N.A. (1988) Pharmaceutical and medical aspects of bioadhesive systems for drug administration. *Drug Development and Industrial Pharmacy*, **14**, 233-318.

Edman, P., Björk, E., Rydén, L. (1992) Microspheres as a nasal delivery system for peptide drugs. *Journal of Controlled Release*, **21**, 165-172.

Fisher, A., Illum, L., Davis, S., Schacht, E. (1992) Di-iodo-L-tyrosine labelled dextrans as molecular size markers of nasal absorption in the rat. *Journal of Pharmacy and Pharmacology*, **44**, 550-554.

Hinchcliffe, M., Illum, L. (1999) Intranasal insulin delivery and therapy. *Advanced Drug Delivery Reviews*, **35**, 199-234.

Hirai, S., Yahika, T., Matsuzawa, T., Mima, H. (1981a) Absorption of drugs from the nasal mucosa of rat. *International Journal of Pharmaceutics*, **7**, 317-325.

Hirai, S., Yashiki, T., Mima, H. (1981b) Mechanisms for the enhancement of the nasal absorption of insulin by surfactants. *International Journal of Pharmaceutics*, **9**, 173-184.

Huang, C., Kimura, R., Nassar, R., Hussain, A.A. (1985) Mechanism of nasal absorption of drugs I: Physicochemical parameters influencing the rate of in-situ nasal absorption of drugs in rats. *Journal of Pharmaceutical Sciences*, **74**, 608-611.

Illum, L. (1998) Chitosan and its use as a pharmaceutical excipient. *Pharmaceutical Research*, **15**, 1326-1331.

Illum, L. (2003) Nasal drug delivery – possibilities, problems and solutions. *Journal of Controlled Release*, **87**, 187-198.

Illum, L., Jorgensen, H., Bisgaard, H. (1987) Bioadhesive microspheres as a potential nasal drug delivery system. *International Journal of Pharmaceutics*, **39**, 189-199.

Junginger, H.E. (1990) Bioadhesive polymer systems for peptide delivery. *Acta Pharmaceutica Technologica*, **36**, 110-126.

Krishnamoorthy, R., Mitra, A.K. (1998) Prodrugs for nasal drug delivery. *Advanced Drug Delivery Reviews*, **29**, 135-146.

Kublik, H., Vidgren, M.T. (1998) Nasal delivery systems and their effect on deposition and absorption. *Advanced Drug Delivery Reviews*, **29**, 157-177.

Lee, W.A., Baldwin, P.A. (1992) Nasal membranes: structure and permeability. In: Junginger H.E. (ed.) *Drug Targeting and Delivery: Concepts in Dosage Form Design*. Ellis Horwood, New York.

Marttin, E., Schipper, N.G.M., Verhoef, J.C., Merkus, F.W.H.M. (1998) Nasal mucociliary clearance as a factor in nasal drug delivery. *Advanced Drug Delivery Reviews*, **29**, 13-38.

McMartin, C., Hutchinson, L.E.F., Hyde, R., Peters, G.E. (1987) Analysis of structural requirements for the absorption of drugs and macromolecules from the nasal cavity. *Journal of Pharmaceutical Sciences*, **76**, 535-540.

Merkus, F.H.W.M., Schipper, N.G.M., Hermans, W.A.J.J., Romeijn, S.G., Verhoef, J.C. (1993) Absorption enhancers in nasal drug delivery: efficacy and safety. *Journal of Controlled Release*, **24**, 201-208.

Merkus, F.H.W.M., Verhoef, J.C., Marttin, E. et al. (1999) Cyclodextrins in nasal drug delivery. *Advanced Drug Delivery Reviews*, **36**, 41-57.

Morimoto, K., Morisaka, K., Kamanda, A. (1985) Enhancement of nasal absorption of insulin and calcitonin using polyacrylic acid gel. *Journal of Pharmacy and Pharmacology*, **37**, 134-136.

Mygind, N., Dahl, R. (1998) Anatomy, physiology and function of the nasal cavities in health and disease. *Advanced Drug Delivery Reviews*, **29**, 3-12.

Ohwaki, K., Ando, H., Kakimoto, F. et al. (1987) Effects of dose, pH, osmolarity on nasal absorption of secretin in rats: histological aspects of the nasal mucosa in relation to the absorption variation due to the effects of pH and osmolarity. *Journal of Pharmaceutical Sciences*, **76**, 695-698.

Pereswetoff-Morath, L. (1998) Microspheres as nasal drug delivery systems. *Advanced Drug Delivery Reviews,* **29**, 185-194.

Sarkar, M.A. (1992) Drug metabolism in the nasal mucosa. *Pharmaceutical Research*, **9**, 1-9.

Schipper, N.G.M., Verhoef, J.C., Merkus, F.W.H.M. (1991) The nasal mucociliary clearance: relevance to nasal drug delivery. *Pharmaceutical Research*, **7**, 807-814.

Su, K.S.E. (1991) Nasal delivery. In: Lee, V.H.L. (ed.) *Peptide and Protein Drug Delivery*. Marcel Dekker, New York.

38

Transdermal drug delivery

B. W. Barry

CHAPTER CONTENTS

INTRODUCTION

The main purpose of this chapter is to show how the physicochemical properties of a drug in a topical dosage form affect the drug's transdermal delivery (or percutaneous absorption). This process and the drug's topical bioavailability depend on the medicament leaving a formulation (cream, ointment, patch, etc.) and penetrating through the stratum corneum into the viable epidermis and dermis. Within the living tissues, the molecule usually produces its characteristic pharmacological response before the blood or lymph circulation removes it (possibly to produce a systemic effect). The ultimate aim in dermatological biopharmaceutics is to design active drugs, or prodrugs, and to incorporate them into vehicles or devices which deliver the medicament to the active site in the biophase at a controlled rate.

The plan of the chapter is:

- to introduce the reader to the structure, functions and topical treatment of human skin
- to deal with the principles of membrane diffusion and skin transport, the properties influencing transdermal delivery, permeation with and without stratum corneum control, and the methods for studying these processes
- to consider how to maximize the bioavailability of a topical drug
- to review the philosophy of transdermal patches

- and to close with a brief discussion of dermatological vehicles and a protocol for producing a dermatological formulation.

The reader may then see that skin therapy is a paradox. At first sight, it appears to be a simple form of treatment, yet closer examination reveals that sound dermatological design represents one of the most difficult aspects of the science of pharmaceutical formulation.

STRUCTURE, FUNCTION AND TOPICAL TREATMENT OF HUMAN SKIN

The skin combines with the mucosal linings of the urogenital, digestive and respiratory tracts to protect the internal body structure from a hostile external environment of varying pollution, temperature, humidity and radiation. The skin safeguards the internal organs, limits the passage of chemicals into and out of the body, stabilizes blood pressure and temperature, and mediates the sensations of heat, cold, touch and pain. It expresses emotions (such as the pallor of fear, the redness of embarrassment and anger, and the sweating of anxiety). The integument identifies individuals through the characteristics particular to humans, e.g. colour, hair, odour and texture.

Skin damages easily: mechanically, chemically, biologically and by radiation. Thus the tissue suffers cuts, bruises, burns, bites and stings; detergents, chemical residues, organic solvents and pollutants attack and pen-

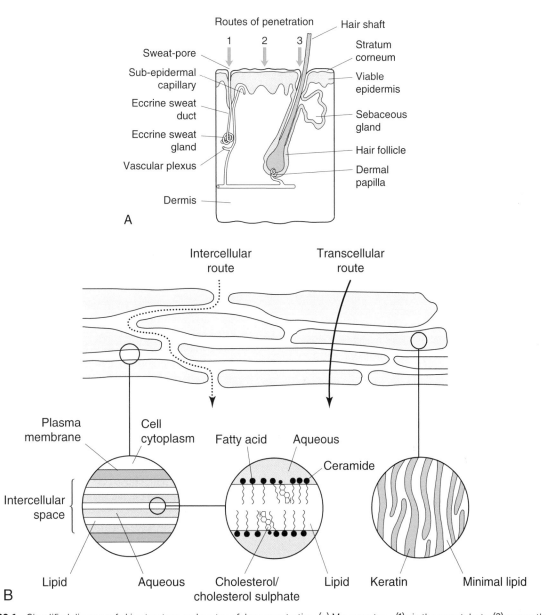

Fig. 38.1 Simplified diagram of skin structure and routes of drug penetration. (a) Macroroutes – (1) via the sweat ducts; (2) across the continuous stratum corneum; or (3) through the hair follicles with their associated sebaceous glands. (b) Representation of the stratum corneum membrane, illustrating two possible microroutes for permeation.

etrate the surface; and microorganisms and plants deliver contact allergens. Topical and systemic drugs, toiletries and cosmetics, and many diseases may all harm the skin.

Anatomy and physiology

The human skin comprises three tissue layers: the stratified, avascular, cellular epidermis, the underlying dermis of connective tissue, and the subcutaneous fat (Fig. 38.1a).

Hairy skin contains hair follicles and sebaceous glands; glabrous skin of the soles and palms produces a thick epidermis with a substantial stratum corneum but there are no hair follicles or sebaceous glands.

Epidermis

The stratum corneum of the multilayered epidermis varies in thickness, ranging from about 0.8 mm on the palms and soles to 0.006 mm on the eyelids. The cells of the basal layer (stratum germinativum) divide and migrate upwards to produce the stratum corneum or horny layer. Humans survive in a non-aqueous environment because of the almost impermeable nature of this dead, dense layer, which is crucially important in controlling the percutaneous absorption of drugs and other chemicals. The stratum corneum may be only 10 μm thick when dry but swells several-fold in water. There are two main types of horny layer: the pads of the palms and soles, adapted for friction and weight bearing, and the remaining flexible, rather impermeable membranous layer. The basal cell layer also includes melanocytes that produce and distribute melanin granules to the keratinocytes. Langerhans cells (important in defence mechanisms operated by the immune system) are prominent in the epidermis.

Dermis

The dermis (or *corium*), at 3–5 mm thick, consists of a matrix of connective tissue woven from fibrous proteins (collagen, elastin and reticulin) that are embedded in an amorphous ground substance of mucopolysaccharide. Nerves, blood vessels and lymphatics traverse the matrix, and skin appendages (eccrine sweat glands, apocrine glands and pilosebaceous units) pierce it. The dermis needs an efficient blood supply to convey nutrients, remove waste products, regulate pressure and temperature, mobilize defence forces and to contribute to skin colour. Branches from the arterial plexus deliver blood to sweat glands, hair follicles, subcutaneous fat and the dermis itself. This supply reaches to within 0.2 mm of the skin surface, so that it quickly absorbs and systematically dilutes most compounds passing the epidermis. The generous blood volume in the skin usually acts as a 'sink' for diffusing molecules reaching the capillaries, keeping penetrant concentrations in the dermis very low, maximizing epidermal concentration gradients, and thus promoting percutaneous absorption.

Subcutaneous tissue

The subcutaneous fat (*subcutis, hypoderm*) provides a mechanical cushion and a thermal barrier; it synthesizes and stores readily available high-energy chemicals.

Skin appendages

The *eccrine sweat glands* (2–5 million) produce sweat (pH 4.0–6.8) and may also secrete drugs, proteins, antibodies and antigens. Their principal function is to aid heat control but emotional stress can also provoke sweating (the clammy palm syndrome).

The *apocrine sweat glands* develop at the pilosebaceous follicle to provide the characteristic adult distribution in the armpit (axilla), the breast areola and the perianal region. The milky or oily secretion may be coloured and contains proteins, lipids, lipoproteins and saccharides. Surface bacteria metabolize this odourless liquid to produce the characteristic body smell.

Hair follicles develop over all skin except the red part of the lips, the palms and soles, and parts of the sex organs. One or more *sebaceous glands*, and in some body regions an apocrine gland, open into the follicle above the muscle that attaches the follicle to the dermoepidermal junction.

Sebaceous glands are most numerous and largest on the face and forehead, in the ear, on the midline of the back and on anogenital surfaces; the palms and soles usually lack them. These holocrine glands produce sebum from cell disintegration; its principal components are glycerides, free fatty acids, cholesterol, cholesterol esters, wax esters and squalene. Abnormal sebaceous activity may lead to seborrhoea (excess sebum), gland hyperplasia without clinical seborrhoea, obstruction of the pilosebaceous canal (acne and comedones – whiteheads or blackheads) and other types of dysfunction – the dyssebacias.

The *nails*, like hair, consist of 'hard' keratin with a relatively high sulphur content, mainly as cysteine. Unlike the stratum corneum, the nail behaves as a hydrophilic matrix with respect to its permeability.

Functions of the skin

The skin performs many varied functions but here we need only consider some aspects of its containment and protective roles.

Mechanical function

The dermis provides the mechanical properties of skin, with the epidermis playing a minor part. Our skin is elastic but once it has taken up its initial slack, it extends further only with difficulty. With age, the skin wrinkles and becomes more rigid. The thin horny layer is quite strong and depends for its pliability on a correct balance of lipids, water-soluble hygroscopic substances (the natural moisturising factor – NMF) and particularly water. The tissue requires some 10–20% of moisture to act as a plasticizer and so maintain its suppleness.

Protective function

Microbiological barrier The stratum corneum provides a microbiological barrier and the sloughing of groups of corneocytes (squames), with their adhering microorganisms, aids the protective mechanism. However, microbes penetrate superficial cracks and damaged stratum corneum may allow access to the lower tissues, where infection may develop. The so-called acid mantle (produced by sebaceous and eccrine secretions, at pH 4.2–5.6) probably does not defend the skin against bacteria via its acidity, as was once thought. However, skin glands also secrete short chain fatty acids that inhibit bacterial and fungal growth. Nitric oxide, produced from nitrates in sweat, may help to prevent infections from skin pathogens, just as acidified nitrite has an antimicrobial action in the oral and gastrointestinal tract. Bacteria are unlikely to enter the tiny opening of the inner duct of the eccrine gland; the entrances to the apocrine gland and the hair follicle are much wider and these appendages may become infected.

Chemical barrier An important function of human skin is to bar the entry of unwanted molecules from outside while controlling the loss of water, electrolytes and other endogenous constituents. The horny layer is very impermeable to most chemicals and usually contributes the rate-limiting step in transdermal absorption. The intact skin is a very effective barricade because the diffusional resistance of the horny layer is large and the permeable appendageal shunt route provides only a small fractional area (about 0.1%).

Radiation barrier For skin exposed to sunlight, ultraviolet light of 290–400 nm is the most damaging. Three main acute reactions follow irradiation: erythema, pigmentation and epidermal thickening. Ultraviolet light stimulates melanocytes to produce melanin, which partially protects the skin. In a severe photosensitive disease such as xeroderma pigmentosum, sunlight may induce changes even in patients whose intense racial pigmentation makes them less susceptible to sunburn. Chronic reactions to sunlight include skin 'ageing', premalignancy and malignancy. Sun-damaged skin may produce solar keratoses, progressing to a squamous cell carcinoma. Bowen's disease, malignant melanoma and basal cell carcinoma may evolve.

Heat barrier and temperature regulation The stratum corneum is so thin over most body areas that it does not effectively protect the underlying living tissues from extremes of cold and heat; it is not an efficient heat insulator. The skin, however, is the organ primarily responsible for maintaining the body at 37°C. To conserve heat, the peripheral circulation shuts down to minimize surface heat loss; shivering generates energy when chilling is severe. To lose heat, blood vessels dilate, eccrine sweat glands pour out their dilute saline secretion, water evaporates and removal of the heat of vaporization cools the body.

Electrical barrier In dry skin, resistance and impedance are much higher than in other biological tissues.

Mechanical shock An acute violent blow bruises and blisters the skin; friction may blister or thicken the epidermis, producing callosities and corns. Accidental minor trauma to patients on corticosteroids may severely damage their skin, when the collagen is thinned by drug overuse.

Rational approach to drug delivery to and via the skin

Three main methods attack the problem of formulating a successful topical dosage form:

- We can manipulate the barrier function of the skin: for example, topical antibiotics and antibacterials help a damaged barrier to ward off infection; sunscreen agents and the horny layer protect the viable tissues from ultraviolet radiation; and emollient preparations restore pliability to a desiccated horny layer.
- Or we can direct drugs to the viable skin tissues without using oral, systematic or other routes of therapy.
- The third approach uses skin delivery for systemic treatment. For example, transdermal therapeutic systems provide systemic therapy for conditions such as motion sickness, angina and pain.

In dermatology, we aim at five main target regions: skin surface, horny layer, viable epidermis and upper dermis, skin glands and systemic circulation (Figs 38.1 and 38.2).

Surface treatment

We care for the skin surface mainly by using a simple camouflage or cosmetic application, by forming a protective layer or by attacking bacteria and fungi. Some examples include protective films, sunscreens and barriers that hinder moisture loss and so avert chapping. For topical antibiotics, antiseptics and deodorants, the surface microorganisms are the target. Then effective surface bioavailability requires that the formulation should release the antimicrobial so it can penetrate the surface skin fissures and reach the organisms. Developmental studies should at least confirm that the formulation releases and does not bind the medicament.

Stratum corneum treatment

The main therapies aimed at the horny layer improve emolliency by raising water content or stimulating sloughing

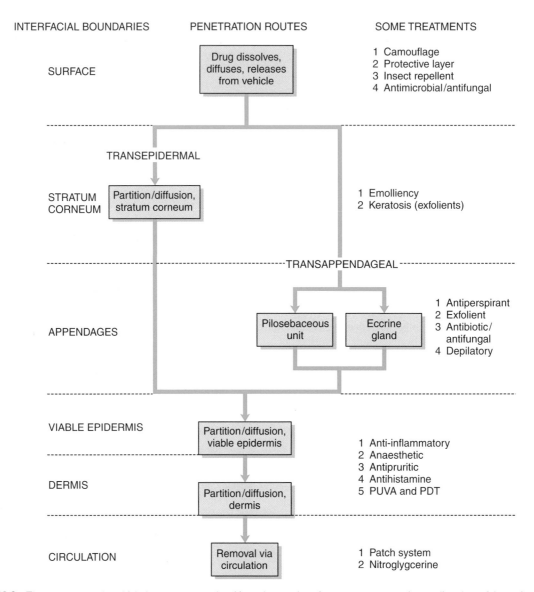

Fig. 38.2 The macroroutes by which drugs penetrate the skin and examples of treatments appropriate to disorders of the various strata (reproduced from Barry 1983 with permission of the copyright owner).

(keratosis) with, for example, salicylic acid. The insertion of moisturizing agents or keratolytics into stratum corneum involves their release from the vehicle and penetration into the tissue. Ideally, the medicament should not enter viable skin; this is difficult to prevent.

Skin appendage treatment

We may reduce hyperhidrosis of the sweat glands with antiperspirants such as aluminium or other metal salts. In acne, we use topical exfolients such as salicylic acid,

tretinoin (retinoic acid) or isotretinoin, and benzoyl peroxide and antibiotics such as erythromycin and clindamycin. Other topical antibiotics applied in skin treatment include framycetin and neomycin sulfates, fusidic acid, polymyxins and mupirocin. Depilatories usually contain strontium or barium sulfides or thioglycolates; male-pattern baldness may be treated with minoxidil and finasteride. Topical imidazoles (clotrimazole, econozole, miconazole, ketoconazole and sulconazole), amoralfine and terbinafine treat fungal diseases of the nails, stratum corneum and hair.

Delivering the medicament to the diseased site is a problem with appendage treatment. For example, it is difficult to achieve a high antibiotic concentration in a sebaceous gland when, as in acne, a horny plug blocks the follicle. When delivered through the skin, the drug may not be sufficiently hydrophobic to partition from the water-rich viable epidermis and dermis into the sebum-filled gland.

Viable epidermis and dermis treatment

We can treat many diseases provided that the preparation efficiently delivers drug to the receptor. However, many potentially valuable drugs cannot be used topically as they do not readily cross the stratum corneum. Hence, investigators may use stratagems such as adding chemical penetration enhancers to diminish this layer's barrier function (discussed later in this chapter). Another approach develops prodrugs, which reach the biological receptor and release the pharmacologically active fragment. The efficacy of many topical steroids depends partly on molecular groups which promote percutaneous absorption but which may not enhance drug-receptor binding.

Drug examples include topical steroidal and non-steroidal antiinflammatory agents; corticosteroids may also be used in psoriasis. Antibiotics include those listed above. Anaesthetic drugs such as benzocaine, amethocaine and lidocaine reduce pain, and antipruritics and antihistamines alleviate itch, but they may cause sensitization. Topical 5-fluorouracil and methotrexate eradicate premalignant and some malignant skin tumours, and treat psoriasis. The psoralens (particularly in conjunction with ultraviolet light – PUVA therapy) mitigate psoriasis, and 5-aminolaevulinic acid (with visible light irradiation – photodynamic therapy) treats skin cancer.

Transcutaneous immunization

The skin has a highly effective immunological surveillance and effector system. A new therapy involves developing transcutaneous immunization via topical application of vaccine antigens. The process uses an adjuvant such as cholera toxin added to a vaccine antigen (e.g. diphtheria toxoid) to induce antibodies to the diphtheria toxoid. The adjuvant and antigen target Langerhans cells, potent antigen-presenting cells in the epidermis. Simple application of the vaccine formulation to the skin of experimental animals and human volunteers has produced positive responses.

Systemic treatment via transdermal absorption

Generally, in the past we have not used healthy skin as a drug route during systemic attacks on disease, with the noteworthy exceptions of nitroglycerin and antileprotics. The body absorbs drugs slowly and incompletely through the stratum corneum and much of the preparation is lost by washing, by adherence to clothes and by shedding with stratum corneum scales. Other problems include marked variations in skin permeability with regard to subject, site, age and condition, which make control difficult. However, in recent years considerable scientific work has led to the route being used to treat several conditions by means of transdermal patches (discussed later in this chapter).

Figure 38.2 illustrates drug penetration routes and examples of treatments appropriate to various skin strata.

DRUG TRANSPORT THROUGH SKIN

Basic principles of diffusion through membranes

A useful way to study percutaneous absorption is to consider, first, how molecules penetrate inert (artificial) membranes and then move on to the special situation of skin transport. An understanding of the basic principles of permeation through membranes is also valuable in all other areas of biopharmaceutics – oral, buccal, rectal, nasal, lung, vaginal, uterine, injection or eye. The underlying mathematics are also relevant to dosage form design, particularly sustained- or controlled-release formulations and drug targeting.

Diffusion process

In passive diffusion, matter moves from one region of a system to another following random molecular motion. The basic hypothesis underlying the mathematical theory for isotropic materials (which have identical structural and diffusional properties in all directions) is that the rate of transfer of diffusing substance per unit area of a section is proportional to the concentration gradient measured normal to the section. This is expressed as Fick's First Law of Diffusion, Eqn 38.1:

$$J = -D\frac{\partial C}{\partial x} \tag{38.1}$$

where J is the rate of transfer per unit area of surface (the flux), C is the concentration of diffusing substance, x is the space coordinate measured normal to the section, and D is the diffusion coefficient. The negative sign indicates that the flux is in the direction of decreasing concentration, i.e. down the concentration gradient. In many situations D is constant but in more complex materials, D depends markedly on concentration; its dimensions are $(length)^2(time)^{-1}$, often specified as $cm^2\,s^{-1}$.

Fick's First Law contains three variables, J, C and x, of which J is additionally a multiple variable, dm/dt, where m is amount and t is time. We therefore usually employ Fick's Second Law, which reduces the number of variables by one. For the common experimental situation in which diffusion is unidirectional, i.e. the concentration gradient is only along the x-axis, Eqn 38.2 expresses Fick's Second Law as:

$$\frac{\partial C}{\partial t} = D \frac{\partial^2 C}{\partial x^2} \qquad (38.2)$$

Many experimental designs employ a membrane separating two compartments, with a concentration gradient operating during a run and 'sink' conditions (essentially zero concentration) prevailing in the receptor compartment. If we measure the cumulative mass of diffusant, m, which passes per unit area through the membrane as a function of time, we obtain the plot shown in Figure 38.3. At long times the plot approaches a straight line and from its slope we obtain the steady flux, dm/dt (Eqn 38.3):

$$\frac{dm}{dt} = \frac{DC_0 K}{h} \qquad (38.3)$$

Here C_0 is the constant concentration of drug in the donor solution, K is the partition coefficient of the solute between the membrane and the bathing solution, and h is the thickness of the membrane.

If a steady-state plot is extrapolated to the time axis, the intercept so obtained at $m = 0$ is the lag time, L:

$$L = \frac{h^2}{6D} \qquad (38.4)$$

From Eqn 38.4, D is estimated provided that the membrane thickness, h, is available. Knowing these parameters and C_0, and measuring dm/dt, Eqn 38.3 provides one way of assessing K. Eqn 38.3 shows why this permeation procedure may be referred to as a zero-order process. By analogy with chemical kinetic operations, Eqn 38.3 represents a zero-order process with a rate constant of DK/h.

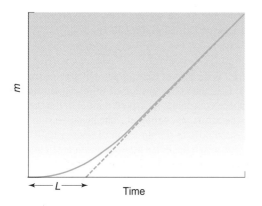

Fig. 38.3 The time course for absorption for the simple zero-order flux case obtained by plotting m, the cumulative amount of diffusant crossing unit area of membrane, as a function of time. Steady state is achieved when the plot becomes linear; extrapolation of the linear portion to the time axis yields the lag time L.

Sometimes with biological membranes (such as skin), we cannot separate the value of D from that of K. We then often employ a composite parameter, the permeability coefficient, P, where $P = KD$ or $P = KD/h$. The latter definition is used when h is uncertain, e.g. diffusion through skin.

Complex diffusional barriers

Barriers in series The treatment above deals only with the simple situation in which diffusion occurs in a single isotropic medium. However, skin is a heterogeneous multilayer tissue and in percutaneous absorption the concentration gradient develops over several strata. We can treat skin in terms of a laminate, each layer of which contributes a diffusional resistance, R, which is directly proportional to the layer thickness, h, and is indirectly proportional to the product of the layer diffusivity, D, and the partition coefficient, K, with respect to the external phase. The total diffusional resistance of all the layers in a three-ply membrane such as skin (stratum corneum, viable epidermis and dermis) is given by the expression:

$$R_T = \frac{1}{P_T} = \frac{h_1}{D_1 K_1} + \frac{h_2}{D_2 K_2} + \frac{h_3}{D_3 K_3} \qquad (38.5)$$

Here R_T is the total resistance to permeation, P_T is the thickness-weighted permeability coefficient, and the numerals refer to the separate skin layers.

If one segment has a much greater resistance than the other layers (e.g. the stratum corneum compared with the viable epidermis or dermis) then the single high-resistance phase determines the composite barrier properties. Then $P_T = K_1 D_1/h_1$, where the subscript 1 refers to the resistant phase.

Barriers in parallel Shunts and pores, such as hair follicles and sweat glands, pierce human skin (see Fig. 38.1). Investigators often idealize this complex structure and consider the simple situation in which the diffusional medium consists of two or more diffusional pathways linked in parallel. Then the total diffusional flux per unit area of composite, J_T, is the sum of the individual fluxes through the separate routes. Thus:

$$J_T = f_1 J_1 + f_2 J_2 \ldots \qquad (38.6)$$

where f_1, f_2, etc., denote the fractional areas for each diffusional route and J_1, J_2, etc., are the fluxes per unit area of each separate route. In general, for independent linear parallel pathways during steady state diffusion:

$$J_T = C_0 (f_1 P_1 + f_2 P_2 + \ldots) \qquad (38.7)$$

where $P_1, P_2,\ldots$ represent the thickness-weighted permeability coefficients.

If only one route allows diffusant to pass, i.e. the other routes are impervious, then the solution reduces to the simple membrane model with the steady-state flux determined by the fractional area and the permeation rate through the open channel.

Skin transport

The skin is very effective as a selective penetration barrier. The epidermis provides the major control element; most small water-soluble non-electrolytes diffuse into the capillary system a thousand times more rapidly when the epidermis is absent, damaged or diseased. Furthermore, in the intact skin, substances penetrate at rates that may differ by 10 000-fold. It is important that pharmaceutical scientists predict and control this selective permeability by relating the physiological and physicochemical attributes of the skin to the properties of the penetrant in a vehicle. We need to correlate the intrinsic properties of the skin barrier with the molecular requirements for breaching it, as modified by interactions with the components of topical vehicles. The eventual aim in dermatological biopharmaceutics is to design drugs with selective penetrability for incorporation into vehicles or devices that deliver the medicament to the active site, at a controlled rate and concentration, for the necessary time.

Several mathematical treatments of various complexities attempt to predict the flux of molecules through the skin, using simple physicochemical attributes. Such assessments typically have accuracies within half a log scale, but occasionally with much poorer agreement for specific molecules.

Routes of penetration

When a molecule reaches intact skin, it contacts cellular debris, microorganisms, sebum and other materials. The diffusant then has three potential entry routs to the viable tissue: through the hair follicles with their associated sebaceous glands, via the sweat ducts or across the continuous stratum corneum between these appendages (see Fig. 38.1). We can summarize relevant features before arriving at a general conclusion.

Sebum and surface material

The layer of sebum mixed with sweat, bacteria and dead cells is thin (0.4–10 μm), irregular and discontinuous; it hardly affects transdermal absorption. This lack of significant effect may seem surprising, particularly as over 300 volatile compounds have been detected on the skin surface, as well as many non-volatiles.

Skin appendages

This route usually does not contribute appreciably to the *steady-state* flux of a drug as the fractional area available for absorption is small (about 0.1%). However, the route may be important for ions and large polar molecules that cross intact stratum corneum with difficulty.

Skin appendages may also act as shunts, important at short times prior to steady-state diffusion, e.g. in bioassays that use pharmacological reactions. Thus minute concentrations of nicotinates or corticosteroids penetrating rapidly down the shunt route may quickly trigger erythema or blanching, respectively.

Although we usually ignore the hair follicle route for molecular flux under steady-state conditions, very large molecules and particles of colloidal dimensions can target the follicle. Thus, 'naked' DNA has been used for immunization by topical application. It was speculated that normal follicles have efficient mechanisms for inducing immune responses to proteins in the follicle. A preparation made from antibodies from transgenic plants, when rubbed into the scalp, neutralized the hair loss effects of toxic chemicals used in cancer chemotherapy. Colloidal particles, such as liposomes and small crystals, are useful for targeting the hair follicle. In general, particles larger than 10 μm remain on the skin surface, those between approximately 3 and 10 μm concentrate in the hair follicle and, when less than 3 μm, they penetrate follicles and stratum corneum alike.

Epidermal route

The epidermal barrier function thus resides mainly in the stratum corneum. This has a 'bricks and mortar' structure analogous to a wall (see Fig. 38.1b). The corneocytes, consisting of hydrated keratin, comprise the 'bricks'. These are embedded in the 'mortar', composed of a complex lipid mixture of ceramides, fatty acids, cholesterol and cholesterol esters, formed into multiple bilayers. Most molecules penetrating through the skin use this intercellular microroute.

Because stratum corneum is dead, it is assumed that there are no active transport processes and no fundamental differences between in vivo and in vitro permeation processes. However, there may be discrepancies in how some substances permeate excised skin and skin in vivo. These differences may arise because we manipulate the skin to insert it into the diffusion apparatus, including possibly damaging it.

Topically applied agents such as steroids, hexachlorophene, griseofulvin, sodium fusidate and fusidic acid may form a depot or reservoir by binding within the stratum corneum.

Diseases that disrupt the horny layer, such as eczema and exfoliative dermatitis, may allow easier access.

The viable layers (particularly the epidermis) may metabolize and inactivate a drug, or activate a prodrug. The dermal papillary layer contains so many capillaries that the average residence time of a drug in the dermis may only be about a minute before it is washed away. Usually, the deeper dermal layers do not influence transdermal absorption, although drugs such as non-steroidal antiinflammatory agents reach as far down as muscle. However, the dermis may bind a hormone such as testosterone, decreasing its systemic removal. If the penetrant is very lipophilic, it crosses the horny layer to meet an aqueous phase in which it is poorly soluble. The chemical potential immediately below the barrier may then become high and approach that in the barrier. The potential gradient (stratum corneum to viable tissue) thus falls, together with the flux. The rate-determining step in percutaneous absorption then becomes barrier clearance, not barrier penetration.

General conclusions on drug transport through the skin

The stratum corneum develops as a thin, tough, relatively impermeable membrane, which usually provides the rate-limiting step in transdermal drug delivery. The entire horny layer, not just some specialized region, provides the diffusional resistance. The membrane allows no drug to pass readily but nearly all low molecular weight molecules penetrate to some extent. The lipid bilayers of the intercellular route provide the main pathway. Diffusion is passive, governed by physicochemical laws in which active transport plays no part.

For electrolytes and large molecules with low diffusion coefficients, such as polar steroids and antibiotics, and for some colloidal particles, the appendages may provide the main entry route.

Once past the horny layer, molecules permeate rapidly through the living tissues and sweep into the systemic circulation.

The fraction of a drug that penetrates the skin via any particular route depends on the:

- physicochemical nature of the drug, particularly its size, solubility and partition coefficient
- timescale of observation,
- site and condition of the skin
- formulation
- how vehicle components temporarily change the properties of the stratum corneum.

PROPERTIES THAT INFLUENCE TRANSDERMAL DELIVERY

When a preparation is applied to diseased skin, the clinical result arises from a sequence of processes:

1. Release of the medicament from the vehicle, followed by

2. Penetration through the skin barriers, and
3. Activation of the pharmacological response.

Effective therapy optimizes these steps as they are affected by three components: the drug, the vehicle and the skin.

Figure 38.4, which represents the movement of drug molecules arising from, for example, a transdermal drug delivery system with a rate-controlling membrane, illustrates the complexity of percutaneous absorption. Any drug particles must first dissolve so molecules may diffuse towards the membrane within the patch. The penetrant partitions into the membrane, diffuses across the polymer and partitions into the skin adhesive. The molecules diffuse towards the vehicle/stratum corneum interface. They then partition into the stratum corneum and diffuse through it. Some drug may bind at a depot site; the remainder permeates further, meets a second interface and partitions into the viable epidermis. For a lipophilic species, this partition coefficient may be unfavourable, i.e. very large. Within the epidermis, enzymes may metabolize the drug or it may interact at a

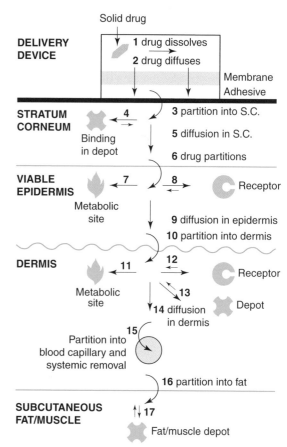

Fig. 38.4 Some stages in drug delivery from a transdermal patch (modified from Barry 1983 with permission of the copyright owner).

receptor site. After passing into the dermis, additional depot regions and metabolic sites may intervene as the drug moves to a capillary, partitions into its wall and out into the blood for systemic removal. A fraction of the diffusant may partition into the subcutaneous fat to form a further depot. A portion of the drug can reach deep muscle layers, as illustrated by, for example, the efficacy of non-steroidal antiinflammatory drugs.

However, there are further complications. The following factors may be important: the non-homogeneity of the tissues, the presence of lymphatics, interstitial fluid, hair follicles and sweat glands, cell division, cell transport to and through the stratum corneum, and cell surface loss. The disease, the healing process, the drug and vehicle components may progressively modify the skin barrier. As vehicle ingredients diffuse into the skin, cellular debris, sweat, sebum and surface contaminants pass into the formulation, changing its physicochemical characteristics. Emulsions may invert or crack when rubbed in and volatile solvents may evaporate.

To discuss this complicated process in a simple fashion, it is necessary to review the material under the headings of biological factors and physicochemical factors. However, because transdermal delivery is a dynamic process, it should be borne in mind that as one variable changes, it usually causes several effects on drug flux. The various factors are separated for our convenience but in practice, this is an artificial distinction, useful only for discussion (and learning) purposes.

Biological factors

Skin condition

The intact, healthy skin is a tough barrier but many agents damage it. Vesicants such as acids and alkalis injure barrier cells and thereby promote penetration, as do cuts, abrasions and dermatitis. In heavy industry, workers' skins may lose their reactivity or 'harden' because of frequent contact with irritant chemicals.

Many solvents open up the complex dense structure of the horny layer. Mixtures of non-polar and polar solvents such as chloroform and methanol remove the lipid fraction, forming artificial shunts through which molecules pass more easily.

Disease commonly alters skin condition; fortunately, for *biopharmaceutical purposes*, we need only an elementary understanding of the gross changes in deranged skin. We are mainly interested in visible damage. Is the skin inflamed, with loss of stratum corneum and altered keratinization? Then permeability increases. Is the organ thickened with corns, calluses and warts, or as in ichthyosis? Drug permeation should now decrease. In diseases characterized by a defective stratum corneum,

percutaneous absorption usually increases. Thus, a psoriatic plaque may take up twice as much 8-methoxypsoralen as does uninvolved skin.

After injury or removal of the stratum corneum, within 3 days the skin builds a temporary barrier that persists until the regenerating epidermis can form normal keratinizing cells. Even the first complete layer of new stratum corneum cells formed over a healing layer can markedly reduce permeation.

Skin age

It is often assumed that the skins of the young and the elderly are more permeable than adult tissue but there is little evidence for any dramatic difference. Children are more susceptible to the toxic effects of drugs and chemicals, partly because of their greater surface area per unit body weight; thus potent topical steroids, boric acid and hexachorophene have produced severe side-effects and death. Premature infants may be born with no stratum corneum. This can be turned to advantage by treating breathing difficulties with caffeine or pain with buprenorphine, via simple topical application instead of intravenous injection through tiny, delicate veins.

Blood flow

Theoretically, changes in the peripheral circulation could affect transdermal absorption; an increased blood flow could reduce the time a penetrant remains in the dermis and also raise the concentration gradient across the skin. *Usually*, the effect is not *clinically* important (although it can be shown experimentally). In clinically hyperaemic skin, any increase in absorption almost always arises because the disease damages the skin barrier. Potent rubefacients such as nicotinic acid esters would also only have a significant effect after damaging the skin. Potent vasoconstricting agents such as topical steroids could reduce their own clearance rate or that of another drug.

Regional skin sites

Variations in cutaneous permeability around the body depend on the thickness and nature of the stratum corneum and the density of skin appendages. However, the absorption rate varies widely for a specific substance passing through identical skin sites in different healthy volunteers; the most permeable regions in some individuals compare with the least permeable sites in others. Investigators produce different rank orders for the permeabilities of skin sites in general; such permeabilities depend on both the intrinsic resistance to permeation per unit thickness of stratum corneum and the overall thickness of the tissue. As an example, plantar and palmar callus may be 400–600 μm thick compared to 10–20 µm for other sites. However, despite this greater thickness, the tissue is less resistant *per unit thickness* so that the flux of diffusing drug is not so decreased compared with other sites as might be expected.

Because of the relatively high permeability and ease of access of the site, the hyoscine Transderm® system employs the postauricular skin (i.e. behind the ear) to insert drugs into the blood stream. Originally this site was selected because it was thought that the layers of stratum corneum are thinner and less dense, there are more sweat and sebaceous glands per unit area and many capillaries reach closer to the surface, increasing its temperature by 4–6°C relative to the thigh. However, facial skin in general is more permeable than other body sites, such as the limbs or torso.

Skin metabolism

The skin metabolizes steroid hormones, chemical carcinogens and some drugs. Such metabolism may determine the therapeutic efficacy of topically applied compounds (particularly prodrugs) and the carcinogenic responses in the skin. It has been estimated that the skin can metabolize some 5% of candidate topical drugs.

Species differences

Mammalian skins differ widely in characteristics such as horny layer thickness, sweat gland and hair follicle densities, and pelt condition. The capillary blood supply and the sweating ability differ between humans and common laboratory animals. Such factors affect the routes of penetration and the resistance to permeation. Subtle biochemical differences between human and animal skin may alter reactions between penetrants and skin.

Frequently, mice, rats and rabbits are used to assess percutaneous absorption but their skins have more hair follicles than human skin and they lack sweat glands. Comparative studies on skin penetration indicate that, in general, monkey and pig skins are most like that of humans. Hairless mouse skin has some similar characteristics. It has been widely used but its stratum corneum is fragile. Hairless rat and fuzzy guinea pig may be better models for humans.

Snake skin has also been used as it has the benefits that no sacrifice is required (the snake sheds its skin), it is readily available and there is little leaching of chemicals to confuse UV assays.

Animal skin has been much used to obtain skin penetration data, but it is best to use human skin whenever possible.

Physicochemical factors

Skin hydration

When water saturates the skin, the tissue swells, softens and wrinkles, and its permeability increases markedly. In fact, hydration of the stratum corneum is one of the most important factors in increasing the penetration rate of most substances that permeate skin. Hydration may result from water diffusing from underlying epidermal layers or from perspiration that accumulates after the application of an occlusive vehicle or dressing. A dramatic example is the use of occlusive plastic films in topical steroid treatment, when the penetration of the steroid often increases 10-fold. Occlusion decreases in the following order: occlusive films = transdermal patches > lipophilic ointments > w/o cream > o/w cream. Powders, applied either as dusting powders or in lotions, provide a large surface area for evaporation and therefore dry the skin.

Commercial products are often promoted as skin softeners with the presumption that they increase the skin's moisture content. However, they may contain humectants such as glycerol, propylene glycol or polyethylene glycol and emulsifiers that actually withdraw moisture from the skin.

Table 38.1 summarizes the effects which skin delivery systems may exert on stratum corneum hydration and permeability.

Temperature and pH

The penetration rate of material through human skin can change 10-fold for a large temperature variation, since the diffusion coefficient decreases as the temperature falls. However, adequate clothing on most of the body would usually prevent wide fluctuations in temperature and penetration rates. Occlusive vehicles increase skin temperature by a few degrees but any consequent increased permeability is small compared to the effect of hydration.

According to the simple form of the pH-partition hypothesis, only unionized molecules pass readily across lipid membranes. Now weak acids and bases dissociate to different degrees depending on the pH and their pK_a or pK_b values (see Chapter 3). Thus, the proportion of unionized drug in the applied phase mainly determines the effective membrane gradient, and this fraction depends on pH. However, ionized molecules do penetrate the stratum corneum to a limited extent. Because they usually have a much greater aqueous solubility than the neutral species, in saturated or near-saturated solutions, they may make a significant contribution to the total flux (i.e. although K may be small for ionized species, C_0 may be very high; Eqn 38.3).

The stratum corneum is remarkably resistant to alterations in pH, tolerating a range of 3–9.

Table 38.1 Expected effects of skin delivery systems on horny layer hydration and skin permeability – in approximate order of decreasing hydration

Delivery system	Examples/constituents	Effect on skin hydration	Effect on skin permeability
Occlusive dressing	Plastic film, unperforated water proof plaster	Prevents water loss; full hydration	Marked increase
Occlusive patch	Most transdermal patches	Prevents water loss; full hydration	Marked increase
Lipophilic material	Paraffins, oils, fats, waxes, fatty acids and alcohols, esters, silicones	Prevents water loss; may produce full hydration	Marked increase
Absorption base	Anhydrous lipid material plus water/oil emulsifiers	Prevents water loss; marked hydration	Marked increase
Emulsifying base	Anhyrous lipid material plus oil/water emulsifiers	Prevents water loss; marked hydration	Marked increase
Water/oil emulsion	Oily creams	Retards water loss; raised hydration	Increase
Oil/water emulsion	Aqueous creams	May donate water; slight hydration increase	Slight increase?
Humectant	Water-soluble bases, glycerol, glycos	May withdraw water; decreased hydration	Can decrease or act as penetration enhancer
Powder	Clays, organics, inorganics, 'shake' lotions	Aid water evaporation; decreased excess hydration	Little effect on stratum corneum

Diffusion coefficient

The diffusional speed of a molecule depends mainly on the state of matter of the medium. In gases and air, diffusion coefficients are large because the void space available to the molecules is great compared to their size, and the mean free path between molecular collisions is big. In liquids, the free volume is much smaller, mean free paths are decreased, and diffusion coefficients are much reduced. In skin, the diffusivities drop progressively and reach their lowest values within the compacted stratum corneum matrix. For a constant temperature, the diffusion coefficient of a drug in a topical vehicle or in skin depends on the properties of the drug and the diffusion medium and on the interaction between them.

However, the *measured* value of D may reflect influences other than intrinsic mobility. For example, some drug may bind and become immobilized within the stratum corneum and this process affects the magnitude of D as determined from the lag time (Eqn 38.4). However, regardless of such complications, the value of D measures the penetration rate of a molecule under specified conditions and is therefore useful to know.

Drug concentration

It was seen previously that the flux of solute is proportional to the concentration gradient across the entire barrier phase (Eqn 38.3). Thus, drug permeation usually follows Fick's Law. One requirement for maximal flux in a thermodynamically stable situation is that the donor solution should be saturated. A formulator can optimize the solubility of a drug such as a corticosteroid by controlling the solvent composition of the vehicle. Then a saturated solution may be obtained at a selected concentration of the drug by experimenting with a series of solvents or, more usually, by blending two liquids to form a miscible binary mixture with suitable solvent properties.

Although the concentration differential is usually considered to be the driving force for diffusion, the chemical potential gradient or activity gradient is actually the fundamental parameter. Often the distinction is unimportant but sometimes we must consider it. Thus, the thermodynamic activity of a penetrant in the donor phase or the membrane may be radically altered by, for example, pH change, complex formation or the presence of surfactants, micelles or cosolvents. Such factors also modify the effective partition coefficient.

Partition coefficient

The partition coefficient (K; see Chapter 2) is important in establishing the flux of a drug through the stratum corneum (Eqn 38.3). When the membrane provides the sole or major source of diffusional resistance, then the magnitude of the partition coefficient is very important; this can differ by a factor of 10^8, drug to drug or (for a given penetrant) vehicle to vehicle. The stratum corneum-to-vehicle partition coefficient is then crucially important in establishing a high initial concentration of diffusant in the first layer of the membrane.

Once it was incorrectly thought that good skin penetration required a K close to unity. However, many congeneric series of molecules display an *optimal K* well below which they are too water soluble to partition effectively into the horny layer. At higher values, the compounds are so lipid soluble that they do not readily pass from the stratum corneum into the water-rich viable tissue. For a drug series, this behaviour produces a parabolic or bilinear relation between pharmacological activity and partition coefficient.

Topical steroids provide a good example of the importance of the partition coefficient. Thus, triamcinolone is five times more active systemically than hydrocortisone but it exhibits only about one-tenth the topical activity. Triamcinolone acetonide, with a more favourable K value, shows a 1000-fold increase in cutaneous activity. Betamethasone possesses only 10 times the topical potency of hydrocortisone, although it is some 30 times stronger systemically. Of the 23 esters of betamethasone tested, the 17-valerate has the highest topical activity and this coincides with the most balanced lipid/water partition coefficient. The antiinflammatory responses to hydrocortisone and its C-21 esters behave similarly. As the side chain lengthens from 0 to 6 carbon atoms, the partition coefficient increases, as does the antiinflammatory index. Thereafter the activity declines as the homologous series extends and the partition coefficient further increases.

Polar cosolvent mixtures such as propylene glycol with water may produce saturated drug solutions and so maximize the concentration gradient across the stratum corneum. However, the partition coefficient of a drug between the membrane and the solvent mixture generally falls as the solubility in the solvent system rises. Thus, these two factors – increase in solubility and decrease in the magnitude of the partition coefficient – may oppose each other in promoting flux through the membrane when the system is not saturated. Hence it is important not to oversolubilize a drug if the aim is to promote penetration; the formulation should be at or near saturation.

Surface activity and micellization affect transdermal delivery. There are two main complicating situations in membrane transport: one where the drug is surface active and forms micelles and the other where additional surfactant is present. When the drug micellizes, its total apparent solubility increases dramatically but its apparent partition coefficient decreases. However, the free monomer concentration remains constant as does the true (monomer) partition coefficient. Then, if the micelle cannot cross the membrane, this aggregate has little effect on the permeation process other than by serving as a reservoir to replace monomers as they leave to enter the skin, and by maintaining a constant donor concentration.

When drug and surfactant are present, the effect of surfactant on drug transport is complicated. The drug in the surfactant solution partitions between the micellar and non-micellar pseudophases. The skin absorption of micellar drug may be negligible and the effective concentration of the unassociated diffusing species may be so lowered that its flux falls drastically. However, all these effects are more important for more permeable membranes such as gastrointestinal or buccal tissue.

Surfactants also have effects on skin which relate to lowering of interfacial tension at the skin surface and in hair follicles, and changes in protein conformation and disruption of intercellular lipid packing in the stratum corneum. They then function as penetration enhancers, discussed later in this chapter.

Complex formation is analogous in many ways to micellar solubilization in the manner in which it affects drug permeation. Thus, when complexes form, the apparent solubility and the apparent partition coefficient of the drug change. An increase in the apparent partition coefficient may promote drug absorption, e.g. some caffeine–drug complexes.

Molecular size and shape

Absorption is apparently inversely related to molecular weight; small molecules penetrate faster than large ones. However, the specific effect of the size of the penetrating molecule on the flux could only be determined if the effect of size could be separated from the resultant change in solubility characteristics. This is difficult to do, as the role of the partition coefficient is so dominant. With rare exceptions, we cannot experimentally increase the size of a molecule without also dramatically changing its partition coefficient.

It is even more difficult to determine the effect of molecular shape, separated from partition coefficient domination, so nothing is known about this factor in skin permeation.

Ideal molecular properties for drug penetration

From the above considerations, we can deduce the ideal properties that a molecule would require so as to penetrate the stratum corneum well. In brief, these are:

- a low molecular mass, preferably less than 600 Da, when the diffusion coefficient will tend to be high
- an adequate solubility in oil and water, so the concentration gradient in the membrane can be high
- a balanced partition coefficient
- a low melting point; this correlates with good ideal solubility.

These features explain why transdermal patches can deliver adequate amounts of nicotine to be effective in smoking cessation therapy because this drug well illustrates all these requirements.

DRUG PERMEATION THROUGH SKIN

Stratum corneum rate controlling

It is useful here to summarize the basic concepts used in considering transdermal drug delivery, when the drug, the skin and the vehicle interact. Usually the relative impermeability of the stratum corneum provides the rate-limiting step in percutaneous absorption. The assumptions made in analysing relevant data include the following:

- Stratum corneum provides the rate-limiting step.
- Skin is a homogeneous intact membrane; appendages are unimportant.
- Only a single non-ionic drug species is important, dissolving to form an ideal solution unaffected by pH, and dissolution is not rate limiting.
- Only drug diffuses from the vehicle. Formulation components neither diffuse nor evaporate and skin secretions do not dilute the vehicle.
- Diffusion coefficient is constant with time or position in the vehicle or horny layer.
- Penetrant reaching viable tissue sweeps into the circulation, maintaining sink conditions below the stratum corneum.
- Donor phase depletes negligibly, i.e. constant drug concentration in the vehicle.
- Vehicle does not alter skin permeability during an experiment by, for example, changing stratum corneum hydration or by acting as a penetration enhancer.
- Drug remains intact and unaltered.
- Flux estimates are steady-state values.

Most analyses use Eqn 38.3, assume that the stratum corneum thickness, h, is constant and relate changes in the penetration rate to variations in the other three parameters.

An important alternative form of Eqn 38.3 uses thermodynamic activities. Thus:

$$\frac{dm}{dt} = \frac{aD}{\gamma h} \qquad (38.8)$$

where a is the thermodynamic activity of the drug in its vehicle and γ is the effective activity coefficient in the skin barrier. To obtain the maximum rate of penetration, we see that we should use the drug at its highest thermodynamic activity. Now the dissolved molecules in a saturated solution are in equilibrium with the pure solid (which by definition is at maximum thermodynamic activity). The solute molecules are also thus at maximum activity. (It is useful in this context to think of thermodynamic activity as 'escaping tendency', i.e. the drive for the drug to escape from the vehicle and enter the skin). The conclusion, therefore, is that all vehicles which contain the drug as a finely ground suspension (in which the solute activity is maximal and equal to that of the solid) should produce the same penetration rate, *provided that the assumptions listed above remain valid*. (The effect of supersaturation is dealt with later.)

If we use the placebo vehicle to dilute, for example, an ointment containing a drug in suspension, the drug flux (and hence the clinical efficacy) will not fall until the concentration decreases below the saturation value. This is why many extemporaneously diluted preparations have essentially the same therapeutic activity as their undiluted form – the dilution process never reached subsaturation.

Stratum corneum not rate controlling

Next we consider situations in which the impermeability of the stratum corneum is *not* important, i.e. we are concerned only with drug and vehicle interactions. Then the release of the drug from the vehicle provides the rate-limiting step and the skin functions as a sink. This could happen to a patient with a disrupted or absent horny layer, or when drug diffusion in the vehicle is exceptionally slow. The vehicle also provides the rate-controlling mechanism in many release studies that use either no membrane or an artificial porous membrane. Such experiments may correlate with clinical treatment only for patients with severely damaged skin.

When diffusion within the vehicle provides the rate-controlling step, our mathematical treatment assumes that the skin is a sink. Thus, it maintains essentially zero concentration of the penetrating material by rapidly passing it to the circulation. Then the concentration gradient develops solely in the applied formulation. Two important situations are absorption from solution and from suspension.

Absorption from solution: skin a perfect sink

We can deduce an equation that applies to the release of penetrant from one side of a layer of vehicle on the skin, under the following conditions:

- Only a single drug species is important, it is in true solution and it is initially uniformly distributed throughout the vehicle.
- Only the drug diffuses out of the vehicle. Other components do not diffuse or evaporate and skin secretions do not pass into the vehicle.
- The diffusion coefficient does not alter with time or position within the vehicle.
- When the penetrant reaches the skin, it absorbs instantaneously.

Under these limitations, Eqn 38.9 represents the relationship between m, the quantity of drug released to the sink per unit area of application, with C_0, the initial concentration of solute in the vehicle, D_v, the diffusion coefficient of the drug in the vehicle, and t, the time after application:

$$m \approx 2C_0\sqrt{\frac{D_v t}{\pi}} \qquad (38.9)$$

Differentiating this equation provides the release rate, dm/dt:

$$\frac{dm}{dt} \approx C_0\sqrt{\frac{D_v}{\pi t}} \qquad (38.10)$$

Figure 38.5 illustrates plots of a typical release experiment for betamethasone 17-benzoate dissolved at various concentrations in a polar gel and diffusing into a chloroform sink. According to Eqn 38.9, a plot of m versus $t^{1/2}$

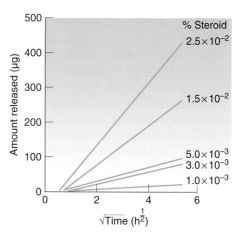

Fig. 38.6 In vitro release of betamethasone-17-benzoate from gel formulations as a function of the square root of time: steroid strength indicated on the plots (reproduced from Barry 1983 with permission of the copyright owner).

should provide a straight line, as Figure 38.6 illustrates. A relationship such as Eqn 38.9, or a modification in which m is still proportional to $t^{1/2}$, often fits data outside the limits used originally to define the equation, i.e. up to 65% release instead of only about 30%.

According to these equations, we may alter the release rate of a drug from solution, and hence its bioavailability, by changing drug concentration or the diffusion coefficient.

Absorption from suspensions: skin a perfect sink

The amount released, and the rate of release, of a drug suspended in a vehicle, such as an ointment, may be related to time and to the variables of the system. The relevant equations are derived for a simple model system under the following conditions:

- The suspended drug is micronized so that particle diameters are much smaller than the vehicle layer thickness.
- The particles are uniformly distributed and do not sediment in the vehicle.
- The total amount of drug, soluble and suspended, per unit volume (A) is much greater than C_S, the solubility of the drug in the vehicle.
- The surface to which the vehicle is applied is immiscible with the vehicle, i.e. skin secretions do not enter the vehicle.
- Only the drug diffuses out of the vehicle; vehicle components neither diffuse nor evaporate.
- The receptor, which is the skin, operates as a perfect sink.

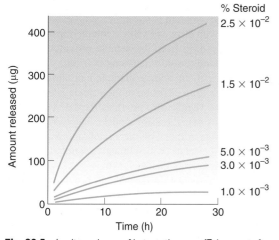

Fig. 38.5 In vitro release of betamethasone-17-benzoate from gel formulations as a function of time: steroid strength indicated on plots (reproduced from Barry 1983 with permission of the copyright owner).

We can then obtain an equation that relates m to t in the form:

$$m = \sqrt{D_v t (2A - C_S) C_S} \qquad (38.11)$$

This equation holds essentially for all times less than that corresponding to complete depletion of the suspended phase. If we differentiate Eqn 38.11 with respect to time, we obtain the instantaneous rate of release, dm/dt, given by:

$$\frac{dm}{dt} = \frac{1}{2} \sqrt{\frac{D_v (2A - C_S) C_S}{t}} \qquad (38.12)$$

For a common condition in which the solubility of the drug in the vehicle is very small and A is appreciable (i.e. $A \gg C_S$), Eqn. 38.11 simplifies to:

$$m \approx \sqrt{2 A D_v C_S t} \qquad (38.13)$$

Then Eqn 38.12 becomes:

$$\frac{dm}{dt} \approx \sqrt{\frac{A D_v C_S}{2t}} \qquad (38.14)$$

These equations indicate that the formulator can manipulate drug bioavailability from ointment suspensions by altering the diffusion coefficient, the total concentration, or the solubility. However, Eqn 38.14 predicts that $dm/dt \propto A^{1/2}$; doubling A only increases dm/dt by about 40%.

For obvious reasons Eqns 38.9–14 are often referred to as 'square root of time' relationships; they may also be called Higuchi equations after the pharmaceutical scientist who developed them. The amount of drug released is proportional to the square route of time; the flux is an inverse function of time$^{1/2}$.

METHODS FOR STUDYING TRANSDERMAL DRUG DELIVERY

Experiments in percutaneous absorption may be designed to answer many questions, such as:

- What is the drug flux through the skin and how do the apparent diffusion coefficient, partition coefficient and structure–activity relationships control it?
- What is the main penetration route – across the stratum corneum or via the appendages?
- Which is more important clinically or toxicologically – transient diffusion (possibly down the appendages) or steady-state permeation (usually across the intact stratum corneum)?
- Does the drug bind to the stratum corneum, the viable epidermis or the dermis? Does it form a depot in the subcutaneous fat or penetrate to the deep muscle layers?
- What is the rate-limiting step in permeation – drug dissolution or diffusion within the vehicle or patch,

partitioning into, or diffusion through, the skin layers, or removal by the blood, lymph or tissue fluids?
- How do skin condition, age, site, blood flow and metabolism affect topical bioavailability? Are differences between animal species important?
- How do vehicles modify the release and absorption of the medicament? What is the optimal formulation for a specific drug – an aerosol spray, a solution, suspension, gel, powder, ointment, cream, paste, tape or other delivery device?
- Are vehicle components inert or do they modify the permeability of the stratum corneum, if only by changing its hydration state?
- To increase drug flux, should we use stratagems such as chemical penetration enhancers, iontophoresis, etc.?
- Is the formulation designed correctly to treat intact stratum corneum, thickened epidermis or damaged skin?
- Should the experimental design produce a pharmacokinetic profile, measuring absorption, distribution, metabolism and excretion in vivo?

No single method can answer all questions and provide a full picture of the complex process of transdermal absorption. We will deal therefore with the important general techniques, dividing them into in vivo and in vitro procedures. The former class uses the skins of living humans or experimental animals in situ, whereas the latter type employs isolated membranes and includes simple release studies.

In vitro methods

These are valuable techniques for screening and for measuring fluxes, partition coefficients and diffusion coefficients because the investigator can closely control laboratory conditions.

Excised skin

Excised skins from rats, mice and guinea pigs (normal and hairless), rabbits, hamsters, pigs, hairless dogs, snake, monkeys, etc., have been mounted in diffusion cells. However, mammalian skin varies widely in stratum corneum properties and the number and density of appendages. Thus, it is best to obtain human skin from autopsies, amputations or cosmetic surgery. Investigators use either stratum corneum, epidermis, dermatomed skin or whole skin clamped in a diffusion cell. They measure the compound passing from the stratum corneum side through to a fluid bath. We can consider two main situations and illustrate just some of the many types of diffusion cell used.

In diffusion cells designed to examine steady-state flux and deduce fundamental parameters, a well-stirred donor solution at constant concentration releases penetrant through a membrane into an agitated 'sink' receptor liquid simulating the blood supply (Fig. 38.7). Figure 38.8 shows how three important quantities vary with time: the amount entering the membrane, that passing through (see also Fig. 38.3 and Eqns 38.3 and 38.4) and that remaining in the membrane.

Diffusion cells aimed more at simulating in vivo or clinical conditions use an agitated receptor solution to correspond to the blood and an unmixed donor phase to represent the formulation (Fig. 38.9). The donor compartment may be closed or open to ambient conditions or to controlled temperature and humidity; the skin may be washed, or materials added during an experiment. The test formulation may be a solid deposited from a volatile solvent, a liquid, a semi-solid, a film or a drug delivery device.

A technique known as attenuated total reflectance spectroscopy (ATRS) may also be used to measure passage across stratum corneum to determine the diffusion coefficient of the penetrating molecule. The measuring technique may employ infrared or Raman spectroscopy.

Artificial membranes

Because human skin is variable and difficult to obtain, workers often use other materials, for example cellulose acetate, silicone rubber or isopropyl myristate, or lamellar systems designed to mimic the intercellular lipid of the stratum corneum. However, these membranes are not as complex as human skin and care has to be taken if the results of such experiments are to be extrapolated to the clinical situation.

Release methods without a rate-limiting membrane

These procedures record drug release to a simple immiscible phase. They measure only those drug/vehicle interactions that affect release characteristics and they

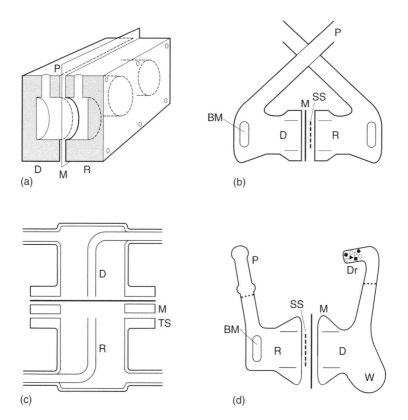

Fig. 38.7 Diffusion cells for zero-order or steady-state flux experiments (not to scale). (a) Bank of two cells drilled from a perspex block. (b) Simple glass diffusion cell suitable for human skin. (c) Glass cell with continuously circulating donor and receptor solutions. (d) Glass cell used for determining vapour diffusion through the skin. *Key:* D, donor compartment; R, receptor compartment; M, membrane, P, sampling port; BM, bar magnet; SS, stainless steel support; TS, teflon support; W, well; Dr, drierite (reproduced from Barry 1983 with permission of the copyright owner).

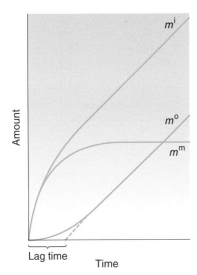

Fig. 38.8 Amount of penetrant entering the membrane (m^i), diffusing through (m^o) and being sorbed (m^m) under zero-order flux conditions (reproduced from Barry 1983 with permission of the copyright owner).

do not determine skin absorption. Such procedures are mainly valuable in quality control protocols. Typical arrangements are shown in Figure 38.10. Eqns 38.9–14 may be used to analyse results.

In vivo methods

Often, in vivo methods use animals. However, most animals differ significantly from humans in features which affect percutaneous absorption: the thickness and nature of the stratum corneum, the density of hair follicles and sweat glands, the nature of the pelt, the papillary blood supply and biochemical aspects. Only a few techniques produce animal diseases that are similar to human afflictions. Thus animal models are valuable for studying the anatomy, physiology and biochemistry of skin, for screening topical agents, for detecting possible hazards and for preliminary biopharmaceutical investigations. However, experience with animals cannot fully substitute for studies in humans; regulatory bodies will usually request additional data from human studies before granting a product licence.

Histology

Experimenters may try to locate skin penetration routes from microscopic sections; however, the cutting, handling and development of skin sections encourage leaching and translocation of materials away from their original sites, a problem with histological methods in general.

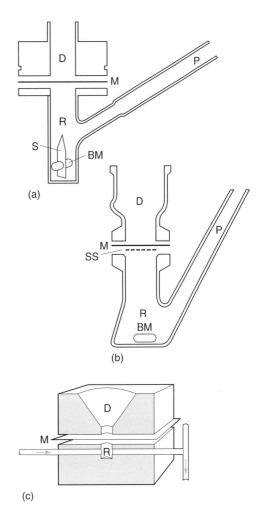

Fig. 38.9 Diffusion cells for simulation of in vivo conditions (not to scale). (a) Teflon and glass cell. (b) Glass cell with stainless steel support for the membrane. (c) Stainless steel cell with flow through receptor solution. *Key:* D, donor compartment; R, receptor compartment; M, membrane; P, sampling port; BM, bar magnet; S, polyethylene sail; SS, stainless steel support (reproduced from Barry 1983 with permission of the copyright owner).

Histochemical techniques have been used for those few compounds that produce coloured endproducts after chemical reaction. A mistake in the past was to colour a penetrant with a dye and examine skin sections to locate the penetrant. However, each chemical species partitions and diffuses separately, and so the dyed complex dissociates and results are valid only for the dye itself. Added dye, or other different tracer molecules, should not be used.

A few compounds fluoresce, revealing their behaviour by microscopy, e.g. vitamin A, tetracycline and benzpyrene. Tumours fluoresce in photodynamic therapy when treated with 5-aminolaevulinic acid.

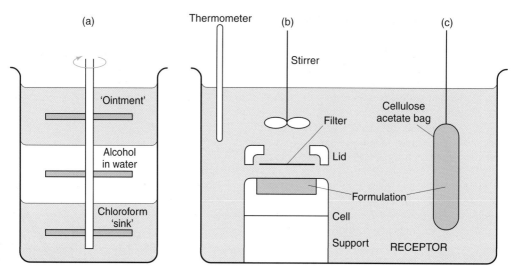

Fig. 38.10 Release methods without a rate-limiting membrane (not to scale). (a) Stirrer agitates three phases, which represent the formulation, the skin and the blood supply. (b) Release from an open container to a stirred immiscible receptor phase. (c) Release through a simple dialysis membrane (reproduced from Barry 1983 with permission of the copyright owner).

Microscopic autoradiography is difficult to apply to diffusable substances without modification. Substances emit α and β rays and there may be considerable scattering on the autoradiogram; reducing substances reacting with the photographic emulsion, or an incorrect technique, can produce shadowing. Tritium-labelled isotopes are useful because of their weak emissions; strong β emitters darken areas up to 2 or 3 mm away, a great distance at the cellular scale.

Confocal microscopy can provide information at different depths in the skin.

Surface loss

In theory, we should be able to determine the flux of material into skin from the loss rate from the vehicle. However, because of skin impermeability, the concentration decrease in the vehicle would generally be small and analytical techniques would have to be sensitive and accurate. Also those differences which could be detected would probably arise because the vehicle changed by evaporation or by dilution with sweat or transepidermal water, and not simply by drug partitioning into the skin. Alternatively, any drug decrease may only reflect deposition on the skin surface or combination with the stratum corneum, rather than penetration to the systemic circulation. Loss techniques have in the past mainly been used to monitor radioactive species; advances in HPLC analysis have made the methods more widely applicable.

Microdialysis

Microdialysis probes are inserted in the dermis and perfused with buffer. Drug molecules pass from the extracellular fluid into the buffer through pores in the membrane, which exclude large molecules, particularly proteins. The resulting drug solution is collected and analysed. For highly protein-bound drugs, the technique requires very sensitive methods of analysis as the drug concentrations in the samples are reduced accordingly.

Analysis of body tissues or fluids

When urinary analysis is used, the entire drug penetrating the skin should be accounted for by 'calibrating' the subject with a slow intravenous injection and a simultaneous determination of blood levels. This procedure allows for the pharmacokinetic factors inherent in drug absorption, distribution, storage, metabolism and excretion. Analysis of circulating blood can present difficulties with dilution, extraction and detection, although we may now routinely detect nanogram (or even lower) drug quantities. Faeces analysis alone has limited use. Sometimes the drug has an affinity for an animal organ, which can be removed and analysed, e.g. for iodine, iodides and mercury. Tissue biopsies may be analysed and even individual sections measured. Adhesive tape can strip sequential layers of the stratum corneum; the individual strips are then analysed for drug content.

Observation of a pharmacological or physiological response

If the drug stimulates a reaction in the viable tissues, we may use this to determine penetration kinetics. Local allergic, toxic or physiological reactions include sweat gland secretion, pigmentation, sebaceous gland activity, vasodilatation, vasoconstriction, vascular permeability, epidermal proliferation and keratinization. The most productive biopharmaceutical technique has been the vasoconstrictor or blanching response to topical steroids. For example, Figure 38.11 illustrates the blanching profiles of betamethasone benzoate in a quick-break aerosol foam, in the foam concentrate and in semi-solids, compared with Betnovate cream. The superiority of the aerosol foam and the inferiority of the benzoate cream are apparent. We use the vasoconstrictor test to screen novel synthetic steroids and develop topical formulations, to test marketed products for bioavailability and clinical efficacy, to perform fundamental studies in percutaneous absorption and to develop dosage regimens.

Other response methods include changes in blood pressure (e.g. topical application of nitroglycerin), reduction in pain threshold and production of convulsions.

Physical properties of the skin

Relevant methods include measurement of transepidermal water loss, thermal determinations (particularly differential scanning calorimetry), mechanical analysis, use of ultrasound, classification of function and dimension, spectral analysis (infrared and Raman) and the use of photoacoustic and electrical properties.

Bioassays

Many specialized bioassays screen topical formulations prior to clinical trial, including those for antibacterials, antifungals, antiyeast preparations, antimitotics, antiperspirants, sunscreen agents, antidandruff, anaesthetic-analgesic formulations, antipruritics, antiwart, poison oak/ivy dermatitis, antiacne and psoriasis. Topical corticosteroid bioassays are the most sophisticated and refined of all such bioassays (discussed previously in this chapter); other steroid bioassays include antigranuloma, thymus involution, inflammation, cytological techniques and psoriasis bioassays.

MAXIMIZING THE BIOAVAILABILITY OF DRUGS APPLIED TO SKIN

Most drugs penetrate human skin poorly and many major research efforts have attempted to maximize the input of such drugs. The great challenge for the future is to deliver the therapeutic peptides and proteins arising from the biotechnology revolution. The fundamental problem has two major aspects: not only is the stratum corneum a resistant barrier to penetration, but there is great biological variability in its impermeability. The next section will therefore consider some ways in which pharmaceutical scientists have attempted to circumvent the horny layer barrier.

Drug or prodrug selection

The easiest way to consider factors that affect the permeation rate of a drug through the stratum corneum is via the simple equation for steady-state flux (Eqn 38.3). When, as is usual, the stratum corneum provides the major source of diffusional resistance of the skin, the partition coefficient of the drug is crucially important in establishing a high initial concentration in the first layer of this membrane. If our drug does not possess the correct physicochemical properties (usually it has too low a partition coefficient), we may be able to design a prodrug with an optimal partition coefficient for entering the skin barrier. After absorption and diffusion to the viable tissues, enzymes convert the prodrug to the active species. Very many steroid derivatives have topical antiinflammatory activity greater than their

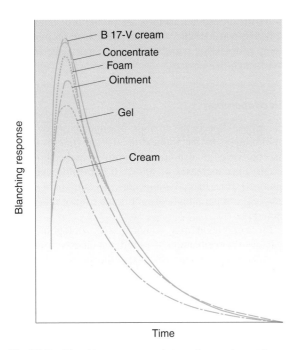

Fig. 38.11 Blanching response to betamethasone benzoate formulations containing 0.025% steroid and 0.1% betamethasone 17-valerate (B 17-V) cream (reproduced from Barry 1983 with permission of the copyright owner).

parent steroids; with their optimized partition coefficients, they act as prodrugs (see earlier in this chapter).

Chemical potential adjustment

One scheme for optimizing the bioavailability of a topical medicament is to ensure that the drug exhibits its maximum chemical potential, and thus its maximum thermodynamic activity, within the vehicle (Eqn 38.8).

Under *ideal conditions*, the drug flux through the skin should be directly proportional to the drug activity in the vehicle, provided that D, γ and h remain constant. This has the important consequence that all saturated solutions of a specific drug in any vehicle (providing it does not modify the properties of the stratum corneum) should provide the same maximal flux.

However, it is possible to produce *supersaturated* solutions, either deliberately or via mixed vehicles evaporating on the skin. The theoretical maximum flux appropriate to thermodynamically stable vehicles may then increase many-fold using such supersaturated systems. Because supersaturated preparations are inherently unstable, manufacturers find it difficult to formulate them. An alternative is to employ controlled supersaturation in the rather special environments of transdermal patches; it is thought that this may offer the best hope of success. In practice, therefore, patients usually only meet the effects of supersaturation from volatile systems evaporating on their skin.

Hydration

Hydration of the stratum corneum is one of the most important factors in increasing the penetration rate of most substances; water opens up the compact layer of the horny layer. Moisturizing factors, occlusive films, hydrophobic ointments and transdermal patches all enhance skin bioavailability (discussed in the Skin hydration section earlier in this chapter and referred to in Table 38.1).

Ultrasound (phonophoresis)

This technique, used primarily in physiotherapy and sports medicine, involves placing the topical preparation on the skin over the area to be treated and massaging the site with an ultrasound source. The ultrasonic energy disturbs the lipid packing in the intercellular spaces of the stratum corneum by heating and cavitation effects, and thus enhances drug penetration into the tissue. A problem with the technique is, of course, the need for an ultrasonic probe, correctly focused to work in the stratum corneum. Thus the method is not readily suitable for home use.

Iontophoresis

Iontophoresis, the electrical driving of charged molecules into tissue, has applications in dentistry, ophthalmology, surgery and general medicine. As usually practised, the procedure involves passing a small direct current (approximately 0.5 mA/cm^2) through a drug-containing electrode in contact with the skin. A grounding electrode placed elsewhere on the body completes the electrical circuit. The transport of the charged molecules is driven primarily by electrical repulsion from the driving electrode. However, polar neutral molecules can also be delivered by a current-induced convective flow of water (electroosmosis). Considerable interest is now being shown in the possible transdermal delivery of therapeutic peptides and proteins, as well as many other drugs.

The Glucowatch device uses reverse electroosmosis to drive glucose from the blood to the skin surface, where it is analysed. Thus the technique can be used for the non-invasive glucose monitoring of diabetes.

A problem with the technique is that, although the apparent current density per unit area is low, nearly all the current penetrates via the low resistance route, i.e. the appendages, particularly the hair follicles. Thus the *actual* current density in the follicle may be high enough to damage growing hair. There is also concern about other possible irreversible changes to the skin.

As for ultrasound, there is the problem of home use, although considerable work has been done on miniaturizing systems for patient use, e.g. paper batteries and wristwatch-like devices.

Electroporation

Electroporation is the creation of aqueous pores in the lipid bilayers by the application of short (micro- to millisecond) electrical pulses of approximately 100–1000 V/cm. Flux increases of up to 10 000-fold have been obtained for charged molecules. Again, there is the problem of instrumentation for home use for this potent technique.

Electroporation may combine with iontophoresis to enhance the permeation of peptides such as vasopressin, luteinizing hormone-releasing hormone (LHRH), neurotensin and calcitonin.

Radiofrequency waves

A technique introduced in 2003 uses the energy of radiofrequency waves to form microchannels through the stratum corneum. A densely spaced array of microelectrodes takes microseconds to form holes through which an applied drug passes easily into the skin.

Stratum corneum removal

Laser ablation uses high-powered pulses from a laser to vaporize a section of the horny layer so as to produce permeable skin regions. The apparatus is costly and requires expert operation to avoid damage such as burns so it is hardly appropriate for home use. Hot needles have also been proposed.

Adhesive tape can remove the horny layer prior to drug application, as can controlled mechanical dermal abrasion. One other method forms a bleb (blister) by suction, an epidermatome removes the raised tissue, after which a morphine solution delivered directly to the exposed dermis produces fast pain relief.

Photomechanical wave

A drug solution is placed on the skin, covered by a black polystyrene target, and irradiated with a laser pulse. The resultant photomechanical wave produces stresses in the horny layer that enhance drug delivery. The technique is likely to remain experimental.

Microneedle array

The stratum corneum can be simply bypassed by an injection and one development of this approach is a device consisting of 400 microneedles to insert drug just below the barrier. The feeling to the skin is rather like a cat's tongue or shark skin. The solid silicon needles (coated with drug) or hollow metal needles (filled with drug solution) penetrate the horny layer without breaking and without stimulating nerves in the deeper tissues. Flux increases of up to 100 000-fold are claimed. The technique may also be combined with iontophoresis.

Chemical penetration enhancers

Substances exist which temporarily diminish the impermeability of the skin. Such materials, known also as *accelerants* or *sorption promoters*, can be used clinically, if they are safe and non-toxic, to enhance the penetration rate of drugs and even to treat patients systemically by the dermal route. The attributes of the ideal penetration enhancer are as follows:

- The material should be pharmacologically inert.
- It should be non-toxic, non-irritating and non-allergenic.
- The action should be immediate and the effect should be suitable and predictable.
- Upon removal of the material, the skin should immediately and fully recover its normal barrier property.
- The enhancer should not cause loss of body fluids, electrolytes or other endogenous materials.

- It should be compatible with all drugs and excipients.
- The substance should be a good solvent for drugs.
- The material should be cosmetically acceptable (such as good spreadability and skin 'feel').
- The chemical should formulate into all the variety of preparations used topically.
- It should be odourless, tasteless, colourless and inexpensive.

No single material possesses all these desirable properties. However, very many substances exhibit several of these attributes and they have been investigated clinically or in the laboratory. A sample summary includes:

- water
- sulfoxides (especially dimethylsulfoxide) and their analogues
- pyrrolidones
- fatty acids and alcohols
- azone and its derivatives
- surfactants: anionic, cationic and non-ionic
- urea and its derivatives
- alcohols and glycols
- essential oils, terpenes and derivatives
- synergistic mixtures.

For safety and effectiveness, the best penetration enhancer of all is water. Most substances penetrate better through hydrated stratum corneum than through the dry tissue. Thus, any chemical which is pharmacologically inactive, non-damaging and which promotes horny layer hydration can be considered as a penetration enhancer. Examples include the natural moisturizing factor and urea.

The literature on the use of skin penetration enhancers is voluminous – entire books have been devoted to considering various theories and examples. One simple way to classify enhancer actions is via the *lipid – protein – partitioning* concept. This hypothesis suggests that accelerants act by one or more ways selected from three main possibilities (see Fig. 38.1b).

Lipid action The enhancer interacts with the organized intercellular lipid structure of the stratum corneum so as to disrupt it and make it more permeable to drug molecules. Very many enhancers operate in this way. Some solvents may act by extracting the lipid components and thus make the horny layer more permeable.

Protein modification Ionic surface-active molecules in particular tend to interact well with the keratin in the corneocytes, to open up the dense keratin structure and make it more permeable. However, the intracellular route is not usually important in drug permeation, although drastic reductions to this route's resistance could open up an alternative pathway for drug penetration.

Partitioning promotion Many solvents can enter the stratum corneum, change its solvent properties and thus increase the partitioning of a second molecule into the horny layer. This molecule may be a drug, a coenhancer or a cosolvent. For example, ethanol has been used to increase the penetration of the drug molecules nitroglycerin and estradiol. Propylene glycol is also widely used, particularly to provide synergistic mixtures with molecules such as azone, oleic acid and the terpenes, i.e. to raise the concentration of these enhancers in the horny layer.

Ion pairs

Charged molecules do not readily penetrate the stratum corneum, so investigators have borrowed a technique used in analytical science. This is to form a lipophilic ion pair, by adding a suitable species of a charge opposite to that of the drug ion. The complex formed then readily partitions into the lipid of the stratum corneum, as the charges temporarily neutralize each other. The ion pair diffuses across the horny layer to meet the aqueous viable epidermis. There the complex dissociates into its component charged species, which are readily soluble in water and thus partition into the epidermis and diffuse onward. However, the magnitude of the enhancement obtained is not great, typically being only about twofold.

Complex coacervates

Complex coacervation is the separation of oppositely charged ions into a dense coacervate oil phase, which is rich in the ionic complex. A coacervate may be thought of in this context as a further development of ion pairs. Similarly to ion pairs, the coacervate partitions into the stratum corneum, where it behaves as ion pairs, diffusing, dissociating and passing into the viable tissues. As for simple ion pairs, the flux enhancement obtained is similarly modest.

Liposomes and transfersomes

Liposomes are colloidal particles, typically consisting of phospholipids and cholesterol, to which other ingredients may be added. These lipid molecules form concentric bimolecular layers in the form of vesicles that may be used to entrap and deliver drugs to and through the skin. How well they transport drugs *through* the skin is controversial, although significant enhanced fluxes, compared to saturated aqueous solution (maximum thermodynamic activity), have been obtained for several drugs. For example, the flux of estradiol has been increased 20-fold using a variety of liposomes. The same vesicles increased 10-fold the deposition of this hormone within the stratum corneum.

Transfersomes are a special type of liposome which incorporate so-called 'edge activators' – molecules such as sodium cholate. The inventors claim that such vesicles are ultradeformable (up to 10^5 times that of an unmodified liposome). As such, they can squeeze through pores in the stratum corneum, which are less than one-tenth the diameter of the liposome. Thus, sizes up to 200–300 nm can penetrate intact skin. Two particular features are claimed to be important when using transfersomes. First, they require a hydration gradient to encourage skin penetration, so they only exhibit their marked delivery abilities when applied to the skin under non-occluded conditions. Then the hydration gradient operating from the (relatively) dry skin surface towards the waterlogged viable tissues drives the transfersomes through the horny layer (Fig. 38.12). Secondly, they work best under in vivo conditions.

Truly remarkable results are claimed for transfersomes. Data indicate that as much as 50% of a topical dose of a protein or peptide (such as insulin) penetrates the skin in vivo in 30 minutes.

Ethosomes are somewhat similar entities, which incorporate a relatively high concentration of ethanol to achieve good drug delivery.

High-velocity particles

The PowderJect system fires solid particles through the stratum corneum into the lower skin layers, using a supersonic shock wave of helium gas travelling at mach 2–3. The claimed advantages of the system include:

- pain-free delivery – the particles are too small to trigger the pain receptors in the skin
- improved efficacy and bioavailability
- targeting to a specific tissue, such as a vaccine delivered to epidermal cells
- sustained release or fast release
- accurate dosing
- overcomes needle phobia

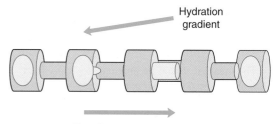

Fig. 38.12 Ultradeformable transfersome squeezing through minute pores in the stratum corneum, driven by the water concentration gradient. The modified liposome thus penetrates from the horny layer surface (relatively dry) to the wet viable tissues.

- safety – the device avoids:
  - skin damage
  - infection from needles or splashback of body fluids, particularly important for HIV and hepatitis B virus.

However, there have been problems with bruising of the skin and particles bouncing off the skin surface. At present, the development work with this technique appears to have ceased.

A similar device is the Intraject, which is a development of the vaccine gun designed to deliver liquids through the skin without the use of needles.

TRANSDERMAL THERAPEUTIC SYSTEMS

Probably the most innovative practical step in the science of transdermal delivery in recent years has been the introduction into medicine of skin patches.

The original transdermal therapeutic system (TTS) or transdermal (drug) delivery system (T(D)DS) was introduced as a device which would release drug to the skin at a controlled rate, well below the maximum that the tissue can accept. Thus, the device, not the stratum corneum, would control the rate at which a drug diffuses through the skin, as the intended flux would be much lower than the maximum skin flux.

A TTS tries to provide systemic therapy in a more convenient and effective way than parenteral or oral therapy. The claimed advantages for the percutaneous over the oral route include the following:

- Drug administration through skin eliminates variables which influence gut absorption, such as changes in pH along the gastrointestinal tract, food and fluid intake, stomach emptying time and intestinal motility and transit time, and the presence of human and bacterial enzymes.
- Drug enters the systemic circulation directly, eliminating the 'first-pass' effect of enzymes in the gut and the liver, the body's main metabolizing organ. (But note that skin has its own enzymes and may thus metabolize some 5% of drug types.)
- Transdermal input may provide controlled, constant drug administration, displaying a single pharmacological effect. The continuity of input may permit the use of drugs with short half-lives and improve patient compliance.
- Percutaneous administration could eliminate pulse entry into the circulation. Peaks in plasma concentrations often produce undesirable effects and troughs may be subtherapeutic.

- The transdermal route can use drugs with a low therapeutic index.
- Patches may be readily removed, although there is a reservoir effect and blood levels do not fall immediately to zero after TTS removal.

Transdermal systems usually contain potent drugs that should not irritate or sensitize the skin; they must be stable and have the correct physicochemical properties to partition into the stratum corneum and permeate to the vasculature.

Device design

Manufacturers design patches in a variety of ways but for simplicity, we may categorize these into one of two main types: the monolith (or matrix) or the rate-limiting membrane configurations. In considering these two designs, it is convenient to accept initially the original assumption that the skin under the patch operates as a perfect sink, even though no TTS produced to date works perfectly on this basis.

Monolith or matrix system

In these patches, the Higuchi Square Root of Time Law is usually obeyed. Equations 38.9–14 illustrate the relationships when the drug is dissolved in the matrix or exists as a suspension; Figure 38.13 illustrates release profiles, plotted both linearly and as square route functions of time. Figure 38.14 illustrates the fundamental construction for a suspension-type TTS. An occlusive backing layer protects the drug matrix, which comprises a suspension of drug in equilibrium with its saturated solution (maximum thermodynamic activity). An adhesive layer contains dissolved drug in equilibrium with that in the matrix and attaches the patch to the skin. A protective strippable film is removed immediately prior to application.

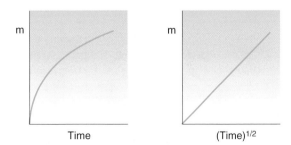

Fig. 38.13 Release profiles, plotted both linearly and as square route functions of time, for matrix or monolith patches operating under Higuchi conditions (see Eqn 38.13).

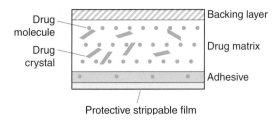

Fig. 38.14 Fundamental construction for a suspension-type transdermal therapeutic system based on a matrix or monolith design (not to scale).

Rate-limiting membrane system

As these patches include a membrane, we might expect that the release profile would follow the simple Fickian conditions considered at the beginning of this chapter. Thus, at steady state we would expect the amount of drug released to the skin to be directly related to time (see Eqn 38.3 and Fig. 38.3). However, such a profile only follows when the membrane is initially free of drug. The lag time then represents the period during which the membrane equilibrates with drug *after application to the sink* (the skin in this case). In practice, this does not happen because the drug equilibrates in all patch components on storage before the patient receives the patch.

Figure 38.15 illustrates the situation; a typical patch in this category consists of a backing layer, a reservoir containing the drug, the membrane, a skin adhesive and the protective film. On storage, the drug equilibrates into the membrane and adhesive. This portion of the drug more readily releases into the skin, as it does not have to permeate through all of the membrane. The result is to produce a so-called 'burst effect' that leads to the type of plot illustrated in Figure 38.16. Such profiles may be confused with Higuchi plots, i.e. with matrix release plots, as illustrated in the first plot of Figure 38.13. An advantage is that the burst component can provide a quick-acting, priming dose of drug.

Future trends

It has become apparent to pharmaceutical scientists how difficult it is to formulate a TTS in such a way that the control of delivery remains within the patch and not in the very impervious skin of the patient. It is also expensive to manufacture complex, multilayered patches, particularly those containing membranes. There is thus a trend to concentrate on simple designs that are also thinner and therefore less obtrusive and so cosmetically more acceptable. The result is a move towards the simple adhesive matrix patch illustrated in Figure 38.17.

Clinical patches

The following section discusses some examples of TTSs used in therapy. Besides their inherent clinical interest and value, each one exemplifies one or more biopharmaceutical features of importance in this mode of disease management.

Transdermal scopolamine (hyoscine)

The first patch brought to market delivered hyoscine through the thin, relatively permeable, postauricular skin via a rate-controlling membrane. The contact adhesive liberates priming drug to saturate horny layer binding sites and thus reduces the time before the clinical effect arises.

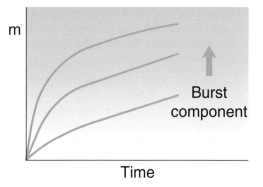

Fig. 38.16 Release profile from rate-limiting membrane patches; effect of increasing amount of drug partitioned into the membrane and adhesive on storage (which provides the 'burst' component).

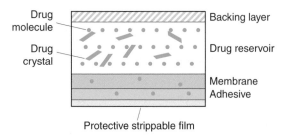

Fig. 38.15 Transdermal therapeutic system based on a rate-limiting membrane design (not to scale).

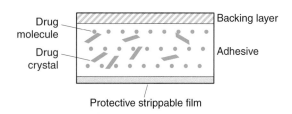

Fig. 38.17 Simple drug-in-adhesive patch (not to scale).

The TTS treats motion sickness and, besides its value to cruise passengers, it was used by American astronauts. Two-thirds of patients still experience a dry mouth but even this has been turned to advantage, by woodwind instrumentalists in orchestras. They have found that application of the patch suppresses salivation.

This patch provides an excellent example of the original basic philosophy of TDDSs. In the conventional dosage form of injections or tablets, hyoscine can produce side-effects such as excitement, confusion and hallucinations, which the controlled input from the TDDS eliminates. About 70% of the control resides in the patch; the variable nature of the patient's skin affects the remainder.

Transdermal nitroglycerin (glyceryl trinitrate – GTN)

A major use of TDDS technology is to deliver nitroglycerin, isosorbide dinitrate and isosorbide mononitrate for the treatment of angina, congestive heart failure and acute myocardial infarction. The nitroglycerin patch can also be valuable for the prophylactic treatment of phlebitis and extravasation secondary to venous cannulation.

The introduction of the first nitroglycerin device led to a vigorous debate as to the relative merits of patches, ointments and tablets. The main arguments revolved around whether or not the patch system delivered suboptimal drug levels to the blood; whether tolerance developed to the nitroglycerin; and if the TDDS or the patient's skin controlled the rate of GTN input. With regard to the last point, it was concluded that only about 50% or less of the control was inherent within the device.

Transdermal estradiol

Several estradiol systems treat females for menopausal symptoms or other results of oestrogen deficiency (hormone replacement therapy – HRT). The claimed benefits of transdermal delivery over oral therapy for such patches include the following:

- First-pass metabolism is avoided; therefore a lower dose is administered.
- Continuous, low-rate transdermal dosing maintains oestrogen plasma levels within physiological limits.
- Such dosing does not affect the blood levels of proteins produced by the liver. In particular, the angiotensin concentration remains the same and therefore the risk of hypertension is minimized. (Oral oestrogen therapy has been likened to hitting the liver with a sledgehammer!) However, as liver enzymes are not stimulated, the beneficial effects on serum lipids are absent.
- Large increases in estrone (the major metabolite of estradiol) are avoided and the estrone:estradiol ratio restores to the premenopausal value.

Originally, the oestrogen patch was marketed only for women who had undergone a hysterectomy, because unopposed oestrogen (that which is given alone) can cause endometrial hyperplasia and increase the risk of endometrial cancer. Now women with an intact uterus can use combination patches that deliver estradiol for 2 weeks, followed by a further 2 weeks of a progestin such as norethysterone acetate or levonorgestrel.

Patches are applied once or twice weekly and are effective in treating menopausal and postmenopausal symptoms such as flushing and vaginal atrophy. They also appear to be valuable in treating osteoporosis. Official medical advice (March 2005) is that for short-term hormone replacement therapy for menopausal symptoms, the balance of risks and benefits is generally favourable. Overall, however, chronic use leads to a net harm.

Transdermal contraceptive

This patch delivers the same hormones as given orally, i.e. ethinyl estradiol and norelgestromin. The woman applies one patch weekly for 3 weeks, with a 1 week patch-free period to allow for a menstrual period.

Transdermal clonidine

This formulation was originally introduced to treat hypertension. It was then reported to ameliorate some of the short-term symptoms associated with stopping smoking (craving, irritability, anxiety, restlessness and hunger).

After its introduction, clinical trials revealed a high incidence of topical irritation to clonidine (up to 50% of patients were affected). This finding emphasizes the importance of screening drug candidates for such side-effects before committing significant resources to a transdermal delivery programme.

Transdermal fentanyl

This opioid analgesic patch treats chronic, intractable pain, such as that produced by cancer, over a 72-hour period. A TTS providing 25 µg of fentanyl per hour is approximately equivalent to oral administration of 90 mg of morphine sulfate daily. The original design of this patch used the reservoir or membrane technology but this has now been superseded by the simpler matrix design.

Transdermal buprenorphine

The Transdec (Napp) matrix patch comes in three strengths for 72-hour use for moderate to severe pain.

Transdermal nicotine

There are several such patches available and commercial competition is intense because of the huge worldwide market for smoking cessation therapy. Within the first year of introduction, total sales exceeded that for any other drug in history! However, as is common to most forms of antismoking treatment, subsequent yearly sales fell dramatically.

The TTSs provide an alternative to treatment via nicotine chewing gum, lozenges, sublingual tablets, nasal spray and inhalers. The patches, designed to be worn for 16 or 24 hours, are available in different strengths so as to provide a weaning process. The concept is to try to match the plasma trough levels of nicotine produced by cigarette smoking but not to mimic the 'hit' arising from tobacco smoke inhalation. A bolus of nicotine reaches the brain within seconds after inhaling from a cigarette and this is the main *physiological* component of addiction.

The nicotine patch can also maintain labour when there is danger of a premature delivery and a Parkinson's patient has claimed that the device had 'restored him to his pre-Parkinson's self'. Tourette's syndrome is a bizarre disorder characterized by jerky motions, rage and a propensity to utter obscenities. Nicotine patches improved the effectiveness of drugs used in the treatment of afflicted children.

Nicotine is an ideal skin penetrant as it has a low molar mass, is liquid (low melting point), has a balanced partition coefficient and is miscible with oil and water (discussed further in the Ideal properties for drug penetration section earlier in this chapter).

Transdermal testosterone

Hypogonadism (arising from pituitary or testicular disorder) affects 1 in 200 men and testosterone deficiency may also arise from accidents and orchidectomy. The first patch developed was applied to the shaved scrotum, as scrotal skin is the most permeable skin site in man. With developments in formulation, more convenient areas, such as the back, abdomen, thigh or upper arm, may be used.

Transdermal testosterone is now being tested on women who have suffered hysterectomies and ovary removals to treat loss of sexual desire. Proponents now propose that it could be used also for women who have not undergone such operations.

Transdermal oxybutynin

This drug is used in the treatment of bladder instability and incontinence. When given orally, oxybutynin has a short half-life, a high first-pass metabolism and a systemic bioavailability that has been claimed to be as low as 6%. These disadvantages make the molecule a good candidate for skin delivery.

General conclusions on the usage of transdermal patches

1. In recent years, the formulation of transdermal patches has been a vibrant developmental area within the pharmaceutical industry.
2. However, the original concept that the patch, not the skin, should control drug input to the patient has not been realized; no marketed patch fully controls the drug flux.
3. There has been a move from a complex patch structure towards a simpler matrix formulation.
4. Future progress will depend on:
   - correct choice of drug
   - synthesis of prodrugs
   - development of suitable penetration enhancers.
5. There is a need to solve problems relating to, e.g.:
   - irritancy
   - sensitization
   - cutaneous metabolism
   - localized body load of drug
   - wearability of the patch for up to 7 days; the device has to:
     – be thin, flexible and unobtrusive
     – adhere well when the patient sweats, exercises and bathes
     – not encourage microbial growth
     – and not collect dirt around the periphery (where the adhesive contacts the environment).

FORMULATION OF DERMATOLOGICAL VEHICLES

People apply many skin preparations, ranging from powders, through semi-solids to liquids. Formulators have often in the past developed such preparations for their stability, compatibility and patient acceptability, rather than considering the influences that the components may have on drug bioavailability. Modern formulation methods nowadays, however, have to concentrate on biopharmaceutical principles.

A valuable approach in designing a vehicle to produce optimum bioavailability is to use fundamental permeation theories, while remembering that the treatment regimen and the diseased skin usually violate the constraints of simple diffusion theory. However, with our present knowledge, such a formal approach may often limit the investigator to a single-phase system such as a polar gel; multiphase systems usually provide intractable theoretical problems. But physicians usually want a topical application to provide several therapeutic effects, as well as good absorption. These aims include antiinflammatory efficacy in acute inflammation, symptomatic relief of pain and itch, protection from irritation, cleansing, lubricant and emollient actions. A single-phase vehicle cannot readily achieve so much; complex multicomponent bases are needed. Patients also tend to favour creams rather than gels or ointments.

This section considers the formulation of vehicles mainly in terms of *unmedicated* preparations. A good base must foster the remarkable recuperative capability of skin. For minor conditions, it is often as important to select a vehicle that promotes healing and does no further damage, as it is to apply a therapeutic agent. A general rule is that for wet lesions, the patient should use an aqueous dressing and for dry skin, a lipophilic base is best. Most vehicles are blended from one or more of three main components – aqueous solvents, powder and oil – together with thickening and emulsifying agents, buffers, antioxidants, preservatives, colours, propellants, etc. Typical examples of the main types of skin preparation will now be considered. The basic structural details of patches have been outlined in the Transdermal therapeutic systems section of this chapter.

Dermatological formulations

Liquid preparations

Liquid preparations for external application include simple soaks or baths, applications, liniments, lotions, paints, varnishes, tinctures and ear drops. A simple soak provides an active ingredient in aqueous solution or suspension, sometimes with water-miscible solvents. Gums and gelling agents may vary the consistency from mobile liquids to stiff ringing gels. Bath additives such as Oilatum emollient deposit a layer of liquid paraffin on the stratum corneum in an attempt to maintain its moisture content by occlusion. Applications may be liquid or viscous preparations and often incorporate parasiticides, e.g. dicophane, benzyl benzoate, γ-benzene hexachloride and malathion. Liniments may be alcoholic or oily solutions or emulsions, which should not be applied to broken skin. Lotions are aqueous solutions or suspensions from which water evaporates to leave a thin uniform coating of powder. Evaporation cools and soothes the skin, making lotions valuable for treating acutely inflamed areas. Alcohol enhances the cooling effect and glycerol sticks the powder to the skin. Lotions may also be dilute emulsions, usually of the oil-in-water type. Paints, varnishes and tinctures present solutions of active ingredients in volatile solvents such as water, industrial methylated spirits, acetone or ether. Ear drops are often aqueous solutions, although glycerol and alcohol may also be used.

Gels (jellies)

Gels are two-component semi-solid systems rich in liquid. Their one characteristic feature is the presence of a continuous structure providing solid-like properties. In a typical polar gel, a natural or synthetic polymer builds a three-dimensional matrix throughout a hydrophilic liquid. Typical polymers used include the natural gums tragacanth, carrageenan, pectin, agar and alginic acid; semi-synthetic materials such as methylcellulose, hydroxyethylcellulose, hydroxypropyl methylcellulose and carboxymethylcellulose; and the synthetic polymer Carbopol (carbomer). Certain clays such as bentonite, veegum and laponite can be used. Provided that the drug does not bind to the polymer or clay, such gels release medicaments well; the pores allow relatively free diffusion of molecules that are not too large.

Powders

Dusting powders for application to skinfolds have finely divided (impalpable) insoluble powders, which dry, protect and lubricate. Examples include talc, zinc oxide, starch and kaolin. Dusting powders should not contain boric acid since abraded skin may absorb it in toxic amounts.

Ointments

Ointments are greasy, semi-solid preparations, often anhydrous and containing dissolved or dispersed medicaments.

Hydrocarbon bases   These usually consist of soft paraffin or mixtures with hard paraffin. Paraffins form a greasy film on the skin, inhibiting moisture loss and improving hydration of the horny layer in dry scaly conditions. This hydration is also a main reason why ointments are so effective in encouraging percutaneous absorption of a drug.

The plastibases are a series of hydrocarbons containing polyethylene, which forms a structural matrix in systems which are fluid at the molecular scale but are typical dermatological semi-solids. They are soft, smooth, homogeneous, neutral, colourless, odourless, non-irritating, non-sensitizing, extremely stable vehicles. Plastibases are compatible with most medicaments and they maintain their consistency even at high concentrations of solids and under extremes of temperature. The bases apply easily and spread readily, they adhere to the skin, imparting a velvety, non-greasy feel, and can readily be removed.

Soap-base greases may be produced by, for example, incorporating aluminium stearate in a heavy mineral oil. A random arrangement of metallic soap fibres weaves throughout the oil, producing a product which changes its consistency only slightly when heated; the base readily incorporates drugs and the addition of lanolin permits the absorption of a little water.

Fats and fixed oil bases   Dermatological vehicles have frequently contained fixed oils of vegetable origin, consisting essentially of the mono-, di- and triglycerides of mixtures of saturated and unsaturated fatty acids. The most common oils include peanut, sesame, olive, cottonseed, almond, arachis, maize and persic. Such oils can decompose on exposure to air, light and high temperatures, and may turn rancid. Trace metal contaminants catalyse oxidative reactions which the formulator combats with antioxidants such as butylated hydroxytoluene, butylated hydroxyanisole or propyl gallate, or with chelating agents such as the salts of ethylenediaminetetraacetic acid (EDTA). However, antioxidants may be incompatible with the drug or they may sensitize some patients.

Silicones Dimethicones, or dimethyl polysiloxanes, have properties similar to hydrocarbon bases. They are water repellent with a low surface tension and are incorporated into barrier creams to protect the skin against water-soluble irritants.

Absorption bases Absorption bases soak up water to form water-in-oil emulsions, while retaining their semisolid consistencies. Generally, they are anhydrous vehicles composed of a hydrocarbon base and a miscible substance with polar groups which functions as a water-in-oil emulsifier, e.g. lanolin, lanolin isolates, cholesterol, lanosterol and other sterols, acetylated sterols or the partial esters of polyhydric alcohols such as sorbitan monostearate or oleate. Bases such as wool alcohols ointment and simple ointment deposit a greasy film on the skin, similar to a hydrocarbon base, but they suppress less the transepidermal water loss. However, they may hydrate the stratum corneum by applying a water-in-oil emulsion, thus prolonging the time during which the horny layer can absorb moisture. Some individuals are sensitive to lanolin. This may be important because the sensitization occurs unexpectedly and physicians frequently overlook it, especially in atopic patients who may apply large quantities of lanolin-containing emollients for protracted periods. Modern purified lanolin preparations are less sensitizing.

Emulsifying bases These essentially anhydrous bases contain oil-in-water emulsifying agents which make them miscible with water and so washable or 'self-emulsifying'. There are three types, depending on the ionic nature of the water-soluble emulsifying agents: anionic (e.g. emulsifying ointment), cationic (e.g. cetrimide emulsifying ointment) or non-ionic (e.g. cetomacrogol emulsifying ointment). Because they contain surfactants, emulsifying bases may help to bring the medicament into more intimate contact with the skin. The bases mix with aqueous secretions and readily wash off the skin; thus they are useful for scalp treatment.

Water-soluble bases Formulators prepare water-soluble bases from mixtures of high and low molecular weight polyethylene glycols (macrogols, carbowaxes). Suitable combinations provide products with an ointment-like consistency, which soften or melt on skin application. They are non-occlusive, mix readily with skin exudates and do not stain sheets or clothing; washing quickly removes any residue. The macrogols do not hydrolyse, deteriorate, support mould growth or irritate the skin. Examples include macrogol ointment and polyethylene glycol ointment. Because they are water soluble, they will not take up more than 8% of an aqueous solution before losing their desirable physicochemical characteristics. To enable a base to incorporate more water, stearyl alcohol can be substituted for some of the macrogol component. Macrogol bases are used with local anaesthetics such as lidocaine but they are incompatible with many chemicals including phenols, iodine, potassium iodide, sorbitol, tannic acid and the salts of silver, mercury and bismuth. The bases diminish the antimicrobial activity of quaternary ammonium compounds and methyl and propyl parahydroxybenzoates, and rapidly inactivate bacitracin and penicillin.

Creams

Creams are semi-solid emulsions for external application. Oil-in-water emulsions are most useful as water-washable bases, whereas water-in-oil emulsions are emollient and cleansing. Patients often prefer a w/o cream to an ointment because the cream spreads more readily, is less greasy and the evaporating water soothes the inflamed tissue. O/w creams ('vanishing' creams) rub into the skin; the continuous phase evaporates and increases the concentration of a water-soluble drug in the adhering film. The concentration gradient for drug across the stratum corneum therefore increases, promoting percutaneous absorption. To minimize drug precipitation, a formulator may include a less volatile, water-miscible cosolvent. An o/w cream is non-occlusive because it does not deposit a continuous film of water-impervious liquid. However, such a cream can deposit lipids and other moisturizers on and into the stratum corneum and so restore the tissue's hydration ability, i.e. the preparation has emollient properties.

Microemulsions are transparent, thermodynamically stable systems that, as their name suggests, have droplet sizes in the sub-micrometer range.

It is difficult to predict the role that an emulsion will play in percutaneous absorption. This is because to all the physiological and physicochemical considerations already discussed in this chapter must be added other factors such as:

- partitioning of the medicament between the emulsion phases
- addition of preservatives
- determination of a true viscosity for the diffusing molecules in the vehicle, and
- the possibility of phase inversion or cracking of the emulsion when applied to the skin.

Drug may also be trapped in the micelles and gel and liquid crystalline phases present in the continuous phase. Emulsions are complex systems and thus all medicaments must be considered individually with respect to emulsion design. There are few worthwhile formulation guidelines additional to the principles already discussed.

Pastes

Pastes are ointments containing as much as 50% powder dispersed in a fatty base. They may be useful for absorbing noxious chemicals in babies, such as the ammonia which bacteria release from urine. Because of their consistency, pastes localize the action of an irritant or staining material, such as dithranol or coal tar. They are less greasy than ointments because the powder absorbs some of the fluid hydrocarbons. Pastes lay down a thick, unbroken, relatively impermeable film that can be opaque and act as an efficient sun filter. Skiers use such formulations on the face to minimize windburn (excessive dehydration) and to block out the sun's rays.

Aerosols

Aerosols may function as drug delivery systems for solutions, suspensions, powders, semi-solids and emulsions.

Solution aerosols are simple products, with the drug dissolved in a propellant or a propellant/solvent mixture. Typical agents incorporated are steroids, antibiotics and astringents. The powder aerosol methodology is useful for difficult soluble compounds such as steroids and antibiotics. Semi-solid preparations, such as ointments and creams, may be prepared in a flexible bag with compressed nitrogen used for expulsion instead of a volatile propellant. Emulsion systems produce foams that may be aqueous or non-aqueous and stable or quick-breaking. Medicinal stable foams are aqueous formulations used, for example, for preoperative shaving and for contraception. The stable foam, which is similar to a medicated shaving cream, varies in stability depending on the selection of surfactant, solvent and propellant.

Cosmetic or aesthetic criteria for dermatological formulations

However well we design a topical vehicle for maximum drug bioavailability, the preparation must still be acceptable to the patient. A product of poor appearance may lead to non-compliance. Patients generally prefer a formulation which is easy to transfer from the container, spreads readily and smoothly, leaves no detectable residue and adheres to the treated area without being tacky or difficult to remove. Dosage of such preparations is typically in the range of 1–5 mg per square cm of skin.

Stiff pastes may be hard to rub into the skin or to apply evenly; application to damaged areas may be painful. However, a thick layer of material can occlude the tissue or protect it from mechanical, chemical or light damage. Ointments and pastes do this and the viscous drag imposed on application may dislodge scales, dead tissue and the remnants of previous doses. The medicament then makes intimate contact with the diseased site. A stiff preparation also helps to delineate the area of treatment.

The sensations of greasiness and tackiness arise from those constituents that form the skin film. For creams, stearic acid and cetyl alcohol produce non-tacky films. Formulations that include synthetic or natural gums should use the minimum amount, as the polymers tend to leave a tacky coating on the skin.

Insoluble solids leave an opaque layer, often appearing powdery or crusty. However, as therapy requires such solids in lotions and pastes, the formulator can do little to vary the film's nature and patients accept the residue as part of the treatment.

Physicochemical criteria for dermatological formulations

The developer of dosage forms must note the physical and chemical characteristics of the drug and the dosage form during preformulation studies, throughout bench-scale work, pilot studies and batch processing, at the manufacturing level and during storage and use of a product. Some general factors that a pharmaceutical scientist evaluates for a new semi-solid during developmental studies and storage include:

- stability of the active ingredients
- stability of the adjuvants
- rheological properties – consistency, viscoelasticity, extrudability
- loss of volatiles, including water
- phase changes – inhomogeneity, bleeding, cracking
- particle size distribution of dispersed phase
- apparent pH
- particulate contamination.

The first difficulty arises in assessing the chemical stabilities of the drug (in its complex vehicle) and the adjuvants. A general method establishes a shelf life by using an accelerated stability test at elevated temperatures and the Arrhenius relationship. However, for a multiphase system such as a cream, heat may change the phase distribution and may even crack the emulsion. Thus, the investigator may have to assess the preparation for a long time at the storage temperature. Because of vehicle complexity, it may be difficult to separate the labile components for analysis.

Many dermatological formulations contain volatile solvents and batches may lose some solvent through the walls of plastic containers or through faulty seams or ill-fitting caps.

Heterogeneous systems may suffer phase changes when stored incorrectly. Emulsions may crack and cream, suspensions can agglomerate and cake, and ointments and gels may 'bleed' as their matrices contract and squeeze out constituents. High temperatures can produce or accelerate such adjustments. Multipoint rheological assessments can readily quantify structural changes in colloidal systems; viscoelastic determinations, such as creep and oscillation, are also valuable.

For suspensions and emulsions, a particle size analysis may often detect a potentially unstable formulation long before any other parameter changes markedly. Emulsion globules may grow through coalescence as gel networks break down on storage; crystals may enlarge or change their habit or revert to a more stable, less active polymorphic form. Such alterations in crystal form may affect the therapeutic activity of the formulation.

The apparent pH of a topical product may change on storage. Although pH measurements of complex vehicles have no fundamental meaning, investigators sometimes use a pH electrode to monitor formulations as they age.

It can be difficult to manufacture creams and ointments completely free from foreign particles. Aluminium and tin tubes may contaminate a topical with 'flashings' – metal slivers and shavings formed during container fabrication. Their presence is particularly undesirable in ophthalmic ointments and various pharmacopoeial tests limit the extent of such contamination. Plastic tubes are now mainly used.

In addition to instrumental tests, the pharmaceutical scientist should note any qualitative changes during product storage. The colour may vary, e.g. natural fats, oils and lanolin brown as they oxidize, becoming rancid with a disagreeable odour. The texture may alter as phase relationships vary.

Microbial contamination and preservation; rancidity and antioxidants

Topical bases often contain aqueous and oily phases, together with carbohydrates and even proteins, and thus bacteria and fungi readily attack them. Microbial growth spoils the formulation and is a potential toxic hazard and a source of infection. Conditions which lower immunity, such as injury, debilitating diseases or drug therapy, may encourage organisms that are usually not highly infectious to infect the host, i.e. to become opportunistic pathogens. In 1969, 33 samples of 169 cosmetics and topical drugs surveyed were microbiologically contaminated, half with Gram-negative organisms which were a health hazard. In the mid-1960s, an outbreak of serious eye infection was traced to an antibiotic ophthalmic ointment contaminated with *Pseudomonas*.

There are many potential sources of microbial contamination. It can occur in raw material and in the manufacturing water, in processing and filling equipment, in packing material, if there is poor plant hygiene or an unclean environment, and if plant operatives fail to comply with good manufacturing procedures.

Because of the complexity of dermatological vehicles and their manufacturing processes, there exists no universal preservative, although the essential requirements for selecting a material to preserve a specific formulation can be summarized. The additive must be compatible with all ingredients; it should be stable to heat, prolonged storage and product use conditions; and it must be non-irritant, non-toxic and non-sensitizing to human tissue.

Many prototype pharmaceutical preparations could deteriorate on storage because some components oxidize when oxygen is present. This decomposition can be particularly troublesome in emulsions because emulsification may introduce air into the product and because of the high interfacial contact area between the phases.

The ideal antioxidant would possess the following properties:

- effective at low concentrations
- it and its decomposition products should be non-toxic, non-irritant, non-sensitizing, odourless and colourless
- stable and effective over a wide pH range
- neutral – should not react chemically with other ingredients
- non-volatile.

PROTOCOL FOR DESIGNING, DEVELOPING AND TESTING A DERMATOLOGICAL FORMULATION

Below are listed steps that may help a pharmaceutical scientist to design a satisfactory formulation. Although condensed, this should be useful for providing a checklist to control the development programme:

1. Identify the disease or condition to be treated.
2. Determine the site for drug action – skin surface, stratum corneum, viable epidermis, dermis, appendages or systemic circulation. Consider the body region, e.g. scalp, trunk, feet, nails, etc.
3. Note the receptor site within the target area (this may be unknown).
4. Estimate the condition of the average patient's skin – thickened (e.g. ichthyosis), broken and inflamed (e.g. acute eczema), pilosebaceous unit blocked (acne), etc. Remember that successful treatment may rapidly change the condition of the skin. For example, a weeping,

wet skin without an intact horny layer may heal quickly to produce a few cell layers with a dry surface.

5. Choose the best drug or prodrug for the disorder; consider its pharmacological and pharmacokinetic profiles, toxicity, sensitizing potential, stability, susceptibility to skin enzyme metabolism and physicochemical properties (particularly the diffusion coefficient and partition coefficient relevant to the horny layer).

6. Evaluate the optimum kinetics for drug delivery to the target site. Consider pulsed or steady-state treatment, amount and strength of dosage form and frequency of application.

7. In the light of points 1–6 above, select the type of formulation needed, e.g. cream, ointment, aerosol or other delivery device.

8. Decide if and where there is a rate-limiting step in the treatment, e.g. solely within the vehicle, permeation across the stratum corneum or clearance from the viable tissues. Concentrate on maximizing this rate.

9. Choose vehicle ingredients that are stable, compatible, and cosmetically and therapeutically acceptable. Be aware that these adjuvants may have their own therapeutic effects, e.g. occlusive vehicles moisturize the skin.

10. If the intention is to promote drug penetration, optimize the formulation to the maximum chemical potential of the drug. Remember that vehicles often change after application to skin as components evaporate or penetrate the skin and secretions mix with the formulation.

11. If the drug is a poor penetrant, consider using a chemical penetration enhancer but remember that a new enhancer will need a full toxicological screen. Regulatory authorities are particularly cautious about the use of such promoters.

12. Perform in vitro tests with trial formulations using a simple synthetic membrane (or no membrane) and a suitable sink; ensure that the drug releases readily from the vehicle.

13. Repeat 12, preferably with human skin, to monitor permeation. Such experiments may include a steady-state design and a scheme that mimics clinical use (the so-called finite dose design).

14. Conduct in vivo studies in animals and human volunteers to check for efficacy, safety and acceptability; determine the pharmacokinetic profile and the topical bioavailability.

15. Do clinical trials.

16. Throughout the programme, review the physicochemical behaviour and stability of the dosage form and package during preformulation studies, scale-up procedures, manufacture, storage and use.

REFERENCE

Barry, B.W. (1983) *Dermatological Formulations: Percutaneous Absorption*. Marcel Dekker, New York. (Provides additional fundamental information and general background.)

BIBLIOGRAPHY

Bronaugh, R.L., Maibach, H.I. (eds) (2005) *Percutaneous Absorption*, 4th edn. Marcel Dekker, New York. (A modern multi-authored text with many relevant chapters.)

Chien, Y.W. (1992) *Novel Drug Delivery Systems*, 2nd edn. Marcel Dekker, New York. (First two chapters provide background on rate-controlled drug delivery.)

Guy, R.H., Hadgraft, J. (eds) (2003) *Transdermal Drug Delivery*, 2nd edn. Marcel Dekker, New York. (Particularly useful for sections on predicting transdermal drug delivery.)

Potts, R.O., Guy, R.H. (eds) (1997) *Mechanisms of Transdermal Drug Delivery*. Marcel Dekker, New York. (Provides information on biophysical methods for determining molecular transport across skin.)

Roberts, M.S., Walters, K.A. (eds) (1998) *Dermal Absorption and Toxicity Assessment*. Marcel Dekker, New York. (A substantial text with much relevant information.)

Smith, E.W., Maibach, H.I. (eds) (2005) *Percutaneous Penetration Enhancers*, 2nd edn. CRC, Taylor and Francis, Boca Raton, Florida. (Chapters deal with chemical and physical enhancement methods and theories, together with analytical techniques.)

Williams, A.C. (2003) *Transdermal and Topical Drug Delivery*. Pharmaceutical Press, London. (A good introductory text with some emphasis on therapy.)

39

Wound dressings

G. M. Eccleston

INTRODUCTION

In the past, traditional fabric wound dressings were used extensively and were assumed to be passive products with only a minor role in the healing process. Their primary function was considered to be to keep the wound as dry as possible by allowing evaporation of exudate. However, it is now realized that a wound heals faster and more success-fully in a moist environment. This has lead to a greater understanding of the influence that wound dressings can have on wound healing and greater attention has been given to the design of more effective dressings. Over the last two decades, a large number of new dressings has become avail-able, based on the concept of creating an optimum environ-ment for the treatment of wounds. However, it is emphasized that there is still no single dressing suitable for the management of all types of wounds or for the treatment of a single wound during all phases of healing.

Many of the newer dressings aim to manage chronic wounds that are difficult to treat because wound physiol-ogy is altered. Such wounds are often a problem of the elderly and bedridden. Chronic wounds, as well as com-promising the quality of life of the patient, place an enor-mous financial burden on health services.

Successful design of wound dressings depends on an understanding of the healing process, the patient condition in terms of health, environment and social circumstance, and the effect that the physical chemical properties of the various dressing materials have on the wound-healing process.

WOUNDS AND WOUND HEALING

Wounds

The protective functions of the skin are compromised by injury. A wound can be defined as a defect or a break in the skin, resulting from either mechanical or thermal damage or as a result of the presence of an underlying medical or physiological condition. Wounds are classified according to the number of skin layers affected and the area of skin involved. *Superficial wounds* involve injury to the epidermis alone, *partial-thickness wounds* involve injury to the epidermis and the deeper dermal layers, including the blood vessels, sweat glands and hair follicles, and *full-thickness wounds* occur when the underlying subcutaneous fat or deeper tissues are also damaged. Wounds are described as *normal (acute)* if they heal rapidly with minimum scarring and *chronic* if they take longer than 8–12 weeks to heal.

Simple mechanical injuries such as cuts, grazes and minor burns are usually treated by the patient, whereas the more severe traumatic injuries caused by surgery, accidents, fires and wars require hospitalization. Chronic wounds require specialist nursing care. Without an understanding of all these factors, dressing selection is potentially ineffective and wasteful in terms of nursing time.

Wound healing

Wound healing may be considered as a dynamic process in which cellular and matrix components act together to reestablish the integrity of damaged tissue and replace lost tissue. Regardless of the source or the extent of tissue damage, under normal conditions the wound-healing process occurs in a predictable fashion as four overlapping stages: inflammation, migration, proliferation and maturation (remodelling). Healing is considered to be complete when the skin surface has reformed and has regained its tensile strength.

Inflammation

Inflammation is the body's initial response to injury and involves both cellular and vascular responses. The release of histamine and a number of other cell-mediated factors into the wound results in vasodilation, increased capillary permeation and stimulation of pain receptors. The release of a protein-rich exudate containing phagocytes and other materials from the blood capillaries onto the wound surface engulfs the debris of dead cells and bacteria (autolytic debridement). Fibrinogen in the exudate elicits the clotting mechanism, producing a clot or scab on the wound which causes bleeding to stop. It also gives strength and support to the injured tissue. This first stage of healing usually occurs within a few minutes to 24 hours of injury, when the wound will be red, inflamed, painful and moist.

Migration

Growth factors in the wound exudate promote the growth and migration of epithelial cells, fibroblasts and keratinocytes to the injured area to replace damaged and lost tissue. These cells regenerate from the margins, rapidly growing over the wound under the dried scab. This epithelial thickening and basal cell proliferation lasts for 2–3 days.

Proliferation

The proliferation phase involves the development of new tissue and occurs simultaneously or just after the migration phase (day 3 onwards), lasting from 5 to 20 days. Granulation tissue is formed by the infiltration of blood capillaries and lymphatic vessels into the wound, and by the supporting collagen network synthesized by fibroblasts. The network is important for developing the tensile strength of the skin. As the proliferation continues, further epithelial cell migration across the wound takes place, providing closure and visible wound contraction. During the proliferation stage, the wound is typically beefy red in colour and moist, but not exuding.

Maturation

This final phase of wound healing (also called the 'remodelling phase') involves the diminution of the vasculature and enlargement of collagen fibres, which increase the tensile strength of the repair. The timescale for wound repair is from about 3 weeks to 2 years. Commonly, the strength of the final scar reverts to 70–90% of that of the preinjured tissue.

Complications in wound healing: chronic wounds

Although wound healing is a natural and predictable phenomenon and most wounds will heal uneventfully, complications can sometimes occur that lead to prolonged healing times or chronic non-healing wounds. A chronic wound fails to heal because the orderly sequence of events is disrupted at one or more of the wound-healing phases. A normal wound may develop into a chronic wound at any time as a result of poor primary treatment, persistent infection or disease. The most common chronic wounds include venous stasis ulcers, diabetic ulcers, ischaemic ulcers, pressure ulcers (bedsores) and ulcers due to systemic infections or malignant disease. Bacteria may gain entry to the deeper tissue of an acute or chronic wound and overcome the body's defence mechanisms, giving rise to infection. Poor nutritional status, disease and other factors regarding the patient's condition may reduce the ability to fight infection, as well as interfere with healing mechanisms (Table 39.1).

Foreign bodies introduced deep into the wound at time of injury can cause chronic inflammatory responses,

Table 39.1 General patient factors that delay healing

Nutritional status	Deficiencies in protein, vitamins (especially ascorbic acid) and minerals impair the inflammatory phase and collagen synthesis and thus prolong healing times
Advancing age	Elderly patients have less effective immune systems, resulting in decreased resistance to pathogens. Potential problems in healing arise from skin changes, slower metabolism and chronic health conditions such as circulatory problems and diabetes
Disease	Poorly controlled diabetes mellitus, renal disease, malignant disease associated with hypoproteinaemia
Compromised circulation	Healing delayed because inadequate nutrients, blood cells and oxygen are delivered to the wound
Treatment	Patients receiving drugs that compromise the immune system (e.g. steroids), chemotherapy or radio-therapy
Mobility	Physical inactivity can result in pressure-related skin damage
Obesity	Excess tension placed on wound and decreased vascularity of adipose tissue delays healing. Mobility may be reduced
Smoking	Decreases oxygen delivery to the wound due to vasoconstriction and coagulation of small blood vessels

delaying healing and sometimes leading to granuloma or abscess formation. Keloid and other scars that are cosmetically unacceptable may result from excess collagen production during the final phases of the wound-healing process. Underlying diseases and drugs that suppress the inflammatory process, e.g. corticosteroids, also interfere with wound healing.

WOUND DRESSINGS

Dressings fall into several categories, depending on their function in the wound (occlusive, absorbent, adherence), the type of material employed to produce the dressing (polyurethane, alginate, collagen, silicone) or the physical form of the dressing (film, foam, gel). Some dressings are impregnated with medicaments such as antibacterial agents (silver, povidone iodine) or wound debridement agents (saline). The incorporation of pharmacological agents such as growth factors into dressings is still in its infancy, although a gel containing human platelet-derived growth factor (PDGF) is now available for treating chronic diabetic ulcers. The properties of the common dressing types in relation to the type of wound being treated are summarized in Table 39.2 and the dressings themselves are discussed in more detail below.

Traditional dressings

Traditional fabric wound dressings, such as natural or synthetic bandages, cottonwool, lint and gauzes, all with varying degrees of absorbency, have been used for centuries in the management of wounds. They can be used as primary or secondary dressings or as a part of a composite of several dressings, each with a specific function.

An example is gauze and cotton tissue (gamgee tissue) that is composed of a tubular cotton gauze wrap surrounding a layer of absorbent cottonwool. It is used to absorb exudate and should be applied over a primary wound dressing to avoid contaminating the wound with cellulose fibres. Many commercially available dressing packs provide a selection of sterile dressings conveniently packaged together. Bandages are used to provide support, act as dressing retention materials or provide protection to clothing following the application of ointments or creams.

Gauze dressings are made from woven and non-woven fibres of cotton, rayon, polyester or a combination of these fibres. Woven products are described as fine or coarse depending on the thread count per inch. Non-woven dressings are generally more absorbent and less likely to shed fibrous material into the wound which will delay healing. Sterile gauze pads are used for packing open wounds to absorb fluid and exudate. The fibres in the dressing act as a filter, drawing fluid away from the wound. The dressing needs to be changed frequently to prevent maceration of the healthy underlying tissue. Such dressings afford some bacterial protection, although this is lost if the outer surface of the dressing becomes moistened by either wound exudate or external fluids. Gauze dressings tend to adhere to wounds as fluid production diminishes, and are painful to remove. Gauze impregnated with soft paraffin is occlusive and easier to

Table 39.2   The key properties of the common types of dressings

Type of dressing	Key features	Uses
Impregnated gauze (soft paraffin or sodium chloride)	Various degrees of absorption. Inexpensive. Needs frequent changing. Dressing may stick to wound, causing pain and damage	Normal or highly exuding wounds. To apply creams or ointments to wound. Infected and necrotic wounds
Films	Non-absorbent. Permeable to moisture vapour, allowing some exudate to evaporate. May be transparent. Conform to contours. Adhere to wound. Impermeable to microorganisms	Later stages of wound healing where little exudate. Loss of water vapour can cause wound to dry out. Not for infected wounds and thin or fragile skin.
Foams	Absorbent. Allow gaseous exchange. Impermeable to water and microorganisms. Can remain on wound for extended times. Thermal insulation. Some are adherent	Performance varies between dressings. Generally low to moderately exuding wounds
Alginates	Form hydrophilic gel on contact with wound exudate to promote moist healing. Absorbent. Physical and thermal protection. Easily washed out of the wound	Performance varies between dressings. Moderate to high exuding wounds. Haemostasis. Suitable for infected wounds. Not suitable for dry wounds
Gels/hydrogels	Maintain moist wound bed by balanced hydration of wound. Absorbent. Non-adherent. Require secondary dressing	Cleansing of necrotic wounds by rehydrating dead tissue and encouraging autolytic debridement
Hydrocolloids	Create moist environment. Absorbent. Initially impermeable to water vapour and air. Adhere to wet and dry wounds. No pain on removal. Can remain on wound for extended times. Provide insulation. Do not require secondary dressing	Performance varies between dressings. Suitable for light to moderately exuding non-infected wounds. Facilitate rehydration and autolytic debridement of sloughy or necrotic wounds

remove from the skin. Antimicrobial agents such as silver and povidone iodine are incorporated into some dressings to control or prevent infection, as are debriding agents such as saline to prevent maceration of healthy tissue.

Traditional fabric dressings provide little occlusion and allow evaporation of moisture, resulting in a dry, desiccated wound bed. Although their unit costs are low, they do not provide a moist environment for wound healing. Consequently, they are being replaced for chronic wounds and burns by the more recently developed dressings described below.

Semi-permeable adhesive films

Semi-permeable adhesive film dressings are sterile, thin films made from polyurethane, usually coated on one side with hypoallergenic acrylic adhesives. These dressings are non-absorbent and permeable to water vapour and gases but not to liquids or microorganisms. Their transparency allows visual observation of the wound without removal of the dressing. The films vary in thickness and size but all are elastic and highly conformable to the anatomy and so suitable for use in flexible areas such as the elbows, knees and sacral areas.

This type of dressing maintains a moist wound-healing environment, promoting the formation of granulation tissue and autolysis of necrotic tissue. However, they are not suitable for use on infected wounds or moderate to heavily exuding wounds where water vapour loss may occur at a slower rate than exudate formation. If the dressing is not changed frequently, the accumulation of exudate under the film may lead to skin maceration and bacterial proliferation. Semi-permeable adhesive film dressings are sometimes difficult to handle and apply as they tend to wrinkle on removal from their packs.

Although the films developed more recently have improved water vapour permeability properties, they are still used mainly as primary or secondary dressings for partial-thickness wounds with little or no exudate, and to prevent and manage the initial stages of pressure ulcers by protecting the fragile skin. The dressings available differ in terms of film thickness and size, vapour permeability, adhesiveness, conformability and extensibility.

Foam dressings

Foam dressings are in the form of sheets of polymer foam, typically polyurethane. Some foams have additional wound contact layers to avoid adherence when the wound is dry and an occlusive polymeric backing layer to prevent excess fluid loss and bacterial contamination. Absorbency is controlled by foam properties such as texture, thickness and pore size. Foam dressings are superior to film dressings because in addition to maintaining a moist environment, they are absorbent and also provide good thermal insulation. The open pore structure also gives a high moisture vapour transmission rate (HVTR).

Commercially available foam dressings vary from products with foam structures that are suitable for partial- or full-thickness wounds with minimal or moderate drainage, to highly absorbent foam structures for heavily exuding wounds. They are used as primary wound dressings for absorption and insulation and as secondary dressings for wounds with packing. Sometimes the foam dressing may be prepared immediately before use and allowed to expand in volume within the cavity of the wound.

Alginate dressings

Alginate dressings are produced from the calcium and sodium salts of alginic acid, a polysaccharide obtained from certain species of brown seaweeds comprising mannuronic and guluronic acid units. They are available as dry woven, fibrous mats and sheets for wound dressings and as thin ribbons and twisted fibrous ropes for packing into wounds. The dressings interact with wound fluid and blood to form a protective film of gel that maintains an occlusive, non-adherent moist healing environment within the contours of the wound. The interaction occurs because a partial ion exchange reaction takes place in situ between calcium ions in the dressing and sodium ions from the wound exudate, resulting in the production of a gel on the wound surface.

The gelling properties of individual dressings depend on both the relative concentrations and arrangements of the mannuronic and guluronic monomers as well as the amounts of calcium and sodium ions. Dressings rich in mannuronic acid tend to react readily with sodium ions, forming soft amorphous gels, whereas those rich in guluronic monomer gel less readily to form firmer gels.

Alginate dressings are generally easy to remove without pain, either by lifting the partially gelled sheet off the wound or by rinsing the gel away with water or physiological saline. They generally need a secondary dressing to prevent the alginate from drying out. Since calcium alginate is a natural haemostat, alginate-based dressings are indicated to control minor wound bleeding.

Alginate dressings are highly absorbent and are used for moderate to heavily exuding wounds. A major disadvantage of alginate dressings is that they cannot be used for dry wounds or those covered with hard necrotic tissue because, to function effectively, they need to absorb exudate from the wound. Different alginate dressings show significant differences in characteristics such as fluid retention, adherence and dressing residues.

Hydrogel dressings

Hydrogel dressings are available in several forms including amorphous hydrogels (that can take up the shape of the wound), saturated gauzes or hydrogel sheets. Hydrocolloid dressings maintain a balanced wound hydration through controlled evaporation.

Hydrogels that are shapeless or amorphous are composed of insoluble non-crosslinked hydrophilic polymers such as polyvinyl pyrrolidone or polyacrylamide in the form of a gel containing 70–95% water. Amorphous hydrogels may be packaged in tubes, spray bottles or foil packs. The gel is applied directly to the wound and is usually covered with a secondary dressing (for example, a foam or gauze). Exudate is absorbed into the gel whilst moisture evaporates through the secondary dressing.

Saturated gauzes, obtained when gauze is impregnated with amorphous hydrogel, are sometimes used to fill the dead space in deeper wounds.

Hydrogel sheets are produced from crosslinked polymers which physically entrap water to form a solid sheet that can be cut to fit the wound. These do not need a secondary dressing as a semi-permeable polymer film backing, which may or may not have adhesive borders, controls the amount of water vapour transmitted through the dressing. The gels and impregnated gauzes are used as primary dressings whereas the hydrogel sheets may be used as primary or secondary dressings.

These three types of hydrogel provide a moist healing environment that promotes granulation and reepithelialization of wounds and absorb small to moderate amounts of exudate. They are particularly suitable for cleansing of dry, sloughy or necrotic wounds as they rehydrate the wound bed and enhance autolytic debridement. They are suitable for use at all stages of wound healing, with the exception of infected or heavily exuding wounds. Hydrogels cannot absorb much exudate and in infected wounds, a foul smell due to skin maceration and bacterial proliferation may occur due to the large water content of the gel. Although the dressings need to be changed frequently, they are relatively inexpensive.

Hydrocolloid dressings

Hydrocolloid dressings are among the most widely used wound management products. The term 'hydrocolloid' has been adopted to describe the family of occlusive or semi-occlusive wound dressings obtained from colloidal gel-forming materials, such as carboxymethylcellulose, gelatin, pectin or alginate, combined with other materials including elastomers and adhesives. The dressings are manufactured in various shapes and sizes and some are in the form of powders, wafers or pastes. They are often applied to a carrier such as a thin waterproof polyurethane film or foam sheet. The composition of the wound contact layer may differ considerably for the different hydrocolloid dressings. Some are transparent, to allow the wound-healing process to be visualized. There are over 60 hydrocolloid dressings currently available that differ in their physical characteristics, such as dressing thickness (some are extra thin), transparency, fluid-handling properties, moisture vapour permeability, conformability, acidity/alkalinity and fluid retention These differences in physical properties govern their specific clinical applications and effectiveness.

In their intact state, the occlusive hydrocolloid dressings are impermeable to water vapour and oxygen but on absorption of wound exudate, a change in physical state occurs with the formation of a gel covering the wound. This seals the wound and provides a moist healing environment that allows clean wounds to granulate and necrotic wounds to debride autolytically. The gel also acts as a barrier to keep bacteria and fluids out. The dressing relieves superficial pain by covering nerve endings with gel and exudate. Angiogenesis (growth of microcapillaries) is stimulated by the dressing initially being impermeable to atmospheric oxygen. The dressing may provide insulation to prevent heat loss from the wound.

Hydrocolloid dressings are particularly useful in paediatric wound care for management of both acute and chronic wounds as they adhere to moist and dry sites and do not cause tissue damage or pain on application or removal. Some hydrocolloid dressings are less occlusive, with higher moisture transmission rates, enhancing their ability to cope with exudate production.

Hydrocolloid dressings are used for light to moderately exuding wounds, including pressure sores, leg ulcers, minor burns and traumatic injuries. They can be left on the wound for up to 7 days provided that leakage does not occur. If leakage occurs and the bacterial barrier is broken, the wound is open to bacterial contamination and may develop an odour. Most of the dressings are not suitable for heavily exuding wounds or infected wounds, as they can encourage the growth of anaerobic bacteria. Some hydrocolloid dressings contain fibres that are deposited in the wound and have to be removed during dressing changes.

Bioactive dressings

Bioactive dressings deliver substances active in wound healing to the wound. They may be prepared from combinations of biopolymers that have a role in the natural wound-healing process, such as collagen, hyaluronic acid, chitosan, alginates and elastin, or may contain materials such as growth factors. Dressings that combine proteins, polymers and cells are generally described as skin substitutes, although there is no strict distinction between them and wound dressings. Technological advances in the fabrication of biomaterials and the culturing of skin cells is driving forward a new generation of engineered skin substitutes.

Tissue-engineered dressings include biodegradable films formed from, for example, collagen as scaffolds onto which skin cells can be seeded for the growth of new tissues. These scaffold dressings possess mechanical properties ideally approaching those of the tissue they are to replace. When introduced into the body, they gradually degrade, leaving behind a matrix of connective tissue with the appropriate structural and mechanical properties. In the future, such scaffolds may also be used for the delivery of additional bioactive materials, such as growth factors, to a wound.

WOUND MANAGEMENT

The design and careful selection of wound dressings represent only a small part of the management of a wound. With chronic wounds, it is essential to treat the underlying cause as well as dressing the wound. Once the underlying condition is controlled and the wound has been cleaned of materials that delay healing, such as dead tissue, extraneous bacteria and debris, an appropriate dressing selection can be made according to the type of wound being treated. Wounds are generally classified by their visual appearance as necrotic, sloughy, granulating or epithelializing, each type having different dressing requirements (Table 39.3). All wounds, regardless of type, may become infected at any stage of the healing process and subsequently develop an unpleasant odour.

The overall aim in the choice of dressing is to provide an environment at the surface of the wound in which healing may take place at the maximum rate consistent with the production of a healed wound with an acceptable cosmetic appearance. Some of the functions that may be required of the dressing are summarized in Table 39.4. The dressing may variously be required to maintain or provide a moist environment, absorb excess exudate,

Table 39.3 Classification of wounds based on appearance. Each type represents the phases that a single wound may go through as it heals. If the wound is infected, dressings may also be required to have antibacterial activity or be able to absorb odour

Wound type	Appearance	Role of dressing
Necrotic	Often olive green or black and dry to the touch, due to presence of necrotic tissue	Remove dead tissue. Rehydrate wound bed. Maintain moist wound bed. Prevent bacterial ingress
Sloughy	Slough is generally yellow in colour	Remove dead tissue. Maintain moist wound bed. Absorb excess fluid. Prevent bacterial ingress
Granulating	Significant quantities of granulation tissue, generally red or deep pink in colour. May produce excess exudate	Maintain moist wound bed. Absorb excess fluid (if present). Provide thermal insulation. Protect from, and prevent, trauma. Prevent bacterial ingress
Epithelializing	A pink margin or isolated pink islands on the surface of the wound. Generally little exudate	Maintain moist wound bed. Provide thermal insulation. Protect from, and prevent, trauma. Prevent bacterial ingress

promote autolytic debridement (the process of natural wound cleaning), provide thermal insulation, relieve pain, protect the wound from trauma, and combat infection and odour. In addition, it should be free from particulate contaminants, sterile and impermeable to microorganisms. To encourage patient compliance, dressings should be cost effective, require infrequent changing and be available in a suitable range of forms.

A simple occlusive/semi-occlusive dressing that prevents the evaporation of exudate is often all that is

Table 39.4 Functions of wound dressings

Dressing function	Clinical significance to wound healing
Provide or maintain a moist wound surface	Prevents desiccation and cell death, enhances epidermal migration, promotes angiogenesis and connective tissue synthesis and supports autolysis by rehydration of desiccated tissue. Enhances migration of leucocytes into the wound bed and supports the accumulation of enzymes
Absorption. Removal of blood and excess exudate	In chronic wounds, there is excess exudate containing tissue-degrading enzymes that block the proliferation and activity of cells and break down extracellular matrix materials and growth factors, thus delaying wound healing. Excess exudate can also macerate surrounding skin
Debridement, i.e. wound cleansing	Necrotic tissue, foreign bodies and particles prolong the inflammatory phase and serve as a medium for bacterial growth
Gaseous exchange (water vapour and air)	Permeability to water vapour controls the management of exudate. Low tissue oxygen levels stimulate angiogenesis. Raised tissue oxygen stimulates epithelialization and fibroblasts
Protect the healing wound from bacterial invasion	Infection prolongs the inflammatory phase and delays collagen synthesis, inhibits epidermal migration and induces additional tissue damage. Infected wounds can give an unpleasant odour
Provision of thermal insulation	Normal tissue temperature improves the blood flow to the wound bed and enhances epidermal migration
Low adherence. Protect the wound from trauma	Adherent dressings may be painful and difficult to remove and cause further tissue damage
Cost effectiveness. Frequency of dressing change	Dressing comparisons based on treatment costs rather than unit or pack costs should be made. Although many dressings are more expensive than traditional materials, the more rapid response to treatment may save considerably on total cost

needed to provide a moist environment at the surface of an acute clean (minimally exuding) wound. Exudate is beneficial to normal wound healing as it contains growth factors that promote the growth and migration of fibroblasts, endothelial cells and keratinocytes. However, some chronic wounds produce excess exudate that may macerate the surrounding skin and delay wound healing (see Table 39.4). Such wounds require dressings that absorb exudate and, if they require frequent changing, should be easy to remove with no tissue trauma or pain.

As mentioned above, there is no single dressing suitable for all types of wounds and often a range of different dressing types is used during the healing of a single wound. Most complex dressing systems are composites of several layers, each layer having a specific role in the wound-healing process. The primary dressing is placed in direct contact with the wound and the secondary dressing is placed over the primary dressing. The central absorbent portion of a composite is called the island

dressing. Some dressings need a bandage or some form of adhesive layer to keep them in position whilst in others there is an adhesive layer incorporated into the dressing itself. Non-adhesive dressings such as gels cause less pain and trauma on removal as they can be washed out of the wound.

BIBLIOGRAPHY

Cockbill, S. (2002) Wounds. The healing process. *Hospital Pharmacist*, **9**, 255-260.

Debra, J.B., Cheri, O. (1998) *Wound Healing. Technological Innovations and Market Overview*, 2nd edn. Technology Catalysts International Corporation.

Drug Tariff (Latest edition) Stationery Office, London (updated monthly).

Hess, C.H. (2005) *Wound Care*, 5th edn. Lippincott, Williams and Wilkins, New York.

Thomas, S. (1990) *Wound Management and Dressings*. Pharmaceutical Press, London.

40

Rectal and vaginal drug delivery

J. J. Tukker

RECTAL DRUG DELIVERY

Introduction

The administration of drugs by routes other than the oral one has to be considered in several circumstances and for many varying reasons. Arguments for choosing the rectal route for drug administration include the following:

- The patient is not able to make use of the oral route. This may be the case when the patient has a problem with their gastrointestinal tract, is nauseous or is postoperative (when the patient may be unconscious or not able to take a dosage form orally). Furthermore, several categories of patients, i.e. the very young, the very old or the mentally disturbed, may more easily be treated via the rectal than the oral route.
- The drug under consideration is less suited for oral administration. This may be so in cases where oral intake results in gastrointestinal side-effects, when the drug may be insufficiently stable at the pH of the GI tract or may be susceptible to enzymatic attack in the GI tract or during the first passage of the liver after absorption. Also drugs with an unacceptable taste can be administered rectally without this inconvenience to the patient. The formulation into suppositories of certain drugs that are candidates for abuse, as in suicide, has also been considered.

Besides these apparent advantages, the rectal route also has several drawbacks. Depending on tradition, there are strong feelings of aversion in certain countries, such as the UK and the USA, to rectal administration of drugs, whereas there is complete acceptance in continental and eastern Europe. More rational points in this respect are slow and sometimes incomplete absorption and the considerable inter- and intrasubject variations that have been reported. The development of proctitis has also been reported. There are also problems with the large-scale production of suppositories and of achievement of a suitable shelf life (the latter demanding stringent storage conditions).

It can thus be concluded that rectal administration is certainly not the route of first choice but can in certain circumstances be of great advantage to the patient.

The rectal route is used in many different therapies, intended either for local or for systemic effect. *Local effect* is desired in the case of pain and itching mostly due to the occurrence of haemorrhoids. Locally active drugs include astringents, antiseptics, local anaesthetics, vasoconstrictors, antiinflammatory compounds and soothing and protective agents. Also some laxatives fall into this category. For the attainment of a *systemic effect,* all orally given drugs can be used and many are, bearing in mind the limitations discussed above. Antiasthmatic, antirheumatic and analgesic drugs are widely administered by the rectal route.

Anatomy and physiology of the rectum

Rectal dosage forms are introduced in the body through the anus and are thus brought into contact with the most caudal part of the GI tract, i.e. the rectum. Anatomically the rectum is part of the colon, forming the last 150–200 mm of the GI tract.

The rectum can be subdivided into the anal canal and the ampulla, the latter forming approximately 80% of the organ. It is separated from the outside world by a circular muscle, the anus. The rectum can be considered as a hollow organ with a relatively flat wall surface, without villi and with only three major folds – the rectal valves. The rectal wall is composed of epithelium, which is one cell layer thick, and contains cylindrical cells and goblet cells which secrete mucus. A part of the rectal wall and the rectum's venous drainage is shown in Figure 40.1.

The total volume of mucus is estimated as approximately 3 mL, spread over a total surface area of approximately 300 cm^2. The pH of the mucous layer is reported as approximately 7.5. Furthermore, there seems to be little buffer capacity. This point will be discussed in relation to drug absorption later in this chapter.

Under normal circumstances the rectum is empty and filling provokes a defaecation reflex under voluntary control. Data comparing drug absorption from freshly prepared and aged (and therefore more viscous) suppositories suggest that there is enough motility to provoke spreading even of rather viscous suppositories.

Absorption of drugs from the rectum

Knowledge of the venous drainage from the rectum is important for the understanding of drug absorption. As can

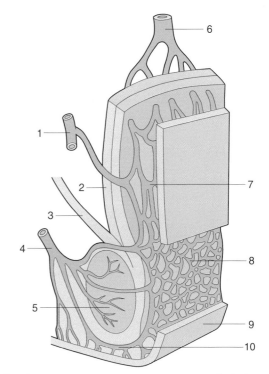

Fig. 40.1 Venous drainage of the human rectum: 1 middle rectal vein; 2 tunica muscularis: stratum longitudinale; 3 m. levator ani; 4 inferior rectal vein; 5 m. sphincter ani externus; 6 superior rectal vein; 7 and 8 plexus venosus rectalis (submucosus); 9 skin; 10 v. marginalis (after Tondury 1981, reproduced by permission of the publishers).

be seen from Figure 40.1, there are three separate veins. The lower and middle haemorrhoidal veins drain directly into the general circulation, while the upper one drains into the portal vein which flows to the liver. This means that drug molecules can enter the general circulation directly or by passing through the strongly metabolizing liver. In the latter case, only a proportion of the drug molecules (if they are of the high clearance type) will enter the general circulation intact. Thus the bioavailability may be less than 100%. Compared to the small intestine, this situation is still more favourable. Recent investigations have shown that avoiding the first passage through the liver is possible; the extent of this effect cannot be generalized since it will depend on the actual part of the rectum through which the drug is absorbed. Thus keeping the drug in the lower part of the rectum would be advisable.

Insertion of a suppository into the rectum results in a chain of effects leading to the bioavailability of the drug. This is represented in a simplified scheme in Figure 40.2.

Depending on the character of its vehicle (see later in this chapter), a suppository will either dissolve in the

RELEASE MECHANISM

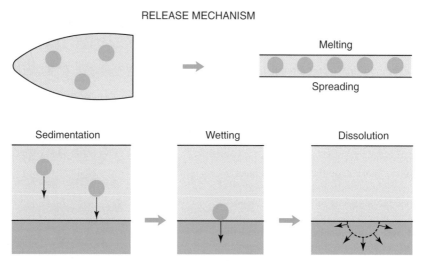

Fig. 40.2 Process of drug release from a suspension suppository.

rectal fluid or melt on the mucous layer. Since the volume of rectal fluid is so small, dissolution of the complete vehicle will be difficult and require extra water. Due to osmotic effects (of the dissolving vehicle) water is attracted, with the unpleasant consequence of a painful sensation for the patient. Independent of the vehicle type, drugs dissolved in the suppository will diffuse out towards the rectal membranes. Suspended drugs will first have to leave the vehicle (if it is water immiscible) under the influence of either gravity or motility movements and then can start dissolving in the rectal fluid. The dissolved drug molecules will have to diffuse through the mucous layer and then into and through the epithelium forming the rectal wall.

The process of absorption will be a passive diffusion process, as it is throughout the whole GI tract for almost all drugs; active transport processes as found in the upper regions of the GI tract have not been shown to be present in the rectal area.

For a generalized discussion on drug absorption, the reader is referred to Part 4 of this book. However, some specific points concerning rectal absorption will be discussed here. Table 40.1 gives a survey of the physiological factors in rectal absorption.

Table 40.1 Physiological factors affecting absorption from the rectum
Quantity of fluid available
Properties of rectal mucus
Contents of the rectum
Motility of the rectal wall

The quantity of fluid available for drug dissolution is very small – approximately 3 mL, spread in a layer of approximately 100 μm thick over the organ. Only under non-physiological circumstances is this volume enlarged, e.g. by osmotic attraction by water-soluble vehicles or during diarrhoea. Thus the dissolution of slightly water-soluble drugs can easily be the slowest step in the absorptive process.

Properties of the rectal fluid, such as composition, viscosity and surface tension, are essentially unknown and have to be estimated from data available for other parts of the GI tract. The pH and the buffer capacity of the rectum have been mentioned earlier in this chapter. The rectum is usually empty except temporarily when faecal matter arrives from higher parts of the colon. This material is either expelled or transported back into the colon, depending on the voluntary control exhibited on the anal sphincter.

The rectal wall may exert pressure on a suppository present in the lumen by two distinct mechanisms. First, the abdominal organs may simply press on to the rectum, especially when the body is in an upright position. This may stimulate spreading and thus promote absorption. The second source of pressure is the motility of the muscles of the rectal wall, which may originate from the normally occurring colonic motor complexes. These are waves of contractions running over the wall of the colon in a caudal direction and are associated with the presence of food residues in the colon.

In contrast with the upper part of the GI tract, no esterase or peptidase activity is present in the rectum, resulting in a much greater stability of peptide-like drugs. Administration of these compounds using the rectal or vaginal route has been satisfactory but only if absorption enhancers such as surfactants are used concomitantly. All kinds of surfactants seem to be effective but polyoxyethylene lauryl alcohol ether seems to be the most powerful. One major drawback of these enhancers, however, is irritation of the rectal mucosa in the long term. Less irritating enhancers are needed to explore this interesting area in greater depth.

Formulation of suppositories

Suppositories are mainly used for the administration of drugs via the rectal route, but not exclusively. Application via other routes, such as the vagina, is less common but of distinct use in the treatment of locally occurring infections. Administration of other suppository-type products (bougies) through other body orifices, e.g. ear, nose and urethra, is used very seldomly and is not discussed here. Alternative dosage forms for the rectal and or vaginal route are tablets, capsules, ointments and enemas. These will be discussed later. Rectal suppositories will be discussed first.

Suppositories are formulated in different shapes and sizes (usually 1–4 g). Their drug content varies widely from less than 0.1% up to almost 40%. A more detailed description, together with the methods of preparation, can be found in *Pharmaceutical Practice* (Winfield & Richards 2004). Generally the suppositories consist of a vehicle in which the drug is incorporated and in some cases additives are coformulated.

Vehicle (suppository base)

There are two main classes of vehicles in use: the glyceride-type fatty bases and the water-soluble ones. Although the ideal vehicle has not been found, the large variety of bases which are available enables a well-considered choice for every drug that has to be formulated as a suppository.

Choosing the optimum base requires much practical experience and can at present only partly be guided by scientifically sound data. Much remains to be learned here. However, some general guidelines can be given.

Requirements of the vehicle There is no doubt that a suppository should either melt after insertion in the body or dissolve in (and mix with) the available volume of rectal fluid. For fatty bases, this means a melting range lower than approximately 37°C (one has to be aware of the fact that the body temperature might be as low as 36°C at night). The melting range should be small enough to give rapid solidification after preparation, thus preventing separation of suspended, especially high-density, drug particles and agglomeration. When the solidification rate is high this may result in fissures in the suppository,

especially when rapid cooling is applied. The melting range, on the other hand, should be large enough to permit easy preparation, which may take a considerable length of time on an industrial scale.

During solidification, a suppository should exhibit enough volume contraction to permit removal from the mould or plastic former. The viscosity of the molten base plays an important role from both a technological and a biopharmaceutical point of view. During preparation the viscosity determines the flow into the moulds but also the separation of drug particles. Clearly, a compromise has to be found here. During and after melting in the rectal cavity, the suppository mass is forced to spread over the absorbing surface, the rate of which may be determined partly by its viscosity. Drug particles that have to be transported through the base to the interface with the rectal fluid and have to pass this interface to be released will evidently also see viscosity as a determining factor in their journey.

A good suppository base should further be chemically and physically stable during storage as a bulk product and after preparation into a suppository. It should have no incompatibility with drug molecules and should permit optimal release of the drug it contains.

Clearly, this list of requirements cannot always be completely fulfilled and often an acceptable compromise is the best that can be expected.

Fatty vehicles The fatty vehicles in use nowadays are almost exclusively semi- or fully synthetic. Cocoa butter is no longer used because of its many disadvantages, such as its well-known polymorphic behaviour, insufficient contraction at cooling, low softening point, chemical instability, poor water-absorptive power and its price.

The semi-synthetic type of fatty vehicles (sometimes termed *adeps solidus*) have few or none of the problems mentioned above. A comparison is made in Table 40.2.

The general composition of both types is mixed triglycerides with C_{12}-C_{18} acids. In the semi-synthetic vehicles these acids are saturated, while cocoa butter contains a considerable amount of the unsaturated oleic acid (see iodine number in Table 40.2, which for reducing drugs should be < 0.5). The presence of oleic acid is almost solely responsible for the special properties of

Table 40.2 Some properties of fatty suppository bases				
	Melting range	Acid content	Hydroxyl number	Iodine number
Cocoa butter	31–34°C	<5	0	34–38
Adeps solidus	33–37.5°C	<2	<5–30	<3

this vehicle. The melting range of the semi-synthetic bases is usually approximately 3°C higher than that of cocoa butter; the acid content is lower (mostly < 0.5) which is one of the reasons why the ageing of aminophylline suppositories is slower when semisynthetic vehicles are used. The hydroxyl number in Table 40.2 refers directly to the amount of mono- and diglycerides present in the fatty base. A high number means that the power to absorb water is high. This may lead to an increased rate of decomposition for drugs that are easily hydrolysed, such as acetylsalicylic acid. It should be realized that this capacity could lead to the formation of a w/o emulsion in the rectum. This is generally to be avoided because of its very low drug release rate. An advantage of high hydroxyl number is the larger melting and solidifying range that permits easier manufacture.

Water-soluble vehicles Water-soluble (or miscible) vehicles are much less used for reasons to be discussed below. They comprise the classic glycerol-gelatin or soap bases which are used exclusively for laxative purposes or in vaginal therapy.

The macrogols are also used. They consist of mixtures of polyethylene glycols of different molecular weight. The melting point is well over body temperature, which means that they mix with the rectal fluid. For true dissolution the available volume of rectal fluid (1–3 mL) is too small. Because of their high melting point they are especially suited for application in tropical climates but several disadvantages have to be considered. They are hygroscopic and therefore attract water, resulting in a painful sensation for the patient. Incorporation of at least 20% water and moistening before insertion can help to reduce this problem. A considerable number of incompatibilities with various drugs has been reported. Due to the solubilizing character of this base (which has a low dielectric constant) drugs may tend to remain in the base and drug release may be slow.

Choice of vehicle A summary of the points which are important for the choice of a suppository base is given in Table 40.3. The parameters mentioned in Table 40.3 are evidently not independent of each other. One interesting parameter can be added to this list – the volume of the suppository. Usually suppositories for adults are 2 mL and for children 1 mL. It has been suggested

that the larger volume may provoke a reaction of the rectal wall, thus helping to spread the melt over a larger area. Indeed, the increase in volume of, for example, paracetamol suppositories results in faster and more complete absorption of the drug.

Drug

Table 40.4 lists the factors that relate to the drug substance that may have possible consequences for the quality of suppositories.

Drug solubility in vehicle The drug solubility in the vehicle is of special interest from the biopharmaceutical point of view. It determines directly the type of product, i.e. solution or suspension suppository. The drug solubility in the rectal fluid determines the maximum attainable concentration and thus the driving force for absorption. When a drug has a high vehicle-to-water partition coefficient, it is likely to be in solution to an appreciable extent (or completely) in the vehicle. This generally means that the tendency to leave the vehicle will be low and thus the release rate into the rectal fluid will be slow. This is obviously unfavourable for rapid absorption. On the other hand, a certain lipid solubility is required for penetration through the rectal membranes (see above under 'Absorption of drugs from the rectum'). The optimal balance between these two requirements is usually found using the rules listed in Table 40.5.

This table assumes that the release from the dosage form is considered as the rate-limiting step. Thus the tendency to remain in the base should be lowered as much as possible (rules 1 and 2). When the solubilities in fat and water are both low, no definite rule can be given. It may well be that the dissolution rate will become the controlling step and thus it seems advisable to use micronized drug particles.

It should be stated as a general rule that w/o emulsion-type suppositories are strongly discouraged. The transfer of drug molecules present in a dissolved state in the inner phase will be very slow and thus drug absorption will be very much retarded.

It seems logical therefore that the first choice of a formulation would be a readily water-soluble form of the drug dispersed in a fatty base. This lays special emphasis on the water solubility of drugs and the methods to

Table 40.3   Formulation parameters of suppository bases
Composition
Melting behaviour
Rheological properties

Table 40.4   Drug substance-related factors
Solubility in water and vehicle
Surface properties
Particle size
Amount
pK_a

Table 40.5 Drug solubility and suppository formulation

Solubility in		Choice of base
Fat	Water	
Low	High	Fatty base (rule 1)
High	Low	Aqueous base (rule 2)
Low	Low	Indeterminate

improve this. The role of pK_a in this respect should also be considered. For a detailed discussion of these points, the reader may refer to Chapters 2, 3, 21 and 24.

Surface properties The surface properties of drug particles are also important as these particles will be transferred from one phase to another (see Fig. 40.2). This happens first when the drug is brought into contact with the vehicle and air has to be displaced from its surface. When this is not achieved particles may form agglomerates. This adversely affects final content uniformity by an increased tendency to separate. If wetting by the vehicle has taken place, displacement by rectal fluid will be required to let the drug go into solution, which is the prerequisite for absorption. This is the underlying reason why formulators have added surfactants to their formulation (see below).

Particle size The particle size of the drug is an important parameter, both technologically and biopharmaceutically. To prevent undue sedimentation during or after preparation, the particle size should be limited. Data from the available literature do not allow us to define an exact limit; however, the use of particles smaller than approximately 150 μm is an indication rather than a rule.

It is, of course, assumed that no agglomeration is taking place. The smaller the particles, the less the possible mechanical irritation to the patient (especially if they are < 50 μm) and the higher the dissolution rate. Therefore drugs with low water solubility should be dispersed in small, preferably micronized particles. One should be aware of the increased tendency of these small particles to agglomerate due to strongly increased van der Waals forces. Also an unnecessary size reduction operation should be avoided when possible.

There are good indications that size reduction is not a good decision for all drugs. It has been shown, especially for readily water-soluble drugs, that large particles give blood levels which are higher than or at least equivalent to small particles. This would lead to the suggestion to use particles in the size range 50–100 μm in that case. The lower limit of 50 μm to increase transport through the molten vehicle (see Fig. 40.2) and the upper limit of 100 μm is a safe protection against undue sedimentation during preparation. There is no clear-cut recommenda-

tion, however, for which solubility class this would be the rule to follow. For example, paracetamol (solubility in water approximately 15 mg/mL) gave the best blood levels when the particle size was smaller than 45 μm.

It should also be borne in mind that the spreading suppository mass should drag the suspended particles along to maximize the absorption surface. For dense particles it has become clear that this is a problem, but so far little or no proof is available that organic drugs (density usually 1.2–1.4 g cm^{-3}) suffer from this disadvantage when dispersed in, for example, 150 μm size particles. Principally this may be expected but care is needed to prevent too rapid formulation decisions in this respect.

Amount of drug A complicating factor is the amount of drug present in a suppository. If the number of particles increases, this would also increase the rate to form agglomerates. This will very much depend on the particle size and on the presence of additives. The theory describing the agglomeration behaviour of dispersed systems (DLVO theory, see Chapter 6) can be applied in the non-aqueous systems described here, but certain refinements are necessary. Another consequence of the presence of suspended particles is the increased viscosity of the molten base. Also in this case the formulator has to rely largely on empirical data rather than on theory. It seems therefore advisable to include a decision on particle size in the development plan of an actual suppository formulation.

Other additives

For several widely varying reasons, formulators of suppositories make use of additives to improve their product. Most of these additions are based on empirical data and are dealt with in the accompanying dispensing volume *Pharmaceutical Practice* (Winfield & Richards 2004). The dispensing aspects include formulations for specific drugs which affect the melting point of the suppository; it may become depressed (by a soluble liquid compound) or increased (by a high amount of soluble high melting active compound). The important point to consider in these situations is the possible influence of formulation changes on the release characteristics.

The inclusion of viscosity-increasing additives (e.g. colloidal silicon oxide or aluminium monostearate, both approximately 1–2%) will create a gel-like system with a slower release rate of the drug. Data from the literature are not consistent on this point. In vitro relationships can be easily established, but whether the actual release in vivo will also be depressed cannot be easily predicted, since rectal motility will in certain cases be able to overcome this problem. The addition of lecithin is a worthy possibility when high amounts of solid drug are used. The reason why can be found in a decreased attraction between the drug particles, altering the flow properties of the dispersion in the positive sense.

The addition of surface-active agents has been practised extensively but still remains a source of great uncertainty. When these compounds are used to create an emulsion system (thus w/o), this has certainly to be discouraged since the release will be unacceptably slow. It may well be, however, that surfactants act as wetting agents. This can influence the release in a positive sense but so far very little convincing information is available showing that wetting (i.e. displacement of base by rectal fluid) exists as a real problem. Surfactants may also act as 'deglomerators', which may prevent the formation of cake in the melting suppository, which in turn would certainly slow down the drug release. No firm conclusions can be drawn since very little research work has been performed on the agglomeration in non-aqueous media. The role of surfactants as spreading enhancers has never been clarified either and this factor is strongly interrelated with the occurrence of rectal motility. There are good indications that the presence of surfactants in a concentration higher than the critical micelle concentration can retard the release from the suppositories.

Finished product

Manufacture

Suppositories are manufactured both on a small scale, in batches of 10–20, and on a (semi) automatic scale in batches up to 20 000 per hour. Essentially the mode of manufacture is similar in both cases and involves melting of the vehicle, mixing the drug and the molten vehicle, dispensing in a shape former, cooling to solidify and packing in the final container. This includes a number of technological processes for which the relevant theory should be considered (see, for example, Chapter 12 for the mixing of semi-solids). Most suppositories are packed individually in a plastic (PVC) or aluminium foil pack. Requirements for good protection against moisture and oxygen can be deduced from the individual needs of the drug and the properties of the packaging material.

Quality control

A list of properties that should be controlled is given in Table 40.6.

The *appearance* of a suppository includes odour, colour, surface condition and shape. These are organoleptically controlled and are discussed in Winfield & Richards (2004). The requirements for *weight* and *disintegration* are given in pharmacopoeias. The melting and dissolution behaviours are in fact reflected in the dis-

Table 40.6   Control parameters of suppositories

Appearance
Weight
Disintegration
Melting (dissolution) behaviour
Mechanical strength
Content of active ingredient
Release

integration test. Many other methods are available, but none of them has been shown to provide more relevant information. The *European Pharmacopoeia* method is rather insensitive and not too much value should be attributed to the passing of this test.

Determination of the *mechanical strength* of suppositories can be valuable to avoid problems with formulations in which the melting range has been depressed. It can be tested by several methods including the use of a tablet crushing strength tester.

No official requirements are published as yet with regard to the *content uniformity*. This, however, has been shown to be a potential problem in semi-automatic manufacture of batches of a few kg. This could result from insufficient mixing leading to a poor uniformity of content. Giving careful attention to the design and control of the filling apparatus could solve most of the problems. However, it is often found that poor uniformity occurs at the beginning and end of the production process, necessitating some degree of rejection.

Drug release from suppositories

Perhaps the most important point to realize is that, for patients, the drug release characteristics are the factor that ensures the success of their therapy. What is really needed is an optimal bioavailability (discussed in detail in Part 4) which, for the formulator, means ensuring optimal and reproducible release in vivo.

Since there are few ways of obtaining in vivo release information, this will usually have to be interpreted from in vitro release data, which introduces the problem of in vitro/in vivo correlation. The present knowledge does not permit the choice of an in vitro method with a high predictive power for in vivo performance. Some aspects can be discussed, however, to give helpful pointers in this respect. Table 40.7 lists the parameters to be examined in testing suppository release in vitro.

The *temperature* to be used for testing rectal dosage forms is easily defined as the body temperature. Although for most practical purposes this temperature can be set at 37°C, this is not so for, especially, fatty

Table 40.7	**In vitro release parameters**
Temperature	
Contact area	
Release medium	
Movements	
Membranes	

suppository testing. Most available vehicles have melting ranges below 37°C but this does not necessarily mean that their viscosity at 37°C is the same. Since the body temperature may be as low as 36°C at night, this implies that the release rate at 37°C may be an overestimate. Also comparing bases at 37°C may lead to erroneous conclusions. The temperature at which testing is performed might be crucial, especially when ageing has occurred. Special attention should therefore be given to the actual testing temperature.

In the set-up shown in Figure 40.3, the temperature at the surface of the water layer inside the tube, where molten suppository material is gathered, may be a few degrees lower than the bulk temperature. By choosing the right dimension and closing the tube at the upper side, this problem is eliminated here.

The *contact area* in the rectum over which spreading occurs cannot be standardized without introducing either an overestimate or an underestimate. In Figure 40.3 the area is relatively small (i.e. approximately 10 cm²) compared to the total surface area of the rectum (approxi-

mately 300 cm²). This type of apparatus is therefore intended to be used for comparative studies only and not for a complete in vivo simulation. At present no method is available which closely mimics the in vivo situation.

Another parameter to be considered is the *release medium*. Whereas not enough information is available on the actual composition and structure of the rectal fluid, a choice is usually made for a relatively large volume of water or buffer solution. Since the rate-limiting step in the bioavailability from fatty suppositories is very often the release from the suppository, it seems reasonable enough not to include mucins which control the viscosity in vivo. The large volume in most in vitro methods would then not be so important either. More difficult is the choice of buffer and especially its strength, since little is known about this factor in the in vivo situation. For water-soluble vehicles the problem is even larger, and essentially no ideal solution has yet been found to the problem of choosing the volume and composition of the release medium. Interest has been directed towards ways of incorporating a *pressure* feature in release testing. It is clear that rectal motility exists and that it may influence the bioavailability. Not yet clear, however, is how to incorporate this knowledge in the design of a release tester. Attempts have been made, but no conclusive answer is possible as yet.

Very often *membranes* have been used in release testers, usually to envelop the suppository in a small volume of release medium. This has the enormous drawback that the release as measured in the outer compartment is not equal to the actual release taking place in the inner compartment. Most results published do not take into account that the membrane may form a resistance to passing drug molecules and that the actual release may be underestimated. By a calculation procedure, it is possible to obtain the actual release if certain conditions can be met. It seems advisable therefore to avoid membranes in a release tester, whenever possible.

The actual true validation of in vitro release testing remains the in vivo performance. Several possibilities exist to obtain such data. Bioavailability determination should consider both rate and extent of absorption. Whenever possible these data should be obtained in humans, since at present no animal model is available which is sufficiently reliable. For a more detailed discussion on the general aspects of bioavailability testing and in vitro/in vivo correlations, Chapter 22 can be consulted.

Rectal formulations other than suppositories

Apart from suppositories, many formulations can be used for rectal administration of drugs. For the treatment of *local* disturbances, like haemorrhoids, fatty ointments are used widely. In the treatment of rectocolitis enemas

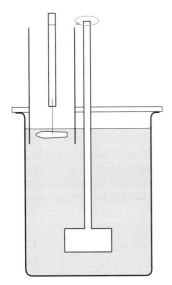

Fig. 40.3 Tube apparatus for testing of sedimentation-controlled release from suppositories.

are used with a rather large volume, e.g. 100 mL. This enables the drug to reach the upper part of the rectum and the sigmoid colon.

For the *systemic* administration of drugs, delivery forms such as tablets, capsules and microenemas are in use.

Tablets

Tablets are not very attractive because they cannot disintegrate rapidly, due to the low amount of water present in the rectum. Tablets releasing CO_2 after insertion can be applied, thus stimulating defaecation.

Capsules

Capsules used to achieve a systemic effect are usually filled with a solution or suspension of the drug in vegetable oil or paraffin. These capsules are mostly of the soft-shell type. With this dosage form limited experience has been obtained, but it seems that no striking differences exist between the bioavailability from rectal capsules and fatty suppositories.

Microenemas

Microenemas are solutions or dispersions of the drug in a small volume (approximately 3 mL) of water or vegetable oil. This form is supplied in a small plastic container, equipped with an application tube. After insertion of the tube, the container is emptied by compression of the bulb. The advantage of this delivery system is obvious, since no melting and dissolution process is necessary before drug release can start, if water is used as a vehicle. Many good results have been obtained with drugs delivered in microenemas but this form is still of limited applicability, because of its relatively high cost compared to, for example, suppositories. Moreover, administration cannot be performed easily by patients themselves, and it is rather difficult to deliver the total content of the plastic container.

Limitations of rectal dosing

Due to the limited rectal area for absorption (in total approx. 300 cm^2) and the limited amount of water (3 mL), the rectum is thought to be unsuitable for absorption of very hydrophilic or very low soluble compounds. However, only scant information is available. After rectal dosing, tamoxifen (which has an aqueous solubility of 400 mg/L, but a solubility in saline of approximately 40 mg/L) showed a marked decrease to 10% of its oral availability. This example illustrates that switching from oral to rectal dosing without proper information, should be discouraged.

VAGINAL DRUG DELIVERY

Vaginal administration of drugs

The vaginal route is mainly used for the achievement of local effects, e.g. in the case of *Trichomonas* and *Candida* infections. Some drugs are, however, administered vaginally to achieve systemic effects. In some cases, drugs given by the intravaginal route have a higher bioavailability compared to the oral route. This is because the drug enters immediately into the systemic circulation without passing the metabolizing liver (as is also the case with drugs absorbed from the lower part of the rectum).

The vaginal wall is very well suited for the absorption of drugs for systemic use, since it contains a vast network of blood vessels. Only a few drugs are administered by this route at present, however. Among these are oestrogens and prostaglandin analogues that are usually administered as vaginal creams or hydrogels. Progesterone has been given as a vaginal suppository (pessary) for some years, and better results are obtained in this way than after oral dosing.

Formulation of vaginal dosage forms

Many different types of formulations have been and are applied vaginally, e.g. tablets, capsules, pessaries, solutions, sprays, foams, creams and ointments. Because of the rather low moisture content under normal physiological conditions, additives are used to improve the disintegration of vaginal tablets, e.g. bicarbonate together with an organic acid, which results in CO_2 release. A good filler for vaginal tablets is lactose, since this is a natural substrate for the vaginal microflora that converts lactose into lactic acid, resulting in a pH value of 4–4.5.

Vaginal suppositories (pessaries) are mostly prepared with glycerol-gelatin bases, since this mixture is well tolerated. Polyethylene glycols are less common, since they are said to promote irritation. Also fatty excipients are not very much used. Most drug delivery forms for vaginal application demand an auxiliary device, in order to obtain deep insertion of the dosage form.

REFERENCES

Tondury, G. (1981) *Angewandte und Topographische Anatomie*, 5th edn. Georg Thieme Verlag, Stuttgart, Germany.
Winfield, A.J., Richards, R.M.E. (2004) *Pharmaceutical Practice*, 3rd edn. Churchill Livingstone, Edinburgh.

BIBLIOGRAPHY

de Blaey, C.J., Polderman, J. (1989) Rationales in the design of rectal and vaginal delivery forms of drugs. In: Ariëns, E.J. (ed.) *Drug Design*, vol. 9. Academic Press, New York.

de Boer, A.G., Molenaar, F., de Leede, L.G.J., Breimer, D.D. (1982) Rectal drug administration: clinical pharmacokinetic considerations. *Clinical Pharmacokinetics,* **7**, 285-311.

Müller, B. (ed.) (1986) *Suppositorien*. Wissenschaftliche Verlagsgesellschaft mbH, Stuttgart, Germany.

Rytting, J.H. (1990) Rectal route of peptide and protein delivery. In: Lee, V.H. (ed.) *Peptide and Protein Drug Delivery*. Marcel Dekker, New York.

Thoma, K. (1980) *Arzneiformen zur rectalen und vaginalen Applikation*. Werbe-und Vertriebsgesellschaft Deutscher Apotheker mbH, Frankfurt am Main, Germany.

Tukker, J.J., Blankenstein, M.A., Nortier, J.W.R. (1986) Comparison of bioavailability of tamoxifen after oral and rectal administration as measured by plasma levels of tamoxifen and its major metabolite N-desmethyltamoxifen. *Journal of Pharmacy and Pharmacology,* **38**, 888-892.

41

Delivery of pharmaceutical proteins

D. J. A. Crommelin, E. van Winden, A. Mekking

INTRODUCTION

Protein structures

Pharmaceutical proteins are built up of amino acid chains (their primary structure). To be pharmacologically active, this amino acid sequence must form a well-defined three-dimensional structure. Parts of the protein will fold in locally identifiable, discrete structures such as α helices or β sheets (known as secondary structures). The overall (tertiary) structure of the protein is established by the proper positioning of the different subunits relative to each other. In some cases individual protein molecules form a quaternary structure, in which the individual protein molecules interact and build a larger, well-defined structure (e.g. haemoglobin).

The formation and stability of the secondary, tertiary and quaternary structures are based on relatively weak physical interactions (e.g. electrostatic interactions, hydrogen bonding, van der Waals forces and hydrophobic interactions) and not on covalent chemical-binding principles. Repulsive energy between apolar parts of the protein and water is responsible for hydrophobic interactions. The physical forces involved are relatively weak which means that protein structures can be rather easily changed, leading to a modification or even loss of their pharmacological characteristics.

Amino acid chains can be modified by covalently attaching non-amino acid sections, such as sugar (glycoproteins), phosphate or sulfate groups. In particular, the sugar part can make up a substantial part of the molecular weight of the (glyco)protein. These groups may be essential for the pharmacological effect of a therapeutic protein, not only while acting at its receptor sites but also to provide the proper pharmacokinetic profile.

Pharmaceutical protein molecules are large and diffusional transport through epithelial barriers such as those encountered in the gastrointestinal tract is slow unless specific transporter molecules are available. Moreover, the conditions in the lumen of the GI tract are extremely hostile to these proteins. Degradation (mainly enzymatic) is fast. Therefore, the large majority of pharmaceutical proteins are delivered via the parenteral route (i.e. via the needle). The issue of alternative routes of administration for proteins is discussed later in this chapter.

Conserving the integrity of these large molecules is essential to ensure an optimal therapeutic effect and to minimize effects such as the induction of unwanted immune responses. An immune response may neutralize the therapeutic activity in chronic dosing schedules and cause serious side-effects. Protein stability concerns both its chemical and physical structure. There are many functional groups in the amino acid chain available for chemical degradation, and the preferred three-dimensional structure is readily irreversibly disturbed (e.g. through heat, changes in pH or ionic strength). Some analytical approaches to monitoring the protein structure are discussed later in this chapter.

The preferred shelf life for pharmaceutical products is a minimum of 2 years. Most proteins degrade too fast when formulated as aqueous solutions, even when kept in the refrigerator. Therefore, they have to be stored in a dry form and be reconstituted before administration. The three-dimensional delicate structures of pharmaceutical proteins are usually dried by freeze drying (see Chapter 30). The choice of proper excipients during this step (e.g. lyoprotectants) has proved to be extremely important.

Sources of pharmaceutical proteins

Nowadays most proteins used in therapy or under development are produced by recombinant DNA or hybridoma technology. They are known as *biotechnology products* or *biotech products* for short. Examples are human insulin, erythropoietin, monoclonal antibodies, cytokines and interferons.

They are all produced in cell cultures by prokaryotic or eukaryotic cells, ranging from *Escherichia coli* to mammalian cells such as Chinese hamster ovary cells, or transgenic animals and genetically modified plants.

From the examples listed above, one may conclude that many of the pharmaceutical proteins are basically endogenous products. However, a number of currently used biotech products are not exactly identical to the endogenous product. For example, the glycosylation patterns of the recombinant form may be reproducibly produced on a large scale, but not completely match the endogenous product. Extensive evaluation of these products in clinical trials has proved their efficacy and safety.

Isolation of the expressed protein from the culture medium is a multistep process consisting of several different (chromatographic/filtration) steps. For every protein a 'tailor-made' purification protocol has to be developed to remove impurities while ensuring integrity.

Biotech-derived molecules may make up the majority of protein drugs, but there are still proteins of major therapeutic importance isolated from blood from humans or animals. Examples are albumin, blood clotting factors (such as Factor VIII from the blood of human volunteers) and antisera from patients or animals such as horses and sheep. Here again, special purification protocols have to be developed, with particular emphasis on reduction of viral contamination (discussed later in this chapter).

Specific challenges

It is clear that pharmaceutical proteins offer special challenges to the pharmaceutical formulator. They are delicate, large molecules with many functional groups. Their three-dimensional structure, being stabilized by relatively weak physical bonds, can be readily and irreversibly changed. In vivo this may directly affect the interaction with the receptor, change their pharmacokinetic characteristics, e.g. their clearance, or make them immunogenic. Moreover, their epithelial penetration capability is very low unless the proper transporter molecules are available. Thus, as a rule, pharmaceutical proteins are administered parenterally.

FORMULATION OF PHARMACEUTICAL PROTEINS FOR PARENTERAL ADMINISTRATION

Stability issues

In the introduction to this chapter it was pointed out that pharmaceutical proteins are high molecular weight molecules with amino acid building blocks that are sensitive to degradation and with a specific three-dimensional structure. Table 41.1 lists the common pathways for degradation of proteins.

Physical instability

Degradation rates depend on environmental conditions and the formulator should carefully select conditions for optimal stability. For example, elevated temperatures can cause denaturation of proteins in aqueous solution. Interestingly, low temperatures may also induce destabilization. Besides, protein aggregation is often initiated by adsorption of the protein monomer on the walls of the container. Proteins may also aggregate by shaking or by exposure to shear forces. This can cause hydrophobic parts of the molecule to be exposed to (hydrophobic)

Table 41.1 Pathways of degradation of protein

Fragmentation

$H_2N \longrightarrow Lys \longrightarrow Ala \longrightarrow COOH \longrightarrow H_2N\longrightarrow Lys + Ala \longrightarrow COOH$

Isomerization

L-form amino acid $\longrightarrow$ D-form amino acid

Deamidation

$H_2N \cdots Asn \cdots COOH \longrightarrow H_2N \cdots Asp \cdots COOH + -NH_2$

Oxidation

$H_2N \cdots Met \cdots COOH \longrightarrow H_2N \cdots \overset{\overset{\textstyle O}{\textstyle \|}}{Met} \cdots COOH$

Disulphide scrambling

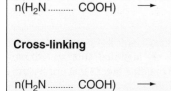

Oligomerization

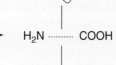

$n(H_2N \cdots Cys \cdots Cys \cdots COOH) \longrightarrow n(H_2N \cdots Cys \cdots Cys \cdots COOH)$

$n(H_2N \cdots Cys \cdots Cys \cdots COOH)$

Aggregation

$n(H_2N \cdots COOH) \longrightarrow (H_2N \cdots COOH)n$

Cross-linking

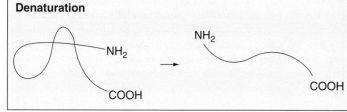

$n(H_2N \cdots COOH) \longrightarrow H_2N \cdots COOH$

$H_2N \cdots COOH$

Key:
Ala = alanine
Asn = asparagine
Asp = aspartic acid
Cys = cysteine
Lys = lysine
Met = methionine

Denaturation

interfaces (air/water). In turn this can result in unfolding of the protein and aggregation occurs.

Chemical instability

Because of the many amino acids involved, full prevention of all chemical degradation reactions is difficult. The formulator should consider which chemical degradation pathways are relevant. Under neutral conditions the peptide bonds between amino acids are stable; only the asparagine–glycine and asparagine–proline bonds are relatively labile.

Deamidation is a rather common degradation reaction in water. Asparagine and glutamine are the amino acids that can be deamidated. Deamidation reaction kinetics depend on pH and neighbouring amino acids.

Oxidation is not limited to methionine and cysteine (see Table 41.1): histidine, tryptophan and tyrosine are also sensitive to oxidation reactions. Oxidation is catalysed by traces of transition metal ions. An oxidative milieu may also cause free cysteine units to form disulphide bridges or disulphide bond scrambling.

Naturally occurring amino acids are in the L form. Isomerization to the D form is possible and will change the structure (and therefore the activity) of the protein.

Incorrect choice of excipients may also cause degradation reactions. For example, sugars are often used as excipients (Table 41.2) but reducing sugars can react with free primary amino groups of the protein molecule via the so-called Maillard reaction (even in the dry state) and form brownish reaction products. Reducing sugars (e.g. lactose) should therefore be excluded from protein-containing formulations.

Excipients used

Table 41.2 lists the excipients used in protein-containing parenteral dosage forms. Not all ingredients listed are always needed, e.g. many pharmaceutical proteins are sufficiently soluble in water. This is in particular true for highly glycosylated molecules. In this case no solubility-enhancing substances are needed. However, if solubility enhancement is necessary, the selection of the proper pH conditions should first be considered. Protein solubility depends on its net charge. In general, as with low molecular weight drugs, uncharged protein molecules (at the pH of their isoelectric point, IEP) have the lowest solubility in water. Therefore, choosing pH conditions 'away' from the IEP can solve the protein insolubility (and thus the problem). Some amino acids (e.g. arginine and lysine) increase protein solubility and reduce aggregation reactions by a poorly understood mechanism. Detergents such as polysorbate 20 and 80 or sodium dodecyl sulfate can also be used to prevent aggregation. These compounds prevent the adsorption of proteins to interfaces (air/water and container/water) and thereby interface-induced protein unfolding. Human serum albumin has a strong tendency to adsorb to interfaces and may therefore be added to therapeutic protein formulations as an antiaggregation agent. Regulatory authorities discourage the use of human serum albumin for this purpose because of the perceived risk of transmitting bovine spongiform encephalopathy agents (BSE).

Oxidation reactions are catalysed by heavy metals. Chelating agents are used to reduce oxidation damage through binding of the ions. This approach cannot be used if the metal ion is necessary as an integral part of the protein structure. Examples are zinc ions in insulin formulations and iron ions in haemoglobin. Then, antioxidants such as sulphites may be added to reduce the oxidation tendency. In the case of vials for multiple dosing, preservatives have to be included in the formulation. Benzyl alcohol and phenol are often used for this purpose.

Buffered aqueous protein solutions may be stable for 2 years under refrigerator conditions. Some monoclonal

Table 41.2 Excipients used in parenteral dosage forms and their function		
Excipient	**Function**	**Examples**
Solubility-enhancing substances	Increase solubility of proteins	Amino acids, detergents
Antiadsorbent/aggregation blockers	Reduction of adsorption and aggregation prevention	Albumin, detergents
Buffer components	Stabilizing pH	Phosphate, citrate
Preservatives	Growth inhibition in vials for multiple dosing	Phenol, benzylalcohol
Antioxidants	Prevent oxidation	Ascorbic acid, sulphites, cysteine
Stabilizers during storage (lyoprotectants)	Preservation of integrity while in dry form	Sugars
Osmotic compounds	Ensure isotonicity	Sugars, NaCl

antibody formulations, for example, are available as aqueous solutions but often the formulation has to be freeze dried in the vials to avoid degradation and to ensure that the product can be readily reconstituted.

During freeze drying (see Chapter 30) water is removed by sublimation. In the freeze-drying process three discrete phases can be discerned. The first is freezing of the solution to temperatures typically around −35 to −40°C, followed by a sublimation phase with temperatures of around −35°C and at very low atmospheric pressures to remove the frozen water (phase 2), and a final, secondary drying stage to remove most residual water. The pressure must remain low but the temperature can rise up to about 20°C without collapse of the porous cake (see below). A lyoprotectant (e.g. sugar) is necessary to stabilize the product as the removal of water may irreversibly affect the protein structure. Moreover, sugar lyoprotectants also happen to form readily reconstitutable porous cakes.

The freezing temperature should be low enough to convert the aqueous solution with the sugar and the protein into a glass. Glass formation in sugar solutions usually occurs around −30°C. Just below the glass transition temperature the sublimation process can begin during the lowering of the pressure in the chamber. The sublimated water is collected on a condenser with a considerably lower temperature (typically −60°C). As sublimation extracts a large amount of latent heat from the system, the temperature in the vials containing the frozen protein solution could fall even lower than the starting temperature, slowing down sublimation. The vials are therefore heated in a controlled way to keep them at temperatures low enough to preserve their glassy texture but high enough to let the sublimation process proceed at a sufficiently high speed.

The mechanism(s) of action of lyoprotectants (non-reducing sugars) is not fully understood. The following may play a role:

- Lyoprotectants replace water as stabilizing agent ('water replacement theory') of the protein.
- Lyoprotectants increase the glass transition temperature in the frozen system and in the dried system, avoiding collapse of the porous cake which would slow down water removal from the frozen cake (during freeze drying) and interfere with a rapid reconstitution of the freeze-dried cake.
- Lyoprotectants slow down the secondary drying process and minimize the chances of overdrying of the product in the secondary drying stage.

Microbiological requirements

Typically, pharmaceutical proteins are administered via the parenteral route. This implies that the product should be sterile. In addition, virus and pyrogen removal steps should be part of the purification and production protocol.

Pharmaceutical proteins cannot be sterilized by autoclaving, gas sterilization or ionizing radiation, because these procedures damage the molecules. Therefore, sterilization of the endproduct is not possible. This leaves aseptic manufacturing as the only option.

All utensils and components must be presterilized (by heat sterilization, ionizing radiation or membrane filtration) before assembling the final formulation to minimize the bioburden. Protein products are manufactured under aseptic conditions in class 100 areas (fewer than 100 particles >0.5 μm per cubic foot). This low-level contamination is reached by filtration of air through HEPA (high-efficiency particulate air) filters. Finally, the product is filled into the containers through sterile filters with 0.22 μm pores before capping or freeze drying/capping.

Pharmaceutical proteins are produced by living organisms. Viruses can be introduced into the product either by the use of contaminated culture media or via infected (mammalian) production cells. It is therefore important that purification and manufacturing protocols contain viral decontamination steps. Viral decontamination can be accomplished by virus removal and/or by viral inactivation. The problem faced when selecting inactivation techniques is that there is often a narrow window between successful viral inactivation and preservation of the integrity of the pharmaceutical protein structure.

Viruses can be removed by filtration, precipitation or chromatography. For virus inactivation, heat treatment (pasteurization), radiation or crosslinking agents (e.g. β-propiolactone) can be used. As no single process guarantees complete virus removal, often several different decontamination steps are introduced in series in the 'downstream' purification process and in the manufacturing of the final formulation.

Gram-negative host cells, such as *E. coli*, are often used as production cells for non-glycosylated proteins. Gram-negative cells contain large amounts of endotoxins in their membranes. These endotoxins are heat stable, amphipatic, negatively charged lipopolysaccharides and are potent pyrogens. Pyrogens have to be removed in order to meet pharmacopoeial criteria and this can be done, for example, through anion-exchange chromatography.

ANALYTICAL TECHNIQUES TO CHARACTERIZE PROTEINS

It is clearly important to be able to guarantee the integrity of a protein. As mentioned earlier, a protein molecule is a complex three-dimensional structure of amino acids, often coupled to saccharide, phosphate or sulfate moieties. The total structure is responsible for the pharmacodynamic (e.g. receptor interaction) and pharmacokinetic (e.g. clearance, targeting) effects. It is not possible to define the structure of a pharmaceutical protein with the same precision as small, low molecular weight molecules, where a combination of analytical techniques provides unequivocal structural evidence.

Therefore, a set of pharmacological, immunological, spectroscopic, electrophoretic and chromatographic approaches is used to characterize the protein as closely as possible. Table 41.3 lists a number of regularly used analytical techniques and the information that is obtained.

Quality assessment used to be based on functional tests in vivo using relevant animal models. An example is the pharmacopoeial test for insulin: the lowering of the blood glucose level in rabbits upon injection of the insulin product to be tested. These tests do not have the sensitivity to identify small changes in molecular structure or detect early degradation products, and they do not provide information on such things as the presence of product immunogenicity. In vitro cell tests, such as those used for cytokine activity assessment, inform us about the functional activity of the molecule, but not its pharmacokinetic behaviour or immunogenicity. ELISA (enzyme-linked immunosorbent assay) and RIA (radioimmunoassay) belong to the class of immunological tests. Here the interaction of a monoclonal antibody with one epitope region on the protein is determined. The rest of the molecule is not 'probed'.

Electrophoretic techniques such as SDS-PAGE (sodium dodecyl sulfate-polyacrylamide gel electrophoresis) and IEF (isoelectric focusing) are powerful tools to assess product purity and to provide molecular weight and IEP information regarding the protein.

Table 41.3 Approaches to confirming protein structure

Approach	Information obtained
In vivo tests, use of test animals	Pharmacological effect
In vitro tests (sensitive cells)	Functional test
Immunological tests	
ELISA	Interaction with one epitope on protein
RIA	Interaction with one epitope on protein
Analytical approaches	
Spectroscopic	
UV spectroscopy	Secondary/tertiary structure
Fluorimetry	Secondary/tertiary structure
CD spectroscopy	Secondary/tertiary structure
Infrared spectroscopy	Secondary/tertiary structure
Mass spectrometry	Secondary/tertiary structure
Electrophoretic approaches	
SDS-PAGE	Molecular weight
IEF	Isoelectric point
High-performance liquid chromatography (HPLC)	
GP (gel permeation)	Molecular weight/aggregates
HI (hydrophobic interaction)	Hydrophobic interactions
Affinity chromatography	Interaction with specific ligand
IEC (ion exchange)	Charge patterns
RP (reversed phase)	

CD, circular dichroism
ELISA, enzyme-linked immunosorbent assay
IEC, ion-exchange chromatography
IEF, isoelectric focusing
HPLC, high-performance liquid chromatography
RIA, radioimmunoassay
SDS-PAGE, sodium dodecyl sulfate polyacrylamide gel electrophoresis

Table 41.3 lists a number of chromatographic techniques that elucidate product characteristics. In particular, impurities and degradation products can be picked up at an early stage. Gel chromatography discriminates mainly on the basis of molecular size and is a powerful technique to monitor aggregate formation. Ion-exchange resins separate on the basis of subtle variations in protein charge patterns and are being used to detect oxidation (e.g. methionine) and deamidated (converted glutamine and asparagine) products. Modern mass spectroscopic techniques such as MALDI-TOF (matrix-assisted laser desorption ionization-time of flight) mass spectroscopic analysis, or a combination of HPLC (high-pressure liquid chromatography) with electrospray ionization-induced mass spectrometry, give detailed information on amino acid sequence and glycosylation patterns.

In conclusion, to ensure pharmaceutical protein quality one must follow a strict protocol regarding the definition of the protein production cell lines used, the chosen culturing conditions and downstream processing conditions, and the filling/(drying)/finishing process. Analytical approaches to confirm the protein structure will always include a long list of techniques, ranging from in vivo tests in animals to information provided by highly sophisticated analytical technologies.

None of these tests tells the whole story; together they tell more but, as stated before, with many high molecular weight molecules it is seldom possible to obtain a full description of the drug, including a detailed impurity profile.

ADMINISTRATION OF PHARMACEUTICAL PROTEINS

Routes of administration

As mentioned in the introduction to this chapter, oral administration of a pharmaceutical protein results in a very low bioavailability. The protein is enzymatically attacked in the gastrointestinal tract and, moreover, penetration through the gut wall will be slow and incomplete. Oral vaccines containing antigenic protein material are an exception to the general rule that proteins should not be administered orally. With vaccines, even low uptake levels may still deliver sufficient material to lymphoid tissue just below the epithelium (in the so-called Peyer's patches) to induce a strong (both local and systemic) immune response.

When a protein is delivered intravenously, clearance from the blood compartment can be fast, with a half-life of minutes, or slow, with a half-life of several days. An example of a rapidly cleared protein is tissue plasminogen activator (tPA), with a plasma half-life of a few

minutes. On the other hand, human monoclonal antibodies have half-lives in the order of days.

Protein drugs are often administered subcutaneously or intramuscularly. These routes of administration are considered to be more patient friendly and the injection process easier than with the intravenous route. Upon intramuscular (i.m.) or subcutaneous (s.c.) injection the protein is not instantaneously drained to the blood compartment. Studies monitoring the fate of a protein upon s.c. injection demonstrate that passage of a protein through the endothelial barrier lining the local capillaries at the site of injection is size dependent. If the protein is too large it will enter the lymphatic system and be transported via the lymph into the blood. Figure 41.1 shows the relationship between molecular size and lymphatic drainage. Lymphatic drainage takes time and a delay in the onset of systemic activity is observed. The protein is also exposed to the local environment containing proteases. Therefore, the bioavailability of protein drugs upon s.c. (and i.m.) administration can be far from 100%. This can have dramatic consequences, e.g. some diabetics become insulin resistant because of high tissue peptidase activity.

There is not always a direct relationship between plasma level and pharmacological response (i.e. no direct pharmacokinetic-pharmacodynamic (PK/PD) relationship). As the mechanism of action of a drug might be complex, involving different sequential steps, fast clearance from the blood compartment may not necessarily mean that drug action is also short-lived. The relationship between a pharmacokinetic profile and the pharmacodynamic result of the presence of the drug can be quite

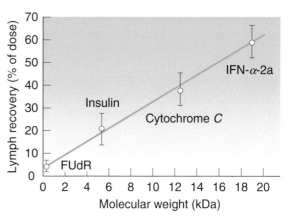

Fig. 41.1 Correlation between the molecular weight and the cumulative recovery of recombinant interferon (IFN α-2a), cytochrome C, inulin and 5-fluoro-2′-deoxyuridine (FudR) in the efferent lymph from the right popliteal lymph node following s.c. administration into the lower part of the right hind leg of sheep (from Crommelin & Sindelar 2002).

complex. A drug may trigger a reaction, which may result in measurable, pharmacological effects much later. As an example, the cytokine interleukin-2 (IL-2) (in its PEG-ylated form) is rapidly cleared from the blood compartment and a pharmacological effect (increase in the number of blood lymphocytes) is observed long afterwards (can be days) (Fig. 41.2).

Finding alternatives to the parenteral route has been an area of interest for many years. Table 41.4 lists different possible routes of delivery for proteins.

With the exception of the pulmonary route, all other options have a low bioavailability. Some bioavailability data on the intratracheal administration of proteins in rats are shown in Table 41.5. The extent of absorption depends strongly on the nature of the protein. An insulin formulation is now marketed for pulmonary delivery to diabetics to mimic the natural physiological response to a meal (postprandial glucose control). Subcutaneous injection gives a relatively slow response; pulmonary uptake is faster. New pulmonary delivery devices (see Chapter 36) not only increase average bioavailability but also reduce variation in uptake.

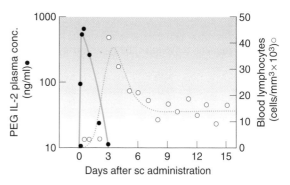

Fig. 41.2 PEG-IL-2 pharmacokinetics and pharmacodynamics (changes in blood lymphocyte count) after subcutaneous adminstration of 10 MIU/kg in rats. PEG = polyethylene glycol (from Crommelin & Sindelar 2002).

Three approaches have been followed to improve the bioavailability of pharmaceutical proteins when exploring alternative routes of administration. First, coadministration of protease inhibitors, such as bacitracin, should

---

Table 41.4   Alternative routes of administration to the oral route for biopharmaceuticals (adapted from Crommelin & Sindelar 2002)

Route	Relative advantage	Relative disadvantage
Nasal	Easily accessible, fast uptake, proven track record with a number of 'conventional' drugs, probably lower proteolytic activity than in the GI tract, avoidance of first-pass effect, spatial containment of absorption enhancers is possible	Reproducibility (in particular under pathological conditions), safety (e.g. ciliary movement), low bioavailability for proteins
Pulmonary	Relatively easy to access, fast uptake, proven track record with 'conventional' drugs, substantial fractions of insulin are absorbed, lower proteolytic activity than in the GI tract, avoidance of hepatic first-pass effect, spatial containment of absorption enhancers (?)	Reproducibility (in particular under pathological conditions, smokers/non-smokers), safety (e.g. immunogenicity), presence of macrophages in the lung with high affinity for particulates
Rectal	Easily accessible, partial avoidance of hepatic first-pass effect, probably lower proteolytic activity than in the upper parts of the GI tract, spatial containment of absorption enhancers is possible, proven track record with a number of 'conventional' drugs	Low bioavailability for proteins
Buccal	Easily accessible, avoidance of hepatic first-pass effect, probably lower proteolytic activity than in the lower parts of the GI tract, spatial containment of absorption enhancers is possible, option to remove formulation if necessary	Low bioavailability of proteins, no proven track record yet (?)
Transdermal	Easily accessible, avoidance of hepatic first-pass effect, removal of formulation is possible if necessary, spatial containment of absorption enhancers is possible, proven track record with 'conventional' drugs, sustain/controlled release possible	Low bioavailability of proteins

Table 41.5 Absolute bioavailability of a number of proteins (intratracheal versus intravenous) in rats (from Crommelin & Sindelar 2002 with permission)

Molecule	MW (kDa)	No. of amino acids	Absolute bioavailability (%)
α–Interferon	20	165	>56
PTH-84	9	84	>20
PTH-34	4.2	34	40
Calcitonin (human)	3.4	32	17
Calcitonin (salmon)	3.4	32	17
Glucagon	3.4	29	<1
Somatostatin	3.1	28	<1

PTH, recombinant human parathyroid hormone

slow down metabolic degradation. Second, excipients (often with an amphipatic character, such as bile salts) can be added to enhance passage through epithelial barriers. The third approach is to prolong the presence of the protein at the absorption surface, e.g. by the use of mucoadhesives.

Intranasal delivery of chitosan and starch microspheres demonstrated enhanced uptake of coadministered insulin. In humans, intranasal delivery of insulin with chitosan results in absolute bioavailabilities of 7%. In conclusion, bioavailability is indeed strongly enhanced when using these approaches, but safety issues must be addressed before these absorption enhancers can be introduced into marketed products.

Release control

Many therapeutic proteins are short-lived in the blood compartment. Assuming there is a direct relationship between blood level and therapeutic effect, it is important to maintain therapeutically relevant drug concentrations in the blood stream. Portable pump systems with adjustable pump rates are available for patients. Catheters provide the link between the pump and, for example, the peritoneal cavity. These systems are particularly useful if a constant dose input is required and the drug is needed over a limited period of time. Otherwise, more flexible delivery systems are preferred. For insulin (with a plasma half-life of 5 minutes) different forms of controlled-release systems for s.c. injection are available. Release control is based on different physicochemical appearances (amorphous/crystalline) of insulin itself and on insulin complexes with Zn^{2+} ions or proteins, such as protamine. Zn^{2+} ions tend to slow down the release of insulin. Amorphous insulin plus Zn^{2+} ions results in

moderate prolongation of drug action. Crystalline insulin plus Zn^{2+} ions gives a long-acting product. The addition of protamine (at neutral pH a positively charged protein) to insulin and Zn^{2+} ion combinations protracts the insulin effects even more (up to 72 hours; and thus can be classified as long-acting). Isophane insulin (NPH: neutral protamine Hagedorn) contains insulin and protamine in isophane proportions (no excess of either component), resulting in intermediate-acting formulations.

At present, efforts are being made to build 'closed-loop' systems in which insulin administration is controlled by:

- a biosensor permanently monitoring blood glucose levels
- an infusion pump with adjustable pump rate, and
- an electronic section with an algorithm linking blood glucose levels to insulin need at any time.

In hospitals such equipment is available to stabilize blood glucose in patients for limited periods, but no portable 'patient-friendly' systems for chronic use are yet available.

In even earlier stages of development are 'artificial pancreases'. Isolated insulin-producing β cells from the islets of Langerhans are introduced into the body in a container system with a wall that allows the passage of glucose, insulin and nutrients. However, the container wall keeps the β cells separated from the patient's immune system. Increasing blood glucose levels will stimulate the secretion of insulin by the encapsulated β cells. The excreted insulin will be released from the container and glucose levels will fall until normal blood levels are reached.

Controlled-release systems containing microspheres (with diameters between 10 and 100 μm) for s.c. administration are currently under development. A 30-day action sustained-release system designed on the basis of biodegradable polylactic-glycolic acid has been formulated for human growth hormone. These microspheres are prepared using a double emulsion technique whereby the proteins are exposed to organic solvents, and protein encapsulation efficiency is rather low. Alternatively, a dextran-based microsphere preparation protocol has been developed without the use of organic solvents and with extremely high loading efficiencies.

SUMMARY

Protein drugs are rapidly gaining in importance, and both market volume and market share are growing. Biotechnological techniques permit the design and synthesis of active proteins. It is the task of the pharmaceutical formulation scientist to turn the pure substance into a stable formulation that can be safely administered to the patient, exerting optimal therapeutic benefits. In this chapter different aspects of this formulation process are described and special attention is given to those aspects where biotech products clearly differ from low molecular weight drugs.

REFERENCE

Crommelin, D.J.A., Sindelar, R.D. (2002) *Pharmaceutical Biotechnology*. Taylor and Francis, London.

BIBLIOGRAPHY

Baudys, M., Kim, S.W. (eds) (1999) Insulin delivery. *Advanced Drug Delivery Review,* **35**, 141-335.

Franssen, O., Vandervennet, P., Roders, P., Hennink, W.E. (1999) Chemically degrading dextran hydrogels: controlled release of a model protein from cylinders and microspheres. *Journal of Controlled Release*, **59**, 219-228.

Manning, M.C., Patel, K., Borchardt, R.T. (1989) Stability of proteins. *Pharmaceutical Research,* **6**, 903-917.

Wang, W. (1999) Instability, stabilization and formulation of liquid protein pharmaceuticals. *International Journal of Pharmaceutics,* **185**, 129-188.

42

Packs and packaging

P. M. Taylor

FUNCTIONS OF PACKAGING

Packaging has been defined as the means of economically providing:

- presentation
- identification and information
- protection
- convenience and compliance
- containment during storage

to a product during all phases of its lifespan. This includes storage, transportation, display and use of the product, and the best pack will enhance the usability and profitability of the product. Packs may be classified as primary packs, which are in direct contact with the product and have a primary role in maintaining product quality, and secondary packs, which contain the product and primary pack and have more of a presentational and protective function.

Pack design

The presentation of a pack and the aesthetics of its design depend very much on the nature of the product. Current medicines regulation in the UK effectively divides pharmaceutical products into those which can only be obtained with a prescription, those that do not require a prescription but can only be purchased from a pharmacy, and generally available or 'over-the-counter' (OTC) medicines. The regulatory agencies require that all pharmaceutical packs provide the same information about the product (e.g. MHRA Guidance Note 25, 2003) – proprietary name, dose, approved name of active components and so on – but the actual design will vary from one type of product to another.

Prescription products tend to have a relatively straightforward design in keeping with their primary market of healthcare professionals, whereas OTC products are more distinctive to attract customers at point of sale and there are also common design features amongst products from the same brand line to enhance the brand identity. Generic prescription products also tend to share a common design, in this case linked to the generic company's overall identity, but concerns have been raised over having too uniform a design as it may lead to confusion between different products in a busy dispensary. Companies are now using variations in visual appearance to distinguish between different products, or different doses of the same product, whilst keeping sufficient common elements to maintain the company identity (e.g. Editorial 2003). Pack design covers more than the decorative aspects, however, and there has been much work in recent years to ensure that good design principles are applied to all the elements of a pack to ensure safety, compliance and convenience for the patient (Wang 2005).

Use of product

The pack should encourage convenience of product use and patient compliance with usage instructions but, apart from maintaining quality, it does not normally affect the functioning of the product. There are some products, however, where the pack is essential to the product's use, a commonly encountered example being an inhaler used to treat asthma. In cases such as this the pack should be considered as an integral part of the delivery system and development of the product should take this into account. Indeed, there is an argument for considering the pack to be part of the product in all cases. The remainder of this chapter, though, will use 'product' to represent the dosage form contained in the pack, except where stated otherwise.

PROTECTIVE FUNCTIONS OF PACKS

One of the main functions of a pack is protection, as this will be of great importance to the quality of the product. Potentially there is a wide array of factors which might adversely affect the product. It is a combination of the pack's format, materials of construction and the type of closure used which gives protection against these.

Environmental protection

Temperature

If a medicine is sold worldwide it can potentially be exposed to an extremely wide range of temperatures. High temperatures increase the rate of reaction and can therefore shorten a product's shelf life, and repeated cycling between high and low temperatures can also cause stability problems (e.g. 'cracking' of creams). In general it is not possible to design a pack which can protect against extremes of temperature for a long time and in cases like this, good labelling to show appropriate storage conditions plays an important role. There are certain subtleties that need to be considered, however. The packaging materials need to be chosen carefully as extremes of temperature may alter the material's properties (e.g. certain plastics become brittle at low temperatures). It should not be assumed that a product intended for temperate climates will not be exposed to extremes of temperature. Transportation during winter may expose the product to prolonged low temperatures, and medicines at home are often stored in the hottest and most humid rooms in the house – the kitchen or bathroom.

Moisture and humidity

Water, in either the liquid or vapour state, can cause a wide variety of problems. Chemical reactions are usually sustained much more easily in aqueous solution, water itself can cause chemical instability via hydrolysis, and an aqueous environment can support the growth of microorganisms. Physical problems at high atmospheric humidity include the caking of powders, dulling or tarnishing of metals and, depending on the difference in moisture levels inside and outside the container, either loss of water from the product or dilution of the product. The pack material and closure are important in preventing problems with moisture, as is the physical design of the container (total surface area and size of opening). For products which have a particular sensitivity to moisture, which can be as diverse as effervescent tablets in metal tubes and dry powder inhalers, sachets of silica gel desiccant are put into the pack to ensure minimal local humidity.

Light

Photodegradation is another major cause of chemical instability, with ultraviolet light being the most damaging. This is easily protected against by using coloured or opaque containers, as well as secondary packs, but care should be taken that labels do not fade or discolour.

Gases and volatile materials

Oxygen is another cause of instability, via oxidation, but carbon dioxide may also cause problems with unbuffered aqueous products as it can dissolve in the water to lower pH by forming carbonic acid. Plastics are permeable to gases and vapours to varying degrees, depending on the type of plastic, but they generally tend to be five times more permeable to carbon dioxide than oxygen.

Volatile compounds may also cause problems with permeable packaging materials. Generally these are present in fragrances or flavouring agents, and permeation of volatile components through the walls of the container can cause a change in taste or odour which may be unpleasant. It is conceivable that volatile components may permeate into the container from the external environment, tainting and possibly harming the product.

Mechanical protection

The product will need to be protected against a variety of mechanical stresses during its life cycle, especially during transportation and storage, and secondary packaging is of particular importance here.

Compression

This is a fairly steady force and occurs most frequency during storage when packs are stacked upon each other. Compression may not directly affect the product but crushing of a pack will affect its appearance and saleability. Protection against compression is afforded by secondary packs made from cardboard of a suitable thickness.

Impact

More sudden and intense forces can happen during movement of the pack or by accident (e.g. dropping). Damage from impact can be minimized by cushioning the primary pack or holding it snugly in the secondary pack, but it is better to prevent damage by careful handling.

Vibration

This frequently occurs during transportation and can lead to physical instability in the product (such as separation of powders) or gradual opening of closures such as screw caps. The stability of the product should be optimized during the formulation and processing development, but improving the performance of the pack requires careful specification of the pack components and full testing of them during development of the product.

Biological hazards

Microbiological

The pack should, as far as possible, minimize contamination by microorganisms, which can cause spoilage of the product as well as pose an inherent health risk. The closure will be the most important component in achieving this end and must provide a reasonable seal and be capable of repeated use. If the product is intended for repeated use then it should also be adequately preserved. Sterile products should be hermetically sealed, use a packaging material capable of supporting the chosen method of sterilization and must be used immediately after opening. Sometimes microorganisms can attack the packaging itself: paper and other fibrous materials are susceptible to attack by fungi (e.g. *Aspergillus* or *Penicillium* species) in damp conditions.

Other infestation

It is possible that insects, rodents or other organisms can contaminate products during storage or transportation. Again, fibrous materials are most vulnerable but, although usually unlikely, infestation is better controlled by good storage conditions than by changing packaging materials.

Humans

Here the concern is to prevent pilferage and tampering with the product. A major stimulus for introducing tamper-proof packaging was the Tylenol tragedy in the US. In 1982 an unknown person, who was never traced, contaminated capsules of Tylenol (an American brand of paracetamol) with cyanide, as a result of which there were several deaths. Subsequent investigations showed how easy it was to remove capsules from the pack, a screw-topped bottle, open the capsule shells, contaminate the contents and then replace the capsules. Since then, medicines have been packed in containers which should prevent tampering or at least show whether tampering has taken place by means of some kind of seal on the closure.

TYPE OF PACK

There are many factors which need to be considered when selecting a suitable type of pack for a product:

- the product or pack contents
- the application of the product
- content stability, and the need for protection from any environmental factors
- content reactivity (with relation to the packaging material)
- acceptability of the pack to the consumer or user
- the packaging process
- regulatory, legal and quality issues.

Each of these factors needs to be addressed when the pack is specified, but over the years the relative importance of these factors has varied. The introduction of new materials and packaging methods has had a great influence, but arguably the single most important change has been the trend of 'original pack dispensing', where the pharmacist dispenses a standard course of medication in the manufacturer's original pack, rather than repacking the medicine from a bulk supply into a generic pack. There are many advantages to this scheme: there should be improved patient safety; manufacturers' original data about the medicine, such as expiry date and batch number, will be preserved; and pharmacists will find it easier to fulfil their legal obligations to provide a patient information leaflet as this will already be present in the pack. From the manufacturer's point of view, original pack dispensing means that a broader variety of pack types needs to be considered and design of the pack must be directed to the patient rather than an intermediate medical professional.

The following sections relate choice of pack to the type of product; it is not an exhaustive review of pack types, rather it highlights various problematic areas of packaging. Packaging materials will be discussed in greater depth in the next section of this chapter.

Solid products

Solid dosage forms such as tablets and capsules are by far the most commonly used today. Traditionally they have been packed in bottles, originally made from glass but latterly from various plastics. The walls of the container are usually amber or completely opaque to minimize the possibility of photodegradation. Effective closure should maintain a reasonable barrier (particularly important for capsules, where excessive moisture can soften the gelatin capsule shells) while still being easy to open and close repeatedly. The mouth of the bottle should be wide enough to allow rapid filling on a high-speed production line and during dispensing.

Powders and granules have a variety of roles when used as the final dosage form and this is reflected in the pack used. A common use of these particulate forms is as a cold or flu remedy which is intended to be dissolved in (often warm) water, and they are usually packed as single doses in flexible sachets to allow convenient carriage of a day's requirements. The sachets will be formed from laminated materials which confer good water-barrier properties (the powders or granules are often effervescent) and allow attractive and informative designs to be printed on them. These dosage forms provide an example where a packaging need influences the formulation and manufacture of the product: the particles should have a reasonably uniform size and density distribution as there could otherwise be segregation of the particles during the packaging stage and irregular doses will result.

A key application of powders is in parenteral products which are reconstituted before injection and such powders are usually lyophilized, or freeze dried. The freeze-drying step is carried out on the powder in its final pack, a glass vial or ampoule that needs to be designed to optimize the drying process as well as performing all the other functions required of the pack.

The preceding discussion has concerned packs used for the final product as presented to the patient or consumer, but the most widespread use of powders and granules is as starting or intermediate materials in the manufacture of other dosage forms. These materials will be packed in bulk, often using temporary packs. More permanent packs are used for raw materials, and the type depends on the quantity and properties of the material. Smaller quantities can be packed in bottles, cartons or tins but larger quantities (5 kg plus) will be packed in sacks made of thick paper, plastic or laminates, or drums of metal or plastic. Again there has to be minimal entry of moisture, which can cause caking of a powder surface as well as chemical stability problems. Metal containers will need to be lined to prevent corrosion problems, although it is usual for bulk powders to be contained within a polyethylene bag as the primary pack. Polyethylene bags are sometimes used for temporary storage of materials in process if the quantity is in the order of tens of kilograms; these packs must be closed and labelled properly – self-adhesive paper labels should be used rather than writing directly on the pack with a marker pen, as components of the ink can migrate into the product.

Semi-solid products

The relevant characteristics of these products for packaging purposes are that they are often too viscous to flow but contain a sufficient amount of water to be classified as 'wet' products, with the usual potential problems of microbial contamination and loss of water from the product. Semi-solid products include creams, emulsions, gels, ointments (which strictly speaking should be free of water as they have hydrocarbon bases) and pastes, and the pack should allow the product to be removed easily. Jars or tubs with wide mouths are frequently used, made from either glass or plastic. The product should be adequately preserved as there will be a relatively large surface area open to contamination.

Flexible tubes are frequently used to contain semi-solids; these can be made from aluminium, although this is not as common as it once was, a plastic such as polyethylene or a plastic-aluminium composite. The latter combination, while being more expensive than plastic alone, has the advantage of deforming permanently, whereas plastic alone tends to spring back into its original position once the deforming force has been removed. This can lead to the phenomenon of 'suck-back', where product which has been exposed to the external environment can be pulled back into the tube and cause contamination problems. Unlike most packs, tubes have two closures, as they are filled through the wider end opposite the cap, which is then sealed by folding and crimping (aluminium) or with heat and pressure (plastics). The product should be formulated to allow it to be easily expelled from the tube without being too fluid.

Liquid products

Traditionally glass has been the material of choice for the packaging of liquids, but a variety of plastics is now also widely used providing they have little or no permeability to the liquid. Aqueous products are the most common type of liquid pharmaceutical formulation and usually materials such as high-density polyethylene are suitable

for short- to medium-term storage without losing water through the walls of the container. Oils may present a problem with plastics, however, as they may be absorbed by the plastic with results that range from altering the strength of the product to a catastrophic weakening of the plastic. Volatile oils may present particular problems if they have an affinity for plastic packaging, as they often give fragrance or flavour to a product and even a minimal sorption of the oil to the plastic may substantially alter the product's taste or smell.

Many liquid products are required to be sterile and the packaging material must be capable of withstanding the rigours of terminal sterilization. Glass is an excellent choice for sterile products as it is not normally affected by sterilization procedures, it can be formed into a wide variety of pack formats (bottles, vials, ampoules, etc.) and it can be hermetically sealed. There is a limited choice of plastics, as there is a much greater potential for the sterilization process to cause interactions between the product and the pack or for the packaging material's properties to alter (e.g. sterilization by radiation could cause the production of highly reactive free radical species). Sterilization may cause other problems if insufficient care has been taken over the pack design – paper labels may come unstuck from glass bottles if the pack is autoclaved, for example.

Unit packs

Unit packs, in which individual doses are separated from each other, are popular for many types of dosage form. They offer a number of advantages over the types of pack discussed above, principally those of convenience to the patient and being well suited to original pack dispensing. The two major forms of unit pack are strip packs (essentially a strip of sachets) and blister packs, which are commonly for tablets and capsules.

Unit packs protect individual doses of the medicine, so any break in the pack should only affect one or two doses, and patients can carry around just the number of doses that they require if the pack is serrated between each dose. A convenient course of medication can be packed into a carton by the manufacturer with a patient information leaflet, and the carton itself provides a more convenient area for giving statutory information than a label on a bottle. A variety of plastics, metals and laminates can be used in forming unit packs and careful selection of these materials will confer any combination of desirable properties on the pack. Unit packs can be more costly to manufacture than a container with the equivalent number of doses, but the unit pack may have a corresponding saving in transportation and storage costs if it is lighter and less bulky than the traditional pack.

Child-resistant packaging

Medicines pose particular dangers to children, because of their potentially greater toxicity and the appearance of some medicines which would entice children into taking them. Packaging to protect children from medicines has been available for over 30 years, and it usually relies on a closure system which is too difficult for the child to open. Standards require that at least 85% of children will be unable to open a child-resistant pack, but that more than 90% of adults should be able to open one. New British and European standards for child-resistant packaging were introduced in 2005 (Wilkins 2005).

Child-resistant containers work on one of two principles: in the first a certain degree of strength will be needed to open the product, and for the second a high degree of manual coordination is required. These translate into three basic types of cap: one which needs to be pushed down before turning; one which needs squeezing before turning; and one where arrows on the cap and container need to be lined up. Blister packs and sachets also have a degree of child resistance. The drawback to some of the systems is that adult patients suffering from disorders like severe arthritis will also be unable to open child-resistant packs.

Guidelines are available to pharmacists informing them when child-resistant containers must be used and when easy-to-open packs may be substituted.

Tamper-resistant packaging

The need for tamper-resistant packaging has been discussed above, although the exact terminology varies, with some authorities using the term 'tamper-evident packaging' and others going further and calling it 'tamper proof'. Tamper resistance can be conferred on a pack by using a Roll-On closure which has a perforated collar which grips onto a lip on the bottle neck, and these perforations must be broken before the cap can be unscrewed. Alternatively a clear plastic film collar can be put around the cap, or a film wrap over the whole container. Blister packs, sachets and similar packs are inherently tamper resistant as the pack must be broken open to gain access to the product.

PACKAGING MATERIALS

Glass

Glass has been used as a packaging material for centuries and has many excellent qualities for pharmaceutical packaging. It is a versatile and attractive material which can be moulded into many shapes, sizes and colours of container, it is hygienic and suitable for sterilization, it has excellent barrier properties (being totally impermeable), it is relatively non-reactive (depending on the grade chosen), it can accept a variety of closures, and glass containers can be used on high-speed packaging lines. In contrast, there are really only two disadvantages to glass as a packaging material: it is relatively heavy and it is fragile in tension, so can shatter easily. The disadvantages can be addressed to a certain extent by careful design of the containers, so the glass walls are thicker where there are greater stresses but thinner elsewhere to reduce weight.

Glass is a supercooled liquid formed after the fusion of silica (silicon dioxide), sodium carbonate and calcium carbonate; the latter ingredients will be transformed to oxides at the high temperatures used. The ratio of these basic ingredients can be changed and other materials added to modify the properties of the glass. For example, lowering the sodium content can increase the chemical resistance of the glass, but this also raises the melting temperature of the mixture. Addition of boric oxide can decrease the melting temperature, making the glass somewhat easier to process. Table 42.1 gives typical compositions for two grades of pharmaceutical glass.

Most glass used for pharmaceutical purposes is either colourless, also known as 'white flint' glass, or amber to prevent ultraviolet light causing photodegradation of the product. The amber colouration results from the addition of iron oxide in the glass. Care must be taken with liquid formulations to ensure that iron oxide does not leach into the product where it can act as a catalyst for some degradation reactions. Other colours have been associated with specific products (e.g. blue glass with certain antacids) but these packs have tended to be superseded in recent years by other materials, and the vast array of possible colours and decorations for glass is now seen in packs for consumer products such as cosmetics rather than pharmaceuticals.

Pharmaceutical glass is grouped into four categories depending on its reactivity (e.g. *British Pharmacopoeia* 2005, Appendix XIXB). Type I, also known as neutral or borosilicate glass, is the least reactive as it contains boric

Table 42.1 Typical final compositions (as weight %) of two grades of pharmaceutical glass		
	Type I glass	Type III glass
Silica	66–74	66–75
Calcium oxide	1–5	6–12
Sodium oxide	7–10	12–19
Aluminium oxide	4–10	1–7
Boric oxide	9–11	None

oxide, which replaces some of the more reactive sodium oxide. This type of glass has higher ingredient and processing costs and is therefore used primarily for more sensitive pharmaceuticals such as parenteral or blood products. Because of the nature and use of these products, most containers made of type I glass are ampoules and vials, and these are formed from lengths of glass tubing rather than being blow-moulded as other glass containers are. Type II, or treated soda-lime glass, also has a high chemical resistance but not as much as type I. It is cheaper than type I glass, however, and is acceptable for most products except blood products and aqueous pharmaceuticals with a pH greater than 7. The low chemical reactivity is actually defined as a high resistance to hydrolysis (it should be noted at this point that the concept of chemical reactivity in glass is a relative one – glass as a whole has little or no reactivity under normal conditions) and is conferred on the glass by a process known as 'sulfating' rather than by altering the chemical composition. Sulfating involves treating the glass surface with sulfur dioxide or ammonium sulfate to neutralize the reactive alkali groups there.

Types III and IV glass have similar compositions and are distinguished from each other by their hydrolytic resistance. Type III has average or slightly better than average resistance and is suitable for non-aqueous parenterals and non-parenteral products; type IV glass has the lowest hydrolytic resistance, which can sometimes be seen as a surface bloom if the glass is stored in damp conditions for prolonged periods, and is suitable for solid products, some liquids and semi-solids, but not for parenterals.

Metals

At one time metals were widely used as rigid containers for many types of solid product. The principal metals used were tin-plated steel and aluminium but in recent years other materials have replaced many of the metals' applications and tin-plate is rarely used now. Aluminium still has many uses as it is relatively light yet strong, totally impermeable and easy to work into a variety of formats, depending on its thickness. The thickest aluminium is used for rigid containers such as aerosol cans and tubes for effervescent tablets; intermediate thicknesses are when mechanical integrity is still important but the pack should be capable of being deformed under a reasonable force (e.g. collapsible tubes for semi-solid preparations or roll-on screw caps); the thinnest aluminium is used in flexible foils that are usually a component of laminated packaging materials.

A major drawback of aluminium is its reactivity in its raw state. Although it does rapidly form a protective film of aluminium oxide, it is still liable to corrosion when exposed to some liquid and semi-solid formulations, particularly at extremes of pH or if the product contains electrolytes. The latter can, in principle, be particularly hazardous as they cause galvanic corrosion which produces hydrogen gas. To prevent these reactions occurring, aluminium that will come into contact with problematic formulations is lined with resins such as epoxide (gives better protection under alkaline conditions), vinyl or phenolic (better under acid conditions) resins. This drives up the cost of the packaging, however. Another disadvantage of aluminium is work-hardening and the remedy for this problem again adds cost to the material. Collapsible tubes are made by impact extrusion, which tends to make the aluminium less flexible and the flexibility has to be restored by an annealing stage. Despite these disadvantages, aluminium will continue to find use in pharmaceutical packaging, mainly because it is a total barrier to both light and chemicals.

Rubbers (elastomers)

Rubbers are excellent materials for forming seals, so they are used almost exclusively to form closures such as bungs for vials or in similar applications such as gaskets in aerosol cans. The two main categories of rubber are natural and synthetic, and the strengths of one group tend to be weaknesses in the other. Natural rubber as it is extracted from the rubber tree is a weak and sticky substance so to make it into a more durable material, it is reacted with sulfur-containing chemicals to crosslink the elastomer molecules ('vulcanization'). Natural rubber therefore has a complex composition: the vulcanization process requires other chemicals to control the reaction and both natural and synthetic rubber contain various additives to aid their processing or modify their properties (e.g. fillers, pigments, antioxidants and plasticizers).

The properties of natural rubber make it particularly suitable for multiple-use closures for injectable products, as the rubber reseals after repeated insertion of a needle. There are several drawbacks to natural rubber, though. It does not age well or tolerate multiple autoclaving, becoming brittle, and the presence of all the additives leads to a relatively high degree of extractable material. There is also the risk of product adsorbing onto or absorbing into the rubber, and there is a certain degree of moisture and gas permeation.

Synthetic rubbers, which include butyl, bromobutyl, chlorobutyl, neoprene, nitrile and silicone rubbers, tend to have the advantages and disadvantages reversed. Synthetic rubbers have fewer additives and thus fewer extractables, and tend to experience less sorption of product ingredients. Silicone is the least reactive of the rubbers but it does experience permeability to moisture and gases. The synthetic rubbers are less suitable for repeated insertion of needles because they tend to fragment or core, pushing small particles of the rubber into the product. An important property of rubbers in this context is their hardness, which is a property determined by the resistance of the rubber to indentation. Softer rubbers experience less coring and reseal better, whereas harder rubbers are easier to process on high-speed packaging lines.

The relative complexity and variety of rubbers mean that full specification of composition should be obtained, and compatability and stability tests conducted before the final selection of material is made.

Plastics

Of all the packaging materials, plastics are the most versatile because of their sheer variety, although they fall into two main categories. The thermosetting resins are made by mixing two or more reactants together and pouring them into a mould where they set; once moulded they cannot be reset, and subsequent heating usually causes their chemical decomposition. Thermosetting resins have few applications in packaging today and they are mostly used for rigid screwcaps. Nearly all the plastics used in packaging are thermoplastics – they can withstand repeated heating, which merely softens and melts the material if kept to reasonable temperatures. This defining property of thermoplastics leads to the first of their many advantages as packaging materials, as they can be formed by techniques such as injection moulding, blow moulding, extrusion or lamination into a huge range of pack types. These packs are usually resistant to breakage and cheap to produce and, providing the right plastic(s) are chosen, will provide the necessary protection of the product in an attractive container.

Like rubbers, plastics are complex materials which may have many constituents apart from the actual polymer, including: residues from the original synthesis of the polymer (e.g. monomer residues, catalysts, accelerators, solvents); additives intended to modify the properties of the polymer (e.g. plasticizers, antioxidants, antistatic agents, colours and whiteners, fillers, UV blockers); or agents to aid some part of the processing (e.g. lubricants, mould release agents). Most plastics will only contain a few of these constituents but, as they are potentially extractable, care should be taken when specifying the plastic for the pack, and full testing of the extractables should be carried out.

Apart from the possibility of extractable material permeating into the product, packaging plastics as a group suffer from a number of drawbacks. Nearly all plastics are permeable to some degree, depending on the storage conditions and the exact nature of the pack and product. Moisture and gases may pass into the containers from the external environment. It has been found that the relative permeability of $CO_2:O_2:N_2$ is approximately 20:4:1. Moisture may also pass out of the pack containing an aqueous formulation. This will alter the strength of the product, and other materials which can migrate out of the product include active ingredients, antioxidants, preservatives, fragrances and flavours. Hydrophobic plastics may encourage permeation of the oily phase from some emulsions and creams. There need not be complete migration of these ingredients to the external environment, and often there is sorption to the plastic itself. Regardless of the exact type and extent of permeation, there will be a consequent loss of function in the product. Migration of substances out of the packs or steam autoclaving can also cause panelling, a deformity of the pack walls. Finally, components of the plastic, notably dyes and plasticizers, may leach into the product. The extent of permeability is temperature and humidity dependent and is also influenced by various properties of the plastic, such as the presence of plasticizer and polymer hydrophilicity, both of which tend to increase permeability.

Other problems are usually linked to specific conditions or groups of plastics. Polyethylene is prone to stress cracking in the presence of surfactants, or vegetable or mineral oils. Chemicals like isopropyl myristate (a common component of skincare creams) produce crazing (a fine network of surface cracks) in polystyrene followed by a weakening and eventually collapse of the container. Rigid polystyrene and PVC have poor impact resistance, which can be improved by adding an elastomer to the plastic although there is an associated increase in the polymer's permeability. Polyethylene and polypropylene are difficult to print to directly unless they have a surface pretreatment, as the ink does not 'key' or take hold. Poor ink keying can also occur when substances migrate to the surface of the plastic.

Polyethylene (PE) and polypropylene (PP)

Polyethylene (polythene) is probably the most commonly used and economical of the packaging plastics. It is graded according to its density – commonly low-density polyethylene (LDPE; approx. 0.915 g/cm³) and high-density polyethylene (HDPE; approx. 0.965 g/cm³) – as many of its applications and properties are related to density. The density increases because of an increase in the length and linearity of the polymer chains, and this leads to the following changes in bulk properties of the material:

- greater rigidity
- higher distortion and melting temperatures
- lower gas and vapour permeability
- increased tendency to stress cracking.

Common additives to polyethylene are antioxidants (e.g. butylated hydroxytoluene at a concentration of hundreds of ppm) and antistatic agents such as polyethylene glycols or long chain fatty amides at concentrations around 0.1% by weight; the antistatic agents minimize accumulation of dust and other small particles on the container's surface.

HDPE is used for more rigid packs, like bottles and tubs, and has a good enough moisture barrier for most purposes and a good chemical resistance. Although a better gas barrier than the lower density polyethylenes, it is still not a particularly good barrier. Lower density polyethylenes are used for more flexible packs such as the ubiquitous polythene bag and as a constituent in laminated films.

Very low-density polyethylene is very flexible and has a high impact and tear strength, so it can confer some degree of puncture resistance to a laminate, and ultra low-density polyethylene and specialized derivatives such as ionomeric PE (Surlyn®) have a role as the heat-sealing layer in laminates.

Polypropylene is not quite as common as polyethylene but is widely used for making closures, and it has similar properties to polyethylene. Polypropylene is also suitable for rigid packs, has good resistance to most chemicals apart from certain organic solvents and similar barrier properties to HDPE. It does not stress crack and has a better resistance to high temperatures, making it more suitable for steam sterilization, although it is more brittle at lower temperatures than polyethylene. In order to make it more suitable for low temperature storage, it can be blended with an ethylene/propylene copolymer.

Polyvinyl chloride (PVC)

This is another of the widely used plastics and, in a similar way to polyethylene, it has a variety of applications depending on the grade used. In this case, the grade of PVC is determined by whether it is plasticized or not, with the former being used for flexible packaging and the latter for rigid packs.

Unplasticized PVC (uPVC) is a clear, colourless material with good chemical resistance and a reasonably good barrier to moisture and gases. The addition of fillers such as titanium dioxide make it opaque to visible and ultraviolet light. Prolonged exposure to UV light or heat will cause the PVC to yellow, so a light stabilizer has to be added. Excessive heat causes PVC to decompose to corrosive products, which means that high temperatures have to be avoided during processing, but it is sufficiently heat stable to allow moulding. The impact resistance of uPVC is relatively poor but this can be improved with the addition of an impact modifier. uPVC is widely used for such diverse pack types as bottles and blister packs, where it is used to form the moulded tray.

Plasticized PVC is used in bags, films, laminates and other flexible packs and is a popular material for tubing, infusion bags and similar medical devices. The plasticizer, usually dioctylphthalate, is added to increase the PVC's flexibility, but it also lowers its strength and melting point and decreases its barrier properties. All PVC must have a very low residual content of the vinyl chloride monomer. This has been implicated in producing serious health problems among plastics workers. There have also been environmental concerns about dioctylphthalate, although it is approved for use in food packaging. PVC has a tendency to ab- or adsorb chemicals and this must be taken into account when drugs are given via PVC infusion sets as the effective dose of the drug might alter.

These concerns about PVC notwithstanding, it has been used for packaging pharmaceuticals and other goods for human consumption for many years and is still widely used today.

Polystyrene

Unlike the previous examples, polystyrene is only used for rigid packs. General-purpose polystyrene is a hard, crystal clear plastic that is used to make attractive and economical bottles or jars, often for containing solid dosage forms. It is not as suitable for liquid or semi-solid formulations as it allows a high transmission of water vapour and oxygen and, as mentioned above, has poor resistance to certain chemicals. Polystyrene is another plastic with poor impact resistance but it can be made tougher with the addition of elastomeric or acrylic compounds, with some loss of clarity. It is not suitable for steam sterilization because of its low melting point.

Other plastics

Polycarbonate is a strong, transparent polymer with a good chemical resistance. It is capable of withstanding sterilization procedures. It is used for rigid packs where other materials will not be as effective, but it is not otherwise widely used because of its cost.

Polyethylene terephthalate (PET) has been used extensively in food packaging for several decades to make drinks bottles. It has good impact strength and provides a good barrier to gases and vapours. It has regulatory acceptance for food products, but is not used as extensively in the pharmaceutical area.

Nylon (polyamide) is more hydrophilic than most other plastics, which means it is a poor barrier to water and has a high incidence of drug–plastic interactions. It is not so useful for the long-term storage of drugs or medicines, but its strength, resistance to chemicals and autoclaving, and ability to form thin sheets make it suitable as a component of laminated packs.

Examples of other plastics which have specialized uses in pharmaceutical packaging are: polytetrafluoroethylene (PTFE, Teflon®), polyester, polyvinylidene chloride (PVdC), styrene acylonitrile (SAN) and acrylontrile butadiene styrene (ABS).

Fibrous materials

Although paper and cardboard, materials based on cellulose fibres, have few applications today as primary packs for pharmaceutical products, they are still widely used for secondary packaging and in subsidiary roles. Cardboard is used for cartons to protect the primary pack and provide an area suitable for decorative design and holding the information required by regulatory authorities. Cartons are convenient for stacking and can hold information leaflets easily. Card can also be used inside secondary packs as dividers or trays. Thicker, corrugated cardboard and fibreboard are used for shipping cartons as these have to tolerate greater mechanical stresses than ordinary cartons.

Paper will be found in most packs as the label on the container and as the patient information leaflet. The paper will usually be printed and may be coated, part of a laminate or adhesive backed. Occasionally, as with sterile sachets for syringes and dressings, paper will be a constituent of the primary pack. Sacks made from thick paper, lined with polyethylene, are used as the primary pack for some bulk powders.

Polymer technology has been used in recent years to introduce more advanced replacements for traditional cellulose-based fibre materials, Tyvek® being a notable example. Tyvek® is made from spun-bonded polyethylene fibres and can be used in most of paper's packaging roles. It has the advantage of being much stronger and more resistant to water and other chemicals.

Foils, films and laminates

These are the main types of thin, flexible packaging. Foils are thin sheets of metal, typically less than 100 µm thick; films are non-fibrous, non-metallic and less than 250 µm thick (technically a thin material is a sheet if it is greater than 250 µm thick); and a laminate is formed when two or more film or foil webs are bonded together.

Foils

The most important metal for this application is aluminium. Foils are primarily used because of their excellent barrier properties. Modern technology enables foils to be produced to thicknesses as low as 10 µm, although below 25 µm gives an increasing risk of pinholes forming, which compromises its barrier properties. The foil can be used by itself or, more often, it is used in combination with other materials in laminates. It has the additional advantage of providing an attractive, reflective surface. Thicker aluminium sheets can be used in more rigid packaging, such as the trays of blister packs, where they are formed by cold-moulding, and are becoming a useful alternative to plastic trays. The problem of work-hardening has been mentioned above and the processing of the aluminium foil or sheet will require an annealing stage to restore its mechanical properties.

Another development using aluminium as part of a thin film is *vacuum dispositioning* in which a thin film of aluminium is effectively 'sprayed' onto a polymer substrate such as polyester. This confers some barrier properties on the polymer but they are not as good as a proper aluminium foil. The film can be printed on one side and have a shiny aluminium coating on the other. This process of metallizing can use paper or card as the base.

Films

The earliest packaging films were made from regenerated cellulose and are what we now call cellophane. Cellophane is an attractive, transparent film which can be coloured and printed upon, so is useful as an outer wrap. It has reasonable barrier properties to vapours but not moisture, although this can be improved by coating the cellophane with various substances. Coated cellophane is also suitable for heat-sealing purposes. Both coated and uncoated cellophane are still in widespread use today in pharmaceutical, food and other types of packaging.

Nowadays many other plastics (e.g. PVC, LDPE, polypropylene and polyester) can be used to make films, a common application being outer wraps for other packs. Some plastics, such as PVC in thicker grades, are suitable for thermomoulding into trays which can be used as part of a blister pack or to hold primary packs inside a secondary pack (e.g. a tray holding several glass ampoules inside a cardboard carton). Plastic films generally have one or two strengths, rather than a range of beneficial properties. This restricts their use as the sole packaging material. If multiple functions are required then films with the desired properties can be selected and combined in a laminate.

The following lists the main properties of the most common plastic films:

- moisture barrier (relative to other plastic films) – PVC, HDPE, polypropylene
- gas barrier (relative to other plastic films) – polyester, nylon, PVC, PVdC
- heat sealers – mainly LDPE, with some nylon and polypropylene
- thermoformable layer – PVC
- printable layers – polyester, nylon, polycarbonate.

Laminates

Laminates are used to combine the properties of individual foils and films, and strictly are made by bonding the layers with adhesive. This can introduce problems as there might be migration of the adhesive through the inner layers of the laminate into the product, especially if the product is a liquid or semi-solid in close contact with the laminated walls of a sachet. As with the other complex packaging materials, it is essential to specify the pack carefully, obtain full specifications from the material's supplier, and thoroughly test compatibility and stability with the intended contents of the pack.

An alternative to adhesive-bonded laminates is coextruded polymers in which the bonding is produced by extruding two or more polymers simultaneously through a single die. This can be cheaper than traditional methods of lamination and allows more control over the final thickness of the web, which can be much thinner than traditional laminates. Coextrusion is only suitable for polymers. Lamination must be used if any of the layers is paper or foil. Although not strictly accurate, coextruded polymers will be considered here under the heading of laminates.

A typical laminate might have many layers to fulfil all the requirements of the pack, so a sachet for a tablet might have the following layers (from the outside in): a layer for decoration and information, a layer for mechanical protection, a layer for light and moisture barrier and a heat sealer layer. Examples of laminated materials are (outer layer given first):

- 'high-performance' plastic laminate – polyester/polyethylene
- coated paper – paper/LDPE
- thermoformed tray for blister packs – nylon/PVC or PVC/polyethylene
- high barrier laminate – paper/polyethylene/Al foil/Surlyn or polyester/Al foil/polyethylene.

The large array of possible functions that laminates can have has led to their widespread adoption in blister packs, bubble packs, strip packs, pouches, sachets and other types of flexible pack.

CLOSURES

The importance of the closure to the proper functioning of a pack, in particular in preventing contamination of the product and enhancing usability by the patient, has already been alluded to. Aside from the considerations of the closure's functioning as part of the pack, the requirements of high-speed packaging lines need to be taken into account. The first consideration when selecting a closure is to ensure that the product is sealed to an appropriate degree.

The most stringent type of closure is a total hermetic seal, which does not allow the passage of any microorganism or gaseous or liquid substances. It is usually achieved by thermal fusion of the material from which the container is made. Hermetic seals are used for single-use sterile products as once the seal is broken, it becomes ineffective.

The next type of closure forms an effective microbiological seal, but there may be some diffusion of other substances and the closure can be reused (e.g. rubber bungs).

Finally, there is the closure which provides an acceptable degree of protection to the product. A cap on a tablet bottle should be a reasonable barrier to moisture, microorganisms and other substances but the pattern of usage is such that the bottle may be opened several times a day and there will inevitably be some exposure to environmental contaminants.

Blister packs, sachets and other flexible packs, as well as ampoules, do not need a separate closure as they are heat sealed. The nature of the packaging material will determine whether the heat seal is truly hermetic, although there is nearly always a good microbiological barrier. Heat sealing is not considered a reliable method for containers holding powder as there is a chance that during the packaging process fine particles will be shaken from the powder surface and lodge in the region of the pack that will be sealed, thus lowering the integrity of the seal.

Other types of container will require a separate closure, usually a cap or bung of some description. Caps are usually made from aluminium, thermosetting plastics (phenol-formaldehyde or phenol-urea) or thermoplastics (polyethylene or polypropylene) which can be retained on the container via a screw thread, an interrupted thread which the cap engages with lugs on its rim or as a crown cap (a single-use closure for glass bottles).

Apart from the mechanism to hold the cap on the container, there will often need to be some kind of lining to give a reasonable seal between cap and container. Metal caps will have a coating of rubber around their circumference to provide the seal, and the metal itself will be lacquered to prevent any interaction with the product. Thermosetting plastics will have a cap insert which is usually a composite of several materials: a backing material made of card coated with a lining of aluminium or plastic film which will form the contact with the product.

One-piece caps are preferred for various quality reasons, such as uniformity and ease of processing, and thermoplastics will be preferred because they can be moulded to give an internal sealing ring. Polyethylene or polypropylene will be the thermoplastics of choice because of their barrier properties, and also because when the caps are screwed onto the container there will be a small degree of 'give' in the plastic which allows an effective seal to be formed.

A specialized type of closure is the roll-on cap, which is formed on the container itself. A plain aluminium cap is pushed over the neck of the container and force is applied from the side to make the aluminium fit the shape of the neck. If the neck has a screw thread then the roll-on cap is pressed to match that thread exactly. This type of closure has the benefit of economy compared to a pre-formed screw cap as well as providing a good seal over the neck. Roll-on closures also permit tamper-evident closures to be formed if the cap includes a strip at the bottom separated from the main cap by perforations. In use this strip will be crimped over a lip at the bottom of the neck, and in order to remove the cap the perforations between cap and strip are broken when the cap is unscrewed. Roll-on closures can also act as a safety device for bungs in vials; if the aluminium is crimped over the bung and the lip of the vial, it prevents the bung being removed. A detachable disc of aluminium on top of the crimp will prevent needles being inserted into the bung unless the disc is removed (if the disc has been unexpectedly removed from the container, it indicates possible interference with the product).

Another type of closure is the bung, which uses either natural or synthetic rubber because of their ability to form a seal. General considerations about rubber have been discussed above, but an important property for its ability to act as a bung is compression set. Compression set is a measure of the rubber's ability to return to its original dimensions after being subjected to a compressive force – a rubber with low compression set is more resistant to being compressed. The effectiveness of a rubber as a bung (and also in other sealing applications such as syringe plungers) needs an intermediate value of compression set:

too high and the rubber does not form an effective seal because it deforms to much; too low and the bung is difficult to apply because it does not compress enough.

REGULATORY AND QUALITY CONSIDERATIONS

Regulatory considerations

Pharmaceutical products are subject to several regulatory and legal regimes. These include the requirements for obtaining a marketing authorization for the product, usage guidelines produced by the local regulatory agency, statutory guidelines for the supply of medicines and any other applicable laws such as Sale of Goods Acts, and Weights and Measures Acts. Regulatory agencies will need evidence on how the pack affects the stability and overall quality of the product, the effect on product usability, validation of manufacturing methods and so on. While the majority of packs will be relatively straightforward and have similarity to many other packs on the market, each marketing authorization application must be judged on its own merits, and there is an increasing recognition that even the simplest of packs makes an important contribution to use and compliance by the patient.

Developers of packs have various resources available to them in the form of national standards, guidelines from the regulatory agencies (e.g. the Best Practice Guidance on Labelling and Packaging of Medicines from the MHRA) and pharmacopoeial specifications. Tables 42.2 and 42.3 respectively show, as examples, the BP 2005 specifications for pharmaceutical containers, and the materials used for manufacturing such containers (Appendix XIX corresponds to Section 3.2 of the *European Pharmacopoeia*, and Appendix XX to sections 3.1.1–3.1.15).

Table 42.2 British Pharmacopoeial specifications for pharmaceutical containers (Appendix XIX, BP 2005)

Section	Contents
A	Pharmaceutical containers introduction (definitions of single-dose, multidose, well-closed, airtight, sealed, tamper proof, child-proof containers)
B	Glass containers for pharmaceutical use
C	Plastic containers
D	Containers for blood and blood components
E	Rubber closures for containers for aqueous parenteral preparations
F	Sets for the transfusion of blood and blood components
G	Sterile single-use syringes

Table 42.3 British Pharmacopoeial specifications for materials used in the manufacture of containers (Appendix XX, BP 2005)

Section	Description
A	Materials for containers of human blood and blood components
B	Polyolefines
C	Polyethylene
D	Polypropylene for containers and closures for parenteral preparations and ophthalmic preparations
E	Polyethylene-vinyl acetate) for containers and tubing for total parenteral nutrition
F	Silicone (liquid and elastomer)
G	Plastic additives
H	Polyethylene terephthalate for containers for preparations not for parenteral use

General quality considerations

The quality control of pharmaceutical packs is ultimately governed by the applicable Good Manufacturing Practice (GMP) and Good Laboratory Practice (GLP) guidelines. The pack developer should first of all ensure that the supplier of the packaging material has a full specification of the required pack, and that identity should be confirmed on delivery. It may be necessary to confirm the identity of the material on receipt from the suppliers, especially for plastics and rubbers where there can be superficial resemblances between materials which are quite different chemically and mechanically. The usual method for identification is infrared spectroscopy.

Pharmacopoeias frequently have monographs for some, but not all, packaging materials. For glass, a typical monograph would describe tests to distinguish between the different types using, for example, hydrolytic resistance to etching by hydrofluoric acid, tests and acceptable levels for extractable materials, and a specification for the absorbance of ultraviolet light by amber glass. Similarly there may be monographs for plastics and rubbers that specify tests and limits for stated extractables and in the case of rubbers, the mechanical properties relevant to their use in closures (e.g. penetrability by a needle, fragmentation) can be given.

Compatibility between the product and pack will be determined during informal and formal stability studies. The regulatory requirements for formal studies require that production-scale batches of the product should be stored in the type of pack, including labels, which will actually be used for the marketed product. Typical storage conditions may be 25°C/60% relative humidity for at least 12 months, plus accelerated stability conditions of 40°C/75% RH for at least 6 months and any others that may be appropriate to the product. Other environmental factors, such as exposure to light and light/dark cycles, will form part of the storage conditions. and there may be exposure to mechanical vibration to simulate transportation conditions (this can affect closure, as poorly specified caps may loosen). If the product is a liquid packed into vials closed with rubber bungs, then part of a stability batch may be inverted at regular intervals to see whether any materials can be extracted from the bung into the liquid.

Compatibility between product and pack will be determined by taking samples of product at regular intervals (3–6 months for long-term stability studies) and testing to see whether product specifications are met and that extractable materials are within acceptable limits. It is prudent when formal stability studies are carried out to include a batch of product in a different pack, for example, a batch of tablets in an amber medicine bottle if it is proposed to market the product in blister packs, so both packs will be approved for use and the second pack can replace the first if there are problems with that one. The formal stability study should be conducted on product made with the validated manufacturing process and one of the validated procedures will be for packing the product using a high-speed packaging line.

There will be a number of quality issues concerning the closure because of its importance to the functioning of the pack. The integrity of the closure can be determined by various tests involving the application of a vacuum or immersion in water (sometimes containing a dye) to see whether there is any movement of material between the outside and inside of the container. Dye tests are useful with heat-sealed packs like sachets, whereby test sachets are filled with a dye solution and exposed to a vacuum to show the path of any interruptions in the seal. The ease of using closures should also be measured, using opening and closing torques for caps, and the various forces required to push doses out of blister packs, insert bungs or tear open sachets.

SUMMARY

The pharmaceutical pack has so many important functions: it should protect the product against many possible sources of harm, it should help maintain the quality of the product, it must contain essential information about the product and it should make the product easy and convenient for the patient to use. Key design points of a pack are its barrier properties and the closure. There is a great diversity of packaging materials and pack designs to ensure the packaging aims are met. The diversity of materials also means that great care should be taken over specifying packs and then testing them. In short, the pack is of such importance to the proper functioning of a medicine that packaging development is an integral part of product development.

REFERENCES

British Pharmacopoeia (2005) British Pharmacopoeia Commission, London.

Editorial (2003) Coloured-pack generic range to expand. *Pharmaceutical Journal*, **271**, 286.

MHRA (2003) *Best Practice Guidance on Labelling and Packaging of Medicines*, Guidance Note 25. Medicines and Healthcare Regulatory Agency, London.

Wang, L-N. (2005) How designer pharmacy could provide the answers to patient issues. *Pharmaceutical Journal*, **275**, 507-508.

Wilkins, S. (2005) Child-resistant packaging: the latest standards and how the industry is responding. *Pharmaceutical Manufacturer and Packaging Sourcer*, **May**, 12-16.

BIBLIOGRAPHY

Ambrosio, T.J. (2002) Packaging of pharmaceutical dosage forms. In: Banker, G.S., Rhodes, C.T. (eds) *Modern Pharmaceutics*, 4th edn. Marcel Dekker, New York.

Bauer, E. (2006) *Pharmaceutical Packaging Handbook*. CRC Press, Boca Raton, Florida.

Dean, D.A., Evans, E.R., Hall, I. (2000) *Pharmaceutical Packaging Technology*. Taylor and Francis, London.

Jenkins, W. A., Osborn, K.R. (1993) *Packaging Drugs and Pharmaceuticals*. CRC Press, Boca Raton, Florida.

43

Microbial contamination, spoilage and preservation of medicines

N. A. Hodges

NEED TO PROTECT MEDICINES AGAINST MICROBIAL SPOILAGE

The need to protect foods against microbial spoilage is well appreciated since microbial growth results in obvious signs of deterioration, but there is a much lower level of awareness among the general public of the need to similarly protect cosmetics, toiletries and medicines. Although most medicines present a less favourable environment for microbial growth than foods, a wide variety of potentially hazardous organisms is nevertheless capable of growing to high concentrations in unprotected products. The subject of preservation is therefore an important aspect of medicine formulation, simply because patients taking medicines are, by definition, unhealthy and so quite possibly more vulnerable to infection.

It is important to distinguish between the terms *contamination* and *spoilage* because they are sometimes used synonymously, which is incorrect.

Contamination, in this context, means the introduction of microorganisms into a product, i.e. it describes microbial ingress. Contaminating organisms can arise from many sources (considered later in this chapter) during the course of both product manufacture and subsequent use of the product. The procedures of good manufacturing practice (GMP, also considered later) are used to limit the first of these, but contamination arising from the patient is largely out of the control of the manufacturer except in the context of container design and labelling. There has been a trend in recent years to adopt containers that minimize contact between the patient's body and the product, e.g. collapsible tubes are used for creams and ointments rather than open-mouthed tubs or jars into which fingers can be inserted. Similarly, single-dose eye drops may be preferred to bottles where the dropper can come into contact with an infected eye and then be replaced in the eye drop solution. Despite this, contamination by the patient is still a problem to be considered in container design and product preservation.

Spoilage follows contamination and describes the process and consequences of microbial growth in the product. Considering the potential for product spoilage and taking appropriate steps to minimize the risk of it occurring are very much the responsibility of the formulation scientist and the manufacturer.

There are three principal reasons why microorganisms should be excluded totally from medicines or their presence subjected to stringent limits set by pharmacopoeias or regulatory agencies like the United States Food and Drugs Administration (FDA) or the UK's Medicines and Healthcare products Regulatory Agency (MHRA):

- Products or raw materials contaminated with pathogenic organisms may be an infection hazard.
- Microorganisms may cause chemical or physical changes in the product that render it less potent or effective.
- Microbial growth is likely to make the product unacceptable to the patient or consumer even if there are no significant infection risks or loss of efficacy.

It is quite obvious that medicines should not contain pathogenic organisms and so represent a source of infection. However, specifying the species and numbers of organisms that represent an infection hazard is not straightforward. Certain pathogens are recognized as 'objectionable organisms' and must be totally excluded from particular raw materials or product types (see Chapter 15), but the risk of infection is influenced not just by the number and type of organism but by other factors too. For example, an organism may be present at a concentration that would be regarded as relatively harmless to a healthy individual but which may pose a problem for patients with impaired immunity.

In the 1960s and 1970s there were several reports in the pharmaceutical literature of infection occurring as a result of medicines containing pathogenic species, e.g. salmonellae, clostridia and *Pseudomonas aeruginosa*, but such reports became far less frequent towards the end of the last century with the adoption of more rigorous quality standards and regulatory control of manufacture. However, contaminated medicines are by no means a thing of the past. The FDA publishes on its website details of product recalls, and there were 45 instances between 1992 and 2004 where microbially contaminated products were recalled from the United States market. It should be emphasized that there is the possibility of an infection arising from the use of a product contaminated with a concentration of organisms that is too low to be detectable by sight or smell. This situation is potentially much more hazardous than that of a patient confronted with a medicine in which microbial growth is clearly evident.

Quite apart from representing an infection hazard, microorganisms may damage the medicine by degrading either the active ingredient or one or more excipients, thus compromising the quality and fitness for use of the product.

Degradation is usually due to either hydrolysis or oxidation but decarboxylation, racemization and other reactions may also occur. Active ingredients known to be susceptible to microbial attack include steroids, alkaloids, analgesics and antibiotics. Much of the literature on this topic has been reviewed by Bloomfield (1990) and Spooner (1996). The numbers and variety of excipients that have been reported to be degraded are at least as great as those of active ingredients. Thus, most categories of excipients contain materials that have been shown to be susceptible to microbial enzymes, acids or other metabolic products.

Common examples of product instability or deterioration include emulsion separation due to surfactant degradation, loss of viscosity due to microbial effects on gums, mucilages and cellulose derivatives employed as thickening agents, and alcohol and acid accumulation following fermentation of sugars. Despite the fact that the very purpose of their use is to restrict microbial growth, even some preservatives are vulnerable to inactivation by microorganisms that, in exceptional cases, use them as a carbon and energy source.

If microbial growth within the product is sufficiently extensive, it is possible for the presence of the organisms to be detectable by:

- their physical presence (cloudiness in liquid medicines, moulds on or in creams and syrups or as discolouration of tablets stored in a damp environment)
- changes in colour (pigment production)
- smell (due, for example, to amines, acetic or other organic acids, or sulfides from protein breakdown)
- gas accumulation without any obvious odour (bubbles of carbon dioxide following sugar fermentation).

Clearly, any product manifesting such changes would be unlikely to be used by the patient. This may result in short-term problems for the patient of obtaining alternative supplies, and possible longer term problems for the manufacturer of customer complaints, product recalls, adverse publicity and possible legal action.

PRODUCTS AND MATERIALS VULNERABLE TO SPOILAGE

Spoilage, in the sense of detectable physical or chemical change within a pharmaceutical product, nearly always follows growth and reproduction of the contaminating organisms. The pharmacopoeial and regulatory limits for the maximum permissible numbers of microorganisms in manufactured products or raw materials are typically not more than 100–1000 colony-forming units per mL or gram. Whilst these concentrations may allow some pathogens to initiate infections, they are not normally sufficient to cause detectable changes in chemical composition, physical appearance or stability. Bacteria and fungi are just the same as all other living organisms in requiring water for growth (although not necessarily for mere survival). This means that only products containing sufficient water to permit such growth are vulnerable to spoilage. Consequently, spoilage is not normally a problem in anhydrous products like ointments and dry tablets or capsules, although hygroscopic materials like gelatin and glycerol may absorb enough water from the atmosphere to enable moulds (but not normally bacteria) to grow. Similarly, cellulosic materials, particularly paper and other packaging, may show mould growth if stored in humid atmospheres, e.g. in tropical climates.

The fact that a product contains water and is obviously a liquid does not necessarily mean that the water is available to participate in chemical reactions and enable microorganisms to grow. Some of the water present in a solution is bound to the solute due to hydrogen bonding or other mechanisms. Thus a parameter that indicates the proportion of 'free' or available water is a useful guide to the ease with which microorganisms might grow in the product. Such a parameter is *water activity* (A_w) which is the ratio of water vapour pressure of a solution to the water vapour pressure of pure water at the same temperature. A_w is expressed on a scale from zero to 1 with a value of 1.00 representing pure water. As the concentration of solute in a solution is increased, A_w falls proportionately and the range of organisms able to grow in the solution progressively diminishes. Thus, it is possible to construct a table indicating the minimum A_w values that permit the growth of different types of microorganism (Table 43.1).

To a certain extent the values of A_w in Table 43.1 are reflective of the natural habitats of the organisms concerned; pseudomonads and other waterborne organisms therefore tend to require high A_w values for optimum growth, whilst skin organisms like staphylococci and micrococci that exist in relatively high salt concentrations (from sweat glands) will tolerate significantly lower values. Pharmaceutical materials that have high solute concentrations, e.g. syrups, may to a large extent be self-preserving just like salted foods. Syrup BP, for example, is 67% by weight sucrose, has an A_w value of 0.86 and so is not susceptible to bacterial growth, but may contain chemical preservatives to protect it from mould spoilage.

Variations in water activity may arise within a single container of a manufactured medicine by, for example,

Table 43.1 Water activity (A_w) minima permitting growth of various organisms

Organism	Approximate minimum water activity
Many common waterborne or soil organisms and non-skin pathogens e.g. *Pseudomonas aeruginosa*, clostridia, *E. coli*	0.95
Staphylococci and micrococci	0.87
Many yeasts, e.g. *Saccharomyces* and *Candida* spp.	0.88–0.92
Many fungi, e.g. *Penicillium*, *Aspergillus*, *Mucor*	0.8–0.9
Osmophilic yeasts, e.g. *Zygosaccharomyces rouxii*	0.65

water evaporating from the bulk liquid during storage in high temperatures and that water vapour condensing on cool glass round the neck of a bottle as the storage temperature drops, then running back to dilute the surface layer of product. It is for this reason that syrups should not be stored in fluctuating temperatures.

The possibility also exists for contaminants to grow and generate water from respiration and so produce localized increases in A_w which allow other, less osmotolerant organisms to grow subsequently. Reducing the water activity of a product as a means of diminishing its susceptibility to spoilage is a formulation strategy that should not be overlooked. However, sugars and glycerol are the only common and acceptable ingredients that may be used in this way in oral products. With topical products, however, alcohols and glycols may also be employed.

SOURCES AND CONTROL OF MICROBIAL CONTAMINATION

In order to manufacture medicines of acceptable microbiological quality, it is necessary to know the common sources of microbial contaminants in the manufacturing environment and the typical organisms that might arise from each source. It is also useful to know how quickly and to what concentration those organisms might grow in pharmaceutical materials in order to put in place good manufacturing procedures that will minimize contamination and spoilage.

Sources and types of contaminating organism

Microbial contamination of medicines arises from three principal sources:

1. The raw materials, including water, from which the product is manufactured.
2. The manufacturing environment including the atmosphere, equipment and work surfaces.
3. Manufacturing personnel.

The relative contributions of these three sources vary depending upon the type of product in question. It has been noted (see Table 15.3) that raw materials of different origin may vary significantly in their extent of microbial contamination. `Natural' materials originating from animals (e.g. gelatin), vegetables (starch, cellulose derivatives, alginates) or minerals (talc, kaolin, magnesium trisilicate, bentonite) usually have much higher bioburdens than synthesized chemicals in which organisms are often killed by heat, extremes of pH or organic solvents. Despite the high levels of microorganisms to be found in locations where many natural materials arise (gelatin, for example, originates in the slaughterhouse where faecal contamination of animal carcasses is not uncommon), the cleaning and purification procedures currently employed mean that contamination levels are only one or two orders of magnitude higher than those for synthesized chemicals. This is reflected in the pharmacopoeial limit of not more than 10^4 cfu of aerobic bacteria per gram for oral products containing materials of natural origin compared with 10^3/g otherwise.

Generally, the types of contaminating organisms are reflective of the origins of the product and this, in turn, is reflected in the objectionable organisms that must be absent. For example, salmonellae and *E. coli* might arise in faeces, so gelatin is subject to tests for the absence of these species. The same organisms might originate from natural fertilizers used on commercial crops and so they must be absent too from vegetable drugs, starches, mucilages, etc. Both vegetable drugs and mined minerals may contain organisms originating from the soil, e.g. *Bacillus* and *Clostridium* species, usually as spores. Vegetable drugs may be contaminated with spores of such fungal plant pathogens as *Cladosporium* that rarely arise in other circumstances.

Water is the most commonly used raw material for manufacturing medicines. Not only is it obviously present in liquid medicines, it may be added, then removed, during manufacture of dry products too, e.g. during tablet granulation. It is also used in the factory for cleaning equipment, work surfaces, mixing vessels and bottles or other product containers. As a consequence, the microbiological quality of both ingredient and cleaning water can have a profound effect on the final bioburden of the manufactured product. To those unfamiliar with methods of water purification, it is a paradox that pharmaceutical purified water is more likely to contain high levels of bacteria (particularly after storage) than the mains water that is used as the source material. This is simply a consequence of the fact that mains water (potable water) is chlorinated, and the chlorine which acts as a preservative is removed during purification. Despite this purification process, purified water still contains sufficient dissolved nutrients to support the growth of several species of Gram-negative bacteria to population levels well in excess of 10^5/mL. Such levels may be attained within days rather than weeks of room temperature storage after chlorine removal. The species commonly found are described as low-demand organisms, i.e. they are metabolically versatile and can efficiently utilize as nutrients low concentrations of a diverse range of carbon-containing compounds. Pseudomonads, i.e. the organisms resembling the pathogen *Pseudomonas aeruginosa,* are good examples of low-demand Gram-negatives, although organisms of other genera like *Flavobacterium* and *Alcaligenes* also arise.

Product contaminants originating from the manufacturing environment all tend to have one characteristic in common, i.e. they survive well in dry conditions. So the Gram-negative bacteria that are prevalent in water are rarely seen in this situation. Most of these environmental contaminants are spore-formers, both bacteria and fungi, or Gram-positive bacteria like micrococci and staphylococci. All of those can persist for long periods whilst attached to dust particles suspended in the atmosphere or settled onto floors, work surfaces or equipment. Modern pharmaceutical factories are supplied with filtered air, so the level of particulate contamination in the atmosphere in a room where there is no activity is usually very low. The main component of the dust in a manufacturing area that is actually in operation is skin scales shed by operational personnel. Humans replace skin constantly and so they are continually shedding particles with attached skin bacteria; these are typically about 20 μm in size and so cannot be seen with the naked eye. The extent to which skin scales are shed depends upon many factors like the design and coverage of protective clothing, general health, personal hygiene and, in particular, levels of activity. Persons standing or sitting still normally shed far fewer particles than those who are in motion. Statistics and estimates of the extent to which humans shed skin vary substantially, but numbers between 10^5 and 10^7 per minute have been quoted (White 1990).

Swabbing with antiseptics or washing with bactericidal soap reduces the numbers of microorganisms on the skin, but is by no means totally effective. Figure 43.1 shows a Petri dish used to take 'finger dabs' from fingers treated in this way. In the upper left segment bacterial

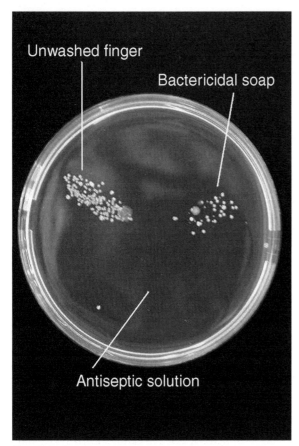

Fig. 43.1 Colonies of bacteria resulting from 'finger dabs' onto agar. Top left: bacteria from unwashed finger; top right: a finger washed with 'bactericidal' soap; bottom sector: no colonies arising from a finger swabbed with antiseptic solution.

colonies were cultured from an unwashed finger; the upper right shows the colonies from a finger washed with bactericidal soap and the bottom sector shows those from a finger swabbed for one minute with cottonwool soaked in antiseptic. It is clear that short periods of exposure to bactericidal soaps cannot be relied upon to eliminate contamination, but a recognized antiseptic is far more effective.

The methods and equipment used for monitoring levels of contaminants arising from water, raw materials and the environment are described in Chapter 15.

Factors influencing the growth of spoilage organisms

In addition to water activity that was considered earlier in this chapter, factors influencing the rate and extent of growth of a contaminant within a pharmaceutical raw material or manufactured medicine include:

- nutrient availability
- temperature
- pH
- redox potential
- the presence and concentration of antimicrobial chemicals.

Microorganisms differ enormously in their metabolic capabilities. Some, like *E. coli, Pseudomonas aeruginosa* and several *Bacillus* species, can synthesize all the amino acids and vitamins they need from a variety of simple carbon and nitrogen sources. The minerals that they require are often present in sufficient concentration as impurities in the ingredients of the medicine. Thus in the absence of antimicrobial chemicals, organisms of this type may grow to concentrations of 10^4 per mL or gram or even higher in products like syrups, linctuses and creams. Products containing glycerol, sugars, amino acids or proteins would clearly represent such ideal media for microbial growth that their preservation is sometimes difficult to achieve even with added preservatives. Even in the absence of these nutritionally rich materials, many bacteria and fungi are still able to utilize other components of the formulation as food sources. Several of these have already been mentioned, but in addition to surfactants and various viscosity-raising agents, the volatile and fixed oils used as flavourings or emulsion components are particularly suitable as nutrients for microorganisms.

The rate of spoilage progression will vary with temperature, although the period of time for which a manufactured medicine is usually stored before use is normally so long that the difference in bacterial growth rate between, say, 15°C and 20°C may become insignificant in the context of a 2-year shelf life. However, there is the possibility of organisms growing during the course of manufacture and so it is important for production scientists to be aware just how rapidly the population of contaminants may rise. Figure 15.1 shows that the concentration of *Pseudomonas aeruginosa* rose 10 000-fold in 44 hours at ambient room temperature in a multidose veterinary injection that was supposedly preserved with benzethonium chloride. Clearly, the potential for a rapid increase in numbers is even greater where there is no antimicrobial agent present at all.

Most bacteria have an optimum pH for growth that is near neutrality, whilst most fungi favour slightly acidic conditions and grow best at pH values of 5–6. Although product pH may markedly influence growth rate itself, it also has a bearing on the activity and stability of any antimicrobial chemicals present, so the magnitudes of these various effects may have to be considered at the product formulation stage and a compromise value selected for the product pH. This is considered further in the next section of this chapter.

Redox potential (oxidation-reduction potential; E_h) is a term that indicates whether oxidizing or reducing conditions exist in a liquid. It is expressed as a positive or negative value on a scale in millivolts. Oxidizing conditions (favouring the growth of aerobic organisms) prevail in culture media or liquids with positive E_h values and reducing conditions (favouring anaerobes) apply at negative values. Facultatively anaerobic organisms such as *E. coli* and many similar intestinal pathogens will grow under both conditions from +150 mV to −600 mV (Dempsey 1996). Most pharmaceutical products possess positive redox potentials and so anaerobic growth is not common. There is the potential for aerobic primary contaminants to utilize the available dissolved oxygen and so render the product vulnerable to secondary spoilage by anaerobes.

Antimicrobial chemicals are usually specifically added as preservatives in multidose sterile and non-sterile medicines. Their properties and the factors influencing their selection are considered later in this chapter. However, it is not uncommon for other ingredients of the product to possess antimicrobial activity or enhance the activity of recognized preservatives. Alcohols used as cosolvents are good examples: ethanol, isopropanol, propylene glycol and glycerol all possess useful antimicrobial activity, although, with the exception of glycerol, their use tends to be limited to topical products. Ethylenediamine tetraacetic acid (EDTA) has a dual role in many pharmaceutical products. It is a chelating agent used to remove metal ions that may catalyse the oxidation of certain active ingredients and, although it possesses little or no antimicrobial activity in its own right, it may markedly potentiate the action of many established preservatives (see below). Indeed, EDTA is present in 29 of the 65 proprietary eye drops currently available on the UK market. In almost every case, one of its functions is to potentiate the activity of benzalkonium chloride used as the preservative.

Control of contamination and spoilage during manufacture

Whilst product contamination during use is largely outside the manufacturer's control, there are many steps that can be taken to minimize contamination whilst the product is made, both by restricting the entry of new organisms into it and limiting the opportunities for growth of organisms that are unavoidably present at the start, from water or raw materials, for example. Many of these procedures and precautions are described in the *Rules and Guidance for Pharmaceutical Manufacturers and Distributors* (the 'Orange Guide'). That publication and other regulatory and pharmacopoeial requirements make it clear that employing good manufacturing practices to limit microbial contamination in the first place is the preferred strategy, rather than, for example, permitting contaminants to enter and proliferate in the product and then attempting to kill them by physical or chemical means.

The factors impacting on the hygienic manufacture of medicines are shown in Figure 43.2. Much of this is self-explanatory, although certain aspects merit more detail. Standards for atmospheric cleanliness in the manufacturing area apply not just for the production of sterile products, but for non-sterile medicines too. Thus, the air supply is invariably HEPA filtered and since air-conditioning plants often act as a breeding ground for microorganisms, filters need to be installed downstream of such equipment. The factors to be considered in the design of premises and equipment are detailed in the Orange Guide, as are the procedures for cleaning and disinfection. There is evidence that persistent use of a single disinfectant might predispose to the development of bacterial resistance to it, although this evidence is far less strong than that concerning antibiotics. Nevertheless, there is a requirement that disinfectants are used on a rotational basis to minimize this risk.

Since human beings are frequently a significant, if not the principal, source of microbial contamination in the atmosphere, their health, hygiene, clothing and training may all have an impact on product contamination. The design of clothing for use in different areas is described in detail in the Orange Guide. Whilst it is an unacceptable practice to use heat, radiation or antimicrobial chemicals to 'clean up' a product which has been allowed to acquire a high level of contaminants that could have been avoided, it is acceptable to use these methods to reduce high bioburdens that are unavoidable, e.g. in raw materials of natural origin. Thus, raw materials may be exposed to radiation or ethylene oxide for this purpose, and filtration units or ultraviolet (UV) light sources employed to reduce the bioburden in water. If the water is to be used as an ingredient of an injectable product, filtration is preferable to UV light because it physically removes the contaminating Gram-negative bacteria that may act as a source of endotoxins, which could cause fever on injection. Although UV light kills the bacteria, the endotoxins remain, because the lipopolysaccharide component of the bacterial outer membrane from which they are derived is not destroyed. Because of the ability of Gram-negative bacteria to grow readily in

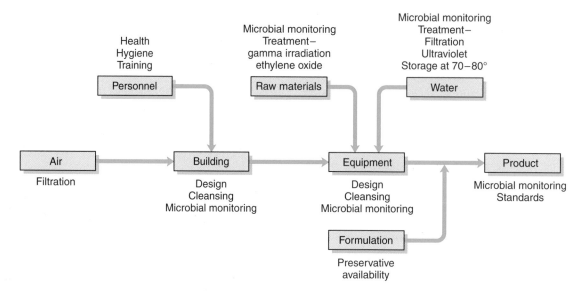

Fig. 43.2 Factors in hygienic manufacture.

stored purified water, it is also common for the water to be maintained at a high temperature, typically 80°C, whenever possible during the manufacturing process in order to prevent such growth.

The final factor shown in Figure 43.2 to impact on hygienic manufacture is that of preservative availability. Whilst the inclusion of a preservative to protect the product from spoilage sounds simple in principle, there are several ways in which the preservative activity may be diminished or virtually abolished as a result of interaction with other components of the formulation or the container. These are considered below.

SELECTION AND USE OF PRESERVATIVES

The antimicrobial chemicals commonly used as preservatives in medicines are described in Chapter 16. The properties that are normally required in such a preservative include the following:

- A broad spectrum of antimicrobial activity covering Gram-positive and Gram-negative bacteria, yeasts and moulds, and no vulnerability to resistance development
- Low toxicity for humans, enabling it to be used in topical, oral and parenteral products
- Good solubility in water; low oil solubility
- Stable and effective over a wide pH range and compatible with common excipients
- Non-volatile, odourless and tasteless.

Not surprisingly, no single preservative satisfies all these criteria; if there were such an agent it would be universally used to the exclusion of all others. Thus, the selection of a preservative (or combination of preservatives) for a newly developed product is inevitably a compromise determined by the formulation characteristics and intended use of the product. Unfortunately, the list of available preservatives is diminishing rather than expanding. This is due both to the high cost of safety testing that would be a prerequisite for the introduction of an entirely new preservative, and to toxicity concerns about some preservatives, causing the use of some agents to be largely discontinued, e.g. phenyl mercury salts and chloroform, which were formerly employed in ophthalmic/parenteral products and in oral medicines, respectively.

Since the function of a preservative is to kill, or at least prevent the growth of, microorganisms, it might be expected that the first item on the above list would be a major determinant in preservative selection, but, in fact, the intended use and route of administration of a product are usually the major factors limiting the choice. The range of potential preservatives is greatest for topical products, and becomes much more restricted when the toxicity considerations applying to oral and parenteral products are applied. Thus, there are several preservatives whose use is restricted largely to topical medicines, e.g. bronopol, isothiazolones and imidazolodinyl ureas.

It has been estimated that fewer than eight preservatives are in common use in the UK (Hiom 2004), with parabens being by far the most frequently selected for topical and oral products, although sodium benzoate is also regularly chosen for the latter. Multidose injections are now rarely used in human medicine but are still common in veterinary practice. Again parabens are used as preservatives with benzyl alcohol, phenol or chlorbutanol being common alternatives. Eye drops are usually, but not invariably, multidose products which, although initially sterile, may require protection against patient-derived contaminants during use. Benzalkonium chloride, often with EDTA, is more common in eye drops intended for the UK market than all other preservatives put together. Despite this popularity, there is increasing concern about the potential for benzalkonium chloride to cause corneal irritation. Single-dose or unpreserved eye drops are also used.

Due to the limited and diminishing range of acceptable preservatives, there has been increasing attention paid in recent years to the possible benefits of using preservatives in combination. Not only is there scope for reducing the concentrations of the agents – which should confer the benefits of reduced toxicity or irritancy – but employing two or more preservatives together might also result in a broader spectrum of antimicrobial cover, a lower risk of resistance development and enhanced activity due to synergy. There are combinations in which each component fills a gap in the antimicrobial spectrum of the other, e.g. parabens and imidazolodinyl ureas which have weak activity against *Pseudomonas aeruginosa* and fungi respectively. The practically useful examples of synergistic combinations have been listed by Hiom (2004). Generally, synergy is most likely to be exhibited when the two agents have dissimilar modes of action. If two agents from the same chemical class or with the same target site in the microbial cell are combined together, the result is commonly found to be additive. Care is required, however, in the investigation and reporting of synergy for two reasons:

- It is well established that synergy might only arise at selected combination ratios so it is unwise to assume that the effects displayed at one ratio will be seen at others.
- Synergy must be divorced from the effects of concentration exponents (see Chapter 16). It is tempting to assume that doubling the concentration of a preservative results in a doubling of its antimicrobial activity, and so two agents together producing more than twice the effect of either one alone must be synergy. This logic is incorrect, however, because some agents that have high concentration exponents, e.g. phenols, exhibit a large change in activity for a small change in concentration. Combining two such agents can result in a dramatic increase in effect that might be erroneously interpreted as synergy whereas, in fact, the increase is only that to be expected from doubling the concentration of either component alone.

PRESERVATIVE INTERACTIONS WITH FORMULATION COMPONENTS AND CONTAINERS

The adequacy with which a formulated medicine is protected from spoilage by the use of a preservative cannot easily be predicted from a study of the activity of the preservative in simple aqueous solutions. A person with limited knowledge of pharmaceutical microbiology might, for example, expect that it would be possible to confirm that a medicine was adequately preserved simply by conducted an assay for the preservative and showing it to be present at a concentration higher than that required to inhibit the growth of common contaminants (i.e. higher than minimum inhibitory concentrations – MIC values – quoted in reference books and explained here in Chapter 15). Not infrequently, however, this logic does not apply because the preservative activity is reduced as a result of it interacting with other components of the formulation or the container, or by a change in the environmental conditions within the product. As a consequence, it is necessary to measure preservative efficacy not by a chemical assay but by a pharmacopoeial preservative efficacy test where the manufactured medicine is inoculated with a range of test organisms whose death rate is measured over a 28-day period (see Chapter 15).

Contaminating microorganisms do not invariably grow uniformly throughout a medicine packed in its final market container; they may be concentrated near the surface as a result of the higher oxygen availability there or, in the case of an emulsion, they grow in the water phase rather than the oil. The concentration of preservative available at the site where the organisms are growing is therefore the principal determinant of how effectively the medicine is protected from spoilage, and the 'free' preservative concentration may be significantly lower than the calculated value. Figure 43.3 shows the major factors that influence preservative activity.

Several groups of common preservatives are affected by pH. This may be a consequence of:

- a change in ionization of the preservative molecule which alters the relative proportions of its undissociated and dissociated forms which possess different intrinsic antimicrobial potencies
- an effect on cell surface charge influencing adsorption of preservative molecules onto the microbial cell
- a change in the solubility or stability of the preservative molecule.

The weak organic acids, e.g. benzoic and sorbic acids, are the most commonly cited examples of preservatives whose ionization and activity are pH dependent, but there are sev-

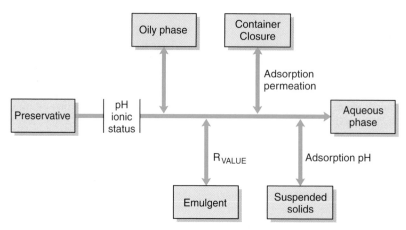

Fig. 43.3 Preservative availability.

eral others. These acids are effective in formulations that are naturally acidic or can be buffered to a low pH. This is because in these conditions they exist as the undissociated molecules which are more lipid soluble and more effective than the ionized forms that predominate when the ambient pH exceeds the molecule's pK_a value. Phenolic preservatives exhibit similar but less marked pH dependence. Parabens are also slightly affected in the same way.

This situation contrasts with that seen with quaternary ammonium compounds which are most effective in neutral or slightly alkaline conditions. Bacterial cells are usually negatively charged, and a rise in pH increases the number of such charges and so promotes the binding of positively charged molecules like quaternary ammonium compounds.

Even though many liquid medicines contain a buffer to restrict pH change, it is not uncommon for the product specification to quote a permissible pH range that is sufficiently large to have a significant impact on preservative activity and for the product pH to drift within that range during its shelf life which may be 2 years or more. Slow precipitation during storage (e.g. parabens precipitating in falling pH) is a further problem that is not necessarily detected by chemical assays because the assay procedure may redissolve the precipitate.

The oil/water partition coefficient is another molecular property that can have a marked influence on preservatives when they are used in emulsions. Since microorganisms grow in the aqueous phase, a preservative that partitions into the oil is essentially inactive, although again, this will not necessarily be apparent because a chemical assay is likely to show that the correct amount of preservative is present in a given weight or volume of sample. This is a factor that makes parabens less useful choices as cream preservatives because they are usually a lot more soluble in vegetable oil than they are in water,

although their partitioning might be reduced by substitution of mineral oil for vegetable oil. Again phenolics and some other preservatives are similarly affected, so when selecting preservatives for multiphase formulations, it is useful to consult publications like the *Handbook of Pharmaceutical Excipients* (Rowe et al 2006) where lists of solubilities and partition coefficients may indicate the likely extent of the problem.

Entrapment of preservatives within micelles of surfactants or emulsifying agents is a related phenomenon where again, the preservative is present but unavailable to inhibit microbial spoilage. Surfactants like lecithin, Tween (polysorbate) 80 and Lubrol W are so effective in removing preservative in this way that they are commonly used as inactivators (neutralizers) to prevent preservative carry-over and erroneous results in bioburden and preservative efficacy determinations (see Chapter 15). Dissolution and dialysis techniques together with mathematical models may provide some indication of the extent of preservative loss in such complex formulations. Complexation between anionic surfactants (e.g. sodium lauryl (docedyl) sulfate) and cationic preservatives (e.g. chlorhexidine and quaternaries) is also a potential problem in emulsion formulation.

Preservatives may be removed from solution by adsorption onto suspended solids like bentonite, kaolin, magnesium trisilicate and talc. Indeed, in the case of bentonite the potential to adsorb cationic drugs has been investigated as a means of retarding drug release to achieve a long-acting formulation. Antacid products, in particular, may prove difficult to protect due to preservative adsorption and there have been several reports of aluminium hydroxide-, magnesium trisilicate- and kaolin-based products being vulnerable to preservative inactivation. This is reflected in the *United States*

Pharmacopeia (2003) that specifies less stringent preservative performance criteria for antacids than for other oral products. The problems posed by adsorption are compounded by the fact that the phenomenon may also be pH dependent, so the most favourable pH for preservative activity itself may be one that promotes adsorption. Other hydrocolloids employed as viscosity-raising agents in oral and topical products, e.g. alginates, tragacanth, cellulose derivatives and polyvinyl pyrrolidone, may also reduce preservative activity. In some cases this is simply a charge effect where an anionic polymer like alginate complexes a cation like a quaternary ammonium compound.

The last major mechanism by which preservative activity may be compromised is interaction with the container or, in the case of volatile agents like chlorbutanol, permeation through the container and loss by evaporation. Preservatives may adsorb onto the internal surface or penetrate into the material of the container itself. This problem has become more significant as plastic has tended to replace glass as a packaging material. Rubber stoppers in vials may also cause preservative loss. Most plastics, but particularly those commonly employed for container manufacture, such as polypropylene and polyethylene, have the potential to remove significant amounts of parabens and other common preservatives. The surface-to-volume ratio of the product in its container is likely to have a bearing on the magnitude of the problem; small containers have a relatively larger surface and may exhibit proportionately greater loss.

REFERENCES

Bloomfield, S.F. (1990) Microbial contamination: spoilage and hazard. In: Denyer, S., Baird, R. (eds) *Guide to Microbiological Control in Pharmaceuticals*. Ellis Horwood, London, pp 29-52.

Dempsey, G. (1996) The effect of container materials and multiple-phase formulation components on the activity of antimicrobial agents. In: Baird, R.M., Bloomfield, S.F. (eds) *Microbial Quality Assurance in Cosmetics, Toiletries and Non-sterile Pharmaceuticals*. Taylor and Francis, London, pp 87-98.

Hiom, S. (2004) Preservation of medicines and cosmetics. In: Fraise, A.P., Lambert, P.A., Maillard, J-M. (eds) *Principles and Practice of Disinfection, Preservation and Sterilization*. Blackwell, Oxford, pp.484-513.

Rowe, R.C., Sheskey P.J., Owen, S.C. (2006) *Handbook of Pharmaceutical Excipients*, 5th edn. Pharmaceutical Press and American Pharmaceutical Association, London and Chicago (or latest).

Rules and Guidance for Pharmaceutical Manufacturers and Distributors (latest edition) Pharmaceutical Press, London.

Spooner, D.F. (1996) Hazards associated with the microbiological contamination of cosmetics, toiletries and non-sterile pharmaceuticals. In: Baird, R.M., Bloomfield, S.F. (eds) *Microbial Quality Assurance in Cosmetics, Toiletries and Non-sterile Pharmaceuticals*. Taylor and Francis, London, pp 9-30.

United States Pharmacopeia (2003) 51 Antimicrobial Effectiveness Testing. US Pharmacopeial Commission, Rockville, Maryland (or latest).

White, P.J.P. (1990) The design of controlled environments. In: Denyer, S., Baird, R. (eds) *Guide to Microbiological Control in Pharmaceuticals*. Ellis Horwood, London, pp 87-124.

44

Product stability and stability testing

A. R. Barnes

STABILITY OF PHARMACEUTICAL PRODUCTS

Pharmaceutical products tend to deteriorate on storage. The shelf life of a pharmaceutical product is the period of time during which, if stored correctly, it is expected to retain acceptable chemical, physical and microbiological stability. The expiry date, or expiration date, is the date given on the product packaging which represents the end of the shelf life.

Chemical stability

Chemical degradation of the drug is often the critical factor which limits the shelf life of a formulation. A reduction of drug content down to 90% of the theoretical value is generally regarded as the maximum reduction acceptable.

A simple means of increasing the shelf life of a product can sometimes be employed, by adding more drug than is declared on the label. This is known as an *overage*. If 110% of the theoretical amount of drug is added to the product when it is manufactured, twice as much degradation will be possible before the product reaches the end of its shelf life. This strategy is only possible for products where the dose is not critical and where the degradation products are not toxic, such as many vitamin products.

However, the nature of the degradation products which form in the product may instead be the factor that limits the shelf life of a product. This may be because the degradation products are toxic. For instance, the antifungal drug flucytosine degrades to fluorouracil, which is cytotoxic (Vermes et al 1999). The degradation products may alternatively give the product an unacceptable appearance. For instance, epinephrine's oxidation products are highly coloured.

The degradation of other ingredients in the formulation other than the drug may be a critical factor in its stability. This can include the degradation of antimicrobial preservatives, fading of dyes used to colour a product or degradation of antioxidants.

Types of chemical degradation reactions

Hydrolysis

Hydrolysis is the breaking of a molecular bond by reaction with water. Water is common in pharmaceutical products, either as an ingredient or as a contaminant, and hydrolysis reactions are the most common cause of chemical degradation. Most hydrolysis reactions involve derivatives of carboxylic acids.

Molecules containing the ester group hydrolyse to produce a carboxylic acid and an alcohol (Fig. 44.1a). The carbon of the carboxyl group of esters is relatively electron deficient, due to bond polarization caused by the adjacent oxygen atoms. Nucleophilic attack by water is therefore promoted at this carbon atom. The ester group is commonly found in drug molecules; examples include aspirin and procaine. For instance, the degradation of aspirin (acetylsalicylic acid) results in the formation of salicylic acid and acetic acid (Fig. 44.2). Aspirin is too unstable to allow the formulation of an aqueous aspirin product with a significant shelf life.

The amide group is also frequently found in drug molecules; it degrades to a carboxylic acid and an amine (Fig. 44.1b). Amides tend to be more stable to hydrolysis than the corresponding esters. This is because the nitrogen atom is less electronegative than the oxygen atom in the corresponding ester. Examples of amide-containing drugs include lidocaine and paracetamol (acetaminophen). The antimicrobial drug chloramphenicol is an amide-containing drug that is relatively susceptible to hydrolysis compared to many amides (Fig. 44.3). This is due to a high degree of polarization of the amide bond by the highly electronegative chlorine substituents which are adjacent. Eye drop preparations of chloramphenicol therefore require storage in a refrigerator.

The lactam group, which is a cyclic amide, is important because it is present in penicillin and cephalosporin antibiotics and this group is very susceptible to hydrolysis.

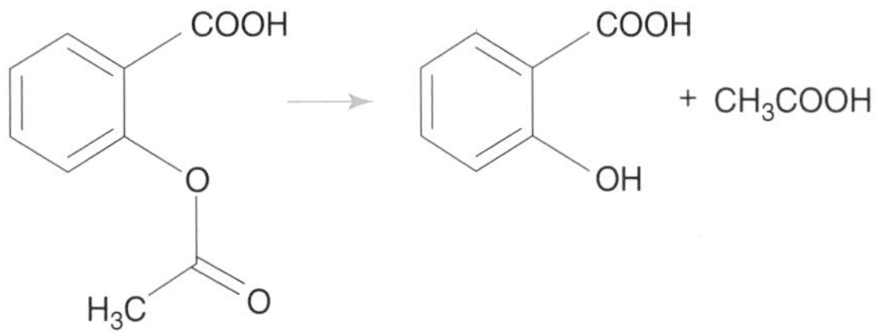

Fig. 44.2 Hydrolysis of aspirin to salicylic acid and acetic acid.

This reactivity is due to bond strain in the four-membered β-lactam ring. A variety of hydrolysis products is formed. In benzylpenicillin, a major one is benzyl penicilloic acid (Fig. 44.4). The amide group of the side chain is less susceptible to hydrolysis.

Hydrolysis is important in the degradation of proteins and polypeptides. Breakdown of the amide bonds which link the amino acids together in the protein or polypeptide chain is known as *proteolysis*. The amino acids glutamine and asparagine possess a side chain linked by an amide bond. Proteins may also degrade by hydrolysis of this side chain; this is known as *deamidation*.

Oxidation

Oxidation reactions involve an increase in the number of carbon-to-oxygen bonds in a molecule or a reduction in the number of carbon-to-hydrogen bonds. These reactions are a common cause of chemical instability of drugs. They are also responsible for the deterioration of

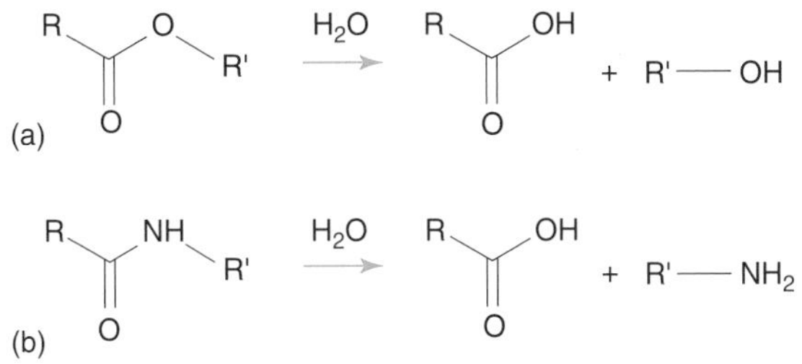

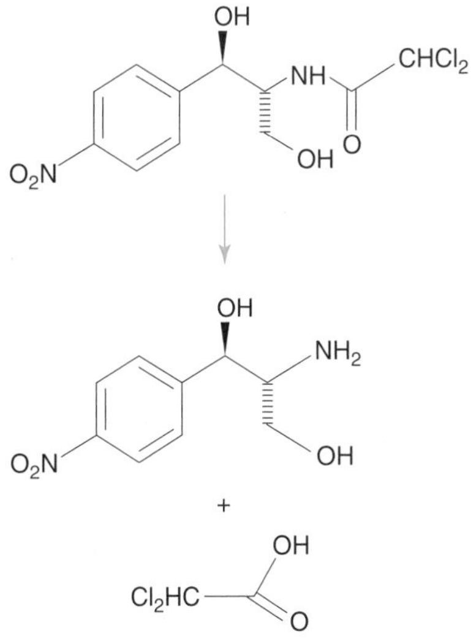

Fig. 44.1 Hydrolysis reactions. (a) Esters. (b) Amides.

Fig. 44.3 Hydrolysis of chloramphenicol to 2-amino-1-(4-nitrophenyl)propane-1,3-diol and dichloroacetic acid.

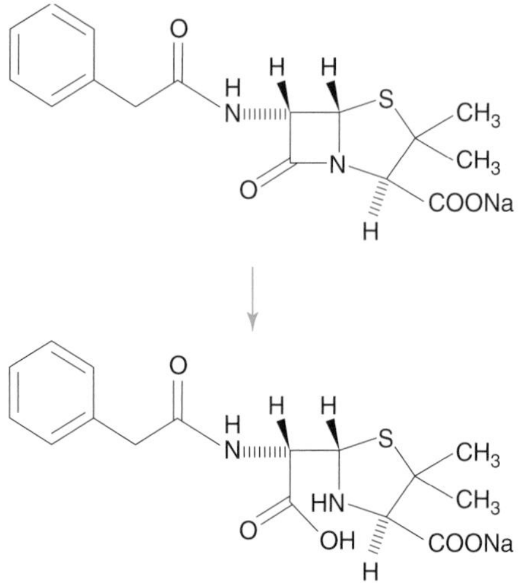

Fig. 44.4 Hydrolysis of the β-lactam ring of benzylpenicillin to give benzylpenicilloic acid.

vegetable oils, which may be used in pharmaceutical products as a solvent or an emollient in emulsions and creams. Oxidation reactions tend to be complex, giving a variety of degradation products. Table 44.1 summarizes common examples.

Oxidation taking place at ambient temperature involving molecular oxygen is known as *autoxidation*. Most such reactions involve free radicals, which are chemical species which possess an unpaired electron. Free radical oxidations are often complex but involve three main phases. The following scheme is a representative summary of the oxidation of many drugs and of vegetable oils.

The *initiation phase* results in the formation of a low concentration of free radicals. For a drug, RH, the generation of free radicals can be represented as:

$$RH \rightarrow R\cdot + H\cdot$$

Initiation is promoted by light and the presence of heavy metals which are inevitably found as trace contaminants of pharmaceutical products.

During the *propagation stage*, the concentration of free radicals increases greatly:

$$R\cdot + O_2 \rightarrow RO_2\cdot$$

$$RO_2\cdot + RH \rightarrow ROOH + R\cdot$$

Oxygen is involved in the propagation stage by forming hydroperoxides (ROOH), which react further to produce stable oxidation products. In this phase, degradation accelerates, with potentially disastrous results for the product.

In the *termination phase*, the availability of oxygen or drug diminishes, the rate of reaction slows and free radicals combine to produce unreactive endproducts. The stable reaction products formed in vegetable oils include carboxylic acids, which are responsible for the rancid smell formed when the oils deteriorate.

Oxidation of some drugs occurs rapidly in solution at room temperature. Ascorbic acid (vitamin C) undergoes a rapid oxidation in solution to dehydroascorbic acid (Fig. 44.5). This reaction is reversible but dehydroascorbic acid is rapidly and irreversibly hydrolysed at the ester linkage to form diketogulonic acid.

Some amino acids, such as cysteine and methionine, possess side chains which contain a thiol group. Oxidation of these groups can be an important factor in the degradation of proteins and polypeptides

Dimerization and polymerization

Reaction of a drug molecule with another molecule of the same drug may result in the formation of a dimer or polymer. Amoxicillin, besides undergoing hydrolysis of the β-lactam ring, also undergoes dimerization by nucleophilic attack on the β-lactam ring by the amino group (Fig. 44.6), especially in more concentrated solutions. The reaction can continue to produce a trimer and tetramer.

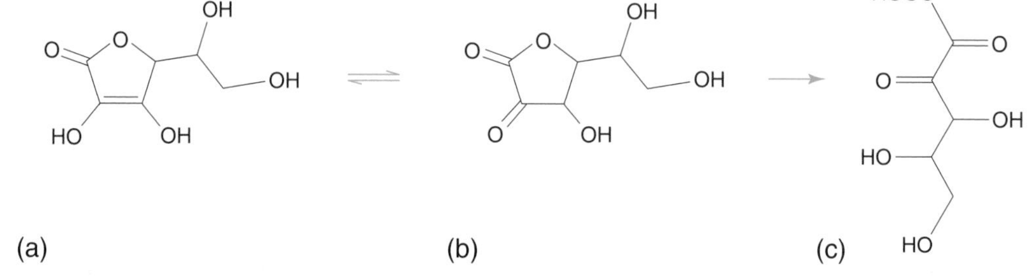

(a) (b) (c)

Fig. 44.5 Oxidation of ascorbic acid (a) to dehydroascorbic acid (b) and subsequent hydrolysis to diketogulonic acid (c).

Table 44.1 Drug oxidation reactions

Functional group undergoing oxidation	Resulting oxidation product	Example drugs
Phenolic OH, catechols	Carbonyl group	Propofol
		Epinephrine and related catecholamines
Phenolic OH	Dimeric product	Morphine
Amine	N-oxide	Morphine
Thioether	S-oxide	Promethazine and related phenothiazines
Thiol	Disulphide	Captopril, 6-Mercaptopurine

Polymerization is a major mechanism of degradation of the disinfectant glutaraldehyde. Its disinfectant activity is optimal at a slightly alkaline pH but at this pH it is subject to polymerization (Fig. 44.7). Because glutaraldehyde undergoes ketoenol tautomerism, an aldol condensation reaction between the keto and enol forms of the molecule results in the production of a dimer (Tashima et al 1987). Further reaction to produce a polymer then occurs. In order to avoid polymerization on storage, glutaraldehyde solution needs to be formulated at an acidic pH, where polymerization does not occur. It is then activated immediately before use by adding an alkaline buffer.

Isomeric change

Different isomers of a drug often have differing pharmacological activity or toxicity so any change in the proportion of isomers on storage of a pharmaceutical product is of importance.

The conversion of an optically active molecule with one chiral centre into its mirror-image is known as

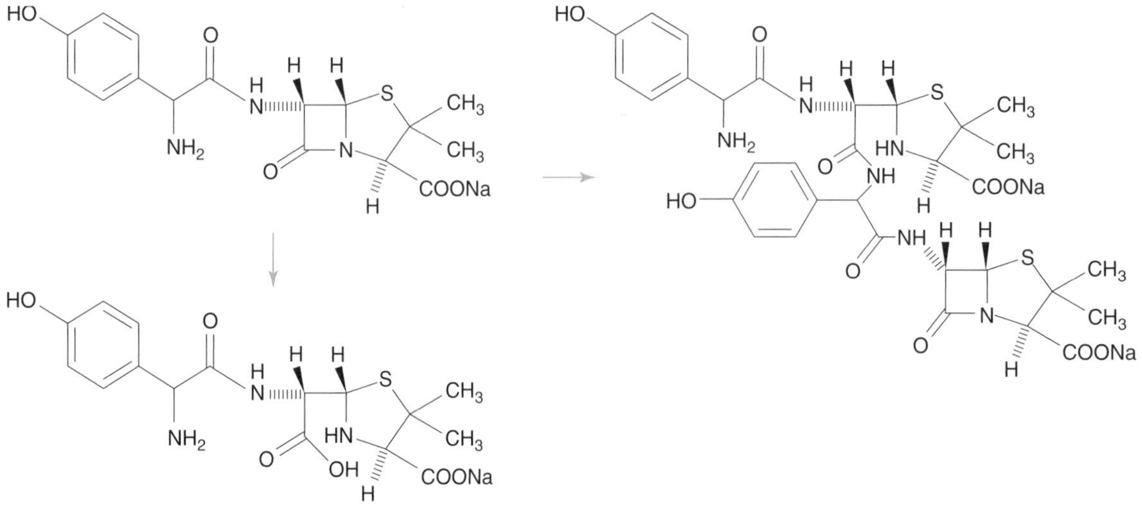

Fig. 44.6 Amoxicillin degrades by both β-lactam ring hydrolysis and dimerization.

racemization. In addition to susceptibility to oxidation, epinephrine may also undergo racemization in aqueous solution. The reaction is acid and base catalysed and involves the formation of an alcoholate anion, which reversibly forms a carbonyl-containing intermediate with no chiral centre (Fig. 44.8). Regeneration of the alcoholate anion in either isomeric form is then possible. If it continued unchecked, this reaction would result in an equilibrium mixture of equal concentrations of each isomer. The R-isomer of epinephrine has much greater pharmacological activity than the S-isomer, so this change would affect the potency of an aqueous epinephrine

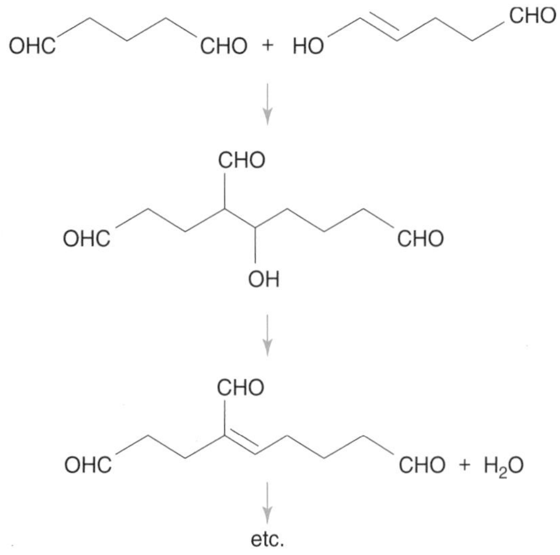

Fig. 44.7 Polymerization reaction of glutaraldehyde. Two molecules of glutaraldehyde are shown in the keto and enol forms respectively.

product. The reason for the difference in potency is that in the R-isomer, the amino and hydroxyl substituents are orientated on the same side of the molecule, allowing them both to hydrogen bond with the epinephrine receptor in vivo. However, in the S-isomer, only one of these substituents can bond with the receptor because they are on opposite sides of the molecule.

In drug molecules with more then one chiral centre, racemization at one of the chiral centres is known as *epimerization*. The antibiotic tetracycline, for instance, forms the 4-epitetracycline epimer (Fig. 44.9), which is not active against microbes and is more toxic than tetracycline.

Geometrical isomers differ in the conformation of groups around a carbon-to-carbon double bond or a cyclic group. Retinol and all other related molecules, which together are known as vitamin A, contain an unsaturated hydrocarbon chain. This makes the molecule susceptible to oxidation but it also undergoes geometrical isomerization. The double bonds in the chain are all in the *trans* configuration. On storage of all-*trans*-retinol or on subjecting it to heat, the molecule changes configuration at the double bond at the 13-position of the molecule, to form 13-*cis*-retinol (Fig. 44.10), which has no activity as a vitamin (Duarte Favoro et al 2003).

Structural isomerization is sometimes a mechanism of drug degradation. The best known example of this is with betamethasone-17-valerate, a potent corticosteroid. A major route of degradation of this drug is by migration of the valerate ester substituent to the side chain, forming betamethasone-21-valerate (Fig. 44.11). The mechanism is promoted by the close proximity of the hydroxyl group in the side chain to the ester sub-

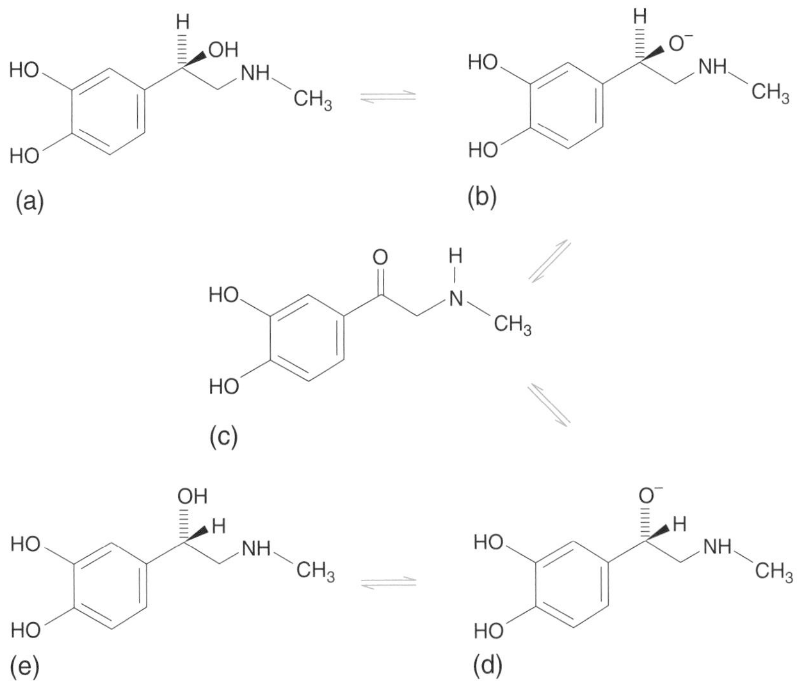

Fig. 44.8 R-epinephrine (a) converts to an alcoholate ion with the R-configuration (b) and then to a carbonyl-containing intermediate (c). This may revert to the original alcoholate ion with R-configuration (b) or to the alcoholate ion with the S-configuration (d), which can then form S-epinephrine (e).

stituent. This reaction is of concern where topical formulations of betamethasone-17-valerate are diluted with an inappropriate diluent.

Photodegradation

Molecules which absorb the wavelengths of light associated with sunlight or artificial light may be susceptible to light-induced degradation (photolysis). The 300–400 nm wavelengths tend to be most damaging. Shorter wavelengths are also damaging but are not of practical concern because they are not found in sunlight or artificial room light.

Many photolysis reactions involve oxidation mechanisms, although other mechanisms may occur. Photodegradation of retinol, as well as promoting oxidative reactions, also results in formation of a *cis*-isomer of the molecule. However, isomerization around the double bond at position 9 tends to occur, in contrast to degradation occurring in the absence of light, where the isomerization occurs at position 13 (see Fig. 44.10).

Conformation of proteins

The therapeutic effect of protein-based drugs depends on the three-dimensional structure of the molecule. Changes

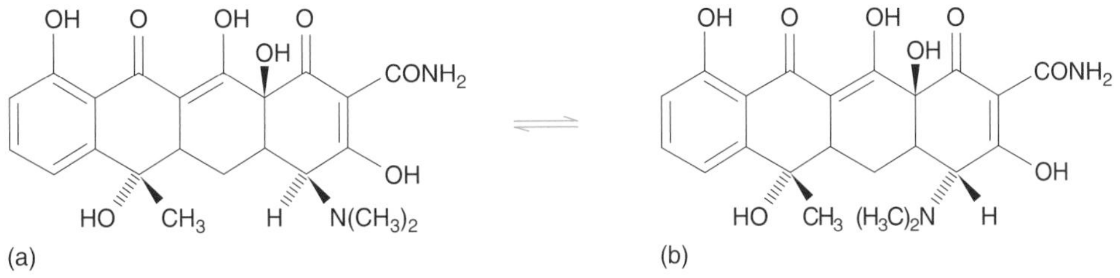

Fig. 44.9 Epimerization of tetracycline (a) to 4-epitetracycline (b).

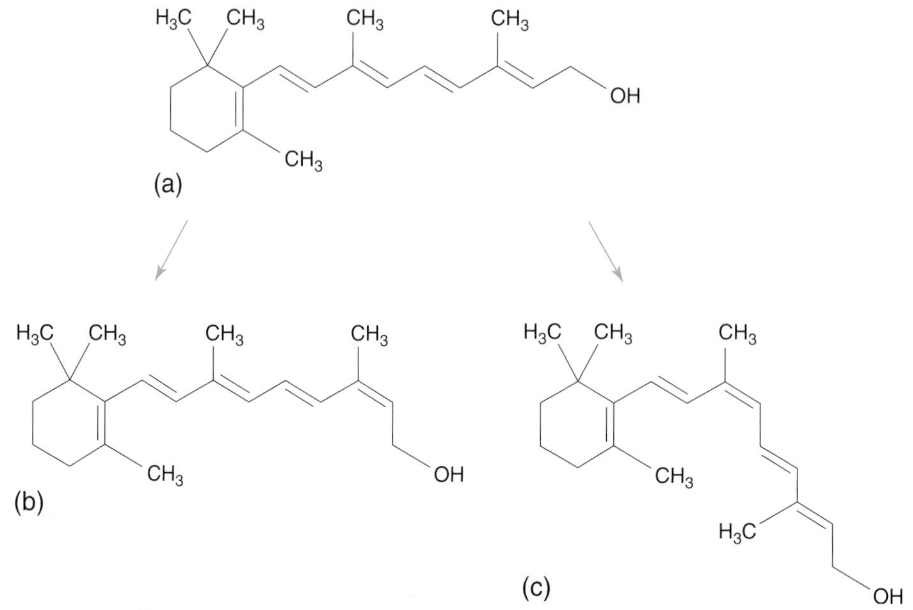

Fig. 44.10 All-*trans*-retinol (a) undergoes thermal degradation to give 13-*cis*-retinol (b) and undergoes photodegradation to form 9-*cis*-retinol (c).

to this on storage or if a protein solution is accidentally frozen lead to a reduction of the protein's efficacy.

Chemical incompatibilities

Degradation of a drug may be caused by reaction with another drug present in the formulation or with a formulation excipient.

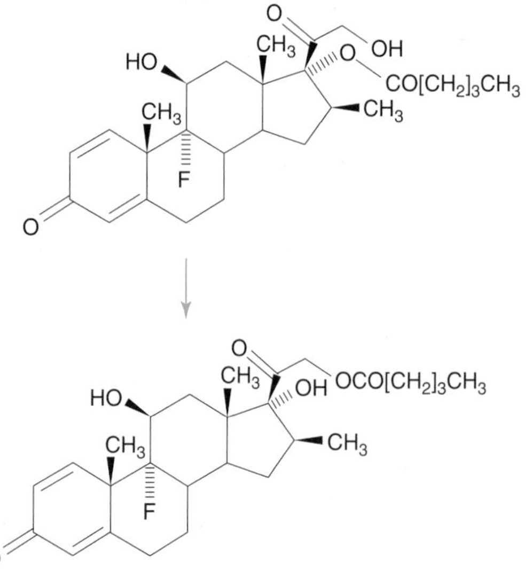

Fig. 44.11 Degradation of betamethasone-17-valerate to betamethasone-21-valerate.

Hydroxybenzoate ester (paraben) antimicrobial preservatives undergo transesterification reactions with sugars and sugar alcohols, which may be present in a formulation as sweetening agents. For instance, methyl hydroxybenzoate undergoes reaction with sorbitol (Fig. 44.12) to produce a variety of sorbitol hydroxybenzoate esters by reaction with sorbitol's various hydroxyl groups (Ma et al 2002).

A related reaction involves the interaction of aminophylline with suppository bases. Aminophylline is a complex of theophylline and ethylenediamine, which is used to increase the aqueous solubility of theophylline. On storage of aminophylline suppositories, the melting point of the base increases to above physiological temperature, preventing release of drug. The mechanism for this is the formation of amide bonds between ethylenediamine and the carboxyl groups of

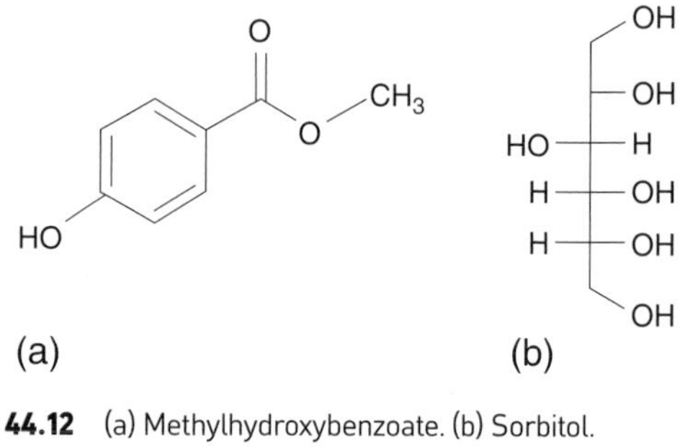

Fig. 44.12 (a) Methylhydroxybenzoate. (b) Sorbitol.

fatty acids present in the suppository base. The reaction is the reverse of the amide hydrolysis reaction shown in Figure 44.1b.

Transacetylation reactions have been reported for some drugs. For instance, in tablet formulations containing both aspirin and phenylephrine hydrochloride (a drug used as a nasal decongestant), the acetyl group is transferred to phenylephrine (Fig. 44.13). A similar reaction occurs between aspirin and paracetamol (acetaminophen). Aspirin also reacts with the polyethylene glycol base of suppository formulations, transferring the acetyl group to the polyethylene glyol.

The Maillard reaction involves a reaction between an amine and a reducing sugar. The reaction is responsible for the browning of cooked foods, where the amino group is provided by the amino acids present in the food. It may also occur between amine-containing drugs and lactose or other sugars when employed as a diluent in tablet or capsule formulations. This reaction results in yellowing of white tablets on storage. The mechanism is reaction of the amine with the sugar to form a glycosyl amine, which rearranges to form a coloured 1-amino-2-keto sugar (Fig. 44.14). The incompatibility can be avoided by replacing the sugar with an alternative diluent. If a sweetening agent is required in a solid dosage form of an amine drug, for instance in a dispersible tablet, sucrose and glucose would tend to undergo the Maillard reaction; however, mannitol can be used, as it does not undergo the reaction.

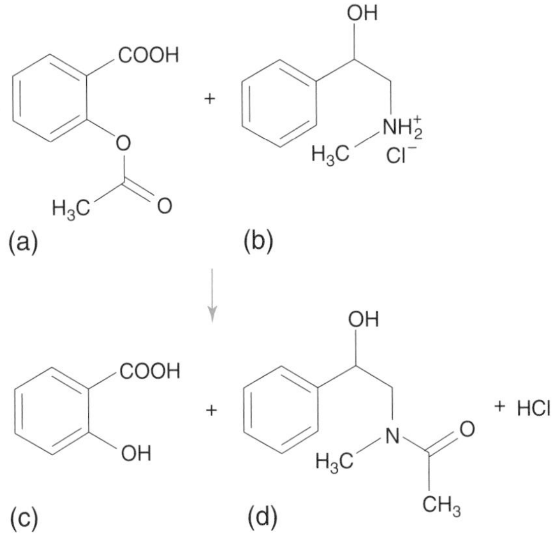

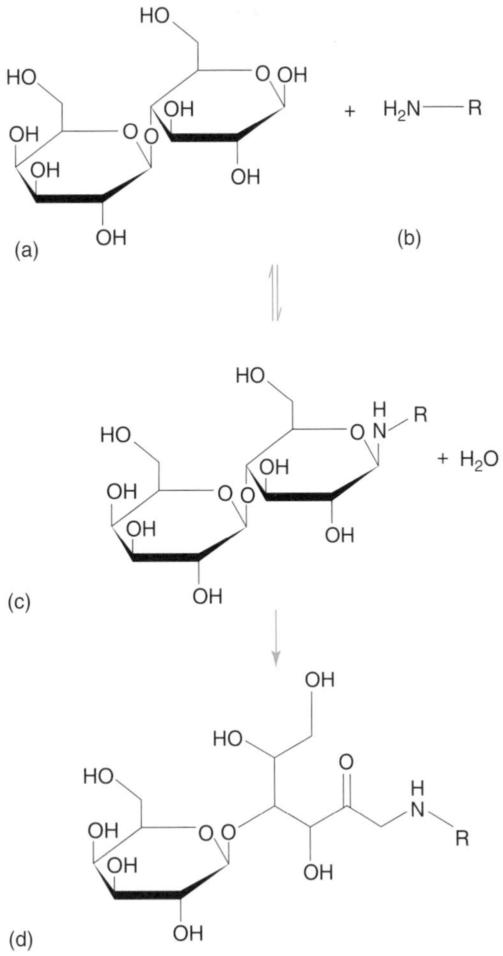

Fig. 44.14 The Maillard reaction between lactose (a) and an amine drug (b) resulting in the formation of a glycosyl amine (c), which rearranges to form a coloured 1-amino-2-keto sugar (d).

Fig. 44.13 Transesterification reaction of aspirin (a) with phenylephrine hydrochloride (b) to give salicylic acid (c) and N-acetyl-phenylephrine (d).

Stabilization of pharmaceuticals

Pharmaceuticals should be formulated and stored in a way that minimizes degradation. The following factors are relevant to most mechanisms of degradation. Oxidation and photodegradation are dealt with separately later in this chapter.

Temperature

The rate of degradation reactions is markedly influenced by temperature. Storage of product in a refrigerator (at 2–8°C) is an option if it is unstable at room temperature.

Using a freezer (at less than −15°C) to store unstable formulations is sometimes adopted; however, this makes storage and distribution of the product inconvenient.

Also, because a liquid product needs to be thawed before administration, there is the risk of degradation occurring if heat is used to achieve this. Amoxicillin is exceptional because it is less stable in solution when frozen than when stored at refrigerator temperature (McDonald et al 1989). Freezing is not applicable for protein-based products and live vaccines.

Formulations are most at risk of exposure to unacceptable temperatures during transportation or storage in vehicles such as ambulances (Helm et al 2003, Lucas et al 2004, Priston et al 2005).

Solvent

Replacing an aqueous solvent in a formulation with a non-aqueous one is a potential means of avoiding hydrolysis.

The dielectric constant of a solvent is related to its polarity, more polar solvents having higher values. The dielectric constant can influence the rate at which charged species react. However, the practical considerations of choosing a solvent for a formulation, such as its toxicity and compatibility with the drug, usually outweigh consideration of any effect due to the solvent's dielectric constant.

Solid dosage forms of a drug, such as a tablet or capsule, are usually more stable than a liquid one. However, reactions can occur in water adsorbed onto the surface of a drug particle or other dosage form component. This is why poorly stored aspirin tablets often smell of acetic acid, formed by the hydrolysis of aspirin. Injection formulations of unstable drugs such as penicillins can be formulated as freeze-dried powders, which are reconstituted with water or saline immediately before administration.

Suspension formulations are often more stable than a solution formulation of the same drug because much of the drug is protected within the insoluble particles.

Acid and base catalysis

A catalyst is a species that accelerates the rate of a reaction without itself being consumed in the reaction. Hydrolysis is often catalysed by hydrogen ion (which exists as H_3O^+ in solution) or hydroxyl ion. The pH of an aqueous formulation is therefore a critical factor which determines its stability. Specific acid catalysis is catalysis by hydrogen ion and specific base catalysis is catalysis by hydroxyl ion.

Investigating the relationship between pH and the degradation rate of a drug is performed during the preformulation phase of drug development (see Chapter 24). Plotting the logarithm to base 10 of the first-order reaction rate constant against pH may yield useful information about the degradation mechanism. A typical curve is shown in Figure

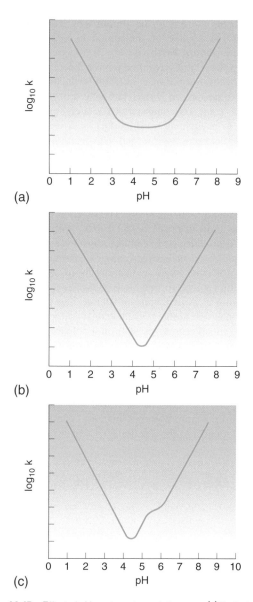

Fig. 44.15 Effect of pH on drug degradation rate. (a) Typical curve where acid catalysed (H_3O^+), base catalysed (OH^-) and uncatalysed (H_2O) hydrolysis occurs. (b) Typical curve with narrow region of maximal stability. (c) Typical curve where the drug molecule ionizes.

44.15a. The increase in degradation rate at low pH is due to specific acid catalysis. The increase in rate seen at high pH is due to specific base catalysis. Straight lines with gradients of −1 in the acidic region and +1 in the basic region are characteristic of specific-acid- and specific-base-catalysed hydrolysis. The flat region of the curve is largely due to uncatalysed hydrolysis. The formulation should be maintained at a pH within this region for optimum stability.

Cefuroxime and other cephalosporin antibiotics typically show this shape of graph.

For some drugs, such as many penicillins, the uncatalysed reaction with water is relatively less important than in the former example, so there is no flat base to the curve (Fig. 44.15b) and a V-shaped graph results. In this case the pH needs to be more precisely controlled than in the previous example because there is a narrower region for optimum stability.

Many drug molecules undergo ionization, depending on the pH. These typically give a curve as in Figure 44.15c. The ionized and unionized forms of the drug degrade at different rates. Therefore the rate of reaction changes as the pH influences the relative proportion of ionized drug present and this gives an inflection point on the graph. Aspirin is an example of a drug which shows this characteristic.

Other species in a formulation besides H_3O^+ or OH^- may act as acids and bases and thus catalyse degradation reactions. This is known as *general acid catalysis* and *general base catalysis* respectively. Buffer ions are a common cause of this so careful selection of buffer for use in a formulation is needed. Hydrolysis of the amide bond of the antimicrobial drug chloramphenicol is catalysed by several common buffers, including phosphate and acetate. Borate buffer, however, does not catalyse degradation and is used to buffer the drug in eye drops.

Ionic strength

The ionic strength of a medium is related to the concentration of ionic species in it. Changing the ionic strength by adding electrolyte to a solution has some influence on the rate of many degradation reactions. This effect is not high enough to be of importance in the formulation of drug solutions. However, it can be important in laboratory experiments to investigate the influence of pH on degradation rate. In this case care should be taken to ensure the ionic strength of the various buffer solutions used is kept the same to avoid interference with the results.

Light

Containers made from tinted materials protect the product from light to some extent because they allow less ultraviolet light to penetrate than untinted materials. Placing the product in an opaque outer container such as a cardboard box is also an option.

Oxygen

Oxidation reactions are less influenced by temperature than most other degradation reactions, so low-temperature storage may be less successful as a stabilization option.

Flushing containers with an inert gas such as nitrogen before they are sealed will reduce the amount of oxygen in the product. However, this technique will not remove all oxygen and is best suited for single-use containers such as ampoules.

Oxidation reactions are generally promoted by high pH, so aqueous products which are susceptible to oxidation should be formulated at as low a pH as possible.

Heavy metal ions such as Cu^{2+} and Fe^{3+} catalyse oxidation reactions, acting at the initiation and propagation stages. These ions are present at trace levels in all formulations. A chelating agent such as ethylenediamine tetraacetic acid (EDTA) or citric acid has a stabilizing effect by binding to the heavy metal ions and preventing them from acting as catalysts.

Chelating agents are usually used in combination with an antioxidant, which acts in one of two ways. It may act as an oxygen scavenger (oxygen is removed from the formulation by reacting preferentially with the antioxidant) or it may terminate free radical reactions. The antioxidant forms a free radical which is relatively unreactive and so cannot contribute to free radical propagation. Sodium metabisulfite and ascorbic acid are examples of water-soluble antioxidants, used in aqueous formulations. Ascorbyl palmitate, butylated hydroxytoluene and α-tocopherol are oil-soluble antioxidants for use in oily formulations.

Physical stability

Common physical causes of instability are summarized in Table 44.2. Most of these are due to changes in the physical properties of the dosage form, either spoiling the product's appearance or reducing its effectiveness. The other potential problems are loss of drug due to sorption or evaporation or contamination of the product by extractives.

Molecules of the drug or other formulation component may be lost from a formulation by *adsorption onto* the surface of the container or closure or by *absorption* of molecules *into* plastic or rubber containers or closures. Adsorption and absorption often operate together and are collectively known as *sorption*. Non-polar molecules are susceptible to sorption to plastics and rubber (see Chapter 42). For instance, diazepam is lost from solutions in contact with plastic packaging. Loss of antimicrobial preservative to rubber closures is a problem with injection dosage forms (see Chapter 43). Sorption is enhanced where the drug (or preservative) is present at low concentration. If the drug molecule ionizes, the pH of the solution may influence the extent of sorption because the unionized form of the molecule, being less polar than the ionized form, may undergo more sorption.

Table 44.2 Physical stability of pharmaceutical products

Formulation type	Physical instability	Effect on dosage form
All liquid products	Sorption of drug to container or closure Extraction of materials into liquid from container or closure Shedding of particles from glass containers Evaporation of chloroform (used as antimicrobial preservative)	Loss of drug Possible toxicity of extractives Change of pH of solution Poor appearance Potential harm to patient with injection products Microbial contamination
Solutions	Precipitation of drug or degradation products	Poor appearance Loss of efficacy
Suspensions	Caking of sediment Particle growth	Inaccurate dose of drug taken by user Poor appearance Grittiness
Emulsions	Creaming and cracking Reduction in viscosity	Poor appearance Non-homogeneous product Increased risk of creaming and cracking Poor application characteristics for topical products
Ointments Solid dosage forms	Separation of liquid onto surface (bleeding) Polymorphic change Change in disintegration time of dosage form Change in crushing strength Cracking of coated tablets Evaporation of glyceryl trinitrate (nitroglycerin)	Poor appearance Reduced drug dissolution rate May affect drug dissolution May cause change in disintegration time of tablets Poor appearance Loss of protection of enteric-coated products from gastric acid Loss of drug
Transdermal patches	Change in drug release rate Change in patch adhesive characteristics	Changed therapeutic effect Patch may not remain adhered to the skin
Inhalation and nasal aerosols	Change in particle size distribution of emitted dose	Reduced therapeutic effect

The evaporation of chloroform from liquid products is one reason why it is unsatisfactory if used as an antimicrobial preservative. Glyceryl trinitrate (nitroglycerin) evaporates from tablets, where it can be lost by sorption to plastic packaging. To avoid this, glyceryl trinitrate tablets need to be packaged in glass bottles with aluminium-lined closures.

Plastic packaging materials may be permeable to water vapour. Aqueous products packaged in plastic containers may therefore lose water on storage and the drug content becomes more concentrated.

The term 'extractive' is used to describe any material which is released from packaging materials into the dosage form.

The common packaging material polyvinyl chloride (PVC) is rendered flexible by the addition of a plasticizer (diethylhexylphthalate; DEHP) which may migrate into injection solutions. This is a particular problem where the solution contains a non-aqueous solvent or surfactant. Paclitaxel, a cytotoxic drug, needs to be administered in dilute solution by slow intravenous infusion. The injection also contains polyoxyethylated castor oil (a material used to solubilize the drug) and ethanol as a cosolvent. Paclitaxel injection therefore cannot be added to infusion fluids contained in PVC because it causes DEHP extraction. Glass or polyethylene infusion containers should be used instead (Allwood & Martin 1996).

Glass containers can release hydroxyl ion into an aqueous product, changing its pH (see Chapter 42). This may occur especially during heating in an autoclave and surface-treated glass is available to minimize hydroxyl ion extraction for formulations where this is of concern.

Microbiological stability

Deterioration due to microorganisms can either render the product harmful to the patient or have an adverse effect on the product's properties (see Chapter 43). Microbiological deterioration is a critical factor in the stability of sterile products once the container is opened. Injection products generally need to be used immediately the container is opened and products for use in the eye have a short in-use life once opened.

STABILITY TESTING

The purpose of stability testing is to define the shelf life of a formulated pharmaceutical product. This needs to be performed on the exact product that will be marketed and ultimately be used by the patient. However, prior knowledge of the drug's stability is needed early in the development process in order to assist with formulating it. Therefore, different approaches to the evaluation of stability are needed at the different stages of product development.

Accelerated stability testing (stress testing)

Preformulation assessment

In the early stages of the development of a new drug, during the preformulation phase, qualitative assessment of the drug's likely susceptibility to hydrolysis, oxidation and light degradation is performed (see Chapter 24). In this stage, potential degradation mechanisms and degradation products are identified and the development of stability-indicating assays is commenced. Susceptibility of the drug to hydrolysis is assessed by heating solutions of it in water, dilute acid and dilute base. Oxidation is investigated by comparing solutions heated with and without flushing with oxygen. The solid-state stability is also studied by storing drug at high temperature, either on its own or combined with potential excipients which might be used in a solid dose formulation. The effect of pH on the drug's stability will be studied by heating solutions which are buffered at a range of pH values. The effect of light on the stability of the drug is discussed later in this chapter.

Prediction of shelf life by stress testing

Determination of the shelf life of a formulated product needs to be performed on the actual product at a realistic storage temperature. However, the shelf lives of commercial pharmaceutical products are typically of several years. Such testing would therefore be too slow to be of use early in product development in order to decide if a particular formulation was of sufficient stability. The Arrhenius equation (see Chapter 7) allows the prediction of reaction rates at proposed storage temperatures, from data obtained at high temperatures. For example, if it is desired to formulate a new drug as a solution dosage form, simple buffered solutions of the drug are stored at a range of elevated temperatures for time periods ranging from minutes to days, depending on the relative stability of the drug. Reaction rates are calculated at each temperature and the Arrhenius equation is used to predict the reaction rate at room temperature, which is used to calculate the estimated shelf life. Later in the development process, prototype formulations may be subject to the same process to allow optimization of the product's stability.

There are a number of pitfalls in the use of this type of testing. The precision of the shelf life estimate is poor, so studies typically give estimates with a wide range of uncertainty. At high temperatures, reactions may take place which are not significant at normal storage temperatures. Alternatively, at high temperatures, the degradation products which are initially formed from the drug (the primary degradation products) may rapidly react to further degradation products (the secondary degradation products) and so not accumulate. Therefore, later in the development process, when the product undergoes stability testing at normal storage temperature, the primary degradation products may accumulate. If these degradation products are not foreseen, they could cause interference with chromatographic analysis of the product or raise questions about the toxicity properties of the formulation. The kinetics of drug degradation may also change at different temperatures. A reduction in the concentration of dissolved oxygen will also tend to occur at high temperatures, so use of the Arrhenius equation may not provide a reliable estimate of shelf life in liquid products which degrade by oxidation. In the case of solid dosage forms, high temperatures often reduce moisture levels associated with drug or excipients, also leading to poor stability prediction. Semi-solid dosage forms are often unsuitable for this type of stress testing due to melting of ingredients at elevated temperature.

Nevertheless, despite these drawbacks, the use of the Arrhenius equation to predict room temperature stability does allow a decision to be made concerning whether a particular formulation type is likely to be sufficiently stable to allow commercial production. It also allows the relative stability of formulations to be studied at an early stage in the development process.

There is, however, no substitute for properly conducted, long-term stability tests carried out under the normal storage conditions required for the product. These are described later in this chapter.

Temperature cycling

Temperature cycling studies involve storing the product at alternating high and low temperatures, often designed to subject liquid products to repeated freezing and thawing. This may reveal stability problems because it potentially accelerates physical deterioration of the product. Temperature fluctuations encourage particle growth in suspensions; cracking of emulsions and precipitation of dissolved drug from solutions. Such studies also allow the effects of extreme temperature variations during distribution of the product to be evaluated (Helm et al 2003, Lucas et al 2004, Priston et al 2005).

Photostability testing

Photostability studies are carried out at various stages of the product development process and involve investigation of the effect of light on drugs and formulated products. Drug or product is exposed to light, provided by artificial-daylight fluorescent lamps, which emit long-wavelength ultraviolet and visible light to simulate indirect, indoor sunlight. The study is performed within a cabinet which has a controlled temperature, typically of 25°C. Initial photostability studies are carried out using pure drug, spread over the base of a shallow container and directly exposed to the light. After a period of storage, the material is chemically analysed to assess the degree of photodegradation. If this reveals that the drug is photosensitive, as shown by a reduction in drug assay, formation of photodegradation products or colour change, the formulated pharmaceutical product is then tested. The product must be stored in the exact same packaging that will be used for marketing the product.

If light exposure causes an unacceptable amount of change in the product, redesign of the packaging is required to increase light protection.

A light dose of 1.2 million lux hours is typically used for photostability studies, which corresponds to an extended period of exposure to indoor light. The light output from the lamps varies as the lamps age and the light dose received by the tested samples also depends on distance from the light source. Frequent measurement of the light energy is therefore required at various positions throughout the light stability cabinet.

Long-term stability testing

Stress testing gives useful information about the likely stability of a formulated product. However, before it can be marketed, it must undergo long-term stability testing. This involves storing the product under realistic worst-case conditions of temperature and humidity in controlled-temperature cabinets or rooms. Samples are removed at intervals and tested. The tests performed will include assay of the drug and other formulation components such as the antimicrobial preservative and determination of drug degradation products. Other tests may be required, such as pH determination, evaluation of the product's physical characteristics (see Table 44.2) and possibly also microbiological tests.

Climatic Zones

The shelf life of a product depends on its storage temperature and, for susceptible products, also on the humidity. These conditions vary from country to country. A pharmaceutical manufacturer may market a product in several countries and to avoid having to carry out long-term stability testing under different conditions for each country, four Climatic Zones have been defined. The four worldwide Climatic Zones (show in Fig. 44.16) recognized by the International Conference on Harmonisation (ICH). They are based on observed temperatures and relative humidities, both outside and inside rooms, from which mean temperatures and average humidity values are calculated.

  I *Temperate climate*, includes Canada, New Zealand, northern Europe, Russia, United Kingdom

  II *Mediterranean and subtropical climate*, includes Japan, southern Europe, USA

  III *Hot and dry climate*, includes Argentina, Australia, Botswana, Middle East

  IV *Hot and humid climate*, includes Brazil, Ghana, Indonesia, Nicaragua, Nigeria, the Philippines

The storage conditions used for stability testing simulate the worst-case average indoor temperature and humidity experienced in that zone (Dietz et al 1993).

Testing protocols

Because the packaging of a product may affect its stability, products which are undergoing long-term stability testing should be stored in the exact packaging that is to be used when the product is marketed. Liquid products packaged in containers with closures need to be stored inverted, to allow any interaction with the closure to be detected, for instance sorption of preservative into rubber

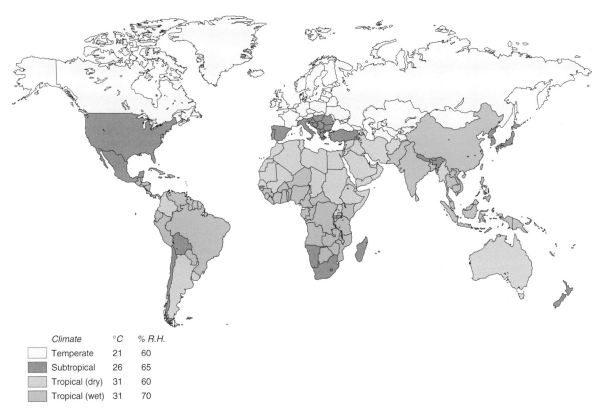

Climate	°C	% R.H.
Temperate	21	60
Subtropical	26	65
Tropical (dry)	31	60
Tropical (wet)	31	70

Fig. 44.16 Distribution of climate-related storage conditions for drug product stability testing

vial closures. This is not necessary where the product has no closure, such as an ampoule.

At least three separate batches should be placed on stability testing. This is to allow any batch-to-batch differences in stability to be detected. A difference might arise, for example, in a liquid product having differing pH between batches. In a solid dosage form, there may be differences in moisture content.

During the development process, smaller batch sizes are made than will be required for full-scale production purposes. However, batch size can have an effect on the stability of the final product. For example, any differences in residual moisture content in solid dosage forms or differing viscosities in semi-solid dosage forms may result in stability differences. Therefore batches of at least pilot scale should be used for stability testing, i.e. batches which, although smaller than the projected batch size for the marketed product, use essentially the same production equipment.

During storage of stability test samples, humidity is controlled because of the potentially harmful effects of moisture on products such as solid dosage forms. However, no humidity control is required for products which are unaffected by humidity, such as aqueous products in glass containers.

A typical testing schedule is shown in Table 44.3. The storage temperatures and humidities required for products to be marketed in the European Union, Japan and the USA, which are all within Climatic Zones I and II, are also shown in this table. There are relatively few countries in Zone I so it is convenient to treat them in the same way as for Zone II. The 25°C storage condition represents a realistic worst-case ambient storage temperature. The product should remain of adequate quality throughout the proposed shelf life at this temperature if the product is intended to be stored at room temperature when it is marketed. Storage at 2–8°C allows adverse effects due to cold to be revealed, such as precipitation of a drug from solution. The 40°C condition is known as the accelerated degradation condition. This represents a moderately stressful environment which will allow stability problems to be detected quickly. Significant degradation at this temperature gives some early warning of stability problems that are likely to develop on prolonged storage at ambient temperature. Reference to accelerated testing in this

Table 44.3 Typical testing schedule for a pharmaceutical product to be marketed in Climatic Zones I or II

Time/months	2–8°C	25°C (60% RH)[a]	40°C (75 % RH)[b]
0	X	X	X
3	X	X	X
6	X	X	X
9		X	
12		X	
18		X	
24		X	
36		X	

[a]30°C (65% RH) for Climatic Zones III and IV.
[b]40°C (75% RH) for Climatic Zones III and IV.

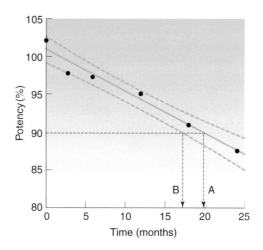

Fig. 44.17 Drug content of hypothetical tablet product. The regression line is shown as a solid line. The time for the regression line to reach 90% of the labelled potency is given by point A. The 95% confidence bounds are shown as dashed lines. The time for the lower 95% confidence bound to reach 90% of the labelled potency is given by point B.

context should be distinguished from stress testing, where more extreme temperatures are used. For products where refrigerated storage temperatures are envisaged, the 2–8°C storage condition represents the realistic storage temperature and the 25°C temperature represents the accelerated degradation condition.

Stability studies for products to be marketed in Climatic Zones III and IV use 30°C as the ambient storage condition (see Table 44.3).

Conditions of low humidity provide a significant stress for aqueous products packaged in plastic containers which allow loss of water vapour, resulting in a more concentrated product. This is especially important within Climatic Zone III (hot and dry). Water loss from plastic containers stored at 30°C is 1.9 times more rapid at 35% relative humidity, representative of a dry climate, compared to 65%, representative of a humid one. An additional stability testing requirement for such products is that they are also stored at very low humidity to detect excessive moisture loss. For instance, for Climatic Zones III and IV, storage at 35% relative humidity at 30°C is required.

Evaluation of results

The results of tests on samples subject to stability studies should remain within the specification set for the product. For instance, degradation of drug should be within allowable limits and the product's appearance, smell and, if relevant, taste should be acceptable.

It is common for the lower acceptable limit for the drug content of a product to be set at 90% of the labelled content of drug. This is not the same as 90% of the original concentration, because this will vary due to manufacturing variation or the presence of an overage.

Various statistical tests are applied to ensure that the amount of drug remaining at the expiry date is above the lower acceptable limit. Figure 44.17 shows hypothetical stability results for a tablet product which, for simplicity, is assumed to degrade by zero-order kinetics. Some scatter is seen in the results due to variability of the analytical technique and non-homogeneity within the product. Linear regression analysis enables the average rate of degradation to be determined and this gives an estimated time of 20 months to reach 90% of the labelled potency. However, linear regression calculates average values, both of the slope of the regression line and of the intercept at the y-axis. Thus it is possible that the true shelf life is less than this estimate. To avoid this possibility, the one-sided 95% confidence bounds for the regression can be determined. These define the region within which there is a 95% probability that the true regression line lies (see Fig. 44.16). The shelf life is determined as the time at which the lower 95% confidence bound crosses the lower specification limit, which in this example is at 17 months. This method of calculating shelf life incorporates a safety margin to allow for the uncertainty in both the degradation rate and the initial drug content (the y-axis intercept value).

In cases where the degradation does not follow zero-order kinetics, appropriate transformation of the data is required before linear regression is performed. For example, for drug degrading by first-order kinetics, logarithmic transformation of the assay data is first performed (see Chapter 7). Knowledge of the order of the degradation reaction is obtained from studies performed at higher (stress) temperatures, which would have been performed earlier. This is because during long-term testing, insufficient degradation would occur to allow accurate determination of the order of reaction.

Because a minimum of three batches are subject to stability testing, the shelf life is calculated for each batch separately and the shortest calculated value is selected as the product's shelf life. Increasing the number of data points available may have the effect of decreasing the width of the confidence bound, making it closer to the average regression line. This would improve the estimate of the shelf life. Pooling the data from all the batches when calculating the 95% confidence bound therefore potentially gives a longer shelf life. This is permitted if the slopes and intercepts of the regression lines for each batch are shown to be statistically equivalent by the statistical technique of analysis of covariance.

Extrapolation of the data beyond the period for which data are available is not advisable because of the possibility that the degradation rate will change.

SUMMARY

Pharmaceutical products tend to deteriorate due to chemical, physical and microbiological causes. Chemical degradation of the drug in a product is influenced by factors such as the presence of water, oxygen, light or incompatible ingredients in the product. Deterioration can be reduced in a number of ways. Careful formulation of the product is necessary to ensure adequate stability. This may be through attention to general factors such as appropriate selection of the solvent or pH or by including specific stabilizing additives such as an antioxidant or antimicrobial preservative. Packaging plays an important role in the prevention of product deterioration, for instance protecting the contents from moisture, but the packaging must avoid interactions such as sorption. Storage conditions of the manufactured product (temperature, humidity and light exposure) need to be appropriate. Adequate stability of the product needs to be demonstrated during its development before it can be assigned a shelf life. Stress testing is valuable in predicting the likely stability of a product but long-term testing is needed before it can be marketed.

In conclusion, stability is an important factor which affects the quality and efficacy of a pharmaceutical product.

REFERENCES

Allwood, M.C., Martin, H. (1996) The extraction of diethylhexylphthalate (DEHP) from polyvinyl chloride components of intravenous infusion containers and administration sets by paclitaxel injection. *International Journal of Pharmaceutics*, **127**(1), 65-71.

Dietz, R., Feilner, K., Gerst, F., Grimm, W. (1993) Drug stability testing: classification of countries according to climatic zone. *Drugs made in Germany*, **36**(3), 99-103.

Duarte Favaro, R.M., Iha, M.H., Pires Bianchi, M. de L. (2003) Liquid chromatographic determination of geometrical retinol isomers and carotene in enteral feeding formulas. *Journal of Chromatography A*, **1021**, 125-132.

Helm, M., Castner, T., Lampl, L. (2003) Environmental temperature stress on drugs in prehospital emergency medical service. *Acta Anaesthesiologica Scandinavica*, **47**(4), 425-429.

Lucas, T.I., Bishara, R.H., Seevers, R.H. (2004) A stability program for the distribution of drug products. *Pharmaceutical Technology*, **July**, 68-73.

Ma, M., Lee, T., Kwong, E. (2002) Interaction of methylparaben preservative with selected sugars and sugar alcohols. *Journal of Pharmaceutical Sciences*, **91**(7), 1715-1723.

McDonald, C., Sunderland, V.B., Lau, H., Shija, R. (1989) The stability of amoxicillin sodium in normal saline and glucose (5%) solution in the liquid and frozen states. *Journal of Clinical Pharmacy and Therapeutics*, **14**(1), 45-52.

Priston, M.H., Grant, I.C., Hughes, J.M., Marquis, P.T. (2005) Pilot study on potential degradation of drug efficacy resulting from Antarctic storage, transport and field conditions. *International Journal of Circumpolar Health*, **64**(2), 184-186.

Tashima, T., Kawakami, U., Harada, M. et al. (1987) Isolation and identification of new oligomers in aqueous solution of glutaraldehyde. Chem Pharm Bull **35**, 4169-4180.

Vermes, A., van der Sijs, H., Guchelaar, H. J. (1999) An accelerated stability study of 5-flucytosine in intravenous solution. *Pharmacy World and Science*, **21**(1), 35-39.

BIBLIOGRAPHY

Barnes, A.R., Nash, S. (1996) Near-patient stability studies. *Journal of Clinical Pharmacy and Therapeutics*, **21**(1), 49-55.

Byrn, S.R., Xu, W., Newman, A.W. (2001) Chemical reactivity in solid-state pharmaceuticals: formulation implications. *Advanced Drug Delivery Reviews*, **48**, 115-136.

Connors, K.A., Amidon, G.L., Stella, V.J. (1986) *Chemical Stability of Pharmaceuticals: A Handbook for Pharmacists*, 2nd edn. Wiley, New York.

International Conference on Harmonization of Technical Requirements for Registration of Pharmaceuticals for Human Use. ICH Harmonized Tripartite Guideline:

Q1A (1993) Stability testing of new active substances and medicinal products

Q1B (1996) Photostability testing of new active substances and medicinal products

Q1E (2003) Note for guidance on evaluation of stability data

Q1F (2003) Stability data package for registration applications in climatic zones III and IV.

World Health Organization 1996 *Guidelines for Stability Testing of Pharmaceutical Products Containing Established Drug Substances in Conventional Dosage Forms*. WHO Technical Report Series No. 863. WHO, Geneva.

45

Pharmaceutical plant design

M. E. Aulton, A. M. Twitchell

CHAPTER CONTENTS

INTRODUCTION

This chapter comprises three separate sections relating to the facilities and equipment in which medicinal products are manufactured. The first part discusses manufacturing facilities and describes the selection, design and utilization of a manufacturing facility and introduces the concept of process validation. The second describes the properties and selection of the materials used in the construction of pharmaceutical facilities. The final part describes the types, causes and prevention of chemical corrosion of pharmaceutical plant.

MANUFACTURING FACILITIES FOR PHARMACEUTICAL PRODUCTS

After considerable investment of both time and money in developing and testing many new chemical entities and medicinal products, some will reach the stage where there is the requirement to manufacture the product in large quantities. The following section summarizes some of the factors that need to be taken into consideration when building a facility for producing pharmaceutical products on a large scale. This is only intended as an overview of this important aspect of product manufacture and the reader is referred to the work of Cole (1998) and Signore & Jacobs (2005) for more detailed descriptions of the design of pharmaceutical production facilities. Further information is also available in the current edition of *Rules and Guidance for Pharmaceutical Manufacturers and Distributors* – 'The Orange Guide'.

Manufacturing site selection

Pharmaceutical manufacturing facilities require considerable capital expenditure and are likely to be used for many years. It is necessary therefore to think very carefully about where the facility is located as well as how it is constructed. One important consideration is whether the company should develop a new site or refurbish an existing one. Upgrading or redesigning an existing site may often be a more cost-effective option but may not always be feasible. For example, there may be insufficient space to expand an existing site or it may be 'outdated' and not suitable for upgrading. The company may also be introducing a new product type where there is no existing plant or the existing site may not be in a suitable location.

Local planning regulations which may delay development of an existing site also need to be considered since even small delays in bringing a pharmaceutical product to market can have considerable cost implications.

Considerations when selecting a new site

Most major pharmaceutical companies are multinational and may have numerous disciplines contributing to the production of the final product (e.g. chemical synthesis, pharmacological and toxicological testing, product development and product manufacture) located in many different countries. Increasingly, however, there is a tendency to concentrate specific disciplines in a small number of sites and this may dictate where the production site is located. If this is not the case, then the advantages and disadvantages of locating in different countries need to be considered. Many countries, particularly developing countries,

offer financial incentives to pharmaceutical companies to attract them to build manufacturing facilities in particular areas. These incentives may take the form of, for example, tax incentives such as no local taxes for a number of years, free land or building grants. Other factors which vary considerably between different countries and which may influence where the site is located include labour costs and availability, energy and construction costs, environmental legislation, likely opposition from local residents and local employment legislation.

The chosen location must also have an acceptable local infrastructure including suitable road and air links, services such as electricity and water, and availability of suitably qualified workforce.

Design and utilization of manufacturing facilities

Aims of manufacturing facility design

The major requirements when designing and using manufacturing facilities should be to ensure the following:

Acceptable product quality

- Each unit dose should contain the correct component(s) in the correct concentration and have the desired release properties. There should be negligible cross-contamination between products or chemical or microbiological contamination from operators. This is particularly important when using highly sensitizing materials (e.g. penicillins), biological preparations (e.g. those made from live microorganisms) and very potent substances (e.g. hormones and cytotoxic drugs). In these latter cases 'dedicated' facilities should ideally be used.
- The facility must be designed to maximize protection against entry of insects/animals.
- Microbiological contamination from all sources (discussed further in Chapter 43) must be acceptably low to both protect the patient and ensure a satisfactory product shelf life.
- The factory should be designed to ensure that no unauthorized personnel can gain entry to production, quality control or storage areas.
- Each product must be correctly packaged and labelled to ensure the patient takes the correct medication and that it reaches the patient in a satisfactory condition.

If the product is not of the required quality and has to be destroyed, this will have considerable cost implications for the manufacturer since, for example, a tablet batch may consist of over a million units and a liquid batch may be as much as 20 000 litres. If the batch has to be recalled after distribution, due to errors such as incorrect labelling, this is very costly both financially and in damage to the company's reputation.

An acceptable working environment

- It is the duty of the pharmaceutical company to ensure that the manufacturing area is designed and operated so that the exposure of personnel to drugs, solvents, etc., is at an acceptably low level. This may be achieved in some circumstances by controlling the air flow and quality in the area but with more toxic materials, special breathing apparatus with appropriate filters may be necessary.
- Comfortable working conditions should be provided for process operators wherever possible, bearing in mind any particular product requirements such as the need to prepare a product at a low temperature or humidity.

Manufacturing efficiency Correctly designed and located facilities within the manufacturing area will improve the efficiency of the manufacturing process and therefore reduce the cost of product manufacture. Careful consideration needs to be given to all the different stages involved in the process and how material will be transferred between stages in order that the production facility layout is optimized. For example, use of gravity feeding of material between stages might require the facility to be sited on different levels, whereas use of pneumatic or vacuum systems allows the facility to be sited on one level.

Achievement of manufacturing aims

Environmental conditions Control of the air temperature, relative humidity and particulate and microbial content is important in order that the aims of the manufacturing process can be met. The specific conditions required depend on the product being manufactured. The following are illustrative examples:

- For a tableting operation, typical environmental conditions might be a temperature of 21°C, a relative humidity of 35–40% and an air filtration target of 95% removal of particles less than 5 μm. These figures are such because powder flow is influenced by both air temperature and, particularly, relative humidity. The specified air cleaning will ensure freedom from dust but sterility is not necessary.
- Hard gelatin capsule filling processes, on the other hand, are typically carried out at a temperature of 24°C and a relative humidity of approximately 30%. These figures are necessary since capsule shells become brittle and crack if the relative humidity and temperature are too low and become soft and sticky and tend to jam the capsule filler if the relative humidity and temperature are too high.

- Air relative humidity is also vital when manufacturing deliquescent products where levels as low as 20% may be required.
- With clean preparation areas, the air particulate level is very important and the filtration target may be for more than 99% removal of particles of 1 μm or less.

Typical 'comfortable' working conditions for operators are 18–24°C and 40–70% relative humidity but the overriding needs of the process will always dictate environmental design conditions.

The temperature of the air may be controlled by passing it either through a steam-based or electrical heating system or over refrigerant coils. The relative humidity of the air may be increased by spraying water (of small droplet size) into the air stream or decreased by using refrigeration systems or desiccant wheels.

In order to maintain the required conditions in the manufacturing area, the stale air must be frequently replaced with conditioned air. The frequency at which this needs to occur will depend on factors such as the nature of the production process, number of operators present and whether the room is 'in use'. It may vary from approximately 20 changes per hour (typical solid dose production) to 500 changes per hour (rooms for sterile production).

Architectural considerations Manufacturing areas should be of a suitable size, construction and location to facilitate proper operation, cleaning and maintenance. They should be laid out in such a way as to allow the production to take place in areas connected in a logical order corresponding to the sequence of the operations and to the requisite cleanliness levels. Working space should be adequate to allow the logical positioning of materials and equipment so as to minimize the risk of confusion between products or their components and to avoid cross-contamination. Any pipe work, light fittings or ventilation points should be designed and sited to avoid the creation of recesses which may collect 'dust' and are difficult to clean. If possible, they should be accessible from outside the manufacturing area for maintenance.

Interior surfaces (walls, floors and ceilings) should be smooth, free from cracks and open joints, should not shed particulate matter and should permit easy and effective cleaning or disinfection. Lighting should be sufficient for easy reading of in-process control systems, equipment dials, etc.

Validation of manufacturing facilities

Validation and why it is required

Detailed coverage of validation is beyond the scope of this chapter due to its complexity and the constantly changing requirements of the regulatory authorities. The following section therefore summarizes the scope of validation with respect to manufacturing facilities and explains why validation is important. In order to be aware of the latest position, the reader should consult information provided by regulatory authorities or other relevant authoritative sources.

Validation is a component of cGMP (current Good Manufacturing Practice). Numerous definitions exist including that of the Food and Drug Administration (FDA, USA) which has defined process validation as 'establishing documented evidence which provides a high degree of assurance that a specific process will consistently produce a product meeting its predetermined specifications and quality characteristics'. In other words, validation is proving that a process works.

Essentially the purpose of validation is to ensure consistent product quality. A new product or an old product manufactured using a modified formulation, process or facility cannot be sold until the 'process' has been adequately validated.

Scope of validation

When manufacturing a product, all aspects of the 'process' need to be validated. This includes the starting materials used, e.g. the bulk drug properties and its method of production, the excipients and the material suppliers. Validated procedures for handling the materials, from the time they are received to the time they are used, should be in place to ensure only materials with the required properties and in the correct amounts are used. The analytical methods used to test starting components, intermediate and finished products and stability samples must be validated to ensure they are capable of both analysing the properties to the required accuracy and detecting unwanted components and degradation products.

Personnel involved in any activity which contributes to the manufacture of a product must be adequately trained and must follow documented procedures. It must be ensured that the manufacturing equipment used complies with the intended specification, that all services and recording equipment function correctly and that any computer systems have been validated.

The manufacturing process must be robust and produce a product with consistent properties. This is usually confirmed by manufacturing three full-scale production batches under specified conditions. In order to minimize cross-contamination between batches, the processes used to clean all equipment in which the product comes into contact must also be validated.

Types of validation

Validation may be divided into four types.

Prospective validation   This is where the validation programme is designed *before* the equipment or facility is used or before the product manufactured by the process being validated is distributed. This is the type of validation employed when producing the data on initial full-scale production batches required in order to obtain a regulatory authorization for manufacture and marketing of that product.

Retrospective validation   This is achieved by reviewing historical manufacturing and testing data of products or processes which are already in operation and working well.

Concurrent validation   This is either ongoing prospective validation or ongoing review with evaluation of historical data.

Revalidation   Revalidation involves repeating all or part of the validation if, for example, a process or facility is modified. Processes and procedures should undergo periodic critical revalidation to ensure they remain capable of achieving the intended results.

Cost/benefits of validation

The cost of validation is considerable with significant resources being required, including personnel (from product development, quality assurance and engineering departments) and significant amounts of materials. Inadequate validation may, however, lead to the rejection or withdrawal of legal authorization for manufacturing and marketing of the product. In other circumstances, it may lead to expensive product recalls. Other benefits of well-designed validation programmes are likely to include a reduction in process support required, fewer batch failures, greater output and speeding up of marketing authorizations.

Cleaning validation as an example of a validation process

It is clearly desirable that a pharmaceutical product contains only those components that are supposed to be present. Since most manufacturing equipment will not solely be used in the production of a single product, there is the possibility that without adequate cleaning procedures cross-contamination between products may occur. Although this should be detected during quality control tests and therefore not endanger the public, it will still lead to costly batch wastage.

Cleaning protocols must therefore be validated to ensure that they are effective. Since equipment can never be 100% clean, the aim of a cleaning procedure is to minimize the possibility of *significant* cross-contamination between batches of different products. A typical specification would be that the contaminant level in the product taken by a patient is not greater than a thousandth of its lowest daily therapeutic dose. The limits set should be verifiable and achievable and the validated analytical methods used must have the sensitivity to detect residues or contaminants at low levels.

Once a piece of equipment has been cleaned following a documented procedure, it is 'analysed' to detect the level of any product residue remaining. This may be achieved, for example, by:

- swabbing the equipment over a 100 cm^2 area at positions likely to be contaminated and analysing the swabs
- collecting and analysing rinsings from final cleaning water (e.g. for cream manufacturing vessels)
- producing a placebo batch of the product in the cleaned container.

Visual and tactile inspection is also useful as an adjunct to the detection of contamination.

It is good practice to select as the product to validate a cleaning procedure the one that is likely to be the most difficult to clean in that particular equipment. Care must also be taken to ensure that any cleaning materials used are pharmaceutically acceptable and that they remain in the equipment in suitably low levels. Once a cleaning process has been validated (this is typically after three consecutive applications of the cleaning procedure have been shown to be effective), operators must then *always* follow the designated procedure to ensure a consistently successful process.

MATERIALS OF FABRICATION

Desirable properties and selection

In selecting materials for the construction of satisfactory plant, the pharmaceutical engineer encounters problems involving chemical, physical and economic factors. The following brief outline of these factors indicates something of the scope and limitations of the choice of materials available.

Chemical factors

Two aspects of chemical action must be considered under this heading: the possible contamination of the *product* by the material of the plant and any effect on the *material of the plant* by the drugs and chemicals being processed.

The importance of the first of these becomes evident when it is realized that impurities often have considerable toxicological effects and that impurities, even in trace amounts, may initiate decomposition mechanisms

in the product. An example of the latter is the inactivating effect of heavy metals on penicillins. The appearance of a product may also be affected by changes in colour due to contamination from the materials of the plant.

It should be remembered that contamination from some materials may be innocuous, the products being non-toxic.

Our increasing knowledge of materials of plant construction is assisting greatly in providing plant that will be resistant to attack and deterioration in use from the effects of acids, alkalis, oxidizing agents, etc. Alloys having special physical and chemical properties have been developed and materials such as plastics have been introduced to meet the problems encountered.

Physical factors

An ideal material of construction would satisfy all the following criteria. In practice, no material is ideal and the selection procedure must be based on compromise.

Strength Sufficient mechanical strength is an obvious necessity and will be suited to the size of the plant and the stresses to which it will be subjected.

Weight In most cases weight should be reduced to a minimum, other factors being satisfactory, and especially in plant that may have to be moved about from place to place.

Wearing qualities These are particularly important where there is a possibility of friction between moving parts, an extreme case in point being the material used for the grinding surfaces of size reduction mills.

Ease of fabrication It must be possible to process the material in order to manufacture the various units of the plant. Properties that enable materials to be cast, welded, bent or machined are of prime importance.

Thermal expansion The design of plant may be greatly complicated by the use of material that has a high coefficient of expansion. This increases the stresses and the risk of fracture with temperature changes, and the temperature range over which the plant will be operated is likely to be considerably restricted.

Thermal conductivity In heat-transfer plant, such as steam or water-heated vessels, good thermal conductivity is desirable. It must be remembered, however, that the bulk of the resistance to heat transfer may lie in the boundary layer films (see Chapter 46).

Cleansing Smooth polished surfaces simplify cleansing processes and materials that can be 'finished' with such surfaces are ideal when scrupulous cleanliness is necessary.

Sterilization Where sterility is essential, the material should be capable of withstanding the necessary treatment, usually steam under pressure. This factor is to some extent bound up with the previous one since cleaning is a normal preliminary to the sterilization of apparatus and plant equipment.

Transparency This *may* be a useful property where it is necessary to observe the process. Borosilicate glass may be used in the construction of some parts of certain pharmaceutical plant.

Economic factors

Cost and maintenance of plant must, of course, be economic. Here the main concern is not simply to obtain the least costly material. Better wearing qualities and lower maintenance may well mean that a higher initial cost is more economical in the long run.

MATERIALS USED IN FABRICATION

A brief description of materials which are suitable for the fabrication or construction of pharmaceutical apparatus and manufacturing plant is given below.

Metals

Ferrous metals – steels

Steel is any alloy of iron and carbon that contains less than 2% carbon. Despite the tendency for this metal to corrode, it is still widely used. The added carbon may exist in the free state (graphite) or in chemical combination as iron carbide, Fe_3C. The phase diagram for the iron/carbon system is complex. Iron can exist in two allotropic forms. At temperatures below 940°C the stable form is α-iron (ferrite). When steel is in a molten condition, the γ form (austenite) is able to dissolve carbon. Various eutectics and solid solutions may form on cooling, giving rise to steels of differing properties. The austenitic form can persist at normal temperatures if other metals such as chromium and nickel are alloyed with the iron. The resulting properties of the steel depend mainly on the content of carbon and other metals that may be added and any heat treatment that the steel may receive.

Mild steel This is the commonest form of steel for general purposes and has a carbon content between 0.15% and 0.3%. It is ductile and can be welded easily to give structures of high mechanical strength. However, its resistance to corrosion is poor.

Cast iron The effect of increasing the carbon content beyond 1.5% is to lower the melting point of iron so that it can be easily melted and cast into sand moulds to form objects of intricate shape. Cast iron is resistant to corrosion (see later in this chapter) but it reacts with materials such as phenols to give coloured compounds.

Cast iron is hard and brittle and can be welded and machined only with great difficulty. The hardness and corrosion resistance can be increased by adding silicon though such high-silicon iron is extremely brittle.

Stainless steels These steels contain a significant amount of nickel and chromium which confer a high degree of corrosion resistance. Stainless steels can be fabricated and polished to a high mirror finish. They are extensively used in the food, pharmaceutical, cosmetic and fermentation industries where their high cost can be fully justified.

The most common type is the so-called austenitic stainless steel where the nickel and chromium content stabilize austenite at normal room temperatures. Austenitic stainless steels contain non-magnetic austenitic grains. Overall, stainless steels are non-magnetic materials and have a basic composition of approximately 18% chromium and 8% nickel: the term '18/8 stainless' refers to this composition. Adding more chromium and nickel increases corrosion resistance but these are expensive metals. The phase diagram for stainless steel (Fig. 45.1) indicates that an alloy containing 18% chromium and 8% nickel (which is more costly than chromium) is the most economical combination of chromium and nickel form to give an austenitic stainless steel. Small amounts of molybdenum greatly increase corrosion resistance.

Stainless steel owes its corrosion resistance to a tenacious oxide layer that forms on the surface. In this case the passivity (see later in this chapter) results from the formation of this oxide film ($Fe O \cdot Cr_2O_3$ in the case of stainless steel) that serves as an impervious protective layer on the surface of the metal. Materials such as nitric acid which are oxidizing agents can be tolerated but

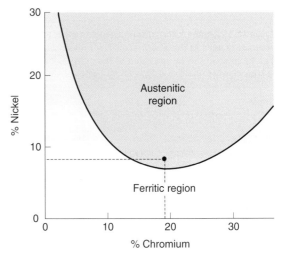

Fig. 45.1 Phase diagram for stainless steel.

chlorides can penetrate the film and stainless steel equipment should not be used for hydrochloric acid.

Some stainless steels contain a low carbon content and have small amounts of molybdenum added. This minimizes carbide precipitation during welding which may lead to corrosion problems – so-called 'weld decay'. This results from the removal of chromium as chromium carbide along the line of any welding which may be performed. Such depleted steel is then prone to corrosion.

The compositions of four grades of stainless steel that are widely used in the pharmaceutical industry are shown in Table 45.1. Those grades with the L suffix are the low carbon with added molybdenum grades referred to above.

One minor objection to stainless steel is the low thermal conductivity (16.3 W m^{-1} K^{-1}) when compared with other metals but this is not usually significant as the main resistance to heat transfer may reside in the boundary layers (as explained in Chapter 46). Other properties of stainless steel are density range: 7861–8082 kg m^{-3}, specific heat: 0.46 kJ kg^{-1} K and coefficient of thermal expansion: 17×10^{-6} m/m per K.

A further problem with stainless steel is a difficulty in welding during fabrication into processing equipment. Stainless steel may be joined using a process known as gas tungsten-arc welding (GTAC), also called TIG (tungsten inert gas) welding. Heating is caused by an arc between the surface of the steel and a tungsten electrode. The electrode is not consumed during the process so filling metal may be needed, depending on the weld. An inert gas (such as argon) is used as a shielding gas to prevent atmospheric contamination of the weld. TIG welding requires a high degree of skill.

Stainless steels can be used for most pharmaceutical laboratory and manufacturing equipment where a smooth surface with high corrosion-resisting qualities is neces-sary. The smooth surface of modern stainless steels is particularly attractive for pharmaceutical operations, both sterile and non-sterile. Various qualities of surface finishes are available. The commonest for pharmaceutical manufacture are listed in Table 45.2. The fabrication costs of producing a smooth surface on stainless steel increases sharply with increasing degree of smoothness.

The high cost of stainless steel can be justified for pharmaceutical manufacture, even on a very large scale. Most manufacturing equipment used in the production of pharmaceuticals is of this material since it is by far the most satisfactory, being strong, corrosion resistant, non-contaminating and readily cleaned and sterilized.

Non-ferrous metals

Copper Copper is malleable and ductile and thus is easily fabricated. It has a thermal conductivity eight times greater than steel but is corroded by a number of substances, particularly oxidizing agents. It is attacked by nitric acid in all concentrations, by hot concentrated hydrochloric and sulphuric acids and by some organic acids. Ammonia reacts with it readily to form blue cuproammonium compounds. Many drug constituents react with it and, for this reason, copper is usually protected by a lining of tin when used for pharmaceutical plant. It was formerly used for evaporators and pans used for sugar coating. Because of its susceptibility to attack by pharmaceutical materials, its usage has been replaced by stainless steel.

Copper piping is easy to make because of the ductility of the metal and it is used extensively for services such as cold water, gas, low vacuum and low-pressure steam. Where necessary, copper piping may be tinned, e.g. for distilled water, but nowadays stainless steel piping is used for this purpose.

Copper alloys These include alloys with zinc, tin, aluminium, silicon and nickel, all of which have their special uses.

Aluminium Aluminium has good corrosion resistance to many substances, although it is attacked by mineral acids (it is resistant to strong nitric acid), caustic

---

Table 45.1 Composition of four stainless steel grades commonly used in the pharmaceutical industry. The balance of the composition of the stainless steel is iron

Grade	304	304L	316	316L
Element		Composition (%)		
Carbon, max	0.08	0.035	0.08	0.035
Manganese, max	2	2	2	2
Phosphorus, max	0.040	0.040	0.040	0.040
Sulfur, max	0.030	0.030	0.030	0.030
Silicon, max	0.75	0.75	0.030	0.030
Nickel	8–11	8–13	10–14	10–15
Chromium	18–20	18–20	16–18	16–18
Molybdenum	None	None	2–3	2–3

Table 45.2 Finishes for pharmaceutical stainless steel

Finish number	Arithmetic mean roughness, R$_a$ (μm)
150	0.68–0.81
180	0.40–0.58
240	0.36–0.45
320	0.21–0.25

alkalis, mercury and its salts. Its resistance is often due to the formation of a film on the surface. For example, pure strong ammonia solutions form a resistant film of aluminium hydroxide. It is also highly resistant to oxidizing conditions since it forms a compact oxide film.

Pure aluminium is soft but more corrosion resistant than most of its alloys such as Duralumin. Alloys combining corrosion resistance with strength are formed with the addition of a small percentage of manganese, magnesium or silicon. Plant is easily fabricated and has excellent thermal conductivity.

Lead   Lead is still used in the chemical industry during the manufacture of active principles because of its remarkable resistance to corrosion and the great ease with which it can be made into complicated shapes. The lead chamber process for manufacturing sulphuric acid is one example from many in the heavy chemical industry. It is little used in pharmaceutical practice, however, because of the risk of product contamination by traces of poisonous lead salts. Pharmaceutical materials must comply with a limit test for lead.

Tin   Tin has a high resistance to a great variety of substances and, since its salts are non-toxic, it has a wide use throughout the food industry. It is, however, weak, its main use being to provide a protective coating for steel, copper, brass, etc.

Non-metals

Inorganics

Glass   Glass is widely used in the laboratory and glass equipment can be obtained for manufacture on a larger scale. Ordinary soda glass is used for bottles and other cheap articles but is not satisfactory for large-scale plant or for containers where alkali contamination might be a serious drawback. For these purposes, borosilicate glass is used, which has several advantages over soda glass. It is, for example, less brittle. It has a low thermal expansion and can be used with safety over wide temperature ranges. However, its thermal conductivity is low and therefore it should be heated gradually to avoid fracturing. Pipe lines may be used with pressures up to 8 bar if the pipe diameter is less than 50 mm and pipe lines with larger diameters are used with pressures up to 400 kPa.

The special advantages of glass are that it can be easily cleaned and sterilized and the contents of vessels can be readily examined for colour and clarity.

A disadvantage is the difficulty of joining sections of glass plant together. Ground-glass joints are sometimes satisfactory, especially in small-scale apparatus, but are rigid. Gaskets of synthetic rubber and plastics are used to form a flexible jointing but these must be chosen with care as they are normally less resistant to attack than glass. For that reason gaskets are now often made from PTFE but careful alignment of the sections is required for their successful use.

Glass pipe line is useful for transporting liquids from stage to stage in various operations. Such pipe line is available from 15 mm to 300 mm in diameter with fittings for the assembly of complete systems.

Fused silica   Fused silica (Vitreosil) has an extremely low coefficient of thermal expansion and vessels made from it can be heated to red heat and plunged into cold water without breaking. It has a high melting point and it is difficult to fuse it completely so that equipment tends to be opaque, though transparent forms are available.

Glass linings and coatings   Metal may be coated with glass to give a protective lining. The dangers of such apparatus are those of uneven expansion of metal and glass and of the glass surface accidentally chipping. Great care must therefore be taken in heating and cooling and in protecting the glass lining from accidental damage.

Vessels of up to 50 000 litres capacity, pipe line and fittings, valves, condensers, columns, pumps, stirrers and mixtures are among the many glass-coated items still in use, although they have been largely replaced with stainless steel vessels.

High resistance to corrosion and case of cleaning make it valuable for pharmaceutical use.

Organics

Plastics   The range of materials known collectively as plastics is so wide that only a brief account can be given. It is convenient to group them under the following headings:

1. rigid materials
2. flexible materials
3. coatings and linings
4. cements and filters
5. special cases.

'Keebush' is an example of a rigid material. It is a phenolic resin with various inert fillers selected for their particular purpose. It may be machined, welded and worked in other ways and is resistant to such an extent that it can be used for gears, bearings and similar items with a noise reduction of two-thirds compared with metal. It is resistant to corrosion except that of oxidizing substances and strong alkalis. Any item may be made from this material – vessels, pipes, fittings, valves, pumps, fans, ducts, filter presses and many others.

Polyethylene and polyvinyl chloride (PVC) are similar materials and are rigid or flexible, depending upon the amount of plasticizer added. These do not withstand high temperatures but are non-resistant only to strong oxidizing acids, halogens and organic solvents.

Rigid or semi-rigid mouldings may be used for tanks, pipes, ducts and other similar items; slightly flexible funnels, buckets and jugs are made which are almost unbreakable.

Polytetrafluoroethylene (PTFE, Teflon) is a semi-rigid plastic with extreme resistance to all agents other than fluorine or molten alkali metals. It is a slippery non-wettable material but it can be bonded to metals as a protective coating. It is also usable at temperatures above 200°C but it is a costly material which prohibits its extensive use.

Metallic surfaces may be protected from corrosion by plastics of the polyethylene or PVC types prepared for coating with suitable plasticizers. Perfect adhesion of plastic to metal is sometimes difficult and other disadvantages are the differences in thermal expansion of plastic and metal and the danger of the coating accidentally chipping.

Uses of these materials include the lining of tanks and vessels and the coatings on stirrers and fans. Plastic cements are used for spaces between acid-resistant tiles and bricks and for similar purposes.

Special cases include transparent plastic guards for moving parts of machinery and asepsis screens. Nylon and PVC fibres may be woven into filter cloths.

Rubber   Hard rubber may be used for purposes similar to those mentioned under plastics. Soft rubber may be used for linings, coatings and valves. Rubber swells in contact with oils; it is subject to oxidation and is attacked by some organic solvents. Synthetic rubbers that have greater resistance have been developed.

CORROSION

General introduction and theory

Corrosion is a complex form of material deterioration as a result of a reaction with its environment. It is the destruction of a material (usually a metal) by means other than mechanical. Most environments are corrosive. Corrosion is not restricted to reactions with strong acids. The following have been shown to cause corrosion:

1. Air and moisture
2. Rural, urban and industrial atmospheres
3. Fresh, salt and distilled water
4. Steam and gases such as chlorine, ammonia, hydrogen sulfide, sulfur dioxide
5. Mineral acids, such as hydrochloric acid, sulphuric acid, nitric acid
6. Organic acids, such as acetic acid, citric acid, formic acid
7. Alkalis
8. Soils
9. Organic solvents
10. Vegetable and petroleum oils.

Importance of corrosion

Corrosion is very important in the chemical and pharmaceutical process industries for a number of reasons. The possibility of any of the following occurring must be considered.

Safety

- Loss of pharmacologically active or toxic substances
- Loss of inflammable or explosive chemicals
- Sudden loss of material being processed at high temperature or high pressure
- Possibility of burns from acids, etc.
- Corroding of equipment is known to have caused fairly harmless compounds to become toxic or explosive.

Financial losses

- Replacement of corroded parts
- Plant shut-down, i.e. stoppage due to unexpected corrosion failures. This leads to loss of revenue
- Loss of expensive chemicals.

Contamination of the product

This is of particular importance in the pharmaceutical industry since the product is usually for human consumption or administration. Metal ions can promote degradation reactions and can be toxic.

Appearance of plant

This is not a minor consideration. Satisfactory factory appearance is an important aspect of good manufacturing practice.

Corrosion mechanisms

The corrosive reaction of metals is generally electrochemical in nature. The relevant points of a simple, acceptable theory of electrochemical corrosion are summarized below:

- An anode (−) and a cathode (+) form a cell in conjunction with an electrically conducting environment (electrolyte). Anodic and cathodic areas can arise on a single piece of metal because of local differences in the outside environment and in the metal itself. Different stresses, scratches and impurities produce varying electrical potential. Cells with far greater electrical potentials are formed between different metals or alloys. Anodes and cathodes may be close (local cells) or far apart.

- Direct current (DC) flows. The current is a flow of electrons within the metal(s) from anode to cathode. Metal ions (positive charge) travel from the anode in the electrolyte; they usually do not reach the cathode but remain in solution.

Single-metal corrosion

Simple electrochemical corrosion is explained diagrammatically in Figure 45.2. It shows the mechanism for corrosion of a single piece of steel (predominantly iron) in water (dissociated by the presence of dissolved chemicals).

The anodic reaction is:

$$Fe \rightarrow Fe^{++} + 2e^-$$

and the cathodic reaction is:

$$2H^+ + 2e^- \rightarrow H_2$$

The overall reaction is therefore:

$$Fe + 2H_2O \rightarrow Fe(OH)_2 + H_2$$

The important consequence of this reaction is that structurally strong metal leaves the anode as a metal ion in solution. The metal is therefore weakened and the solution contaminated with corrosion product.

Corrosion between metals

This is important because joints, flanges, seals, bolts, etc., are often constructed of different metals. A cell is set up between the metals, one becoming the anode and the other the cathode. The potential difference between the metals depends on their electrode potentials. Knowledge of the electromotive series of metals is therefore important. These are summarized in Table 45.3.

The following points can be noted from Table 45.3:

1. A negative sign in the fourth column implies that the reaction in the direction of element to ion is spontaneous, i.e. it requires negative energy to proceed in that direction.
2. A metal higher in the series will be the anode and one lower will act as the cathode when two metals are coupled or in indirect contact with each other via the electrolyte.
3. Metals high in the table have less corrosion resistance. For example, metals above copper readily oxidize. This also explains why gold and silver are found as free metals in their native state whilst aluminium and iron are found only combined as oxides.

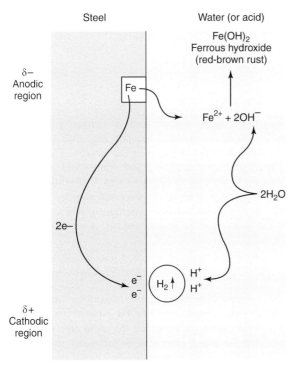

Fig. 45.2 Diagrammatic representation of the electrochemical corrosion of steel (iron) in water.

Table 45.3 The electromotive series of some commonly used metals

	Element	Ion produced	Standard electrode potential (V)
Active end	Na	Na$^+$	-2.71
	Mg	Mg^{2+}	-2.34
	Al	Al3$^+$	-1.67
	Zn	Zn^{2+}	-0.76
	Cr	Cr^{3+}	-0.71
	Fe	Fe^{3+}	-0.44
	Ni	Ni^{2+}	-0.25
	Sn	Sn^{2+}	-0.14
	Pb	Pb^{2+}	-0.13
Reference zero	H	H$^+$	0.000
	Cu	Cu^{2+}	+0.35
	Cu	Cu$^+$	+0.52
	Ag	Ag$^+$	+0.80
	Pt	Pt^{2+}	+1.20
Noble end	Au	Au^{3+}	+1.42

4. The greater the difference in potential between two metals, the greater will be the rate of corrosion. For example, sodium reacts violently with water, iron slowly rusts yet lead is not attacked by water.
5. When two metals are in contact, the corrosion rate of the anodic member of the couple is accelerated.
6. A metal will replace another metal in solution if the latter is lower in the series. This is best understood by examination of Figure 45.3.
7. The table therefore indicates whether or not a metal is attacked by acids or water, since metals above hydrogen are attacked because they replace hydrogen in solution, e.g.:

$$Al + HCl(\text{in solution}) \rightarrow AlCl_3(\text{in solution})$$

$$Fe + H_2O(\text{in solution}) \rightarrow Fe(OH)_2(\text{in solution})$$

Cathodic protection

This term is used to describe the technique whereby a structurally important metal is forced to become wholly cathodic (and therefore protected from corrosion) by attaching to it a more electronegative second metal. An example is galvanization in which steel is coated with a layer of zinc. The zinc becomes the anode, thus protecting the steel. The advantage of this technique over normal coatings is that even if the galvanized coating is scratched, the exposed metal surface will remain cathodic. Metal objects can be protected in a similar way by attaching to them replaceable pieces of a more electronegative metal (e.g. aluminium block attached to a steel object).

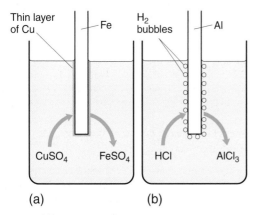

(a) (b)

Fig. 45.3 (a) Reaction of iron in copper sulfate solution. The copper ions in solution are being replaced by iron ions (lower in table) at the same time as the copper from solution is being deposited as copper metal on the iron sheet. (b) Similarly the hydrogen in the HCl solution is replaced by aluminium ions and the hydrogen is evolved as bubbles of gas.

Passivity

This is the phenomenon in which a metal appears in practice to be much less reactive than would be predicted by its position in the electromotive series. For example, one would expect aluminium to be extremely reactive since its electrode potential is -1.67 volts, yet it is commonly used in construction because of its lack of reactivity. The explanation is that aluminium does in fact react quickly with air but an aluminium oxide coating is produced which is very resistant to further atmospheric attack.

Lead, which has a small electronegativity and would therefore be expected to react, at least with strong inorganic acids, is in fact used in the production of sulphuric acid (lead chamber process). In this example an impervious, unreactive layer of lead sulfate is formed on the outside of the lead sheets.

Types of corrosion

The various types of corrosion can be classified by the form in which the corrosion manifests itself. The eight most common types of corrosion are:

1. uniform attack or general, overall corrosion
2. galvanic or two-metal corrosion
3. concentration-cell corrosion
4. pitting
5. intergranular corrosion
6. parting (or dezincification)
7. stress corrosion
8. erosion corrosion.

Uniform attack

This is the most common form of corrosion. It is normally an electrochemical reaction in which the anode and cathode move slowly over the surface of the metal. The metal becomes thinner and thinner and eventually fails, e.g. sheet-iron roof, zinc in acid. Uniform corrosion is the easiest to predict, discover and stop by means of the use of (i) more suitable materials, ii) inhibitors either in the metal or in the product and (iii) protective coatings (paint, plastic, etc.).

Galvanic corrosion

This is corrosion between two dissimilar metals (see above). An example could be the case of a concentric pipe heat exchanger in which the main structure is of steel but the heat exchange pipes are made of copper to improve heat transfer. In domestic central heating systems, the commonest situation is to have steel radiators joined by copper piping.

Control of galvanic corrosion Use only one metal if this is possible. If not:

1. select combinations of metals as close together as possible in the electrochemical series
2. avoid combinations where the area of the more active metal (i.e. the anode) is small, since this increases the anodic reaction rate. It is therefore better to have the more noble metal or alloy for fastenings, bolts, etc.
3. insulate dissimilar metals completely wherever possible
4. apply coatings such as paint or plastic but with caution. Small holes in the coating over an anodic region will result in rapid attack. Therefore, it is important to keep the coating in good repair
5. add chemical inhibitors to the corrosive solution. The nature of these inhibitors depends on the specific nature of the solution to be inhibited. Particular care must be taken in their selection when the corrosive solution is the pharmaceutical product or is an intermediate for drug synthesis
6. avoid joining metals with threaded connections since the threads will deteriorate excessively; spilled liquids or condensates can concentrate in thread grooves. Welded joints (using welds of the same alloy) are preferred.

Concentration-cell corrosion

Cells can form because of differences in the environment rather than differences in the metal itself. These are known as concentration (or solution) cells. There are two types: metal-ion cells and oxygen cells.

Metal-ion cells These can form in areas where stagnant liquid collects. Metal ion concentration cells are caused, as their name suggests, by differences in metal ion concentration in the corroding solution. A build-up of metal ions can occur in stagnant conditions caused by holes, gaskets, lap joints, surface deposits (scale, dirt) and crevices under bolt heads and rivet heads. They can also be caused by material, such as plastic, rubber, etc., lying on the surface of the metal.

Oxygen cells These are similar to metal-ion cells in a number of ways but here the corrosion is caused by differences in the dissolved oxygen content of the solution.

Control of concentration-cell corrosion This can be achieved in the following ways:

1. Use welded butt joints instead of riveted or bolted joints in new apparatus.
2. Existing lap joints should be welded, sealed or soldered to close the crevices.
3. Design vessels for complete drainage, avoid sharp corners and stagnant areas.

4. Inspect and clean deposits frequently.
5. Use solid, non-absorbent gaskets, such as Teflon, wherever possible.
6. Use welded pipes rather than the rolled-in type.

Pitting

This is a form of extremely localized attack where the anode remains as one spot. This results in rapid corrosion and deep penetration (small anode area, large cathode). Pits may be isolated or close together, the latter appearing as a rough surface. The pits usually occur at impurities in the metal, grain boundaries, small scratches, rough surfaces, etc. Pitting is one of the most destructive forms of corrosion. It is difficult to detect in a laboratory corrosion test because the pits are very small and there will be little loss in weight.

Pitting is responsible for more unexpected plant equipment failures than any other form of corrosion. Additionally, the liquid in the pit becomes stagnant, resulting in metal-ion and/or oxygen concentration-cell corrosion. Furthermore, metal ions from the corrosion will accumulate in the pit. The process is therefore self-accelerating.

Control of pitting This is very difficult but most of the points mentioned under concentration cells will help. If a test material shows the slightest signs of pitting in a laboratory test using microscopy, it must never be used.

Intergranular corrosion

Solid metals consist of a large number of grains (actually metal crystals) and thus have a granular (or polycrystalline) structure. Intergranular corrosion is localized attack at grain boundaries, with relatively little corrosion of the grains themselves. Due to stresses and structural imperfections at the grain boundaries (plus the increased concentration of impurities there), they are usually anodic. As corrosion proceeds, the grains fall out and the metal or alloy disintegrates. This type of corrosion occurs in stainless steel, particularly after welding (know as *weld decay*).

Control of intergranular corrosion This can be achieved in the following ways:

1. High-temperature postweld heat treatment (solution quenching) can be used. This involves heating the metal to about 1000 K and then cooling it rapidly by quenching in water. This reduces the precipitation of carbon at the grain boundaries.
2. Add stabilizers to the metal, such as columbium, tantalum or titanium. These combine strongly with free carbon to form carbides, leaving no free carbon at the grain boundaries.

3. Lower the carbon content of the steel to below 0.03%. Below this figure carbon is usually completely soluble.

Parting (or dezincification)

This is a general term referring to selective corrosion of one or more components from a solid solution alloy. Removal of zinc, particularly from brass (a 70/30 copper/zinc alloy), is common.

Control of parting This is not easy. Reduction of the corrosive environment and cathodic protection are suggested. Small amounts of arsenic, antimony or phosphorus can be used as 'inhibitors'. The addition of 1% tin to brass (Admiralty brass) results in good resistance to sea water.

Stress corrosion

Generally a high stress in a piece of metal tends to make it more anodic. The greater the stress, the greater this effect. There are two main categories.

Stress-accelerated corrosion This is a decrease in corrosion resistance due to continuous static stress such as applied stresses or residual stresses after welding (as occurs in pressure vessels).

Stress corrosion cracking This is an increase in the tendency of the metal to crack or show brittle fracture. It is usually caused by alternating stresses (i.e. vibrations).

Erosion corrosion

Erosion is a mechanical process, corrosion is electrochemical. They combine in situations where corrosive products which might have protected metals from further corrosion are eroded by mechanical wear or rapid fluid flow. This maintains a fresh metal surface in contact with the corrosive environment.

REFERENCES

Cole, G.C. (1998) Pharmaceutical Production Facilities – Design and Applications, 2nd edn. Taylor and Francis, London.

Rules and Guidance for Pharmaceutical Manufacturers and Distributors (latest edition) Pharmaceutical Press, London.

Signore, A.A., Jacobs, T. (2005) Good Design Practices for GMP Pharmaceutical Facilities. Taylor and Francis, London.

46

Heat transfer and the properties and use of steam

A. M. Twitchell

HEAT AND HEAT TRANSFER

Introduction

Heat is a form of energy associated with the disordered and chaotic movement of molecules and ions. A substance will have no heat content only if it is at a temperature of absolute zero (0 K). Although heat is intangible, it is a form of energy and can be accurately measured and expressed in (preferably) joules (J). The joule represents a very small quantity of heat; for example, 1 J will raise the temperature of 100 mL of water by only approximately 0.002°C. A more practically useful quantity is the kilojoule (kJ) or the megajoule (MJ), which denote 1000 and 1 000 000 joules, respectively. It requires about 65 kJ of heat to raise 200 mL of water from room temperature to its boiling point. The temperature of a material is an indication of its internal energy: the greater the molecular motion, the greater the internal energy and the higher the temperature.

Heat transfer is the exchange or movement of heat energy and will occur spontaneously wherever there is a temperature gradient. The *rate* of heat transfer indicates how quickly heat is exchanged and is expressed in $J\ s^{-1}$ or watts (W).

Many pharmaceutical processes involve the transfer of heat energy. These include:

- melting materials
- creating an elevated temperature during cream, suppository or ointment production
- controlled cooling of the same products
- heating of solvents to hasten dissolution processes, e.g. dissolution of preservatives in the manufacture of solution products
- sterilization of products, e.g. using steam in autoclaves
- evaporation of liquids to concentrate products
- heating or cooling of air in an air-conditioning plant

- drying granules for tablet production
- heating air to facilitate coating processes
- spray-drying and freeze-drying processes.

It is therefore important to have a basic understanding of how materials may be heated and what influences the rate at which they can be heated (so that the heating or cooling can be controlled). This chapter considers the methods by which heat is transferred and the factors that influence the rate of heat transfer. Particular emphasis will be given to the properties and use of steam, as heat energy provided by steam remains as a major source of heating in pharmaceutical production processes. This chapter is only intended as an introduction to this complex subject; the reader is referred to texts by Long (1999) and Holman (2001) if more detailed information is required.

Methods of heat transfer

Conduction

Heat transfer by conduction in solids results from the movement of heat energy to adjacent molecules by vibrational energy transfer and the motion of free electrons. The molecule/electron donating the heat energy will subsequently vibrate to a lesser extent and therefore cool down, whereas the molecule receiving the heat energy will vibrate to a greater extent and therefore increase in temperature.

In the case of a solid, no appreciable movement of the molecules occurs. Heat transfer due to electron movement is generally a greater effect than that due to vibration of the atomic lattice; therefore metallic solids are good conductors and non-metallic solids are not (as they contain few free electrons).

In *static* fluids (and therefore through boundary layers; see Chapter 4) the mechanism is virtually the same. Heat is transferred between molecules as a result of molecular collisions. When a faster-moving molecule from a region of higher energy (or temperature) collides with a slower-moving molecule from a region of lower energy, energy transfer takes place. The molecule with the lower energy gains energy from the high-energy molecule, and the higher-energy molecule loses energy. As a consequence, the temperature of the initially high-energy molecule falls and that of the low-energy molecule rises.

Gases become better conductors at higher temperatures owing to the faster movement of the molecules, whereas most liquids (with the notable exception of water) become poorer conductors at higher temperatures.

Heat transfer by conduction is the main way in which heat is transferred through solids and through fluid boundary layers. It is slow compared with heat transfer by convection.

Convection

Heat transfer by convection is due to the movement of molecules and their associated heat energy on a macroscopic scale. It involves the mixing of molecules and occurs within fluids, where the molecules are free to move around.

Heat transfer by natural convection occurs when there is a difference in density within the fluid arising from the greater expansion and hence the lower density of the fluid in the hotter region. Convection currents are set up as the warm, less dense fluid rises and mixes with colder fluid. As the molecules move, heat transfer *between* molecules can occur by conduction.

Heat transfer by forced convection occurs when the fluid is forced to move, for example by the movement of a mixer blade or disruption caused by baffles. Heat transfer usually occurs more quickly by forced convection than by natural convection, owing to the greater intensity of movement and therefore the increased velocity of the fluid. If forced convection also induces turbulent flow (Chapter 4) then the heat transfer process is aided, as there will be a reduction in the fluid boundary layer thickness.

Radiation

The energy emitted by the sun is transmitted in the form of electromagnetic waves through empty space. These waves can be reflected, transmitted or absorbed. When they are absorbed by a material on which they fall, energy reappears as heat and the material increases in temperature. All hot materials radiate energy in this way. Heat transfer by radiation is only of pharmaceutical practical importance during microwave drying (see Chapter 30).

Heat transfer by conduction and practical heat transfer

Of the three mechanisms of heat transfer described above, the one that will be considered in most detail is heat transfer by conduction. Heat transfer by convection, although important in pharmaceutical processing, is a complex process that is not completely understood and is difficult to define mathematically. More importantly, as far as calculating the rate of heat transfer is concerned, it is the slower heat transfer by conduction that will be the rate-limiting step in the overall heat transfer process. If natural convection is inadequate then forced convection can be induced, e.g. by the use of a stirrer.

Many of the principles to be discussed in this chapter can be illustrated in the first instance by the operation of a laboratory 'water bath', as shown in Figure 46.1.

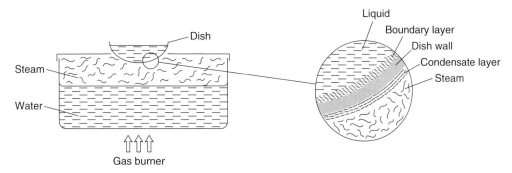

Fig. 46.1 Heating a liquid using a steam bath.

Heat energy from the gas burner is transferred by conduction through the container wall to the water in the bath, which therefore increases in temperature until its boiling point is reached. The heat gained is referred to as *sensible heat*, as it produces an appreciable rise in temperature and the change can be detected by the senses.

When the boiling point of the water has been reached, further heating generates steam without further increase in temperature. This heat gain by the steam is termed *latent heat of evaporation* or *latent heat of vaporization* and is used to change the water from liquid into vapour at constant temperature. The steam produced rises and contacts the dish wall, which initially is at room temperature. The steam condenses on the cool outer surface of the dish and, in doing so, gives up its latent heat and forms a layer of condensate on the dish that runs down over the surface and drops back into the water bath. Fresh condensate is continually formed to take its place so that a layer of condensate will always be present. The latent heat that is liberated by the condensation passes by conduction through the wall of the dish and into the contents to be heated. Heat is then transferred through the fluid by natural convection and conduction.

The term 'water bath' is therefore a misnomer and the equipment is described more accurately as a 'steam bath'. The steam functions as a heat transfer agent whereby the heat from the gas burner is transferred by the liberation of the latent heat into the liquid in the dish. There are advantages in this indirect heating in that the temperature can never exceed 100°C (at atmospheric pressure) and therefore there is less chance of localized overheating and damage to the product being heated. In addition, because the steam circulates over the whole dish surface, heating is much more uniform than it would be if the dish were heated directly over the gas flame.

The insert in Figure 46.1 shows a section of the dish wall in greater detail. If this is considered to be rotated into a vertical position and straightened, it would appear as in Figure 46.2.

A temperature drop occurs from the temperature of the condensing steam to the lower temperature of the liquid in the dish. If this liquid is assumed to be of a lower boiling point than water, then eventually it will boil at this lower constant temperature and temperature gradients would appear as indicated in Figure 46.2. T_S denotes the steam temperature, T_L the temperature of the boiling liquid and T_O and T_I are the temperatures of the outer and inner surfaces of the dish.

In many pharmaceutical processes it is important to know or control the rate at which heat can be transferred. The rate of heat transfer is the quantity of heat transferred in unit time and must be distinguished from the total quantity of heat that needs to be supplied. Consider heating a beaker of water using a Bunsen burner flame. Under a low flame it might take 20 minutes to boil, whereas using a full flame it may only take 5 minutes. To illustrate the point, if heat losses to the environment are neglected and the initial water temperature were the same each time, the total quantity of heat required to boil the water would be the same in each case. The rate of heat transfer, however, would be four

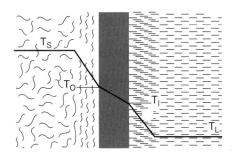

Fig. 46.2 Temperature gradients between steam and a boiling liquid.

times greater over the full flame, i.e. the water will reach boiling point in a quarter of the time.

In the heating situation depicted in Figure 46.1 there are three barriers to the flow of heat energy from the steam to the liquid bulk, namely the condensate layer, the dish wall and the liquid side boundary layer adjacent to the dish wall. The origin and nature of this type of boundary layer are discussed in Chapter 4.

The same quantity of heat must pass through each layer in turn at the same rate. Initially we will consider the factors that affect heat transfer through a single layer of material, in this case the dish wall. Conduction is governed by Fourier's Law, which states that 'the rate of conduction is proportional to the area measured normal to the direction of heat flow and to the temperature gradient in the direction of heat flow'. The rate of heat transfer, i.e. the quantity of heat transferred (Q, joules) in unit time (t, seconds), will therefore depend on the difference in temperature (ΔT or $T_O - T_I$) between the outer and inner surfaces of the dish (the driving force for the heat transfer process), the dish thickness L_D and the area available for heat transfer, A. The proportionality constant is termed the thermal conductivity of the material and is denoted by the symbol K (K_D in the case of the dish). It gives an indication of the ability of the material to conduct heat: the higher the value, the more easily heat is conducted.

Combining all these factors gives:

$$\frac{Q}{t} = \frac{K_D A (T_O - T_I)}{L_D} \tag{46.1}$$

Eqn 46.1 indicates that to increase the heat transfer rate (i.e. conduct heat more quickly) through a layer of material, the value of A, ΔT or K may be increased or the value of L decreased.

By rearranging Eqn 46.1 and using appropriate SI units, thermal conductivity can be shown to have units of W/mK. Table 46.1 gives some typical representative thermal conductivity values. It shows that metals are the best conductors, followed by non-metallic solids, liquids and gases. It should be noted that the value of K will vary with temperature and also with the composition of the material (e.g. from 13 to 19 W/mK in the case of stainless steel).

Illustrative calculation for heat transfer by conduction

Q Calculate the quantity of heat passing in a period of 4 minutes through a stainless steel dish whose effective heating surface area is 25 cm² and whose thickness is 1 mm if the temperatures at the outer and inner surfaces of the dish are 90°C and 80°C, respectively.

A The first step is to convert all values into SI units. Thus:

Table 46.1 Thermal conductivity values of some materials encountered during pharmaceutical processing

Material	Thermal conductivity (W/m K)
Copper (pure)	386
Aluminium (pure)	204
Mild steel	43
Stainless steel (typical)	17
Glass	0.86
Water (at 20°C)	0.60
Water (at 80°C)	0.67
Boiler scale	0.09–2.3
Glass wool insulation	0.04
Air	0.03

$A = 25$ cm² $= 25 \times 10^{-4}$ m², $L_D = 1$ mm $= 1 \times 10^{-3}$ m, $K = 17$ W/mK (typical value for stainless steel; see Table 46.1), $T_O - T_I = 10$ K or 10°C (note because it is a temperature *difference* the numerical value is the same whether expressed in K or °C) and Q/t is expressed in watts.

The converted values can then be inserted into Eqn 46.1, thus:

$$Q/t = (17 \times 25 \times 10^{-4} \times 10)/1 \times 10^{-3} \text{ W} = 425 \text{ W}$$

Therefore, 425 J of heat energy will be transferred every second, and in 4 minutes (240 s) the total heat transferred will be 425×240 J $= 102\,000$ J $= 102$ kJ.

Heat transfer through multiple layers

In most practical circumstances heat needs to be transferred through multiple layers (as illustrated in Fig. 46.1). In order to calculate the rate of heat transfer through more than one layer, the thermal conductivity and thickness values of each layer need to be taken into account. It is not possible, however, to generate a value for the overall conductivity simply by adding the individual K values, as each layer offers a different *resistance* to heat transfer. The overall thermal conductivity (K_O) of a system is inversely proportional to the overall thermal resistance (R_O), which in turn is the sum of the thermal resistance of the individual layers.

Thus:

$$K_O = 1/R_O \tag{46.2}$$

and:

$$R_O = R_1 + R_2 + R_3 + \ldots R_N \tag{46.3}$$

This situation is analogous to the flow of electricity, where the total resistance to flow needs to be quantified in order to calculate the current flowing at any particular voltage.

To find the thermal resistance of an individual layer, Eqn 46.1 can be rearranged so that it becomes:

$$\frac{Q}{t} = \frac{\Delta T}{L/KA} \qquad (46.4)$$

This represents the general form of an equation for any rate process, where the rate at which the process occurs is expressed as a driving force divided by a resistance. In the case of heat transfer, the driving force is the temperature difference across the layer and the group L/KA represents the thermal resistance of that layer. Other rate processes that can be expressed in this form include the rate of the dissolution (see Chapter 2) and the rate of filtration (see Chapter 26).

Film heat transfer coefficient

Referring back to the situation illustrated in Figure 46.1, it can be seen that heat has to pass three layers (condensate, C, the dish wall, D, and the liquid boundary layer, L) in order to reach the liquid to be heated. The total thermal resistance for this heating process can be calculated by adding the thermal resistance of each layer (or film), i.e:

Total thermal resistance

$$= L_C/K_C A + L_D/K_D A + L_L/K_L A \qquad (46.5)$$

$$= 1/A (L_C/K_C + L_D/K_D + L_L/K_L) \qquad (46.6)$$

as the area term is generally the same for each layer.

Substituting this back into Eqn 46.4:

$$\frac{Q}{t} = \frac{A\Delta T}{L_C/K_C + L_D/K_D + L_L/K_L} \qquad (46.7)$$

where ΔT is the temperature difference across all the layers, i.e. the difference between the temperature of the steam and that of the boiling liquid.

Overall heat transfer coefficient

Eqn 46.7 now accounts for the resistance of multiple layers and can be used to calculate the rate of heat transfer through layers of known thickness and thermal conductivity. It is useful for assessing the effect of individual layers on the overall heat transfer process, as indicated in the illustrative calculations at the end of this chapter.

The overall conductivity is represented by U and is known as the overall heat transfer coefficient (OHTC), which gives an indication of the ability of a combination of layers to conduct heat. When heat has to be transferred through n layers, U can be calculated as:

$$U = 1/(L_1/K_1 + L_2/K_2 + L_3/K_3 + ...L_n/K_n) \qquad (46.8)$$

and thus for the situation shown in Figure 46.1:

$$U = 1/(L_C/K_C + L_D/K_D + L_L/K_L) \qquad (46.9)$$

Substituting this into Eqn 46.7 gives:

$$Q/t = U A \Delta T \qquad (46.10)$$

U has units of W/m^2 K and is only affected by factors that change the thermal conductivity or thickness of the layers through which heat is transferred; it is not affected by A. The value of the OHTC provides a useful indication of the overall conductivity of a heating system and can be estimated using practically obtained data (calculation 6 at the end of this chapter is an illustration of this). Estimation is necessary as it is not possible to determine the thermal conductivity and/or thickness of all the layers through which heat has to be transferred.

STEAM AS A HEATING MEDIUM

In pharmaceutical processes at anything other than laboratory scale, the most commonly used heating medium is steam. Steam is also very important as a sterilizing medium. The reasons for the continued widespread use of steam include the following:

- The raw material (water) is cheap and plentiful.
- It is easy to generate, distribute and control.
- It is generally cheaper than viable alternative forms of heating, e.g. electricity.
- It is clean, almost odourless and tasteless, and accidental contamination of the product is less likely to be serious.
- It has a high heat content (in the form of latent heat) and can heat materials very quickly.
- The heat is given up at a constant temperature, which is useful in controlling heating processes and in sterilization.

One disadvantage of the use of steam is that it is used at pressures that are typically 2–3 times higher than atmospheric, and thus steam presents potential safety problems and necessitates the use of high-strength piping and equipment.

To appreciate why steam is used in pharmaceutical processing and the principles of heat transfer using steam, it is necessary to consider how steam is produced, its heat content, and how the heat content varies with pressure and temperature.

Heat content of steam

Consider heating 1 kg of ice-cold water in a closed container at atmospheric pressure. Initially all the heat supplied will be sensible heat used to raise the temperature of the water to the boiling point (100°C in this case). The quantity of heat (Q, joules) required to raise the temperature of a material can be calculated using Eqn 46.11:

$$Q = M \, S \, \Delta T \tag{46.11}$$

where M is the mass heated (kg), S is the specific heat capacity of the material (J/kg K) and ΔT is the change in temperature (K or °C). The specific heat capacity is therefore the quantity of heat (J) required to raise 1 kg by 1°C or 1 K.

The value of S for water varies slightly with changes in temperature and pressure. For water at atmospheric pressure (1.013 bar/101.3 kPa) $S = 4.2$ kJ/kg K and therefore the quantity of heat required to raise the temperature from 0°C to 100°C $= 4200 \times 1 \times 100$ J $= 420\,000$ J (420 kJ).

Once the water has reached boiling point, further heat energy input will not raise the temperature of the water but will convert the boiling water at 100°C to water vapour at 100°C, i.e. steam at 100°C. Steam at a temperature corresponding to the water boiling point at that pressure (as in this case) is referred to as *saturated steam*.

The energy required to change unit mass from a liquid to a vapour at constant temperature is called the latent heat of vaporization (L, J/kg). For water at atmospheric pressure $L = 2.26 \times 10^6$ J/kg. L is not a constant value and depends on the steam pressure and temperature, e.g. L is 2.20 MJ/kg at 120°C and 2.14 MJ/kg at 140°C. The quantity of heat required to cause vaporization is calculated using Eqn 46.12:

$$Q = M \, L \tag{46.12}$$

where M is the mass vaporized (kg).

To convert 1 kg of water at 100°C to steam at 100°C, $Q = 1 \times 2.26 \times 10^6$ J $= 2.26$ MJ, i.e. the steam now contains 2.26 MJ of latent heat energy. Steam in this state is referred to as *dry saturated steam*, as *all* the liquid water has been converted to steam. This form of steam should ideally be used for heating and sterilization processes, as it contains the maximum latent heat energy and no associated air or water.

If only half the water had been converted to steam, the latent heat content would have been $0.5 \times 2.26 \times 10^6$ J $=$ 1.13 MJ. Steam in this state is said to have a *dryness fraction* of 0.5, where dryness fraction is defined as the weight fraction of steam in a steam/water mixture. The dryness fraction is important because it governs the latent heat content of the steam, this being at a maximum when the dryness fraction $= 1$.

Once all the water has been converted to steam, any further heat energy input increases the *steam* temperature, i.e. the steam gains sensible heat. Steam at a temperature above the saturation temperature is called *superheated steam*. It only takes about 50 kJ of heat

energy to raise the temperature of 1 kg of steam from 100°C to 200°C at atmospheric pressure.

The changes in the properties of water or steam, as appropriate, with increasing heat input at atmospheric pressure are shown in Figure 46.3. The total heat content is measured from a datum at 0°C and is the sum of the sensible heat, latent heat and superheat.

If superheated steam at 200°C (A on Fig. 46.3) is cooled (e.g. if it contacts a colder surface) then it will lose heat energy. First, the steam will decrease in temperature until the small amount of superheat is given up and the steam reaches the saturation temperature. Only when the steam temperature has reduced to 100°C (B on Fig. 46.3) will the steam condense and the latent heat energy be released. When half the steam (0.5 kg) has condensed (C on Fig. 46.3), 1.13 MJ of latent heat energy will have been given up and the saturated steam will have a dryness fraction of 0.5. While there is still steam present, the temperature of the steam and any condensate formed that is in contact with the steam will remain at 100°C. Once all steam has condensed (D on Fig. 46.3) the condensate will lose sensible heat and decrease in temperature until the temperature gradient is reduced to zero. If the temperature of the surface in contact with the condensate is at 0°C then point E on Figure 46.3 will be reached.

It is important to note that most of the heat energy of steam (over 80%) is in the form of latent heat and that when latent heat energy is released there is no drop in temperature. This latter point is important in sterilization processes and in maintaining temperature gradients when heating.

Effect of pressure on steam properties

The temperature at which water boils depends on the pressure exerted on the water surface. If the pressure is

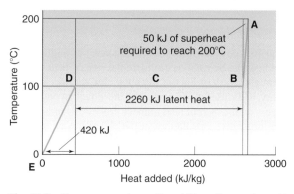

Fig. 46.3 Changes occurring on the addition of heat to ice–cold water at atmospheric pressure.

above atmospheric water will boil above 100°C and if it is below atmospheric, for example if a vacuum is applied, water boils at a temperature below 100°C. The saturation temperature (and the temperature at which steam condenses) will also therefore be dependent on pressure. This is utilized in sterilization processes where adjustment of the pressure allows selection of the temperature at which steam condenses and therefore the temperature at which the articles to be sterilized are exposed. Similarly, in heat transfer processes the desired temperature gradient can be achieved by adjusting the steam pressure. Some examples of how steam temperature changes with increasing pressure are given in Table 46.2.

Steam tables

The values in Table 46.2, along with temperatures at other steam pressures and values for the sensible and latent heat content at different pressures, can be found in *steam tables*. It should be noted that there is not a linear relationship between steam pressure and steam temperature and that the increase in steam temperature becomes less pronounced as the pressure increases.

Adverse effects of air in steam

There are two potential ways in which air may contaminate steam. First, water always contains dissolved air and this air will be driven off when the water is converted to steam. Second, air will be present in equipment in the steam space when the process is started and incoming steam may not entirely flush this air out.

Air is a permanent gas which remains when the steam condenses to form a condensate layer and therefore an air layer forms in contact with the condensate.

The adverse effects caused by the contamination of air are twofold:

1. Air is a very poor conductor of heat (see Table 46.1) and forms a formidable barrier to heat flow. A very thin layer of air can markedly reduce the overall heat transfer coefficient (calculations 4 and 5 at the end of this chapter) and the presence of as little as 1% of air in steam can result in a 50% reduction in the OHTC. Because the rate of heat transfer is proportional to the OHTC, there will be a corresponding reduction in the rate of heat transfer and thus an increase in heating-up times, process times and process costs.

2. Air will cause the steam temperature at any measured pressure to be lower than that of air-free steam. Steam containing air will therefore not be saturated. This arises from Dalton's Law of Partial Pressures that states that the total pressure in a system is the sum of the partial pressures of each of the components. Thus in an air/steam mixture the total pressure (P_T) is the sum of the partial pressure of the steam (P_S) and the partial pressure of the air (P_A). Therefore if P_T is 200 kPa and the steam contains 10% air, then P_A will be 20 kPa and P_S will be 180 kPa. The steam temperature, however, depends solely on the partial pressure exerted by the steam (not the total pressure) and will be 117.3°C. It would be 120.4°C if no air were present and the pressure were 200 kPa. Thus 10% of air has caused a reduction in the steam temperature at 200 kPa of 3.1°C. This is important in heating processes where the temperature gradient will be lower than expected and thus the heating-up rate will be lower. Note that this detrimental effect will be in addition to that caused by the poor thermal conductivity of air.

Both of the effects described above may also have potentially serious consequences if air contaminates steam in autoclaves. Its presence will give rise to an increase in the heating time required for the heating-up phase and the required sterilization temperature will not be reached. Sterilization processes use steam at a specific pressure with the implicit assumption that the steam will be saturated (i.e. no air is present) and therefore at the saturation temperature. If this does not occur the material may not be exposed to a sufficient temperature for a sufficient time and the material may not be sterilized. Steam pressure alone should therefore never be used as an indirect measure of sterilization temperature.

Steam generation and use

Manufacturing installations for liquid and semi-solid products

A diagrammatic representation of a steam-jacketed installation typical of that used for the preparation of liquid and semi-solid products is shown in Figure 46.4.

Table 46.2 Relationship between steam pressure and steam temperature	
Steam pressure (kPa)	**Steam saturation temperature (°C)**
101.3	100.0
200	120.4
300	133.7
400	143.8

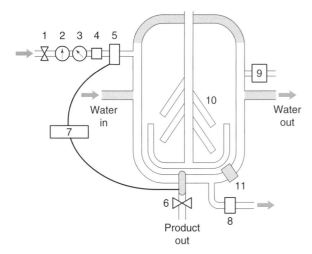

Fig. 46.4 Diagrammatic representation of an industrial steam-jacketed vessel. 1. Reducing valve; 2. pressure gauge; 3. temperature gauge; 4. safety valve; 5. control valve; 6. temperature probe; 7. temperature controller; 8. steam trap; 9. air vent; 10. stirrer; 11. homogenizer.

This type of installation is available in sizes capable of manufacturing products from development scale (approximately 20 L) up to full production-scale batches of 20 000 L. It is constructed from a suitable grade of stainless steel (typically 316; see Chapter 45), as this has acceptable thermal conductivity, is strong and easily fabricated, resists corrosion and is easily cleaned and sterilized. These further properties of stainless steel are also discussed in Chapter 45. The outer surface of the jacket may be suitably lagged with materials having poor thermal conductivity in order to protect the operators and reduce heat loss to the environment. In installations used for heating products using steam, the steam is usually generated in a remote boiler that supplies steam to many different locations and pieces of equipment. The steam is usually generated at high pressures and temperatures (typically 600–800 kPa and 160–170°C). This enables it to be delivered to the equipment where required. Suitably strong pipes are used which need to be well lagged to avoid heat loss and condensation.

The ancillary equipment shown in Figure 46.4 is now discussed.

Most heating installations use steam at about 150–300 kPa and a temperature of 110–135°C. This usually gives a sufficient temperature gradient to heat the product at the required rate, but reduces the chances of localized overheating. A *reducing valve* (1 on Fig. 46.4) is used to reduce, adjust and control the pressure to the desired level. This may be operated manually or, on larger equipment, controlled automatically via a *control panel*

(7 on Fig. 46.4) and electronic signals from the *pressure gauge* (2 on Fig. 46.4).

A *control valve* (5 on Fig. 46.4) regulates the entry of steam into the jacket. As with the reducing valve, this may be either manually operated, for example on smaller development units, or automatically controlled on larger production units so that the product is heated to the desired temperature and at the desired rate. An automatically operated system may function by selecting on the control panel the heating-up rate required, e.g. 2°C/min, and the final product temperature. A temperature probe in contact with the product sends a signal to the control panel, which in turn will cause the control valve to open if the product temperature is below the set value. When the control valve opens, steam enters the jacket and the product starts to heat up. The panel will continuously monitor the product temperature, and the extent to which the control valve is opened will be controlled so that the product heats up at the required rate. When the desired temperature is reached a signal from the control panel closes the control valve and so no further steam enters. After a short time the product will start to cool slowly, as it is at a higher temperature than the surrounding environment. The temperature control system will detect this drop and reopen the control valve, so that more steam enters and the process is repeated. Using this type of control system, the temperature of the product may be maintained within ±2–3°C of the required value. Examples of where this may be used include maintaining a fixed temperature (usually somewhere between 60 and 70°C) during cream manufacture, or a temperature of 80–90°C when preparing solution products where poorly soluble preservatives are employed.

The *pressure* and *temperature gauges* (2 and 3 on Fig. 46.4) allow the monitoring and recording of the steam properties. As mentioned previously, the latter may be used to control the pressure of the steam entering the system.

Because steam is generated at high pressures there is the potential to expose the equipment to pressures higher than it can safely withstand. To prevent this, a *safety valve* (4 on Fig. 46.4) is positioned before the control valve. This valve will open and direct steam away from the installation if the pressure reaches a value above the safe operating pressure of the system.

When steam first enters the jacket surrounding the product, it contacts the cooler surface, condenses and releases latent heat. In turn this is then transferred through the various layers (condensate, vessel wall, etc.) to the product. On condensing, steam contracts to a small volume (e.g. at 121°C, 850 mL of steam will condense to approximately 1 mL of condensate). This creates an area of lower pressure within the jacket into which more steam will then flow. Unless the control valve is closed, steam will therefore continue to enter the jacket to maintain the desired pressure until the product temperature reaches the steam temperature and no further condensation occurs.

If products are heated to temperatures above 60°C (as is often the case in cream or solution manufacture) and then left to cool naturally, they will take a considerable time to cool to ambient temperature. This will be exacerbated when the volume in the vessel is large and if the vessel is efficiently lagged. Some products will need to be cooled before volatile components (e.g. flavourings) are added. To use the manufacturing vessels efficiently, the cooling of these products will need to be accelerated. This can be achieved by circulating a cold fluid, e.g. water or 'brine' (a concentrated salt solution), through the vessel jacket. The brine can be at a temperature below 0°C and so will give a greater temperature gradient and faster cooling if required. However, if the rate of cooling is important (e.g. to avoid the formation of 'lumps' of higher melting-point components in cream and ointment manufacture) then the inlet and outlet of the cooling fluid can be controlled by a system similar to that used to control the heating rate.

The presence of a *stirrer* (10 in Fig. 46.4) helps to ensure that the product is evenly heated. The flow created will reduce the thickness of the boundary layer adjacent to the heating surface and thus speed up the heating process, and will mix the components of the product. If more intense mixing is required, as will be the case in the manufacture of emulsion, lotion and cream products, then a homogenizer (see Chapter 12) can be used. This will normally be sited at the bottom of the vessel, as shown in Figure 46.4. Where aqueous and oily phases need to be mixed when they are both at elevated temperatures, two jacketed vessels need to be sited close together and the appropriate phase pumped into the vessel containing the homogenizer.

The presence of a vessel lid protects the product from the operator and environment and vice versa. In addition, if the lid can be sealed then negative or positive pressures can be applied above the product's surface. A negative pressure (by application of a vacuum) is useful to minimize the incorporation of air during the manufacture of viscous products, especially when the homogenizer is used. This can avoid the manufacture of a product with an unsightly appearance and can reduce stability problems. A positive pressure can be used to aid emptying of the vessel.

Steam traps

To ensure maximum heating efficiency the apparatus should minimize the amount of air and condensate liquid present in the jacket. If the condensate is allowed to build up it will gradually reduce the area over which steam can condense and therefore progressively slow down the heating process. If the condensate completely fills the jacket then heating will stop. The consequences of not removing the air from the jacket are described above. Fitting a simple drainage pipe to the jacket would be ineffective as this, as well as removing condensate and air, would also allow steam to escape and this would be both wasteful and potentially dangerous. Condensate and air can be removed and steam retained by using a suitably designed device known as a *steam trap*.

The simplest form of steam trap is a mechanical device, an example of which is shown in Figure 46.5.

These devices rely on the fact that condensate is more dense than water and will thus tend to collect at the bottom of the jacket. When sufficient condensate has entered into the trap, the float will rise and open the outlet, allowing the condensate to drain away. Mechanical traps are robust but have the major disadvantage that they do not allow air to escape, as there will always be condensate in contact with trap outlet. The alternative type of steam traps are referred to as thermostatic devices, and these rely on the fact that condensate can lose sensible heat and thus be at a temperature which is lower than the steam.

A common form of thermostatic steam trap is the *balanced pressure thermostatic steam trap* shown diagrammatically in Figure 46.6. This contains a capsule in the form of bellows that contain a liquid having a boiling point a few degrees below that of water. Thus, when the capsule is surrounded by steam the liquid in the capsule boils and causes the bellows to expand and close the outlet. When condensate enters the trap it will lose sensible heat and decrease in temperature. The trap is usually constructed of a material with good thermal conductivity, e.g. copper, to hasten this heat loss. The condensate then cools the capsule, the liquid in the capsule ceases to boil (and condenses) and the bellows contract, thereby opening the outlet and discharging the condensate. When the condensate is removed steam surrounds the bellows, causing the trap to

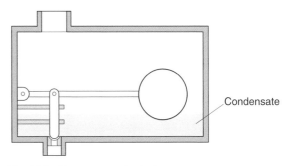

Condensate

Fig. 46.5 Float-type mechanical steam trap.

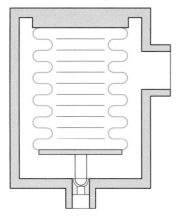

Fig. 46.6 Balanced pressure thermostatic steam trap.

close again. These traps will operate over a wide pressure range as any increase in steam pressure not only raises the boiling point of water but, because the same pressure acts on the surface of the bellows, will elevate the boiling point of the liquid in the bellows by a similar amount. Hence the alternative title applied to this type – *balanced pressure expansion trap* – as it will always operate a few degrees below the saturation temperature of the steam.

Although these devices tend to be less robust than mechanical traps they have one major advantage in that they will also vent air from the jacket. Because air is denser than steam, it will tend to collect at the bottom of the jacket and enter the steam trap. Contamination of steam with air will cause the steam temperature to be lower than the water boiling point at any operating pressure (see above). Once sufficient air is in the trap to reduce the steam temperature to below the boiling point of the liquid in the bellows, the bellows will contract and the air-contaminated steam will be removed.

Generally there are at least two traps on a heating installation: one at the bottom of the jacket to remove condensate and air generated during the heating process and one towards the top of the jacket on the opposite side to which steam enters. This latter trap (which is of the thermostatic type) acts as an air vent and will be open when the equipment is started and therefore help to flush out the air initially present in the jacket. It will close when the temperature of the steam exiting the vent is sufficient to cause the liquid in the bellows to boil.

The condensate released from the jacket will possess significant heat energy and may be fed back to the steam boiler or used for other manufacturing plant, such as air-conditioning systems.

Illustrative calculations involving the use of steam

This chapter concludes with some calculations that illustrate various points raised in the text.

1. **Q** What is the energy requirement to produce 13 kg of dry saturated steam at a pressure of 200 kPa (2 bar absolute/1 bar gauge) from water at 18.4°C? Assume the specific heat capacity of water is 4.21 kJ/kg K and the latent heat of evaporation is 2.20 MJ/kg.

   A The saturation temperature at 200 kPa is 120.4°C. The heat energy required to raise 13 kg of water to 120.4°C = $13 \times 4210 \times 102$ J = 5.58×10^6 J or 5.58 MJ.
   The heat energy required to convert 13 kg of water at 120.4°C to steam at 120.4°C = $13 \times 2.2 \times 10^6$ J = 28.6×10^6 J or 28.6 MJ.
   The total heat energy required therefore = $5.582 \times 10^6 + 28.6 \times 10^6$ J = 34.18×10^6 J (34.18 MJ).

2. **Q** What temperature would be reached if the steam produced in Question 1 was used in a steam-jacketed vessel to heat 150 kg of water whose initial temperature was 21.8°C? Assume there are no heat losses to the environment.

   A The 28.6×10^6 J of heat energy required to convert water to steam will be released as latent heat when the steam condenses during the heating process.
   From $Q = M\,S\,\Delta T$, the increase in temperature of the water = $28.6 \times 10^6 \div (4210 \times 150)$°C = 45.3°C. The final water temperature therefore = 45.3 + 21.8°C = 67.1°C.

3. **Q** If the steam produced in Question 1 was passed through unlagged pipes on its passage to the steam-jacketed vessel and the dryness fraction reduced from 1.0 to 0.94, what temperature would the water reach?

   A Because some steam has condensed in the unlagged pipe work, the latent heat content of the steam has been reduced and now = $0.94 \times 28.6 \times 10^6$ J = 26.9×10^6 J.
   The increase in temperature of the water therefore = $26.9 \times 10^6 \div (4210 \times 150)$°C = 42.6°C and the final temperature = 64.4°C.

4. **Q** The data in the table below represent the different layers through which the latent heat from steam has to be conducted in a stainless steel steam-jacketed vessel when scale and air are present and water is heated. What is the overall heat transfer coefficient of the system?

	Thickness (mm)	K (W/m K)
Air film	0.2	0.03
Condensate film	0.1	0.60
Scale	0.2	1.00
Pan wall	3.0	17.0
Water boundary layer	0.4	0.60

A Using Eqn 46.8:

$$U = 1/\left[\left(\frac{0.2}{0.03} + \frac{0.1}{0.6} + \frac{0.2}{1.0} + \frac{3.0}{17} + \frac{0.4}{0.6}\right) \times 10^{-3}\right]$$

(The factor 10^{-3} is required to convert from mm to m.)
In this case, $U = 1/(7.88 \times 10^{-3})$ W/m^2 K = 127 W/m^2 K.

5. Q What would happen if:
 (a) the vessel described in Q4 was made of copper (K = 386 W/m^2 K)?
 (b) the scale was removed?
 (c) the air film was halved?
 (d) the air film was removed?
 (e) the air film was removed, the scale layer eliminated and the water boundary layer halved?

A
 (a) U = 130 W/m^2 K (U was 127 W/m^2 K in Q 4). Even though copper conducts heat over 20 times more easily than stainless steel, this alone has little effect on the overall conductivity.
 (b) U = 130 W/m^2 K. Removing the scale alone similarly has little effect.
 (c) U = 220 W/m^2 K. Removing just 0.1 mm of air gives rise to an approximate 75% increase in thermal conductivity.

 (d) U = 827 W/m^2 K. If the air film is completely removed there is a huge increase in U, the value being over six times greater than when air was present.
 (e) U = 1478 W/m^2 K. Reducing the film layers that offer the largest resistance to heat conduction has the greatest effect on increasing heat transfer.

6. Q A steam-jacketed vessel of heated area 2.0 m^2, using steam at 200 kPa, was found to evaporate 11.2 kg of water in a 5-minute period. Assuming the latent heat of vaporization is 2.20×10^6 J/kg, what is the value of U, the overall heat transfer coefficient (OHTC) of the system?

A The heat energy used to evaporate the water = $11.2 \times 2.2 \times 10^6$ J = 24.64×10^6 J. The rate of heat transfer occurring is 24.64×10^6 J in 300 s = 8.213×10^4 W (or 82.13 kW).
From Eqn 46.10: $Q/t = U A \Delta T$
The temperature of steam at 200 kPa = 120.4°C and therefore the temperature difference between the steam and the boiling water, ΔT = 120.4 − 100°C = 20.4°C.
Therefore $U = 8.213 \times 104 \div (2 \times 20.4)$ W/m^2 K = 2013 W/m^2 K.

REFERENCES

Holman, J.P. (2001) *Heat Transfer*. McGraw-Hill Education, London.

Long, C.A. (1999) *Essential Heat Transfer*. Pearson Education, Harlow.

Index

Note: Page numbers in *italics* refer to diagrams and tables.

interfacial reaction, 18
nature of, 26–7
solubility, 343
solvent power of, *343*
transdermal drug delivery, 574
using to avoid hydrolysis, 658
vapour pressure, 34
Solvolysis, 353
Solvolytic breakdown, 12
Sonication, 248–9
Sorbents, 454
Sorbitan esters, 95, 386, 397
Sorbitan monolaurate, *394*
Sorbitan monooleate, 86, 93, 394, *394,*
395
Sorbitan monostearate, *394*
Sorbitan trioleate, *394*
Sorbitol, 13, 363, 369, 656, *656*
Sorption, 67, 659
see also Absorption; Adsorption
Sorption promoters, 586–7
Soya oil, 367, 392
Spacers, metered-dose inhalers, *545,*
545–6
Sparingly soluble, 24
Species differences, effect on heat
resistance, 230
Specific adsorption, 77
Specific viscosity, 43–4
Spectrophotometers, 198, 210
Spectroscopy, *621, 622*
ultraviolet, 338, 350
Spheronization, 419–21, *421*
Spheronized granules, 512
Spheronizers, 419, 420, *420*
Spin fluid, 134
Spinhaler®, 546, *547*
Spirillum, 187, *187*
Spirits, 372
Spirochaetes, 187, *187*
Spironolactone, 9
Spiros®, 548, *548*
Splenic flexure, 274
Spoilage *see* Microbial spoilage
Spongiform encephalopathies, 228, 244,
516, 619
Spore formation, 203, 229
Sporulation, 190, *191*
Spotted fevers, 186
Spray coating, 503, *504*
Spray dryers, 418–19, 432–5, *433*
Spray drying, *434,* 434–5, 448
Spreading, 61, 65
Spread plates, 198–9
Springs, 55
Sputtering time, 551
Squeezed bottles, nasal, 562
Stability, 12–13, 351–4
assessment of, 354
of emulsions, 400–1
kinetics of product, 99–107
of pharmaceutical products, 650–61
of pharmaceutical proteins, 617–19
of softgels, 531
of solutions, 373
of suspensions, 385, 399–400

testing for, 661–4
testing of emulsions, 402–3
see also Chemical stability
Stabilization of pharmaceuticals,
657–9
Stabilizers
nebulizer fluids, 550
protein, *619*
used in powder-filled capsules, *522*
Staining of bacteria, 191–3
Staining tests, 391, *391*
Stainless steels, 671, *672, 682*
Standard deviation, 157–8
Staphylococci, *187,* 188, 195, 200, *642*
Staphylococcus aureus, 213, 219
growth promotion test, 222
recommended tests for, *220*
resistance to ethylene oxide, 234
Staphylococcus epidermis, 188
Starch, *358, 389, 432,* 451, 452
Static disc method, 22–3
Steady state, 105, 328, 484, 585
factors influencing, 329–34
Steam
adverse effects of air in, 685
effect of pressure on, *684,* 684–5,
685
generation and use of, 685–8
heat content of, 683–4
as a heating medium, 683–9
in restrictive calculations involving the
use of, 688–9
Steam baths, 680–1, *681*
Steam-jacketed vessel, 685–7, *686*
Steam sterilization, 227, 228–31, 244–5,
245, 253, *256, 263*
see also Moist heat
Steam tables, 685
Steam traps, *687,* 687–8
Stearic acid, 138, *358,* 453, *495*
Steels, 671–2
Steric effects, 345
Steric repulsion, 82
Steric stabilization, 81, 82–3
of suspensions, 91
Sterile products, 251, *252–3*
microbiological quality of, 220–3
Sterility assurance level (SAL), 221,
259
Sterility testing, 221–3, 259
Sterilization, 242–9, 251–63
chemosterilants, 247, 258–59, *263*
determination of protocols, 251–53
filtration, 247, *263*
gaseous, 245–6, *253,* 257,
263
heat, 244–5, *253,* 256, *256, 263*
limitations of methods, 262,
263
monitoring, 221
need for sterility, 243
new technologies, 248–9
non-terminal, 242
parameters, 243–4
process principles, 244–8
process selection, 253, *254*

radiation *see* Radiation sterilization
recommended pharmacopoeial
processes, 253–8
statistical considerations of sterility
testing, 258
steam, 227, 228–31, 244–5, *245,* 254,
256
sterile products, 251
tests for sterility, 259
validation of processes, 260–2, *263*
Stern layer, 76, 88
Stern plane, 76, 77, 78
Stern potential, 77
Steroids, 89
bioassays, 585
topical, 576, 578, *584,* 585
Sterol-containing substances, 398
Sticking, 358, 454
Stirred-vessel methods, 463
Stokes diameter, 124, 133
Stokes-Einstein equation, 40, 132–3
Stokes' equation, 73, 133, 134, 148
Stokes' Law, 48, 73, 96–7, 133, 134
Stomach, 272–3, *273*
Stomach acid, 272
Storage conditions, 477, *477*
adverse, 402
adverse temperatures, 402–3
Strain, 54
Strain differences, effect on heat
resistance, 230
Strain energy release rate, 476
Strain gauge, 446
Straining, filtration by, 375
Strain rate sensitivity, 471–2
Strains of species, 206
Stratum corneum, 567, *567,* 568, 569,
573
hydration, 585
not rate controlling, 579–80
rate controlling, 578–9
removal of, 586
Streaking methods, 195–6, *196,* 199
Streaming potential, 78
Streamlined flow, 45–6
Streptococci, *187,* 188, 200, 222
Streptococcus faecalis, 231
Streptococcus mutans, 188
Streptomyces, 187, *187*
Streptomycin, 291
Stress, 137–8
powder arch, 175
Stress conditions, *352*
Stress corrosion, 678
Stress relaxation, 55, 477
Stress testing, 661–2
Strip packs, 630
Structure-activity prediction, 343–5
Structure-activity relationships (SAR),
343–5
Styrene acylonitrile (SAN), 635
Subcoating sugar coatings, 509
Subcutaneous administration, 8
pharmaceutical proteins, 622
see also Parenteral administration
Subcutaneous implants, 8

The Art of
Card Making

Published in the UK in 2005 by
Apple Press
7 Greenland Street
London NW1 0ND
United Kingdom

www.apple-press.com

ISBN 978-1-84543-030-6

Reprinted 2007

10 9 8 7 6 5

Grateful acknowledgment is given to Claire Sun-ok Choi for her work from *Designing Handcrafted Cards* (Quarry Books, 2004) on pages 10-57, 78-109, and 271-277; to Ricë Freeman-Zachery for her work from *Stamp Artistry* (Rockport Publishers, 2003) on pages 170-171; to Gail Hercher for her work from *Crafting with Handmade Paper* (Quarry Books, 2000) on pages 228-237; to Susan Jaworski-Stranc for her work from *Garden Greetings* (Rockport Publishers, 2003) on pages 146-169, 172-179, 196-227, 256-270, and 281; to Lisa Kerr for her work from *The Paper Card Book* (Quarry Books, 1997) on pages 8-9, 110-145, 180-195, 242-255, and 286-302; to Laura McFadden and April Paffrath for their work from *The Artful Bride: Wedding Invitations* (Quarry Books, 2004) on pages 58-77; and to Jessica Wrobel for her work from *The Paper Jewelry Book* (Quarry Books, 1997) on pages 303-304.

Printed in China

The Art of Card Making

APPLE

Contents

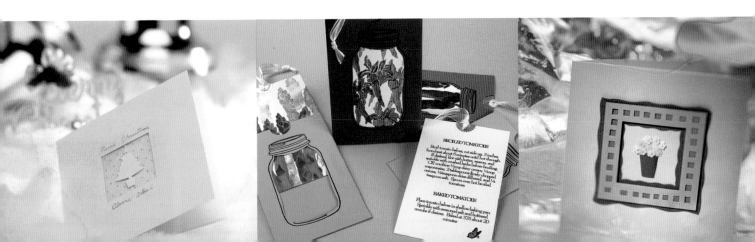

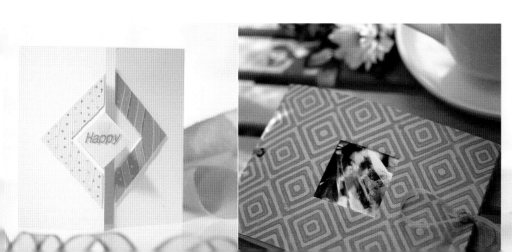

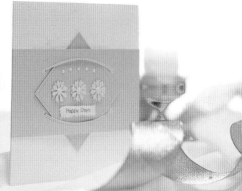

Introduction

These days, we can deliver our thoughts to our loved ones through ready-made cards or email quickly and easily. Somehow, despite their ease, these are not always completely fulfilling modes of communication. In contrast, sending a hand-made card allows you to tailor the message, the style, and the content while keeping a special person in mind.

In this book, there are wonderful cards made with simple tools, colorful papers, uncomplicated techniques, and a world of ideas and inspiration. All projects found in this book are easily adapted for many special occasions, thoughts, or wishes. Seasonal celebrations offer perfect opportunities for incorporating elements of nature into your designs, such as pressed flowers and leaves. Holidays such as New Year's, Valentine's Day, and Christmas invite traditional styles and colors to merge with new interpretations.

Each project can be viewed as a source of inspiration—a starting point for your own personal expressions—or work that can be created exactly as described. The charm of making a card lies

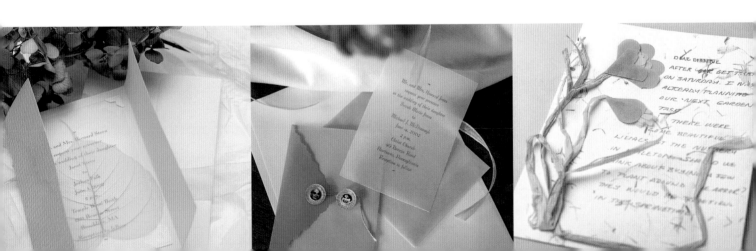

in its process—creating a fresh design, using an exquisite combination of colors, enjoying the delicate cutting and folding—that holds our concentration throughout.

After exploring all these pages have to offer, you may feel inclined to create original designs on your own. Experiment with creative approaches, dabble in exquisite color combinations, unearth new papers and embellishments, and crystallize them into a new idea. You are bound only by your creativity!

We hope that you enjoy making and giving these beautiful projects, and that they will create a lasting impression on all who have the pleasure of receiving them. May this book guide you in the art of designing handmade cards and help you expand your artistic repertoire.

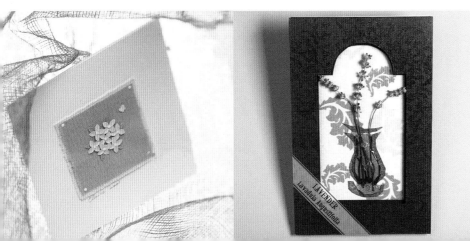

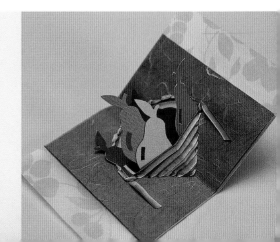

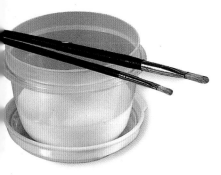

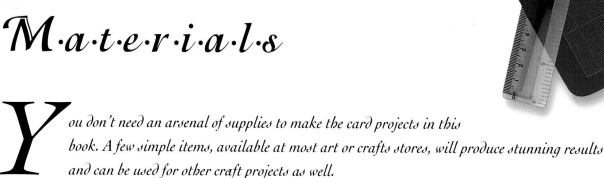

M·a·t·e·r·i·a·l·s

Y ou don't need an arsenal of supplies to make the card projects in this book. A few simple items, available at most art or crafts stores, will produce stunning results and can be used for other craft projects as well.

Tools

Polyvinyl acetate glue (PVA glue) is a white glue that dries clear. It will spread easier when diluted with water (use a ratio of four parts glue to one part water, and adjust as necessary), but be careful that it is not too watery or the wetness will damage the paper. Transfer the glue to a plastic container with a lid to make it easier to dilute the glue, and to dip larger brushes into the glue more quickly.

Use inexpensive brushes to apply PVA glue because it can harden and destroy them. Cheap, wooden-handle brushes, in sizes of 1" (2.5 cm) to 2" (5 cm), are available at hardware stores. For smaller tipped brushes, look for sets of children's brushes. To extend the life of your brushes, wash them with hot water after each use and let dry, or leave them in water overnight.

A craft knife is essential for these projects because it gives you control over the edges you wish to create. Buy extra blades and change them often. A metal ruler makes cutting paper much easier. The cork underside of the ruler keeps it from moving, and elevates it to keep the craft knife aligned against the ruler. A self-healing cutting mat protects your work surface from knife cuts, won't slip as you cut, and helps to produce crisp, clean edges in your card projects.

A bone folder is a carved piece of bone or plastic, rounded at one end and pointed at the other, that helps to fold paper. Use the pointed edge to score folds in thick paper, or the round end to smooth out wrinkles after glue has been applied. Be careful not to rub the paper surface too much, or the bone folder will impart a sheen to the paper.

Paper

Today there is a abundance of papers to choose from in a
range of prices. Thicker papers, such as handmade or
mold-made papers, are better for folding and for serving as the card
base. Decorative papers such as marbled, block-printed, silk-screened, or printed papers
are ideal for layering onto card bases. Before buying paper for your card base, gently bend, fold, or
crease it to see if it will crack along the fold. Some papers have a grain, which is often parallel to the
longest dimension of a sheet. Papers fold or tear easily with the direction of the grain.

Decorative Elements

Experiment with grosgrain ribbon, soft satin, or voluptuous velvet to enhance your cards or envelopes.
Twine, string, rawhide, gimp, raffia, lace, and woven trims add texture and dimension. Tie, weave, or
sew them by hand or machine.

Collect old buttons from yard sales and flea markets. Kitchen supply stores
are filled with cake-decorating treasures to adorn your cards. Look for shells
and dried flowers on your next trip to the beach or woods. Ask family and
friends to save stamps from foreign countries for your collage collection. And
tell them to save last year's calendars to tear up for collage elements or fold into
handmade envelopes.

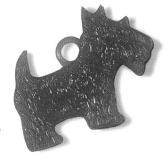

Look for printing inks in art supply stores. I prefer water-based inks because they are easy to clean,
take less time to dry, and are very vibrant. The rubber ink roller or brayer is a fairly inexpensive tool
that you will use often. You can print from any object with a relief surface, from vegetables to keys,
Styrofoam, or coins.

You will need photo corners for a few of the projects. Traditional black corners lend an air of antiquity
to your design, but white photo corners and self-adhesive clear corners are also available at paper
specialty stores and office supply stores.

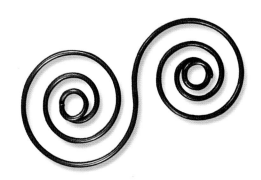

Tools and Supplies

PATTERNS

Using tracing paper to transfer images and characters onto another paper has long been the most common pattern-making method. However, it can be time-consuming. Many people now find it easier to use a photocopier to reproduce—even reduce or enlarge—images. The copied patterns can then be placed on top of the project paper and used as a cutting guideline.

PAPER

Because paper is a very important material in making cards, use moderately thick, good quality paper that is easy to cut. It is good to use crinkle paper in various colors with moderate thickness and a soft surface that can be hand-torn and works well with punches, craft knives, and scissors.

PUNCH WHEEL

A punch wheel is one of the most useful tools for making the cards in this book. It can be used to transform an even surface into a three-dimensional one. A punch wheel can add elegance to your cards by creating lace-style and stitching borders.

SCISSORS

Generally speaking, there are two types of scissors: those that simply cut and those that cut and add style at the same time. These days, we can easily obtain a variety of decorative scissors: ripple, lace, wave, stamp, sunshine, seagull, bubbles, and so much more. No matter which pair you are looking for, it is important to choose lightweight and comfortable scissors.

ADHESIVE

It is important to choose adhesive suitable for use with paper. PVA adhesive is suitable, because it is permanent, firm, and transparent when it dries. Spray adhesive is good for preventing wrinkles when using thin paper, and it won't cause stains when paper is detached and reattached. However, it can be quite messy, so surrounding table areas should be protected.

TAPE

Foam tape is good for creating a three-dimensional effect on cards. Transparent tape is suitable for the temporary attachment of paper.

AWL AND NEEDLE TOOLS

An awl can be used as a pencil substitute when drawing lines or marking sections to cut. Also, you can use an awl to create lace-style patterns in paper. Quilling needles with grips are perfect for making paper-quilling flowers or for applying small quantities of adhesive.

CUTTING MAT

Use a cutting mat to protect the blades of craft knives and the surface you are working on. Cutting mats prevent papers from curling and can be used as measurement tools instead of rulers because they have horizontal and vertical lines every centimeter.

CRAFT KNIFE

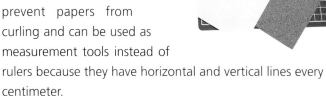

It would be hard to make cards without using a craft knife. It's best to choose a knife that is not shaky, is easy to grip, and has changeable blades. Use a knife at a 45-degree angle to ensure crisp cuts.

TWEEZERS

Many of the cards included in this book require delicate work. Sometimes it is difficult to move tiny pieces with your bare hands. Fine-pointed tweezers can help you handle small paper-quilling shapes.

CORKBOARD

When using an awl or a punch wheel, it's best to work on a ¹⁄₁₀" (2 mm)-thick corkboard. This allows the awl and punch wheel to function properly.

PUNCHES

Using various types of punches—stars, hearts, flowers, snowflakes, butterflies—will provide you with many design options for your cards. A punch with a variety of shapes to choose from is convenient for all projects.

METAL RULER

Metal rulers are more accurate and safer to use than plastic rulers when cutting papers with a craft knife.

EMBOSSING TOOLS OR PRESS PENS AND TRACING PENS

These tools, with round-tipped metal ends, can be used to press designs into the paper. When they are used from the front of the paper, you are pressing, since the design is pushed into the paper. When they are used from the back of the paper, it's called embossing, since the design appears raised from the front view. Press pens are good for making indented patterns, and tracing pens are good for embossing patterns. Embossing tools can be used for both.

PENS

Gel pens in various colors work well for decorating cards.

GRAPH PAPER AND TRACING PAPER

Graph paper with measurements makes it easy to design shapes. Because tracing paper is soft and transparent, it can create elegant pastel tones when layered over paper. Tracing paper can also make special effects when used for printing computer images.

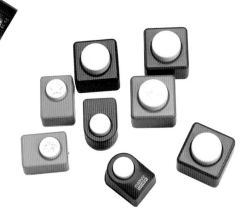

Techniques

To make a card, we usually purchase one that is partially ready-made at a stationery store or an art shop. However, if you learn basic techniques, such as measuring and cutting, and make one entirely on your own, you can double your satisfaction.

The following sections will help beginners learn how to make the basic shapes of cards. If it is your first time using craft knives and you have trouble making the shape you want, don't give up. Continue practicing and you will learn the proper way before long.

Basic Card I

This card is a basic 5" (12.5 cm) square card.

① Position the paper on a cutting mat.

② Using a ruler and craft knife, cut a 10" x 5" (25 cm x 12.5 cm) rectangle.

③ Fold the rectangle in half to make a 5" x 5" (12.5 cm x 12.5 cm) square.

Basic Card II

This card opens like a set of doors.

① Follow Step 1 and 2 of Basic Card I to create a rectangle.

② Measure and mark a line 2½" (6.25 cm) in from each short side.

③ Fold along each marked line toward the center, where the edges should meet. Be careful not to make a gap between the two doors on the front cover.

Paper-Quilling

Paper-quilling flowers add a special touch to birthday, wedding, and congratulation cards. Use 1/10" (2 mm)-wide paper ribbon, a paper-quilling needle, paper glue, and scissors. Below are the quilling methods for the shapes used in this book.

TIGHT CIRCLE

Grab one end of paper ribbon with your fingers. With the other hand, rub the paper ribbon with the needle to make the ribbon soft. (Be careful not to make the ribbon curl up.) Coil the ribbon with the needle while your fingers press the ribbon firmly to ensure a tight coil. After coiling the ribbon with the needle two or three times, pull out the needle and carefully roll the ribbon to the end. Glue the end to complete a tight circle.

TEARDROP

Coil paper ribbon into a tight circle, and then loosen the coil, controlling the size with your fingers. Hold the center of the roll with your fingers or tweezers and pinch the opposite side to make a point. Press the opposite side of the roll and glue it with paper adhesive to complete a teardrop.

MARQUISE

Coil paper ribbon into a tight circle, and then loosen the roll to make a loose circle. Pinch opposite points of the circle with your fingers to complete a marquise shape.

APPLICATION

Depending on the length of paper ribbon or the number of petals (one teardrop per petal), you can make flowers of varying sizes. Most flowers can be completed with five or six teardrops placed around a tight circle center. Marquise-shaped quillings can also be used for petals.

MATERIALS

white card stock,
  10" x 5" (25 cm x 12.5 cm)
white paper
graph paper
light box
awl
metal ruler
pencil
transparent tape
cutting mat
craft knife
embossing tool or press pen

BASIC CARDS Pressing

1. With a pencil, mark a 3⅕" x 3⅕" (8 cm x 8 cm) square at the center of 5" x 5" (12.5 cm x 12.5 cm) graph paper.

2. Place the graph paper on 5" x 5" (12.5 cm x 12.5 cm) white paper and use an awl to poke the four corners of the 3⅕" x 3⅕" (8 cm x 8 cm) square through the white paper.

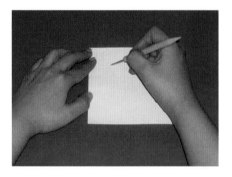

3. Remove the graph paper and make sure the four points appear on the white paper.

4. Use a metal ruler and craft knife to cut out the 3⅕" x 3⅕" (8 cm x 8 cm) square marked by the points on the white paper.

5. Place the frame-shaped paper created in Step 4 on 10" x 5" (25 cm x 12.5 cm) white card stock. Use transparent tape to attach the 3⅕" x 3⅕" (8 cm x 8 cm) square back into the center of the frame. Then, lift the frame; the square should be exactly at the center of the white card stock. Detach the external rectangle 5" x 5" (12.5 cm x 12.5 cm). You should be able to see the inner rectangle exactly at the center of the white card paper.

6. Put the white card stock on a light box. Make a square by using an embossing tool to draw lines two or three times along the lines of the square. When you turn the card stock over, you should see a pressed square border at the center.

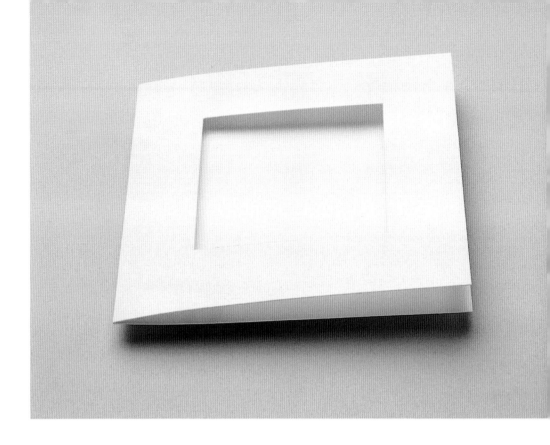

MATERIALS

white card stock,
  10" x 5" (25 cm x 12.5 cm)
graph paper
awl
metal ruler
pencil
cutting mat
craft knife

Basic Window-Shaped Card I

1. With a pencil, draw a 3⅕" x 3⅕" (8 cm x 8 cm) square on 5" x 5" (12.5 cm x 12.5 cm) graph paper.

2. Put the graph paper on white card stock and use an awl to poke the four corners of the 3⅕" x 3⅕" (8 cm x 8 cm) square through the card stock.

3. Remove the graph paper and make sure the four points appear on the card stock.

4. Cut out the square using a metal ruler and craft knife.

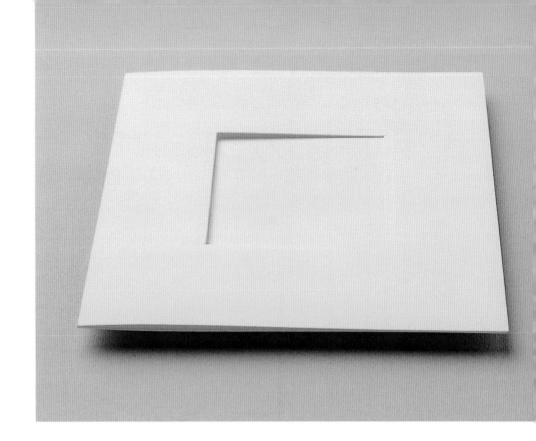

MATERIALS

white card stock,
  10" x 5" (25 cm x 12.5 cm)
white paper
graph paper
awl
metal ruler
pencil
transparent tape
light box
cutting mat
craft knife
embossing tool or press pen

Basic Window-Shaped Card II

1. With a pencil, draw a 2¼" x 2¼" (6 cm x 6 cm) square on 5" x 5" (12.5 cm x 12.5 cm) graph paper. Mark a smaller 2⅛" x 2⅛" (5.8 cm x 5.8 cm) square within the 2¼" x 2¼" (6 cm x 6 cm) square.

2. Put the graph paper on top of 5" x 5" (12.5 cm x 12.5 cm) white paper and use an awl to poke through the papers at the eight corners of the squares.

3. Remove the graph paper and make sure the eight points appear on the white paper.

4. Use a metal ruler and craft knife to cut out the 2¼" x 2¼" (6 cm x 6 cm) square from the white paper.

5. Spread 10" x 5" (25 cm x 12.5 cm) white card stock on the front side and put the frame-shaped white paper made in Step 5 on the white card stock. Use transparent tape to attach the 2¼" x 2¼" (6 cm x 6 cm) square into the center of the frame and then remove the frame.

6. Place the white card stock on a light box. Make a square by using an embossing tool to draw lines two or three time along the lines of the square. When you turn the card stock over, you should see a square press at the center.

7. Cut out the 2⅛" x 2⅛" (5.8 cm x 5.8 cm) square on the front side of the white card stock.

MATERIALS

white card stock,
  10" x 5" (25 cm x 12.5 cm)
white paper
graph paper
awl
metal ruler
cutting mat
craft knife
transparent tape

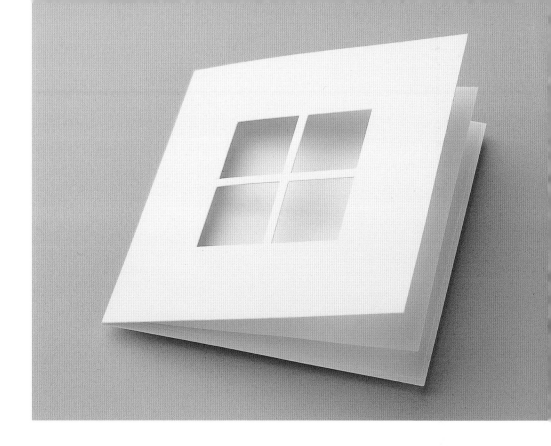

Basic Window-Shaped Card III

1. Follow the instructions for Pressing (p. 14) and Basic Window-Shaped Card I (p.15).

2. Design four 1¹⁄₁₀" x 1¹⁄₁₀" (2.8 cm x 2.8 cm) squares on graph paper or use the pattern on page 271.

3. Put the patterns on the front side of the white card stock and use an awl to poke the four corners of each of the four squares through the card stock. Cut out the four squares with a metal ruler and craft knife.

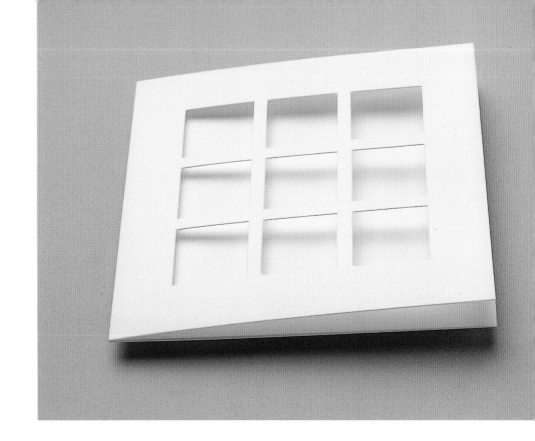

MATERIALS

white card stock,
  10" x 5" (25 cm x 12.5 cm)
white paper,
  5" x 5" (12.5 cm x 12.5 cm)
graph paper
awl
metal ruler
transparent tape
pencil
cutting mat
craft knife

Basic Window-Shaped Card IV

1. Follow the instructions for Basic Window-Shaped Card III (p.17).

2. Design nine 1" x 1" (2.5 cm x 2.5 cm) squares on graph paper with a pencil or use the pattern on page 271. The spaces between the squares should be ⅕" (5 mm).

3. Put the graph paper on the front side of white card stock and use an awl to poke the four corners of each of the squares through the card stock.

4. Remove the graph paper and use a metal ruler and craft knife to cut out the nine squares.

MATERIALS

white card stock,
  10" x 5" (25 cm x 12.5 cm)
white paper,
  4¾" x 2" (12 cm x 5 cm)
flower stencil pattern
light box
pencil
cutting mat
craft knife
embossing tool or press pen

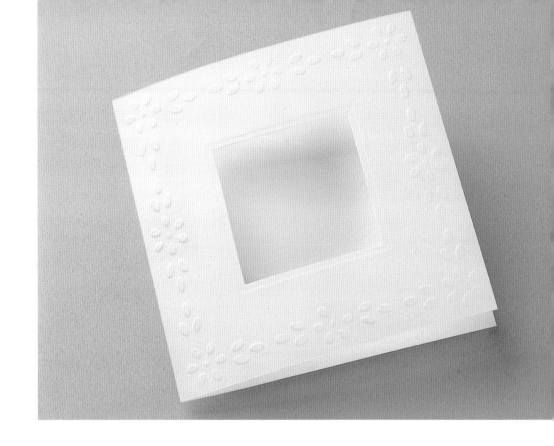

Basic Embossing

1. Use the flower stencil pattern on page 271. Place the pattern on a 4¾" x 2" (12 cm x 5 cm) sheet of white paper and trace the shapes with a pencil. Place the paper on a cutting mat and cut out the flower shapes.

2. Place the flower stencil pattern on a light box and spread the back side of white card stock on it. Rub each flower shape with an embossing tool two or three times so the shapes appear on the card stock. Continue around all four edges to complete the design.

3. Turn the white card stock to the front cover. Follow the instructions from Pressing (p. 14) and Basic Window-Shaped Card I (p.15).

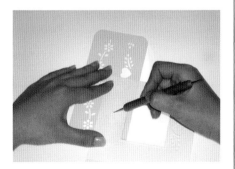

New Year

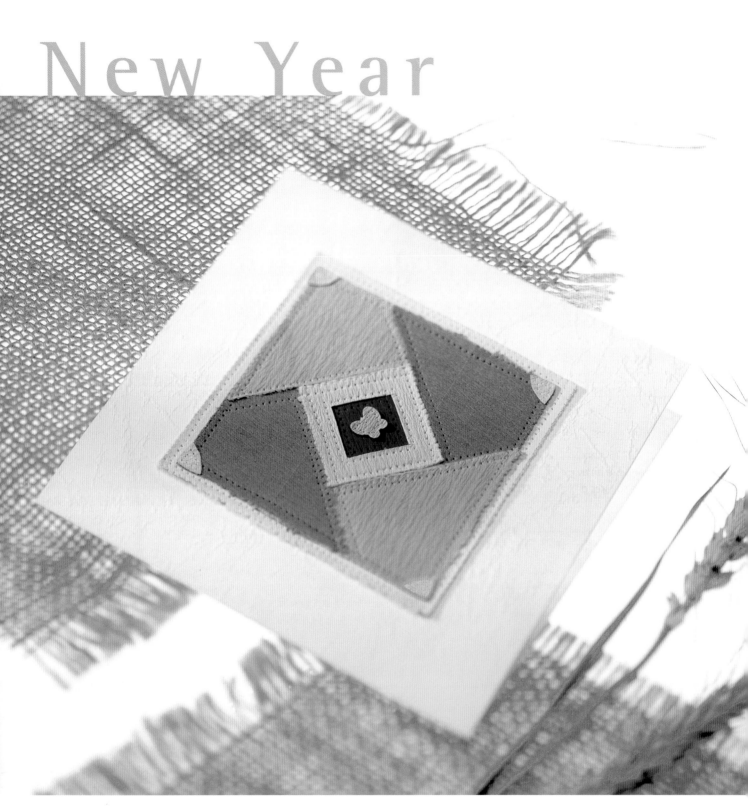

MATERIALS

white wrinkled card stock,
  10" x 5" (25 cm x 12.5 cm)
jade, brown, taupe, red, pink,
  and orange crinkle paper
thick white paper
graph paper
awl
metal ruler
pencil
PVA adhesive
corkboard
punch wheel
craft knife
heart punch

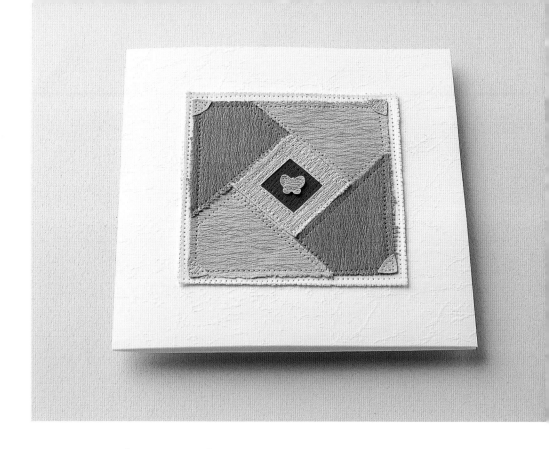

Traditional Pattern Card I

1. Draw two 2" x 2" (5 cm x 5 cm) squares on graph paper and use an awl to mark the four corners of the squares on the jade and brown crinkle paper.

2. Remove the graph paper and mark a diagonal line with an awl and a metal ruler from one corner to the opposite corner.

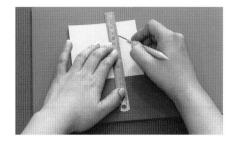

3. Put the jade paper on a corkboard and roll a punch wheel along the edges and along the diagonal line for a stitched appearance.

4. Cut the jade paper in half diagonally to make two triangles. Do the same with the brown paper.

5. Repeat Steps 1 and 2 to make a 1⅕" x 1⅕" (3 cm x 3 cm) square on taupe crinkle

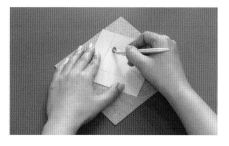

paper. Cut out a ⅖" x ⅖" (2 cm x 2 cm) square window with a craft knife. Attach a red 1" x 1" (2.5 cm x 2.5 cm) square to the back side of the taupe paper.

6. Cut four rounded quarter-circle shapes out of orange paper. Poke the edges of the pieces with an awl for a stitched appearance.

7. Follow Steps 1 through 4 to make a 3⅕"

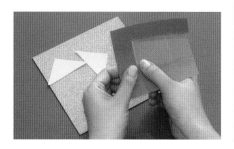

x 3⅕" (8 cm x 8 cm) square of thick white paper.

8. Attach the four jade and brown triangles to the white square in the shape of a square. The ends of the triangles should overlap. Attach the taupe 1⅕" x 1⅕" (3 cm x 3 cm) square to the center of the triangles and attach the orange quarter-circles to each corner of the brown and jade triangles.

9. Punch a butterfly out of pink paper and attach it to the center of the red square.

10. Use a punch wheel to add a stitched appearance to the overlapped areas of the triangles. Attach the entire square to the white card stock.

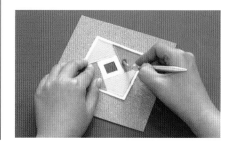

MATERIALS

rice card stock,
  10" x 5" (25 cm x 12.5 cm)
thick pale gray paper
white, pale pink, pale red, brown,
  and ocher crinkle paper
graph paper
awl
metal ruler
pencil
small flower punch
corkboard
punch wheel

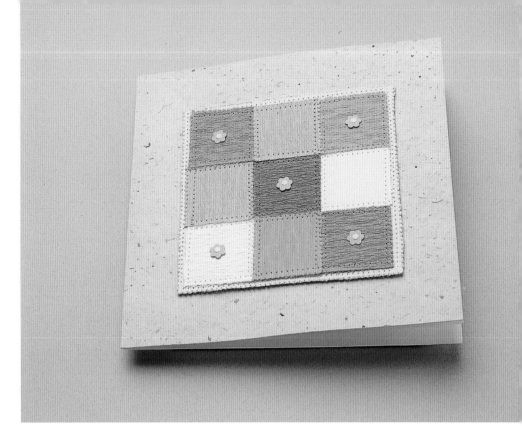

Traditional Pattern Card II

1. Draw two 1" x 1" (2.5 cm x 2.5 cm) squares on graph paper with a pencil.

2. Place one of the squares on pale red crinkle paper and mark the corners with an awl. Remove the graph paper and cut the square out with a metal ruler and craft knife.

3. Put the pale red crinkle square on a corkboard and roll a punch wheel along the edges to create a stitched appearance.

4. Follow Steps 1 through 3 to make two squares each of white, pale pink, brown, and ocher crinkle paper. You should then have nine squares in total.

5. Make a 3⅕" x 3⅕" (8 cm x 8 cm) square with a thick pale gray paper.

6. Attach the nine small squares to a 2¾" x 2¾" (7 cm x 7 cm) square of graph paper so they are lined up next to each other like quilt squares. (Using graph paper helps ensure the squares are attached straight.)

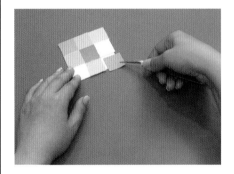

7. Attach the graph paper with the nine squares to the thick pale gray square and add stitching to the edges with a punch wheel.

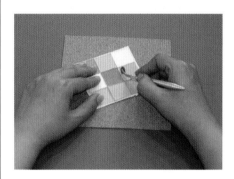

Punch out five flowers and attach white circles at the center of each flower. Attach the flowers to the center of five of the squares. Adhere the pale gray paper to rice card stock.

MATERIALS

ivory card stock,
  10" x 5" (25 cm x 12.5 cm)
thick ivory paper
jade, orange, beige, brown,
  and red crinkle paper
graph paper
seven khaki paper ribbons,
  ¹⁄₁₀" x 3¹⁄₅" (2 mm x 8 cm)
six orange paper ribbons,
  ¹⁄₁₀" x 9½" (2 mm x 24 cm)
two brown paper ribbons,
  ¹⁄₁₀" x 9½" (2 mm x 24 cm)
pencil
PVA adhesive
cutting mat
craft knife
metal ruler
punch wheel

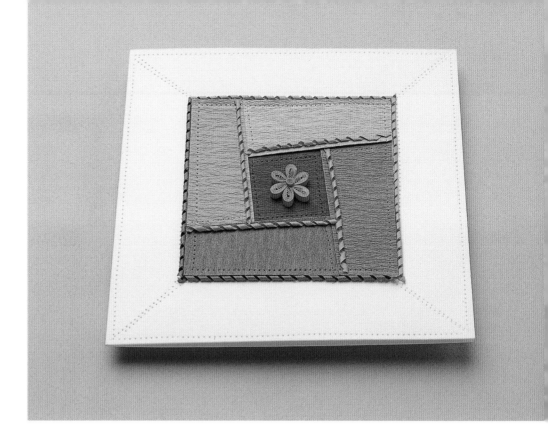

Traditional Pattern Card III

1. Design a trapezoid ²⁄₅" x 1¹⁄₅" x 3" (2 cm x 3 cm x 7.5 cm) on graph paper or use the pattern on page 272. Stack jade, orange, beige, and brown papers together and use an awl to mark the four corners of the trapezoid.

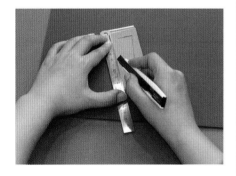

2. Remove the graph paper and cut the trapezoid shape out of all the paper at once.

3. Adhere the four trapezoids to a 2¾" x 2¾" (7 cm x 7 cm) piece of thick ivory paper. The trapezoids should form a 3" x

3" (7.5 cm x 7.5 cm) square with a smaller 1" x 1" (2.5 cm x 2.5 cm) square opening in the center.

4. Attach a 1³⁄₅" x 1³⁄₅" (4 cm x 4 cm) square of red paper in the center space.

5. Attach the entire square to the center of ivory card stock.

6. Wind brown and orange paper ribbons around a paper-quilling needle so that the ribbons become long spirals. Attach the spiral ribbons to the long edges of the

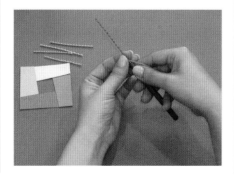

trapezoids. Use a small amount of adhesive so the spirals will not unwind.

7. Make a teardrop petal flower using seven khaki paper ribbons and attach it to the red square.

8. Roll a punch wheel along the edges of the ivory card stock and from each corner of the card inward to each corner of the decorative square.

MATERIALS

white card stock,
  10" x 5" (25 cm x 12.5 cm)
purple, lavender, and
  pale blue paper
four white paper ribbons,
  ¹⁄₁₀" x 1¹⁄₅" (2 mm x 3 cm)
awl
yellow highlighter
pencil
flower stamp
ink
corkboard
punch wheel
silver embossing powder
heat gun

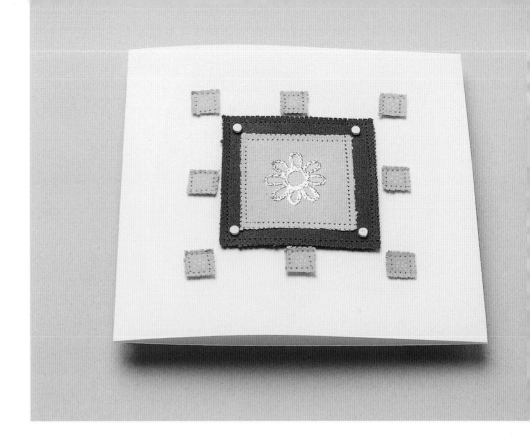

Traditional Pattern Card IV

1. Make a basic white card using the instructions for Pressing (p. 14).

2. Use an awl to draw a 2⁷⁄₁₀" x 2⁷⁄₁₀" (5.5 cm x 5.5 cm) square on purple paper and a 1³⁄₅" x 1³⁄₅" (4 cm x 4 cm) square on lavender paper.

3. Put the purple paper on a corkboard and use a punch wheel along the edges to give the appearance of stitching.

4. Tear the purple paper along the awl lines. Tear the marked square out of the lavender paper in the same way.

5. Attach the lavender rectangle to the center of the purple paper with PVA adhesive. Place it on a corkboard and use a punch wheel along the edges for a stitched appearance.

6. Attach the square to the center of the white card stock and attach eight ²⁄₅" x ²⁄₅" (1 cm x 1 cm) pale blue squares to the card stock around the purple square.

7. Stamp a flower at the center of the lavender square. While the ink is still wet, spread silver embossing powder, shake off any excess powder, and then melt it with a heat gun. Paint the flower petals with a yellow highlighter. Use the highlighter to add dots in a flower pattern to each of the blue squares. Make tight circles using white paper ribbon and attach them to the corners of the purple square.

MATERIALS

white card stock,
  10" x 5" (25 cm x 12.5 cm)
taupe rice paper
brown, coral, red, and
  beige crinkle paper
thick pale gray paper
tracing paper
awl
metal ruler
spray adhesive
PVA adhesive
cutting mat
craft knife
corkboard
punch wheel
heart punch

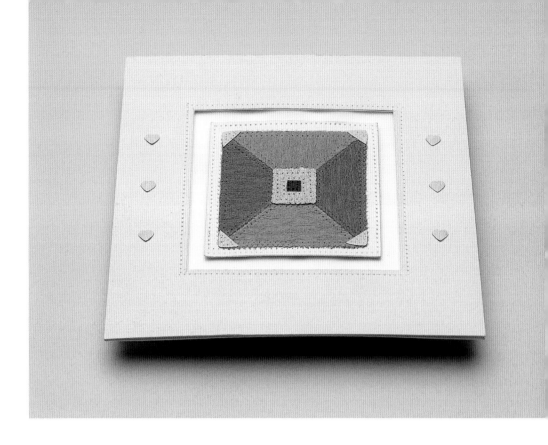

Traditional Pattern Card V

1. Use spray adhesive to attach a 5" x 5" (12.5 cm x 12.5 cm) square of taupe rice paper to one half of the white card stock and proceed to make a Basic Window-Shaped Card (p. 15). Use a punch wheel to add a stitched appearance around the window.

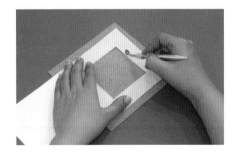

2. Attach tracing paper between the covers as an interior page.

3. Cut a 2¼" x 2¼" (6 cm x 6 cm) square out of thick pale gray paper.

4. Use a craft knife and metal ruler to cut two 1⅖" x 1⅖" (3.5 cm x 3.5 cm) squares out of brown and coral crinkle paper.

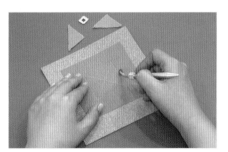

5. Place the crinkle paper on a corkboard and use a punch wheel to create a stitched appearance.

6. On the graph paper used to design the 1⅖" x 1⅖" (3.5 cm x 3.5 cm) squares, draw an X from corner to corner to divide the square into four isosceles triangles. Place the graph paper on the brown and coral squares and mark the corners of the triangles with an awl. Use a craft knife and metal ruler to cut out two triangles.

7. Make a ½" x ½" (1.5 cm x 1.5 cm) square of beige crinkle paper with a ⅕" x ⅕" (5 mm x 5 mm) window in the center. Attach a ½" x ½" (1.5 cm x 1.5 cm) square of red crinkle paper behind the beige frame.

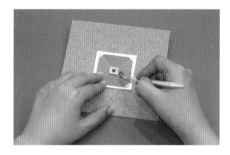

8. Adhere the four isosceles triangles to the 2¼" x 2¼" (6 cm x 6 cm) pale gray square so that the same color isosceles triangles face each other. Attach the square from Step 7 to the center of the triangles.

9. Punch four hearts out of beige paper and cut the pieces in half horizontally. Attach the bottom pieces of the hearts to the corners of the square made by the triangles. Poke the pieces with an awl for a stitched appearance.

10. Attach the rectangle to the center of the card stock window and add three beige punched hearts to each side of the window.

Anniversary

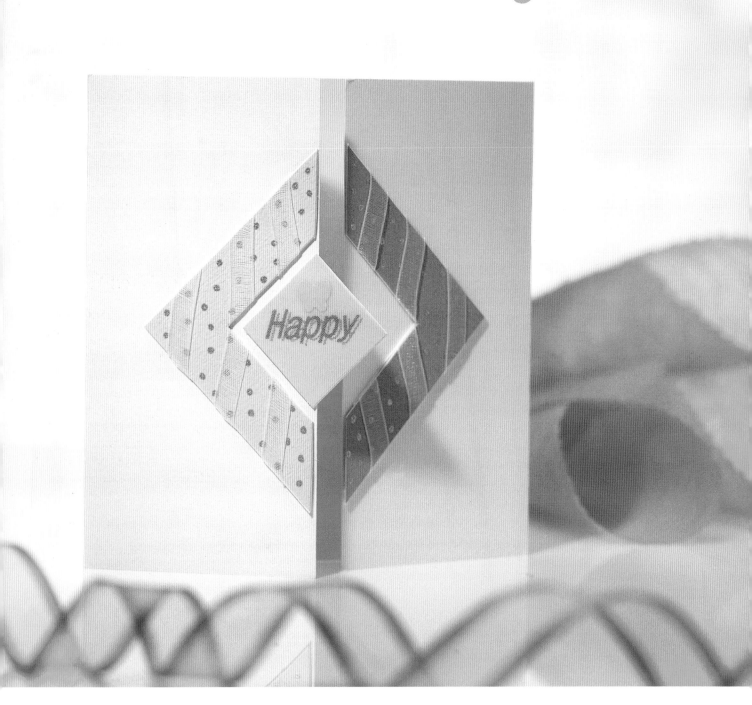

MATERIALS

white card stock,
  10" x 5" (25 cm x 12.5 cm)
thick white, lavender,
  and gray paper
lavender-pearl paper
tracing paper
two translucent white
  ribbons, 8" (20 cm) long
foam tape
metal ruler
butterfly punch
spray adhesive
PVA adhesive
cutting mat
craft knife

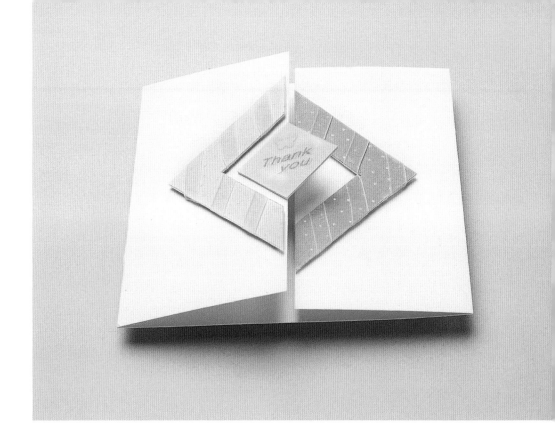

Diamond and Lace Ornament

1. Make a door-shaped card using the instructions for Basic Card II (p. 12).

2. Print "Happy" lettering on tracing paper with a computer printer.

3. Cut a 2½" x 2½" (6.5 cm x 6.5 cm) square out of thick white paper. Cut two 2½" x 2½" (6.5 cm x 6.5 cm) squares each out of lavender and gray paper and cut them in half to make triangles. Attach a lavender triangle and a gray triangle to the thick white paper with spray adhesive and cut a 1³⁄₁₀" x 1³⁄₁₀" (3.3 cm x 3.3 cm) window in the center to make a frame shape.

4. Cut the lavender and gray frames diagonally so they form arrows. Use a silver gel pen to draw dots on the arrows and wrap ribbon around both arrows.

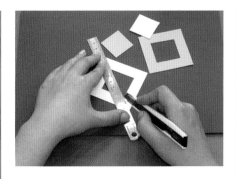

5. Cut a 1¹⁄₁₀" x 1¹⁄₁₀" (2.7 cm x 2.7 cm) square out of lavender-pearl paper. Cut a 1¹⁄₁₀" x 1¹⁄₁₀" (2.7 cm x 2.7 cm) diamond around "Happy" on the tracing paper.

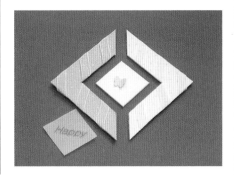

6. Punch out a butterfly and attach it to the lavender-pearl square together with the "Happy" diamond.

7. Attach the square (turned to be a diamond so "Happy" is horizontal) at the center of the white card. Use foam tape to adhere the lavender arrow on the left side of the "Happy" square and the gray arrow on the right side.

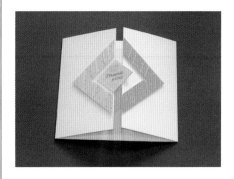

Variation: Make thank-you cards by following the same steps and replace "Happy" with "Thank you."

MATERIALS

blue card stock,
  10" x 5" (25 cm x 12.5 cm)
green, orange, pale green,
  red, and white paper
graph paper
foam tape
metal ruler
multicircle punch
decorative-edge scissors
small flower punch
PVA adhesive
cutting mat
craft knife
tweezers

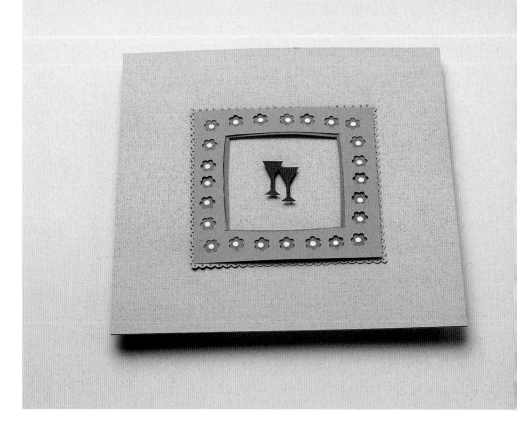

Wine Glasses in a Frame

1. Put a 2¾" x 2¾" (7 cm x 7 cm) green square on a cutting mat and use a craft knife to cut out a 1⅗" x 1⅗"(4 cm x 4 cm) square from the center or use the frame pattern on page 272.

2. Mark six holes on each side of the frame with an awl and punch them with a small flower punch.

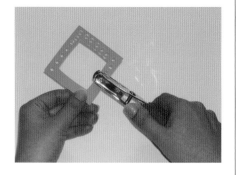

3. Use foam tape to attach a 2⁷⁄₁₀" x 2⁷⁄₁₀" (6.8 cm x 6.8 cm) orange square to the back side of the green frame and place it on a cutting mat. Use a craft knife

to cut out the orange paper that shows in the center of the frame, but leave a ¹⁄₂₀" (1 mm) margin.

4. Make a pale green 3" x 3" (7.5 cm x 7.5 cm) square and attach the frame to the center of it. Trim the outer margin of the pale green square with decorative-edge scissors, leaving a ¹⁄₁₀" (2 mm) margin. Use a craft knife to cut out the center of the pale green square.

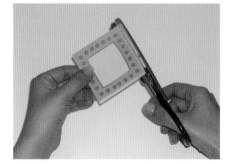

5. Make twenty-four ¹⁄₂₀" (1 mm) circles and use PVA adhesive to attach them to the centers of the flower-shaped holes in the frame.

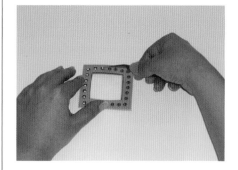

6. Use the pattern on page 272 to cut two wine glasses out of red paper.

7. Use PVA adhesive to attach the frame to the center of the blue card stock and use foam tape to attach the wine glasses in the center of the frame.

MATERIALS

white card stock,
  10" x 5" (25 cm x 12.5 cm)
pale green, lavender, white,
  dark gray, and blue-gray paper
gray-pearl paper
spray adhesive
PVA adhesive
metal ruler
silver and white gel pens
cutting mat
craft knife
small heart punch

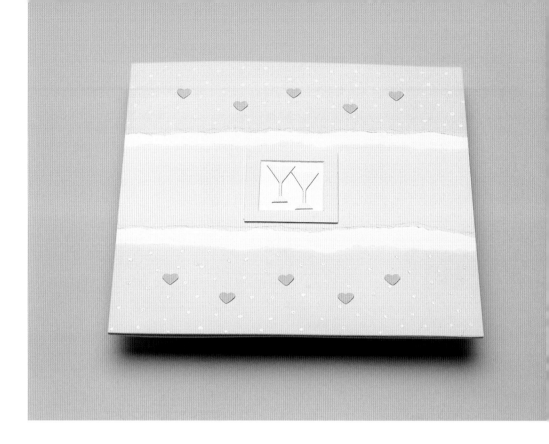

Wine Glasses

1. Roughly tear both long edges of a 2¾" x 5⁹⁄₁₀" (7 cm x 15 cm) lavender rectangle. Tear only one side of 2¾" x 5⁹⁄₁₀" (7 cm x 15 cm) pale green and blue-gray rectangles.

2. Use spray adhesive to attach the lavender strip in the middle of white card stock, the pale green strip on the top edge of the card stock, and the blue-gray strip on the bottom edge.

3. Cut a square frame (outer edge 1³⁄₁₀" x 1³⁄₁₀" [3.3 cm x 3.3 cm], inner edge ⁹⁄₁₀" x ⁹⁄₁₀" [2.3 cm x 2.3 cm]) out of dark gray paper and attach a 1³⁄₁₀" x 1³⁄₁₀" (3.3 cm x 3.3 cm) white paper to the back side of it.

4. Use the pattern on page 272 to cut two wine glasses out of white-pearl paper and attach them in the center of the dark gray frame. Attach the frame in the middle of the light purple strip.

5. Use a silver gel pen to make dots on the blue-gray strip and a white gel pen to make dots on the pale green strip.

6. Punch ten hearts out of dark gray paper and attach five each to the blue-gray and the pale green strips.

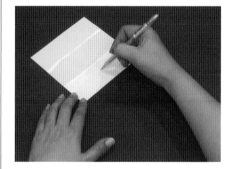

MATERIALS

white card stock,
  10" x 5" (25 cm x 12.5 cm)
pale gray, pale blue, and
  white paper
awl
small heart punch
spray adhesive
foam tape
PVA adhesive
corkboard
punch wheel
tweezers

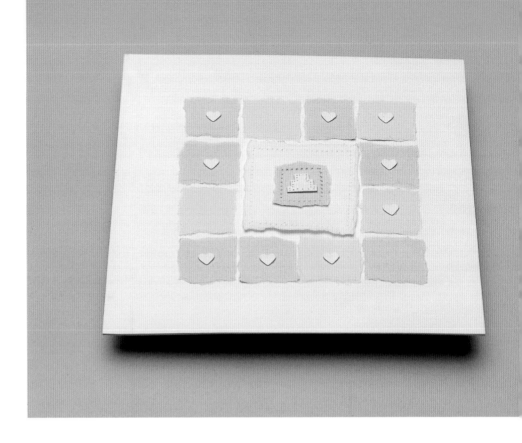

Cake and Heart

1. Cut five ⅖" x ⅖" (2 cm x 2 cm) squares out of pale gray paper and seven ⅖" x ⅖" (2 cm x 2 cm) squares out of pale blue paper. (See pattern on page 272.) Roughly tear by hand the edges of all the squares.

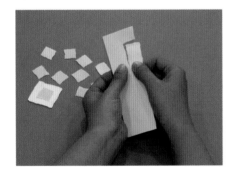

2. Use spray adhesive to attach the squares to white card stock as shown in the picture.

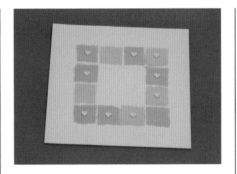

3. Punch nine hearts out of white paper and attach them to the squares.

4. Cut a 1⅗" x 1⅗" (4 cm x 4 cm) square out of white paper, then roughly tear all the edges. Place the square on a corkboard and use a punch wheel to create a stitched appearance. Cut a ⅖" x ⅖" (2 cm x 2 cm) square out of pale blue paper, then tear the edges, and use a punch wheel around the edges. Attach it to the center of the white paper.

5. Cut a three-tiered cake out of white paper and use an awl to create a stitched appearance along the outer edges. (See the pattern on page 272.) Use foam tape to attach the cake to the center of the pale blue square.

6. Attach the white square decorated with the cake to the center of the larger white card stock.

MATERIALS

white card stock,
   10" x 5" (25 cm x 12.5 cm)
lavender and white paper
6 mm circle punch
awl
spray adhesive
foam tape
PVA adhesive
corkboard
white gel pen
embossing tool or press pen
tracing paper
"Anniversary" lettering
   printed on tracing paper with
   a computer printer

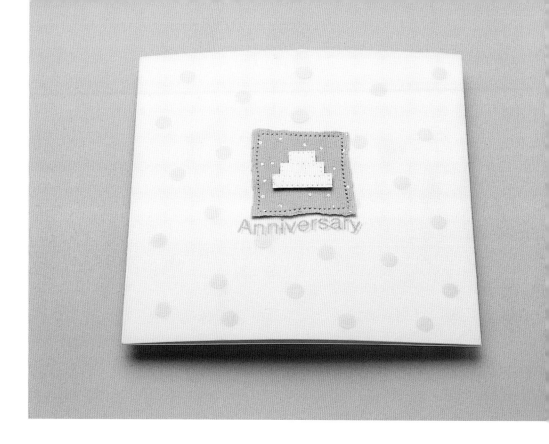

Anniversary Cake

1. Punch approximately thirty ²/₁₀" (6 mm) circles out of lavender paper and place them on a corkboard. Add a three-dimensional effect with an embossing tool and attach them to white card stock.

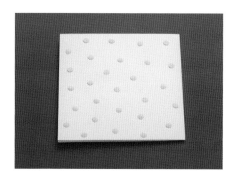

2. Cut a 1³/₅" x 1³/₅" (4 cm x 4 cm) square out of lavender paper, then roughly tear the edges. Use a white gel pen to make dots on it, and use a punch wheel to create a stitched appearance along the outer edges.

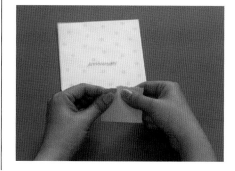

3. Cut a three-tiered cake shape out of white paper and use an awl to create a stitched appearance. (See the pattern on page 272.)

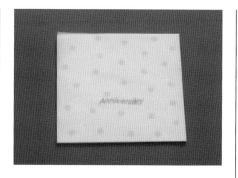

4. Attach the cake shape to the lavender square with foam tape, then attach the square to the center of the white card stock.

5. Adhere the "Anniversary" lettering to the card stock just below the lavender square.

Mother's Day

MATERIALS

white card stock,
  10" x 5" (25 cm x 12.5 cm)
lavender, yellow, pale
  gray-pearl, and white paper
tracing paper
heart and leaf stencil patterns
paper crimper
flower punch
light box
foam tape
metal ruler
cutting mat
craft knife
tracing pen
tweezers

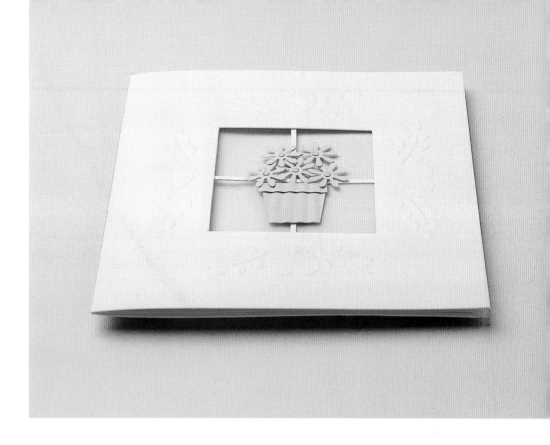

A Flower Vase in a Window

1. Make a card using the instructions for Pressing (p.14) and Basic Window-Shaped Card I (p.15).

2. Put the heart and leaf stencil patterns on a light box and put the back side of the white window card on it.

3. Center the stencil patterns on one side of the white frame and use a tracing pen to press the pattern into the card. Do the same on the other sides of the frame.

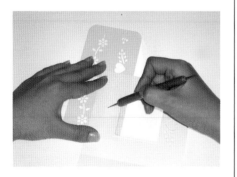

4. Attach a 4¾" x 4¾" (12 cm x 12 cm) tracing paper square to the back side of the 2⁷⁄₁₀" x 2⁷⁄₁₀" (5.5 cm x 5.5 cm) window of the white card.

5. Use a paper crimper to create a corrugated effect on pale gray paper, then cut a flowerpot shape from it. Punch five flower-shaped pieces out of lavender paper. Punch tiny circles out of yellow paper and attach them to the centers of the five flowers.

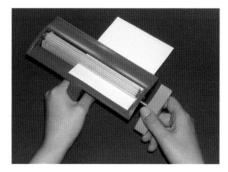

6. Use a metal ruler and craft knife to cut two thin strips out of white paper. Attach them in a cross shape to the back of the window.

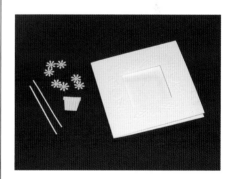

7. Use foam tape to attach the flowerpot to the bottom center of the window. Use tweezers to arrange and adhere the flowers above the flowerpot.

MATERIALS

white card stock,
  10" x 5" (25 cm x 12.5 cm)
white designer's paper
pale red, yellow, green,
  and white crinkle paper
foam tape
awl
metal ruler
decorative-edge scissors
PVA adhesive
cutting mat
craft knife
tweezers

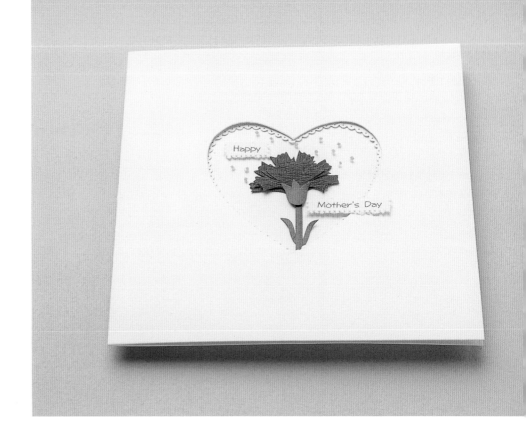

Carnation and Lace Heart

1. Make a card using the instructions for Pressing (p. 14).

2. Use the pattern on page 273 to make a heart-shaped piece of paper, then use a pencil to trace the heart onto the center of the white card stock. Place it on a cutting mat and cut out the heart shape.

3. Place the heart cut out in Step 2 at the center of a 2¾" x 2¾" (7 cm x 7 cm) white square and trace the outer edge with an awl.

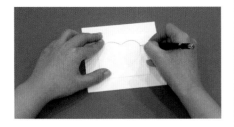

4. Use decorative-edge scissors to cut out the heart just inside the awl line. Poke the center of each rounded section with an awl.

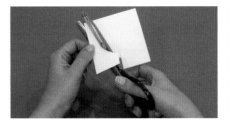

5. Attach the lace heart to the back side of the white card stock and attach a 3⁹⁄₁₀" x 3⁹⁄₁₀" (10 cm x 10 cm) white square behind the lace heart.

6. Using the patterns on page 273, cut three carnations out of red paper. Attach the smaller carnations on top of the bigger carnations. Cut out a calyx and a stem for the flower, attach them to the flower, and attach the entire flower to the center of the heart-shaped space.

7. Make thirteen small rectangles out of yellow paper. Place foam tape on the backs and use tweezers to attach them to the space around the carnation.

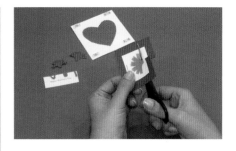

8. Print "Happy Mother's Day" lettering on white paper with a computer printer and then cut the strip of paper between "Happy" and "Mother's Day." Tear the edges of the strips of paper and use a punch wheel around the edges of both strips. Attach the words to the card.

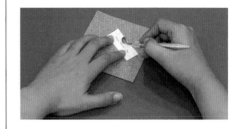

MATERIALS

gray card stock,
  10" x 5" (25 cm x 12.5 cm)
white, lavender, purple, jade,
  and brown paper
foam tape
multicircle punch
decorative-edge scissors
small flower punch
large flower punch
punch wheel
PVA adhesive
tweezers
"Thank you" letters printed
  with a computer printer

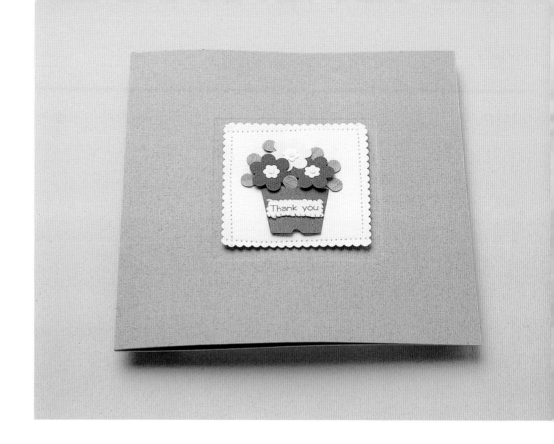

Purple Flowers and Flower Vase

1. Make a 2¼" x 2¼" (6 cm x 6 cm) gray card using the instructions for Pressing (p. 14).

2. Cut a 2" x 2" (5 cm x 5 cm) square out of white paper and trim the edge of it with decorative-edge scissors. Use a punch wheel along the outer edges of the square.

3. Use the pattern on page 273 to cut a flowerpot out of brown paper.

4. Make a lavender flower and two purple flowers with a large flower punch. Make three white flowers with a small flower punch and attach them to the larger flowers. Punch three small circles out of yellow paper and attach them to the small white flowers. Make a flower out of jade paper with a large flower punch and cut apart the petals. These will be used as leaves around the flowers.

5. Use tweezers to place and adhere the flowerpot and flowers to the white square. Arrange the jade petal-shaped pieces around the flowers.

6. Attach the white square to the center of the front cover of the gray card stock.

7. Tear the edges of the "Thank You" strip and use a punch wheel or awl along the edges. Attach the strip to the flowerpot.

MATERIALS

pale gray card stock,
   10" x 5" (25 cm x 12.5 cm)
purple, lavender, yellow, pale
   yellow, jade, and white paper
sixteen white paper ribbons,
   ¹⁄₁₀" x 2¼" (2 mm x 6 cm)
three pale yellow paper ribbons,
   ¹⁄₁₀" x 2¼" (2 mm x 6 cm)
scissors
small heart punch
large flower punch
foam tape
transparent tape
PVA adhesive
cutting mat
craft knife
punch wheel
tweezers

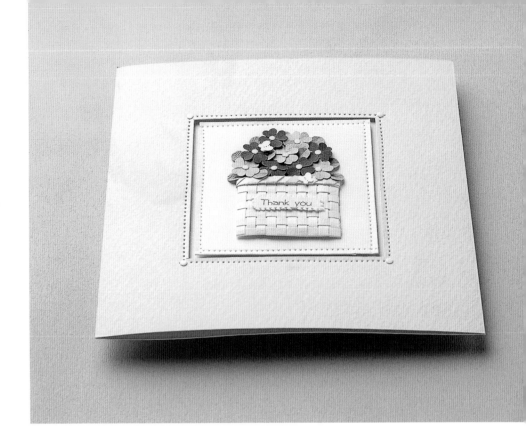

A Flower Basket

1. Make a card using the instructions for Basic Window-Shaped Card I (p. 15). The window should measure 2½" x 2½" (6.5 cm x 6.5 cm). Use a punch wheel along the edges of the window.

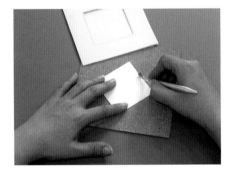

2. Punch out twenty purple hearts and sixteen lavender hearts. Use tweezers to attach four hearts together in a circle to make a flower. Punch nine tiny circles out of yellow paper and attach them to the flower centers.

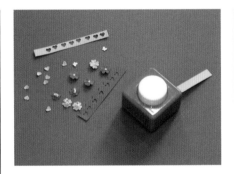

3. Attach the ends of the white paper ribbons parallel on transparent tape. Interweave the row of white strips with the ends of four white strips and two light yellow strips, alternating the colors. Attach a thick paper at the backside of the interwoven strips for preventing them from being loosened.

4. Trim the excess strips from the woven section to create a basket shape. Attach foam tape on the back side of it, to give it dimension, and attach it to the white square. Arrange the flowers above the basket.

5. Punch two flowers out of jade paper and cut apart the petals to be used as leaves around the flowers.

6. Use a punch wheel along the edges of the white 2¼" x 2¼" (6 cm x 6 cm) square and then attach the square to the interior paper with foam tape.

Valentine's Day

MATERIALS

white card stock,
  10" x 5" (25 cm x 12.5 cm)
eighteen papers in various colors
silver paper
foam tape
metal ruler
spray adhesive
cutting mat
craft knife
large heart punch

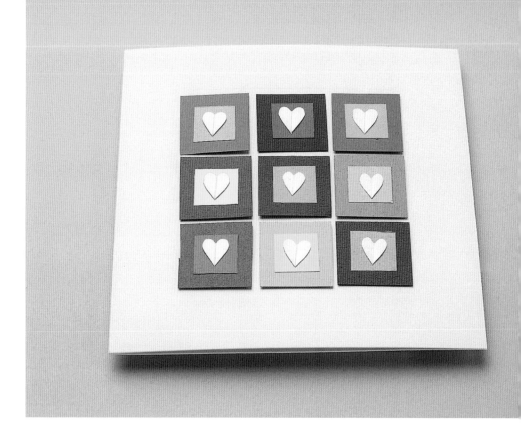

Rectangle and Heart

1. Make a card using the instructions for Pressing (p. 14).

2. Categorize the various colored papers into darker-tone and lighter-tone groups and attach the papers in each category together with a stapler. Use a metal ruler and craft knife to cut nine 1" x 1" (2.5 cm x 2.5 cm) squares out of the darker-tone papers and nine ½" x ½" (1.5 cm x 1.5 cm) squares out of the lighter-tone papers.

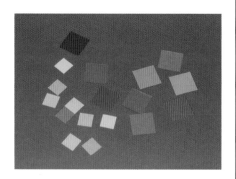

3. Place the nine lighter-tone squares on corrugated cardboard and apply spray adhesive to them.

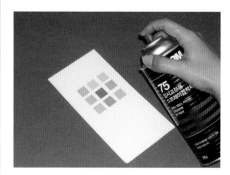

4. Attach the smaller squares to the larger squares.

5. Punch or cut nine hearts out of silver paper.

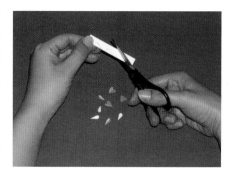

6. Attach the hearts to the center of each square.

7. Use foam tape to attach the nine squares to the white card stock.

MATERIALS

white card stock,
  10" x 5" (25 cm x 12.5 cm)
red and silver paper
decorative-edge scissors
foam tape
silver gel pen
PVA adhesive
cutting mat
craft knife
awl or pencil

Lace and Silver Heart

1. Make a card using the instructions for Basic Window-Shaped Card I (p. 15).

2. Use an awl or pencil to mark lines for a 3⅕" x 3⅕" (8 cm x 8 cm) inner square on a 4¾" x 4¾" (12 cm x 12 cm) sheet of red paper.

3. Mark four strips ½" x 3⁹⁄₁₀" (1.5 cm x 10 cm) on the back side of silver paper and cut the strips out with decorative-edge scissors.

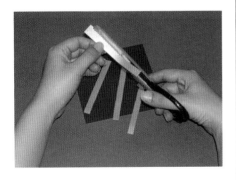

4. Attach the strips with PVA adhesive along the marked lines of the inner square on the red paper.

5. Cut a 1⅕" x 8" (3 cm x 20 cm) strip of silver paper and mark a vertical line down the center of it with an awl. Fold the strip along the awl line and design small and large half heart shapes on it to make ten hearts when unfolded.

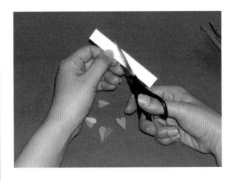

6. Write "I," "LOVE," and "YOU" on the smaller hearts by poking them with an awl and attach them to the larger hearts with foam tape.

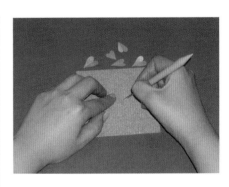

7. Attach the red paper to the inside of the white card stock and attach the five hearts to the red square with foam tape. Use a silver gel pen to draw dots around each heart.

MATERIALS

dark blue card stock,
  10" x 5" (25 cm x 12.5 cm)
white, red, and gold paper
PVA adhesive
scissors
awl
metal ruler
craft knife
foam tape
tweezers
embossing tool or press pen

Red Heart

1. Cut out one red 3" x 3" (7.5 cm x 7.5 cm) square and one white 2¾" x 2¾" (7 cm x 7 cm) square.

2. Use an embossing tool to create sixteen small circles in a grid pattern on the back side of the white square. When turned over, the circles should be slightly raised.

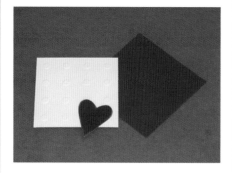

3. Cut a heart out of a red 2" x 2" (5 cm x 5 cm) sheet of red paper and poke around the edges with an awl.

4. Use foam tape to attach the red heart to silver paper. Trim the silver paper around the heart, leaving a ¹⁄₂₀" (1 mm) margin of silver.

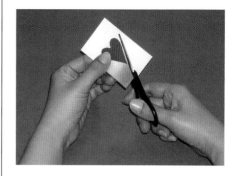

5. Attach the white square to the red square and attach the heart to the center of the white square.

6. Adhere the red square to the center of the dark blue card stock.

MATERIALS

white card stock,
  10" x 5" (25 cm x 12.5 cm)
red and silver paper
scissors
foam tape
awl
metal ruler
PVA adhesive
cutting mat
craft knife
corkboard
punch wheel
tweezers

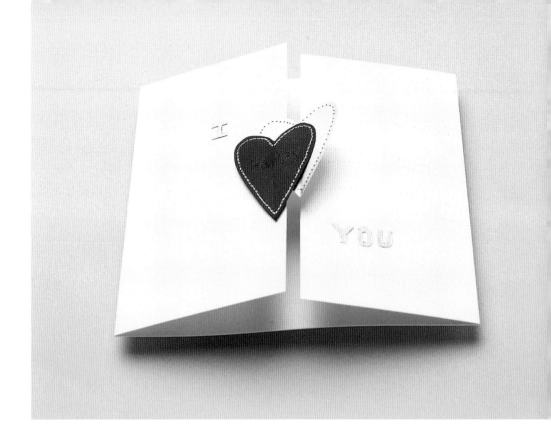

Silver and Red Heart

1. Make a card using the instructions for Basic Card II (p. 12).

2. Place the card on corkboard and roll a punch wheel horizontally across the card to add approximately ten wavy lines.

3. Use an awl to mark a vertical line down the center of a 3½" x 2" (8 cm x 5 cm) sheet of red paper. Fold the paper along the line and design a half heart shape on it with a pencil. Cut the heart out. Do the same with a 3½" x 2" (8 cm x 5 cm) sheet of silver paper. (See the pattern on page 273.)

4. Put the hearts on corkboard and poke the outer edges with an awl.

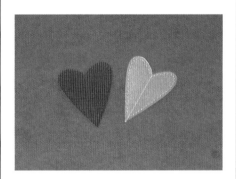

5. Attach foam tape on the back side of the red heart and attach it to the silver heart, allowing some of the silver heart to be seen.

6. Use a craft knife to cut "I," "LOVE," and "YOU" letters out of silver paper.

7. Attach the heart to the left flap of the white card with foam tape. (The right side of the heart should overlap the right flap of the card.) Attach "I," "LOVE," and "YOU" characters to the white card stock with PVA adhesive.

Invitation

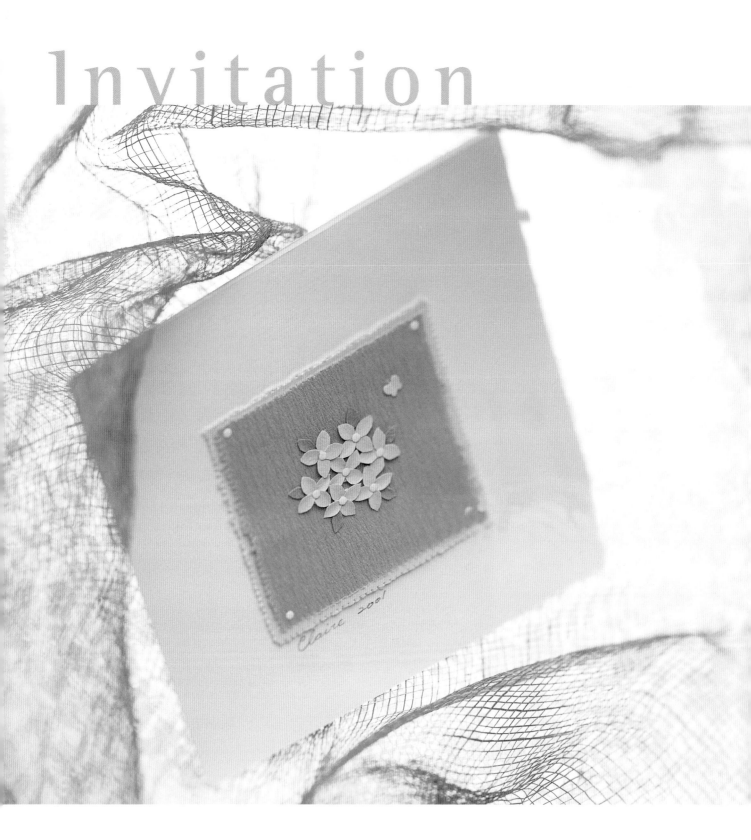

MATERIALS

white card stock,
   10" x 5" (25 cm x 12.5 cm)
tan, pale pink, green,
   and gray paper
small butterfly punch
circle punch
foam tape
multicircle punch
awl
metal ruler
scissors
PVA adhesive
corkboard
punch wheel

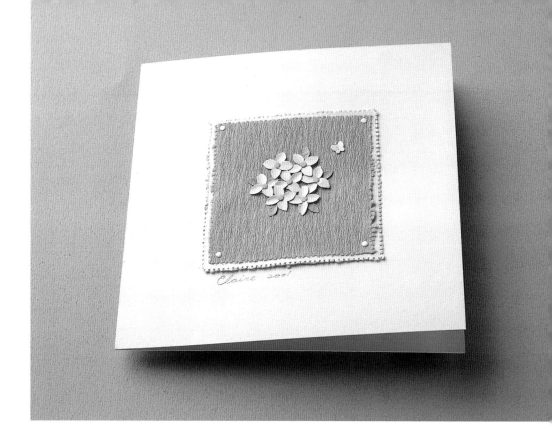

Flowers and a Butterfly

1. Use an awl and a metal ruler to mark a 2½" x 2½" (6.5 cm x 6.5 cm) square at the center of gray paper and a 2¼" x 2¼" (6 cm x 6 cm) square at the center of tan paper.

2. Place them on a corkboard and roll a punch wheel along the inside edges of the squares to create a stitched appearance.

3. Fold the paper along the marked lines and tear off the margins by hand.

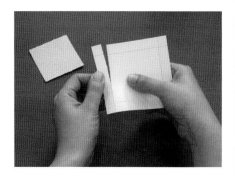

4. Fold a pale pink paper in half twice and punch out four circles. Trim each circle into a petal shape.

5. Attach four petal-shaped pieces together to make a flower and attach a yellow circle at the center of the flower. Make six more flowers in this way.

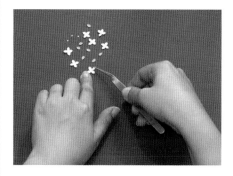

6. Cut leaf-shaped pieces out of green paper and punch a butterfly out of gray paper.

7. Layer the tan square onto the gray square and attach them both to the card stock with foam tape.

8. Attach the flowers, leaves, and butterflies to the tan square with foam tape.

9. Punch out four small circles and attach them to the four corners of the tan square.

MATERIALS

white card stock,
  10" x 5" (25 cm x 12.5 cm)
jade crinkle paper
red, gray, and white paper
wave-edge scissors
foam tape
metal ruler
small butterfly punch
PVA adhesive
cutting mat
craft knife
tweezers

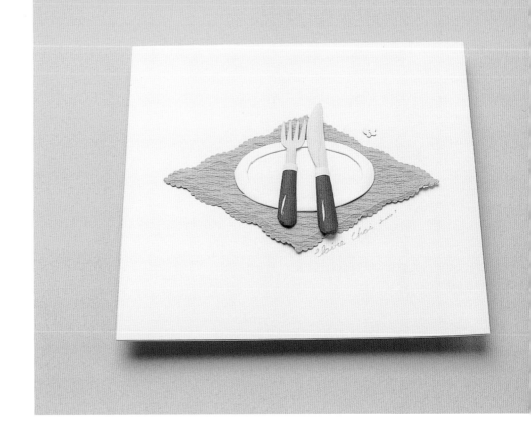

Fork and Knife

1. Design a 3⁹⁄₁₀" x 2¼" (10 cm x 6 cm) diamond shape (or use the pattern on page 273) with a pencil on jade crinkle paper and cut it out with a wave-edge scissors. Mark lines just inside the edge of the diamond with an awl and make a slight fold to add a three-dimensional effect.

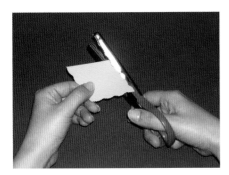

2. Copy the fork and knife patterns and attach the tops to gray paper and the handles to red paper.

3. Use a craft knife to delicately cut out the fork and knife shapes.

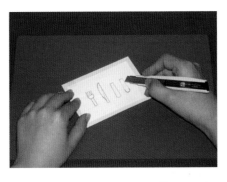

4. Add a three-dimensional effect to the fork and knife by slightly curling them with an awl.

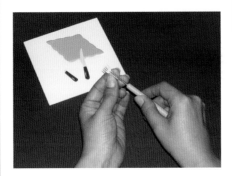

5. Attach the tops and bottoms of the fork and knife together.

6. Make a dish-shaped piece out of white paper and add a three-dimensional effect by slightly curling it with an awl.

7. Use foam tape to attach the diamond at the center of the white card stock and use PVA adhesive to attach the dish to the diamond. Attach the fork and knife to the dish. Punch a small butterfly out of white paper and attach it to the white card stock.

MATERIALS

white card stock,
  10" x 5" (25 cm x 12.5 cm)
red crinkle paper
white, pale green,
  and orange paper
wave-edge scissors
foam tape
awl
metal ruler
PVA adhesive
cutting mat
craft knife

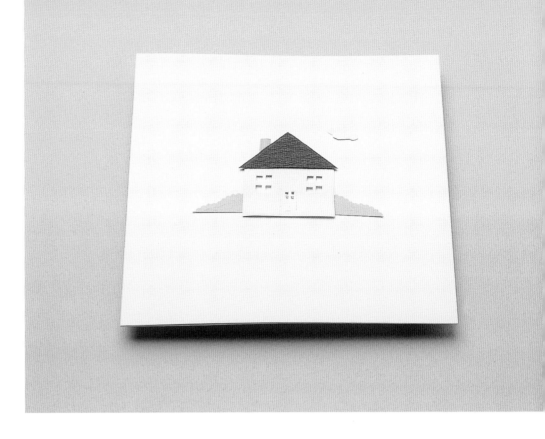

A Red Roof

1. Use the pattern on page 274 to design a roof (a 1⅗" x 1¹⁄₁₀" [4 cm x 2.7 cm] isosceles triangle) and a wall (a 1⅕" x ⁹⁄₁₀" [3 cm x 2.3 cm] rectangle) on graph paper, allowing ⅖" (1 cm) for attaching the pieces together.

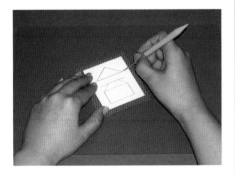

2. Put the roof on red crinkle paper, trace it with an awl, and cut the shape out. Cut out a white wall the same way, being careful when cutting out the windows.

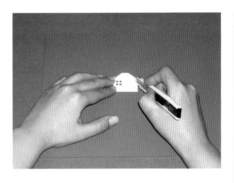

3. Attach the roof and wall together with foam tape and adhere the house to white card stock.

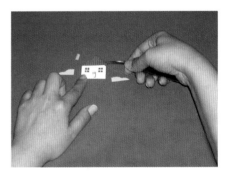

4. Cut a 3" (7.5 cm)-long shrubbery-shaped piece out of pale green paper with wave-edge scissors and cut it in half. Attach one piece of shrubbery to each side of the house. Make a chimney-shaped piece out of orange paper and attach it to the roof.

MATERIALS

pale gray card stock,
  10" x 5" (25 cm x 12.5 cm)
khaki crinkle paper
white, pale gray,
  and pale blue paper
graph paper
wave-edge scissor
multicircle punch
foam tape
awl
metal ruler
pencil
cutting mat
craft knife
PVA adhesive
tweezers

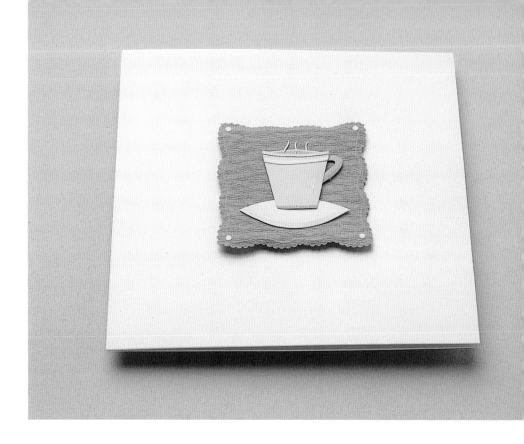

A Coffee Mug

1. Use the pattern on page 274 to design a coffee mug, saucer, and handle on graph paper. Place it on pale gray paper and trace the pattern with an awl.

2. Place the gray paper on a cutting mat and cut out the shapes with a craft knife.

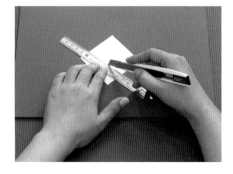

3. Add a three-dimensional effect to the mug, saucer, and handle by slightly curling them with an awl. Attach them together with foam tape.

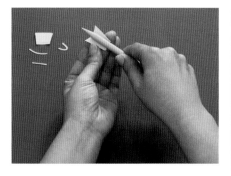

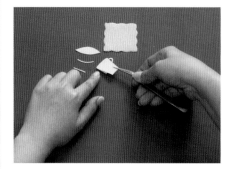

4. Cut a 2⁷⁄₁₀" x 2⁷⁄₁₀" (5.5 cm x 5.5 cm) square out of khaki crinkle paper with wave-edge scissors. On the back side, use an awl to mark lines ¹⁄₁₀" (2 mm) inside the edges and fold the edges slightly.

5. Attach the khaki square to the center of white card stock with foam tape, then attach the saucer and coffee mug to the center of the khaki square.

6. Attach four small white circles to the four corners of the khaki square. Cut out small wavy pieces to act as steam rising from the mug.

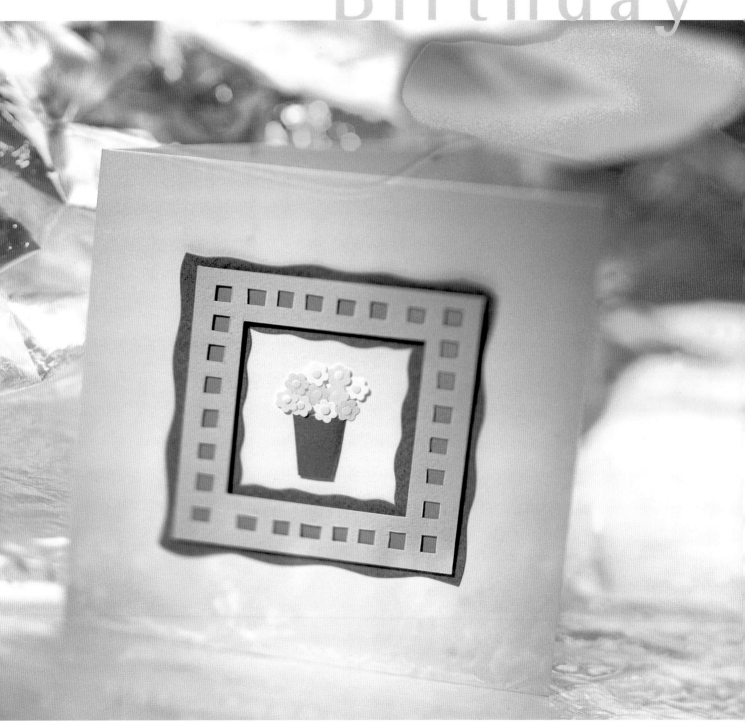

MATERIALS

white card stock,
   10" x 5" (25 cm x 12.5 cm)
dark gray, lavender, green,
   pale green, yellow, pale
   yellow, and white paper
foam tape
small flower punch
awl
metal ruler
PVA adhesive
cutting mat
craft knife
tweezers

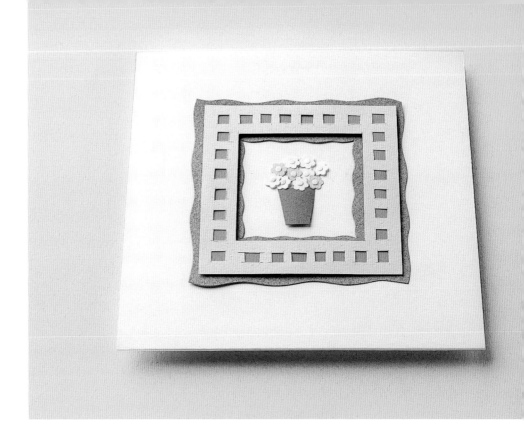

Flowers in a Frame

1. Place a lavender 3" x 3" (7.5 cm x 7.5 cm) square on a cutting mat and cut out a 1⅘" x 1⅘" (4.5 cm x 4.5 cm) square from the center to make a frame. (See the pattern on page 274.)

2. Use an awl to mark eight ⅕" x ⅕" (5 mm x 5 mm) squares on each side of the frame and cut out the small squares.

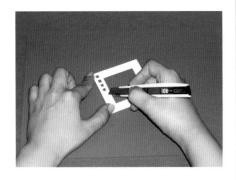

3. Use foam tape to attach the frame to a pale green 2⁹⁄₁₀" x 2⁹⁄₁₀" (7.3 cm x 7.3 cm) square. Place it on a cutting mat and cut out the pale green paper that shows through the frame's window.

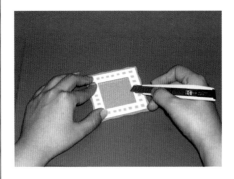

4. Attach the frame to the center of a dark gray 3³⁄₁₀" x 3³⁄₁₀" (8.5 cm x 8.5 cm) square and trim the inner and outer edges of the dark gray square into wavy lines.

5. Make three yellow, four pale yellow, and three white flowers with a small flower punch and attach small pale yellow

circles to the centers of the flowers with tweezers. Cut a flowerpot shape out of green paper and curl it slightly with an awl to add a three-dimensional effect.

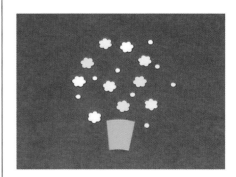

6. Use PVA adhesive to attach the frame to the center of white card stock, and use foam tape to attach the flowers and flowerpot in the center of the frame.

MATERIALS

white card stock,
 10" x 5" (25 cm x 12.5 cm)
white paper
flower stencil pattern
light box
transparent tape
cutting mat
craft knife
tracing pen

Embossed Flowers and Happy Birthday

1. Copy the "Happy Birthday" lettering from the pattern on page 94 and attach them to a white 5" x 5" (12.5 cm x 12.5 cm) square. Cut out the characters with a craft knife.

2. Place the "Happy Birthday" lettering backwards on a light box and center white card stock on top.

3. Trace the letters with a tracing pen several times to ensure that the characters appear on the surface of the white card stock.

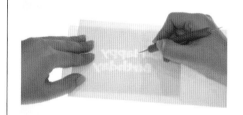

4. Use the same technique to transfer the flower pattern on page 271 to the card stock.

MATERIALS

white card stock,
   10" x 5" (25 cm x 12.5 cm)
pale green, white, yellow,
   and jade paper
scissors
circle punch
spray adhesive
PVA adhesive
metal ruler
craft knife
punch wheel
tweezers

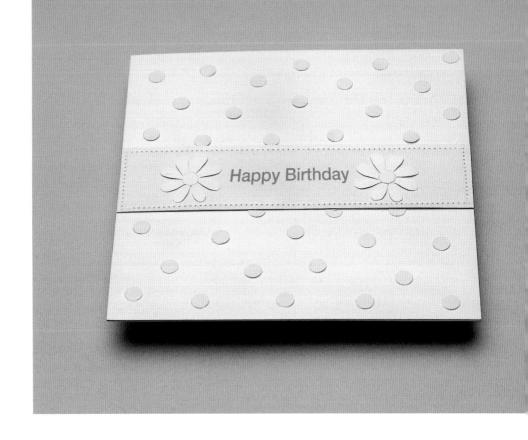

White Flowers and Circles

1. Print "Happy Birthday" lettering on a ⅖" x 2¼" (1 cm x 6 cm) sheet of jade paper.

2. Fold pale green paper in half and punch it thirty times with a circle punch for a total of sixty ⅕" (6 mm) circles. Attach the circles on the front cover of white card stock with PVA adhesive.

3. Use the pattern on page 274 to make two white flowers with yellow centers.

4. Cut a 1⅕" x 5" (3 cm x 12.5 cm) rectangle out of the jade paper around "Happy Birthday" and use a punch wheel along the edges.

5. Attach the rectangle across the center of the white card stock and attach one flower to each end of "Happy Birthday."

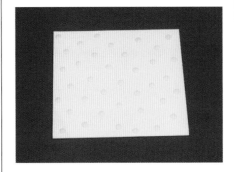

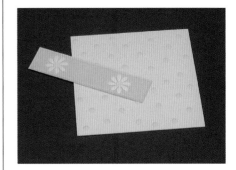

MATERIALS

green card stock,
  10" x 5" (25 cm x 12.5 cm)
pale jade and lavender paper
tracing paper
scissors
circle punch
PVA adhesive
stapler
pencil
spray adhesive

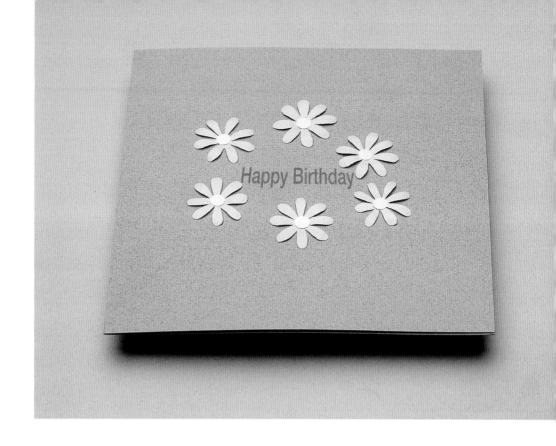

Card Embellished with Flowers

1. Print "Happy Birthday" lettering ⅖" x 2 ¼" (1 cm x 6 cm) on tracing paper with a computer printer.

2. Attach the two flower patterns on page 274 to a stack of three pale jade sheets of paper and cut out six flowers with a pair of scissors by cutting twice.

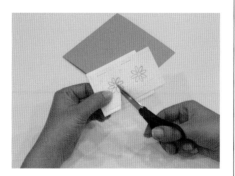

3. Punch six small circles out of lavender paper and attach them to the centers of the flowers.

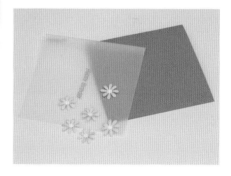

4. Use spray adhesive to attach "Happy Birthday" to the center of green card stock.

5. Adhere the flowers to the card stock around the words.

MATERIALS

lavender card stock,
  10" x 5" (25 cm x 12.5 cm)
thick white paper
lavender paper
tracing paper
butterfly punch
metal ruler
silver gel pen
PVA adhesive
cutting mat
craft knife
spray adhesive

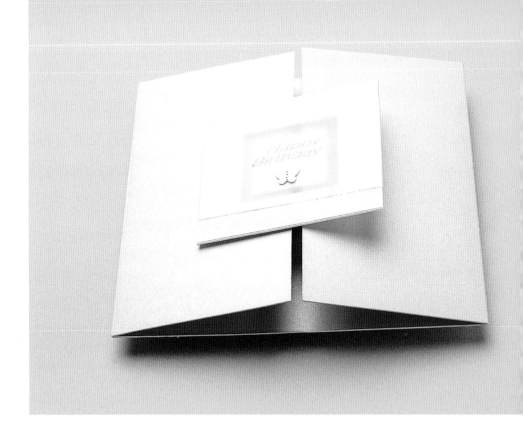

A Butterfly and A Frame I

1. Make a card using the instructions for Basic Card II (p. 12).

2. Print "Happy Birthday" lettering on tracing paper with a computer printer and cut it onto a 1⅗" x 3⁹⁄₁₀" (4 cm x 10 cm) rectangle.

3. Attach lavender paper to thick white paper and cut it to make a 2½" x 2½" (6.5 cm x 6.5 cm) square. Cut out a 1⅕" x 1⅕" (3 cm x 3 cm) inner square at the center.

4. Use a silver gel pen to make dots on the frame and attach the "Happy Birthday" rectangle across the center of the frame with spray adhesive, trimming the excess tracing paper.

5. Cut out a white 1" x 1" (2.5 cm x 2.5 cm) square and attach it to the back side of the characters. Punch out a butterfly and attach it below "Happy Birthday."

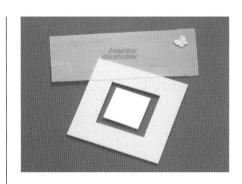

6. Attach the left half of the frame to the left flap of the card with PVA adhesive.

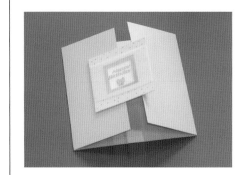

Wedding

MATERIALS

white card stock,
   10" x 7 1/10" (25 cm x 18 cm)
four white, pale green,
   and ivory paper ribbons
   1/5" x 5 1/2" (6 mm x 14 cm)
twenty-four white paper ribbons,
   1/10" x 4 3/4" (2 mm x 12 cm)
four pale green paper ribbons,
   1/10" x 2" (2 mm x 5 cm)
scissors
paper-quilling needle
flower-shaped beads
foam tape
silver gel pen
PVA adhesive
cutting mat
craft knife
tracing pen
tweezers

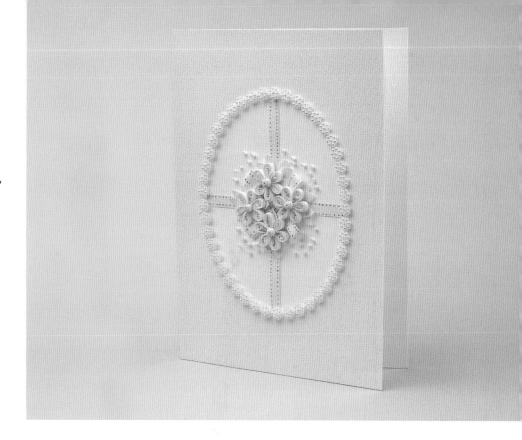

Wedding Card

1. Place the white card stock on a cutting mat with the front side up. Put an oval pattern in the center of it and mark it with a tracing pen. Cut out the oval center. (See the pattern on page 275.)

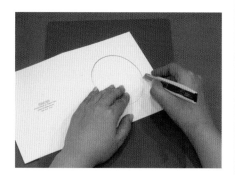

2. Attach a 4 4/5" x 6 9/10" (12.3 cm x 17.5 cm) white rectangle to the back side of the front cover with PVA adhesive.

3. Make a cross with two ivory paper ribbons and attach it to the center of the card.

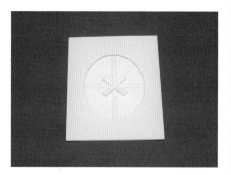

4. Fold in half two 5 1/2" (9 cm) ivory paper ribbons. Attach both of these folded strips to the center of the cross in the shape of an X.

5. Make twenty-four teardrop quilling pieces using white paper ribbon. Assemble six teardrop pieces to make a flower (four flowers total). Make four tight circles using four pale green paper ribbons and attach them to the centers of the flowers.

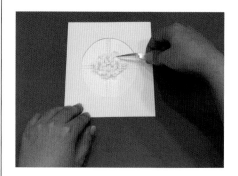

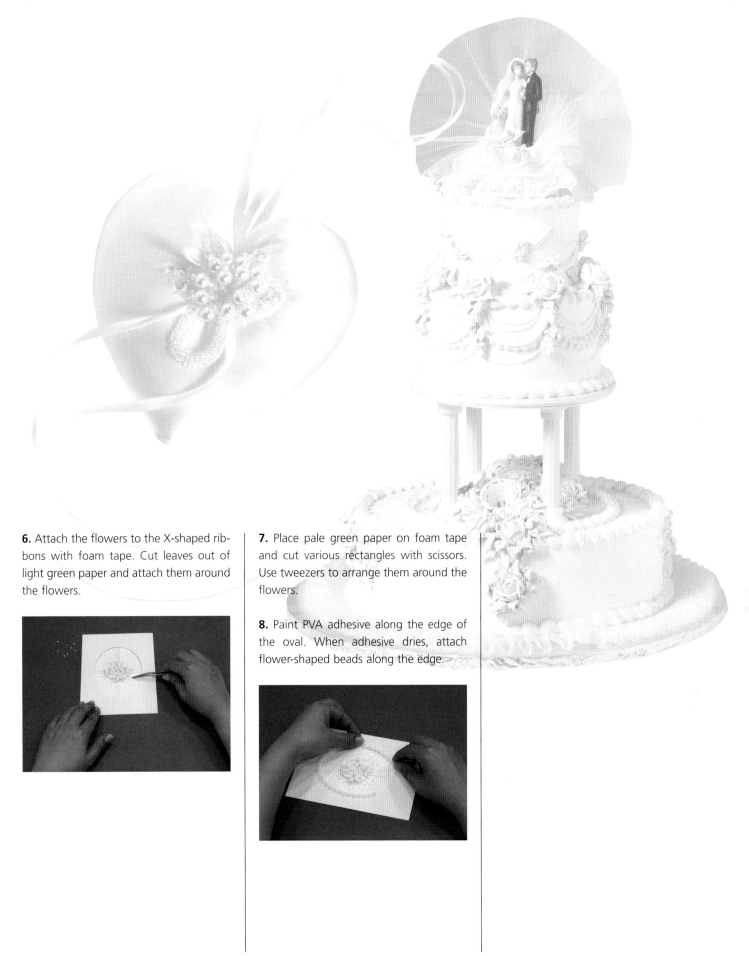

6. Attach the flowers to the X-shaped ribbons with foam tape. Cut leaves out of light green paper and attach them around the flowers.

7. Place pale green paper on foam tape and cut various rectangles with scissors. Use tweezers to arrange them around the flowers.

8. Paint PVA adhesive along the edge of the oval. When adhesive dries, attach flower-shaped beads along the edge.

MATERIALS

white card stock,
    10" x 5" (25 cm x 12.5 cm)
jade paper
thirteen white paper ribbons,
    1/10" x 2¾" (2 mm x 7 cm)
thirteen pale green paper ribbons
    1/10" x 2¾" (2 mm x 7 cm)
metal ruler
PVA adhesive
cutting mat
craft knife
tweezers

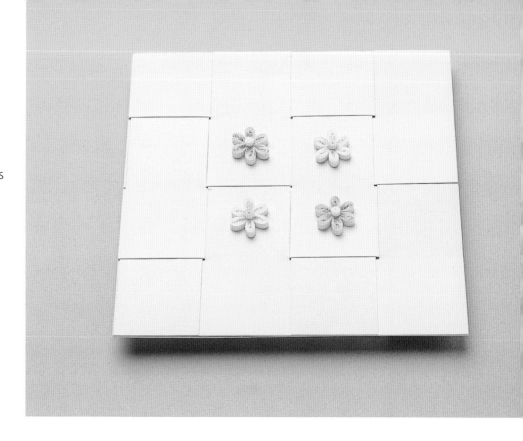

Cross Strips and Paper-Quilling Flowers

1. Place white card stock on a cutting mat and cut the front cover into four even rectangular sections. Trim the rectangles 1/20" (1 mm) more so there is room for weaving.

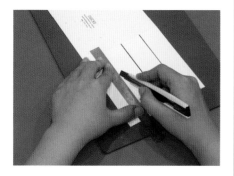

2. Cut four 1⅕" x 5" (3 cm x 12.5 cm) strips out of jade paper.

3. Weave the jade strips with the white card stock.

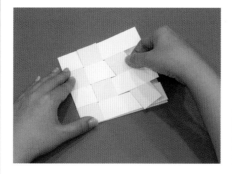

4. Glue the woven strips together with PVA adhesive.

5. Make four teardrop petal flowers using twelve white paper ribbons and twelve pale green paper ribbons. Make four tight circles with white paper ribbon and attach them to the centers of the flowers.

6. Attach the flowers to four woven squares on the card.

MATERIALS

white card stock,
  10" x 5" (25 cm x 12.5 cm)
white and white-pearl paper
twenty-four white paper ribbons,
  $\frac{1}{10}$" x 5$\frac{1}{2}$" (2 mm x 9 cm)
four pale green paper ribbons,
  $\frac{1}{10}$" x 2" (2 mm x 5 cm)
two ivory paper ribbons,
  $\frac{1}{10}$" x 5$\frac{9}{10}$" (2 mm x 15 cm)
scissors
foam tape
awl
multicircle punch
metal ruler
decorative-edge scissors
PVA adhesive
cutting mat
craft knife
tweezers

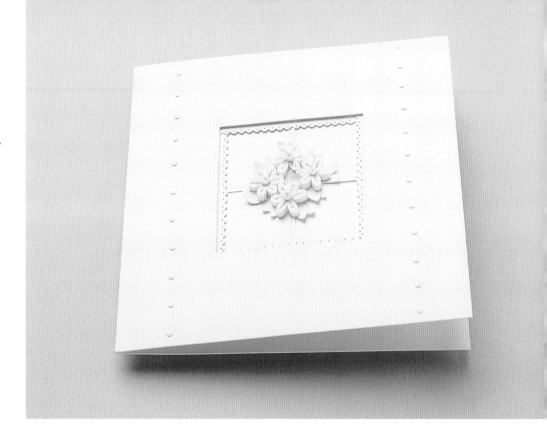

A White Flower on Lace

1. Make a card using the instructions for Pressing (p. 14) and Basic Window-Shaped Card II (p. 15).

2. Cut a white 2$\frac{3}{4}$" x 2$\frac{3}{4}$" (7 cm x 7 cm) square and mark a smaller 2$\frac{7}{10}$" x 2$\frac{7}{10}$" (5.5 cm x 5.5 cm) square at the center of the white square with an awl.

3. Cut out the inner square with decorative-edge scissors, leaving a $\frac{1}{10}$" (2 mm) margin. Poke the lace-shaped edges with an awl for embellishment.

4. Attach the lace frame to the back side of the white card stock. Attach a 3$\frac{9}{10}$" x 3$\frac{9}{10}$" (10 cm x 10 cm) white-pearl square to the back side of the lace frame. Use a punch wheel in the center of two ivory paper ribbons and position a cross shape at the center of the frame. Attach the ribbons to the back of the window.

5. Make four teardrop petal flowers with white paper ribbons. Make tight circles with pale green paper ribbons and attach them to the centers of the flowers.

6. Use foam tape to attach the four flowers to the center of the ribbon cross. Cut leaves out of white paper and attach them around the flowers.

7. Punch approximately twenty-two $\frac{1}{10}$" (2 mm) circles out of white paper and attach them in a vertical line on the left and right sides.

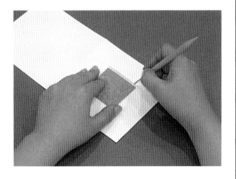

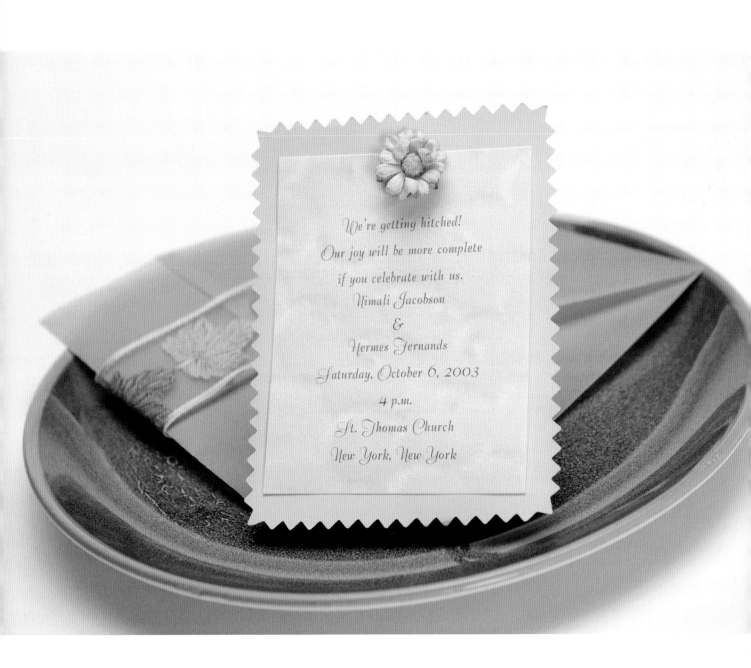

We're getting hitched!
Our joy will be more complete
if you celebrate with us.
Nimali Jacobson
&
Hermes Fernands
Saturday, October 6, 2003

4 p.m.

St. Thomas Church
New York, New York

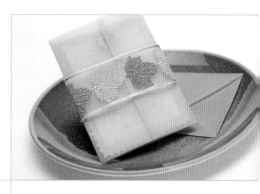

Green and Lovely

SPRINGY, RIBBONED INVITATION

Spring is in the air, in your heart, and in your step. Why not let it show? Go on, spread the green and wrap up this leafy invitation. The layers of different, but coordinating, green create a translucent effect like light filtering through the tree canopy in your neighborhood park. The effect mimics the growth of a new season.

DIRECTIONS

1. Using your favorite page layout program, create a new document 8 ½" × 11" (22 cm × 28 cm).

2. Draw a box 3 ½" wide × 4 ½" deep (9 cm × 11 cm). Set the type for your invitation in the box, leaving about ¾" (2 cm) on top blank for the flower. We used 14 point Bernhard Tango Swash type on leading of 25 points. We chose a coordinating dark green for the type.

3. Once you've perfected the first invitation, copy and paste an additional one right next to the original and two below. This way, you'll be able to run four up on the 8 ½" × 11" (22 cm × 28 cm) sheet.

4. Print onto 8 ½" × 11" (22 cm × 28 cm) scroll cream paper and trim.

5. Center printed scroll paper invite onto ric-rac card. Place a needle through the two cards about ¼" (0.5 cm) down from top of scroll paper and pierce through the two layers.

6. Place flower in through hole and twist the wire around the back in a coil.

7. Draw a rectangle, 9" wide × 5 ¾" deep (23 cm × 14.5 cm), onto sage vellum. Trim paper to size with craft knife.

8. Center assembled invite onto sage rectangle. Fold left side of sage vellum over right so ends meet in the middle. Score edges with bone folder.

9. Wrap with leaf ribbon and insert in chroma lime vellum envelope.

VARIATION *For autumn wedding colors, replace the greens with russet, burnt sienna, orange, and yellow colors.*

MATERIALS

8 ½" × 11" (22 cm × 28 cm) scroll cream paper

4 ¼" × 5 ½" (10.5 cm × 14 cm) A2 butter colored ric-rac cards

heavy-duty embroidery needle

green and yellow silk favor flowers with metal stems

coordinating 2"-wide (5 cm) leaf ribbon

8 ½" × 11" (22 cm × 28 cm) sage-colored vellum

4¼" × 6 ½" (12 cm × 17 cm) chroma lime vellum envelopes

personal computer

page layout software (such as Quark or PageMaker)

color printer

pencil

metal ruler

drafting triangle

craft knife

bone folder

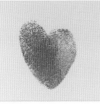

No Two Alike

THUMBPRINT CARD

MATERIALS

11" × 17"
(28 cm × 43 cm) white
cover-weight stock

personal computer

page layout software
(such as Quark or
Page Maker)

color printer

bone folder

craft knife

4 ½" × 6"
(11 cm × 15 cm)
red envelopes

Obviously, you and your intended are stylish and individual. Give your invitations your own personal mark—literally. Of course, you can enlist some friends to help you make these invitations and no one will care if the thumbprints belong to you two or not, unless you have an FBI agent on your guest list. (Would we assume that you don't? Never!) However, it is much more fulfilling and, indeed, sweet to spend a little quality time together when it may be a scarce commodity. Talk about your plans, the red ink you've accidentally smeared across your face, or why the dog loves it when you play bossa nova music. Just cherish the time and know that you have sent an inimitable mark of your union to all of your guests.

DIRECTIONS

1. Using your favorite page layout software, create a document 16" wide × 5 ½" deep (41 cm × 14 cm).

2. Divide the layout into four sections and mark with vertical rules, 4" (10 cm) wide for each section.

3. In the first section, set the type for the first name to appear on the invitation, approximately 3 ¼" (8.5 cm) from the top and centered left to right. We used 9 point Garamond on 13 point leading.

4. Do the same in the second and third sections, setting the type for the second name and subsequent names together accordingly.

5. In the fourth section, set the invitation with all the pertinent information.

TIP *If you are new to the scanning and layout game, have no fear (OK, less fear). You can go a more low-tech, but somewhat messier route, and stamp each invitation with your lovely prints. Technology makes this project swifter, but don't forget that you have the basic tools, literally, at your very fingertips.*

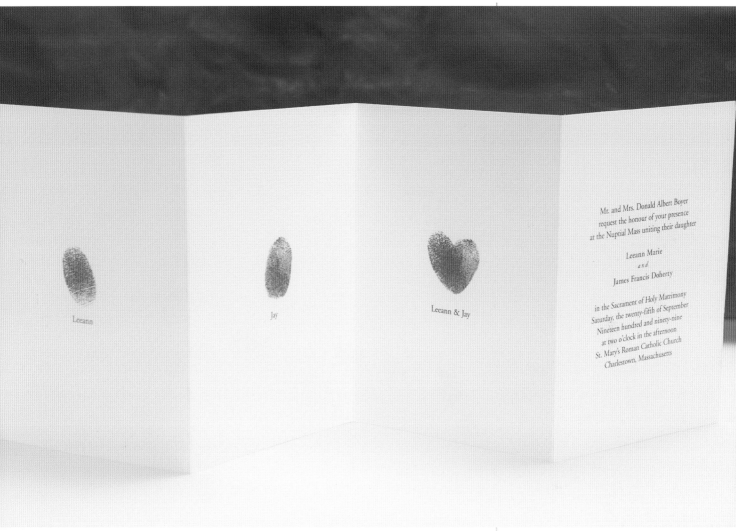

Mr. and Mrs. Donald Albert Boyer
request the honour of your presence
at the Nuptial Mass uniting their daughter

Leeann Marie
and
James Francis Doherty

in the Sacrament of Holy Matrimony
Saturday, the twenty-fifth of September
Nineteen hundred and ninety-nine
at two o'clock in the afternoon
St. Mary's Roman Catholic Church
Charlestown, Massachusetts

Leeann

Jay

Leeann & Jay

6. Remove the vertical lines from the four sections.

7. Place your thumbs on a red inkpad, press stamp onto white paper in the patterns shown, and scan into your computer.

8. Place thumbprint images in document and then print out on a white textured 11" × 17" (28 cm × 43 cm) cover-weight stock. If you don't have a large-format printer, bring it on a disk to a copy center and have them print it.

9. Fold the card into four sections and score with a bone folder.

10. Place in red envelopes.

VARIATION *If you don't own a large-format printer, you could make a small card and attach it into the last panel of the card and handprint the names under the thumbprints.*

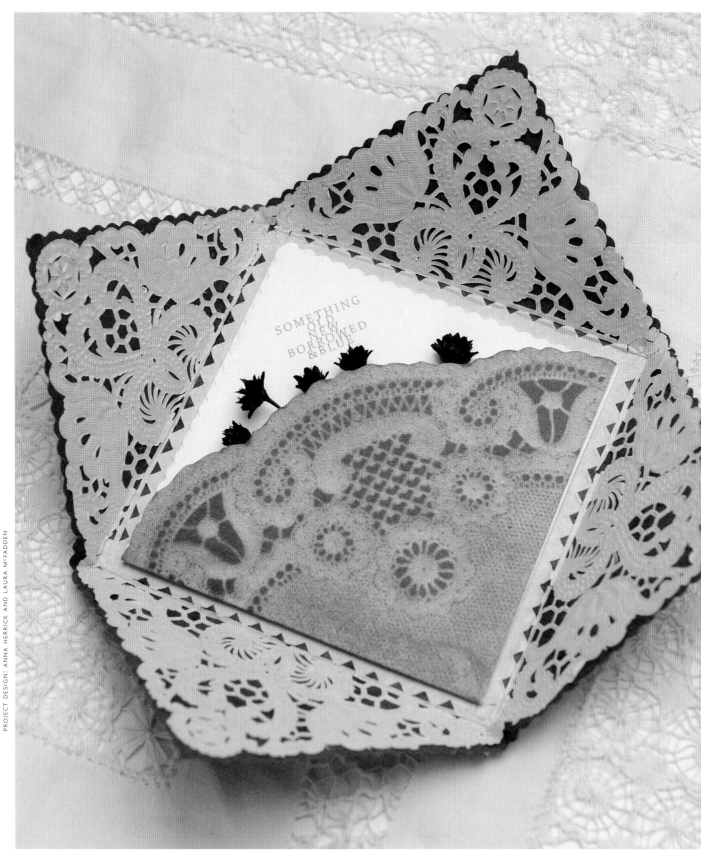

SOMETHING
OLD
NEW
BORROWED
&BLUE

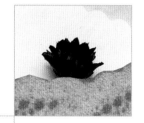

Something Blue
SUN-PRINT LACY INVITE

Who says lace needs to be white and frilly? This lace is blue, baby! Sun prints are made by placing an object on light-sensitive paper. As the sunlight strikes the paper, the lace blocks and leaves its design behind. And while you make the print, you'll be dosing up on vitamin D: essential for energy and good moods (OK, that may or may not be true, but it sure sounds good to us). The diamond shape of this invitation creates a pocket for all the elements of the invitation.

DIRECTIONS FOR THE LACE ENCLOSURE

1. Place sun-print paper on a piece of cardboard and place circular doily on top of sunprint sheet. Expose to sunlight anywhere from 1 to 5 minutes or until the sheet starts to turn white.

2. Rinse sheet with water and let dry. It may take some experimentation to get the print looking the way you want it, so you may want to try doing several at once, pulling them out of the sunlight at different times.

3. Scan the photo into your computer. If this is not an option, bring it to a graphics shop, have them scan it for you and place it onto a disk.

4. Create a document in your layout program 10 ½" wide × 5 ¾" deep (27 cm × 14.5 cm). Place digital image on right side of page and scale up photo until it measures 5 ¼" (13.5 cm) square. Align image on top and right edges.

5. Output image onto white card stock.

VARIATION *If you have difficulty rotating the type on the 45° angle, just set it in the square on the page.*

MATERIALS

Sun-print kit with 4 ¼" (10.5 cm) square sheets

circular doily

scanner

personal computer

page layout program (such as Quark or PageMaker)

color printer

8 ½" × 11" (22 cm × 28 cm) white laser or inkjet card stock

craft knife

metal ruler

triangle

bone folder

craft glue

Obonai white laser or inkjet rice paper

spray adhesive

small blue dried flowers

thin gauge wire

scalloped paper edgers or rotary trimmer with scalloped-edge rotary blade

scissors

8" × 8" (20 cm × 20 cm) white paper doilies

sheet of decorative blue paper cut down to 8 ¼" (20.5 cm) square

daisy wafer seals

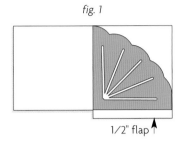

fig. 1

1/2" flap

6. Trim image to size leaving a ½" (1 cm) flap under the image side of the printed card *(see fig. 1)*.

7. Using scissors or craft knife, cut around shape of doily *(see fig. 2)*.

8. Cut 45° angles in on flap as shown *(see fig. 3)*.

9. Fold card in half and burnish with bone folder. Reopen card and fold left square half behind scalloped half.

10. Using craft glue, adhere the ½" (1 cm) flap to inside back of card *(see fig. 4)*.

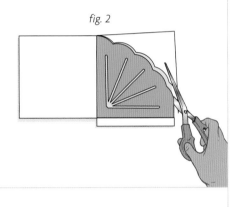

fig. 2

DIRECTIONS FOR THE INVITATION, DIRECTIONS, AND RSVP PAGES

1. Create a new document 4 ¾" (11.5 cm) square.

2. Set the type for your invitation and rotate text on a 45° angle *(we used 8 point Chaparral Display type on leading of 13 points)*.

3. Create a new page and set the type for your directions, rotating text on a 45° angle as well.

4. Create another new page and set the type for your RSVP, also rotating that text.

5. Print out invitation and directions onto the Obanai white laser paper and set aside.

6. Print the RSVP onto the white laser card stock.

7. Trim all edges of each page with scalloped paper edgers or rotary trimmer.

8. Place a postcard stamp on your RSVP card and handwrite your return address on it.

9. Stuff enclosure with all four sheets.

10. Fan out five dried flowers and join together at base by wrapping a piece of wire at base of bouquet.

11. Place dried flowers in enclosure.

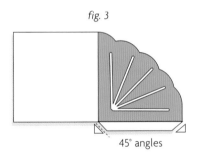

fig. 3

45° angles

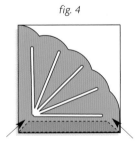

fig. 4

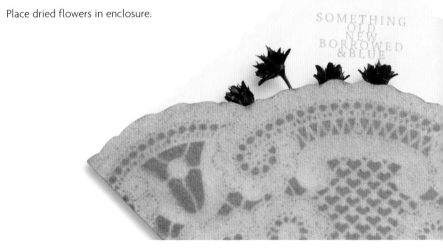

SOMETHING
OLD
NEW
BORROWED
&BLUE

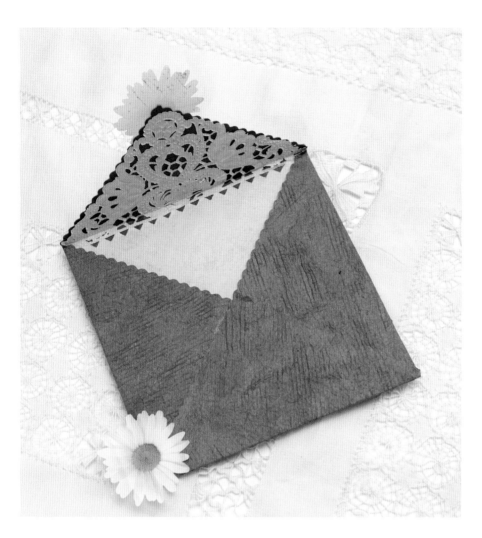

DIRECTIONS FOR THE ENVELOPE

1. Cut out an 8 ½" (22 cm) square of the decorative blue paper.

2. Spray adhesive on the back of one of the 8" (20 cm) square doilies and adhere to the blue paper.

3. Trim edges of the blue paper with the scalloped paper edgers or rotary trimmer with the scalloped attachment.

4. Fold in edges of lace doily and burnish edges with the bone folder.

5. Glue three edges with craft glue.

6. Place enclosure into envelope and seal with a daisy sticker.

7. Address the envelope with a white gel marker.

"Princely" Frog Invite

ASIAN-STYLE FROG ENCLOSURE

MATERIALS

20" × 28"
(51 cm × 71 cm)
decorative
Chinese-style paper

5" (13 cm) square
white petal envelope

red Chinese
frog closure

salmon-colored laser
or inkjet card stock

spray adhesive

craft knife

metal ruler

sewing needle

red thread

bone folder

personal computer

page layout software
(such as Quark or
PageMaker)

color printer

Small pieces of gorgeous paper and some braided frogs (those twisted pieces of shiny cord) are all you need to transform a simple petal envelope into a classic and elegant invitation enclosure. Choose coordinating paper and frogs, but don't go too matchy-matchy; contrast within the realm of coordination will make the frog stand out. When finished, this invitation makes a dazzling impression of sophistication; so if you're secretly hoping to keep attendance numbers down, don't send this invitation—people won't be able to resist the event that goes with this card.

This invitation is a great way to use the wide array of handprinted, or otherwise gorgeous, papers. Why decide on just one pattern? Use the papers that appeal to you and avoid the difficult decision of choosing just one.

DIRECTIONS FOR THE ENCLOSURE ENVELOPE

1. Place the Chinese paper decorative side down on your work surface and cut it down to 12" (30 cm) square.

2. Spray adhesive on the nondecorative side of the paper and adhere to the front of the petal envelope. Burnish entire surface by rubbing the bone folder across the surface several times.

3. Trim around petal edges with craft knife *(see fig. 1)*. Cut off two of the petals *(see fig. 2)* and put aside. Fold in remaining petals and burnish to make edges crisp.

TIP *You can make several layers to go into the enclosure. Make an RSVP card and a directions card and output onto the salmon-colored card stock.*

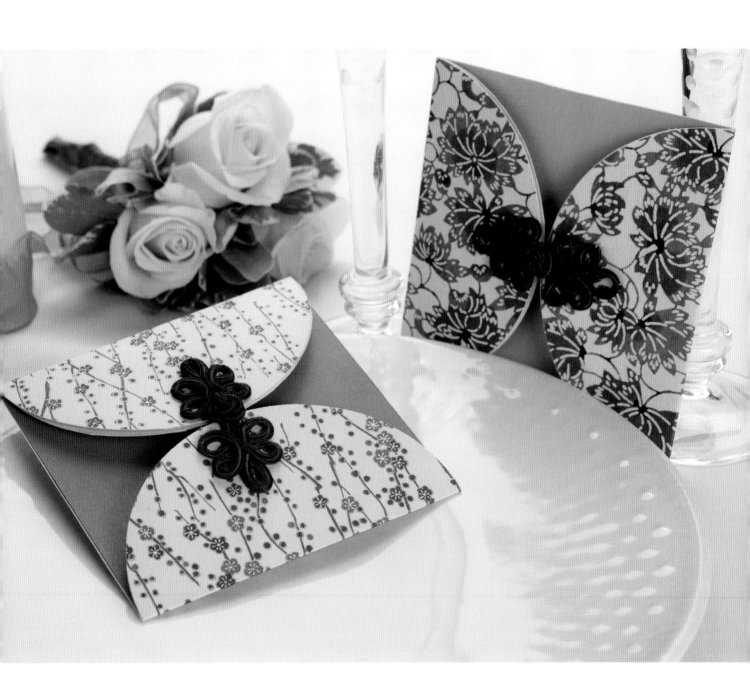

fig. 1

fig. 2

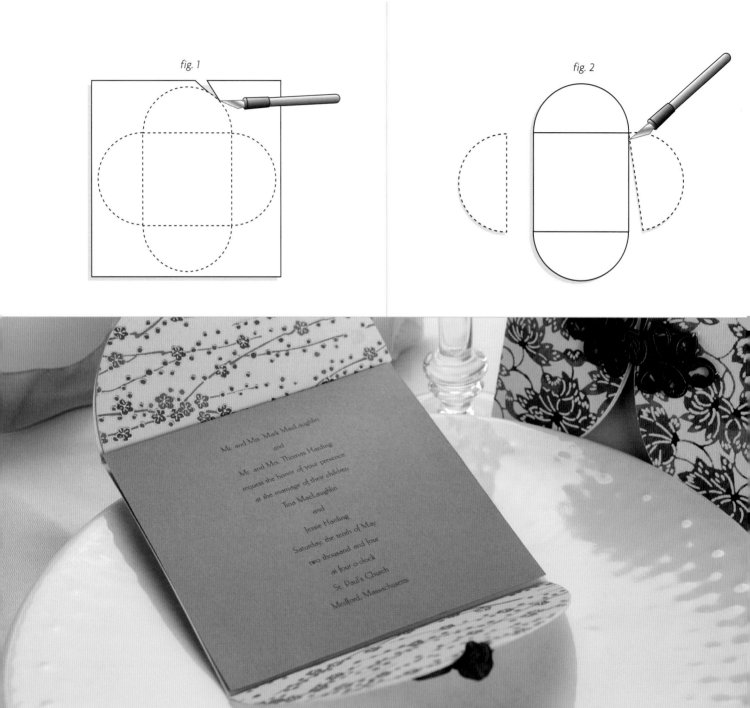

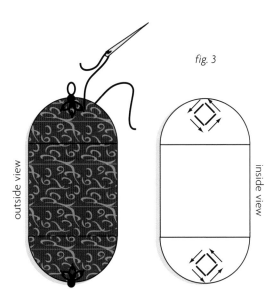

fig. 3

outside view

inside view

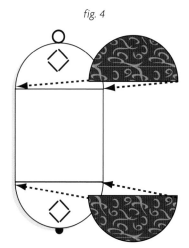

fig. 4

4. Sew frogs onto the front top and bottoms of the petal envelope *(see fig. 3)*, stitching in and out from plain to decorative sides of envelope.

5. Open enclosure and place decorative side down on your work surface.

6. Spray adhesive onto nondecorative side of the petals that had previously been put aside. Adhere petals to inside of enclosure, covering the nondecorative side with the sewn petals *(see fig. 4)*.

7. Cut any excess overlap away around petal shape.

DIRECTIONS FOR THE INVITATION

1. Create a new document in your page layout software that is 5 ¼" (13.5 cm) square.

2. Set the text for your invitation (we used 12 point Carlton Letter on leading of 22 points).

3. Print out onto salmon-colored card stock and trim so edges are flush with edges of closure.

4. Place into envelope.

VARIATION *If the petals do not cover your typography, consider making an invitation that folds in half with a blank cover and fits inside the petal enclosure.*

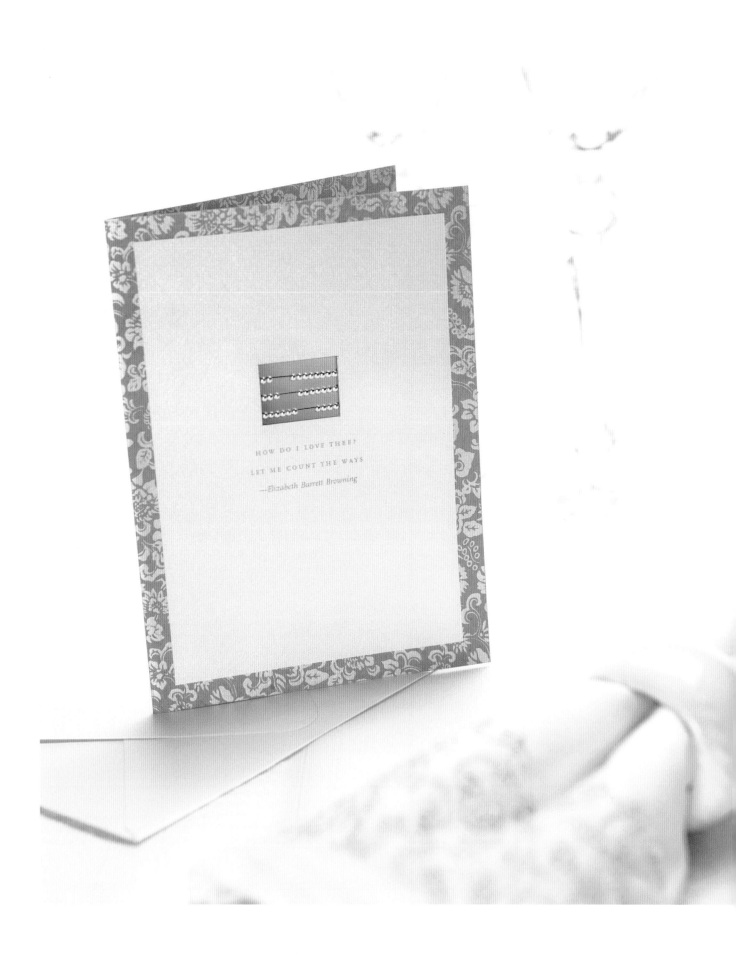

HOW DO I LOVE THEE?

LET ME COUNT THE WAYS

—Elizabeth Barrett Browning

Count Us In

ABACUS CARD

The light rattle of this elegant and poetic invitation gives people advance notice of something special as they open the envelope. This invitation is inspired by an abacus necklace engraved with the first words of Elizabeth Barrett Browning's evocative and love-filled poem. That necklace was given decades ago from a thoughtful man to his wife (Laura's father to her mother) and sweetly connects the traditional Chinese counting instrument with one of the best-loved poems in the English language. Here's a twist on that idea.

DIRECTIONS FOR CARD

1. With your favorite page layout software, create a 3 ¾" wide × 5 ½" deep (9.5 cm × 14 cm) document.

2. Draw a window 1" wide × ¾" deep (3 cm × 2 cm). Center horizontally on page and 1 ½" (4 cm) from top of page.

3. Set type under box "How do I love thee? Let me count the ways."—*Elizabeth Barrett Browning*. Quote is set in 8 point Scala caps type on leading of 17 points. Author's name is 8 point Scala Italic. Type color: 60 percent black.

4. Print document onto 8 ½" × 11" (22 cm × 28 cm) pearlescent cover stock and trim.

5. Using decorative paper, draw and cut out two rectangles 9" wide × 6 ¼" deep (23 cm × 15.5 cm).

6. Spray mount two sides together, decorative sides facing out, and fold in half width-wise, using a bone folder to score the edges.

7. Spray mount printed pearlescent sheet to front of card, centering within decorative rectangle.

8. Unfold and lay card flat facing up and cut out window.

MATERIALS

8 ½" × 11"
(22 cm × 28 cm)
pearlescent
cover stock

8 ½" × 11" (22 cm × 28 cm), or larger, sheet decorative paper

three 2"-long (5 cm) dressmaker's pins

adhesive tape

repositionable spray mount adhesive

personal computer

page layout program (such as Quark or PageMaker)

color printer

triangle

pencil

metal ruler

craft knife

bone folder

silver-colored seed beads

4 ¼" × 6 ½" (12 cm × 17 cm) pearlescent envelope

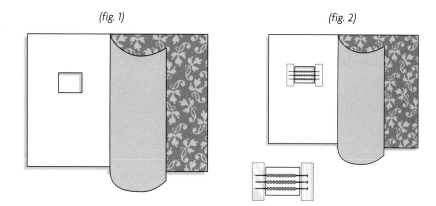

(fig. 1)   *(fig. 2)*

9. Flip card over so inside spread faces up. Temporarily pull apart the two decorative paper layers on left side of the card *(see fig. 1)*.

10. Take three straight pins and gather up ten seed beads onto each pin.

11. Place and center horizontally in cut-out window. Tape sides of pins to back of card and reposition decorative paper back over left hand side of the card *(see fig. 2)*.

12. Burnish with bone folder until all of the air bubbles have disappeared.

DIRECTIONS FOR INVITATION INSERT

1. With your favorite page layout software, create a new document 4 ½" wide × 6 ¼" deep (11 cm × 15.5 cm).

2. Set invitation type. Type should start roughly 3" (8 cm) down from top of page. Ours is set as follows: 8 point Scala caps on leading of 17 points. Type color: 60 percent black.

3. Print out on pearlescent paper and trim.

4. Insert in center of card.

5. Insert card in pearlescent envelope.

VARIATION *For a more translucent look, the invitation insert can also be printed on vellum (shown right), which comes in either laser or inkjet varieties. For best results, make sure the vellum matches your printer type.*

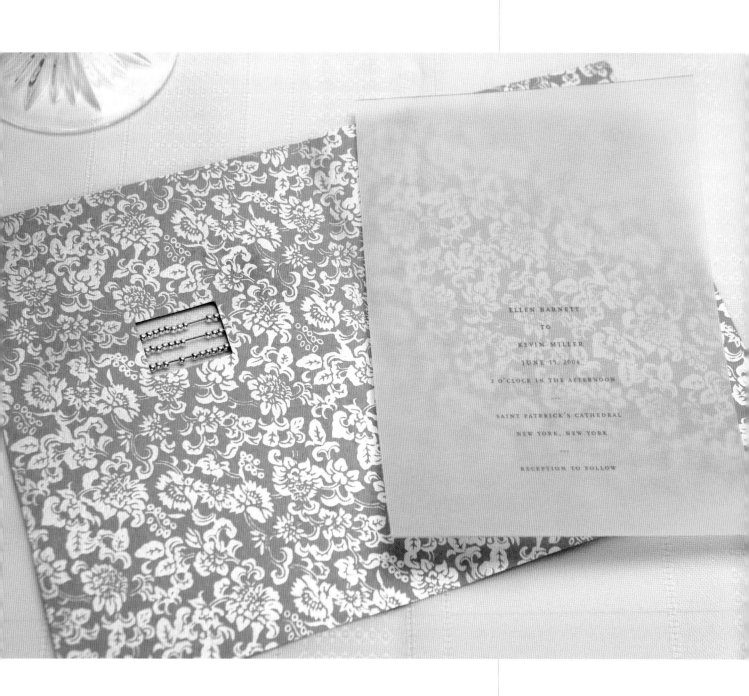

ELLEN BARNETT
TO
KEVIN MILLER
JUNE 15, 2004
2 O'CLOCK IN THE AFTERNOON
···
SAINT PATRICK'S CATHEDRAL
NEW YORK, NEW YORK
···
RECEPTION TO FOLLOW

All Zipped Up and Ready

ZIPPER-PULL PHOTO INVITATION

Two halves join together to become one entirely neat invitation. Print your picture on one side, your sweetheart's photo on the other, and sew on a zipper. Instead of sending an invitation that just sits there, yours can have moveable parts! You need not have latent punk rock tendencies or a pedigree in the fashion industry to use this invitation to great effect. The invitation card sits inside the zippered enclosure, waiting to be uncovered.

ZIPPER ENCLOSURE DIRECTIONS

1. Create a document in your page layout program 6 ¼" wide × 7 ⅛" deep (15.5 cm × 18.3 cm).

2. Import the digital photo into document and enlarge to fill the page.

3. Create a black strip down the center of the page ½" wide × 7 ⅛" deep (1 cm × 18.3 cm).

4. Print out page onto glossy photo paper and trim to size, also trimming center strip *(see fig. 1 on page 50)*.

5. Place photos about ⅛" (0.3 cm) to left and right sides of zipper and glue with the craft glue. Let it set for about 10 minutes.

6. Sew left and right sides of photo with red thread on sewing machine. Use the zipper foot on a sewing machine to get as close as you can to the zipper edge.

7. Cut out a rectangle of the black card stock 11 ¾" wide × 7 ¼" deep (29.3 cm × 18.5 cm).

VARIATION *Fond of your campground courtship? Change the tag on the lanyard of the zipper. Or replace the pull tab with something else: a yin-yang symbol, a heart, a wedding bell, or your initials on a tag.*

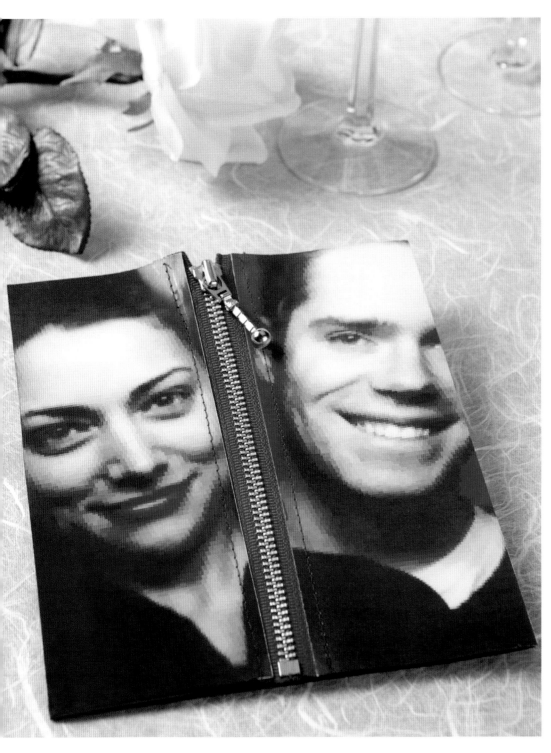

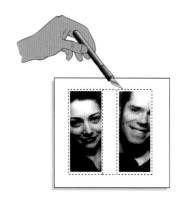

(fig. 1)

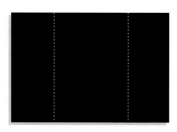

(fig. 2)

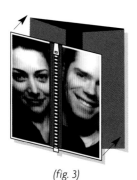

(fig. 3)

8. Draw pencil lines 2 ¾" (6.5 cm) in from ends of wide side of the paper *(see fig. 2)*.

9. Fold in at pencil lines and burnish with a bone folder at fold.

10. Use a glue stick to adhere front to backing as shown *(see fig. 3)*.

INVITATION INSERT DIRECTIONS

1. Create a document in your page layout program 5 ⅛" wide × 5 ¾" deep (13.3 cm × 14.5 cm).

2. Set type for invitation (we used 11 point AgencyFB-Light Wide on leading of 24 points. We set the red squares in 7 point Zapf Dingbats, letter "n" on leading of 24 points.)

3. Output from printer onto a sheet of the white text weight paper and trim.

4. Cut out a sheet of wavy red card stock 6" wide × 6 ¾" deep (15 cm × 17.5 cm).

5. Place printed white invitation on top of wavy red card stock and center.

6. Punch a hole through the two layers centering it left to right and 1" (3 cm) from the top of the wavy card stock.

7. Place silver grommet in hole and set with eyelet setting tool.

8. Insert invitation into zipper enclosure.

9. Slip into large red envelope.

RSVP DIRECTIONS

1. Create a document in your page layout program 4" wide × 2 ½" deep (10 cm × 6 cm).

2. Set type for "RSVP."

3. Print onto a sheet of the white text-weight paper and trim.

4. Cut out a sheet of wavy red card stock 4 ½" wide × 3" deep (11 cm × 8 cm).

5. Place printed white invitation on top of wavy red card stock and center.

6. Punch a hole through the two layers centering it left to right and 1" (3 cm) from the top of the wavy card stock.

7. Insert silver grommet in hole and set with eyelet setting tool.

8. Slip into small red envelope, stamp red envelope, and handwrite your address.

9. Place in larger red envelope behind invitation.

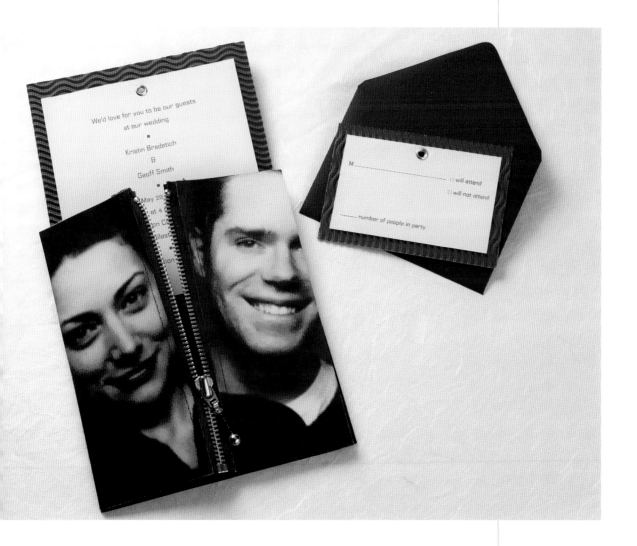

Christmas

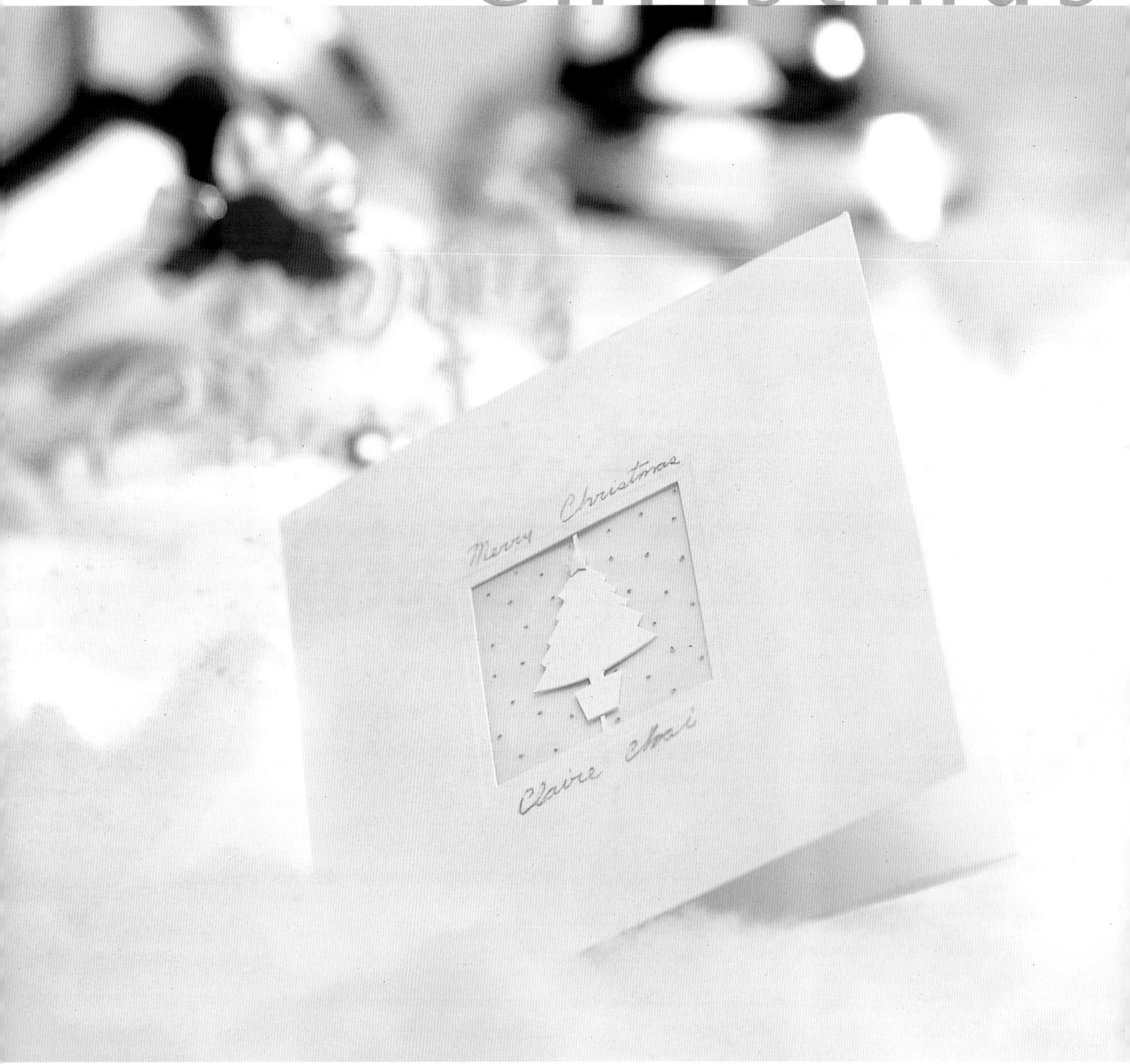

MATERIALS

white card stock,
  10" x 5" (25 cm x 12.5 cm)
white paper
tracing paper
PVA adhesive
metal ruler
silver gel pen
cutting mat
craft knife
tweezers

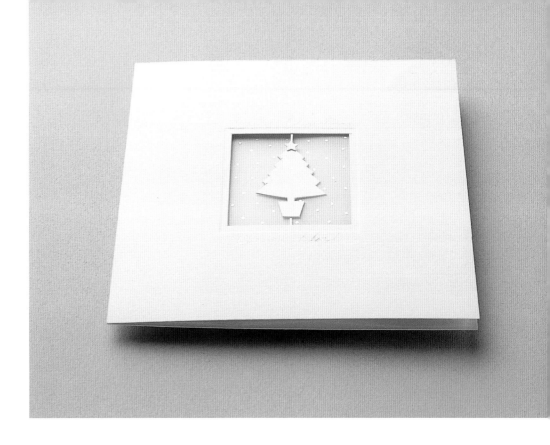

A Christmas Tree Covered by Snow

1. Make a card using the instructions for Pressing (p. 14) to make a 2" x 2" (5 cm x 5 cm) square and the instructions for Basic Window-Shaped Card I (p. 15) to make a 1⅘" x 1⅘" (4.5 cm x 4.5 cm) square window.

2. Reduce the Christmas tree pattern on page 275 by 50% and cut the shape out of white paper.

3. Attach a 2" x 2" (5 cm x 5 cm) square of tracing paper behind the front cover and embellish it by dotting with a silver gel pen.

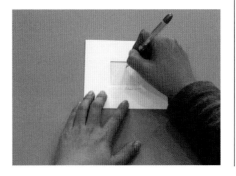

4. Attach a 2" (5 cm)-long paper ribbon vertically through the center of the window and attach the Christmas tree to the ribbon.

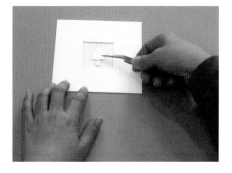

5. Use a silver gel pen to write "Merry Christmas" above the window and your signature below it.

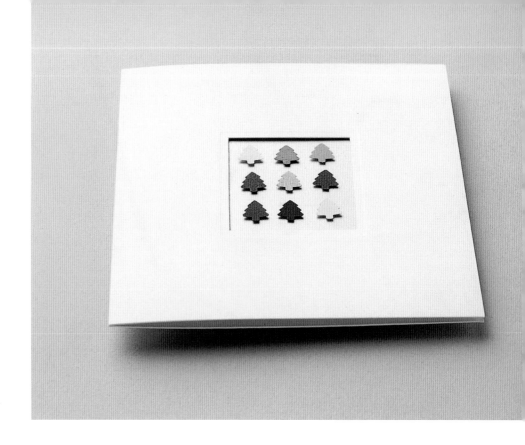

MATERIALS

white card stock,
  10" x 5" (25 cm x 12.5 cm)
red, orange, yellow, green, pale
  green, lavender, blue, dark
  blue, purple, and silver paper
tree punch
foam tape
metal ruler
cutting mat
craft knife
tweezers

Christmas Trees

1. Make a card using the instructions for Pressing (p. 14) to make a 2" x 2" (5 cm x 5 cm) square and the instructions for Basic Window-Shaped Card I (p. 15) to make a 1⅕" x 1⅕" (4.5 cm x 4.5 cm) square window.

2. Cut one tree each out of red, orange, yellow, green, pale green, lavender, blue, dark blue, and purple paper (nine trees in total).

3. Cut out a silver 2¾" x 2¾" (7 cm x 7 cm) square and attach it to the back side of the front cover with foam tape.

4. Use foam tape and tweezers to attach the nine trees in a grid pattern to the silver square.

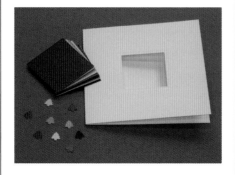

MATERIALS

red card stock,
   10" x 5" (25 cm x 12.5 cm)
silver, gold, green, red,
   and white paper
scissors
metal ruler
multicircle punch
small circle punch
paper-quilling needle
PVA adhesive
cutting mat
craft knife
punch wheel
tweezers

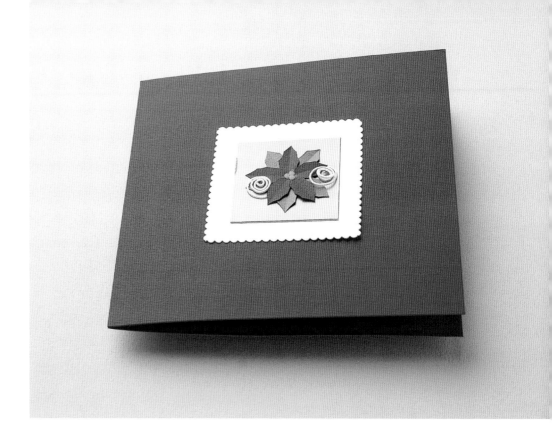

Poinsettia

1. Cut a 2¼" x 2¼" (6 cm x 6 cm) square out of silver paper with decorative-edge scissors.

2. Cut a 1⅗" x 1⅗" (4 cm x 4 cm) square out of gold paper.

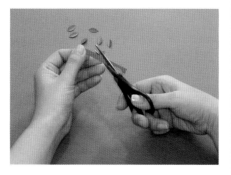

3. Fold red paper in half and draw five half poinsettia petals on it. Do the same with green paper and cut out all the petals.

4. Use PVA adhesive to attach the five green flower petals in a circle arrangement. Attach the five red petals between the green petals.

5. Attach the gold square to the silver square and then the silver square to the center of the red card stock.

6. Punch out three ¹⁄₁₀" (2 mm) green circles and attach them to the center of the poinsettia. Wind two thin, white paper ribbons around a paper-quilling needle and attach them to the poinsettia.

Love

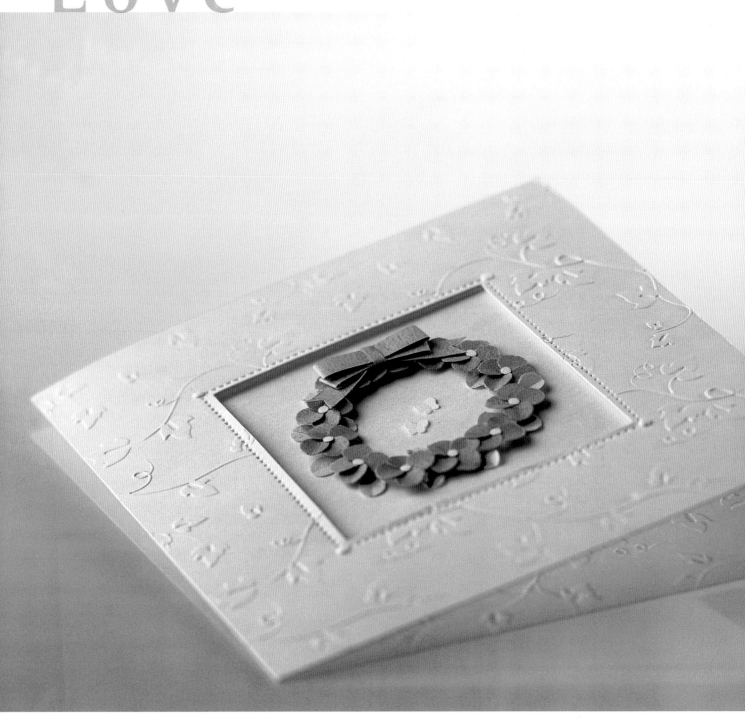

MATERIALS

ivory card stock with
  embellished surface,
  10" x 5" (25 cm x 12.5 cm)
three purple paper ribbons,
  ¹⁄₁₀" x 2" (2 mm x 5 cm)
pink-purple, blue-purple, pale
  green, yellow, and white paper
scissors
large flower punch
multicircle punch
butterfly punch
foam tape
PVA adhesive
⅕" (6 mm) circle punch
cutting mat
craft knife
corkboard
punch wheel
tweezers

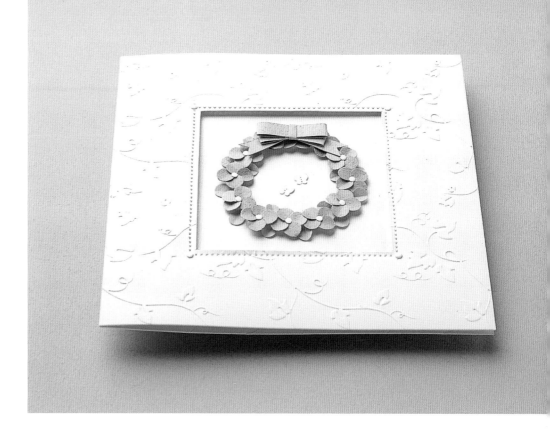

Purple Flower Garland

1. Make a card using the instructions for Basic Window-Shaped Card I (p.15) to make a 2½" x 2½" (6.5 cm x 6.5 cm) square out of ivory paper with embellished surface and use a punch wheel along the edges of the window.

2. Punch thirty ⅕" (6 mm) circles out of pink-purple and blue-purple papers and twelve ¹⁄₁₀" (2 mm) circles out of yellow paper.

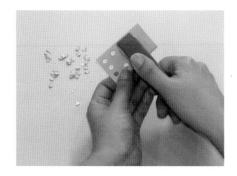

3. Attach four ⅕" (6 mm) circles in a circle with tweezers to make six pink-purple flowers and six blue-purple flowers.

Attach the yellow circles to the centers of the flowers.

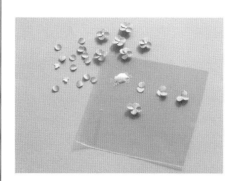

4. Punch two flowers out of pale green paper and cut apart the petals to be used as leaves.

5. Using the photo for reference, take a strip of purple paper and fold each end into the center to make a ribbon shape. Make another ribbon shape and stack the two ribbons together. Bind them with a strip of paper across the center. Trim the extending ends into a fish tail shape. (See the pattern on page 275.)

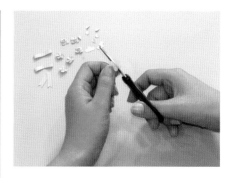

6. Mark a 1⅗" (4 cm) circle guideline on a white 3⁹⁄₁₀" x 3⁹⁄₁₀" (10 cm x 10 cm) square and use foam tape to attach the twelve pink-purple flowers and the twelve blue-purple flowers along the circular line.

7. Attach the ribbon to the top of the flower garland. Punch two butterflies out of yellow paper and attach them in the center of the wreath.

8. Attach the white rectangle with the wreath to the window on the back side of the cover.

MATERIALS

white card stock,
   10" x 5" (25 cm x 12.5 cm)
lavender and pale blue paper
twelve pale blue paper ribbons,
   ¹⁄₁₀" x 2¾" (2 mm x 7 cm)
twelve lavender paper ribbons,
   ¹⁄₁₀" x 2¾" (2 mm x 7 cm)
four white paper ribbons,
   ¹⁄₁₀" x 2" (2 mm x 5 cm)
tracing paper
graph paper
metal ruler
spray adhesive
transparent tape
PVA adhesive
cutting mat
craft knife
tweezers

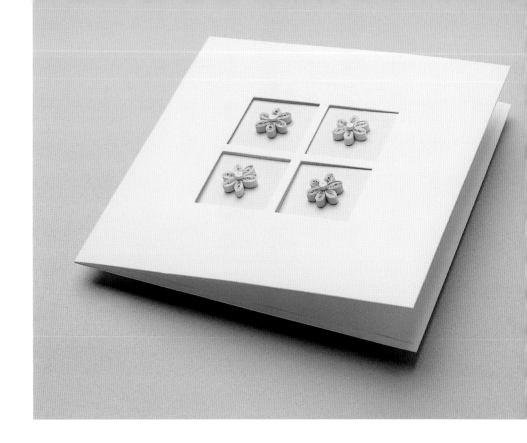

Window and Paper-Quilling Flowers

1. Make a card using the instructions for Basic Window Shape III (p. 17) and attach a tracing paper square behind the front cover. (See the pattern on page 271.)

2. Make four paper-quilling teardrop petal flowers using twelve lavender paper ribbons, twelve pale blue paper ribbons, and four white paper ribbons.

3. Design a 1⅖" x 1⅖" (3.5 cm x 3.5 cm) square on graph paper. Put it on lavender paper and trace it twice with an awl to make two squares. Do the same on pale blue paper.

4. Attach the four squares together with transparent tape to make a 2¾" x 2¾" (7 cm x 7 cm) square. Attach it to an interior paper with spray adhesive. (To attach it accurately, use a light box.)

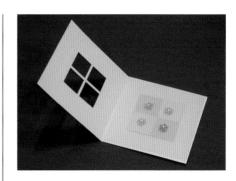

5. Use tweezers to attach the teardrop flowers to the center of each coordinating colored square.

MATERIALS

white card stock,
   10" x 5" (25 cm x 12.5 cm)
nine pieces of various
   colored paper
six paper ribbons of nine
   various colors,
   $\frac{1}{10}$" x 2$\frac{3}{4}$" (2 mm x 7 cm)
nine white paper ribbons,
   $\frac{1}{10}$" x 2$\frac{3}{4}$" (2 mm x 7 cm)
paper-quilling needle
metal ruler
spray adhesive
PVA adhesive
cutting mat
craft knife
tracing paper
tweezers

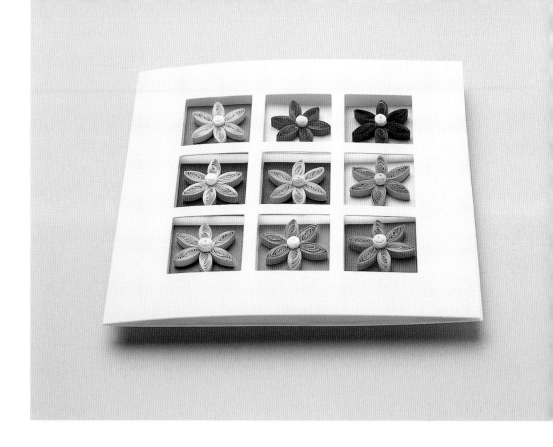

Beautiful Paper-Quilling Flowers

1. Make a card using the instructions for Basic Window-Shaped Card IV (p. 18) and attach a 4$\frac{9}{10}$" x 4$\frac{9}{10}$" (12.3 cm x 12.3 cm) square of tracing paper behind the front cover. (See the pattern on page 276.)

2. Make one 1" x 1" (2.5 cm x 2.5 cm) square out of each shade of paper, totaling nine squares.

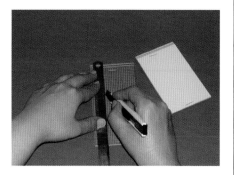

3. Put the nine squares on corrugated cardboard and apply spray adhesive.

4. Use tweezers to attach each of the nine squares to tracing paper in a grid pattern.

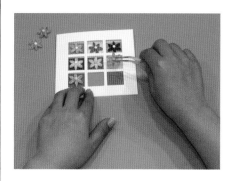

5. Make nine marquise petal flowers using each color of paper ribbon. (Each flower should have six same-color petals.) Make nine tight circles using white paper ribbon and attach them to the centers of the flowers.

6. Attach one flower to the center of each square.

MATERIALS

white card stock,
  10" x 5" (25 cm x 12.5 cm)
lavender, gray, yellow, dark jade,
  white, and pale blue paper
white corrugated board
flower punch
circle punch
metal ruler
multicircle punch
decorative-edge scissors
PVA adhesive
cutting mat
craft knife
spray adhesive

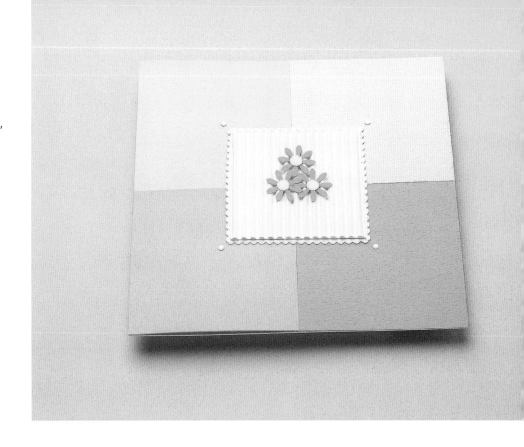

Flowers on Corrugated Cardboard

1. Cut four 2½" x 2½" (6.25 cm x 6.25 cm) squares out of lavender, gray, yellow, and dark jade paper and attach them to white card stock with spray adhesive.

2. Cut a 2" x 2" (5 cm x 5 cm) square out of white corrugated paper and attach it to white paper. Trim the edges of the white square with decorative-edge scissors to add a lace embellishment.

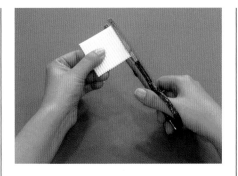

3. Punch out three pale blue flowers. Punch out three yellow circles and attach them to the centers of the flowers.

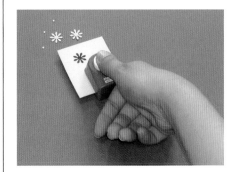

4. Attach the corrugated board square to the center of the card stock and attach the three pale blue flowers to it.

5. Make four small circles and attach them outside of each outer corner of the white squares.

MATERIALS

white card stock,
 10" x 5" (25 cm x 12.5 cm)
white, pale jade, lavender,
 and purple-pearl paper
butterfly punch
awl
multicircle punch
PVA adhesive
punch wheel
tweezers

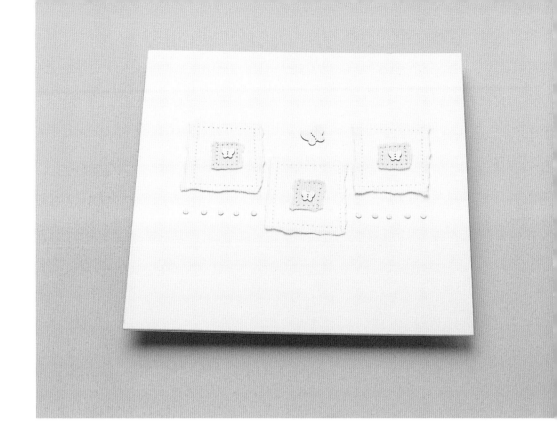

Butterflies and White Rectangle

1. Tear by hand three white 1⅕" x 1⅕" (3 cm x 3 cm) squares. Use a punch wheel to add a stitched appearance to the edges.

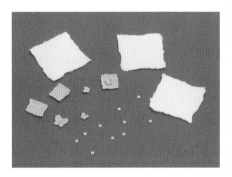

2. Repeat Step 1 to make three pale jade ⅖" x ⅖" (1 cm x 1 cm) squares. Attach these smaller squares to the centers of the white squares and attach the white squares to white card stock.

3. Punch out three small butterflies and one large butterfly. Attach the small butterflies to the centers of the pale jade

squares and the large butterfly to the white card stock.

4. Punch out ten ⅒" (2 mm) circles and attach them in two lines to the white card stock with tweezers.

Friendship

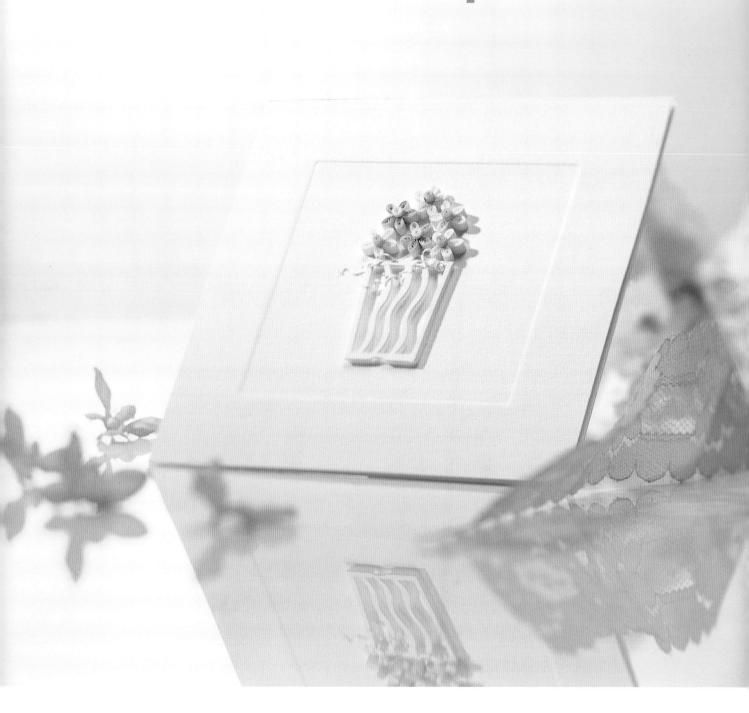

MATERIALS

white card stock,
  10" x 5" (25 cm x 12.5 cm)
fifteen white paper ribbons,
  $\frac{1}{10}$" x 2$\frac{7}{10}$" (2 mm x 5.5 cm)
ten pale blue paper ribbons,
  $\frac{1}{10}$" x 1$\frac{7}{10}$" (2 mm x 4.4 cm)
five pale yellow paper ribbons,
  $\frac{1}{10}$" x 1$\frac{1}{5}$" (2 mm x 3 cm)
foam tape
paper-quilling needle
PVA adhesive
cutting mat
craft knife
tweezers

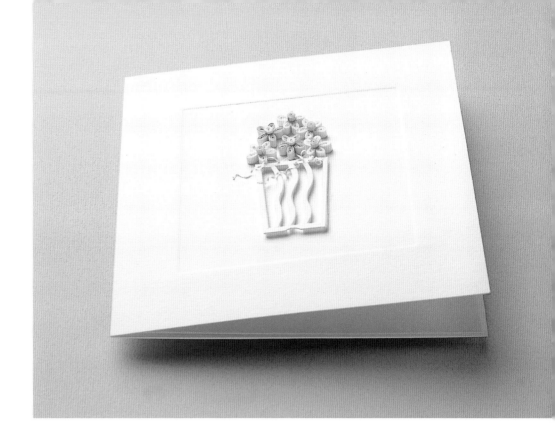

A Vase and Flowers

1. Make a card using the instructions for Pressing (p. 14).

2. Use the flower pattern on page 275 to cut a flowerpot out of white paper.

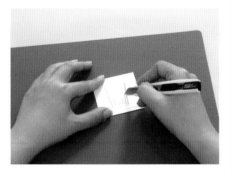

3. Make six teardrop petal flowers using white paper ribbons and ten pale blue paper ribbons. (Each flower should have five teardrop petals.) Make tight circles using pale yellow paper ribbons and attach them to the centers of the flowers.

4. Use thin foam tape and tweezers to attach the flowerpot and the five flowers to the front.

5. Make three creeper stems by winding white paper ribbons around a paper-quilling needle and attach them around the flowers.

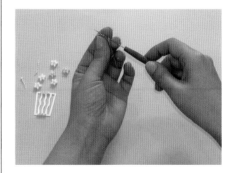

MATERIALS

white card stock,
  10" x 5" (25 cm x 12.5 cm)
pink and white crinkle paper
yellow, lavender, and jade paper
scissors
circle punch
spray adhesive
PVA adhesive
cutting mat
craft knife
tracing paper
tweezers
"Thank You" characters
  printed on tracing paper

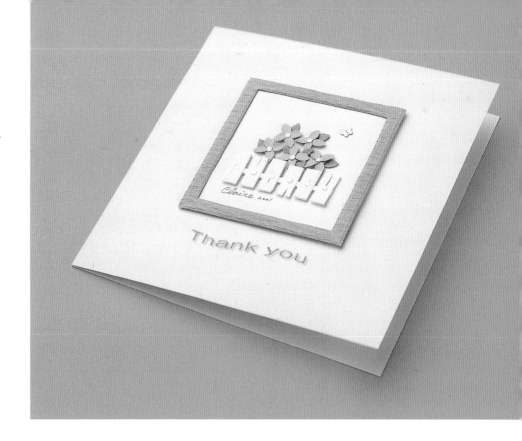

Fence and Flowers

1. Use spray adhesive to attach the "Thank You" tracing paper to the front of the card so that the words are at the bottom center.

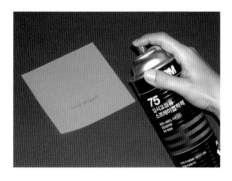

2. Cut a 2⅗" x 2⅗" (6.7 cm x 6.7 cm) frame (⅕" [6mm] wide) out of pink crinkle paper. Use an awl to mark lines along the outer edges of the rectangle and fold slightly along the marks to add a three-dimensional effect.

3. Fold lavender paper in half twice and punch out five circles. Fold jade paper in half twice and punch out a circle.

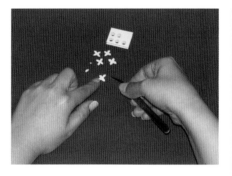

4. Stack four lavender circles together and cut them into a flower petal shape. Add a three-dimensional effect to the petals by curling them slightly with an awl.

5. Attach four petals together to make each flower and attach one yellow circle at the center of each.

6. Use the pattern on page 275 to cut six ⅕" x ½" (5 mm x 1.5 cm) fence posts out of white crinkle paper. Cut them partially up the centers to make them look more natural. Attach the white posts to a thin

1⅘" (4.5 cm)-long white paper strip to complete the fence.

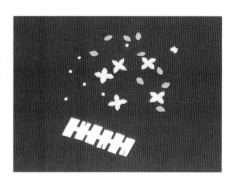

7. Attach the frame to the printed tracing paper with foam tape. Attach the fence, the five flowers, and the leaves in the center of the frame.

8. Punch out a butterfly and attach it inside the frame above the flowers.

MATERIALS

white card stock,
   10" x 5" (25 cm x 12.5 cm)
green, yellow, and red paper
six khaki paper ribbons,
   1/10" x 3 1/5" (2 mm x 8 cm)
white paper ribbon
foam tape
metal ruler
multicircle punch
PVA adhesive
decorative-edge scissors
cutting mat
craft knife
punch wheel
tweezers

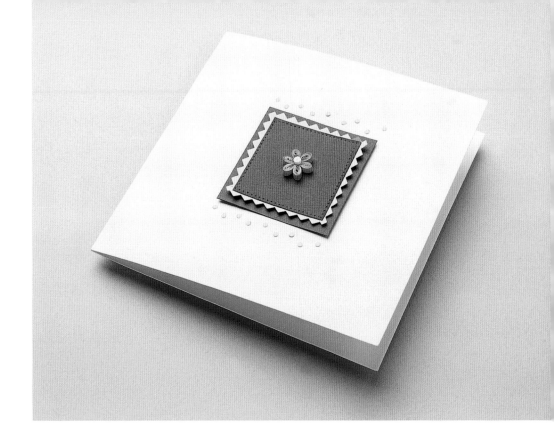

Flowers and Embellishment

1. Attach a red 1 3/5" x 1 3/5" (4 cm x 4 cm) square to yellow paper and trim the yellow edges with decorative-edge scissors.

2. Use a punch wheel along the outer edges of the red square to create a stitched appearance.

3. Attach the yellow square to a dark green 2" x 2" (5 cm x 5 cm) square with foam tape.

4. Attach the square to the front cover with foam tape.

5. Make one teardrop petal flower using six khaki paper ribbons. Make a tight circle using white paper ribbon and attach it to the center of the flower. Attach the flower to the center of the red square.

6. Punch sixteen 1/10" (2 mm) circles out of yellow paper and attach them in jagged lines to the upper and lower edges of the square.

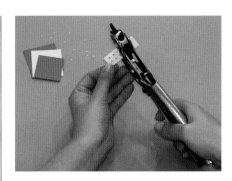

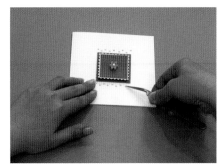

MATERIALS

white card stock,
  10" x 5" (25 cm x 12.5 cm)
yellow, white, gray, blue, purple,
  lavender, and jade paper
flower punch
foam tape
awl
PVA adhesive
tracing paper
punch wheel
tweezers

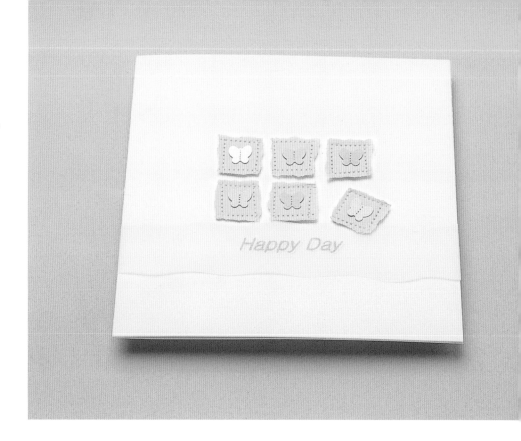

Butterflies on a Rectangle

1. Tear six ½" x ½" (1.5 cm x 1.5 cm) squares out of yellow paper and use a punch wheel to create a stitched appearance.

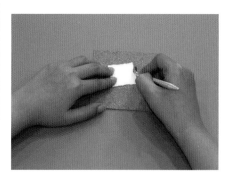

2. Punch six butterflies out of various colored paper and use an awl to poke lines down the centers of them.

3. Attach the butterflies to the squares with foam tape and attach the squares to white card stock in two lines of three squares each.

4. Print "Happy Day" characters on tracing paper with a computer printer. Cut the phrase out and attach it below the squares.

Thank You

Spring

MATERIALS

white card stock,
  10" x 5" (25 cm x 12.5 cm)
brown crinkle paper
purple, yellow, green,
  and jade paper
butterfly punch
wave-edge scissors
foam tape
awl
metal ruler
stapler
PVA adhesive
cutting mat
craft knife

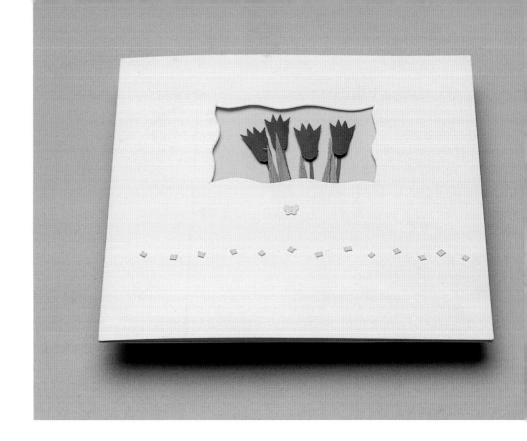

Purple Flowers and a Butterfly

1. Use the window pattern on page 276 to mark with an awl the shape to cut on white card stock.

2. Cut out the rectangle with a craft knife.

3. Cut a rectangle out of yellow paper with wave-edge scissors, making the rectangle ⅖" (1 cm) larger than the window in the card stock. Attach the yellow sheet to the interior card stock.

4. Cut four flowers out of purple paper using the pattern on page 276. Fold the flowers in half slightly to add a three-dimensional effect. Cut stems out of green paper and leaves out of jade crinkle paper.

5. Cut a flower vase out of brown crinkle paper. Slightly fold the vase down the center to add a three-dimensional effect.

6. Attach the purple flowers to the yellow rectangle with foam tape and then attach the stems, the leaves, and the vase.

7. Punch out a butterfly and attach it to the front of the white card stock. Cut fifteen small squares out of yellow paper and attach them to the white card stock in a jagged line.

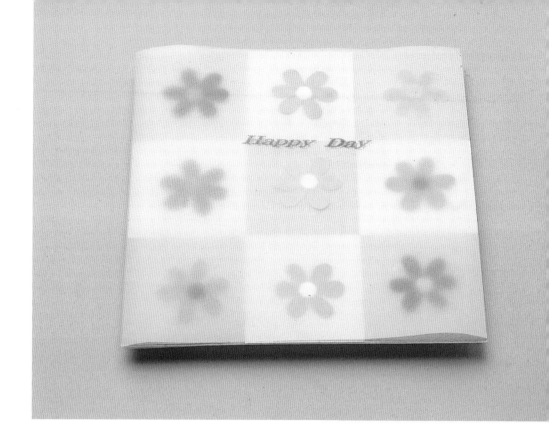

MATERIALS

white card stock,
  10" x 5" (25 cm x 12.5 cm)
pink, pale pink, orange, pale
  blue, purple, yellow, lavender,
  dark blue, dark purple, pale
  green, and dark green paper
scissors
metal ruler
spray adhesive
transparent tape
PVA adhesive
cutting mat
craft knife
tracing paper
tweezers

A Bundle of Flowers

1. Print "Happy Day" characters on tracing paper with a computer printer.

2. Stack together pink and pale pink papers. Trisect and cut them vertically and horizontally to make nine 1⅗" x 1⅗" (4.1 cm x 4.1 cm) squares on each paper. Arrange nine of the squares so that the colors alternate and attach them together with transparent tape.

3. Attach the checkered square to white card stock with spray adhesive.

4. Use the pattern on page 276 to cut out one flower each from orange, pale blue, purple, yellow, lavender, dark blue, dark purple, pale green, and dark green paper.

5. Cut out different colored circles and attach them to the centers of flowers.

6. Use tweezers to attach the nine flowers to each of the nine checkered squares on the front of the card.

7. Place the "Happy Day" tracing paper on top of the white card stock with a ⅖" (2 cm) overhang on the left side of the card. Fold the ⅖" (2 cm) overhang and attach it to the back side of the card stock with spray adhesive.

MATERIALS

white card stock,
  10" x 5" (25 cm x 12.5 cm)
yellow, green, pale green,
  orange, and white paper
decorative-edge scissors
foam tape
awl
metal ruler
PVA adhesive
corkboard
cutting mat
craft knife
punch wheel

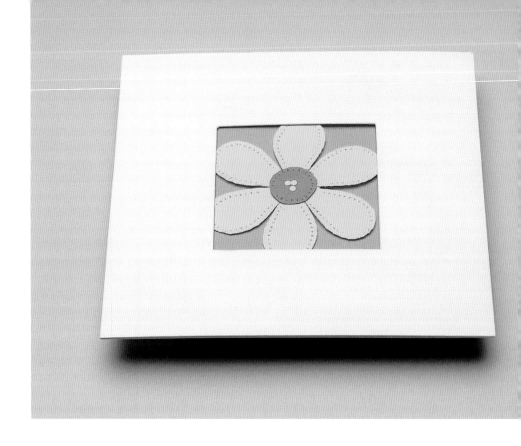

Yellow Spring Flowers

1. Make a card using the instructions for Pressing (p. 14) and Basic Window-Shaped Card I (p. 15).

2. Stack three pieces of yellow paper and cut out the teardrop pattern on page 276. Do the same once more to make six flower petals in total.

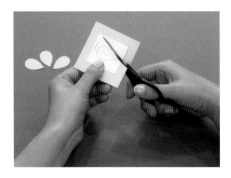

3. Cut a ⅖" (1 cm) circle and attach the flower petals to it with PVA adhesive and tweezers. Cut a ½" (1.5 cm) orange circle and press it slightly with an embossing tool to add a three-dimensional effect.

Attach the circle to the center of the yellow flower. Put the flower on corkboard and use an awl to add stitching around the edges of the center circle and each petal.

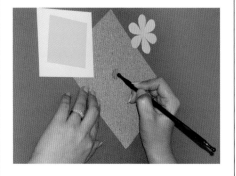

4. Make a 2½" x 2½" (6.5 cm x 6.5 cm) square out of green paper and attach it to pale green paper. Trim the pale green paper with decorative-edge scissors.

5. Attach an interior paper between the covers and attach the pale green square to it. Attach the flower to the center of

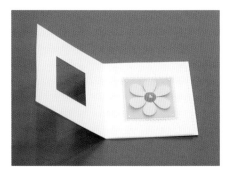

the pale green square with foam tape. Cut out small circles and attach three to the flower center and one to each corner of the green square.

MATERIALS

white card stock,
   10" x 5" (25 cm x 12.5 cm)
white, lavender, and purple paper
tracing pen
two ivory paper ribbons,
   ¹⁄₁₀" x 3 ¹⁄₅" (2 mm x 8 cm)
graph paper
cutting mat
craft knife
foam tape
awl
metal ruler
snowflake punch
multicircle punch
small flower punch
decorative-edge scissors
PVA adhesive
corkboard
punch wheel
tweezers

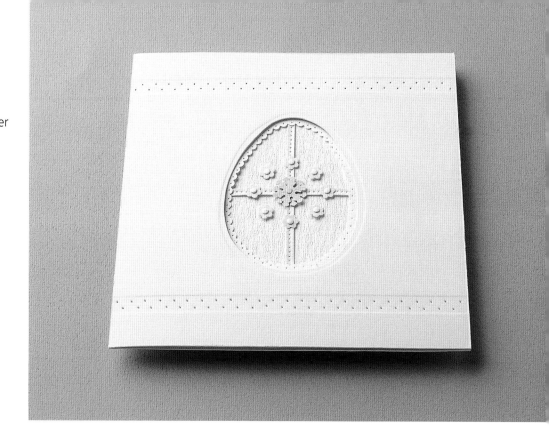

An Egg Embellished with Flowers

1. Use the pattern on page 276 to cut an egg-shaped window in white card stock. If you want to add a three-dimensional effect to the window, see Pressing (p. 14).

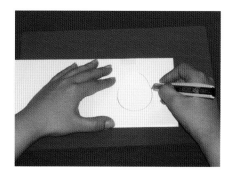

2. Put the egg-shaped piece on a white 3 ¹⁄₅" x 3 ¹⁄₅" (8 cm x 8 cm) square and trace the shape on it. Use decorative-edge scissors to cut out the egg just inside the traced line. Use an awl to poke the lace trim and attach the lace frame to the back side of the front cover.

3. Place a sheet of graph paper ½" (1.5 cm) below the upper line of the white card and mark dots with a ¹⁄₅" (5 mm) gap. Slide the graph paper down to create another row of dots offset from the first. Add a three-dimensional effect by pressing the opposite side of it with a tracing pen.

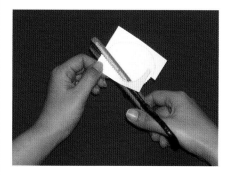

4. Use foam tape to attach a white 3 ⁹⁄₁₀" x 3 ¹⁄₅" (10 cm x 8 cm) rectangle behind the lace frame on the back side of the front cover.

5. Place two ivory paper ribbons on corkboard and roll a punch wheel up the center. Attach the ribbons in a cross shape at the center of the egg-shaped hole.

6. Punch out two snowflakes and stack them so they do not line up evenly. Punch out eight small flowers and attach them around the snowflake in the egg-shaped window.

Thank You
Summer, Autumn, Winter

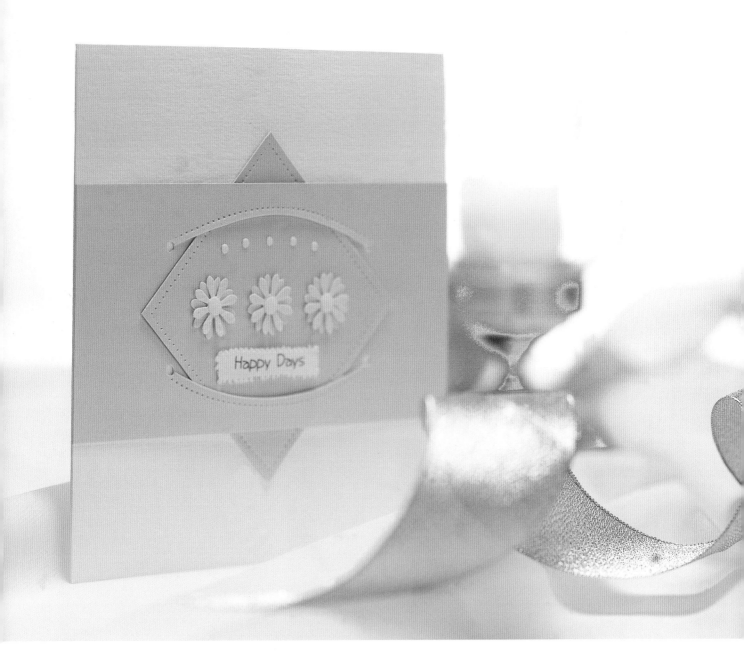

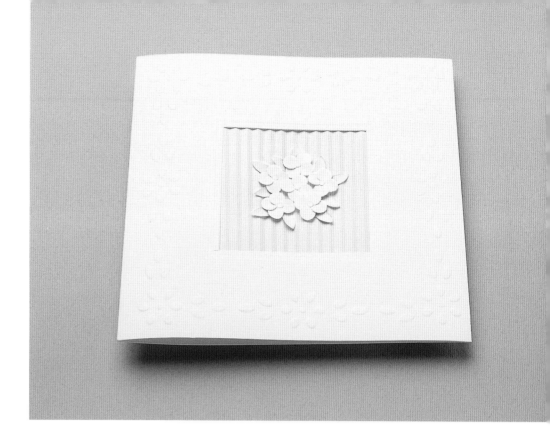

MATERIALS

white card stock,
  10" x 5" (25 cm x 12.5 cm)
pale green, white, and
  yellow paper
scissors
paper crimper
flower stencil pattern
circle punch
foam tape
metal ruler
PVA adhesive
cutting mat
craft knife

Cute White Flowers

1. Make a card using the instructions for Pressing (p. 14) and Basic Window-Shaped Card I (p. 15).

2. Put pale green paper through a paper crimper to make a corrugated effect on the surface and cut it into a 3⅕" x 3⅕" (8 cm x 8 cm) square.

3. Fold white paper in half twice and punch out a circle. Attach the four resulting circles together to make a white flower. Attach a small yellow circle at the center of the flower. Make five more flowers in the same manner.

4. Fold the yellow paper in half and cut out ten leaves.

5. Attach the pale green square to the back side of the front cover.

6. Attach one white flower to the center of the pale green square with foam tape and attach the other five flowers around the center flower. Attach the leaves around the flowers.

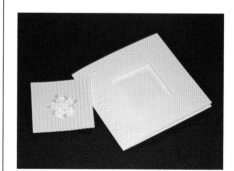

MATERIALS

white card stock,
  10" x 5" (25 cm x 12.5 cm)
white and yellow paper
scissors
PVA adhesive
cutting mat
craft knife
punch wheel
stapler

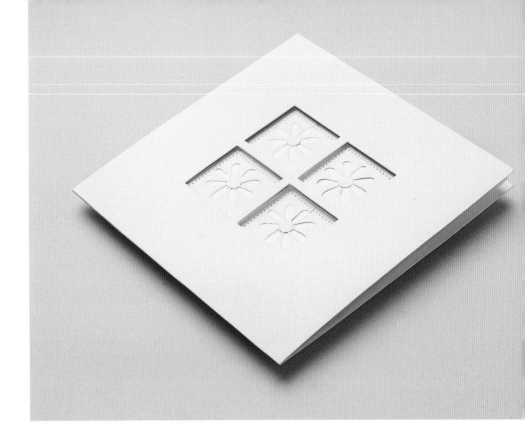

Yellow Flowers Behind a Window

1. Make a card using the instructions for Basic Window-Shaped Card III (p. 17). Attach tracing paper to the back side of the front cover.

2. Stack four pieces of white paper together, with the square and flower pattern from page 277 on top. Use a craft knife to cut the flowers out of the paper and then cut along the edges of the square. You should end up with four 1⅕" x 1⅕" (3 cm x 3 cm) squares with empty flower shapes in the centers.

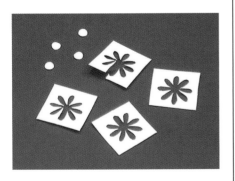

3. Use a punch wheel along the outer edges of the squares and attach yellow paper to the back sides of the squares with PVA adhesive. Cut out four white circles and attach them to the centers of the flowers.

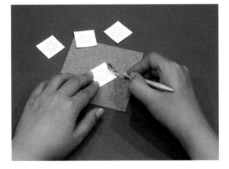

4. Attach the four squares to the interior paper with PVA adhesive, making sure they line up with the windows in the front cover.

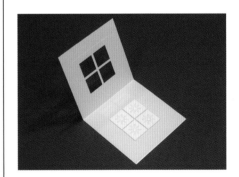

MATERIALS

white card stock,
  10" x 5" (25 cm x 12.5 cm)
white, bright green, lavender,
  yellow, pale blue, jade, and
  purple paper
flower punch
circle punch
foam tape
metal ruler
PVA adhesive
cutting mat
craft knife
tweezers

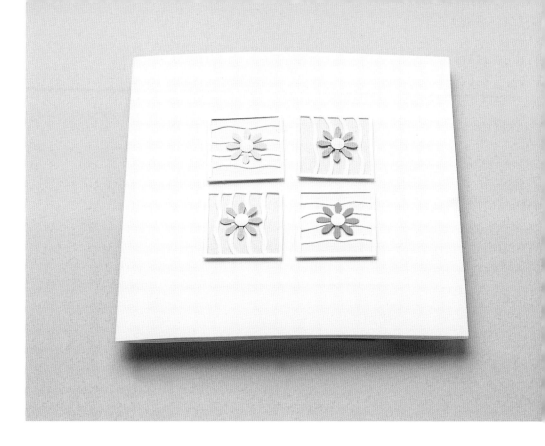

Flowers and Waves

1. Make a card using the instructions for Pressing (p. 14).

2. Copy the wave pattern on page 277 and place it on white paper. Use a craft knife to cut out the squares and the waves within each one.

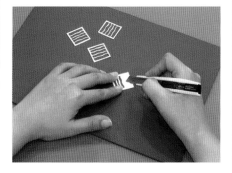

3. Make two 1" x 1" (2.5 cm x 2.5 cm) squares out of lavender and bright green paper and attach the squares to the back sides of the wave squares.

4. Punch four flowers out of the lavender, yellow, pale blue, jade, and purple paper. Attach the flowers to the centers of the wave squares.

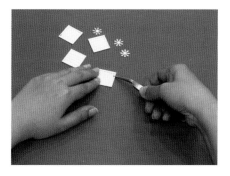

5. Attach the wave squares to the front cover with foam tape.

MATERIALS

- white card stock, 10" x 5" (25 cm x 12.5 cm)
- pale pink, pale blue, lavender, dark jade, and jade-pearl paper
- five white paper ribbons, $\frac{1}{10}$" x 1$\frac{4}{5}$" (2 mm x 4.5 cm)
- metal ruler
- stapler
- PVA adhesive
- cutting mat
- craft knife
- corkboard
- punch wheel
- awl

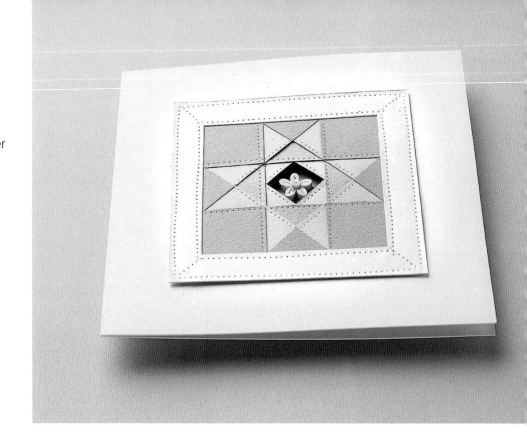

Patterns and Flowers I

1. Cut a 1$\frac{1}{5}$" x 1$\frac{1}{5}$" (3 cm x 3 cm) diamond out of white card stock.

2. Cut 3$\frac{9}{10}$" x 3$\frac{9}{10}$" (10 cm x 10 cm) squares out of pale pink, lavender, pale blue, and dark jade paper.

3. Make four copies of the quilt pattern on page 277 and attach it to each of the squares with a stapler. On the pale pink paper, use an awl to mark the points of the $\frac{1}{2}$" x $\frac{1}{2}$" (1.5 cm x 1.5 cm) diamond in the center of the pattern. On the purple paper, mark the points of the $\frac{2}{5}$" x $\frac{2}{5}$" (2 cm x 2 cm) square around the center diamond. On the pale blue paper, mark the points of the 1$\frac{1}{5}$" x 1$\frac{1}{5}$" (3 cm x 3 cm) diamond. On the dark jade paper, mark the points of the outer cross shape with the fish-tailed ends.

4. Remove the patterns and use a craft knife to cut the shapes out of each paper.

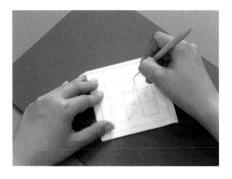

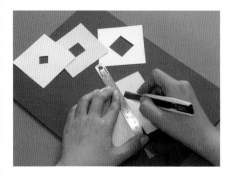

5. Layer the frames created in Step 4 starting with the pale pink frame and continuing each layer with the next largest shape. Use a punch wheel around the edges of each shape.

6. Cut a 3$\frac{3}{10}$" x 3$\frac{3}{10}$" (8.5 cm x 8.5 cm) frame ($\frac{2}{5}$" [1 cm] wide) out of jade-pearl and attach the frame on top of the completed piece made in Step 5.

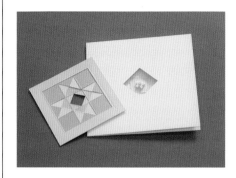

7. Attach the completed frame to the white card stock so that the pale pink cutout diamond is centered in the diamond cut out in Step 1.

8. Make a white teardrop petal flower using five white paper ribbons. Attach the flower to the interior page in the center of the diamond window.

MATERIALS

white card stock,
   10" x 5" (25 cm x 12.5 cm)
gray, jade, white, and
   pale green paper
thick white paper
flower punch
foam tape
metal ruler
multicircle punch
PVA adhesive
cutting mat
craft knife
punch wheel
tweezers

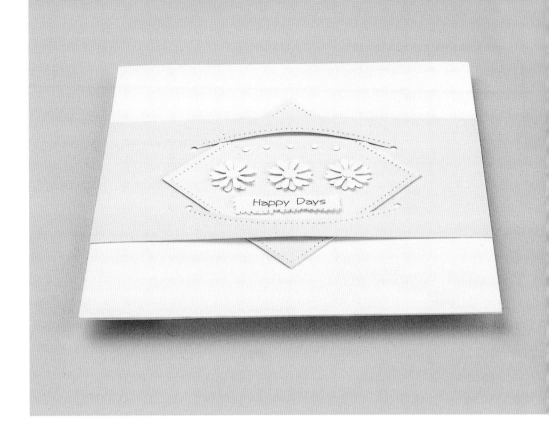

White Flowers on a Rectangle

1. Cut a 2¼" x 5" (6 cm x 12.5 cm) rectangle out of gray paper and attach to a piece of thick white paper of the same size. Use a multicircle punch to make a hole at a point ½" (1.5 cm) below the top edge and 1⅕" (3 cm) from the right edge. Make three other holes using the same measurements on the other edges of the rectangle. (See the pattern on page 277.)

2. Put the rectangle on a cutting mat and cut curved lines between the two holes on the top and the two holes on the bottom. Use a punch wheel to create a stitched appearance just above the top curved line and just below the bottom line.

3. Cut a 2¼" x 2¼" (6 cm x 6 cm) square out of jade paper and roll a punch wheel along the outer edges. Slide two corners of the square through the curved lines in the rectangle so the jade square is positioned as a diamond.

4. Punch out six large flowers. Attach two pieces together to make three flowers. Attach the flowers in a line to the center of the jade diamond. Make five ⅒" (2 mm) circles with a multicircle punch and attach them in a line above the flowers.

5. Print "Happy Days" characters with a computer printer. Use an awl to mark a rectangle around the phrase, roll a punch wheel over the lines, and then tear along the lines. Attach the rectangle below the flowers.

MATERIALS

white card stock,
   10" x 5" (25 cm x 12.5 cm)
red paper
twelve pink paper ribbons,
   ¹⁄₁₀" x 4¾" (2 mm x 12 cm)
six pale pink paper ribbons,
   ¹⁄₁₀" x 4¾" (2 mm x 12 cm)
three white paper ribbons,
   ¹⁄₁₀" x 2" (2 mm x 5 cm)
foam tape
awl
metal ruler
PVA adhesive
cutting mat
craft knife
corkboard
punch wheel
heart punch

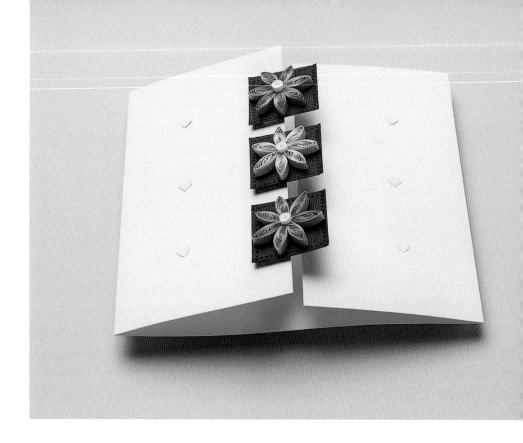

Three Paper-Quilling Flowers

1. Make a card using the instructions for Basic Card II (p. 12).

2. Cut three 1¹⁄₁₀" x 1¹⁄₁₀" (2.7 cm x 2.7 cm) squares out of red paper. Place the squares on corkboard and roll a punch wheel along the outer edges.

3. Make marquise petal flowers using seven pale pink paper ribbons and fourteen pink paper ribbons. Make tight circles using three white paper ribbons and attach them to the centers of the flowers.

4. Use foam tape to attach the left sides of the red squares to the left flap of the front cover. (The right sides of the squares will overlap the right flap of the cover.)

5. Attach flowers to the red squares. Punch six hearts out of pale pink paper and attach them in two vertical rows on the right and left flaps.

MATERIALS

jade card stock,
   10" x 5" (25 cm x 12.5 cm)
jade crinkle paper
orange, dark green, lavender,
   pale green, jade, and pale
   blue paper
gold gel pen
snowflake punch
foam tape
metal ruler
multicircle punch
decorative-edge scissors
PVA adhesive
punch wheel
tweezers

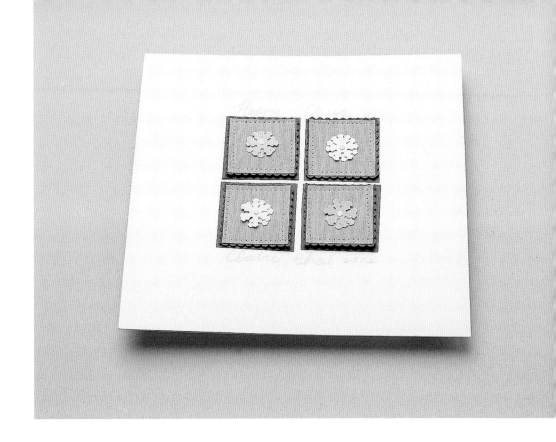

Patterns

1. Cut four 1" x 1" (2.5 cm x 2.5 cm) squares out of jade crinkle paper and roll a punch wheel along the edges.

2. Attach the jade squares to orange paper and use decorative-edge scissors to trim the orange paper, leaving a ¹⁄₂₀" (1 mm) margin. Attach the orange squares to dark green 1⅕" x 1⅕" (3 cm x 3 cm) squares with foam tape.

3. Punch two snowflakes out of lavender, pale blue, and jade paper and attach the matching color snowflakes together with

foam tape. Cut out four yellow circles and attach them to the centers of the snowflakes.

4. Attach the snowflakes to the jade squares and attach the completed squares to the white card stock. Use the gold gel pen to write a signature or message below the squares.

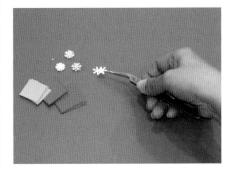

MATERIALS

jade card stock with
  embellished surface,
  10" x 5" (25 cm x 12.5 cm)
pale jade rice paper
white and pale yellow paper
four ivory paper ribbons,
  ¹⁄₁₀" x 2½" (2 mm x 6.5 cm)
foam tape
spray adhesive
metal ruler
small flower punch
PVA adhesive
cutting mat
craft knife
corkboard
large flower punch
punch wheel
tweezers

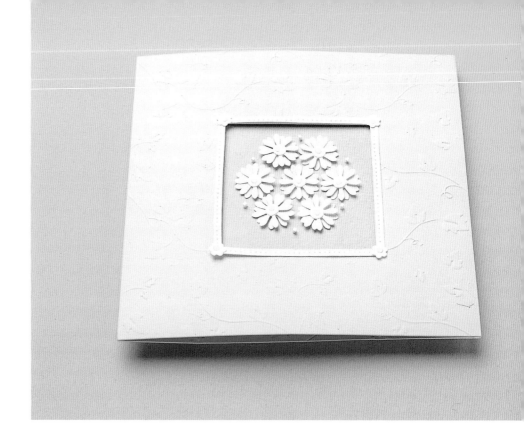

Daisy

1. Make a card using the instructions for Basic Window-Shaped Card I (p. 15).

2. Place four ivory paper ribbons on corkboard and roll a punch wheel up the center. Attach the ribbons to the edges of the window, overlapping each other at the corners.

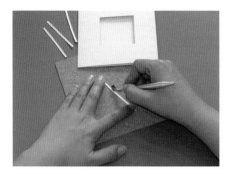

3. Punch out four white flowers with a small flower punch and attach them to the corners where the ribbons meet.

4. Punch out fourteen white flowers with a large flower punch. Attach two flowers together with foam tape and add white and yellow circles to the center to make a daisy. Repeat this process for a total of seven daisies.

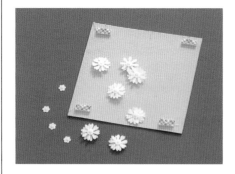

5. Apply spray adhesive to the back side of the front cover and attach a 3⁹⁄₁₀" x 3⁹⁄₁₀" (10 cm x 10 cm) square of pale jade rice paper.

6. Attach one daisy to the center of the square window and arrange the other six daisies around it.

7. Place white paper on foam tape and cut small rectangles out of it. Attach the small rectangles between the six outer daisies.

MATERIALS

white card stock,
  10" x 5" (25 cm x 12.5 cm)
thick white paper
lavender paper
tracing paper
white translucent fabric ribbon,
  3⅕" x 2¼" (8 cm x 6 cm)
star punch
metal ruler
spray adhesive
PVA adhesive
cutting mat
craft knife

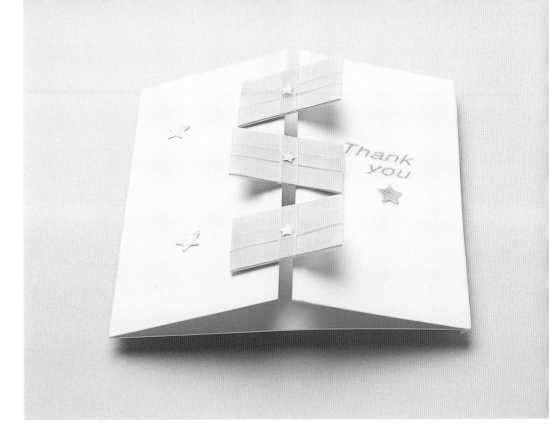

A Wrapped Gift Box

1. Make a card using the instructions for Basic Card II (p. 12).

2. Print "Thank you" characters with a computer printer and use spray adhesive to attach it to the right flap of the card cover.

3. Attach lavender paper to thick white paper and cut three 1⅒" x 1⅗" (2.7 cm x 4 cm) rectangles out of it.

4. Attach 1⅒" x 2¾" (2.7 cm x 7 cm) tracing paper rectangles to the lavender

rectangles so that there is a ⅟₂₀" (1 mm) margin on each end. Fold the margins and attach them to the back side of the lavender rectangles.

5. Use PVA adhesive to attach white fabric ribbon horizontally and vertically to the lavender rectangles. Punch out stars and attach them to the center points where the ribbons overlap.

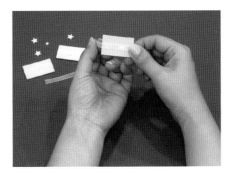

6. Attach the right side of one rectangle to the right cover flap. Attach the left sides of the other rectangles to the left cover flap above and below the center rectangle.

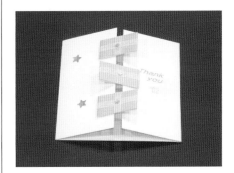

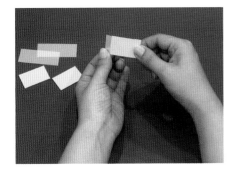

MATERIALS

white card stock,
  10" x 5" (25 cm x 12.5 cm)
thick white paper
bright green and lavender paper
four white paper ribbons,
  ⅕" x 4¾" (6 mm x 12 cm)
four bright green paper ribbons,
  ¹⁄₁₀" x 4¾" (2 mm x 12 cm)
metal ruler
butterfly punch
yellow highlighter
PVA adhesive
cutting mat
craft knife

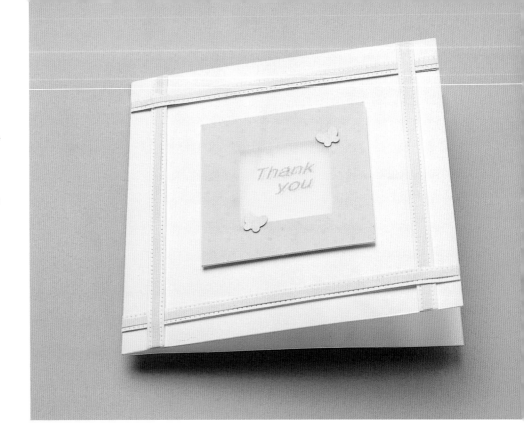

Butterflies and a Frame II

1. Print the "Thank you" characters on tracing paper with a computer printer.

2. Attach one bright green paper ribbon to each of the white paper ribbons, then attach the four ribbons along the outer edges of white card stock with PVA adhesive.

3. Attach bright green paper to thick white paper and cut a 2½" x 2½" (6.5 cm x 6.5 cm) square out of it. Cut a smaller 1⅕" x 1⅕" (3 cm x 3 cm) square from the 2½" x 2½" (6.5 cm x 6.5 cm) square.

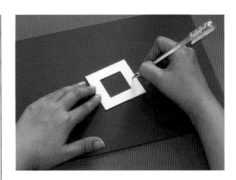

4. Use a yellow highlighter to make dots on the bright green frame. Cut a 2½" x 2½" (6.5 cm x 6.5 cm) square around the "Thank You" characters and attach it on top of the frame.

5. Punch out two butterflies and attach one to the upper part of the frame and one to the lower part of it.

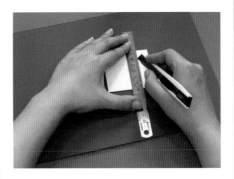

MATERIALS

white card stock,
   10" x 5" (25 cm x 12.5 cm)
gold, pale green, and
   dark green paper
twenty-six white paper ribbons,
   ¹⁄₁₀" x 4¾" (2 mm x 12 cm)
one pale green paper ribbon,
   ¹⁄₁₀" x 1⅕" (2 mm x 3 cm)
gold gel pen
foam tape
metal ruler
small flower punch
cutting mat
craft knife

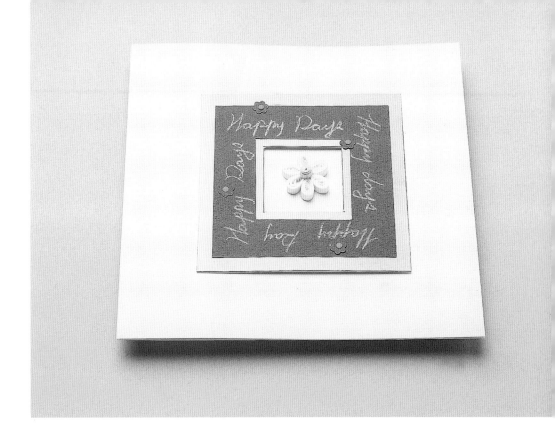

A White Flower in a Frame

1. Cut a 1⅖" x 1⅖" (3.5 cm x 3.5 cm) square out of a dark green 2½" x 2½" (6.5 cm x 6.5 cm) square to create a frame. Attach it to a gold ⅕" x 3" (5 mm x 7.5 cm) rectangle.

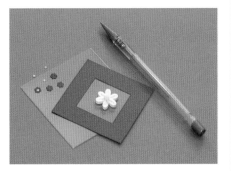

2. Trim the gold paper from the center of the frame, leaving a ¹⁄₁₀" (2 mm) margin.

3. Write "Happy Day" with a gold gel pen on each side of the frame.

4. Make a teardrop petal flower using white paper ribbons.

5. Use foam tape to attach the frame to the center of white card stock and attach the paper-quilling flower to the center of the frame. Make a tight circle using pale green paper ribbon and attach it to the center of the white flower.

6. Punch four small flowers out of dark green paper. Cut small circles out of pale green paper and attach them to the centers of the punched flowers. Attach the flowers to the frame.

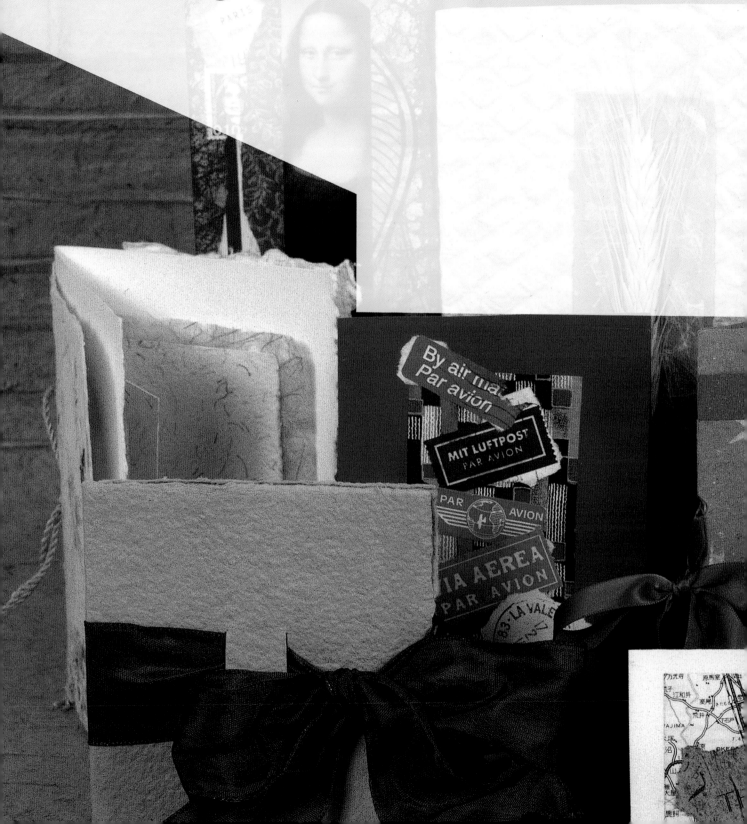

C·o·l·l·a·g·e C·a·r·d·s

*U*sing your imagination — and a little glue — you can create a card featuring a paper collage customized for any occasion. Collage combines texture, color, and shape to achieve a balanced visual presentation. The colors, patterns, and textures of your papers will inspire the basic design. Enhance the card with objects from your everyday travels or color photocopies of your favorite images, photographs, or postcards to add a personal touch. For a travel theme, incorporate maps, stamps, and postcards. Use dried flowers and handmade papers for a soft, natural effect. To add texture and to achieve a festive feeling, weave ribbon through slits in the card. Layer papers to create a multipaged card that holds a special message in the innermost layer. The possibilities are almost endless and depend on the occasion, the recipient, and the materials you have available.

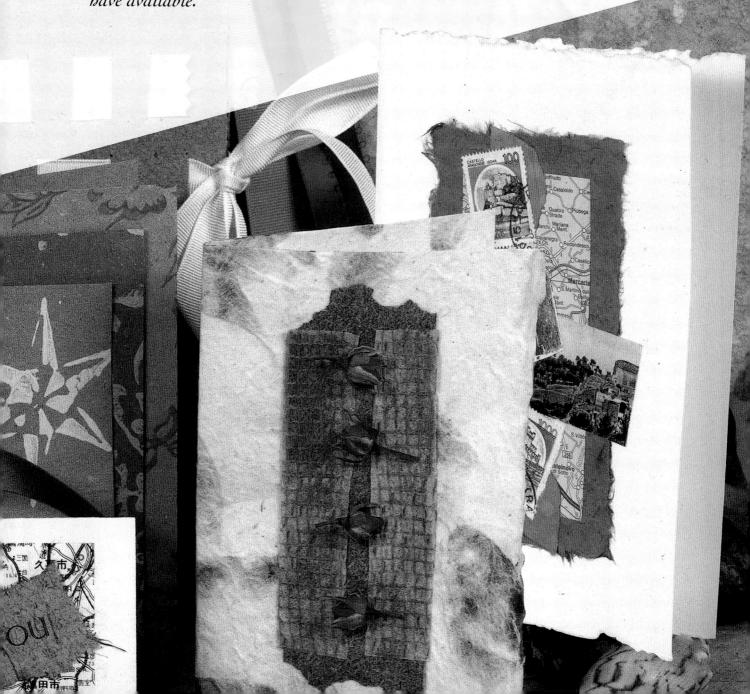

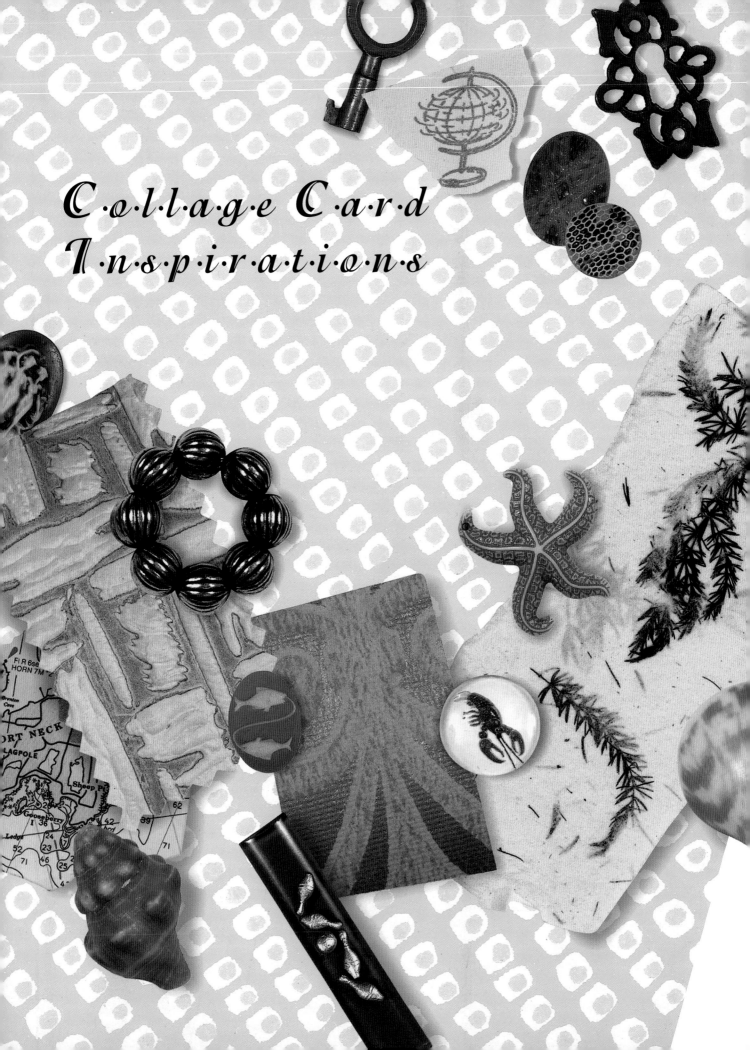

Collage Card Inspirations

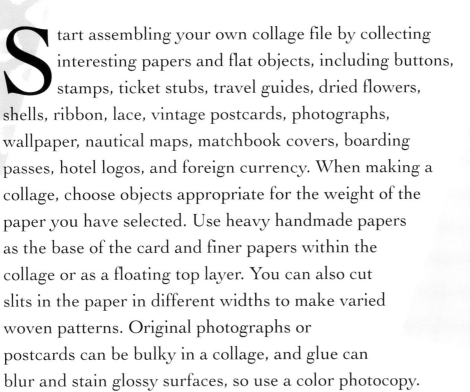

S tart assembling your own collage file by collecting interesting papers and flat objects, including buttons, stamps, ticket stubs, travel guides, dried flowers, shells, ribbon, lace, vintage postcards, photographs, wallpaper, nautical maps, matchbook covers, boarding passes, hotel logos, and foreign currency. When making a collage, choose objects appropriate for the weight of the paper you have selected. Use heavy handmade papers as the base of the card and finer papers within the collage or as a floating top layer. You can also cut slits in the paper in different widths to make varied woven patterns. Original photographs or postcards can be bulky in a collage, and glue can blur and stain glossy surfaces, so use a color photocopy.

Weave dried flower stems, paper strips, fabric, plastic, wood, or wire through slits in your card.

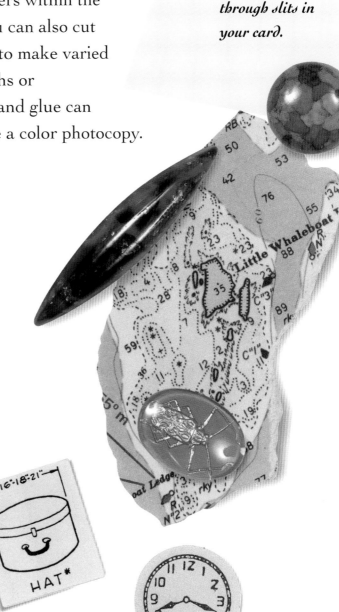

A n easy way to get started is to buy pre-cut blank cards. These can be found at stationery or art supply stores. You will have a larger selection of color and textured papers, however, if you create your own card base from the paper you have on hand.

Travel Collage

Collect items related to a destination. Arrange the collage pieces first to help determine the color and weight of the paper. Begin with more collage elements than you may actually use. Glue the smaller elements together before attaching them to the card. Pick coordinating colors from the map to use for the collage papers. Center the background paper and map on the card. Then layer the torn paper and photo, followed by the stamps and travel motif.

Materials

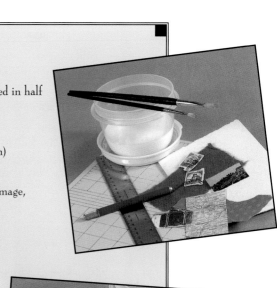

- Piece of heavyweight paper, 10" x 7" (25 cm x 18 cm), folded in half
- Piece of background paper, 3" x 5" (8 cm x 13 cm)
- Piece of map, 2" x 4" (5 cm x 10 cm)
- Piece of decorative paper, torn to 4½" x 1" (11 cm x 2.5 cm)
- Two postage stamps
- Color photocopy of a postcard, magazine, or photographic image, 2" x 1" (5 cm x 2.5 cm)
- Travel motif (i.e., suitcase, airplane, train, building, statue)
- Craft knife
- Metal ruler
- PVA glue
- Glue brush
- Cutting mat

❖*1* Apply glue with a brush to the back of the background paper, stroking from the center of the paper out to the edges. Do not use too much glue or it will wrinkle and stain the card. Adhere each layer to the card firmly before applying the next layer.

❖2   Center the background paper on the heavyweight paper with a 1" (2.5 cm) border on all sides, and adhere it to the front of the card. Place the paper down gently at first in case you need to adjust it. Press the paper flat with your fingers, starting at the center and moving out to the edges.

❖3   Apply glue to the back of the map. Center it on the background paper, and adhere it. To avoid bubbling, press the paper down from the center out to the edges.

❖4   Apply glue in a band that is approximately ⅛" (.3 cm) wide to the front left side of the postcard, magazine, or photographic image. Adhere the image to the center of the right side of the torn paper strip to create a unit.

❖5   Apply glue to the back of the torn paper strip and postcard, magazine, or photographic image. Cover the entire surface, including the edges. Center the unit and adhere it to the map, so that the top and bottom edges of the torn paper extend beyond the map.

❖6   Apply glue to the back of the travel motif, and adhere it to the center of the torn paper strip, overlapping the postcard, magazine, or photographic image.

❖7   Apply glue to the back of the stamps. Position one at the top left corner of the map, overlapping the torn paper and the edge of the map. Place the other at the lower left corner of the map on top of the torn paper. Make sure all edges of both stamps are firmly glued.

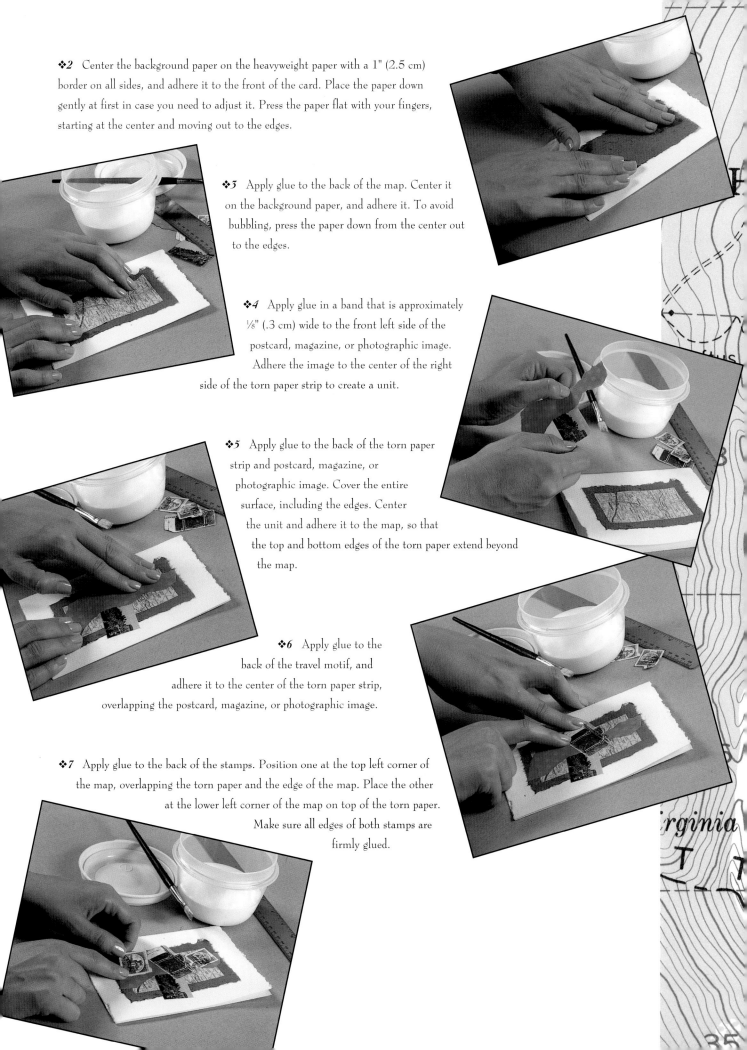

Dried Flower Collage

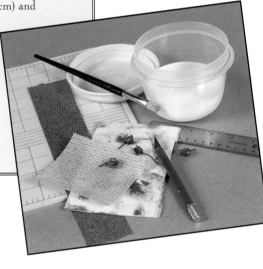

H andcrafted papers made with dried herbs and flowers are ideal for this project because the texture is as important as the collage elements. Apply two textured papers to a base card, add roses, scent the card with rose oil, and send it to a friend. Wrapping the finished card in tissue or lightweight paper protects the flowers and adds a nice surprise when the envelope is opened.

Materials

- Piece of handmade paper with pressed flowers or leaves, 8" x 6" (20 cm x 15 cm), folded in half
- Two pieces of textured paper, 3 ½" x 4" (8.5 cm x 10 cm) and 1 ¾" x 4 ½" (4.5 cm x 11 cm)
- Miniature dried roses or other small dried flowers
- Craft knife
- Metal ruler
- PVA glue
- Glue brush
- Cutting mat

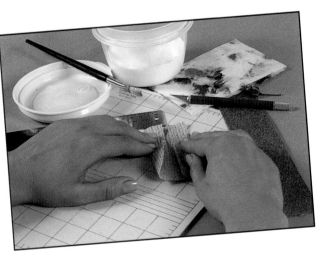

❖*1* Lay the piece of 3 ½" x 4" (9 cm x 10 cm) textured paper flat on the work surface. Measure ¾" (2 cm) from the left edge and make a fold. Measure ¾" (2 cm) from the right edge and make a fold.

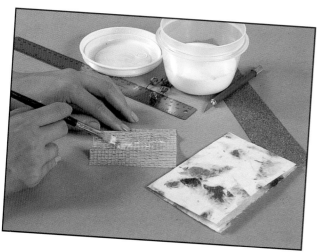

❖*2* Apply glue to the back of the textured paper in the center panel only (between the folds). Be careful not to apply glue over the folded edges, as it will show on the finished side of the panel.

❖*3* Center the panel on the front of the card and adhere it. Press firmly

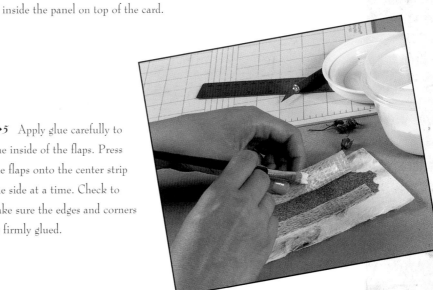

along the folded edges to create a flap on each side. If any of the flowers in the handmade paper fall off, stick them back on with a dab of glue.

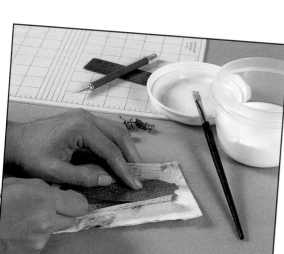

❖*4* Create a ragged edge on each end of the strip of 1 ¾" x 4 ½" (4.5 cm x 11 cm) textured paper by tearing no more than ¼" (.5 cm) from the top and bottom edges. Glue this strip inside the panel on top of the card.

❖*5* Apply glue carefully to the inside of the flaps. Press the flaps onto the center strip one side at a time. Check to make sure the edges and corners are firmly glued.

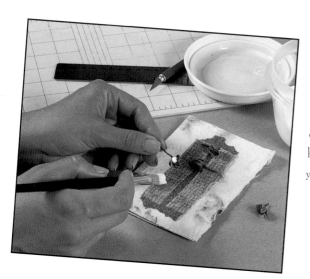

❖*6* Apply a small dab of glue to a flower and gently place it on the center strip. Hold the flower with your finger for a minute until the glue sets. Space the flowers evenly down the center strip. Dried flowers are brittle and often crumble, so handle them gently and always have a few more than you think you need.

Woven Ribbon Collage

Create an elegant card by weaving paper and ribbon. Use stiff paper so the card will not sag from the weight of the ribbon. Cut slits in the card using the ribbon and paper strips as a guide. Weave the ribbon and paper strips through the slits, and glue the paper to the back of the card. Add a surprise by tying the ribbon in a bow.

Materials

- Piece of heavyweight or printmaking paper, 6" x 8" (15 cm x 20 cm), folded in half
- Piece of ½" to 1" (1 cm to 2.5 cm) cloth ribbon, 30" (76 cm) long
- Assorted handmade paper scraps, ¾" x 7" (2 cm x 18 cm) each
- Masking tape
- Pin, push pin, or sewing needle
- Craft knife with extra blades
- Metal ruler
- Pencil
- PVA glue
- Glue brush
- Cutting mat

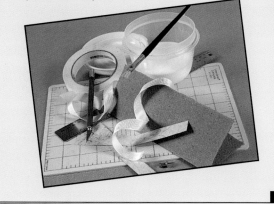

❖1 Open the card flat and secure the edges with masking tape. Lay the ribbon horizontally across the middle of the card. Tape one end of the ribbon to the work surface. Pull it taut to make it straight, then tape the other end. Using a pin to mark the distance, measure ½" (1 cm) in from both sides of the card along the top and bottom edges of the ribbon. From those points, measure and mark four 1" (2.5 cm) intervals along the edges of the ribbon.

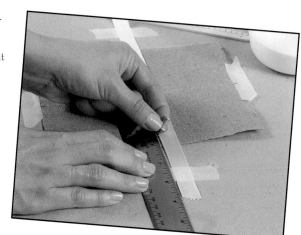

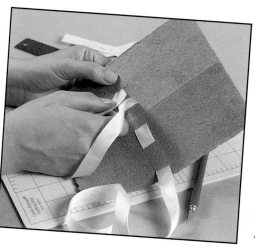

❖2 Carefully remove the tape and the ribbon. Place the card flat on the cutting mat. With the metal ruler, align the pin holes vertically. Slowly cut slits from top to bottom, using the tip of the craft knife along the edge of the ruler. For clean, precise slits, use a new blade. Cut both ends of the ribbon on a diagonal. Use one end to thread the ribbon through the slits.

❖3 Place the card on your work surface. Measure ½" (1 cm) above and below the edges of the ribbon. Mark the spots lightly with the pencil. Place two ¾" (2 cm) paper strips horizontally on the ½" (1 cm) marks above and below the ribbon. Secure the ends with tape so the strips will not move.

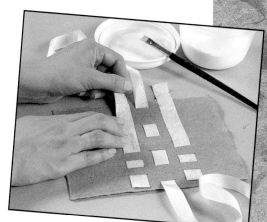

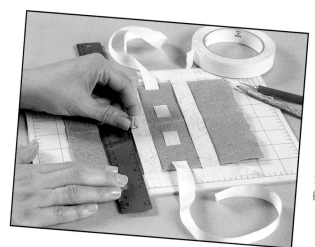

❖4 Measure and mark with the pin 1" (2.5 cm) from the right edge of the card at the top and bottom edges of the paper strips. Then make holes at ½" (1 cm) intervals along the edges of the paper strips only as far as the folded edge of the card.

❖5 Remove the tape and the paper strips. Open the card flat on the cutting mat. With the metal ruler, align the pin holes vertically. Slowly cut slits from top to bottom, using the tip of the craft knife along the edge of the ruler.

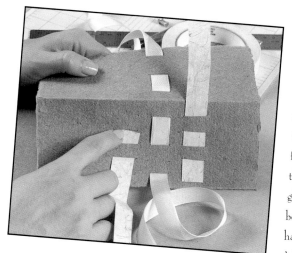

❖6 Weave the paper strips through the slits above and below the ribbon. The edges of the paper strips should extend about ¼" to ½" (.5 cm to 1 cm) beyond the front right edge of the card. Apply glue to the back of the paper strips from the fold to the left edge of the card. Be careful not to apply glue beyond the edge of the card because that piece of the strip will hang over the edge of the card. Adhere the strips to the back of the card.

Lavishly Layered Card

T his design highlights the beauty of handmade
paper. Use four different textures or colors to
create a theme. Cut the papers to different sizes,
fold them, and bind them together. Do not make the holes on the fold too
large or the layers will be loose. If the ribbon is too wide, fold it in half lengthwise and use pliers to pull it
through. Complete the card by writing a special message on the innermost page or even a single word on
every layer.

Materials

- Piece of handmade flower paper, torn to 8 ½" x 5 ¾" (21 cm x 14.5 cm)
- Piece of heavyweight or printmaking paper, 9" x 6 ¼" (23 cm x 16 cm)
- Piece of colored lace paper, 8" x 5" (20 cm x 13 cm)
- Piece of handmade or textured writing paper, torn or cut to 4" x 7" (10 cm x 18 cm)
- Cord, string, or thin ribbon for binding
- Toothpick, knitting needle, or awl
- Craft knife
- Metal ruler
- Pencil
- Bone folder
- Cutting mat

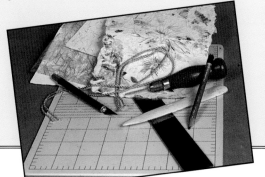

❖1 Fold each paper in half separately in the following way:
Take the top left corner of the paper and fold it over to the top right corner,
matching the corner edges exactly; holding the edges together with your right
hand, make a small crease at the top left edge with your left hand; press with your
thumb firmly to crease the fold. If any edges are not even, carefully trim them
with the ruler and knife.

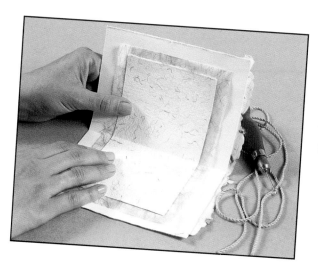

❖*2* Lay the 8 ½" x 5 ¾" (21.5 cm x 14.5 cm) handmade paper flat on the work surface. Place the 9" x 6 ¼" (23 cm x 16 cm) sturdy paper on top of it. Center the 8" x 5" (20 cm x 13 cm) lace paper on top of the sturdy paper. Then center the 4" x 7" (10 cm x 18 cm) handmade paper on top of the lace paper. Stack the fold lines directly on top of each other.

❖*3* Open all the layers, center them, and hold them in place. From the top of the outermost paper, measure 2" (5 cm) down the card on the fold line and mark lightly with the pencil. From the bottom of the outermost paper, measure 2" (5 cm) up the card on the fold line and mark lightly with the pencil.

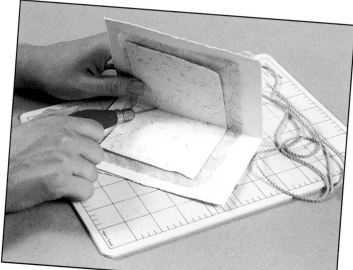

❖*4* Fold the card halfway shut, holding all the layers together. With the sharp tool (toothpick, knitting needle, or awl), puncture a small hole through the marks on the fold line. Make sure you go through all the layers before you remove the tool.

❖*5* Thread the ribbon through the holes, starting from the inside of the card. Use the sharp object to help thread it through. Tie the ribbon in a knot or bow along the spine of the card.

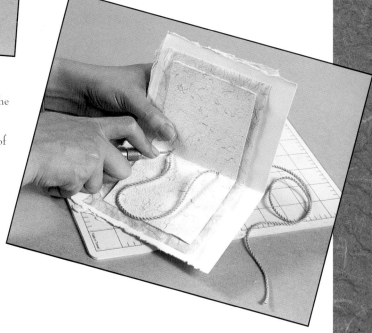

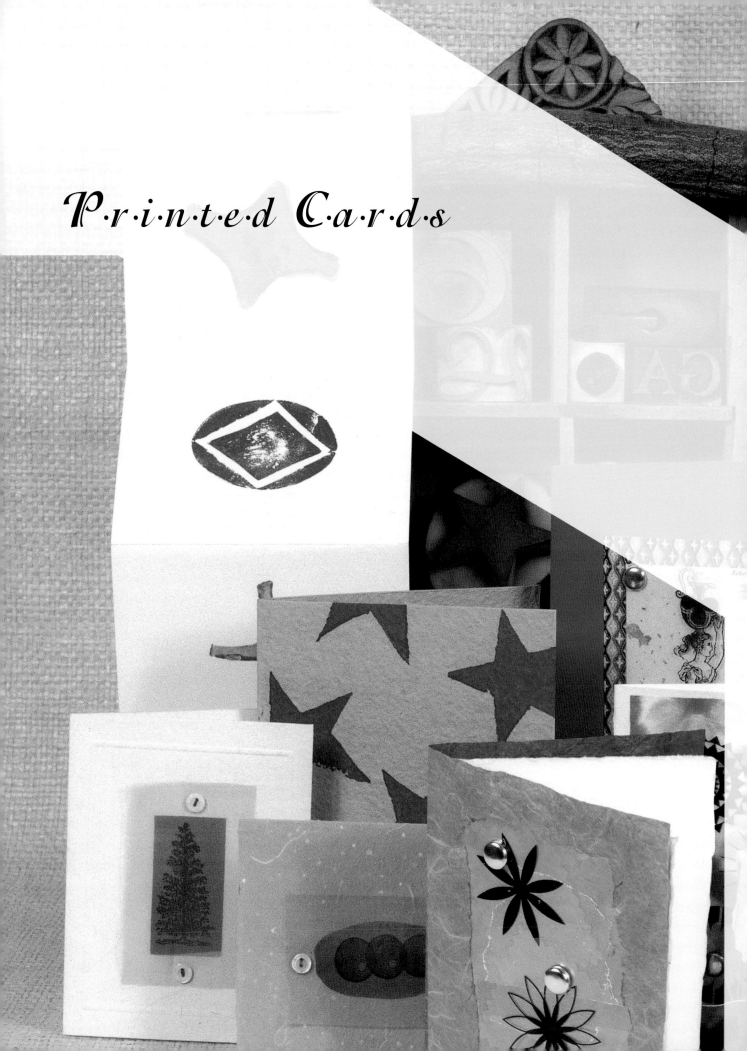

P·r·i·n·t·e·d C·a·r·d·s

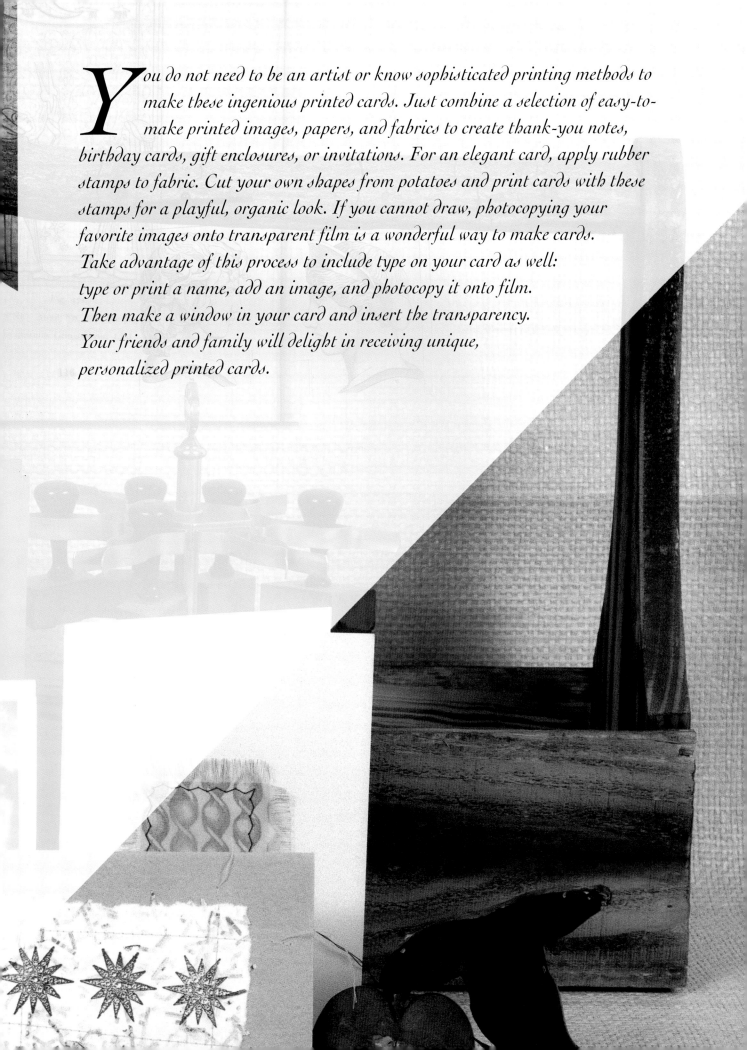

Y ou do not need to be an artist or know sophisticated printing methods to make these ingenious printed cards. Just combine a selection of easy-to-make printed images, papers, and fabrics to create thank-you notes, birthday cards, gift enclosures, or invitations. For an elegant card, apply rubber stamps to fabric. Cut your own shapes from potatoes and print cards with these stamps for a playful, organic look. If you cannot draw, photocopying your favorite images onto transparent film is a wonderful way to make cards. Take advantage of this process to include type on your card as well: type or print a name, add an image, and photocopy it onto film. Then make a window in your card and insert the transparency. Your friends and family will delight in receiving unique, personalized printed cards.

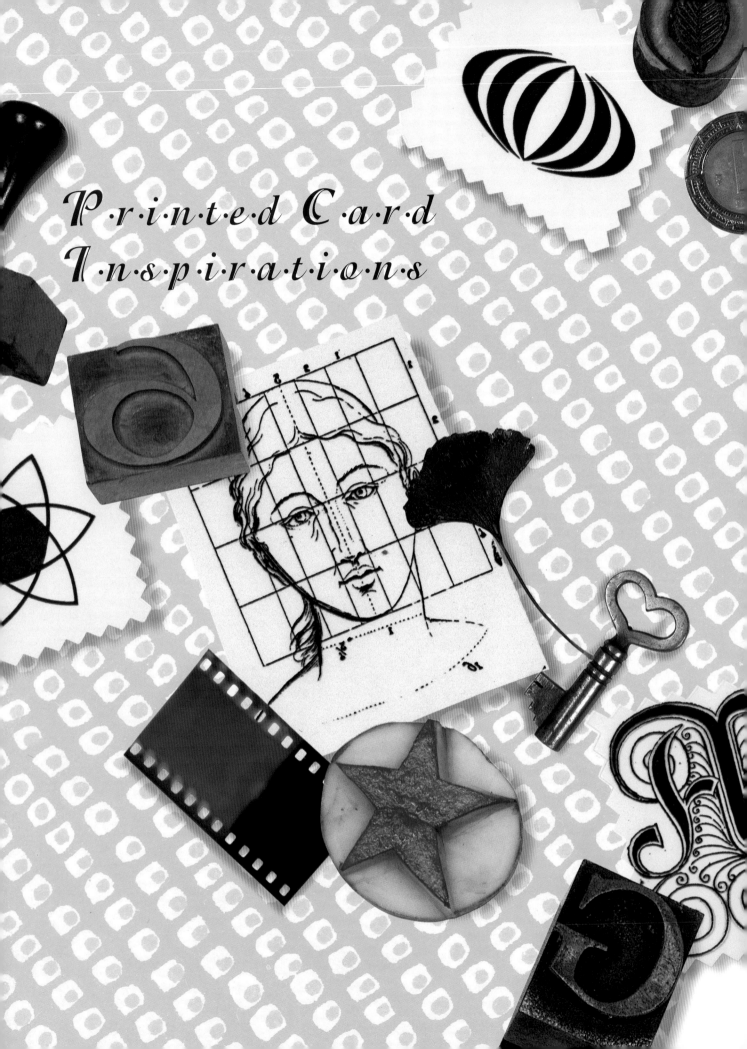

Printed Card Inspirations

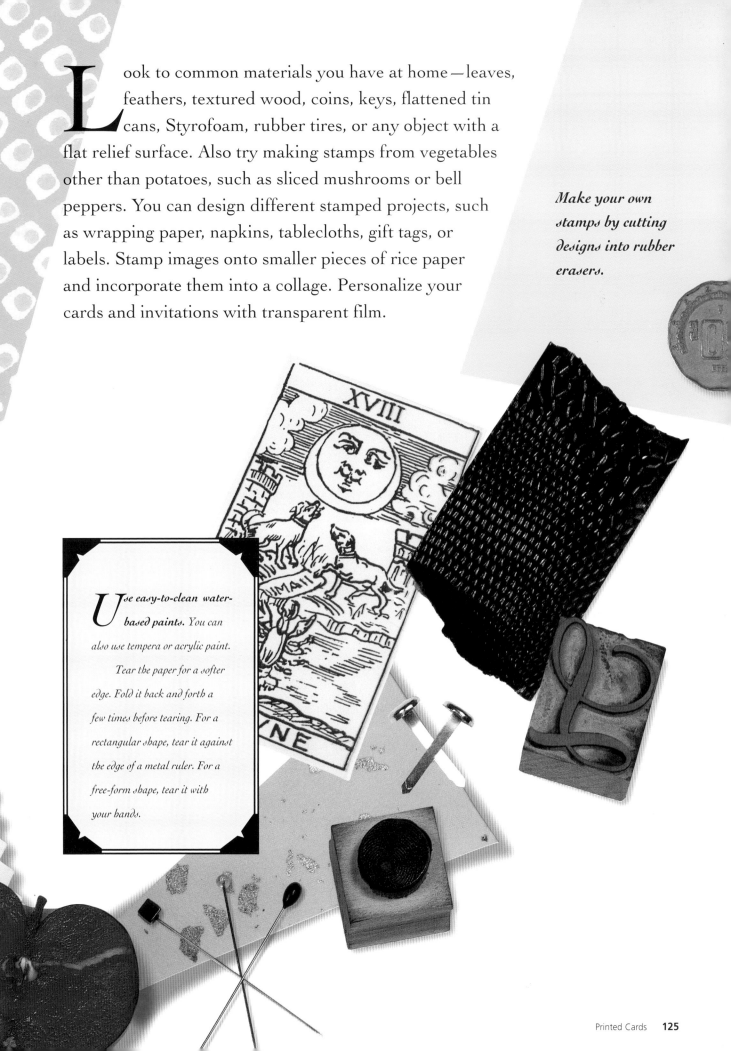

L ook to common materials you have at home—leaves, feathers, textured wood, coins, keys, flattened tin cans, Styrofoam, rubber tires, or any object with a flat relief surface. Also try making stamps from vegetables other than potatoes, such as sliced mushrooms or bell peppers. You can design different stamped projects, such as wrapping paper, napkins, tablecloths, gift tags, or labels. Stamp images onto smaller pieces of rice paper and incorporate them into a collage. Personalize your cards and invitations with transparent film.

Make your own stamps by cutting designs into rubber erasers.

U se easy-to-clean water-based paints. You can also use tempera or acrylic paint.

Tear the paper for a softer edge. Fold it back and forth a few times before tearing. For a rectangular shape, tear it against the edge of a metal ruler. For a free-form shape, tear it with your hands.

Rubber Stamp Card

Cut a window for your stamped image in the front of the card. Stamp the image onto sheer fabric, placing a piece of scrap paper under the fabric to keep the ink from bleeding through. Let the ink dry. Glue gold paper on the inside of the card under the stamped fabric. Sew the buttons on to fasten the fabric to the card, and then fray the edges of the fabric.

Materials

- Piece of fibrous handmade paper, cut or torn to 8" x 4 ½" (20 cm x 11.5 cm) and folded in half
- Piece of sheer fabric (polyester or silk organza), 2" x 3" (5 cm x 7.5 cm)
- Piece of gold or decorative paper, cut or torn to 2" x 2 ½" (5 cm x 6.5 cm)
- Rubber stamp with an image not larger than 1 ½" (4 cm)
- Ink pad with dark ink
- Needle and thread or sewing machine
- Two small, flat buttons
- Craft knife
- Metal ruler
- Pencil
- PVA glue
- Glue brush
- Bone folder
- Cutting mat
- Scrap paper

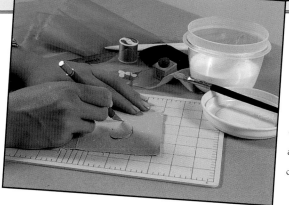

❖**1** Lay the folded handmade paper on your work surface and measure and mark 1 ¼" (3 cm) from the middle of the top and bottom edges. Then measure and mark 1 ½" (4 cm) from the middle of the left and right edges. Open the card flat on the cutting mat. Cut through the marks, angling the knife to make an oval hole approximately 1 ½" x 1" (4 cm x 2.5 cm) in the center of the card. Erase any pencil marks left on the card.

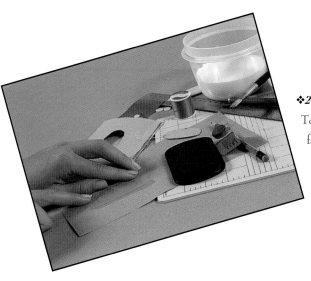

❖*2*   Trace the shape of the hole onto the scrap paper. To determine exactly where to stamp the image on the fabric, center the fabric over the traced hole.

❖*3*   Place the rubber stamp on the ink pad and tap gently two or three times. Press the stamp flat onto the fabric, applying an even amount of pressure on all sides. Be careful not to rock the stamp from side to side, as this will cause the ink to smear. Lift the stamp straight up from the fabric. Let the ink dry before attaching the fabric to the card.

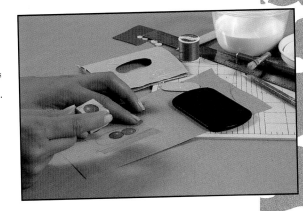

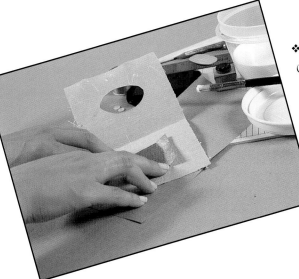

❖*4*   Open the card. Apply glue to the back of the gold paper. Center the paper behind the oval cutout on the front of the card, and adhere it to the inside of the card. It is best to use gold, silver, or light-colored papers for the background to the stamped fabric—stamped images tend to disappear against a dark background.

❖*5*   Center the stamped fabric over the hole on the front of the card. Sew the buttons above and below the oval to secure the fabric to the paper. Fray the edges of the fabric to create a frame around the oval.

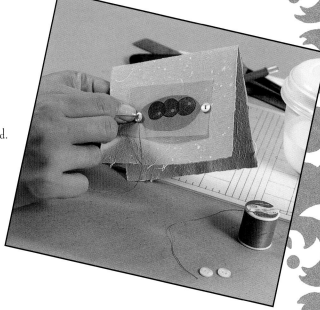

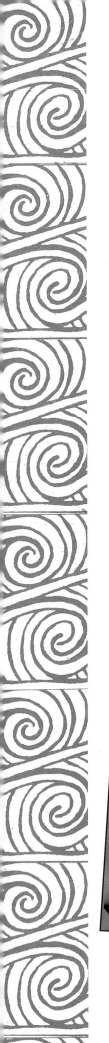

Potato Print Card

To create a star stamp, make a cutting guide by tracing the shape of the potato and drawing a star, or by pressing a cookie cutter star into the potato. Cut out around the star. Let the potato sit face down on a paper towel to drain for fifteen minutes before printing. Tap the stamp in ink on an inking slab or roll ink onto the relief surface. Then stamp the card. Repeat or overlap the stamps to make a pattern.

Materials

- Washed and uncooked large, firm potato
- Piece of heavyweight or printmaking paper, 10" x 7" (25 cm x 18 cm), folded in half
- Tracing or scrap paper
- Craft or paring knife
- Pins
- Scissors
- Metal ruler
- Pencil
- One or two colors of water-soluble printing inks
- Rubber ink roller
- Inking slab (smooth, nonabsorbent, easy-to-clean surface such as glass, sheet metal, plastic, or Formica)

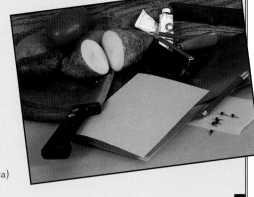

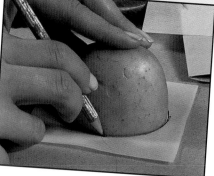

❖1 Cut the potato in half. To make a pattern for your stamp, place the cut edge of the potato on the tracing or scrap paper. Use the pencil to trace the shape of the potato. You can also cut the potato freehand—experiment with different shapes.

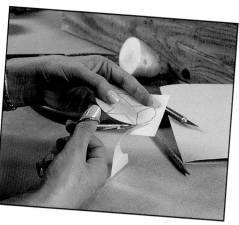

❖*2* Make a five-point star in the paper circle; simple shapes are easier to execute than intricate patterns. Mark the pieces you will cut away with an X. Cut out the circle using the scissors.

❖*3* Pin the paper pattern to the surface of the potato in the spaces marked with an X. Use the knife to cut away the five marked sections of the potato. For the best results, cut from the center of the potato out to the edge, approximately ½" (1 cm) deep, then along the side of the potato. Cut straight up and down in one motion, and clean any loose edges with your knife, as they will appear in the printed image.

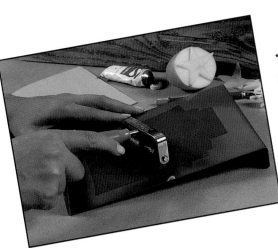

❖*4* Squeeze a dollop of ink onto the inking slab. Use the rubber roller to spread the ink to a thin consistency. You can roll two colors side by side, but be sure to wash the roller before changing colors to avoid mixing ink colors.

❖*5* To ink the stamp, tap the potato a few times on the freshly spread ink or run the roller over the relief image. Wash the stamp before changing colors to avoid mixing ink colors. Be sure to cover the entire surface of the potato with ink, filling in any blank spots with your finger.

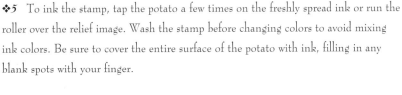

❖*6* Use both hands to press the stamp firmly onto the paper. Be careful not to smudge the ink. Lift the stamp up and away from the paper. If the potato print is watery, stamp the potato a few times on scrap paper before re-inking. Reapply ink to the stamp each time you print.

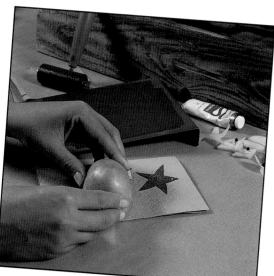

Transparent Film Card

Rummage through books for images you would like to use, or make an original drawing. For the best results, select images printed in black, such as old playing cards, etching plates from an opera libretto, and mod Japanese graphic design images. Photocopy the images onto transparent film or acetate; reproduction businesses provide this service for a small fee. Then cut the paper for the card and background papers to place behind the image. Assemble the card with brass fasteners.

Materials

- Transparent film with photocopied image
- Piece of Japanese handmade paper, 8" x 5" (20 cm x 13 cm), folded in half
- Piece of medium-weight cardstock for the inside, 7 ½" x 4 ½" (19 cm x 11.5 cm)
- Piece of background paper, 2 ¾" x 3 ½" (7 cm x 9 cm)
- Piece of gold or silver paper
- Brass paper fasteners (found in stationery stores)
- Craft knife
- Metal ruler
- PVA glue
- Glue brush
- Cutting mat

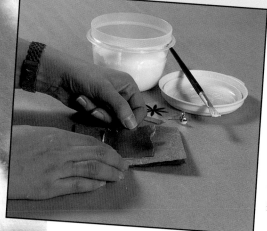

❖1 Place the folded card on the work surface. Apply glue to the back of the background paper. Center the background paper and adhere it to the front of the card. Adhere the other layers of paper you will use as a backdrop for the acetate image. Use gold, silver, or light-colored background paper to enhance the image.

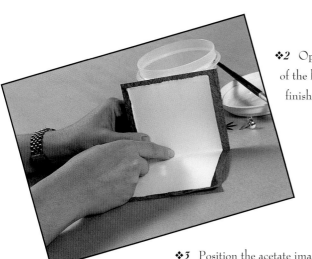

❖*2*　Open the card. Align the fold of the inside paper with the fold of the base card. Position the papers as they will appear in the finished card.

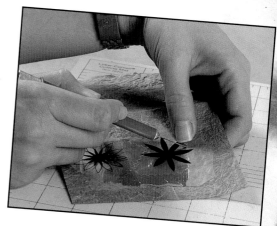

❖*3*　Position the acetate image on the front of the card over the background papers. With the knife, cut a small slit in the upper left corner through the acetate and all the layers of paper. Be careful not to scrape the transparent film or acetate, because the image may flake off or become damaged.

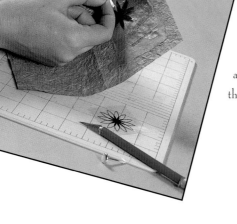

❖*4*　Slide the brass fastener through the slit. You could also attach the acetate by sewing it to the paper, or using clear picture corners to hold the image.

❖*5*　If desired, put a second acetate image or text through the prongs of the fastener on the inside of the card. Spread the prongs open to secure the images and the papers. Use more than one fastener if needed.

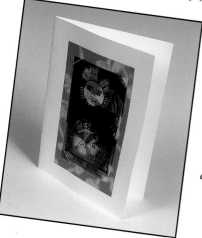

Variation

If you don't have any brass fasteners on hand, attach the acetate to the paper by sliding it into four slits cut into the card, as shown in this variation.

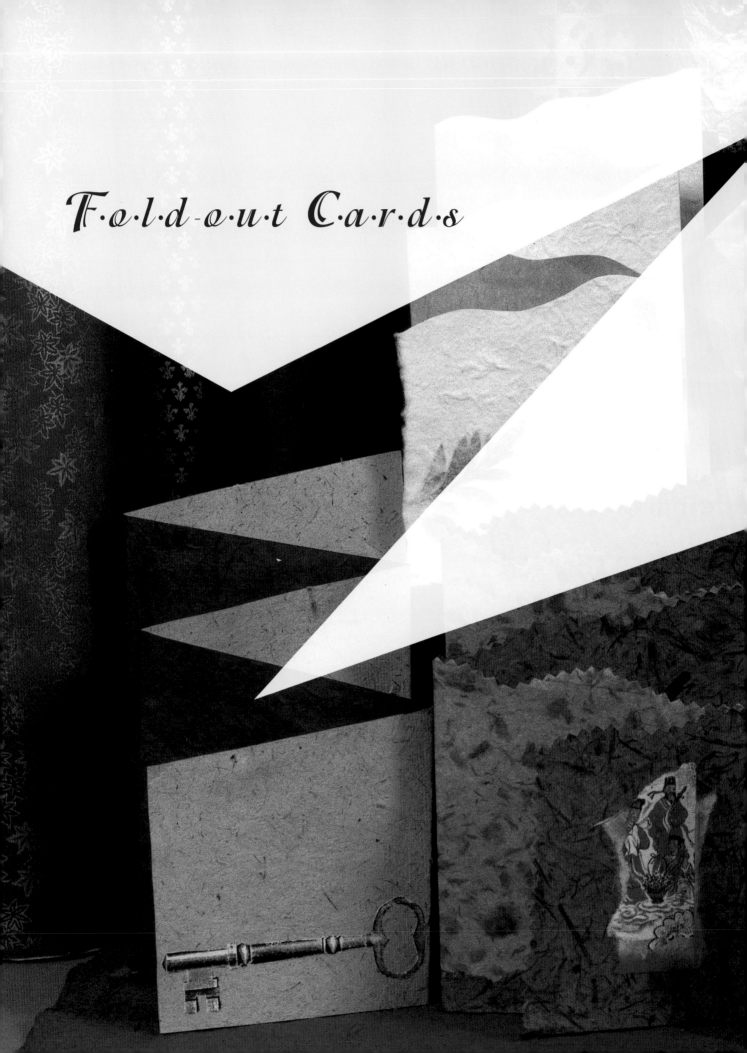

F·o·l·d-o·u·t C·a·r·d·s

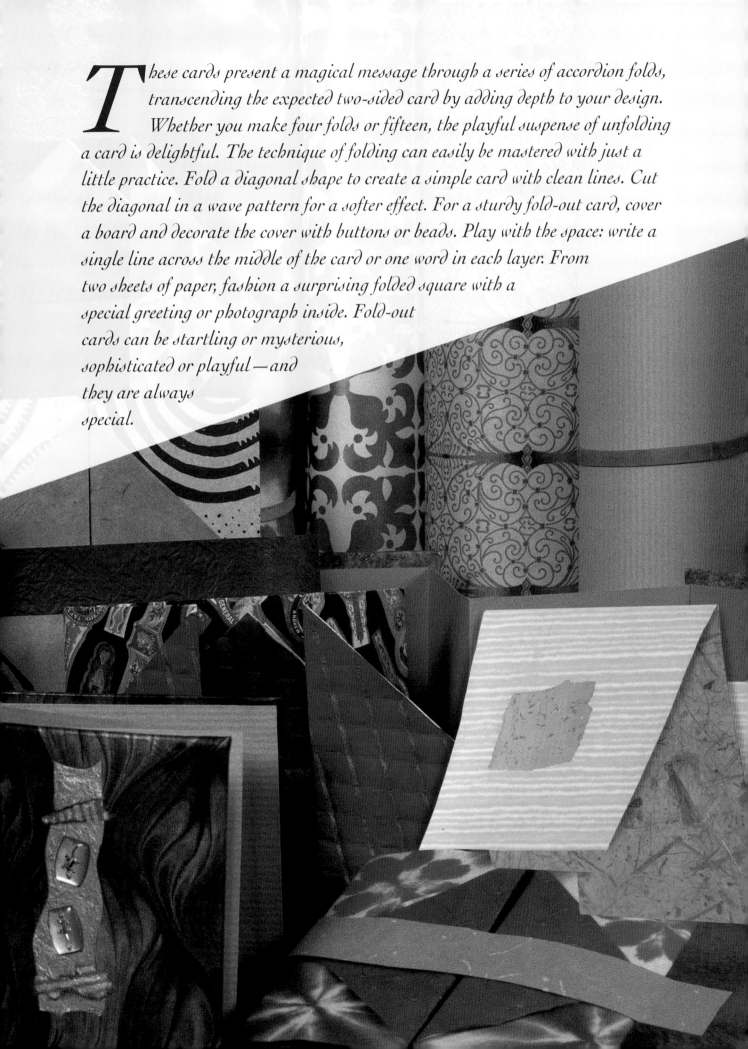

*T*hese cards present a magical message through a series of accordion folds, transcending the expected two-sided card by adding depth to your design. Whether you make four folds or fifteen, the playful suspense of unfolding a card is delightful. The technique of folding can easily be mastered with just a little practice. Fold a diagonal shape to create a simple card with clean lines. Cut the diagonal in a wave pattern for a softer effect. For a sturdy fold-out card, cover a board and decorate the cover with buttons or beads. Play with the space: write a single line across the middle of the card or one word in each layer. From two sheets of paper, fashion a surprising folded square with a special greeting or photograph inside. Fold-out cards can be startling or mysterious, sophisticated or playful—and they are always special.

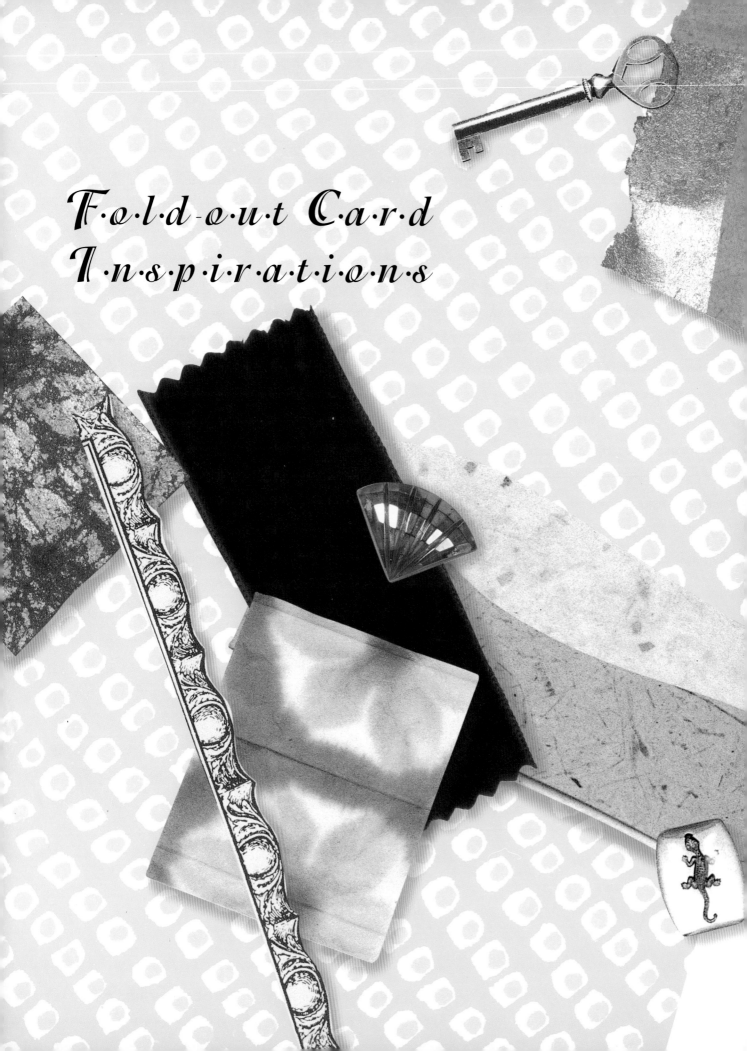

F·o·l·d-o·u·t C·a·r·d
I·n·s·p·i·r·a·t·i·o·n·s

Design a fold-out birthday card that has a panel for each year to be celebrated. These elongated cards can also be used to send a poem or write a letter. Use pinking shears to create a zigzag edge, or sew a pattern on the diagonal edge with embroidery thread. Run a gold marker along the edge to highlight the shape. Add a third dimension to your card by gluing objects onto the inner fold that pop up when the card is opened. Announce a birth or congratulate a graduate with a personalized message in a surprising folded square.

Make a miniature art gallery by putting a photo or collage in each panel.

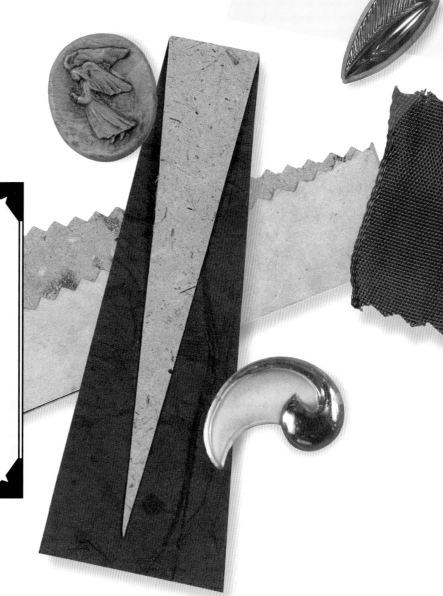

Mark the paper carefully and fold it accurately the first time. Refolding leaves unwanted lines. Practice on a piece of scrap paper first.

Some papers are not suitable for writing, so select a paper with a smooth surface and test it with your pen before you write the final copy.

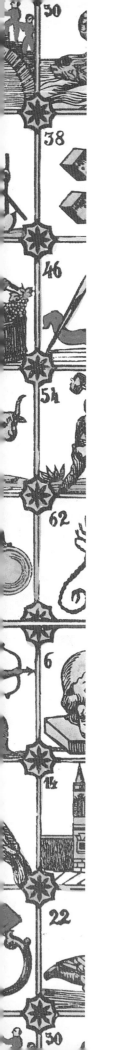

Classic Fold-out Card

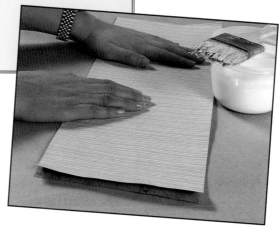

Classic lines and contrasting papers make this card striking. The construction is simple, with the different papers folded on top of each other in a diagonal line. Cut the papers, glue them together, and fold. Try a pattern and a solid color together or two solid colors. Personalize your card with words or images. You can also make this card with one sheet of paper, but adhering two sheets makes the card sturdier and the design more interesting.

Materials

- Two pieces of paper in contrasting colors and textures 7 ½" x 20 ½" (19 cm x 52 cm) each
- Craft knife
- Metal ruler
- Pencil
- PVA glue
- Glue brush
- Bone folder

❖**1** Apply glue to one sheet of paper. Align the edges and adhere the glued piece to the other sheet of paper. Smooth the papers with your hands to press out any wrinkles. Trim the edges to 7" x 20" (18 cm x 51 cm).

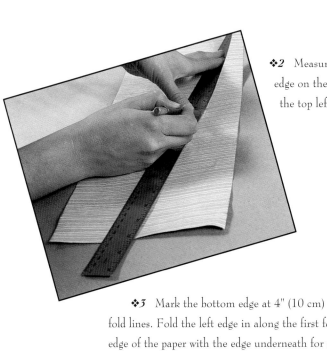

❖2   Measure and mark with the pencil 3 ½" (9 cm) up from the bottom edge on the right side of the paper. Cut the top edge in a diagonal from the top left corner to the 3 ½" (9 cm) mark on the right side.

❖3   Mark the bottom edge at 4" (10 cm) intervals to indicate the fold lines. Fold the left edge in along the first fold line. Align the top edge of the paper with the edge underneath for a straight fold line.

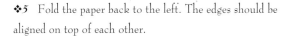

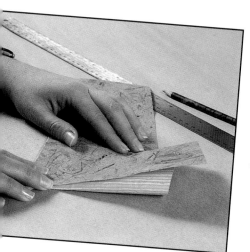

❖4   Turn the paper over. Fold the paper back, align it with the bottom edge underneath, and crease the paper with your thumb or the bone folder.

❖5   Fold the paper back to the left. The edges should be aligned on top of each other.

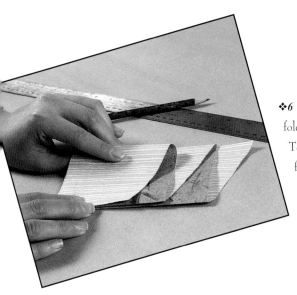

❖6   Fold the last flap to the right. Crease all the folds with the bone folder for a crisp fold. Trim any excess paper. To personalize the card, glue decorative paper or images to the front of the card.

Accordion Fold Card

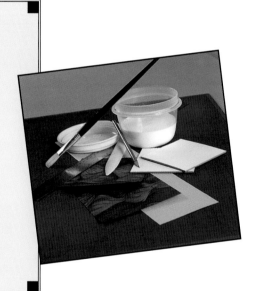

Be the master of many folds. Cover two pieces of illustration board with decorative paper. This provides a protective case for the folded paper inside and is also sturdy enough for attaching beads or buttons. Glue the paper to be folded to the inside of one board, then fold it an even number of intervals to achieve the accordion effect. You can make more than four folds but, to ensure the card folds properly, remember to use an even number of folds.

Materials

- Two pieces of illustration board, 4" x 4" (10 cm x 10 cm)
- Two pieces of decorative paper for the outside, 5" x 5" (13 cm x 13 cm)
- Piece of text paper for the inside, 3 ¾" x 15 ½" (9.5 cm x 39 cm)
- Metal ruler
- Pencil
- PVA glue
- Glue brush
- Bone folder

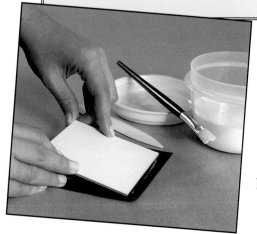

❖*1* On the back of one piece of the 5" x 5" (13 cm x 13 cm) decorative paper, measure and mark ½" (1 cm) from the edge on all sides. Apply glue within the lines. Center one piece of illustration board on the paper. Turn the card over and use your hand to smooth the paper from the center to the edges.

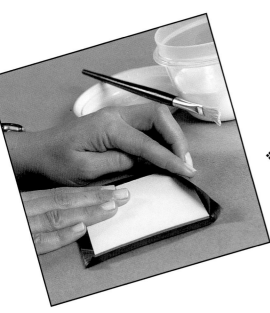

*Always work in a clean
area, with scrap paper
under your projects.*

❖**2** Turn the card over again. Apply glue to the right and left flaps
with the brush. Fold the flaps over the illustration board and smooth
them with your fingers. Do not press the paper together at the top
and bottom of the flaps where the paper extends beyond the board;
the corners are handled in the next step.

❖**3** Apply glue to the flaps at the top corners. In each corner,
pull the top piece of folded paper to a 45-degree angle and crease.
Angle the fold so the paper will not hang over the edges of the board.
Tuck any excess paper toward the edge of the board. Repeat on the
bottom corners.

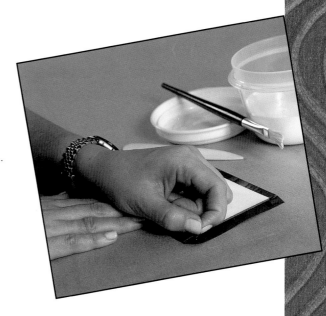

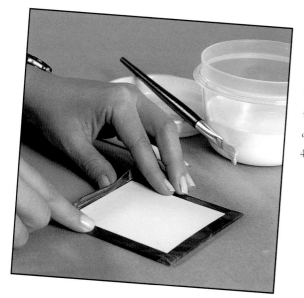

❖**4** Apply glue to the top and bottom flaps and fold them
onto the board. Make sure that the angled corners are attached
to the inside edge of the board or you will see them on the
outside of the card when it is closed. Repeat steps 1 through
4 for the other side of the cover.

❖5 Center the inside paper ¼" (.5 cm) from the top, bottom, and left edges of one board. Make a fold in the paper ¼" (.5 cm) from the right edge of the board. Make sure, as you fold, to align the folded paper on top of the bottom portion of the paper.

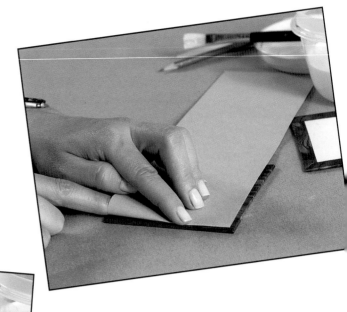

❖6 Turn the paper over. Apply glue from the fold line to the edge of the paper. Center the paper and adhere it to the board ¼" (.5 cm) from the edges. Let the glue dry for a few minutes, then fold the paper to the left. Crease the fold with a bone folder.

Be careful not to glue beyond the fold line on the inside paper, as it will show on the finished card.

❖7 Make a fold along the left edge of the paper, starting at the top left corner. Align the fold with the left edge of the paper on the board underneath.

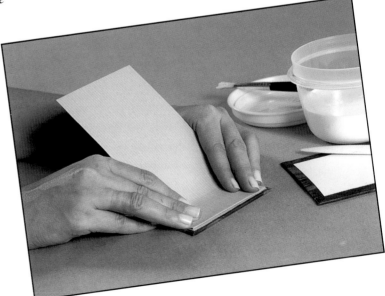

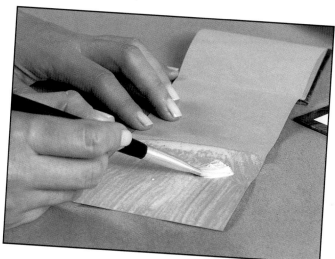

❖8 Slide the board under the paper beside the other board to use as a guide for paper placement. Turn the folded paper and glued board over, and apply glue from the last fold line to the outside edge.

❖9 Center the paper and adhere it to the second board ¼" (.5 cm) from the right edge. Smooth the paper with your fingers and with the bone folder. Align the boards on top of each other at the right edge, and press down evenly toward the left edge.

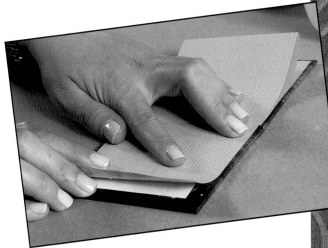

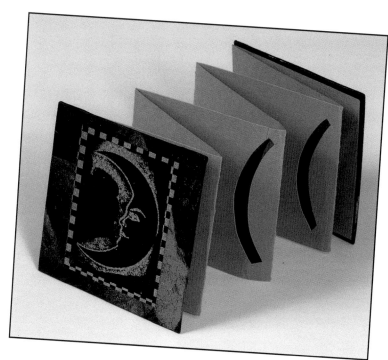

Variation
A smaller card, with more folds and shapes cut from the folded inside paper, adds light and shadow to the greeting.

Surprising Square Card

The Surprising Square is perfect to give as an invitation or graduation card. Words of welcome or congratulations surprise and delight as they emerge from colorful layers of paper. The challenge of this card is in the alignment; it may take a few attempts to get it right. Use black, red, and gold paper to make a traditional Japanese card. Cover the card in layers of tissue for a softer feeling, or clear patterned acetate or plastic wrapping paper for a more sophisticated message.

Materials

- Piece of patterned paper, 10" x 10" (25 cm x 25 cm)
- Piece of solid color paper, 10" x 10" (25 cm x 25 cm)
- Piece of card stock or heavy paper, 4" x 4" (10 cm x 10 cm)
- Strip of paper for closure, 11 ¼" x 1 ½" (28.5 cm x 4 cm)
- Craft knife
- Double stick tape
- PVA glue
- Glue brush
- Metal ruler
- Bone folder

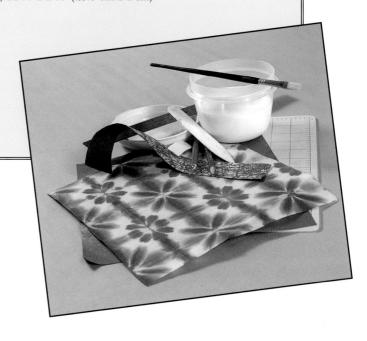

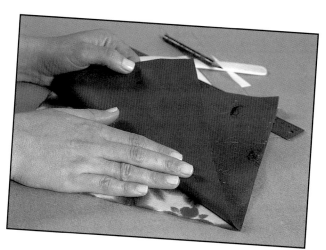

❖1 Position the two sheets of 10" x 10" (25 cm x 25 cm) paper back to back with the wrong sides together. Align the edges. Fix the papers in place with a piece of double stick tape. Trim the edges if they aren't even.

❖2 Turn the paper on a diagonal. Measure and mark 4 ¾" (12 cm) intervals along the vertical, dividing the paper into three parts. Use the metal ruler and bone folder to score horizontal lines at the marked intervals.

Fold along the edge of a ruler for clean lines.

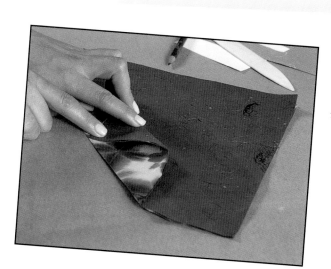

❖3 Fold the paper on the bottom score line. Then fold the point back down evenly to the bottom edge. The point should meet the edge of the bottom fold. Crease the folds with the bone folder.

❖4 Fold the paper on the top score line. Then fold the point back to the upper edge. Use the bottom point fold as a guide. The folds should be flush with one another. Crease the folds with the bone folder.

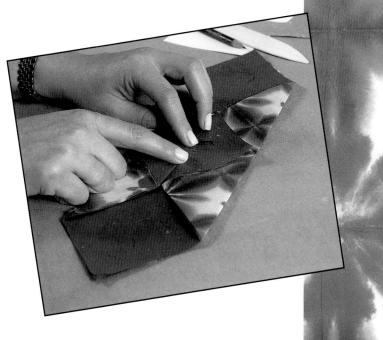

❖**5** Score the horizontal lines at each end of the folded triangles to make the square shape.

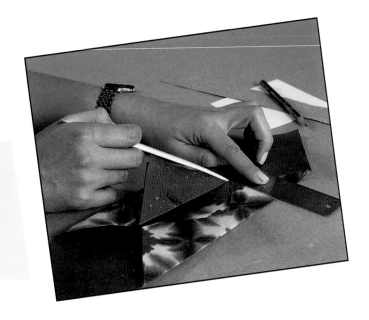

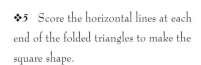

For best results, measure twice and cut accurately.

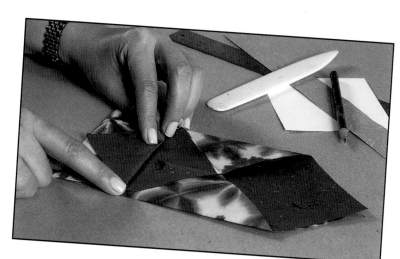

❖**6** Fold the left flap in. Align the left and right edges with the edges underneath for an even square. Fold the flap point back to the left edge. Crease well.

❖**7** Repeat the last two folds on the right side.

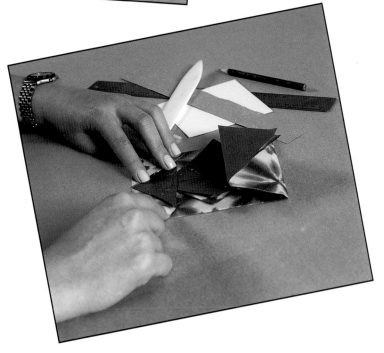

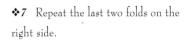

❖*8* Insert the 4" x 4" (10 cm x 10 cm) message card or a photograph inside.

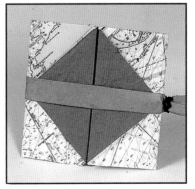

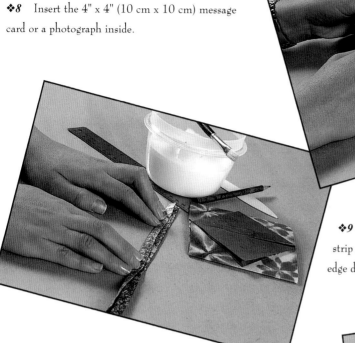

❖*9* To make the paper closure, lay the paper strip right side down. Fold one-third of the upper edge down. Then fold the lower edge up one-third.

❖*10* Wrap the paper strip around the card so that the edges of the strip meet evenly on one side. Apply glue to the lower half of the strip and press the strip ends together. The band should be able to slide on and off easily.

For a different closure, wrap thread several times around the end of the paper bands. Trim ends.

Variations

Experiment with different papers and patterns, to dramatically alter the square design. Try centering strong geometric patterns them on the square shape. Or mix the pale pastels of old maps with darker, solid colors.

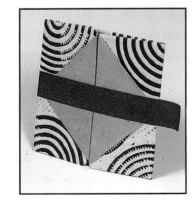

Movable Cards
Flowers in Motion

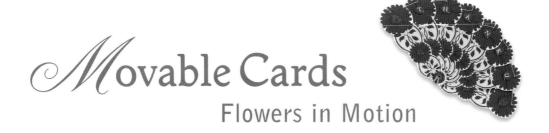

There is a life force flowing through nature. The sun illuminates and the plants grow. The rain comes down and nourishment is taken up. Honeybees buzz, aspen leaves flutter, pine branches sway, flower buds open, ripe seeds fall. The garden is energized with continuous movement, change, and flux. Re-create the magic with the enchantment of energized garden greetings that pop up, swirl, and unfold. Engaging and intriguing, these projects bring alive the power of the wind, the mystery of growth, and the motion of flowers unfolding.

Projects allow recipients to:

- *Unfold a flower to reveal a hidden message*
- *Open a card with whimsical pop-up posies*
- *Spread out a fan and behold a bouquet*
- *Gather seeds to cultivate in the future*

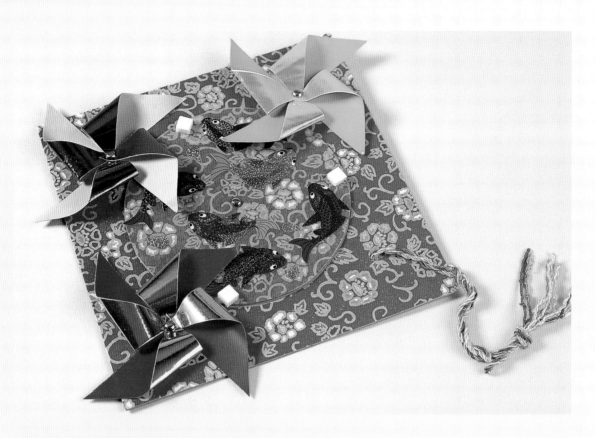

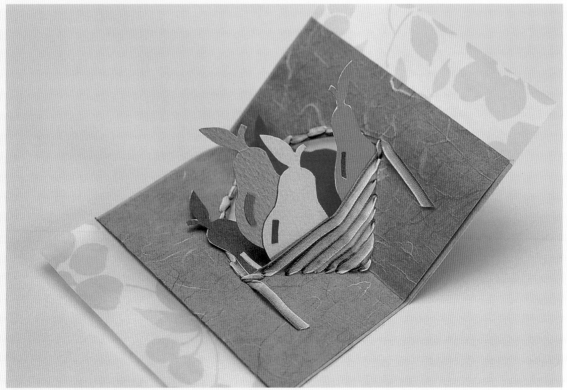

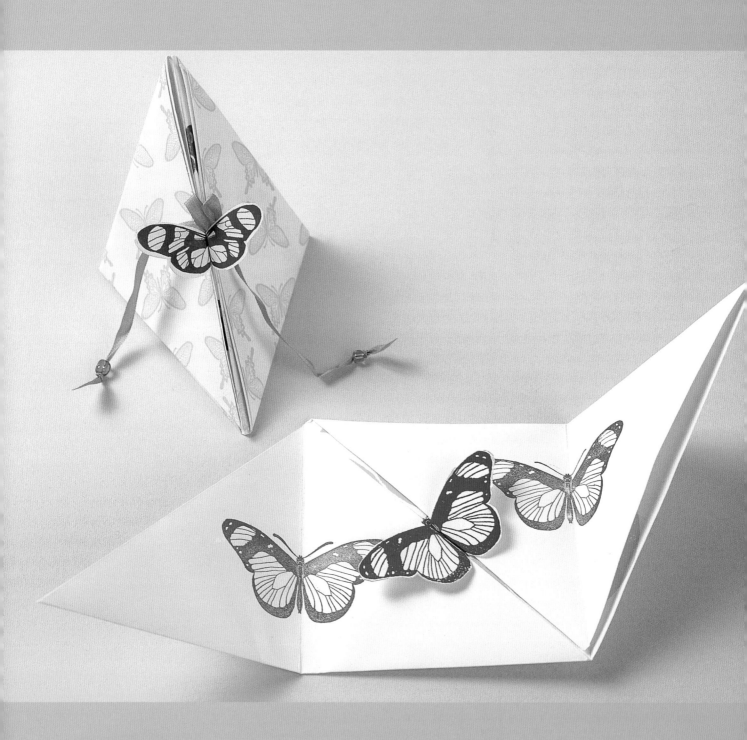

Flutter Bug Origami Greeting

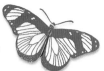

What can be more delightful to the gardener's eye than the graceful journey of a butterfly flitting from flower to flower? After alighting on a bloom, it sips nectar while its wings gently open and close. This card's geometric design simulates the butterfly's triangular shape, while the folding and unfolding patterns mimic the movement of the wings. Feel free to write a bright and cheerful note along an imaginary curving line, expressive of the butterfly's serendipitous flight through the garden.

MATERIALS

- 4½" x 9" (11.4 cm x 22.9 cm) medium weight paper
- large motif stamp
- flower stamp
- butterfly stamp
- blue, yellow, and red ink pads
- craft knife
- bone folder
- pencil
- ruler

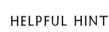

HELPFUL HINT

For critical placement of the butterfly stamp on the centerline, place a dot on the stamp's edge using an indelible marker, marking the top and bottom center-line of the butterfly design. Use these marks to position the stamp on the centerline. A right angle ruler can also be helpful in proper placement.

The card's size can be amended with a 2:1 proportion of length to width: 11" x 5½" (28 cm x 14 cm), 18" x 9" (46 cm x 23 cm), etc.

INSTRUCTIONS

1. Score the centerline to divide the paper into two squares. Score four diagonal lines dividing the two squares into eight triangles; the lines create an "X" in each square. Find and mark the center point of the centerline by placing a ruler along the two points of intersection where the diagonals meet.

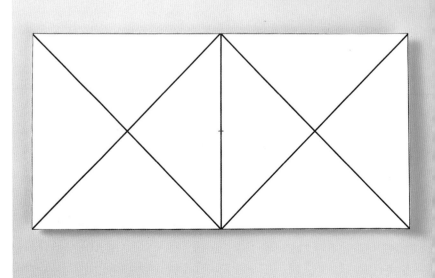

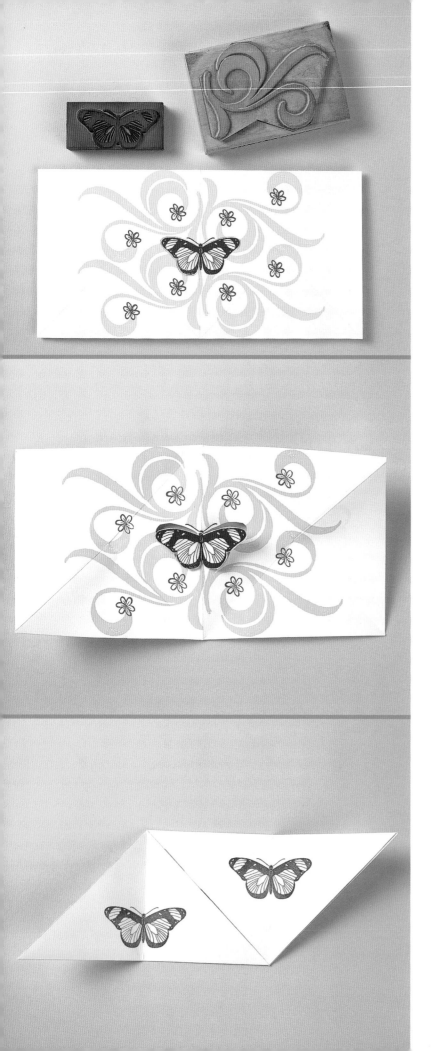

2. Stamp a butterfly exactly on the centerline and center point. Stamp a decorative motif around the butterfly using other stamps. Using a craft knife, cut along the outline of the wings only, leaving the body and antennas uncut along the fold line.

3. With the paper horizontal on your work surface, take the lower left corner and match it with the top point of the centerline, creasing along the scored diagonal. Take the upper right corner and match it with the bottom point of the centerline, creasing gently along the scored diagonal line. Take the lower left corner and match it with the top point of the centerline. Take the top right corner and match it with the bottom of the centerline. You should have a folded piece of paper in the shape of a square.

4. Unfold the paper and repeat directions starting with step 3, except this time, fold the butterfly wings upward and perpendicular to the paper while folding. Fold the wings down flat against the square to present the card.

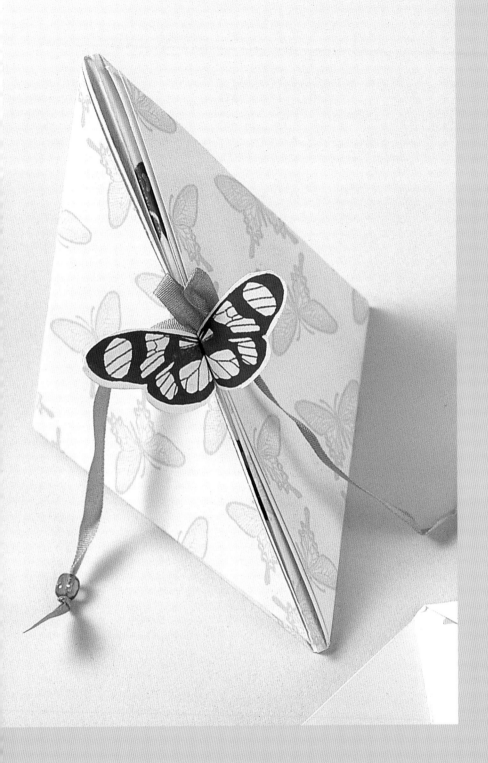

 GOING ONE STEP FURTHER

The card can be tied shut with the aid of an 8" (20 cm) length of $1/8$" (3 mm)-wide silk ribbon. After completing step 4, fold the square along the centerline to create a triangular shape. With the butterfly wings out and away from the fold, mark a point $1/4$" (6 mm) away from and just below the butterfly's abdomen. Center this point within the paper punch's opening and cut a hole through all of the card layers. Fold the ribbon in half and slip the loop through the hole. With the loop placed at the butterfly's head, pull the ribbon ends through the loop. Tie a bow at the butterfly's head to mimic the look of antennas.

Pop-up Potted Posies

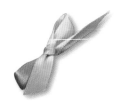

In late winter, gardening catalogs arrive almost everyday in the mail. While perusing those beautiful catalogs, select a few beautiful photos and make one or two pop-up greeting cards. Also, if you order bulbs or other plantings to give as gifts, this is a great card to give to the recipient. The card will illustrate nicely what she has to look forward to come spring and summer.

INSTRUCTIONS

1. Score a parallel line 2" (5.1 cm) from the 6" (15.2 cm)-long edge of the blue paper. Crease along the scored line. Unfold the paper and lay flat.

2. Along the fold line, mark dots at the following six locations starting from the left edge: $^5/_8$" (1.6 cm), $1^5/_8$" (4.1 cm), $2^3/_8$" (6 cm), $3^3/_8$" (8.6 cm), $4^3/_8$" (11 cm), and $5^3/_8$" (13.7 cm).

3. Draw three pairs of parallel lines centered on the fold line. The first pair consists of 2" (5.1 cm) lines at the $^5/_8$" (1.6 cm) and $1^5/_8$" (4.1 cm) marks. The second pair consists of $2^1/_2$" (6.4 cm) lines at the $2^3/_8$" (6 cm) and $3^3/_8$" (8.6 cm) marks. The third pair consists of 2" (5.1 cm) lines at the $4^3/_8$" (11 cm) and $5^3/_8$" (13.7 cm) marks. Using a craft knife, cut all six lines.

4. Turn the blue paper over. Run a strip of double-sided tape along the two 6" (15.2 cm)-long edges.

5. Turn the paper over. Place the blue paper over the yellow vellum with $^1/_4$" (6 mm) of vellum extending beyond the blue paper's top. Remove the tape's backing. Adhere the sheets together.

6. Fold the paper at a 90° angle. Reverse the folds of the three 1" (2.5 cm)-wide strips. They should look like tables jutting out. The flowerpots will be attached to these three strips. Flatten paper.

MATERIALS

- three 2" (5.1 cm) square catalog blooms
- 4" x 6" (10.2 cm x 15.2 cm) metallic copper card stock
- 24" (61 cm) length of $^3/_8$" (1 cm)-wide ribbon
- $5^3/_4$" x 6" (14.6 cm x 15.2 cm) blue paper
- $6^1/_2$" x 6" (16.5 cm x 15.2 cm) yellow vellum paper
- roll of $^1/_4$" (6 mm)-wide double-sided tape
- 4" x 6" (10.2 cm x 15.2 cm) sheet of double-sided tape
- flowerpot template (page 268)
- craft knife
- bone folder
- ruler
- white glue

HELPFUL HINT

The card can be mailed either flat or folded. Include a brief description to the recipient on how to pop up her flowers if mailing flat. A simple description would be: Fold your card at a 90° angle and enjoy!

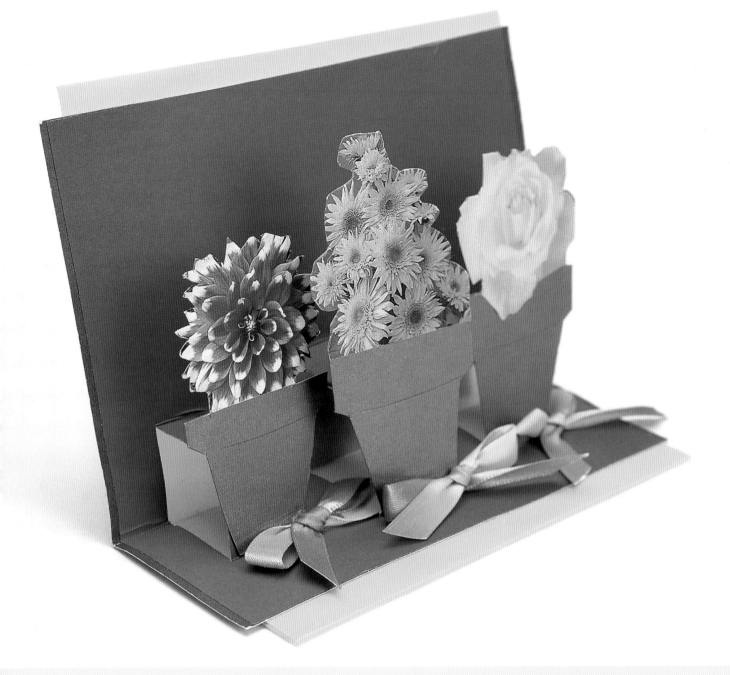

7. Cut the metallic paper into three 4" x 2" (10.2 cm x 5.1 cm) strips. Trace the flowerpot shape at the bottom of each copper paper strip. Adhere the catalog blooms onto the sheet of double-sided tape. Using a craft knife, cut out the blooms. Cut one side of bloom to have a flat edge. This edge will be placed on the traced flowerpot rim. If preferred, a petal can overlap the rim, so trim accordingly.

8. Remove the tape's backing from the blooms. Adhere the blooms to the metallic paper with the flat side at the flowerpot rim. Using a craft knife, cut along the outline of the potted blooms.

9. Run a strip of double-sided tape down the middle of the bottom half of the three 1" (2.5 cm) strips. Remove the backing. With the bottom of the pots lined up with the bottom fold of the 1" (2.5 cm) strips, adhere the flowerpots to each strip.

10. Fold the card at a 90° angle, easing the flowerpots to stand up and away from the blue paper. Cut the ribbon into three 8" (20 cm) lengths. Tie each length into a bow. Glue each bow at the bottom corner of each pot on the blue paper.

Bouquet Fanfare

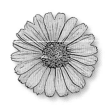

Unfold a rainbow of colors with this bouquet of bright and sassy zinnias. Each panel of the fan can be ornamented with a letter of your message, such as T-H-A-N-K-U or M-I-S-S-Y-O-U.

INSTRUCTIONS

1. On a copy machine, reproduce the flower panel on medium weight paper six times.

2. Hand color each panel as desired.

3. Stack the flower panels together and clip with a binder clip. Punch a $^{3}/_{16}$" (4.8 mm) hole at the bottom of the fan.

4. Set an eyelet in the hole.

5. With the panels stacked together, pierce a hole through all panels using an awl at the center/top of the fan about $^{1}/_{2}$" (1.3 cm) from the edge.

6. Open the fan. Begin sewing from the back. Pull the needle and thread through to the front of the first panel. Then loop the thread over the top edge and return to the back of the panel. Secure the ends with a knot. Return the thread to the front by passing the needle through the hole. Position the second panel with a slight overlap over the first panel. Push the needle and thread through the back of the second panel to the front. Then loop over the top edge, push the needle and thread from the back to the front again. Position the third panel with a slight overlap of the second panel. Repeat the sewing sequence until all panels have been tied together. Tie off the threads to the back of the last panel.

7. Slip the ribbon through the eyelet and pull it through until the ribbon has equal amounts on either side of the eyelet. Slip one end through the eyelet again and pull.

MATERIALS

- flower panel template (page 268)
- $^{3}/_{16}$" (4.8 mm) paper punch
- 18" (46 cm) length of ribbon
- 36" (92 cm) length of thread
- $^{3}/_{16}$" (4.8 mm) eyelet
- eyelet punch
- needle
- awl
- binder clip
- colored markers

HELPFUL HINT

Be sure to check the thickness of the stacked panels against the depth of the eyelet being used. Too many panels will cause the eyelet to malfunction and the fan to fall apart. If a large number of panels are desired, use an album post to secure the panels together.

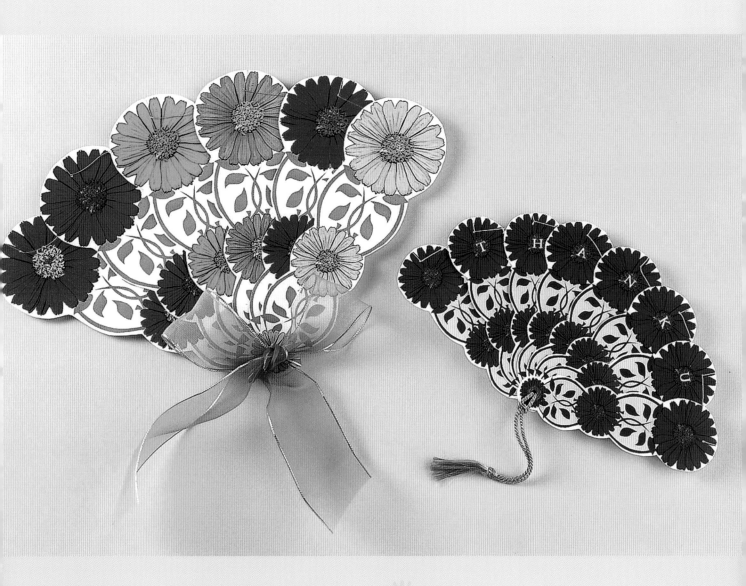

 ## GOING ONE STEP FURTHER

While the fan is spread out, turn the card over and write a message or note on the back. Also a very simple message such as "THANK U" can be revealed during the unfolding of the fan. Simply stamp individual letters onto each flower disk spelling out a greeting. The example on the right has the addition of two, nonlettered panels: one at the beginning and the other at the end with a total of eight panels.

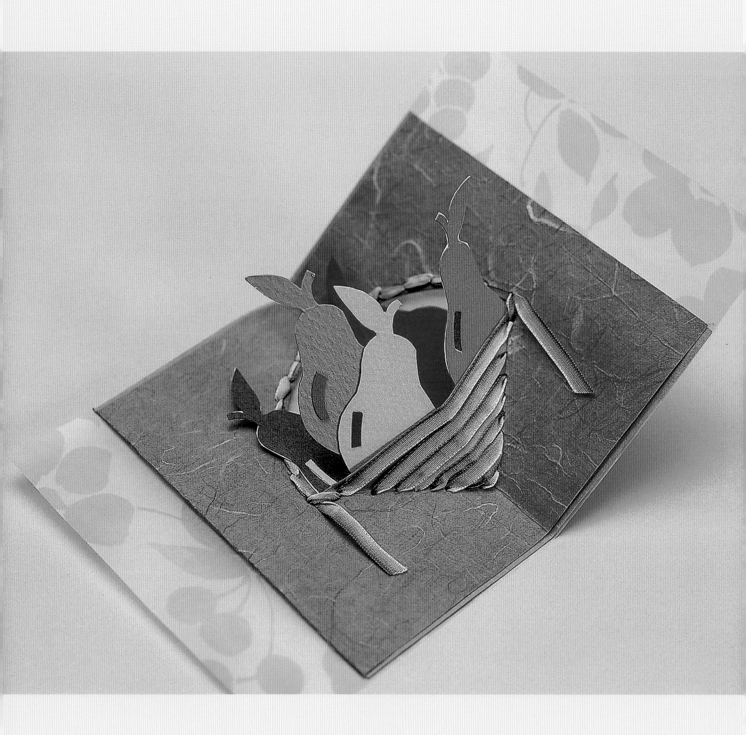

$\mathcal{F}$ruit Basket Pop-Up

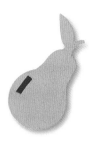

This greeting card delivers a bountiful harvest. Create a pretty, hand-woven ribbon basket and fill it with rainbow-colored pears. The fruit collection pops up into view when the card is opened. When placed on a shelf, the shapely forms stay fresh for a very long time.

MATERIALS

- 5" x 12" (12.7 cm x 30.5 cm) card stock
- 5" x 8½" (12.7 cm x 21.6 cm) decorative paper
- five cut out paper fruits, approximately 2½" (6.4 cm) high
- 1 yard (90 cm) of ¼" (6 mm)-wide ribbon
- roll of ¼" (6 mm)-wide double-sided tape
- ¹⁄₁₆" (1.5 mm) paper punch
- craft knife
- needle
- ruler
- hammer
- compass
- bone folder
- scissors
- pencil

INSTRUCTIONS

1. Fold the card stock into quarters. Unfold and lay the paper flat. On the last fold, place a ruler and make a pencil mark 2½" (6.4 cm) and 1¼" (3.2 cm) from the bottom. Draw a 3½" (8.9 cm)-long line centering it on the 2½" (6.4 cm) mark, parallel to the bottom edge. Using a bone folder, score two lines connecting the end points of the 3½" (8.9 cm) line to the 1¼" (3.2 cm) mark. Place a compass point on the 2½" (6.4 cm) mark. Open the compass until it reaches the end of the 3½" (8.9 cm) line. Draw a half circle above the triangle. Using a craft knife, cut along the 3½" (8.9 cm) line. Next, reverse the fold of the triangle by pulling down the cut edge of the triangle while pressing down on the scored lines. Fold closed along the fold line. Open.

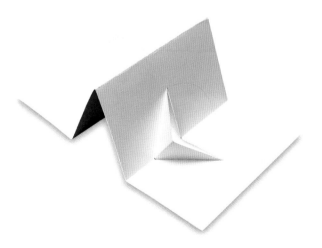

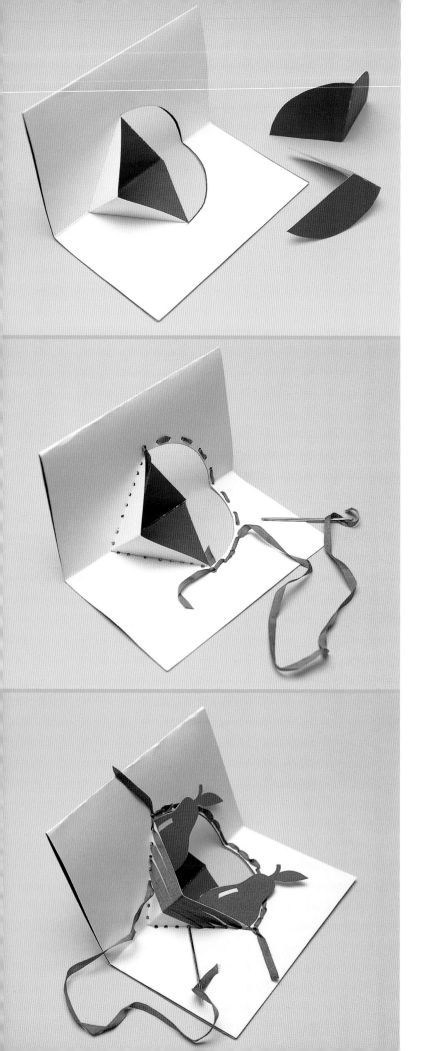

2. Fold the paper in half with the drawing side up. Using a craft knife, cut along the circle line, cutting through both paper layers. Remove the half circle shape from the top layer. In the half circle area, place a ruler on the fold and mark 1" (2.5 cm) up from circle's center. Using a craft knife, cut two lines, each radiating down from the 1" (2.5 cm) mark to each of the half circle's corners. Remove the shape. Place a strip of double-sided tape on the inside edge of one of the short sides. Remove the backing and adhere to sides.

3. Using a paper punch, punch out seventeen holes along the outside edge of the circle. Next, punch out eight holes on each scored line of the triangle. Fold the ribbon in half and cut into two pieces. Take one piece and cut it in half. Thread a needle with a short length of ribbon. Begin on the right side of the card and weave the ribbon through the holes of the basket handle. The weaving will look like a broken line. To complete the weaving of the handle, thread the other short ribbon onto the needle and begin weaving from the other end of the basket handle.

4. Place one fruit in each corner of the basket. Re-punch the holes, making new holes through the paper fruit. Place a 2" (5 cm) strip of double-sided tape to the top edge of the triangle. Remove the backing. Thread the needle with the long length of ribbon. Begin weaving the basket from the back side of the card, coming up through the first hole and going to the opposite side of the basket, and passing the needle and ribbon through hole number two. From the back, come up through the third hole, just below the last hole, across the basket to its opposite side. Continue weaving back and forth until the basket is complete. To be sure the weaving is done correctly, the back side of the card should have a broken line of ribbon along the two scored lines.

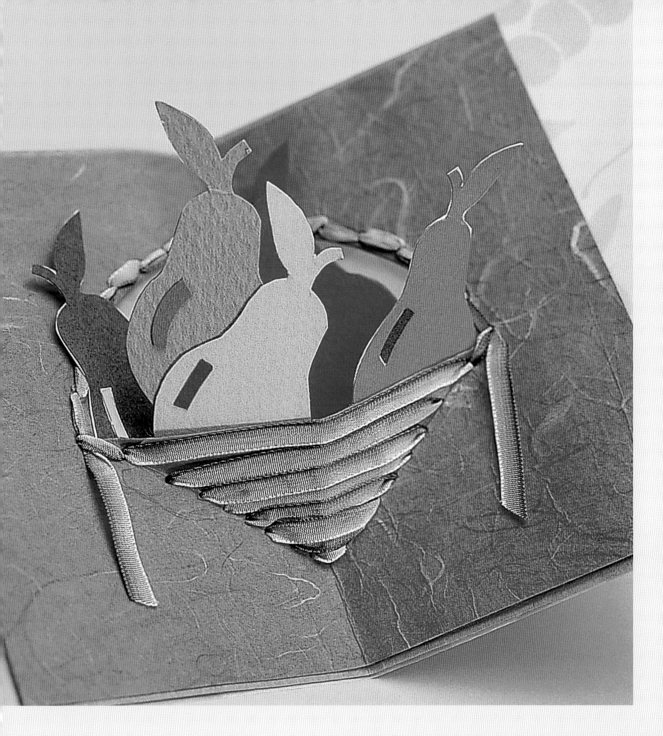

5. Arrange the remaining paper fruits in the basket.
They can be placed either to the inside back of
the basket or to the inside front of the basket.
The fruits should be positioned to either side of
the fold. The card will only close properly if the
pieces are not placed directly on the fold. Test
their positioning before taping by folding the card
in half and observing how the paper fruits fall
into position when the card is closed. Use double-
sided tape to adhere the pieces in place. Fold the
decorative paper in half and attach to the back of
the pop-up card using strips of double-sided tape.

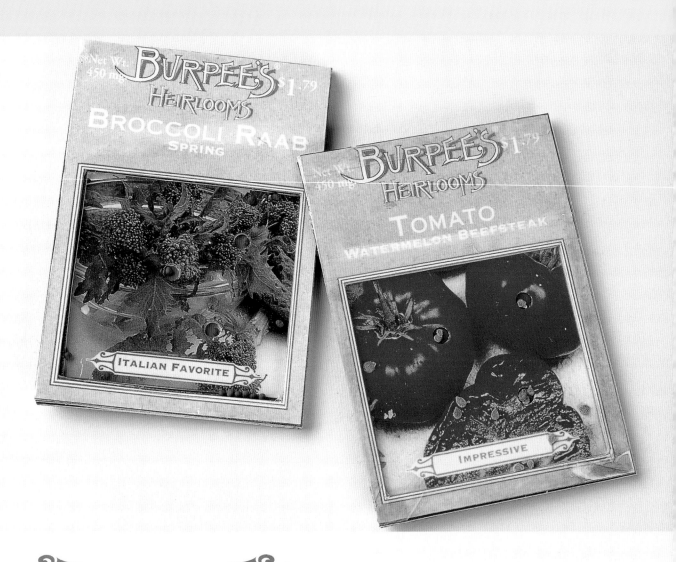

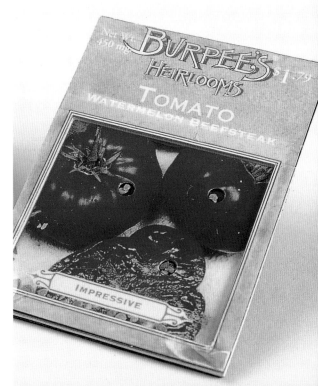

HELPFUL HINT

When adhering two boards together with double-sided tape, begin by lightly cutting a line through the tape backing, approximately 1" (2.5 cm) from an edge. Do not remove backing material. Put the two surfaces together, lining up the sides. Attach a binder clip to the bottom, opposite the cut line. Separate the boards slightly at the top and remove the 1" (2.5 cm)-wide backing strip from the double-sided tape. Adhere the boards together. Remove the binder clip. Slightly separate the boards at the bottom and remove the remaining backing. Adhere the boards together. Using this technique, it is far easier to take the boards apart if they need to be realigned.

Seed Packet Game

Turn a collection of beautiful seed packets into pocket games for children. While playing these simple games, children can visually associate a particular vegetable with its seed. Also, the games are great illustrations, demonstrating the wide variety of seed shapes and sizes. For adults, the game cards become handsome shadow boxes when placed on a shelf.

MATERIALS

- front of 4½" x 3¼" (11.4 cm x 8.3 cm) seed packet
- fifteen seeds
- 4½" x 3¼" (11.4 cm x 8.3 cm) piece of clear acetate
- two 4½" x 3¼" (1.4 cm x 8.3 cm) pieces of mat board (one marked A, one marked B)
- 4½" x 3¼" (11.4 cm x 8.3 cm) colored paper
- 10" x 10" (25 cm x 25 cm) sheet of double-sided tape
- ³/₁₆" (4.8 mm) paper punch
- mat knife

INSTRUCTIONS

1. Place double-sided tape on the back of the seed packet, on both sides of mat board A, and on one side of mat board B.

2. Cut a 2½" x 2½" (6.4 cm x 6.4 cm) area from the seed packet, which highlights the vegetable or flower.

3. Trace the opening of the seed packet on mat board A and on the untaped side of mat board B. Using a mat knife, cut out the marked area from mat board A only.

4. Adhere the acetate to the back of the seed packet. Adhere the acetate and seed packet panel to mat board A.

5. Remove the backing from the 2½" x 2½" (6.4 cm x 6.4 cm) seed packet illustration and adhere to mat board B within the area previously traced.

6. Using the paper punch, punch out three or four holes within the seed packet illustration. Adhere the colored paper to the back of mat board B.

7. Place seeds into the holes.

8. Remove the tape backing from mat board A and adhere it to mat board B.

Posy Packets

These six-sided bundles hold a surprise greeting. As each petal is unfolded, a hand-stamped note is revealed within the flower's interior. And with a few twists of the elastic band, the cheery posy can bloom and reign on the end of a pencil.

INSTRUCTIONS

1. Trace the posy template shape onto the plain side of the paper. Stamp your message multiple times on the paper surface. Cut out the flower shape.

2. Place the colored paper circle in the center of the flower. Punch a hole through both pieces of paper. Insert and set the eyelet in the hole.

3. Fold the elastic cord in half and tie an overhand knot at the ends. With printed side up, slip the loop down through the eyelet opening and pull the elastic knot up against the eyelet.

4. Close the flower by folding over each petal, one on top of the other. Secure the bundle by slipping the elastic loop over the closed form.

MATERIALS

- 5" x 5" (12.7 cm x 12.7 cm) decorative paper
- 1½" (3.8 cm)-wide color circle
- 6" (15 cm)-long metallic gold elastic cord
- ¼" (6 mm) paper punch
- ¼" (6 mm) eyelet
- posy template (page 269)
- eyelet setter
- small letter stamping blocks
- ink pads
- hammer
- ruler
- craft knife
- scissors

HELPFUL HINT

To stamp a word instead of individual letters, group the stamps side by side and tape them together. If you would like the word to appear in an arc, hold the grouping in your fingers in a curved position while stamping. If a word has a letter appearing twice, such as the word "soon," and you have only one letter available, place any letter block upside down to hold the space open while printing. Later, remove the needed letter from the grouping and stamp it in the open space.

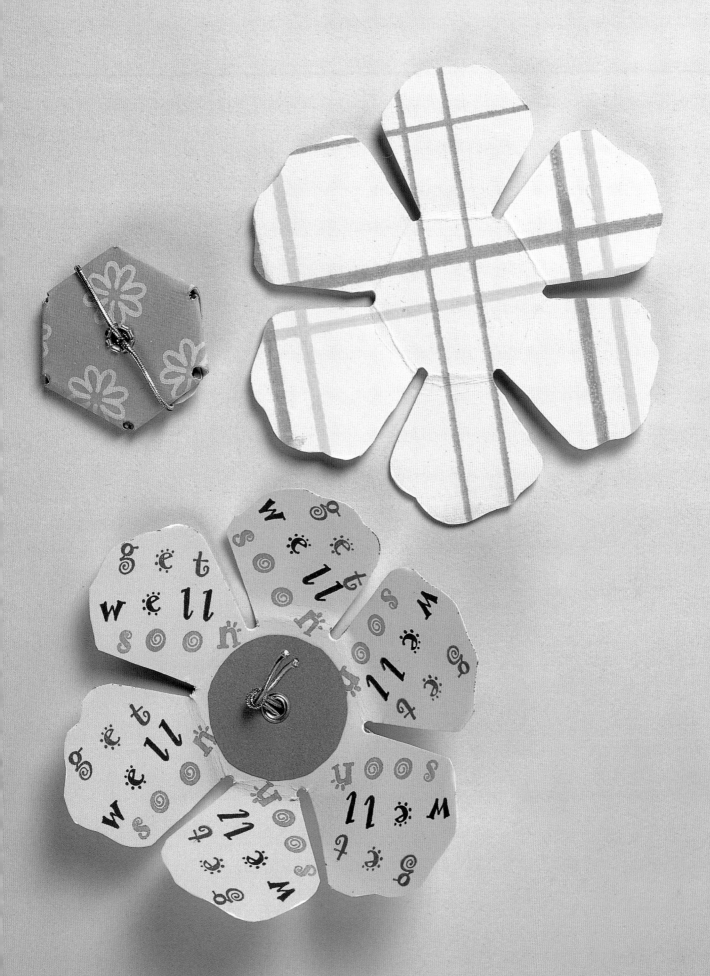

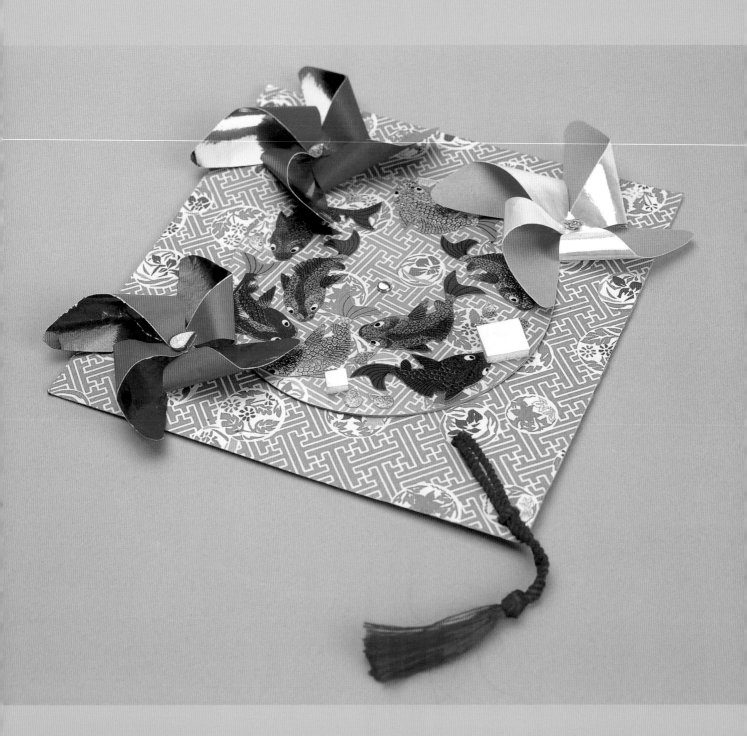

$\mathcal{K}$oi Fish Pond

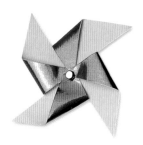

MATERIALS

- two 6" x 6" (15.2 cm x 15.2 cm) pieces of thin cardboard
- 6" x 6" (15.2 cm x 15.2 cm) decorative origami paper
- three 6" x 6" (15.2 cm x 15.2 cm) foil origami papers
- 6" x 6" (15.2 cm x 15.2 cm) clear contact paper
- 6" x 6" (15.2 cm x 15.2 cm) sheet of double-sided tape
- fish stickers
- tassel
- four tiny paper brads
- three $1/4$" (6 mm) foam sticky squares
- compass
- $1/8$" (3 mm) paper punch
- craft knife
- scissors
- ruler

HELPFUL HINT

The tricky part of this project is positioning the pinwheels so they'll rotate when the sticky squares come in contact with the blades. The squares push the pinwheels into rotation when the circle is rotated by hand.

Energize this water garden greeting card with twirling pinwheels and whirling fish, by spinning the inner circle. In Chinese culture, the fish symbolizes wealth and success. Write your well wishes on the back of this movable card and mail it to a friend for the start of the New Year or a new planting season.

INSTRUCTIONS

1. Place a sheet of double-sided tape on the back of the decorative origami paper. Mark the center of the paper. Place the point of the compass on the center mark and draw a 4" (10.2 cm)-wide circle. Using a craft knife, cut out the circle. Adhere the paper circle to one of the square cardboard pieces. Cut out the circle and cover it with the clear contact paper. Trim away the excess contact paper. Arrange the fish stickers on the circle. Place the three $1/4$" (6 mm) sticky squares near the edge of the circle, dividing the circle into thirds.

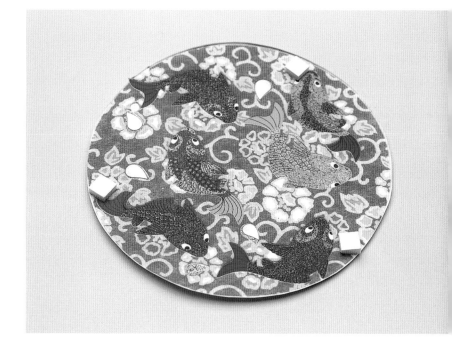

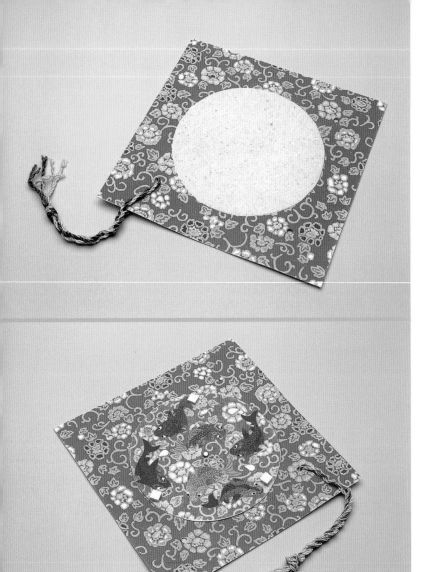

2. Adhere the decorative paper with the circular hole onto the other cardboard square. Turn the square over, wrong side up. Draw a $1\frac{1}{8}$" (2.9 cm) square in each corner of the cardboard. Punch a hole in the corner of each small square that is nearest the center of the board. Turn the square over, right side up. Insert the tassel into one of the corner holes.

3. Position the fish circle within the circular area of the cardboard square. Place the paper punch on the compass point, mark and cut through the two boards. Insert a paper brad in the hole.

4. To make the pinwheels, cut three $2\frac{5}{8}$" (6.7 cm) squares from the origami paper. Stack the paper squares and pierce through all layers at the center with the compass point. Cut a diagonal line from each corner to the center, stopping about a $\frac{1}{8}$" (3 mm) from the center point. Fold every other paper point to the center of the square. With the point of the craft knife, make a tiny center cut through all layers. Pass a paper brad through the cut.

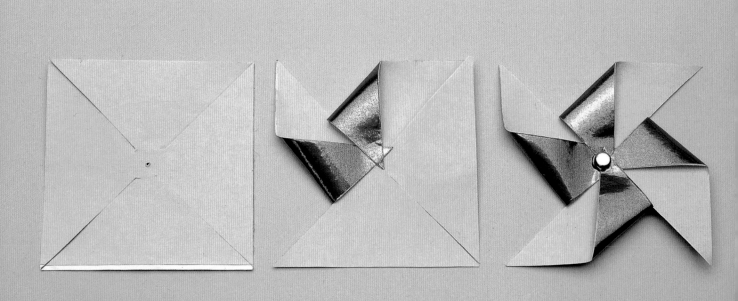

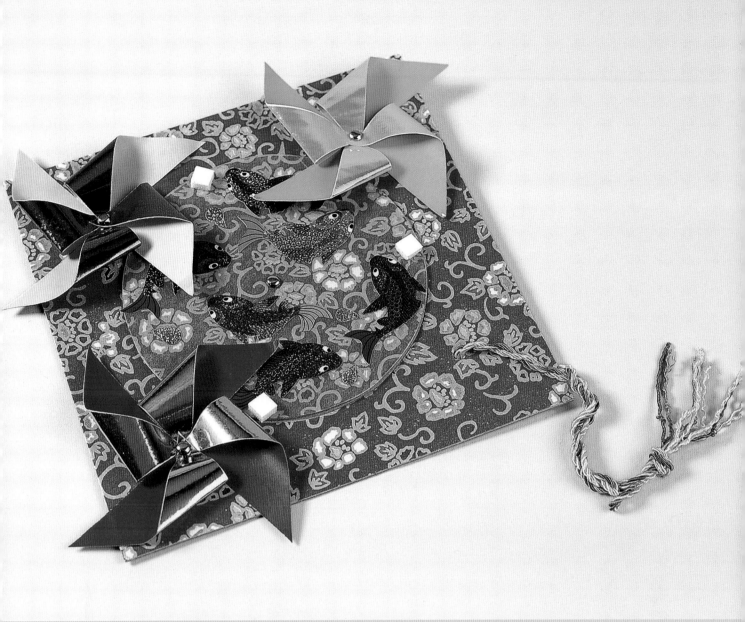

5. Place the pinwheel's paper brad through a corner hole of the decorative square. Fasten it to the back of the board. Repeat this step with the two remaining origami squares. Check to see if all pinwheels rotate easily before rotating the inner circle.

 GOING ONE STEP FURTHER

If you like double-sided colored paper for the pinwheels, adhere two sheets together using a sheet of double-sided tape.

Decorated Photo Corner Frame

Create an elegant frame for garden photos with a contemporary twist on the old-fashioned photo corner theme. A variety of stamped or transfer designs can be used to create decorative corners. Metallic inks work nicely to add a delicate sheen to the final frame design.

INSTRUCTIONS

1. Using a bone folder and ruler, measure, then score a line 2½" (6.4 cm) from each short edge of the translucent paper.

2. Fold up each 2½" (6.4 cm) section at the score lines to create panels. Position the paper horizontally with the panels folding up and toward the center of the paper.

3. Rub one triangular transfer or stamp a triangular motif in each corner of folded panels. Place the designs ¹/₁₆" (1.6 mm) away from the edges of the paper.

4. Open the panels flat. For each corner, cut an opening ¹/₁₆" (1.6 mm) outside of the stamp or transfer's diagonal line, beginning and ending ¹/₁₆" (1.6 mm) from the fold and the edge of the paper.

5. Fold panels over again and slip the corners of a 4" x 6" (10.2 cm x 15.2 cm) photo into the openings.

MATERIALS

- 11" x 4¼" (27.9 cm x 10.8 cm) colored translucent paper
- triangular transfer or rubber stamp (shown here: Chartpak transfers, Victorian lace, silver)
- silver ink pad (if using a stamp)
- transparent ruler
- craft knife
- bone folder

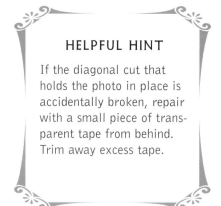

HELPFUL HINT

If the diagonal cut that holds the photo in place is accidentally broken, repair with a small piece of transparent tape from behind. Trim away excess tape.

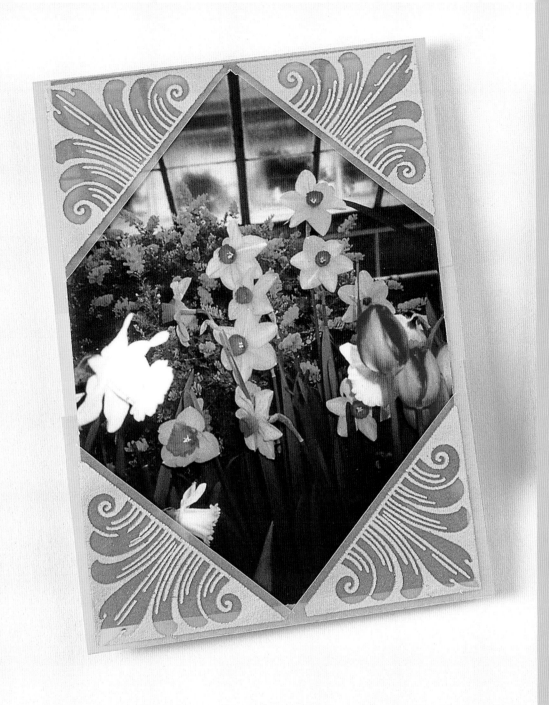

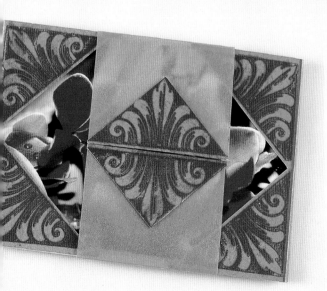

 GOING ONE STEP FURTHER

For an element of intrigue when you present your photo frame, create a paper band, $2\frac{3}{4}"$ x $8\frac{1}{2}"$ (7 cm x 21.6 cm) to partially screen the photo. Slip the decorated band between the paper and the back of the photo. Then fold each end of the band over the photo. Adhere the band closed with a sticker.

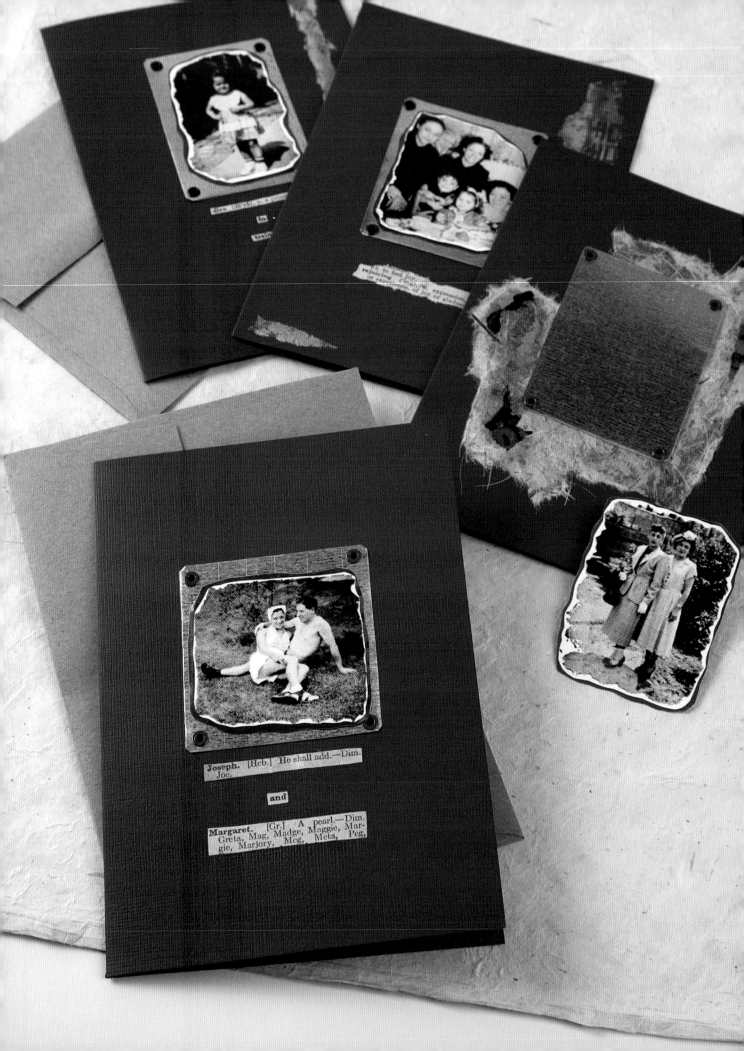

Joseph. [Heb.] He shall add.—Dim. Joe.

and

Margaret. [Gr.] A pearl.—Dim. Greta, Mag, Madge, Maggie, Maggie, Marjory, Mcg, Meta, Peg.

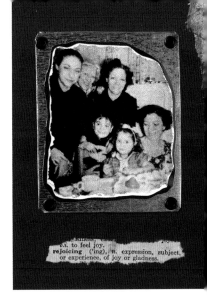

ARTIST: *Linda O'Brien*

mailable photo note cards *These*

note cards are the perfect combination of card and gift. They are not only mailable, but also magnetic: you can make a card and send it through the mail to your aunt or your sister-in-law, and she can remove the magnet and put it on her refrigerator to hold artwork or recipes. Perfect!

1 Stamp images on glossy paper with permanent black ink.

2 Trim the paper, and then laminate the fronts and apply magnetic sheeting to the back. (This is easiest to do with a Zyron machine, but you can do it all by hand.)

3 Use the tin snips to cut a rectangle from the roofing tin, just a little larger all around than the laminated images. File the edges to smooth them.

4 Drill a hole in each corner of the roofing tin.

5 Lay the tin over the note card, and use the pencil to mark the holes. Punch holes in the note card.

6 Attach the tin to the note card with the eyelets, one in each hole. Set with the setting tool.

7 Place the magnet on the tin.

8 Embellish the card as desired.

MATERIALS

- galvanized roofing tin
- blank note cards
- four ⅛" (3 mm) short eyelets
- eyelet setter
- glossy paper
- photo rubber stamps
- permanent ink
- drill with ⅛" (3 mm) bit
- pencil
- awl or ⅛" (3 mm) paper punch
- hammer
- metal file
- laminating sheets
- magnetic sheets

TIP

- *Add captions to your cards with words and phrases that you have cut from old, discarded books—textbooks are especially fun for this—or simply stamp captions below the photos.*

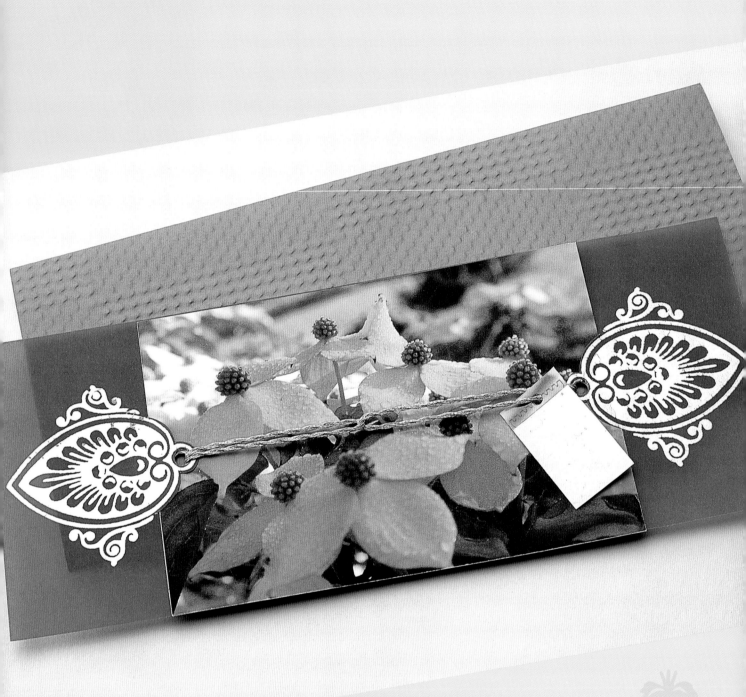

 GOING ONE STEP FURTHER

Want to add a personal message? Punch a hole in a small tag, add your greeting, and thread it onto the ribbon strand before looping the ribbons together.

Victorian Locket Photo Holder

MATERIALS

- 4" x 10" (10.2 cm x 25.4 cm) piece of colored translucent paper
- locket-shaped transfers or rubber stamp (shown here: Chartpak transfers, Victorian lace, locket design, silver)
- silver ink pad (if using a stamp)
- 18" (46 cm) length of metallic ribbon or cord
- 1½" (3.8 cm)-wide round sticker
- paper punch
- pencil
- craft knife
- ruler

This photo project is based on the locket—a small, ornamental case designed to hold a cherished photo or keepsake. Slip one of your favorite photos under the locket tabs. Then link the two lockets together with metallic threads and mail to a special friend.

INSTRUCTIONS

1. Lightly mark the center points of the short edges of the translucent paper. With a pencil, lightly draw a line between these two points, dividing the paper in half.

2. Center the transfer or stamped image on this line with each design positioned about ⅛" (3 mm) from the opposite ends of the paper. Adhere the transfer following the manufacturer's instructions or apply your stamped design.

3. Next, lightly draw a line parallel to and 2" (5 cm) inside of each short edge, skipping over the stamped image.

4. Using a craft knife, cut along the edge of the design that extends past this drawn line into the center section of the paper. Slip a 4" x 6" (10.2 cm x 15.2 cm) photo under the cut area of the locket.

5. Using a punch, make a hole through one end of the locket and the photo. To create a link between lockets, thread the ends of the 18" (46 cm) length of ribbon up through card holes to the front. Loop the ribbons around each other in the center, and then return each ribbon end back through its original hole. Adhere the ribbon ends to the back of the card using stickers.

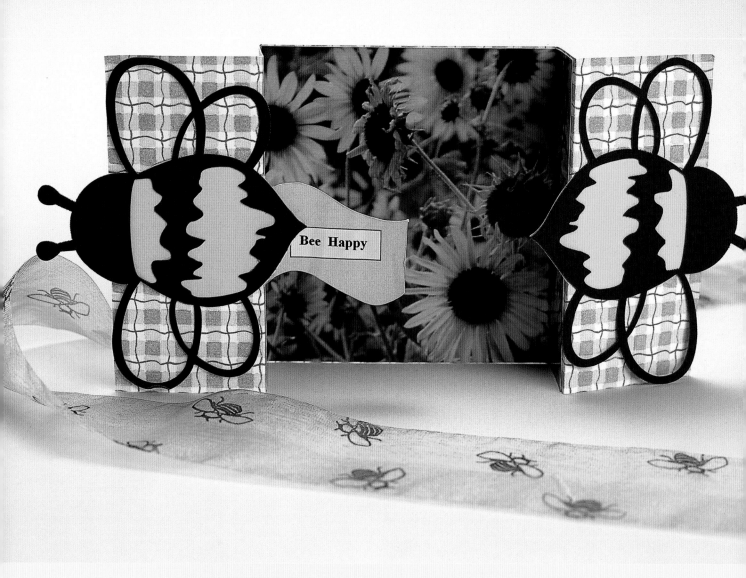

$\mathscr{B}$ee Happy Photo Card

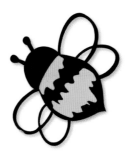

This folded card creates a stagelike setting for a favorite garden photo. The photo is the backdrop and the bees the main characters. The recipient of this charming, freestanding card will want to display it where it will receive rave reviews.

MATERIALS

- 4" x 10" (10.2 cm x 25.4 cm) medium weight decorative paper
- bee template (page 266)
- 4" x 6" (10.2 cm x 15.2 cm) photo, landscape format
- roll of ¼" (6 mm)-wide double-sided tape
- pencil
- ruler
- craft knife
- bone folder

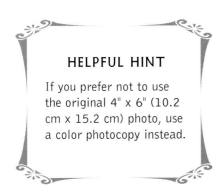

HELPFUL HINT

If you prefer not to use the original 4" x 6" (10.2 cm x 15.2 cm) photo, use a color photocopy instead.

INSTRUCTIONS

1. With the paper right side up, measure 2" (5 cm) in from each short edge of the paper, and draw two parallel pencil lines.

2. Photocopy, then cut out the bee template from a piece of yellow card stock. Adhere a strip of double-sided tape to the wrong side of each bumblebee. Position the bumblebee's wings within the 2" (5 cm)-wide panel. Antennas and stinger should extend beyond the panel on both sides. Remove the tape backing and adhere each bee in the correct position.

3. Using a craft knife, cut along the bumblebee's stinger, beginning and ending at the pencil line. Fold the panels toward the back of the card along the pencil line. Turn the card over, keeping the panels folded back.

4. Run doubled-sided tape along the top and bottom of the photograph. Center and adhere the photo in the middle section of the card.

5. Using a bone folder and ruler, score a line on the photo, which measures 1¼" (3.2 cm) from each folded edge. Fold along the scored line, returning bumblebee panels to the front of the card.

Garden Gate Greeting

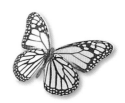

At the garden gate, an opportunity full of promise and wonder awaits. Crossing over the threshold, you can wander along the garden paths, marveling over each and every flower that catches your eye. Designed as a simple paper cut out, let your recipient open the gate onto a beautiful garden photograph.

INSTRUCTIONS

1. Cut a 6" x 8½" (15.2 cm x 21.6 cm) section from the card stock. Fold it in half.

2. Stamp the floral design onto the remaining 5" x 8½" (12.7 cm x 21.6 cm) section of card stock. Sprinkle with embossing powder. Apply heat with the heat gun to melt the powder.

3. Trace the contour of the garden gate template onto the stamped paper. Using a craft knife, cut out the design. Cut the design into two pieces by cutting along the left side of the gate.

4. On the back of the last picket of each unit, run a strip of double-sided tape.

5. Place the two picket units on the photograph, lining up the bottom edges. The left unit should extend one picket under the gate picket. Fold over the extra pickets, which extend beyond the photograph edges to the back of the photograph. Remove the tape backing and adhere.

6. On the back of the photograph, run a strip of double-sided tape along the top and bottom. Remove the tape's backing and adhere to the front of the folded card stock.

7. Adhere the butterfly onto the first picket of the garden gate. Fold the wings up.

MATERIALS

- garden gate template (page 267)
- 4" x 6" (10.2 cm x 15.2 cm) photograph
- 8½" x 11" (21.6 cm x 27.9 cm) off-white card stock
- 1½" (3.8 cm) paper butterfly cut out
- embossing powder, clear
- roll of ¼" (6 mm)-wide double-sided tape
- floral design rubber stamp
- light green ink pad
- heat gun
- craft knife
- ruler

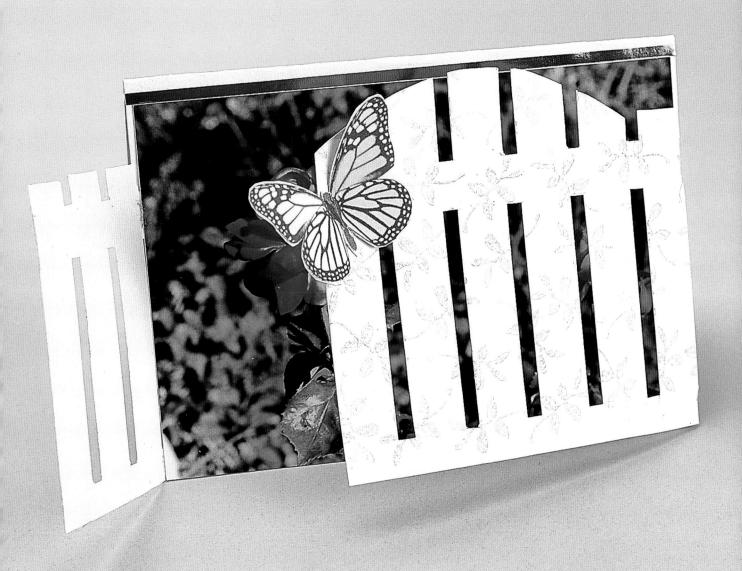

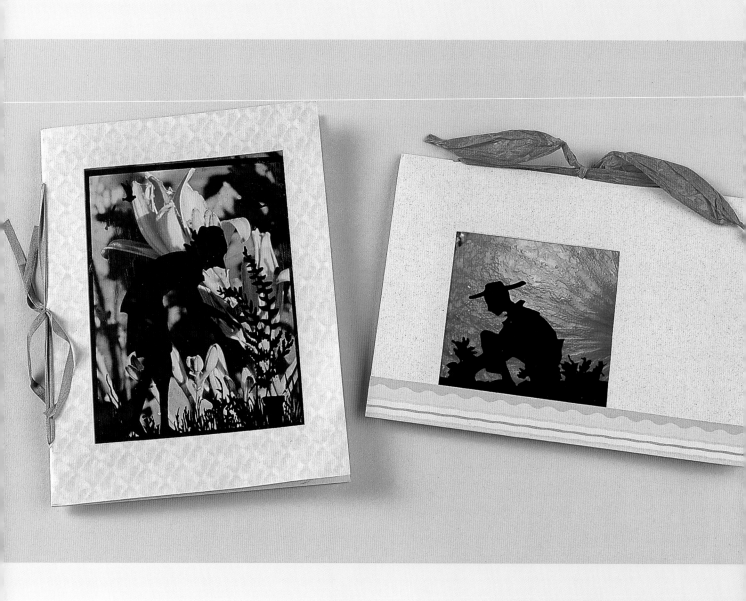

$\mathcal{G}$arden Silhouettes

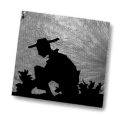

MATERIALS

- 7$\frac{1}{8}$" x 11" (18.1 cm x 27.9 cm) colored paper

- silhouette-style clip art or other black and white art

- plastic window decal sheet (shown here: Avery window decals #3276)

- 4" x 6" (10.2 cm x 15.2 cm) photo

- blank greeting cards & envelopes (shown here: Strathmore KIDS Series)

- ribbon or paper ribbon

- roll of $\frac{1}{4}$" (6 mm)-wide double-sided tape

- craft knife

- transparent ruler

- paper punch

- needle

- ink-jet printer

HELPFUL HINT

If you don't have access to a computer, your local printer can transfer your silhouette design to a transparency. Be sure to tell the printer that the black design needs to be opaque. The transparency can then be adhered to the back of the card window to create the same effect.

Close-up shots of flowers and vegetables make great fantasy backdrops for cut paper silhouettes. The illustrated silhouettes were transferred to decal sheets using an ink-jet printer. Decals stick to photos and are easily removed and replaced without causing harm to the photos.

INSTRUCTIONS

1. Transfer the silhouette design to the decal sheet using an ink-jet printer. Position the decal over the photo and adhere. Trim excess decal from the edges using a craft knife. On the back of the photo, place strips of double-sided tape along the top and bottom.

2. Fold the colored paper in half. Unfold. Center the photo on one half of the paper. Use a needle to mark the four corners of the photo by piercing the paper. Remove the photo. To create the window opening, cut an area that is $\frac{1}{8}$" (3 mm) greater than the photo markings using the craft knife and a transparent ruler.

3. Place the blank card inside the folded colored paper and clip the papers together. Open the card. On the fold, use a needle to pierce three tiny holes denoting the center, 1" (2.5 cm) from the top edge, and 1" (2.5 cm) from the bottom edge. Use a paper punch to create $\frac{1}{8}$" (3 mm) holes.

4. Thread a paper ribbon through the holes and tie a bow on the outside of the card.

5. On the blank card, position the photo within the window opening. Remove the tape backing and adhere.

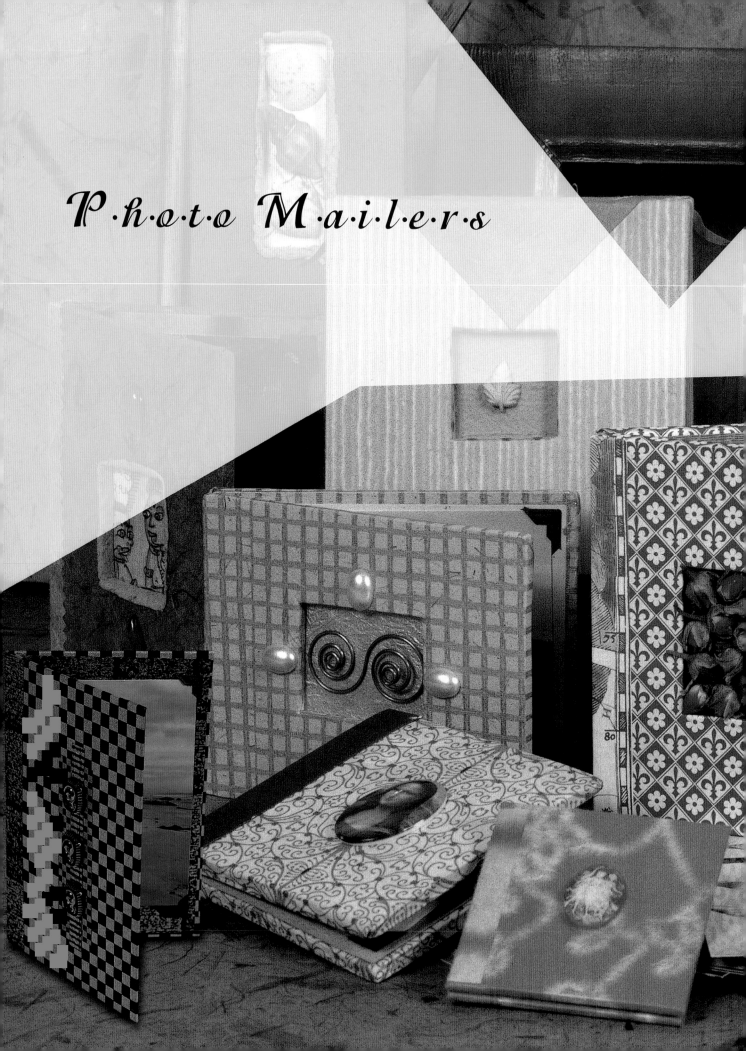

P·h·o·t·o M·a·i·l·e·r·s

Although photo mailers appear complicated, they are easy to make; think of them as paper packages holding wonderful images inside. This unique style of card works as both a card and a photograph frame. Small photo mailers are perfect as baby announcements and can be made to the size of any picture. Tailor this card to many different occasions by choosing various papers. Do not limit yourself to photographs when designing a photo mailer. Window photo mailers take a little more work to construct, but can be used to frame small three-dimensional items, such as seashells, keys, or dried flowers, depending on the occasion.

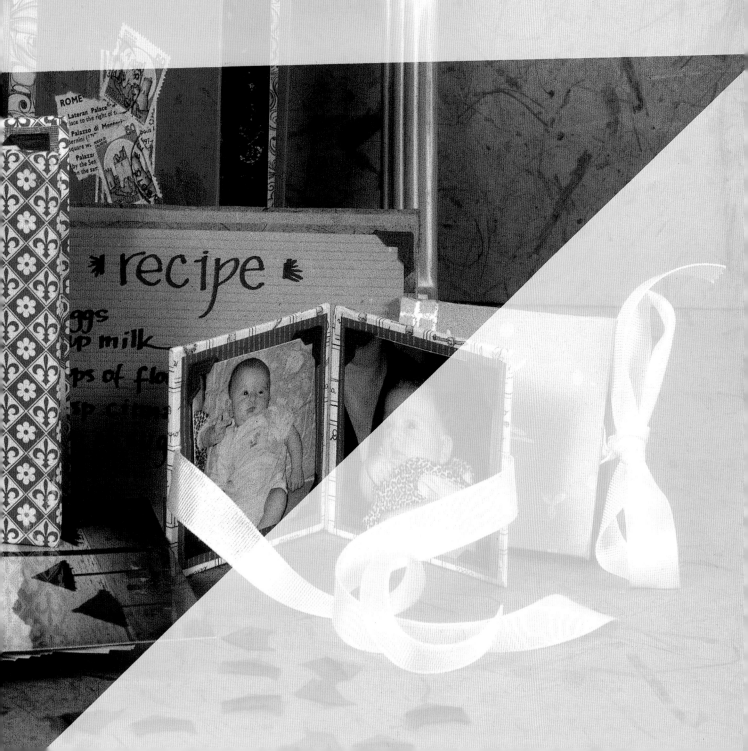

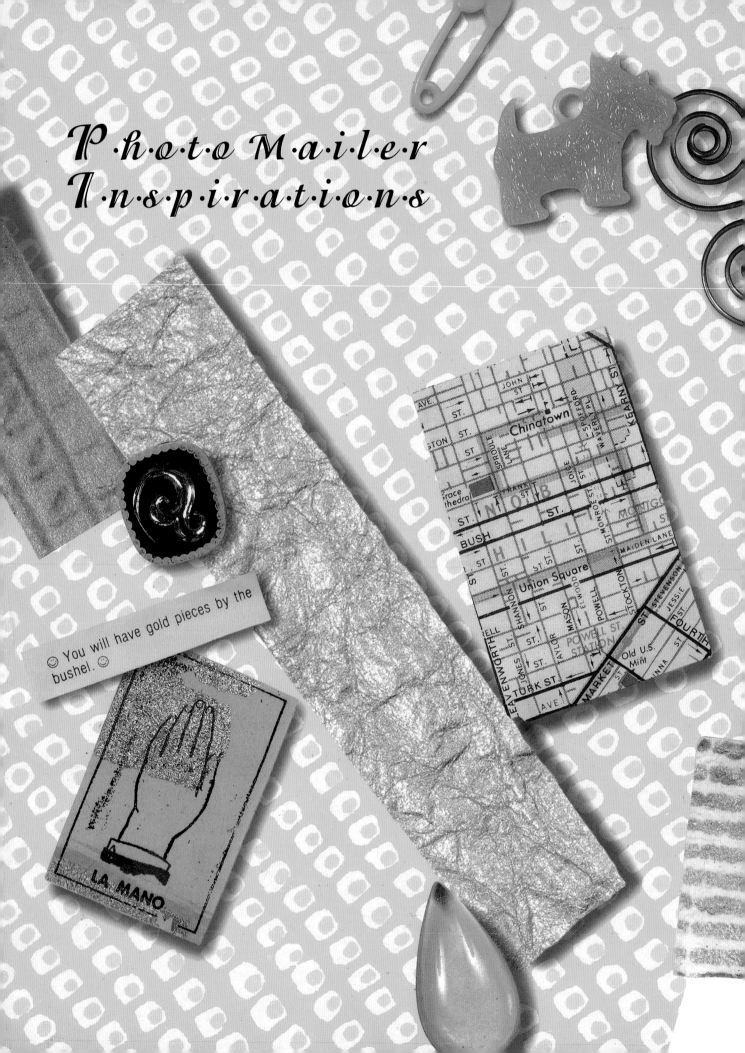

P·h·o·t·o M·a·i·l·e·r I·n·s·p·i·r·a·t·i·o·n·s

☺ You will have gold pieces by the bushel. ☺

LA MANO

U se festive paper to create a birthday theme, or white and gold papers for an elegant wedding invitation. Decorate the cover of the photo mailer with a collage, special mementos, or images cut from books and magazines. You can build a paper "inspirations" file by collecting everyday items such as stamps, photographs, ticket stubs, playbills, subway maps, wine labels (especially exotic ones), cookie fortunes, travel brochures, road maps, shopping bags, and calendars.

Other finds—buttons, flat beads, coins, dried flowers—are treasures that can double as decorations.

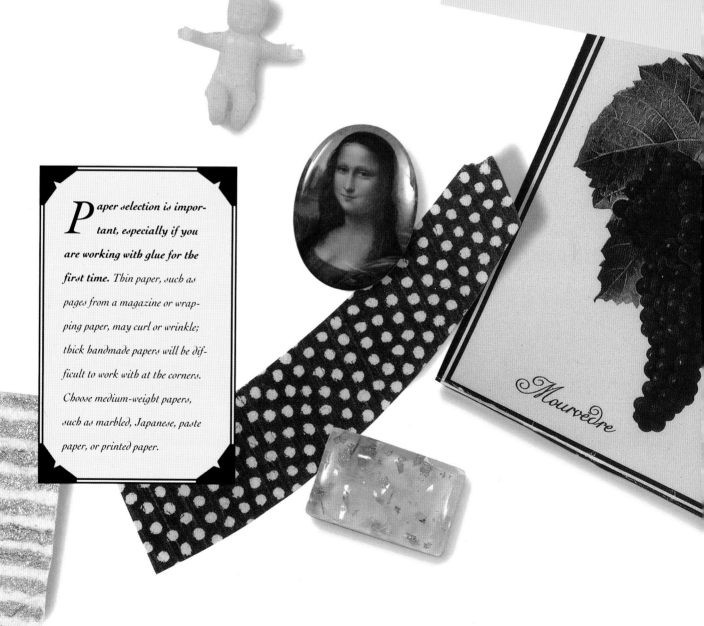

P aper selection is important, especially if you are working with glue for the first time. Thin paper, such as pages from a magazine or wrapping paper, may curl or wrinkle; thick handmade papers will be difficult to work with at the corners. Choose medium-weight papers, such as marbled, Japanese, paste paper, or printed paper.

Basic Photo Mailer

This special card combines many of the techniques already presented in the previous chapters. Prepare all the materials before you start to glue. Choose papers for the outside of the cover, the interior, and the binding strip. Measure the papers and then cut out each piece. Once the first few steps have been completed, the corners require special attention. You may want to practice making them a few times before attempting the final project.

Materials

- Two pieces of illustration board, 4" x 6" (10 cm x 15 cm)
- Two pieces of decorative paper for the outside, 5" x 7" (13 cm x 18 cm)
- Two pieces of decorative paper for the inside, 3 ¾" x 5 ¾" (9.5 cm x 14.5 cm)
- Piece of paper for the binding strip (use the same paper as on the inside), 1 ¼" x 6" (3 cm x 15 cm)
- Piece of writing paper or a photograph, 3 ½" x 5 ½" (9 cm x 14 cm)
- Black photo corners
- Craft knife
- Metal ruler
- Pencil
- PVA glue
- Glue brush
- Bone folder
- Cutting mat

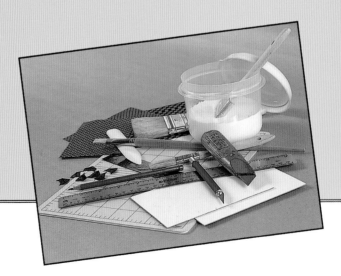

❖*1* Lay the paper for the outside cover pattern-side down. Measure ½" (1 cm) from all edges and mark this border with the pencil. Apply glue to cover the square area inside the pencil lines, then center the illustration board and gently adhere it to the glued surface, using the pencil marks as a guide.

❖*2* Turn the glued piece over. With the side of your thumb or the bone folder, press firmly from the center out to the edges to create a smooth surface. Rub the entire surface with your fingers until the paper is flat and wrinkle-free.

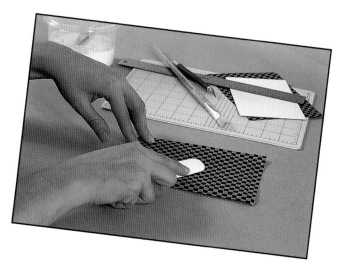

❖*3* Turn the card back over. Apply glue to the long flaps of paper on the right and left edges. Fold the flaps firmly over the illustration board and smooth them with your thumb or the bone folder. Press the paper flat only to the top and bottom edges of the illustration board. Be careful not to press the paper together at the corners where it extends beyond the board.

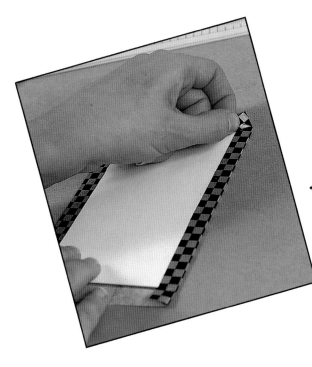

❖*4* Apply glue to the top corners of the paper. Fold the corner paper at a 45-degree angle toward the center of the board. Crease the paper and press down. Press in the excess paper created by the angle fold along the top edge of the illustration board. Repeat with the bottom corners.

❖5 Apply glue to the remaining short strips of paper at the top and bottom edges of the boards. Fold them over the illustration board and smooth them with a bone folder or your fingers. Make sure that the paper does not hang over the edge of the board.

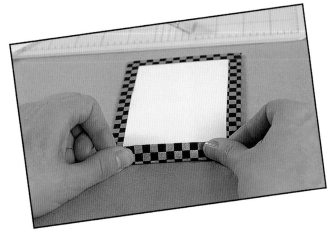

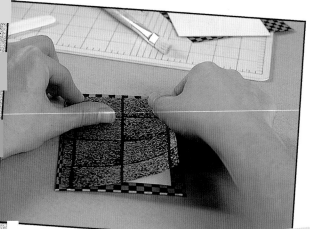

❖6 Apply glue to the back of the contrasting paper. Work from the center out, covering the entire surface and all edges. Center the paper on the illustration board and press to adhere. One half of the card is now complete. Repeat steps 1 through 6 to make the other side of the card.

To prevent the illustration board from warping as the glue dries, put a sheet of paper between the sides of the finished card so they will not stick to each other, and press the card under a pile of heavy books.

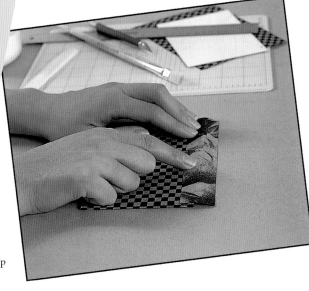

❖7 Place one card on top of the other, with the contrasting papers facing each other. Apply glue to the back of the binding strip, covering the entire surface. Place one half of the glued strip on the left side of the top card.

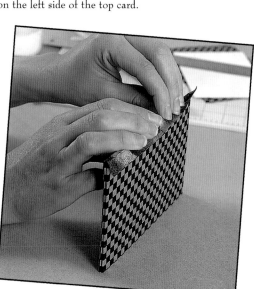

❖8 Stand the card upright on its right edge. Square the covers, matching the edges evenly all the way around. Use your thumb and forefinger to roll the binding strip firmly around the two boards to the back card.

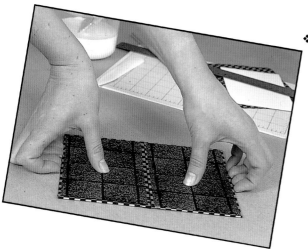

❖9 Open the card and lay it flat, with the outside covers facing down. Press the right and left edges of the card toward the center to catch the glued strip between the two boards. Hold the cards for about a minute until the glue sets. The card should open and close easily as if on a hinge.

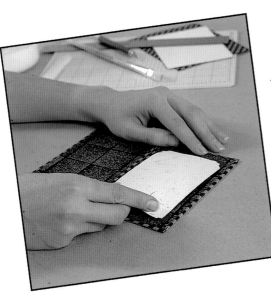

❖10 Position two photo corners on the left and right top corners of the 3 ½" x 5 ½" (9 cm x 14 cm) paper. Apply glue to the back of the corners. Press the corners onto the inside of the card at an equal distance from the top edges. Slide the paper out and repeat this procedure with the bottom corners. If you want a double frame, apply corners to the other side of the card as well.

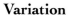

❖11 Insert a 3 ½" x 5 ½" (9 cm x 14 cm) piece of writing paper or photograph into the photo corners to complete your card. To personalize the card, make a paper or photo collage on the front cover with items from your collage file.

Variation

Choose paper to complement the photograph you want to send. Dress up a child's photo with playful, colorful papers from different countries and glue tiny toys or objects to the front of the card.

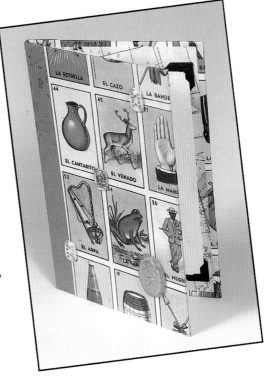

Baby Photo Mailer

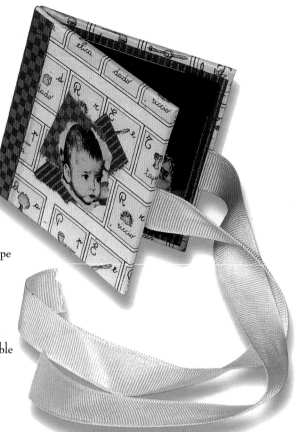

The baby photo mailer is a perfect card to welcome a little one into the world, but this type of card can be used for any occasion. Select papers and ribbon appropriate for your design, and cut them to the required sizes. Glue the paper to the boards, add the ribbon, and bind the boards together. For a double frame, you can apply picture corners on both sides of the card.

Materials

- Two pieces of illustration board or cardboard, 3" x 3" (7.5 cm x 7.5 cm)
- Two pieces of decorative paper for the outside, 4" x 4" (10 cm x 10 cm)
- Two pieces of contrasting decorative paper for the inside, 2 ¾" x 2 ¾" (7 cm x 7 cm)
- Piece of paper for the binding strip (use the same paper as on the inside),
  1" x 3" (2.5 cm x 7.5 cm)
- Piece of writing paper, 2 ½" x 2 ½" (6.5 cm x 6.5 cm)
- Length of ribbon, 8 ½" (21 cm)
- Picture corners
- Craft knife
- Metal ruler
- Pencil
- PVA glue
- Glue brush
- Bone folder
- Cutting mat

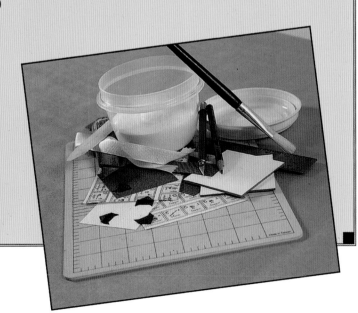

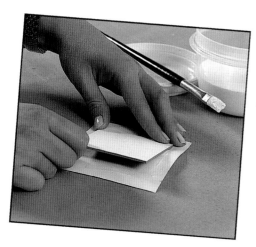

❖**1** Apply glue to the back of the paper for the outside cover. Center the illustration board on the paper, leaving approximately ½" (1 cm) on all sides. Turn the card over. Use your fingers to smooth the paper over the board. Start at the center and work out to the edges.

Brush the glue evenly, taking care not to use too much because it will cause the paper to tear, especially in the corners. Also, if the glue leaks out, it will stain the ribbon and paper.

❖**2** Turn the card over again. Apply glue to the right and left flaps. Fold the flaps over the illustration board and smooth the paper with your fingers. Do not press the paper at the top and bottom edges together; they will be folded at an angle for the corners in the next step.

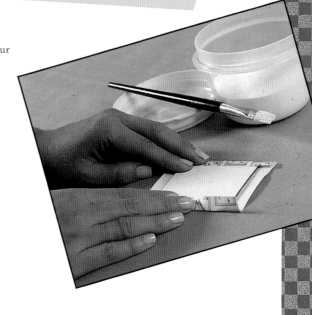

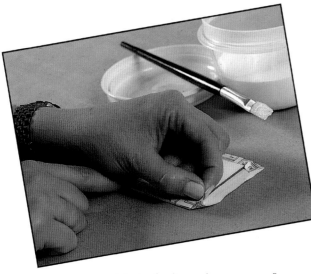

❖**3** Apply glue to the top corner flaps. For each corner, pull the top piece of folded paper to a 45-degree angle. It is important to angle the fold so that the paper will not hang over the edge. Tuck any excess paper toward the board edge. Repeat on the bottom corners.

❖**4** Apply glue to the top and bottom flaps and adhere them to the board. Make sure that the folded corner is glued on the inside of the board edge. Now repeat steps 1 through 4 for the other side of the card.

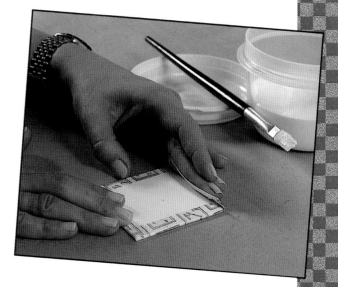

❖5 Lay the card pieces side by side with the outside covers facing down. Cut the ribbon in half, and add glue to one of the pieces of ribbon, ¼" (.5 cm) away from its end. Glue the ribbon to the middle of the outside edge of one card. To position the ribbon in the same place on the other card, close the card, lay the second piece on top of the first, and make a mark. Glue the second length of ribbon to the other card.

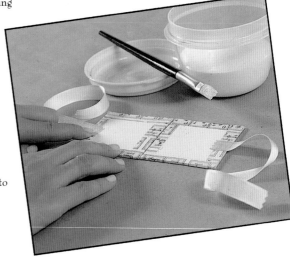

❖6 Lay the contrasting papers right side down. Brush glue from the center out to the edges. Center and adhere the papers to the inside of the cards. Use your thumb or a bone folder to smooth the paper flat.

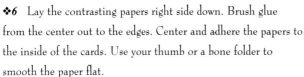

Match the placement of the ribbons, one on top of the other, so the card will tie properly.

❖7 Place one card on top of the other, with the outside covers facing out and all the edges meeting. Apply glue to the back of the binding strip. Place half of the glued strip evenly on the front left side of the top card. Roll the paper over the edges and adhere it to the back of the card.

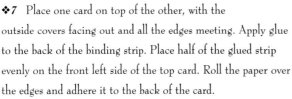

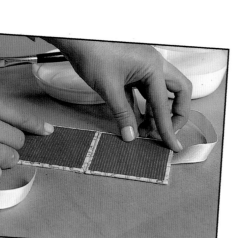

❖8 Open the card flat. Press the left and right edges of the card toward the center to catch the binding strip between the boards. Hold the cards about a minute until the glue sets.

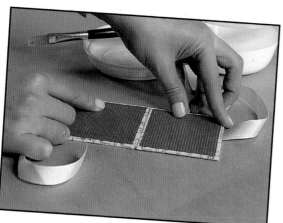

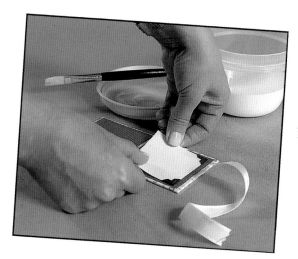

❖**9** Place the photo corners on the left and right top corners of the 2 ½" x 2 ½" (6.5 cm x 6.5 cm) writing paper. Apply glue to the back of the corners, center them, and press them onto the inside of the card. Slide the paper out and repeat the procedure with the bottom corners.

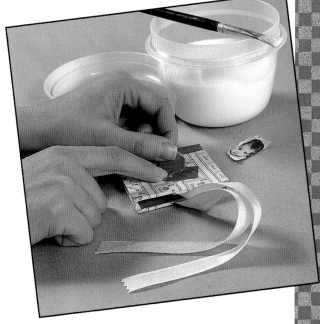

❖**10** Make a collage on the front cover with complementary papers. Glue a baby photo for a final layer over the collage.

Variations

For more sophisticated photo mailers, make the paper and the binding all the same color. Add a button that closes the photo mailer with string. Simply glue the button to the top of a glass bead that is then glued to the card. The bead gives the button height to wrap the string around the base.

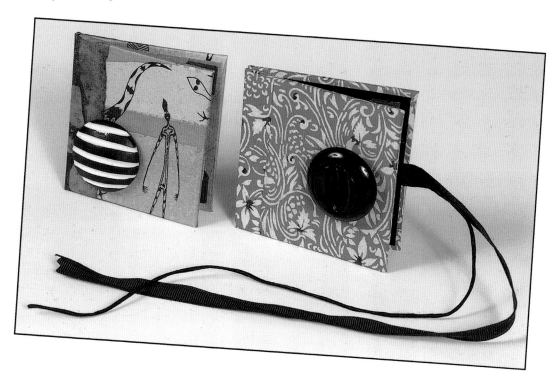

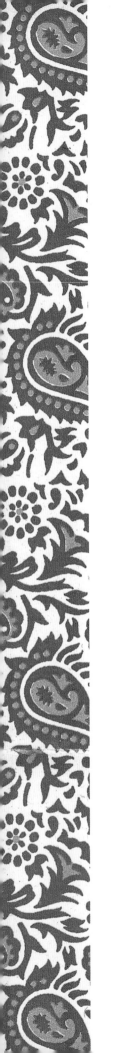

Keepsake
Photo Mailer

T ailor this versatile card to suit almost any occasion.
Measure the foam core and outside paper to make the
window, then remove the window. Cover the foam core and line the
window frame with paper. Glue a piece of paper or a photograph behind the window
to serve as a backdrop for your object. Cover the other piece of foam core, then bind the two pieces
together. Add picture corners and decorate the window.

Materials

- Two pieces of ¼" (.5 cm) foam core, 4" x 5" (10 cm x 13 cm)
- Two pieces of decorative paper for the outside, 5 ½" x 6 ½" (14 cm x 16 cm)
- Two pieces of decorative paper for the inside, 3 ¾" x 4 ¾" (9.5 cm x 11.5 cm)
- Strip of paper for window lining, ¼" x 7" (.5 cm x 18 cm)
- Piece of card stock or firm paper for behind the window, 3 ½" x 4 ½" (8.5 cm x 12 cm)
- Piece of decorative paper, photograph, or image for the window, 2" x 2 ½" (5 cm x 6.5 cm)
- Piece of paper for the binding strip (use the same paper as on the outside), 4" x 2" (10 cm x 5 cm)
- Object for the window and four picture corners
- T-square
- Eraser
- Craft knife
- Metal ruler
- Pencil
- PVA glue
- Glue brush
- Bone folder
- Cutting mat

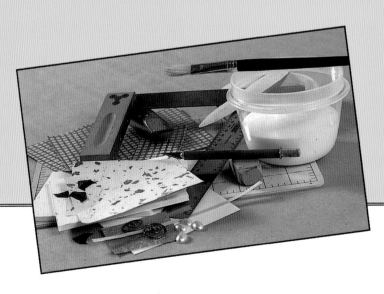

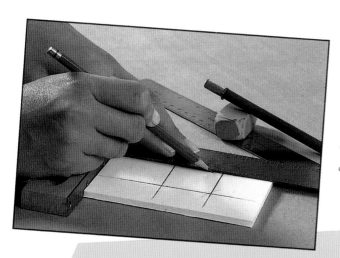

❖*1* Lay one piece of the foam core on your work surface. Measure and mark with the pencil 1 ¼" (3 cm) from the left and right edges, then measure and mark 1 ½" (4 cm) from the top and bottom edges. Make straight lines with the T-square at the marks to form the shape of the window. Use the T-square as a guide as you cut out the window with the craft knife.

Cut the foam core several times before moving the ruler to ensure that the blade is all the way through.

Draw arrows on the paper and the foam core to use as placement guides.

❖*2* Make a line ¾" (2 cm) from all edges on the back of the outside paper. Position the foam core within the lines. Hold the foam core in place and use the pencil to trace around the inner edges of the window. Center the piece of card stock under the window and trace around the inner edges of the window again.

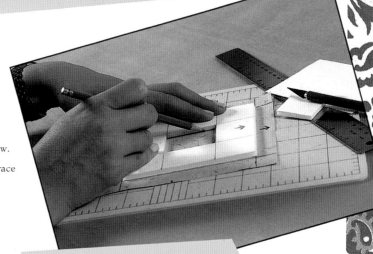

Cut from corner to corner for clean edges.

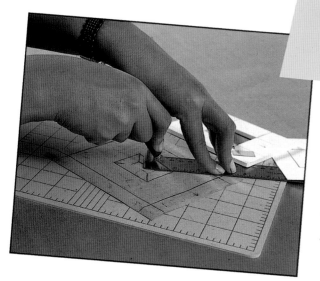

❖*3* Remove the foam core and the card stock. On the outside paper, measure ½" (1 cm) from each side of the window outline to form a smaller square. Use the metal ruler and craft knife to cut out the inner square. Then cut a diagonal from each window corner to the corner of the inner square to create flaps.

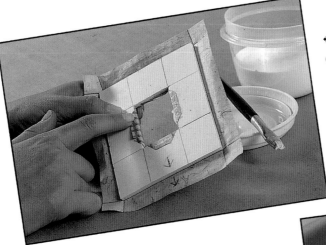

❖4 Apply glue to the back of the outside paper. Center the foam core on the paper within the marked lines and adhere it. Turn the foam core over and smooth the paper with your hand. Pull the flaps gently through the window in the foam core toward the back of the card.

❖5 Apply glue to the left and right flaps along the length of the card. Fold the flaps over the edges and adhere them to the foam core. Glue only as far as the top and bottom edges of the foam core. Glue the paper between the folded flaps at the corners onto the top edge of the foam core.

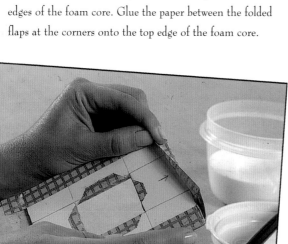

❖6 Glue the back flap over the top edge toward the front flap. Apply glue and fold both flaps over the top edge toward the back of the foam core. Repeat these steps at the bottom edge of the card.

❖7 Apply glue to the back of the ¼" (.5 cm) paper strip. Insert the paper strip at the lower left corner and along the edges of the window. Push it into the corners tightly for an accurate fit. Trim any excess. Use the bone folder to work the paper into the corners and smooth the edges.

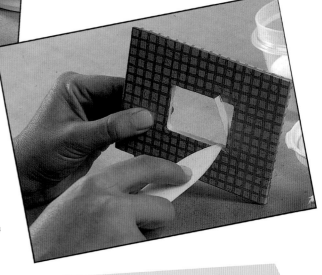

Check the length of the paper strip to make sure it fits before applying the glue.

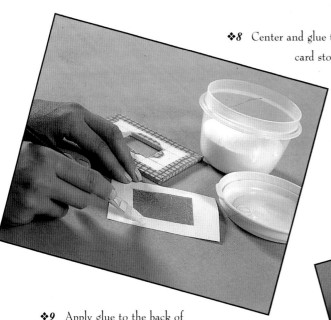

❖8 Center and glue the 2" x 2 ½" (5 cm x 6.5 cm) window paper onto the card stock over the pre-traced square. Apply glue to the front of the card stock around the window paper. Adhere the front of the card stock to the back of the foam core, so that the window paper appears in the window.

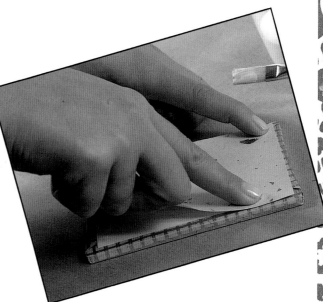

❖9 Apply glue to the back of the inside paper. Center the paper over the card stock on the foam core and adhere it. Smooth the paper flat with your hands. Create the other side of the card following the previous steps, eliminating the construction of the window.

❖10 Place one side of the card on top of the other, with the inside papers facing each other. Apply glue to the back of the binding strip. Put half of the glued strip on the front left side of the top card. Pull the other half of the binding strip around the foam core edges to the outside edge of the bottom card.

❖11 Open the card and lay it flat with the outside covers facing down. Press the right and left edges of the card toward the center to catch the glued strip between the two pieces of foam core. Let the glue set for about a minute. To finish the card, add the picture corners (see the instructions given for the Basic Photo Mailer on page 234) and your window object.

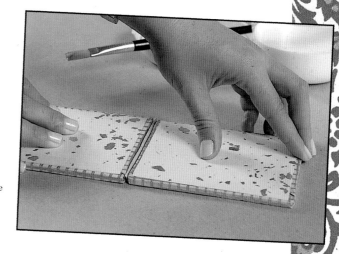

Greeting Cards and Stationery: Seasons Handmade

Each season, distinct and unique, offers a plenitude of garden gifts.

Share your garden's abundance and experience the pleasure of enriching other people's lives. The simple act of creating one of these cards holds the promise of touching another's heart by sharing the connections you feel to the garden's earthly riches. Pass along a sense of well-being, wholesome thoughts, and feelings through the creation of handsome cards and stationery that weave the beauty of soft textures, herbal scents, and floral colors.

- *Compose a letter with the beauty of Japanese leaves layered beneath your writing.*

- *Gather a few sprigs of lavender that, upon the card's opening, release a delightful fragrance.*

- *Share a favorite garden recipe.*

- *Give the gift of relaxation with homemade tea.*

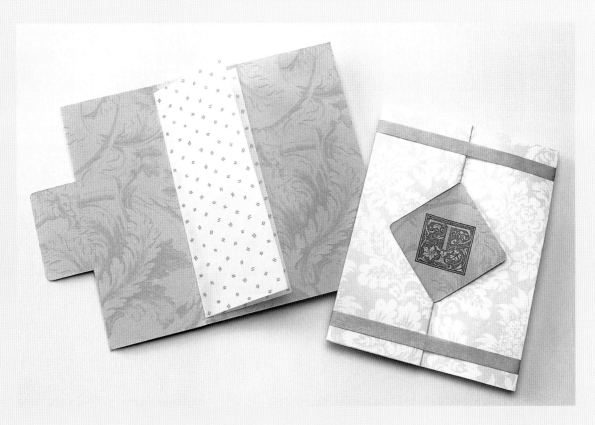

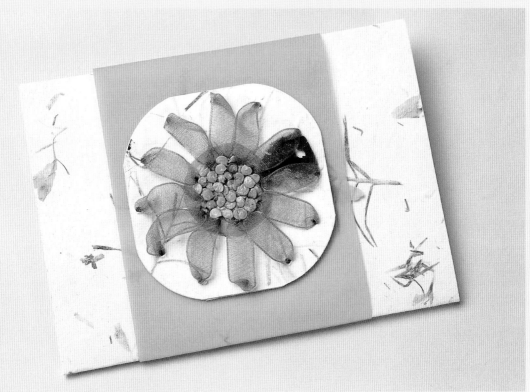

Dear Anne,

What a treat to visit with you in your beautiful garden.

The roses were so fragrant and th delphiniums so sky blue.

To sip tea among such beau birds hum, sing and n always delight in doing

Let us always fir strength to conti. and godly work divinely grow +

Your I Mar.

Garden Motif Stationery

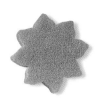

Design personal stationery as unique as your garden. Easily made with the stamping of large, simple garden forms onto paper, the design's soft boldness is sure to dance with delight under your printed words.

MATERIALS

- 12" x 18" (30 cm x 46 cm) best quality paper
- scrap paper
- sponge stamps—garden motifs, such as birds, trowel, watering can
- stamp pads—red, yellow, blue, and green
- ruler

INSTRUCTIONS

1. Tear the paper into four 6" x 9" (15 cm x 23 cm) sheets using the ruler as a tearing edge.

2. Gently press the sponge stamp onto the selected stamping pad. Place the stamp into position on the surface of the stationery. Cover the stamp with a piece of scrap paper and press down with the palm of your hand. Remove the scrap paper and stamp.

3. Repeat stamping process until a satisfactory design is complete.

HELPFUL HINT

If a stronger edge is desired after printing, use a colored pencil to redraw the outline of the stamped motif.

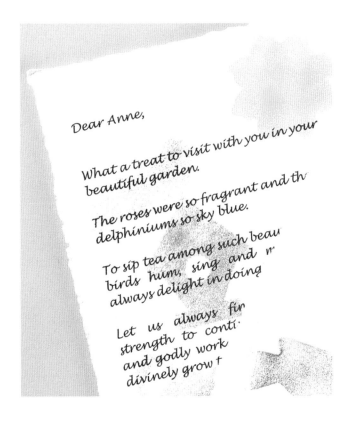

Pressed Leaves Stationery

Leaf types come in a wide variety of forms. Many are quite beautiful to behold, such as the Red Japanese Maple. Their elegant shape makes an attractive "falling leaf" background to letter writing. Lift the translucent notepaper to have a closer look at each leaf's rich intricacies of vein and toothed edge.

INSTRUCTIONS

1. Arrange five or six leaves on the stationery into a pleasing composition.

2. Brush small amounts of white glue onto the back of a leaf, including the stem. Reposition the leaf on the stationery. Repeat with the remaining leaves.

3. Place a sheet of waxed paper over the stationery. Then place a heavy book over the project and leave it in position overnight.

4. Remove the waxed paper and the book.

5. Place a strip of double-sided tape across the top of the stationery. Remove the backing from the tape. Position the translucent paper over the stationery and adhere it into position.

MATERIALS

- 5½" x 8½" (14 cm x 21.6 cm) bright white stationery with matching envelope
- 5½" x 8½" (14 cm x 21.6 cm) translucent paper
- five or six assorted pressed maple leaves
- roll of ¼" (6 mm)-wide double-sided tape
- white glue
- #1 brush
- 5½" x 8½" (14 cm x 21.6 cm) waxed paper
- heavy book

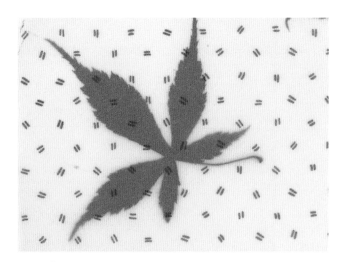

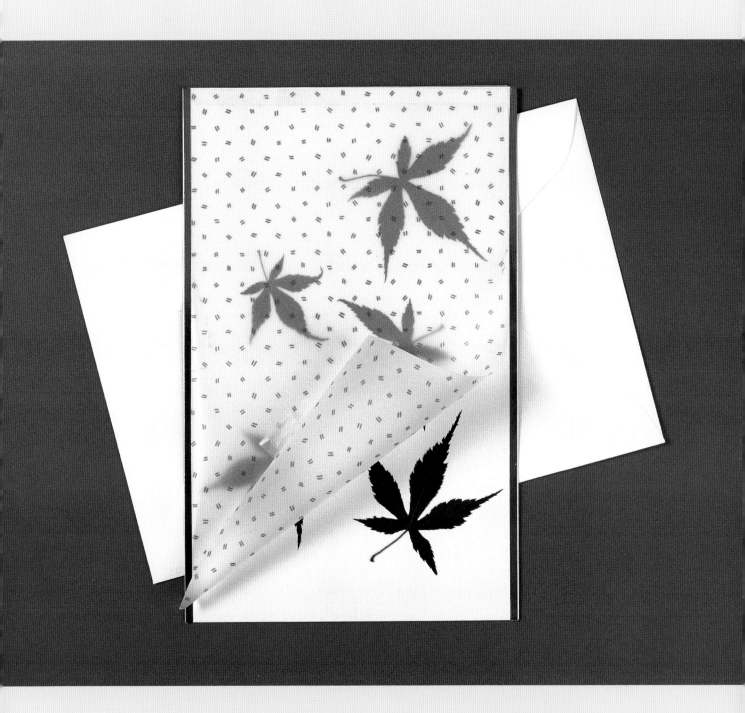

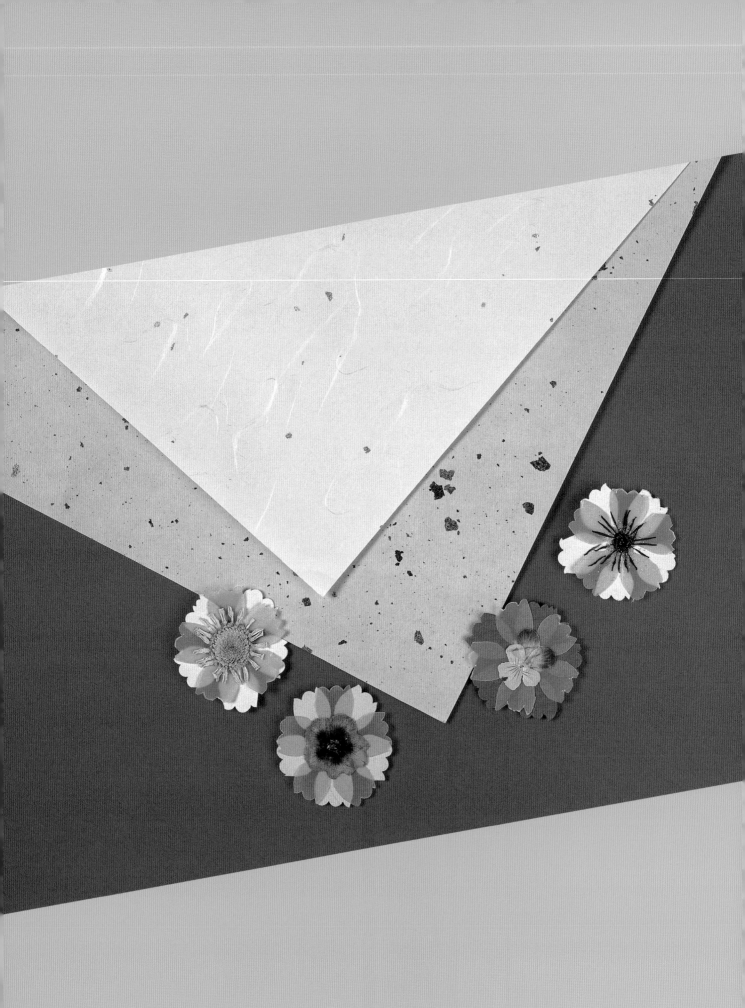

Dried Flower Medallions

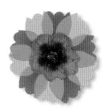

Accentuate your pressed flowers with these colorful paper medallions. Fashion a colorful collection to use year round as "dash of summer" embellishments for your letters. Freely combine different sorts of papers to generate whimsical blooms.

MATERIALS

- pressed flowers
- assortment of 2" (5 cm) squares of colored and translucent paper
- flower template (page 262)
- white glue
- craft knife
- scissors with a decorative edge, such as scalloped

HELPFUL HINT

Place the finished medallions back into the flower press for safekeeping.

INSTRUCTIONS

1. Stack papers in the following order: flower template, translucent paper, and colored paper.

2. Use a craft knife to cut along the inside edges of the flower petals. Next, use the decorative-edged scissors to cut out the flower.

3. Remove the template design. Rotate the translucent paper design until its petals are over the spaces between the colored paper petals.

4. Place a drop of glue in between the paper layers and in the center of the top paper.

5. Press a dried flower into the drop of glue.

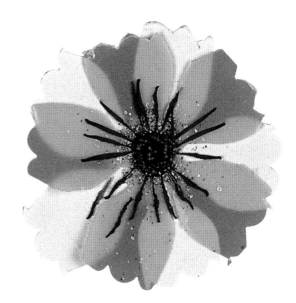

Garden Recipe Cards

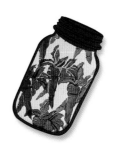

These recipe cards feature dancing chili peppers, a forest of asparagus, and intertwined carrots—a delightful feast for the eyes. Each card is decorated on one side with stamps and the other with a recipe. They slide in and out of windowed envelopes that are made using folded paper. The cards make thoughtful and inexpensive presents, especially when printed with friends' and family members' favorite recipes.

INSTRUCTIONS

1. Fold the colored paper in half. Using a bone folder, score a line ¹/₂" (1.3 cm) from each of the open edges opposite the fold. Open the paper. Trim the ¹/₂" (1.3 cm) strip from the right edge. Run a strip of double-sided tape along the left edge. Fold the paper in half. Fold over the ¹/₂" (1.3 cm) strip to the back. Do not remove tape backing.

2. Transfer or trace the Mason jar shape onto the front of the paper. Open the paper and cut out the inside of the Mason jar. Don't cut directly on the outline of the jar, but rather make the cut ¹/₈" (3 mm) inside the line.

3. Cut out a half circle, 1" (2.5 cm) wide, at the top and center of the paper, above the Mason jar. This will be the pull slot.

4. Fold the paper in half again. Fold over the ¹/₂" (1.3 cm) strip to the back of the sleeve. Remove the tape backing and adhere the edges together.

5. Practice the basic printing techniques of the veggie foam rubber stamps on a piece of scrap paper. When you are confident with the techniques, begin printing on the white card stock. When the print is dry, enhance it using colored pencils.

MATERIALS

- 6" x 10" (15.2 cm x 25.4 cm) colored paper
- 3³/₄" x 6" (9.5 cm x 15.2 cm) white card stock
- 12" (30 cm) length of ¹/₄" (6 mm)-wide ribbon
- 1" (2.5 cm) circle sticker
- 4¹/₂" (11 cm) Mason jar template (page 262) or similar rubber stamp
- black marker or ink pad
- press set of veggie stamps
- craft knife
- paper punch
- roll of ¹/₄" (6 mm)-wide double-sided tape
- acrylic paint set
- colored pencils
- watercolor brushes
- water cup
- bone folder
- ruler
- scrap paper

HELPFUL HINT

Other printing techniques can be just as effective as printing with foam rubber veggie shapes. Stencils or rubber stamps are great alternatives.

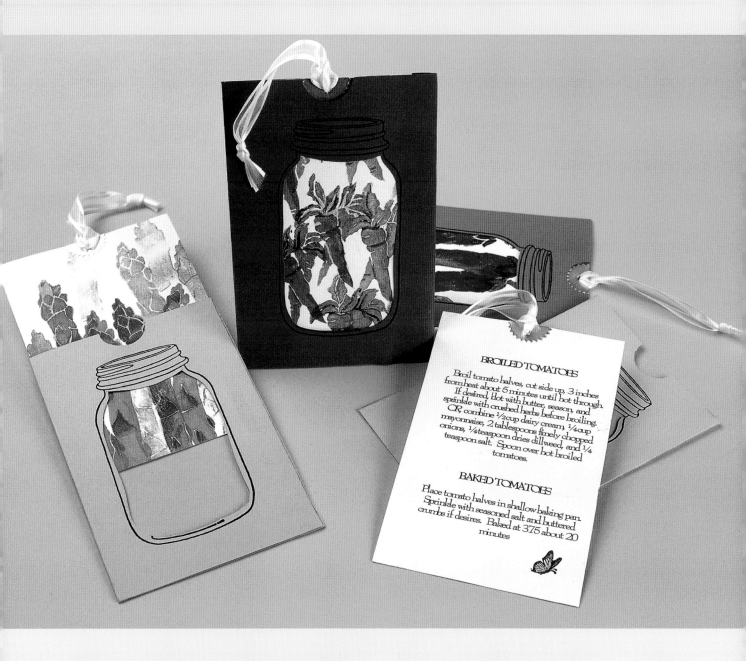

6. Turn the card over and write or type the recipe on the back of the card.

7. Adhere one half of the circle sticker to the top and center of the printed side. Fold the rest of the sticker to the back. Punch a hole through the sticker. Fold the ribbon in half. Slip the fold through the hole from the back of the card. Pull the ribbon ends through the loop and pull tight.

8. Slip the recipe card into the Mason jar sleeve.

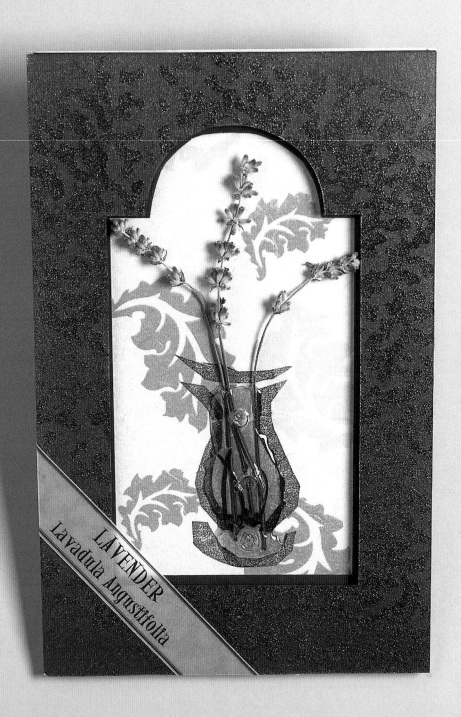

Lavender and Vase

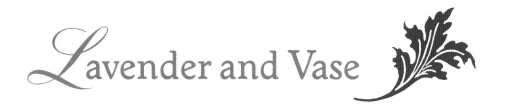

MATERIALS

- four to six stems of fresh lavender
- 5¹/₂" x 8¹/₂" (14 cm x 21.6 cm) heavy weight, metallic rose paper
- 5¹/₂" x 8¹/₂" (14 cm x 21.6 cm) decorative paper
- 5¹/₂" x 8¹/₂" (14 cm x 21.6 cm) mat board
- 5¹/₂" x 8¹/₂" (14 cm x 21.6 cm) sheet of double-sided tape
- 1" x 5" (2.5 cm x 12.7 cm) label
- ten ¹/₂" (1.3 cm) foam sticky squares
- large rubber stamp of a vine background
- claret embossing powder
- water-based craft lacquer
- 2¹/₂" (6.4 cm)-high rubber stamp vase
- black and maroon ink pads
- craft knife
- compass
- heat gun
- ruler

Dried lavender keeps its aromatic qualities for a long time. Create a simple floral arrangement using freshly cut or dried lavender stems and a stamped vase design. Any small leaf herb, such as thyme, can be used as well.

INSTRUCTIONS

1. Stamp the metallic paper with an overall design using the large stamp block. Sprinkle with claret colored embossing powder and adhere with heat gun.

2. Using a compass, draw a 2¹/₂" (6.4 cm) circle on the back of the metallic paper, 1" (2.5 cm) from the top. Next, draw a 3¹/₂" x 5" (8.9 cm x 12.7 cm) rectangle, 2" (5 cm) from the top. Using a craft knife, cut along the drawn lines, creating a frame.

3. Adhere ten sticky squares to the back—one in each corner and the remainder placed equally around the perimeter. Write the name of the herb on the label and adhere it to the front.

4. Adhere the sheet of double-sided tape to the mat board. Remove the backing and place the decorative paper on top.

5. Remove the backing paper from the sticky squares on the metallic paper and place the metallic frame onto the decorative paper. Stamp the vase and arrange plant stems within the vase.

6. Fill the inside area of the vase with a thin layer of craft lacquer, tacking down the stems. Let dry. Repeat this step until the vase looks three-dimensional.

Floral Monogram Tab Cards

With the use of subtle colors and a large floral block letter, this elegant card spells sophistication. The design could easily be adapted as an invitation for a special event, or fashion a set of five and give them as a gift to a newly wedded couple.

INSTRUCTIONS

1. Turn the floral paper face down. Adhere the contrasting floral paper to one half of the larger paper using the sheet of double-sided tape. Fold the large sheet of paper in half with the contrasting paper on top and facing up.

2. With the fold to your left, draw a vertical line dividing this section in two. Next, center the square template on the drawn line. Trace the sides of the square to the right of the dividing line.

3. Unfold the paper. Using a craft knife, cut the traced lines. Fold along the drawn line, creating a square. Unfold and place a strip of double-sided tape along the 5½" (14 cm) edge. Fold over again and adhere.

4. Stamp a letter in the newly created square.

MATERIALS

- 5½" x 8½" (14 cm x 21.6 cm) floral paper
- 5½" x 4¼" (14 cm x 10.8 cm) contrasting floral paper
- roll of ¼" (6 mm)-wide double-sided tape
- 5½" x 4¼" (14 cm x 10.8 cm) sheet of double-sided tape
- 2" (5.1 cm) square template cut from card stock
- craft knife
- floral alphabet block letters
- ink pad
- ruler

HELPFUL HINT

Nervous about stamping on your newly created card? Experiment by stamping letters on extra floral paper. Trim away the chosen block letter and adhere to the card using double-sided tape or glue.

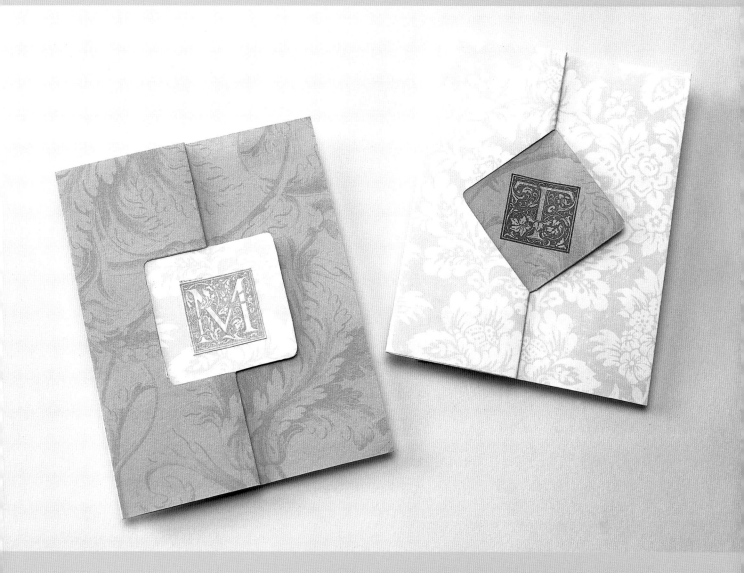

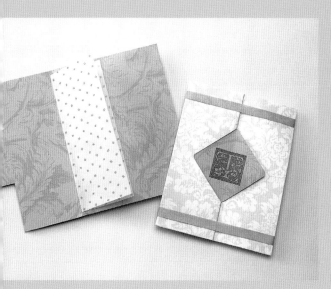

 GOING ONE STEP FURTHER

Insert a $5\frac{1}{2}$" x $4\frac{1}{4}$" (14 cm x 10.8 cm) note paper folded in half and adhere with a strip of double-sided tape to the inside of the folded card. Also, $\frac{1}{4}$" (6 mm)-wide paper bands can give the card an added decorative element as well as a means of keeping the card closed.

$\mathscr{S}$haring Seeds Greeting

If you are a seed saver, here's a creative way to package seeds and share them with your friends. The textural qualities of the packaged seeds are highlighted through the cut out stenciled letters. Although the illustrated design uses the aid of a computer to create an overall design, any decorative or brightly colored paper can be used just as effectively.

INSTRUCTIONS

1. To fold a spine in the colored paper, position the sheet on a flat surface with the 8½" (21.6 cm) sides at the top and bottom. Fold the top edge down, leaving ¼" (6 mm) of the bottom edge of paper extending beyond the top edge, and then crease the fold. Turn the paper over, keeping the fold along the top. Lift the top edge and reposition it ¼" (6 mm) above the bottom edge, and crease it to make a second fold. These two folds should be ¼" (6 mm) apart, creating a spine in the center of the paper.

2. Decide the general area in which the stenciled letters will be placed. To create a guide for letter placement, use a pencil and draw a straight line.

3. Place the letter stencils along the pencil line. Trace the letters onto the paper. Use a craft knife to cut out the individual letters.

4. Refer to the five enlarged folding diagrams on page 263 (also on facing page) to assist with this step. On all four sides of the acetate, score a line ¼" (6 mm) from the edge. Score another set of four lines, ¼" (6 mm) in from the first set. Cut away a ½" x ½" (1.3 cm x 1.3 cm) square from each corner. To create the box shape, fold the inside scored sections in toward the center of the acetate. Next, fold the outside scored sections out away from the box. For each side, gently pull the

edges upward making a right angle section. Place a strip of doublesided tape along the outer folded lip of each of the four sides of acetate that will come in contact with the card. Turn the box over.

5. Position the box under the cut out letters of colored paper. With a pencil, mark the corners onto the colored paper. Remove the backing from along one edge. Place into proper position on the back of the card and adhere. Repeat with the other two sides, leaving one short edge open.

6. Fill the box with seeds through the open side. Remove the backing from the tape and adhere the remaining side closed.

MATERIALS

- 8½" x 11" (21.6 cm x 27.9 cm) colored paper
- 2½" x 6¼" (6.4 cm x 15.9 cm) clear acetate
- roll of ¼" (6 mm)-wide double-sided tape
- 8½" x 11" (21.6 cm x 27.9 cm) colored paper
- 1⅛" (2.9 cm-high) letter stencils
- seeds
- craft knife
- pencil
- bone folder
- ruler
- folding diagrams (page 263)

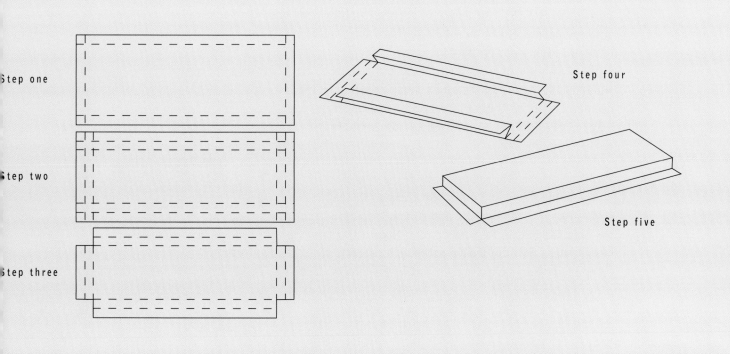

Step one

Step two

Step three

Step four

Step five

Seeded Center Flower Cards

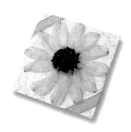

When store-bought seeds are past their prime and you are ready to throw them out, use them to make textural centers for these ribbon-pierced flowers. Just about any leftover seeds can be used. Try small seeds, such as lettuce seeds or radish seeds. Garlic chive seeds (dark) and pepper seeds (light) are used in the illustrated cards.

INSTRUCTIONS

1. Photocopy the template onto card stock and cut out around the 4" (10.2 cm) square. Pierce the center dot of the template using a needle. Turn the paper over.

2. Place a strip of double-sided tape on the back of the $1^1/_4$" (3.2 cm) yellow circle. Remove the backing and adhere the circle to the center of the paper. Turn the paper over. Pierce the remaining dots on the circle template.

3. Thread the 36" (91 cm) length of organza ribbon onto the needle. Push the needle up from the back, through a dot on the template's inner circle. Pull the ribbon through, leaving a ribbon end of $1/_2$" (1.3 cm) on the other side. Push the needle and ribbon through the opposite dot of the outer circle. Pull the needle and ribbon through to the template side.

4. Push the needle and ribbon through the next dot on the outer circle and pull them through to the other side. Push the needle and ribbon through the opposite dot on the inner circle. Repeat the sewing steps until all twelve petals have been completed. Trim excess ribbon end to the length of $1/_2$" (1.3 cm).

MATERIALS

- weaving template (page 264)
- $1^1/_4$" (3.2 cm) yellow construction paper circle
- 36" (91 cm) length of $3/_4$" (2 cm)-wide silk organza ribbon
- 6" (15.2 cm) length of $3/_8$" (1.3 cm)-wide silk organza ribbon
- $5^1/_2$" x $8^1/_2$" (14 cm x 21.6 cm) card stock
- 4" x 4" (10 cm x 10 cm) paper
- $3^1/_4$" x $3^1/_4$" (8.3 cm x 8.3 cm) tag board
- roll of $1/_4$" (6 mm)-wide double-sided tape
- seeds
- needle
- white glue

HELPFUL HINT

The template can be enlarged or reduced to any size. The alternate design on page 213 was reduced to a $2^1/_2$" (6.4 cm) circle and was sewn using a $3/_8$" (1 cm)-wide ribbon. The $1^1/_4$" (3.2 cm) yellow circle remained the same.

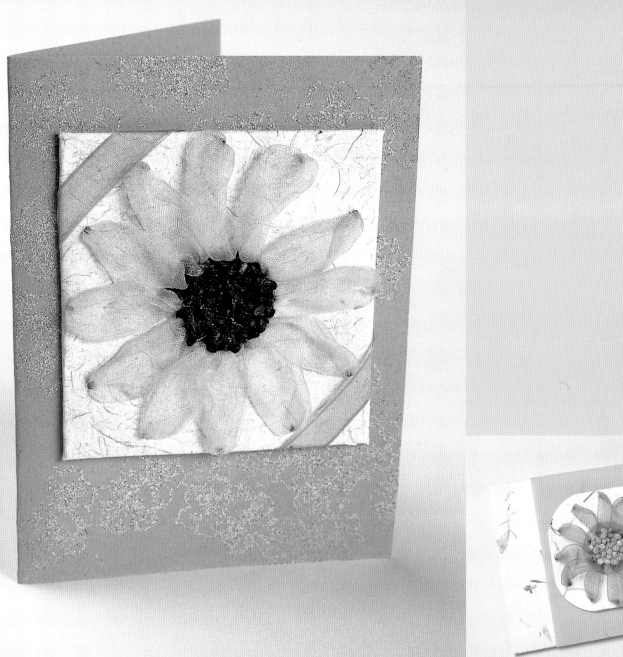

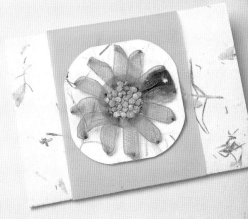

5. Place strips of double-sided tape along the edges of 3$\frac{1}{4}$" x 3$\frac{1}{4}$" (8.3 cm x 8.3 cm) tag board. With tape side up, center the tag board over the template side of the flower design. Remove the backing of the double-sided tape, and fold over and adhere the edges of the flower design onto the tape strips. Run another set of the double-sided tape strips along the edges of the square. Remove the backing paper.

6. Cut the 6" (15.2 cm) length of organza ribbon in half. Place ribbons on the diagonal in opposite corners of the flower design. Fold over the ribbon ends to the other side and adhere to the tape.

7. Fold the card stock in half. Center the flower design on the card stock and press down.

8. Fill the center of the flower with white glue. Sprinkle seeds into the glue. Shake off any excess seeds.

Trellis and Tendrils

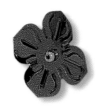

Garden structures, such as trellises, provide necessary support as well as interesting architecture in the garden. The strong linear lines of the trellis and the curvy lines of the flowers give this card a bold geometric look.

INSTRUCTIONS

1. Cut the decorative paper into a $3^1/_2$" x $8^1/_2$" (8.9 cm x 21.6 cm) length. Along the short edges of the wrong side, run strips of double-sided tape. Turn the paper to the front. Lightly draw a line $^1/_2$" (1.3 cm) from the top and bottom edge of the short edges.

2. Cut the ribbon into three lengths of 9" (23 cm). Starting $^3/_8$" (1 cm) from the long edge of the paper, lay down one ribbon strip. Mark the ribbon's width on the top and bottom lines. Lay the ribbon down next to the pencil mark and mark the ribbon's width again. Repeat this step until there are six marks on each line.

3. On the bottom line, use a craft knife to cut a total of three lines, which lay between marks 1 and 2, 3 and 4, and 5 and 6. Slip the ribbon ends into the cuts. Turn the paper over and remove the tape backing. Secure the ribbon ends to the tape. Turn the paper over.

4. On the top line, cut an inverted "V" between marks 1 and 2, 3 and 4, and 5 and 6. Insert the ribbon ends into the cuts. Turn the paper over and remove the tape backing. Secure the ribbon ends to the tape. Turn the paper over.

5. Cut the remaining ribbon length in half. Run a length of tape along one edge of the ribbon. Remove the tape's backing. Reduce the ribbon's width by half by folding it in half lengthwise. Adhere the ribbon closed with the tape.

6. At the top, tuck the $^1/_4$" (6 mm) ribbon end behind the left side of the middle vertical ribbon. Cross over the center ribbon and weave the $^1/_4$" (6 mm) ribbon over and under the vertical ribbons. The $^1/_4$" (6 mm) ribbon should be angled downward in a zigzag manor when weaving. To finish, tuck the $^1/_4$" (6 mm) ribbon end under the left side of the middle ribbon.

MATERIALS

- 9" x $10^3/_4$" (22.9 cm x 27.3 cm) yellow, textured craft paper
- 6" x $8^1/_2$" (15.2 cm x 21.6 cm) decorative paper
- 50" (127 cm) length of $^5/_8$" (1.6 cm)-wide black ribbon
- roll of $^1/_4$" (6 mm)-wide double-sided tape
- nine assorted shapes of sequin flowers
- nine glass beads
- 36" (90 cm) length of craft wire
- bone folder
- scissors
- ruler
- pencil

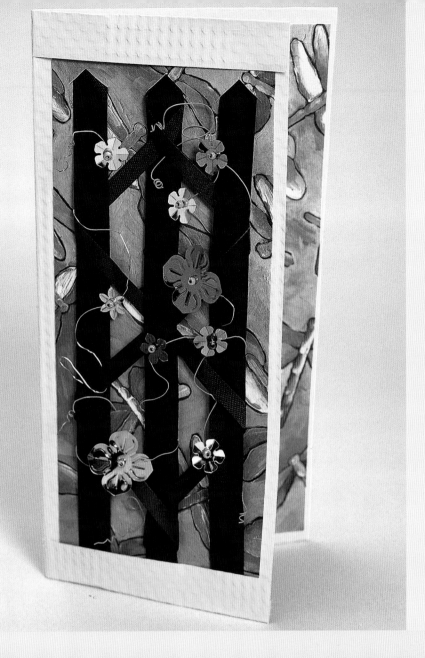

7. Using the other ribbon length, repeat the design but in the other direction. Secure the ribbon ends behind the middle vertical ribbon. Using a bone folder, burnish the folds flat.

8. Cut five lengths of wire. Secure the flowers to the wire by inserting the wire from behind the flower, up through the hole. Slip a glass bead onto the wire and pass the wire back through the flower hole. Pull the ends tight. If the length of wire is long, put a flower sequin at the other end. Bend the wire into curves and slip it between the

ribbons. Continue creating flower vines with the remaining wire.

9. Remove the tape backing and adhere the trellis to the yellow craft paper, about $1/4$" (6 mm) from the edge. Fold over $5/8$" (1.6 cm) of the top and bottom edge of the yellow paper toward the trellis side. Next, fold the yellow paper in half approximately $1/4$" (6 mm) from the decorative paper's edge.

10. Run strips of tape along the long edges of the remaining piece of decorative paper. Adhere the paper to the inside of the card.

Teacup Card

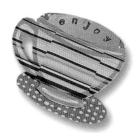

If you grow herbs, such as chamomile, sage, or lemon mint, you can make your own tea for brewing. Dry a select group of herbs, package them into store bought tea bags, and send them off to a friend or two to warm themselves on a cold winter's day. Write a note of cheer or an herbal remedy associated with the tea on the hangtag.

INSTRUCTIONS

1. Copy the teacup template design onto white card stock. With right side up, cover the card stock paper with double-sided tape. Remove the backing. Place a 4" x 4" (10.2 cm x 10.2 cm) sheet of translucent paper over the teacup design, then cut it out. Copy the two oval shapes onto contrasting paper and cut them out.

2. Glue one oval to the bottom back of the teacup, as a saucer, and the other to the top back of the teacup, as the interior of the cup.

3. Using a craft knife, cut along the inside rim of the teacup, starting and ending ¹/₄" (6 mm) from the outside edge. Slip the tag from behind the teacup and push it up and through the opening. If the tag does not fit through the opening, cut a little more along the rim until the opening is large enough to accommodate the tag's width. Remove the hangtag.

4. Stamp a one word greeting such as "enjoy" at the top of the tag.

5. Fold 12" (30.5 cm) of colored string in half. Slip the loop through the tag's grommet. Then slip the string's ends through the loop. Pull to tighten. Knot the ends and staple them to the tea bag.

MATERIALS

- 2¹/₂" x 5" (6.4 cm x 12.7 cm) hangtag
- 12" (30.5 cm) length of colored string
- 8¹/₂" x 11" (21.6 cm x 27.9 cm) white card stock
- 4" x 4" (10.2 cm x 10.2 cm) translucent paper
- 1³/₄" x 8" (4.4 cm x 20.3 cm) contrasting paper
- 4" x 12" (10.2 cm x 30.5 cm) purple embossed paper
- 6" x 8" (15.2 cm x 20.3 cm) sheet of double-sided tape
- teacup template (page 265)
- oval template (page 265)
- tea bag
- small alphabet letter stamps
- craft knife
- stapler
- glue

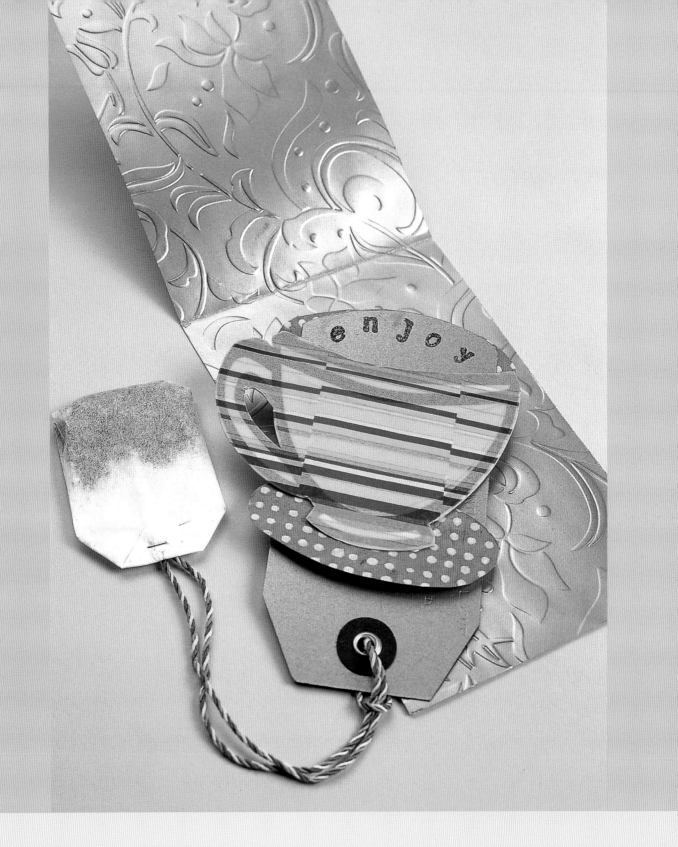

6. Fold the 4" x 12" (10.2 cm x 30.5 cm) embossed paper in half. Open the paper. Run a small length of double-sided tape on the top back of the teacup. Remove the backing and adhere the teacup to the bottom half of the embossed paper. Slip the tag through the teacup opening.

Special Occasion Cards:
With Every Leaf a Miracle

New life, life in motion, always evolving, life ending.

We observe transitions and passages, growth and renewal, through rituals and celebrations that enrich our lives throughout the year. There is a strong desire to honor, sanctify, and memorialize these momentous events and to bring special attention to special occasions. We feel connected with others and our world when we take part in customs that enable us to express appreciation, celebration, generosity, comfort, and foremost, love. Bless these celebratory events through the generous act of creating a very special card. Make your card one of lasting endurance, because special occasions create special memories that are treasured over and over again.

- *Herald a life passage with a flight of birds making their way to their new abode*

- *Celebrate continual growth and renewal with the upward curve of flower petals in an iris bouquet.*

- *Illuminate a special event, such as a wedding, through the creation of a paper lantern card*

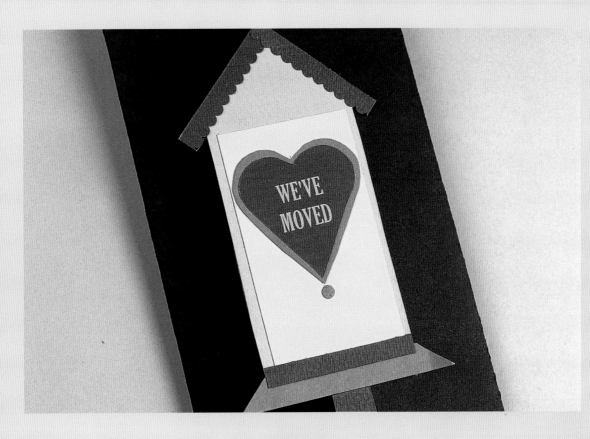

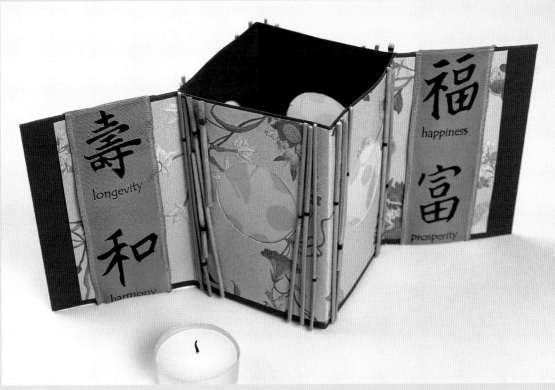

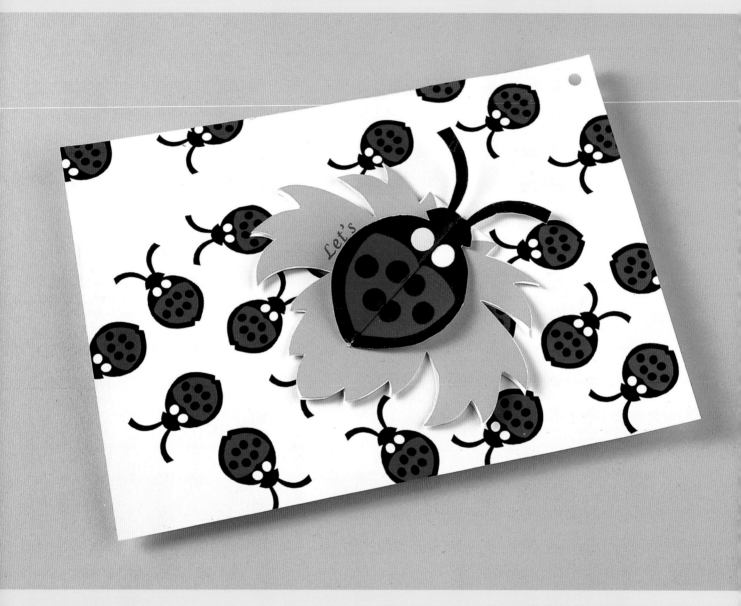

Ladybug Invite

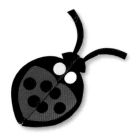

MATERIALS

- twenty-five small ladybug stickers
- two large ladybug stickers
- 8" x 5½" (20.3 cm x 14 cm) white medium weight paper
- 7½" x 5" (19.1 cm x 12.7 cm) green medium weight paper
- leaf template (page 270)
- craft knife
- ruler

HELPFUL HINT

If you need many invitations, have color copies made of the small ladybug arrangement. Then proceed with step 2.

One grand ladybug sits upon a leaf, while her many neighbors wander in all directions. The leaf slips out from under her and opens to reveal a handwritten message: "Let's get together soon, away from the business of daily life." Easily adapted for any occasion, this card makes a great summer party invite too!

INSTRUCTIONS

1. Make a random arrangement of twenty-five ladybug stickers on white paper.

2. Measure the large ladybug body, not including the length of antennas. With this measurement, cut a straight line at an angle anywhere in the middle of the white paper. Cut another line, parallel to previous cut, approximately ¹⁄₃₂" (.8 mm) apart.

3. Take both large ladybug stickers and fold in half. Unfold. Remove the right antenna of one and the left from the other. Turn the stickers over. Using the craft knife, gently cut just the paper backing of stickers along the fold line. Fold in half again.

4. Ease one half of the ladybug sticker (the side without an antenna) through the cut of the white paper. Repeat with the remaining sticker. Turn the paper over. Remove the sticker backing and adhere to the back of the paper.

5. Trace the leaf template onto the green paper and cut it out. Along its outline, fold in half.

6. Use the craft knife to cut two parallel lines, approximately ¹⁄₁₆" (1.6 mm) apart, down the leaf's center. The line length equals the length of the ladybug as measured in step 2.

7. Write a message on the inside of the leaf. Close the leaf and slide it under the ladybug.

Cut Flowers for a Special Couple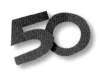

In Europe during the eighteenth century, there was a system invented by Lady Mary Montague called the Language of Flowers. It was a list associating flowers with romantic and heartfelt meanings. For instance, the rose had the meaning of love, the daisy was innocence, and the ivy symbolized fidelity. Someone sending a bouquet of flowers to a lover or dear friend could communicate intimate or sentimental feelings to the other.

In this card, the two golden irises send a beautiful "message" of happiness to a very special couple celebrating their fiftieth wedding anniversary.

INSTRUCTIONS

1. Trim a 1¼" x 11" (3.2 cm x 27.9 cm) strip from the dark gold metallic paper. Fold the larger sheet in half.

2. Lightly stamp the corners of the maroon paper with the flower design. Sprinkle with embossing powder. Apply heat with a heat gun to melt the powder.

3. Place the stencil on the paper and dab the ink in the open areas. Wipe the stencil clean and turn it over. Position the turned over stencil in an open area and dab with the copper color.

4. Using a craft knife, cut along the stenciled lines, but leave a hinged area so the petals and leaves are still attached in places. Bend, curl, or lift the flowers and leaves creating a three-dimensional look.

5. Turn the paper over and run strips of tape along the edges. Remove the tape's backing and adhere the paper to the light gold paper. Turn the paper

MATERIALS

- 8½" x 11" (21.6 cm x 28 cm) dark gold metallic card stock
- 5³⁄₈" x 6" (13.7 cm x 15.2 cm) light gold metallic paper
- 5⁷⁄₈" x 5¼" (14.9 cm x 13.3 cm) maroon card stock
- roll of ¼" (6 mm)-wide double-sided tape
- three ¼" (6 mm) sticky squares
- 5" (12.7 cm) iris stencil
- flower stamp
- colonial blue ink pad
- champagne and copper metallic ink daubers
- gold embossing powder
- heat gun
- craft knife

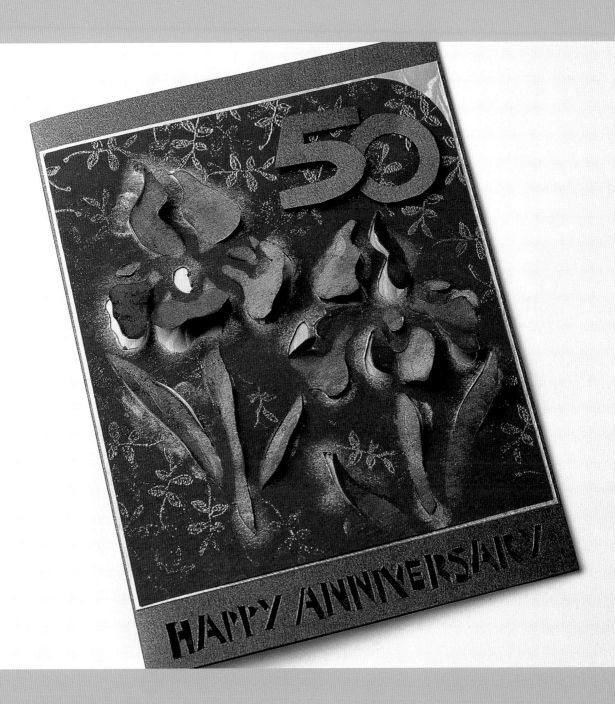

over and run strips of tape along the paper edges. Remove the tape's backing and place it $^7/_8$" (2.2 mm) from the bottom of the dark metallic paper.

6. Draw the numbers "5" and "0" on the strip of dark metallic paper. Using a craft knife, cut out the numbers. Adhere two sticky squares to the back of the "5." Adhere one sticky square to the bottom right of the "0." Adhere the numbers to the upper right corner of the maroon paper, slightly overlapping the "5" over the "0."

7. In the space below the irises, hand cut stencil-like letters for the card's message. Stamping small block letters is another method for creating the card's message.

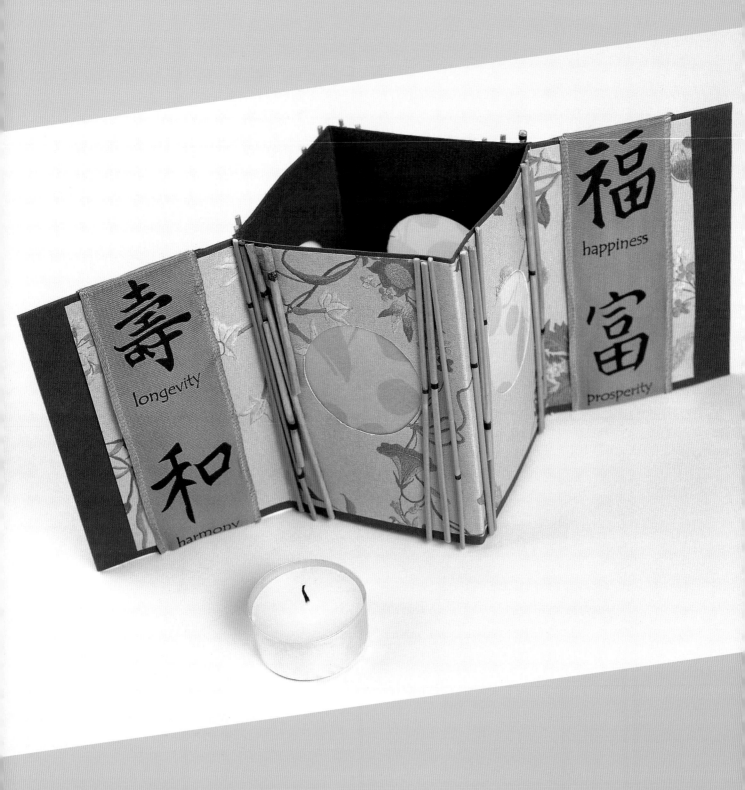

Chinese Paper Lantern Card

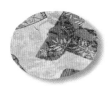

MATERIALS

- 9" x 12" (23.9 cm x 30.5 cm) maroon paper
- two 4¼" x 11" (10.8 cm x 27.9 cm) pieces of decorative paper
- four 2½" (6.4 cm) square pieces of translucent paper
- 18" (46 cm) length of 1½" (3.8 cm)-wide ribbon
- six marsh reed stems
- compass
- roll of ¼" (6 mm)-wide double-sided tape
- two 3" x 5" (7.5 cm x 12.5 cm) sheets of double-sided tape
- craft knife
- glue

HELPFUL HINT

It will be necessary to flatten the card before slipping it into an envelope. If you would like to mail this card, reduce the lantern's length to fit a 4¾" x 11" (12.1 cm x 27.9 cm) business size envelope.

In the summer, garden lanterns are bright, dancing illuminations, swaying in a gentle breeze. For a newly wedded couple, this specialized card lights up the good fortunes you're sending their way. Designed as a small table lantern, a small votive can be placed within the opened center. The light shining through the portals will dance like a full moon in a bamboo grove.

INSTRUCTIONS

1. Fold the maroon paper in half. Unfold the paper. Fold the paper in half in the other direction. Fold the paper in half one more time. Unfold the paper. The paper should be divided into eight sections. Place the paper in the landscape/horizontal format. Using a craft knife, cut the center horizontal fold between the first and last vertical fold. Fold the paper in half.

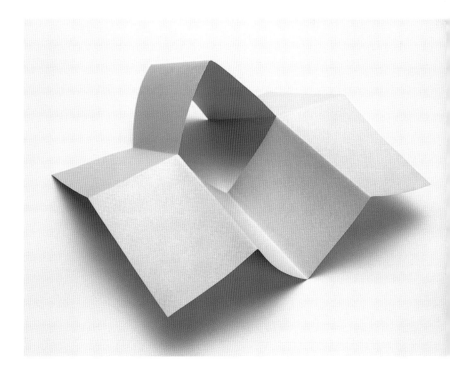

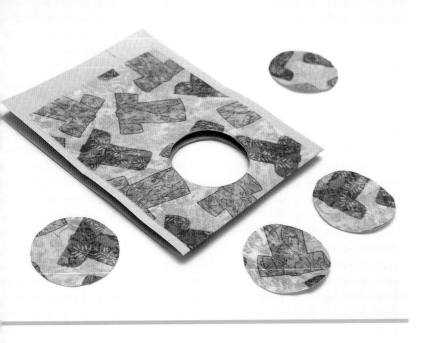

2. On the back of the decorative papers, run a strip of double-sided tape along the top and bottom edges. Remove one strip of tape backing from each sheet of paper. Center and adhere the papers in each half of the folded maroon paper. Keep the project paper folded. Using a compass, draw a $1^3/_4$" (4.4 cm) circle in each of the two center panels, $1^1/_4$" (3.2 cm) from the paper's top edge. Using a craft knife, cut out four circles.

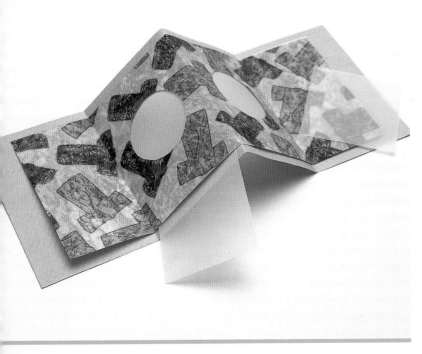

3. Run a strip of double-sided tape along one edge of the four translucent papers. Remove the tape backing. Slide the papers between the decorative and maroon paper, covering the four circular areas. Adhere the squares into place. Remove the tape backing from the strip that runs along the bottom back edge of the decorative paper. Adhere the papers together.

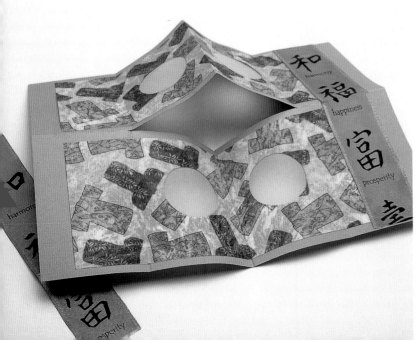

4. Cut the ribbon into two equal lengths. Run each length down the middle of the end panels. Adhere the ribbon ends to the paper with double-sided tape. Turn the maroon paper over with the wrong side up. Cover the end panels with double-sided tape. Fold the paper in half, securing the end panels together.

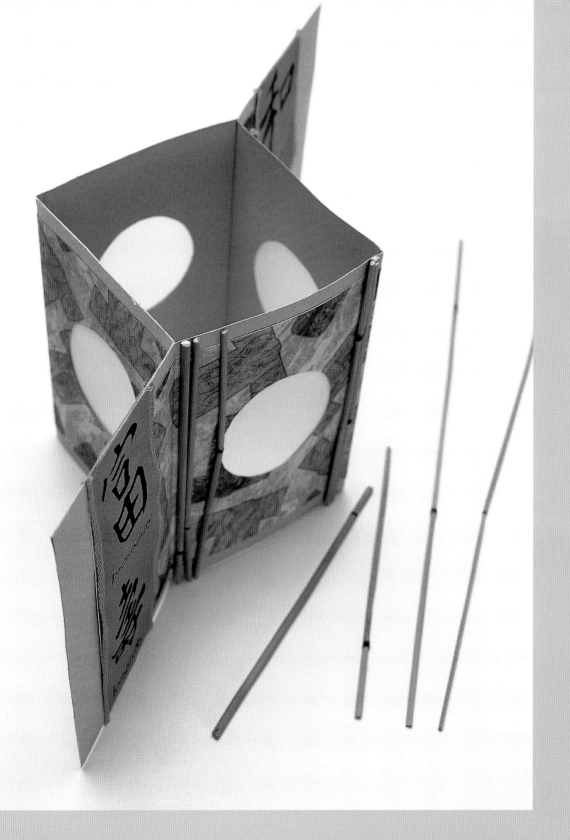

5. Flatten the lantern. Using a craft knife cut the marsh reeds into 4¹/₂" (11.4 cm) lengths. Glue the reeds to the circle panels. When the glue is dry, push the lantern's side panels toward each other and crease the middle folds to form the lantern.

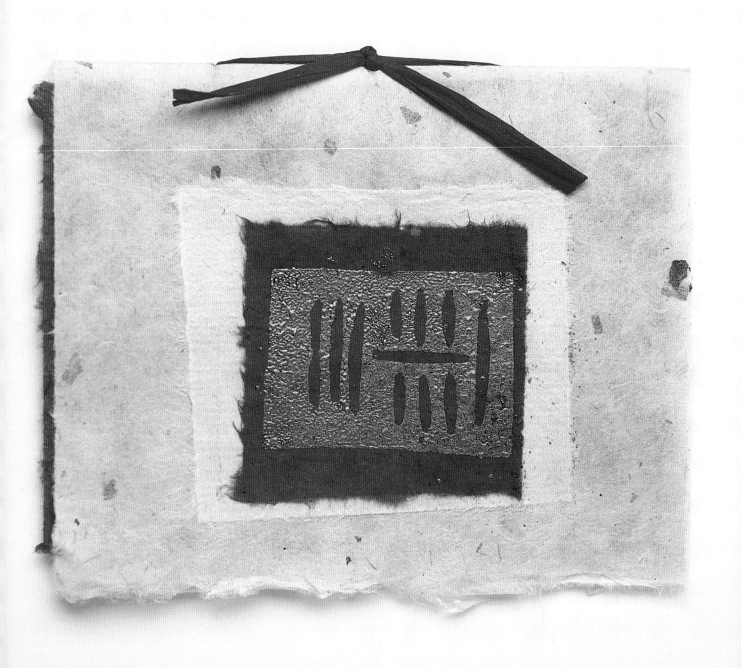

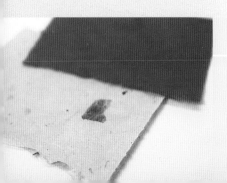

Choosing the Paper

This simple style can be very elegant. Choose a good-quality stock for the inside sheet, a handmade cover sheet, and a thin tissue for the inside. Use computer graphics to add images. Make the envelope first, using the same paper as either the inside sheet or the cover sheet. Make the invitation to fit the envelope.

the PAMPHLET-STYLE *invitation*

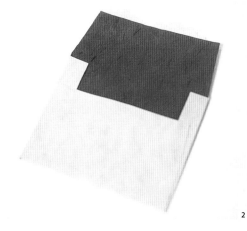

1

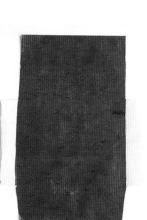

2

Materials · *makes two invitations and two envelopes* · 1 sheet 8 ¹/₂" x 11" (22 cm x 28 cm) good-quality computer printer paper or a smooth, thin handmade paper (for invitation) · 2 sheets 8 ¹/₂" x 11" (22 cm x 28 cm) thick tan Bhutanese paper (for cover of invitation and envelope) · 1 sheet 8 ¹/₂" x 11" (22 cm x 28 cm) thin pink Bhutanese paper (for invitation and envelope liner) · glue stick · 2 feet waxed linen thread, embroidery thread, or narrow ribbon · metal ruler for measuring and tearing · scissors · pencil · sewing needle · computer printer (or your own handwriting)

TIP
One quarter of an 8 ¹/₂" x 11" (22 cm x 28 cm) sheet fits into an A2 envelope.

STEP 1 Using the template from the back of this book (see Template, pg. 278), trace an A2 envelope shape onto envelope paper and cut out. Trace this pattern again onto contrasting paper to make the envelope liner. Remove side flaps from pink liner paper. **STEP 2** Glue liner onto envelope with glue stick (not wet glue, as paper will wrinkle). Fold in flaps; glue envelope into shape with glue stick. **STEP 3** Cut one sheet of cover paper in half. Take one half sheet, 5 ¹/₂" x 8 ¹/₂" (14 cm x 22 cm), and fold in half to make the invitation cover. **STEP 4** Print text by running invitation paper through computer. Two invitations will fit on one sheet. Cut in half. Fold so that text is on the inside. **STEP 5** Cut a piece of envelope liner paper to the same size as the invitation, 4 ¹/₄" x 5 ¹/₂" (11 cm x 14 cm).

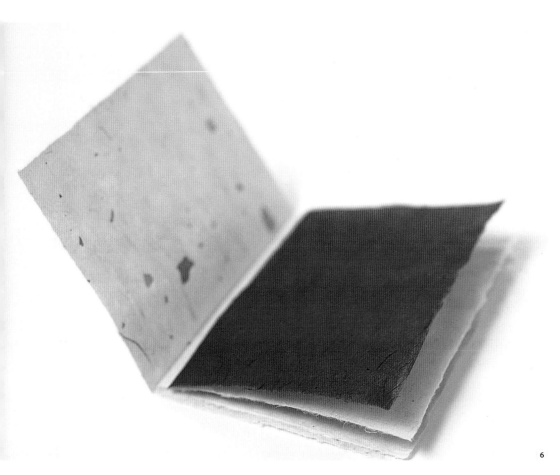

6

Pamphlet Stitch

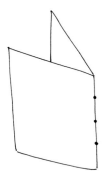

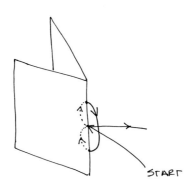

START

STEP 6 Assemble in the following order from inside to outside: invitation, thin paper, thick cover paper. Sew together with pamphlet stitch according to diagram.
STEP 7 Tear two rectangular shapes of tan and pink. Glue onto cover with glue stick.

Use a hand-carved eraser stamp or commercial rubber stamp to create an embossed design on the front of the invitation. Using Color Box Ink, stamp image onto cover. Sprinkle with embossing powder. Melt with heat gun.

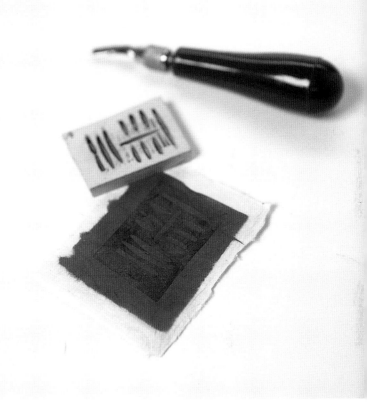

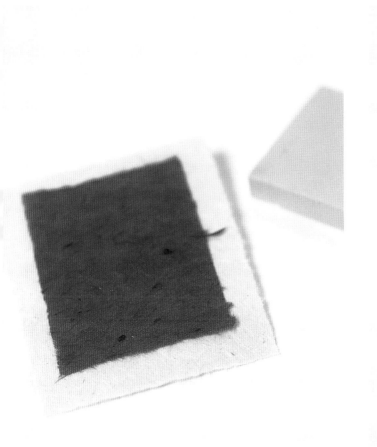

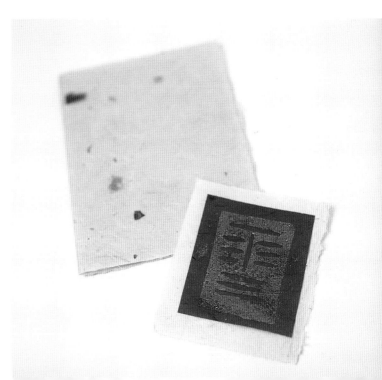

the LAYERED invitation

Materials · *makes three invitations and three envelopes* · 1 sheet Indian floral paper, 22" x 30" (56 cm x 76 cm) · 1 sheet Japanese unryu paper, 22" x 30" (56 cm x 76 cm) · 1 sheet card stock, 8 ½" x 11" (22 cm x 28 cm) · raffia · pencil · scissors · glue stick · needle · bone folder

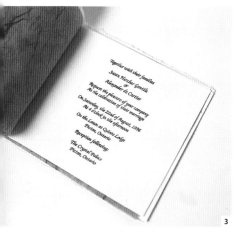

1

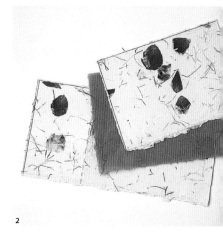

2

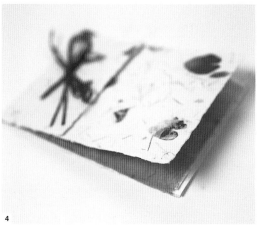

3

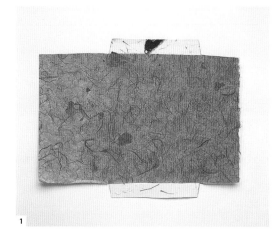

4

STEP 1 Trace A6 envelope pattern (see Template, pg. 279) onto Indian floral paper and Japanese unryu paper (for liner). Cut out; remove side flaps from unryu liner. Crease with bone folder and glue together into envelope shape. **STEP 2** Cut out two pieces of Indian floral paper, one the size of the envelope and the other about 3" (8 cm) longer. Cut Japanese unryu paper the size of the envelope. **STEP 3** Print text on card stock or paper the size of the envelope. **STEP 4** Stack in the following order, top to bottom: smaller floral paper, unryu, text paper, longer piece of floral paper. Wrap extra length around to front. Sew pamphlet stitch (see page 230).

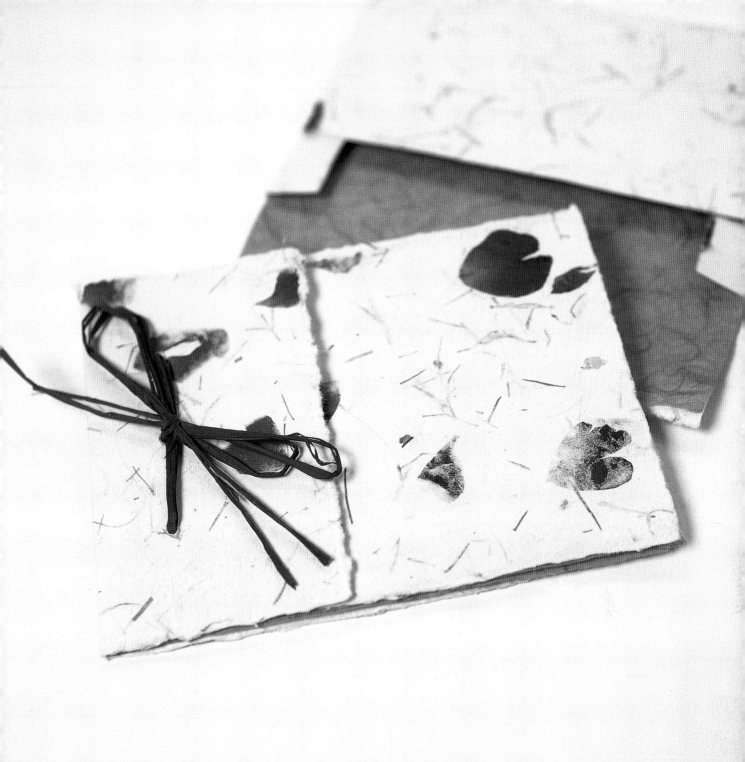

Choosing the Paper

This style of invitation uses the pamphlet stitch on the top surface of the invitation instead of the spine. It offers many opportunities to go wild with sheer and opaque papers, ribbons, raffia, and cutout designs. The key is an imaginative choice of papers and a sensitivity to the juxtaposition of ragged and straight edges.

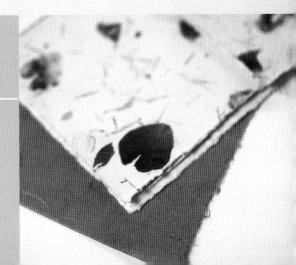

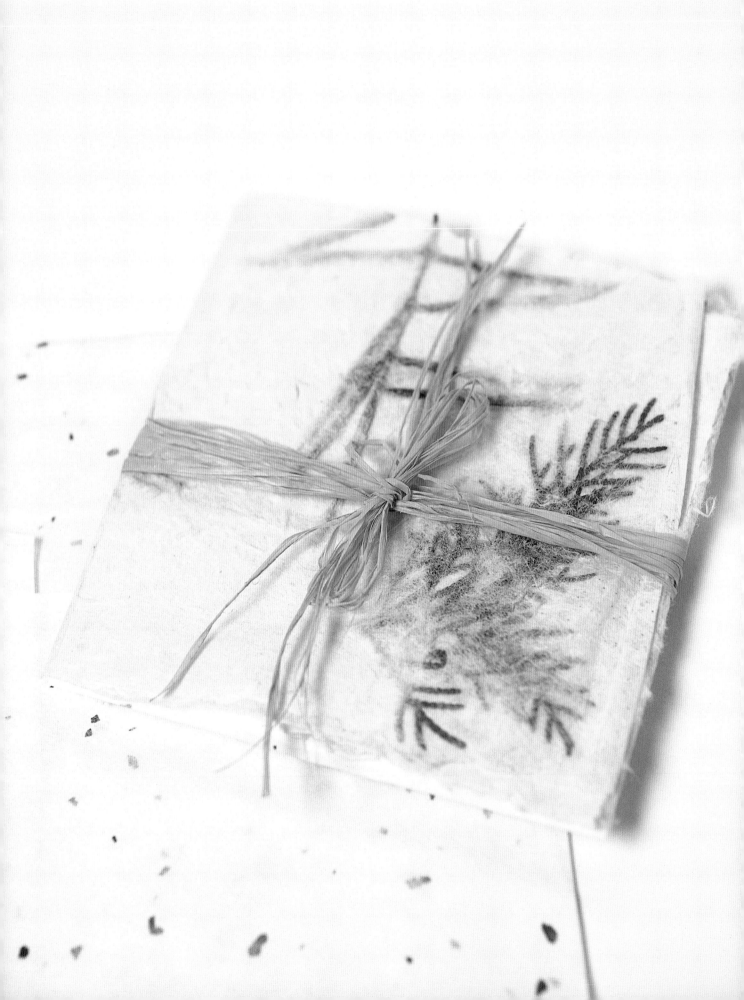

the WRAPPED *invitation*

Materials · *makes four invitations and four envelopes* • 1 sheet Thai floral paper for outside wrapping, 22" x 30" (56 cm x 76 cm) • 1 sheet Japanese coordinating lightweight paper for liner and envelope, 22" x 30" (56 cm x 76 cm) • 1 sheet card stock for invitation printing, 8 ½" x 11" (22 cm x 28 cm) • raffia • pencil • scissors • glue stick • bone folder

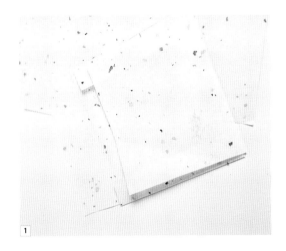

STEP 1 Cut out square envelope template (see Template, pg. 280) and trace onto lightweight paper. Cut out envelope and glue into shape with glue stick. **STEP 2** Print invitation text on card stock the same size as envelope.

Choosing the Paper

This invitation uses the simplest technique-wrapping-no sewing or gluing necessary. The text is surrounded by beautiful handmade paper, tied with raffia, and placed inside an exquisite envelope made of lightweight bark paper. Another piece of bark paper veils the invitation inside. This technique can be utilized on any scale.

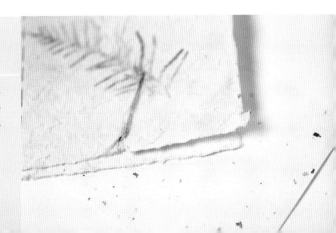

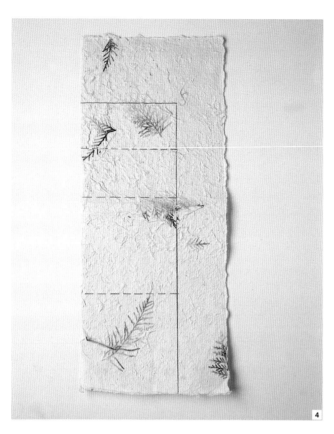

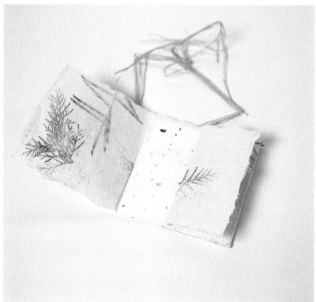

STEP 3 Cut invitation veil (liner) out of the same paper as the envelope. The liner should be the same size as envelope. **STEP 4** Cut a piece of Thai floral paper three times as long as the invitation. Fold into thirds. Fold the first third in half as shown on dotted line. This designates the front of the invitation. Place veil on top of invitation, wrap floral paper around the text with the veil, and tie with raffia.

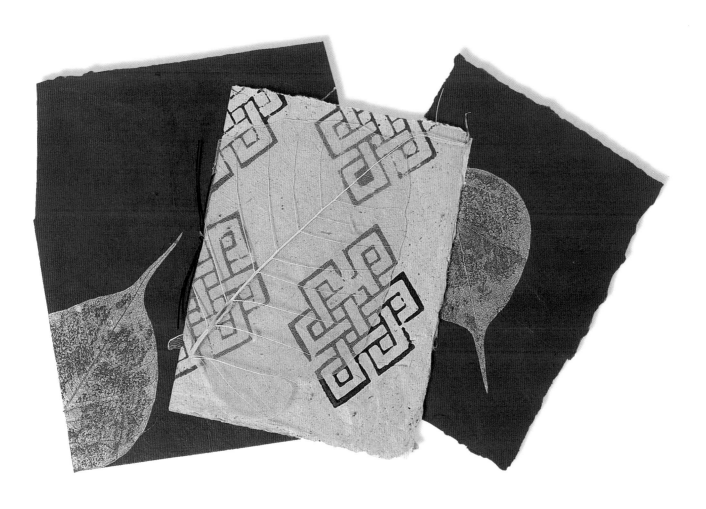

An Invitation for Any Occasion

Create unique invitations to coordinate with a theme, be it an Asian dinner party, a black-tie affair, or a simple get-together. Experiment with different textures of paper, ribbons, and cords.

"We've Moved" Birdhouse

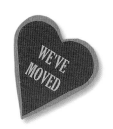

Oh, the migratory life of birds! When spring comes around, our feathered friends return. They begin their search for a protective place to build a new nest. Next, they begin the arduous task of raising their young. At summer's end, they are off for warmer parts of the country with a promise to return next year.

If your future plans consist of a moving adventure, why not make a card collection to send to your favorite friends and relatives. Use removable labels so the recipients can adhere your new address right into their address books.

INSTRUCTIONS

1. Place the black paper in the landscape format. Using a bone folder, score a line 2^1/$_4$" (5.7 cm) from the left edge. Score another vertical line 4^1/$_2$" (11.4 cm) from the previously scored line. Fold the edges to the center with the short flap on top. Lightly draw a pencil line along the flap's edge onto the flap underneath.

2. Cut a variety of shapes to create a birdhouse approximately 5^1/$_2$" (14 cm) high and 2^1/$_2$" (6.4 cm) wide. Use a glue stick to adhere all the pieces together. Place the birdhouse on a sheet of double-sided tape. Using a craft knife, cut along the outline of the birdhouse, trimming away the excess tape.

3. Center the birdhouse along the pencil line and 1" (2.5 cm) from the top of the black paper. Mark with a pencil the top and bottom of the bird-house. Remove the tape's backing from the back of the birdhouse and re-deposit the house on the black paper.

4. Cut a strip of colored paper approximately ^{5}/$_8$" (1.6 cm) wide. Run a strip of tape on the back.

Remove the tape's backing. Place the paper strip at the bottom and center of the birdhouse. Trim away excess paper from the bottom edge of the black paper.

5. Open the black paper with the birdhouse facing up. Using a craft knife, trim along the pencil line and the left side of the bird-house. Photocopy and cut out the heart template from colored paper. Adhere the heart to the

MATERIALS

- 9" x 11" (23 cm x 27.9 cm) black card stock
- assortment of bright colored paper
- printed address labels
- 6" x 6" (15.2 cm x 15.2 cm) sheet of double-sided tape
- roll of ^{1}/$_4$" (6 mm)-wide double-sided tape
- flying bird templates (page 277)
- heart template (page 277)
- paper punch
- glue stick
- bone folder
- craft knife
- ruler
- pencil

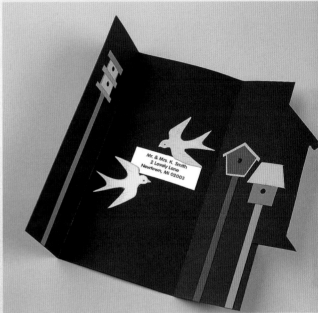

front of the birdhouse with double-sided tape. Turn the paper over.

6. Create three small birdhouses from the bright colored paper. Use the glue stick to adhere all the shapes together. Adhere double-sided tape to the backs. Punch holes for the house openings. Remove the tape's backing and place the houses at varying heights on the side panels. Cut strips of colored paper ¼" (6 mm) wide. Adhere strips of double-sided tape to the backs, beneath the houses and to the bottom of the paper. Trim away any excess paper.

7. Copy the bird templates. Color them with markers. Adhere double-sided tape to the backs of the templates. Using a craft knife, cut out the birds. Place the address label in the center of the card. Place the birds with their wings slightly overlapping the label. Mark the bird's position with a pencil.

8. Remove the label. Remove the tape's backing from the birds and re-deposit the birds on the black paper. Using a craft knife, cut along the bird where they overlap the label. Insert the label into the cuts.

*L*ittle Sprout Birth Announcement

Plant markers are used to identify newly planted seeds. They're used to record planting dates and specific names of plants. Here the plant marker becomes a birth announcement, recording the baby's name, date of birth, and weight. These make great bookmarks for grandparents.

INSTRUCTIONS

1. Using a bone folder, score two lines 2$\frac{1}{4}$" (5.7 cm) from the long sides of the yellow card stock. Fold the panels to the center. Unfold the paper.

2. Stamp a number of medium and small daisies in the upper two-thirds of the center panel.

3. Draw a pencil line 2" (5 cm) from the bottom of the yellow card stock and another line 2$\frac{1}{4}$" (5.7 cm) from the previously drawn line.

4. To make the orange flowerpot, use a craft knife to cut two angled lines. Begin the lines on the first drawn line, 2" (5 cm) apart. Angle the lines outward and upward stopping at the second drawn line. Take the 2$\frac{1}{4}$" x 5$\frac{1}{2}$" (5.7 cm x 14 cm) orange paper and slip the ends through the two paper slits.

5. To make the flowerpot rim, use a craft knife to cut two $\frac{1}{2}$" (1.3 cm)-long lines $\frac{3}{8}$" (1 cm) away from the orange pot. Slip the ends of the $\frac{1}{2}$" x 5$\frac{1}{2}$" (1.3 cm x 14 cm) orange paper through the paper slits.

6. On the 4" x 4" (10.2 cm x 10.2 cm) yellow card stock, stamp a large daisy. Cut out the flower. Adhere double-sided tape to the back of the photograph. Remove the tape's backing and adhere the photograph to the center of the daisy. Adhere the daisy to the marker using double-sided tape.

MATERIALS

- 8$\frac{1}{2}$" x 10" (21.6 cm x 25.4 cm) yellow card stock
- 4" x 4" (10.2 cm x 10.2 cm) yellow card stock
- 2$\frac{1}{4}$" x 5$\frac{1}{2}$" (5.7 cm x 14 cm) orange paper
- $\frac{1}{2}$" x 5$\frac{1}{2}$" (1.3 cm x 14 cm) orange paper
- 1$\frac{3}{8}$" (3.5 cm) circle photograph
- 8" (20.3 cm) planting marker
- small, medium, and large daisy rubber stamps
- yellow, red, and blue ink pads
- small daisy sticker
- 2" x 2" (5 cm x 5 cm) sheet of double-sided tape
- bone folder
- craft knife
- ruler
- permanent marker, ultra-fine

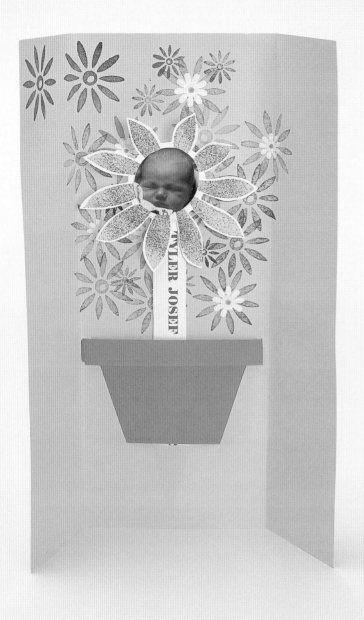

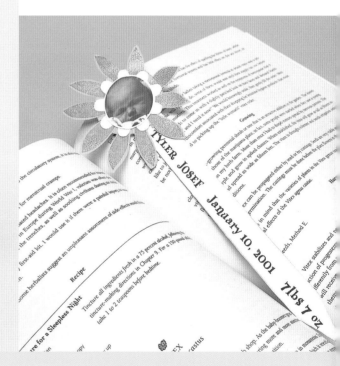

HELPFUL HINT

Use a computer to save time writing out the announcements. Adhere a sheet of double-sided tape to the back of the paper. Cut the paper into strips. The computer paper can then be adhered to the plant markers. Trim the excess paper with a craft knife.

7. Write the baby's birth information on the plant marker using an ultra-fine permanent marker.

8. Using a craft knife, cut a 1" (2.5 cm)-long line along the bottom of the pot.

9. Insert the plant marker into the flowerpot. Then push it through the paper slit at the bottom of the pot to the back of the yellow card stock.

H·a·n·d·m·a·d·e E·n·v·e·l·o·p·e·s

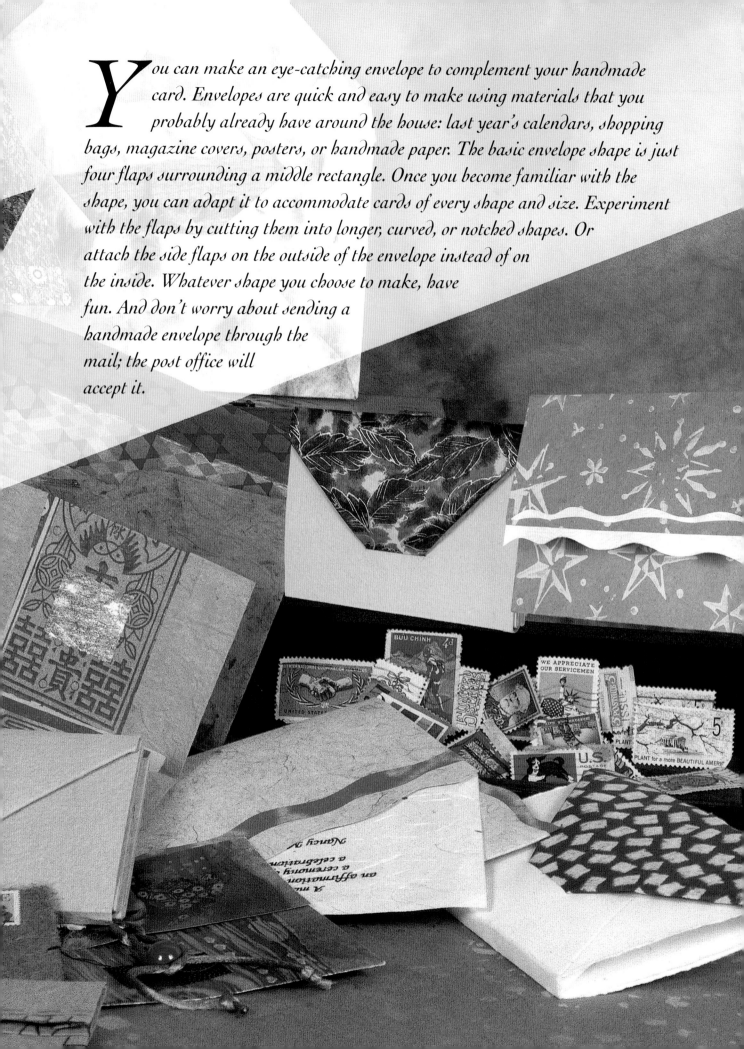

*Y*ou can make an eye-catching envelope to complement your handmade card. Envelopes are quick and easy to make using materials that you probably already have around the house: last year's calendars, shopping bags, magazine covers, posters, or handmade paper. The basic envelope shape is just four flaps surrounding a middle rectangle. Once you become familiar with the shape, you can adapt it to accommodate cards of every shape and size. Experiment with the flaps by cutting them into longer, curved, or notched shapes. Or attach the side flaps on the outside of the envelope instead of on the inside. Whatever shape you choose to make, have fun. And don't worry about sending a handmade envelope through the mail; the post office will accept it.

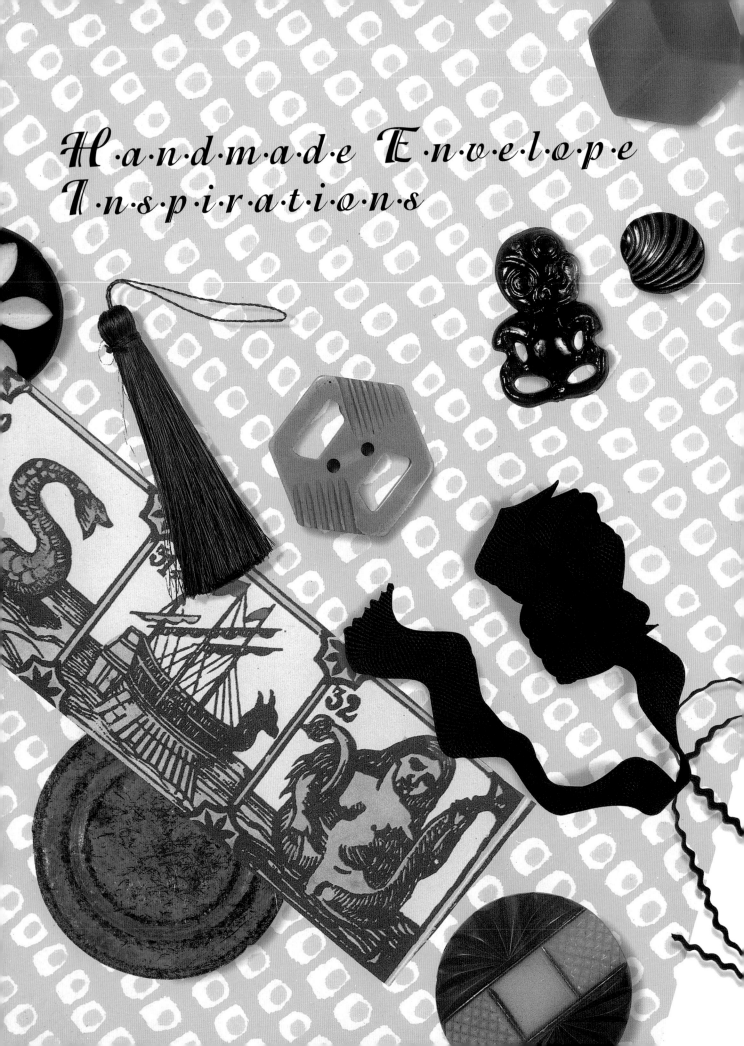

H·a·n·d·m·a·d·e E·n·v·e·l·o·p·e I·n·s·p·i·r·a·t·i·o·n·s

The simplest way to seal an envelope is with glue, but you can also punch a hole through the top flap and close it with a string or ribbon. Sew the side flaps or the edges of the envelope together with different colors of thread. Use cutouts from magazines or catalogs to create collages. Line the inside with a collection of postage stamps, newspaper comics, or astrological charts. Rubber stamps are great for adding printed images or patterns. However you choose to design your envelope, it will be happily received.

Glue a piece of ribbon along the top flap or sew on buttons for clasps.

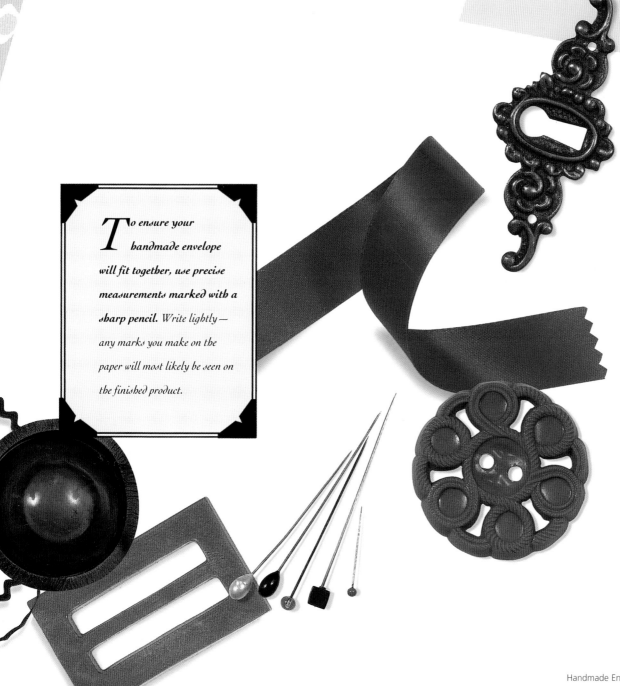

To ensure your handmade envelope will fit together, use precise measurements marked with a sharp pencil. Write lightly — any marks you make on the paper will most likely be seen on the finished product.

Easy Handmade Envelope

Using the card to be enclosed in your handmade envelope as a guide, add 4 ½" (11 cm) to the length and 2" (5 cm) to twice the width. To make a pattern, trace lines out from all four edges of the card. The lines divide the paper into five sections: the top flap, main body, bottom flap, and side flaps. Make crisp folds on each line because refolding will leave creases on the outside of the finished piece.

Materials

- Scrap paper for the envelope pattern
- Decorative or solid-color paper for the finished envelope
- Craft knife
- Metal ruler
- Pencil
- PVA glue
- Glue brush
- Bone folder
- Cutting mat or dense cardboard

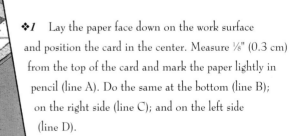

❖1   Lay the paper face down on the work surface and position the card in the center. Measure ⅛" (0.3 cm) from the top of the card and mark the paper lightly in pencil (line A). Do the same at the bottom (line B); on the right side (line C); and on the left side (line D).

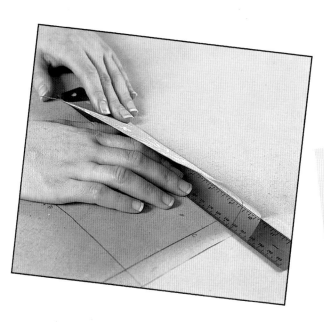

❖2   Remove the card. Place the metal ruler on line A and fold down to make the top flap. Crease the fold with your thumb or the bone folder.

If your enclosed card is a standard size, such as 4" x 6" (10 cm x 15 cm) or 5" x 7" (13 cm x 18 cm), take apart a standard envelope and use it as a pattern.

❖3   Place the metal ruler on line B and fold the paper up to make the bottom flap. Crease the fold.

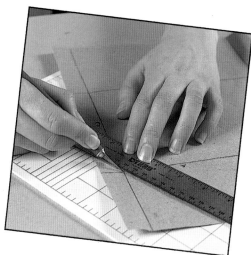

❖4   Unfold lines A and B. Use the metal ruler to fold lines C and D toward the center of the paper. Crease the folds. You now have the basic shape of the envelope.

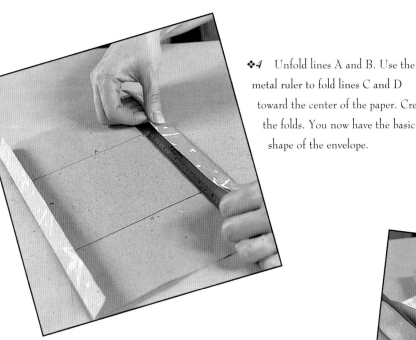

❖5   Position the metal ruler on a diagonal at a 45-degree angle through the intersection of lines A and C. For sharp corners and crisp lines, cut from the intersection of the folds out to the edge of the paper.

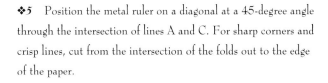

❖**6** Position the metal ruler on a diagonal at a 45-degree angle through the intersection of lines A and D. Cut from the intersection to the edge of the paper.

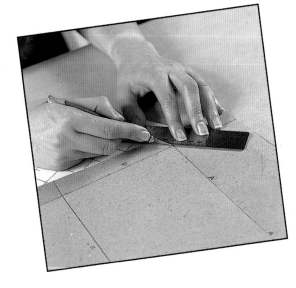

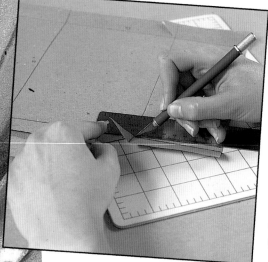

❖**7** At the top edge of the paper, measure and mark ¼" (0.5 cm) to the left of line C (toward the center). Place the ruler on a diagonal through the intersection of lines A and C to the ¼" (0.5 cm) mark. Cut from the intersection to the mark.

❖**8** As in the previous step, measure and mark ¼" (0.5 cm) to the right of line D (toward the center). Place the ruler on a diagonal through the intersection of lines A and D and cut from the intersection to the mark.

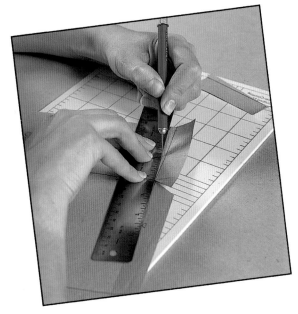

❖**9** Position the metal ruler on a diagonal at a 45-degree angle through lines B and C. Cut from the intersection up to the edge of the paper.

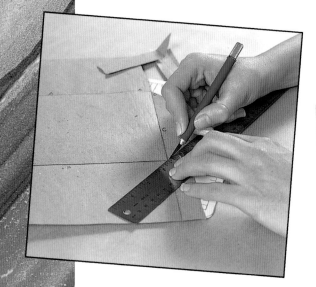

For added decoration, line the inside with contrasting paper. Glue together the wrong sides of two contrasting papers. If the papers begin to warp, put them under a pile of books until the glue dries. Then trace the envelope pattern onto the paper that will serve as the inside of the envelope and construct the envelope.

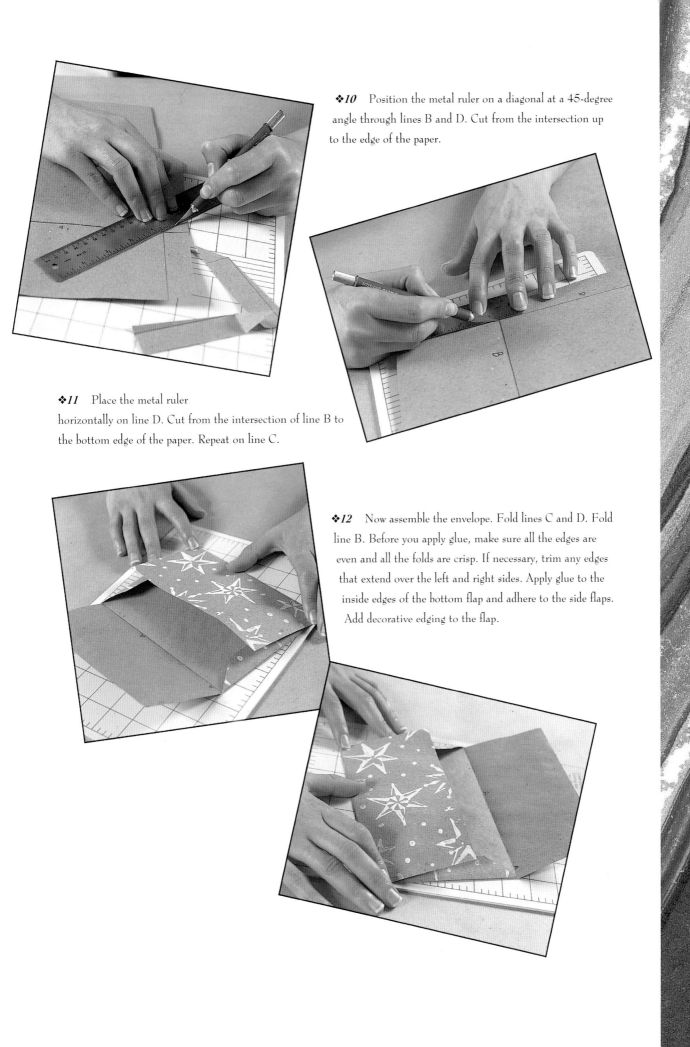

❖*10* Position the metal ruler on a diagonal at a 45-degree angle through lines B and D. Cut from the intersection up to the edge of the paper.

❖*11* Place the metal ruler horizontally on line D. Cut from the intersection of line B to the bottom edge of the paper. Repeat on line C.

❖*12* Now assemble the envelope. Fold lines C and D. Fold line B. Before you apply glue, make sure all the edges are even and all the folds are crisp. If necessary, trim any edges that extend over the left and right sides. Apply glue to the inside edges of the bottom flap and adhere to the side flaps. Add decorative edging to the flap.

Letter Envelope

The beauty of the letter envelope is that you can write notes, glue or draw in pictures, or paste in a collection of stamps or small objects, then fold it up and send your correspondence in style. Cut the paper and add embellishments before you begin to fold. Then measure and mark the paper at intervals to use as a folding guide. Fold the end edges under to create a flap, and make a slit for the flap to fit into. Or try weaving papers through the flap, as shown in the Woven Ribbon Collage project

Materials

- Piece of handmade or heavyweight paper, 5 ½" x 30" (14 cm x 76 cm)
- Piece of solid or patterned paper, 3 ¼" x 5 ½" (8.5 cm x 14 cm)
- Craft knife
- Metal ruler
- Pencil
- Bone folder
- Cutting mat

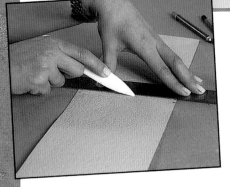

❖1 Measure and lightly mark with pencil 7 ¼" (18.5 cm) and 7 ½" (19 cm) away from the left side of the paper at the top and bottom edges. Use the metal ruler and bone folder to score the fold lines. Begin at the 7 ½" (19 cm) mark to measure the remainder of the paper at 3 ¾" (9.5 cm) intervals. Use the ruler and bone folder to score the fold lines.

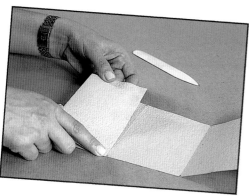

❖*2* Fold the right edge of the paper at the first fold line. Align the top edge of the paper with the edge underneath and crease it with the bone folder.

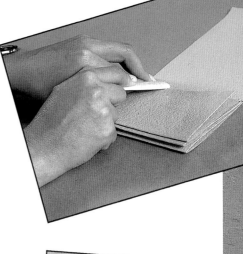

❖*3* Turn the paper over. Fold the next section over and crease the paper to make a crisp fold. Repeat to make two more folds.

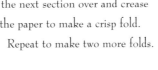

❖*4* Measure and mark 3 ¼" (8.5 cm) from the left edge of the paper. Score and fold the paper. This last section is the envelope flap.

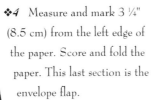

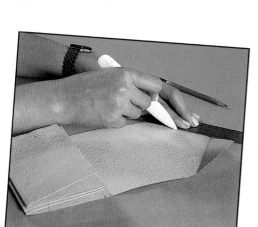

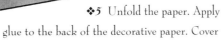

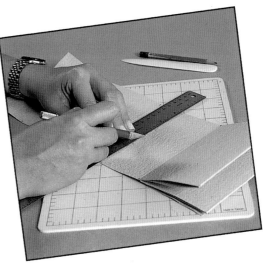

❖*5* Unfold the paper. Apply glue to the back of the decorative paper. Cover the envelope flap with the paper. Lay the paper along the fold line and press out to the edge with the bone folder. Trim any excess.

❖*6* To finish the envelope flap, measure 2 ½" (6.5 cm) down and 2 ½" (6.5 cm) over from the corners of the flap. Place the metal ruler on the diagonal of each corner at the 2 ½" (6.5 cm) mark. Score and fold the paper.

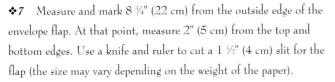

❖*7* Measure and mark 8 ¾" (22 cm) from the outside edge of the envelope flap. At that point, measure 2" (5 cm) from the top and bottom edges. Use a knife and ruler to cut a 1 ½" (4 cm) slit for the flap (the size may vary depending on the weight of the paper).

M·a·k·i·n·g Y·o·u·r O·w·n P·a·p·e·r

Making paper is a magical experience that takes you back to the basics of paper craft. It is fun, easy, and rewarding, and requires only a few household items and readily available art supplies. Once you discover how quickly you can make beautiful paper from scraps of junk mail or papers in your recycling pile, you will find yourself with a growing stack of handmade papers to make into cards, wrapping paper, bookbinding, or any other project.

Most of the supplies you will need for making your own paper are already at hand. You will need a large shallow vat such as a plastic wash basin or a cat litter box, a blender, and the material to make the paper. The best source for this is junk mail and other paper recycling that so easily collects at home. These used papers can be reduced down to paper pulp—a mixture of paper fibers and water—to produce fresh, new sheets of paper. To make existing paper into pulp, remove staples, cellophane, or other miscellaneous materials from the paper. Tear the paper into small pieces and soak in water to soften and break down the fibers. Then put the soaked bits of paper into a blender, with water, to make into pulp.

The other supplies you will need to make paper are a deckle and mold, felts, and pressing boards, all of which can be found at artist's supply stores.

The deckle and mold form and determine the size of the final sheet of paper. The deckle looks like a picture frame with a screen covering it. It captures the paper pulp, separating the fibers out from the water as it is removed from the vat. On top of the deckle is the mold, which shapes the sheet of paper. The deckle and the mold are slipped beneath the surface of the pulp in the vat and then lifted out, capturing the paper fibers while allowing the water to drain away.

After you remove the deckle and mold from the vat, you have what is essentially a very soggy piece of paper. To remove the moisture from the paper, press the sheet between felts and boards. The felts absorb some of the extra water, allow you to move the paper in progress from one work station to another, and prevent the paper from sticking to the pressing boards. If you can't find felts, wool blankets cut to size work just as well. Press as much water as possible out of the sheet of paper, then move it to a smooth surface, such as foam core, glass, or Formica, to dry.

Once you understand the basic paper-making techniques, you can easily produce numerous variations and styles of paper. At the pulp stage, add dyes to make colored papers, or mix in found objects such as petals, lace, or string to become an integral part of the paper. Add another sheet of handmade paper, or press shapes into the paper. To turn out larger sheets of paper, use larger deckles and molds and correspondingly bigger vats. If you do not have the room to set up a bigger vat, create larger sheets by overlapping smaller ones. After a sheet of paper has been placed on the pressing board, do not press it, but add another sheet of unpressed paper right next to and touching the first. Continue adding these unpressed sheets until the paper is the size you want, and then place the second felt and pressing board on top of the paper and press as usual. The resulting sheet is a composite of all the smaller sheets you placed together.

How to Make Paper

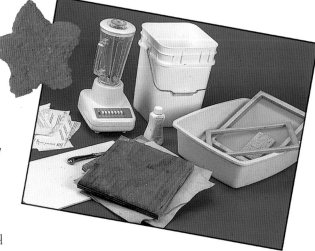

This recipe for navy colored paper is quick, easy, and produces beautiful results. To create a different color paper, simply substitute the blue dye with another color, or after you have made a few blue sheets of paper, add some yellow or red dye to the pulp to make either green or purple sheets of paper. Take your time, have fun, and experiment. The result will be your own unique papers you can use to add a more personal touch to your paper projects.

Materials

- Paper scraps
- Blender
- Water
- Blue dye
- Large shallow vat (large enough to contain deckle and mold)
- 8 ½" x 11" (21.5 cm x 28 cm) deckle and mold
- 2 pieces of felt just larger than the paper you are making
- Pressing boards
- Sheet of foam core or other smooth surface
- Towels and sponges
- Bucket
- Putty or butter knife

❖1 Tear the paper into small pieces, measuring no more than 1" (2.5 cm) square, and place them in the bucket. Add enough water to cover

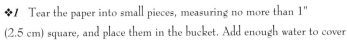

the paper and let it soak overnight to soften the fibers. The next day, put a small handful of the paper pieces into the blender with a little bit of water and blend until the pulp is smooth, with no lumps. It should resemble the consistency of cooked oatmeal. Repeat until all of the soaked paper bits have been made into pulp. Pour it all into the shallow vat and add several tablespoons of the blue dye until you have created a rich, blue-colored mixture.

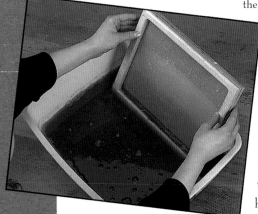

❖2 Mix enough water into the pulp so that it has a soupy consistency (the more water you add to the pulp, the thinner the sheet of paper will be). Agitate the mixture to ensure an even dispersion of the pulp. Stack the mold on top of the deckle and, beginning at one side of the vat, slip the deckle and mold beneath the surface of the pulp solution in one smooth movement.

❖3 Lift the deckle and mold straight up out of the vat and gently shake them to ensure an even dispersion of the paper pulp. Allow as much water as possible to drain off, and remove the mold from the top of the deckle.

❖4 To prevent the pulp from sticking to the felts, soak them in water and then wring them out. Place one pressing board on the work surface with a piece of felt on top of it. In a quick, smooth motion flip the deckle over onto the felt so that the sheet of paper you are forming is trapped between the screen of the deckle and the felt. With a towel or sponge, press against the screen of the deckle to squeeze out as much water from the pulp sheet as possible. Gently remove the deckle, leaving the pulp sheet on the felt. If the pulp starts to tear as you lift off the deckle, press out more water before continuing.

❖5 Lay the other felt on top of the pulp sheet and the other pressing board on top of that. Press the sheet firmly between the two boards to remove more water. You may find that standing on the boards is the easiest way to do this. Carefully remove the top board and felt.

❖6 Lift the felt that the sheet of paper is on and turn it over onto the foam core, pulp side down. Press the sheet against the foam core and gently peel the felt away from the sheet of paper. If the paper starts to tear, press it back against the foam to remove more moisture before continuing to peel off the felt. Leave the newly formed sheet of paper on the foam for several hours to dry.

❖7 When the edges of the paper sheet start to pull away from the foam core, and the center of the sheet feels dry to the touch, slip a putty or butter knife between the paper and the foam core, and gently pry the paper from the surface.

Paper-Making Tips

To make your own deckle and mold set, use two matching picture frames and enough window screening (available at any hardware store) to cover the opening of one frame. Remove the glass, backing, and stands from the frames so that only the front portion of the frame remains. Wrap the screening around one frame and staple or glue it in place. This frame is now the deckle. Stack the other frame on top of the deckle to use it as the mold for your paper.

Use cookie cutters as molds on top of a deckle to make small, fun shaped pieces of paper to use for invitations or name tags.

To make a thick sheet of paper, add only a little water to the pulp before forming the sheet. For a thin sheet of paper, dilute the pulp considerably with water.

Artist Gallery

The following group of artist friends exchange cards as a sort of visual poetry, often creating and giving them at holiday time or simply sending them off with "Just been thinking of you" or "Have you heard the news?" Ideas, thoughts, and feelings are exchanged, while, love and devotion are expressed toward one another. With a handmade card, we honor the recipient, and, in return, the sender is rewarded in knowing that the card will be cherished. Artists know that the time spent in hand-making something is a reason for loving it more. Stored in a special box, stuck between the wall and doorframe, or pinned to a bulletin board, they are messengers gently calling us back to the people we love.

Mother's Day
Luncheon Invitation

Terry Peterson

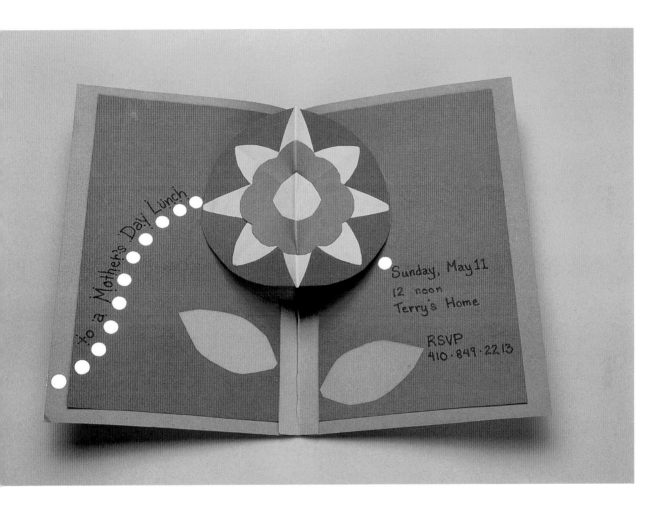

Fold two sheets of different colored papers in half. Trim ½" (1.3 cm) from all sides of the inside paper. Open the paper and, on the fold, cut a large circle leaving it attached at the 3 and 9 o'clock positions. Decorate the circle to create a flower design. Adhere both papers together. Reverse the circle's fold to create the pop-out. Add a flower stem, two leaves, lettering, and other embellishments to the inside of the card.

Party Invites in the Round

Nancy Marculewicz

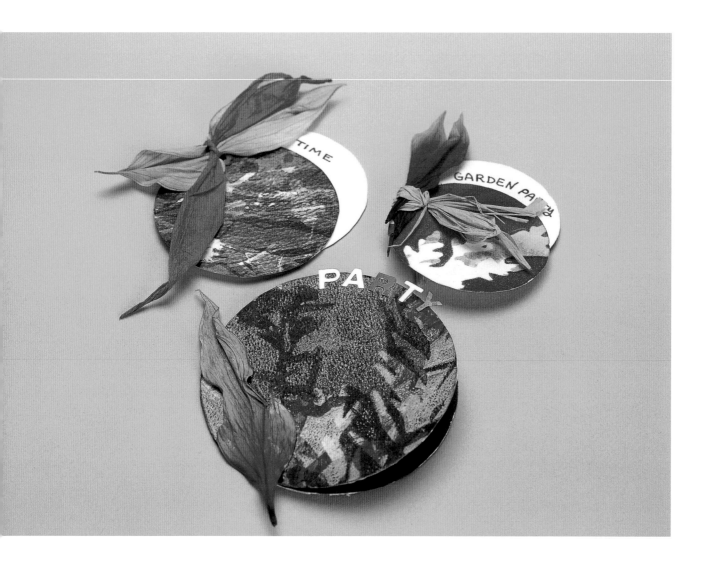

Step out from the square and make these charming circular invites. For card covers, Nancy cuts different sized circles from her handmade gelatin nature prints. Attach the covers together by gluing a small area to the left side or by punching a hole and inserting a small eyelet. Decorate the hinged area with brightly colored paper ribbon and dried leaves. For lettering pizzazz, glue letter confetti along the invite's circumference.

ᴀutumn Greeting Notes

Mary Byrom

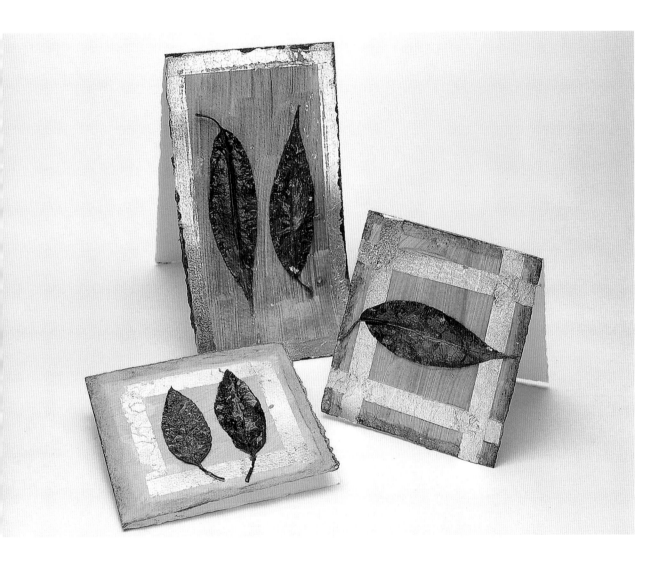

Ah, the warm, golden colors of autumn are richly represented in these gorgeous leaf notes framed with gold leafed lines. Begin by painting with a wide brush, the front of folded artist paper (100% cotton) with a matte medium mixed with yellow ochre acrylic paint. Let dry. Follow the manufacturer's instructions for gold leafing to make the gold frame. Place newly collected autumn leaves between waxed paper and dry with a hot iron. Paint both sides of the leaves with orange acrylic colors. When the leaves are dry, glue them on the card.

Budding Friendship Note Paper

Barbara Frake

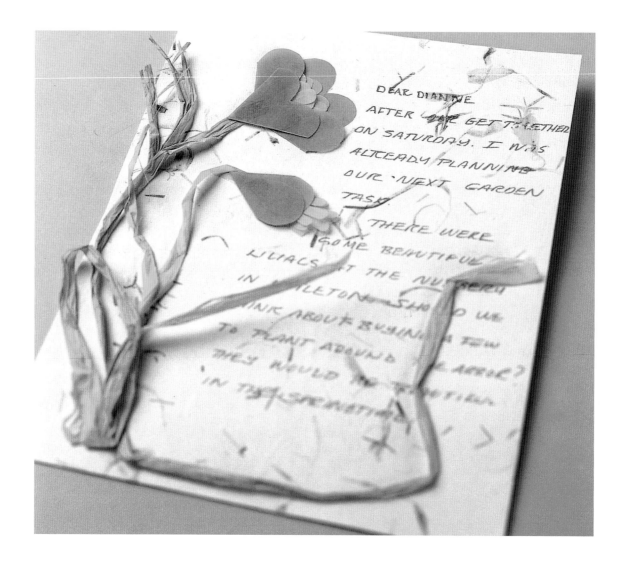

Using simple materials and scissors, charm your friends with this handmade paper stationery. Make the flower petals by cutting heart shapes on the paper fold, varying the length and width of each heart. Construct the flower head by inserting the largest heart shape with progressively smaller hearts. The flower stamens are cut into very long, narrow heart shapes then inserted into the flower. Glue the flowers to the far left side of a sheet of handmade paper. Use paper ribbon or raffia for the stems.

A long the Garden Fence

Susan Keller

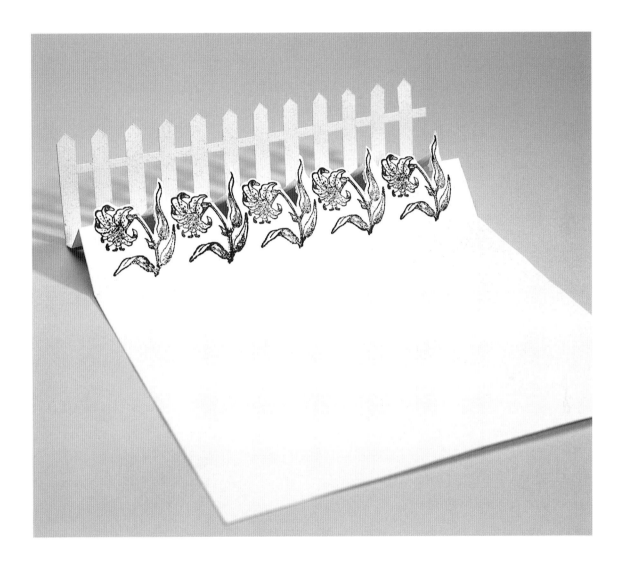

Do you wish for the old days of leaning over a fence and chatting leisurely with a neighbor? Here's an old-fashioned idea in a contemporary letter writing form. Cut a picket fence design along the top of your stationery. Score two parallel lines ¹/₂" (1.3 cm) apart just below the fence bottom. Fold and crease along each line. Unfold. Stamp a line of flowers about 1" (2.5 cm) below the fence. Using a craft knife, cut along the flowers' contour leaving the space between the flower and the paper edge untouched. Score a line along the bottom of the flowers design. Fold the flowers design so they stand upright along the fence pickets.

Templates

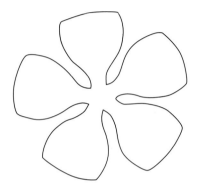

Dried Flower Medallions, page 202
Flower Template

Garden Recipe Cards, page 204
Mason Jar Template

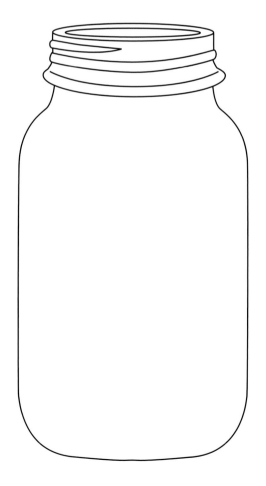

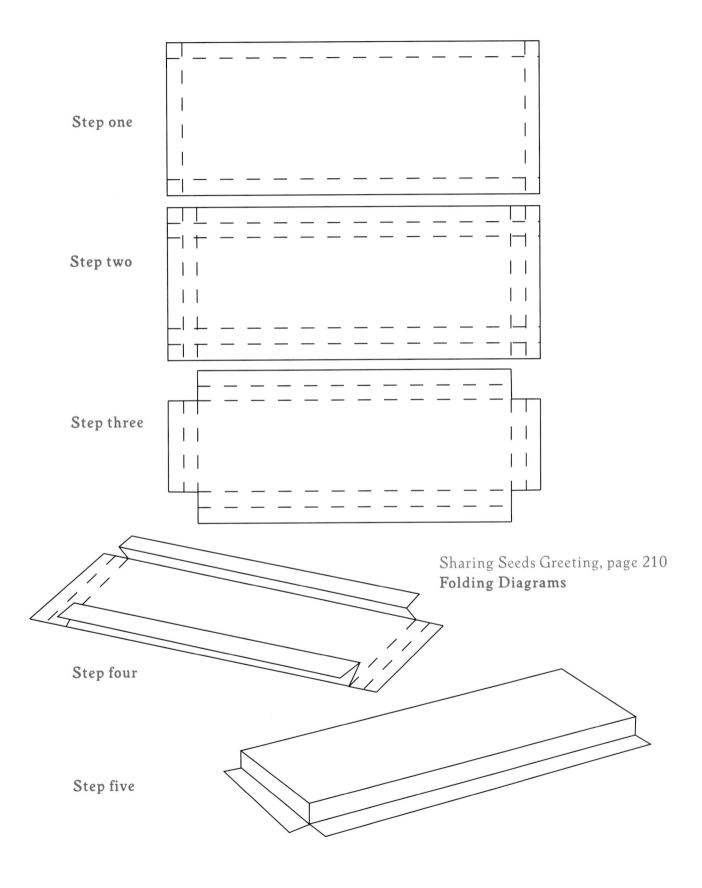

Step one

Step two

Step three

Sharing Seeds Greeting, page 210
Folding Diagrams

Step four

Step five

Seeded Center Flower Cards, page 212
Weaving Template

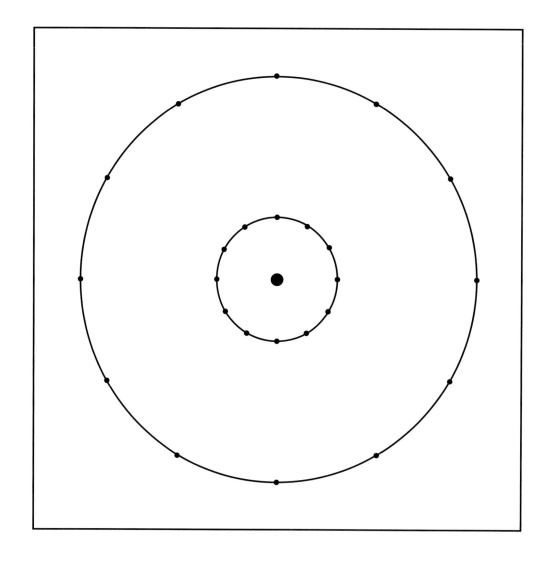

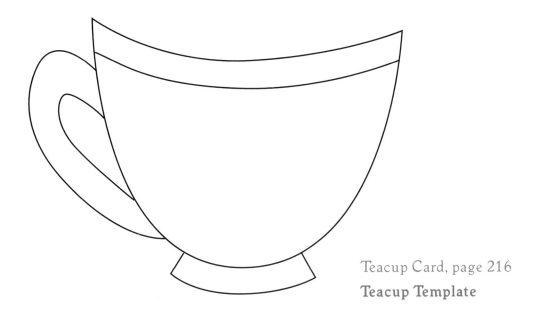

Teacup Card, page 216

Teacup Template

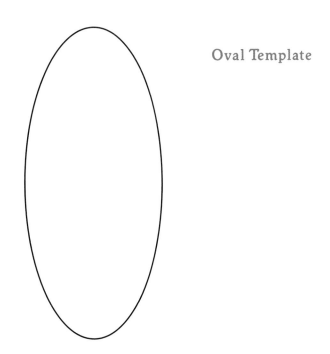

Oval Template

Bee Happy Photo Card, page 174
Bee Template

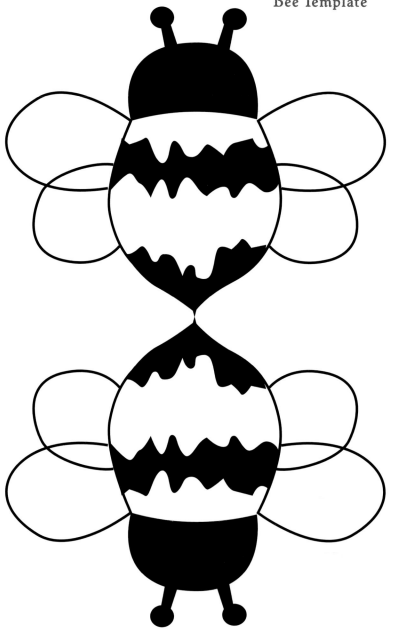

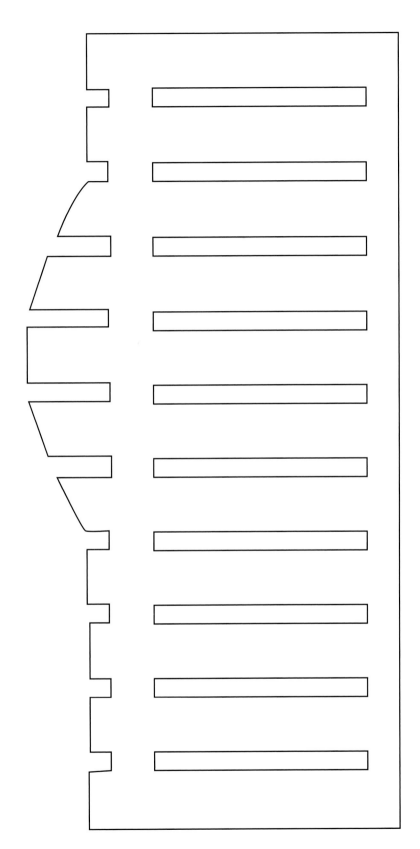

Garden Gate Greeting, page 176

Garden Gate Template

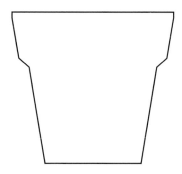

Pop-up Potted Posies, page 152

Flower Pot Template

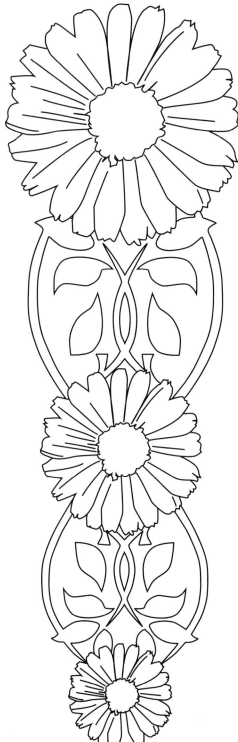

Bouquet Fanfare, page 154

Flower Panel Template

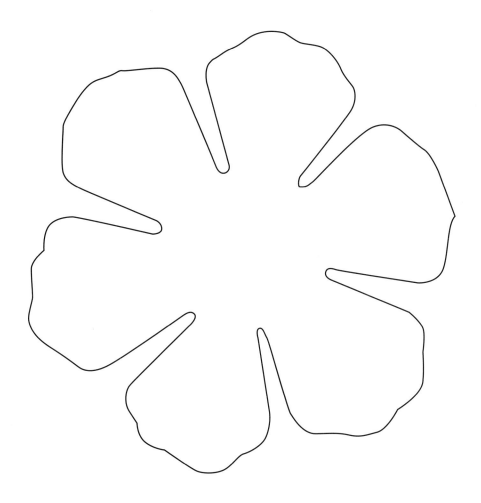

Posy Packets, page 162

Posy Template

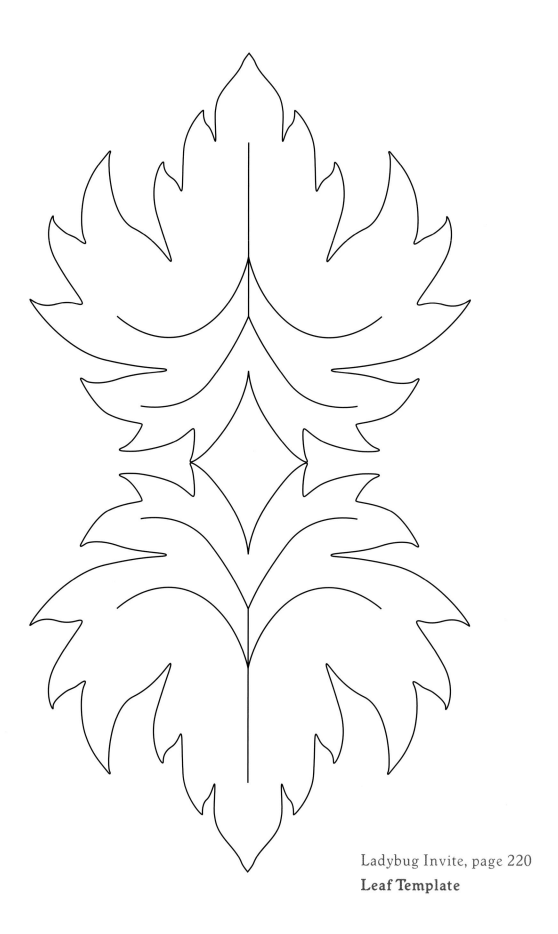

Ladybug Invite, page 220
Leaf Template

↓ **P. 17 | BASIC WINDOW-SHAPED CARD III**

↓ **P. 18 | BASIC WINDOW-SHAPED CARD IV**

→ **P. 19 | BASIC EMBOSSING**

↓ **P. 23 | TRADITIONAL PATTERN CARD III**

↓ **P. 28 | WINE GLASSES IN A FRAME**

↓ **P. 29 | WINE GLASSES**

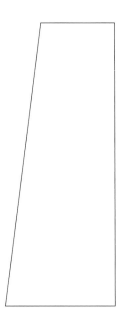

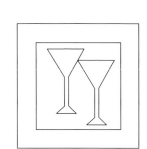

↓ **P. 30 | CAKE AND HEART**

→ **P. 31 | ANNIVERSARY CAKE**

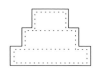

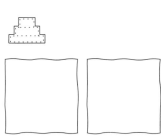

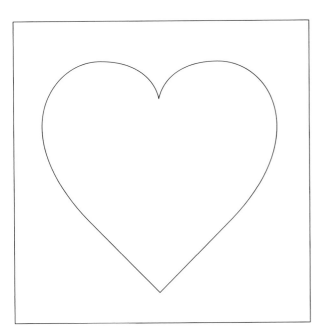

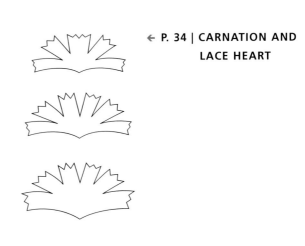

← **P. 34 | CARNATION AND LACE HEART**

Happy   Mother's Day

↓ **P. 35 | PURPLE FLOWERS AND FLOWER VASE**

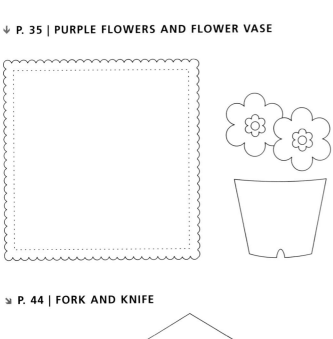

I

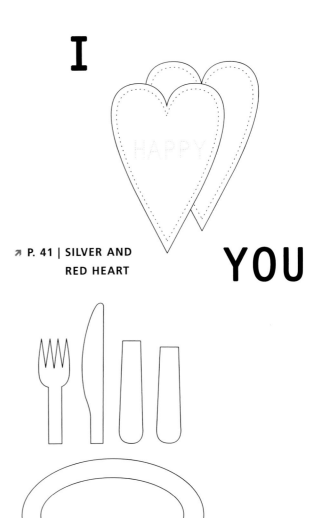

YOU

↗ **P. 41 | SILVER AND RED HEART**

↘ **P. 44 | FORK AND KNIFE**

↓ **P. 45 | A RED ROOF**

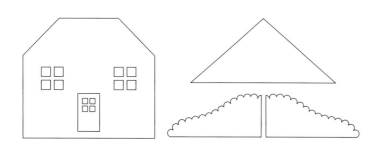

↘ **P. 46 | A COFFE MUG**

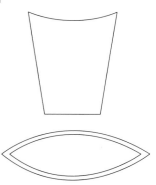

↓ **P. 48 | FLOWERS IN A FRAME**

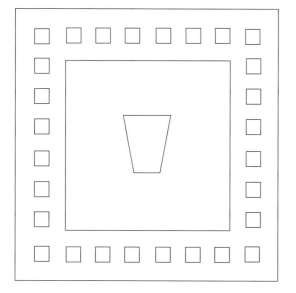

↘ **P. 49 | EMBOSSED FLOWERS AND HAPPY BIRTHDAY**

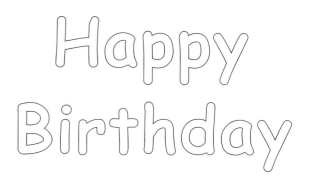

↓ **P. 51 | CARD EMBELLISHED WITH FLOWERS**

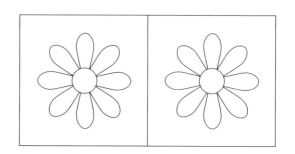

↘ **P. 54 | WEDDING CARD**

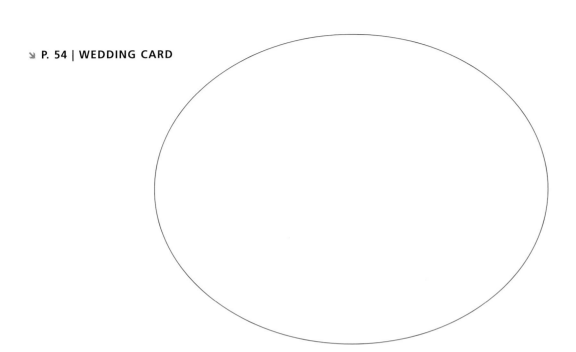

↓ **P. 83 | PURPLE FLOWER GARLAND**

↓ **P. 89 | A VASE AND FLOWERS**

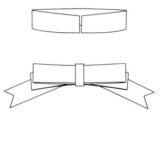

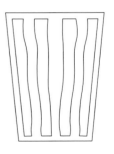

↓ **P. 90 | FENCE AND FLOWERS**

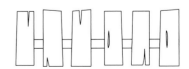

↘ **P. 79 | A CHRISTMAS TREE COVERED BY SNOW**

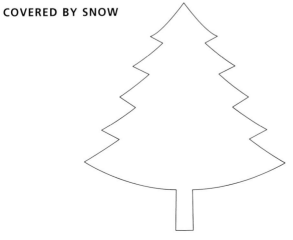

↓ **P. 94 | PURPLE FLOWERS AND A BUTTERFLY**

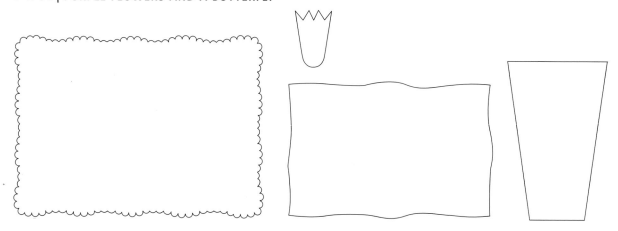

↓ **P. 95 | A BUNDLE OF FLOWERS**

↙ **P. 96 | YELLOW SPRING FLOWERS**

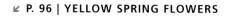

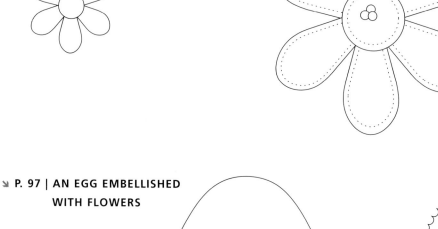

↘ **P. 97 | AN EGG EMBELLISHED WITH FLOWERS**

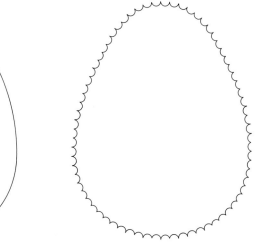

⤷ P. 100 | YELLOW FLOWERS BEHIND A WINDOW

→ P. 101 | FLOWERS AND WAVES

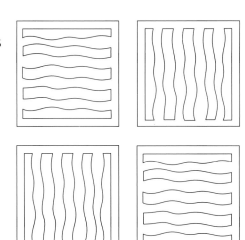

⬇ P. 103 | WHITE FLOWERS ON A RECTANGLE

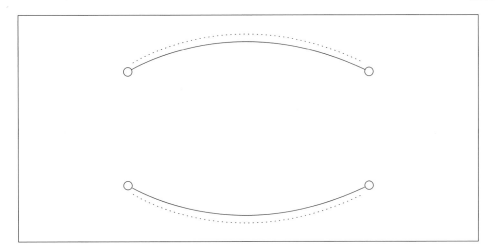

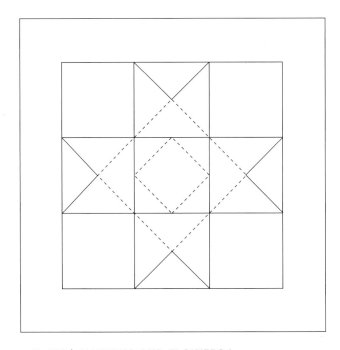

⬆ P. 102 | PATTERNS AND FLOWERS I

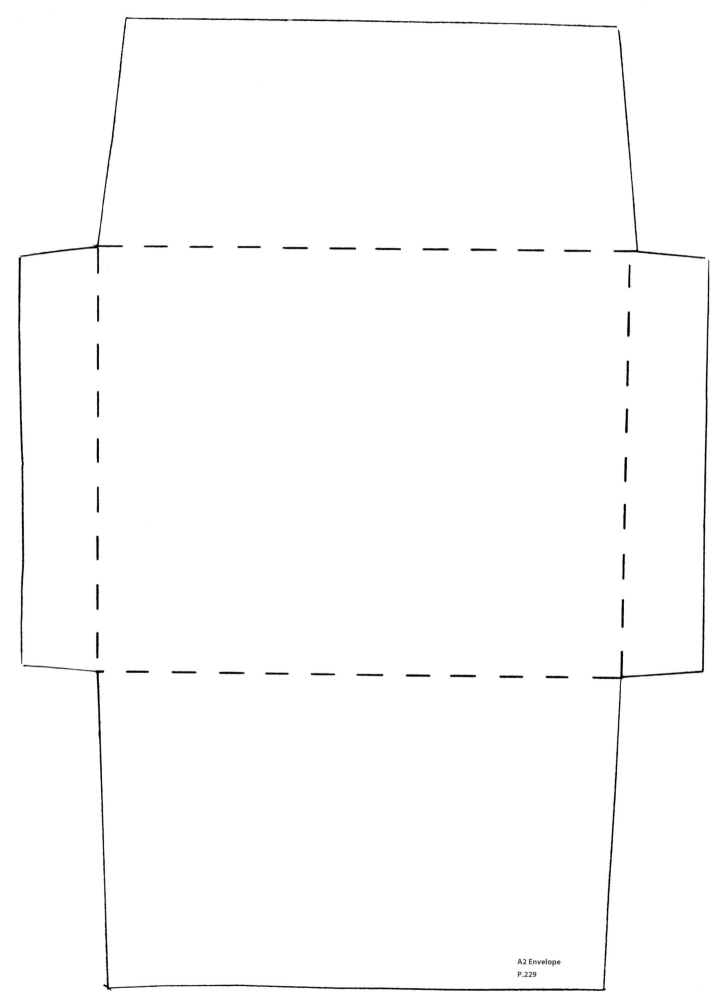

A2 Envelope
P.229

278

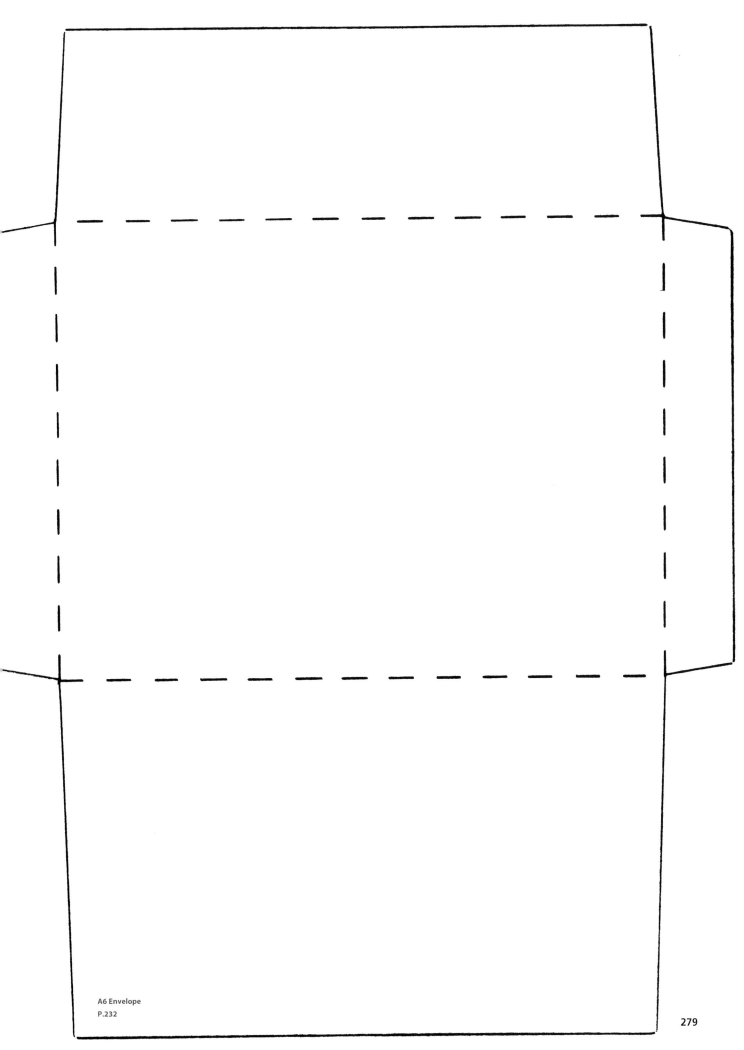

A6 Envelope
P.232

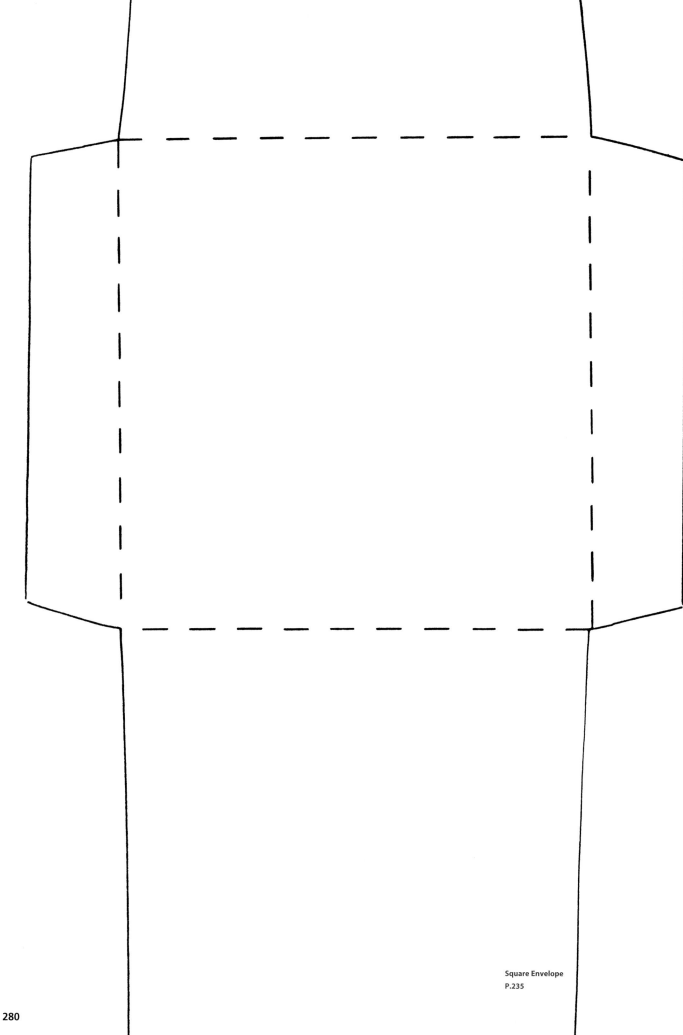

Square Envelope
P.235

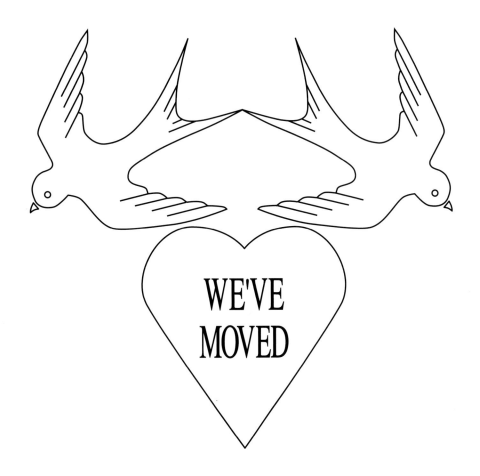

WE'VE
MOVED

"We've Moved" Birdhouse, page 238
Flying Bird Template
Heart Template

Resources

Handmade Papers, Papermaking Supplies, and Assorted Art Supplies

Aiko's Art Materials Import, Inc.
3347 North Clark Street
Chicago, IL 60657 USA
(312) 404-5600

Amsterdam Art
1013 University Avenue
Berkeley, CA 94710 USA
(510) 649-4800

Arnold Grummer
(800) 453-1485
www.arnoldgrummer.com

Aussie Stamps & Crafts
4 Brougham Place
Golden Grove SA 5125 Australia
+61 08 82898871
mwo@lweb.net.au

Black Cat Creations
P.O. Box 489
Everton Park QLD 4053 Australia
+61 07 3354 4411

Black Ink
5 Brattle Street, Harvard Square
Cambridge, MA 02139 USA
(617) 497-1221

Bonnie's Best
3314 Inman Drive NE
Atlanta, GA 30319-2428 USA
(404) 869-0081
www.coilconnection.com

Bumble Bee Crafts
7 Toolara Street
The Gap QLD 4061 Australia
+61 07 3511 0068
buzz@gil.com.au

Carriage House Paper / New York
79 Guernsey Street
Brooklyn, NY 11222 USA
(718) 599-7857

Cherry Pie Art
Via Antica Romana
33A/4, 16166 Quinto al Mare
Genova, Italy
www.cherrypie.theshoppe.com

Coffee Break Design
P.O. Box 34281
Indianapolis, IN 46234 USA
(317) 290-1542

Create an Impression
56 East Lancaster Avenue
Ardmore, PA 19003 USA
(610) 645-6500

Creative Crafts
11 The Square
Winchester, Hampshire SO23 9ES UK
+44 01962 856266
www.creativecrafts.co.uk

Daniel Smith
4150 First Avenue South
P.O. Box 84268
Seattle, WA 98124-5568 USA
(800) 426-6740
www.danielsmith.com

David Reina Designs, Inc.
79 Guernsey Street
Brooklyn, NY 11222 USA
(718) 599-1237

Dick Blick
P.O. Box 1267
Galesburg, IL 61402-1267 USA
(800) 447-8192
www.dickblick.com

Dieu Donné Papermill, Inc.
433 Broome Street
New York, NY 10013 USA
(212) 226-0573
ddpaper@cybernex.net

Eckersley's Arts, Crafts, and Imagination
+61 (300) 657-766
www.eckersleys.com.au
Store locations in New South Wales, Queensland, South Australia, and Victoria, Australia

The Fabric Place
www.fabricplace.com
(800) 556-3700

Fascinating Folds
(800) 968-2418
www.fascinating-folds.com

Fine Paper Company
www.finepaperco.com

Heindesign
Expressby Road 76
58091 Hagen, Germany
+49 0 23 32/7 22 11
www.heindesign.de

HobbyCraft
Head Office
Bournemouth, UK
+44 1202 596 100
Stores throughout the UK

Inkadinkado
61 Holton Street
Woburn, MA 01801 USA
(800) 888-4652
www.inkadinkado.com

JoAnne Rossman Design
No. 6 Birch Street
Roslindale, MA 02131 USA
(617) 323-4301

John Lewis
Flagship Store
Oxford Street
London W1A 1EX UK
+44 207 629 7711
www.johnlewis.co.uk

Kate's Paperie
561 Broadway
New York, NY 10012 USA
(212) 941-9816
www.katespaperie.com

Legion Paper Corp.
11 Madison Avenue
New York, NY 10010 USA
(800) 278-4478

Lee Scott McDonald, Inc.
P.O. Box 264
Charlestown, MA 02129 USA
(617) 242-2505

Littlejohns Art & Graphic Supplies Ltd
170 Victoria Street
Wellington, New Zealand
+64 04 385 2099

Loose Ends
P.O. Box 20310
Salem, OR 97307 USA
(503) 390-7457
www.looseends.com

Magenta Style
2275 Bombardier
Sainte-Julie QC J3E 2J9 Canada
(450) 922-5253
www.magentastyle.com

Magnolia
2527 Magnolia Street
Oakland, CA 94607 USA
(510) 839-5268

Michael's
www.michaels.com

New York Central Art Supply
62 Third Avenue
New York, NY 10003 USA
(212) 473-7705

Oblation Papers & Press
www.oblationpapers.com

Paper Connection International
Lauren Pearlman
208 Pawtuxet Avenue
Cranston, RI 02905 USA
(401) 461-2135
www.paperconnection.com

The Paper Crane
280 Cabot Street
Beverly, MA 01915 USA
(978) 927-3131
www.papercrane.com

The Paper Cut
www.thepapercut.com

Paper Source
232 West Chicago Avenue
Chicago, IL 60610 USA
(800) 248-8035
www.paper-source.com
Store locations also in Evanston, Kansas City, Philadelphia, and Cambridge

The Papertrail
170 University Avenue West
Waterloo, ON N2L 3E9 Canada
(800) 421-6826

Pearl Art & Craft
www.pearlpaint.com

Platypus Creek Stamping & Craft
Shop 3 Stanto Place (Cnr Stanton Rd & Captain Cook Hwy)
Smithfield QLD Australia
+61 07 4038 1013
platycreek@bigpond.com

Rivendell Cottage
109 Ryrie Street
Geelong VIC 3220 Australia
+61 03 5224 1911

Rock Paper Scissors
78 Main Street
Wiscasset, ME 04578 USA
(207) 882-9930

Rugg Road Paper Company
105 Charles Street
Boston, MA 02114 USA
(617) 742-0002

Snazzy Bags
www.snazzybags.com

Staples
www.staples.com

T N Lawrence & Son Ltd.
208 Portland Road
Hove BN3 5QT UK
+44 0845 644 3232
www.lawerence.co.uk

Timothy Moore Paper Molds and Bookbinding Tools
14450 Behling Road
Concord, MI 49237 USA
www.timothymooretools.com

Twinrocker
P.O. Box 413
Brookston, IN 47923 USA
(800) 757-8946

Contributors

Mary Byrom
102 Wells Street
North Berwick, ME 03906 USA
mbyrom@maine.rr.com
page 259

Barbara Frake
Currierville Road
P.O. Box 273
Newton, NH 03858 USA
www.frakefineart.com
page 260

Susan Keller
8 Summit Place
Newburyport, MA 01950 USA
page 261

Nancy Marculewicz
P.O. Box 177
Essex, MA 01929 USA
jellyroller@earthlink.net
page 258

Linda O'Brien
Burnt Offerings Studio
2170 Evergreen Road
North Perry Village, OH 44081 USA
www.burntofferings.com
page 171

Terry Peterson
523A Epping Forest Road
Annapolis, MD 21401 USA
page 257

About the Authors

Claire Sun-ok Choi, named simply Sun-ok Choi in Korean, was born in South Korea. She worked as a quilling paper craft instructor at Hyundai Culture Center and the Education Center for the Quilling Paper Craft Association for five years in Korea. In 2000, she had her first solo exhibition at Insadong Gallery in Seoul entitled, "Paper Wanting to Be Flower," and was invited by Ferry Building Gallery to a group exhibition held in Vancouver, Canada, in 2002. She is currently living and studying in Vancouver, Canada. Since 2000, she has been devoting the majority of her time to the creation of quilling paper crafts and card design.

Ricë Freeman-Zachery was teaching college English classes in 1992 when she began writing regularly for *Rubberstampmadness*, the original rubber-stamp magazine. Since then she has also written for *Belle Armoire*, *Legacy, Personal Journaling*, and the *Studio*. Her projects and articles have also been featured in galleries and shops in New Orleans, Denver, Taos, Santa Fe, Albuquerque, Seattle, and Tacoma. She teaches stamping and art workshops as well as a variety of other media.

Gail Hercher, a paper artist and teacher, is the owner of The Paper Crane, a studio/gallery in Beverly, Massachusetts, that offers exhibits, workshops, and supplies for the paper arts. She has taught for more than twenty years in schools, museums, and colleges and currently gives workshops throughout New England. She exhibits her work and has received several awards and grants, including a Fulbright Fellowship to study in Europe.

Susan Jaworski-Stranc of Apple Cider Press & Prints Studio is an established printmaker, teacher, lecturer, and gardener. She lives and works in Newbury, Massachusetts. She is a professional member of the American Craft Council and her book work is exhibited annually at the council's craft shows in Charlotte, North Carolina, and West Springfield, Massachusetts. She exhibits her handcrafted books and prints in numerous fine juried craft shows, and her one-of-a-kind artist books reside in gallery, library, and museum collections. She has contributed artwork to several books, magazines, and websites.

Lisa Kerr, a Boston-based author and artist, has been making cards for more than twenty years. In 1990, her one-time hobby developed into Monolisa Worldwide, a successful business that creates cards, blank journals, and photo albums, and distributes them through gift stores in the U.S. and Europe. Kerr has traveled all over the world, gathering unique papers and techniques to use in her card making.

Laura McFadden is a freelance art director living in Somerville, Massachusetts. She is a former design director for *Inc.* magazine. She currently runs her own graphic design studio, Laura McFadden Design, Inc., and has contributed to various craft books for publishers such as Rockport Publishers and Martingale & Company, and to magazines such as *Handcraft Illustrated*. She is coauthor, with April Paffrath, of *The Artful Bride: Simple, Handmade Wedding Projects* (Rockport Publishers, 2003).

April Paffrath is a freelance editor and writer in Cambridge, Massachusetts. In addition to book and magazine editing, she has written architecture profiles, travel pieces, cooking articles, and craft how-tos for magazines such as *Scientific American Explorations* and *Martha Stewart Living*. She is coauthor, with Laura McFadden, of *The Artful Bride: Simple Handmade Wedding Projects* (Rockport Publishers, 2003).

Jessica Wrobel began her professional life as a costumer and paper and fiber artist, retailing her handcrafts in boutiques throughout New England and teaching art to the students of the ARC of Haverhill, Massachusetts, and Second Step/YMCA of Lawrence, Massachusetts. She was further able to explore the rich world of decorative techniques when she authored *The Paper Jewelry Book* (Quarry Books, 1997), *The Crafter's Recipe Book* (Quarry Books, 1998), and *Quick and Easy Flower Design* (Quarry Books, 2005).

P·a·p·e·r S·a·m·p·l·e·s

The beautiful paper samples provided here are for you to cut out and create cards of your own. The heavier card stock papers can be used as card bases; cut and fold them so that the solid colors lie inside the card—or reverse the pattern for a color surprise inside. Use the smaller images to glue to the card bases. Create card collages with a travel or horticultural theme. Or attach a layer of transparent film, photocopied with a rubber stamp image, over vibrant patterned paper. With the easy card-making instructions inside and these companion papers, you will be well on your way to making original card designs that you can give to your friends and family.

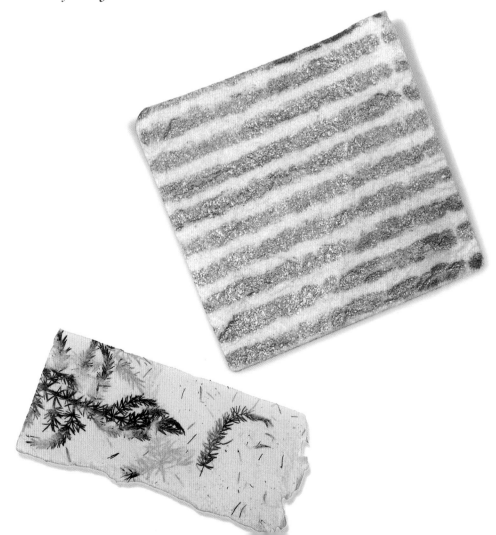

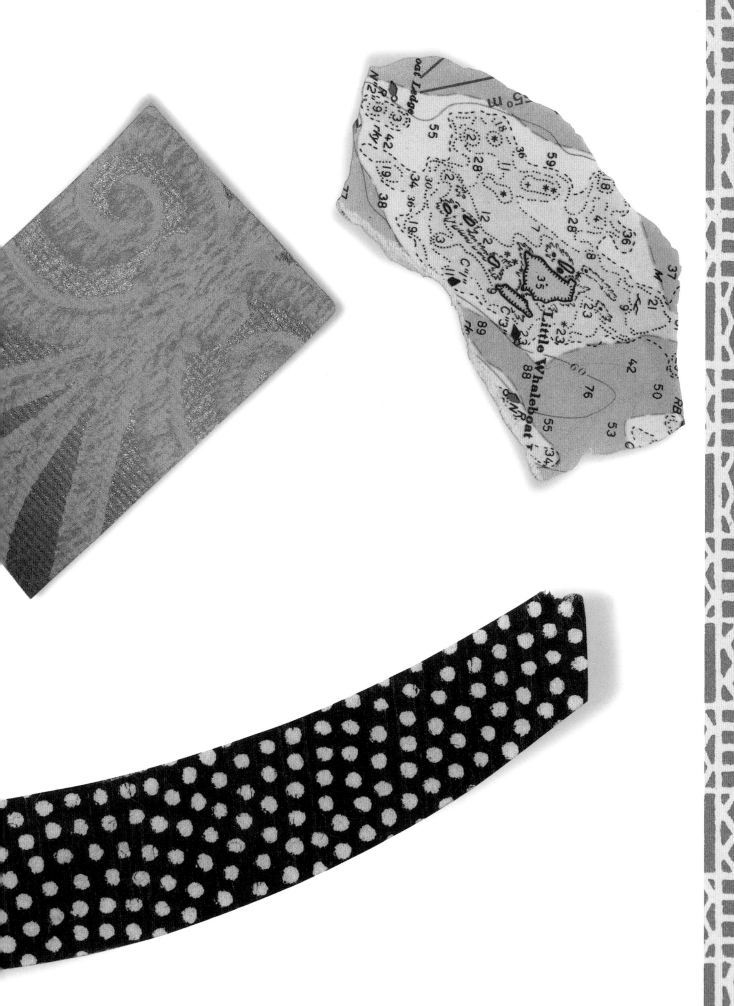

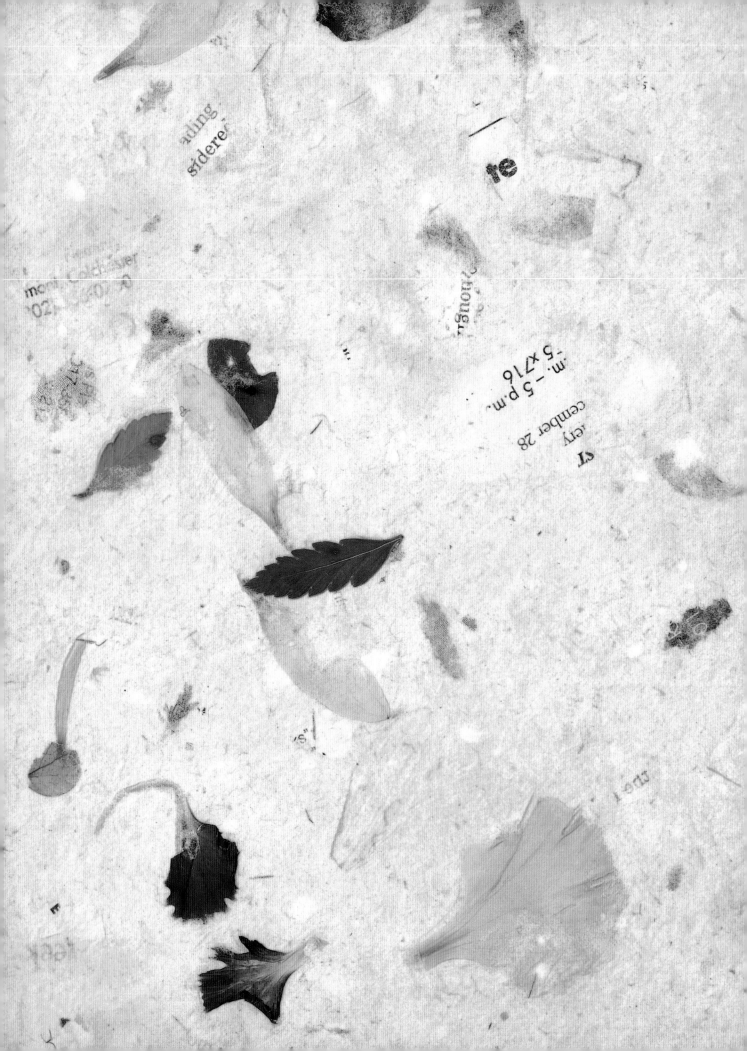

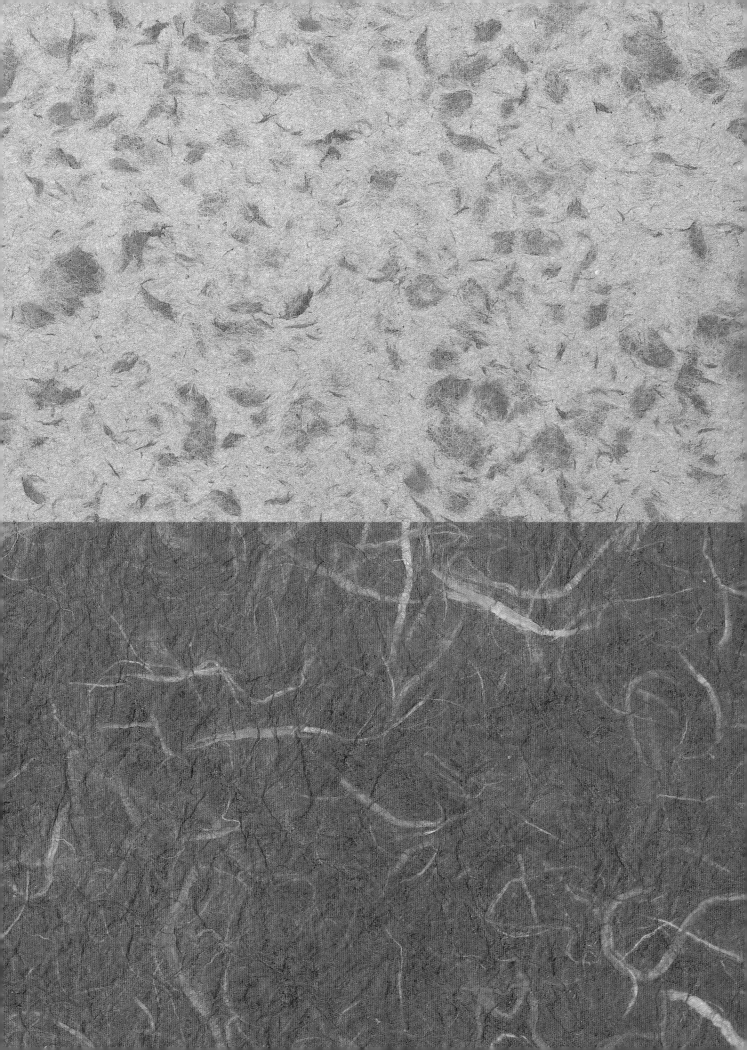

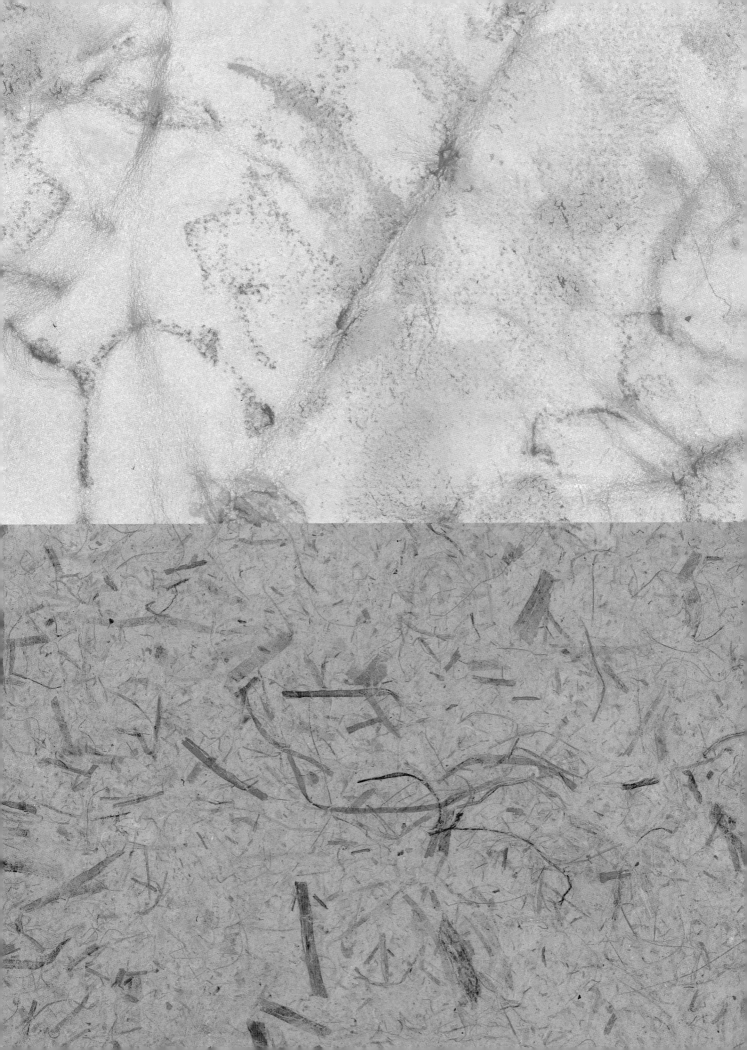

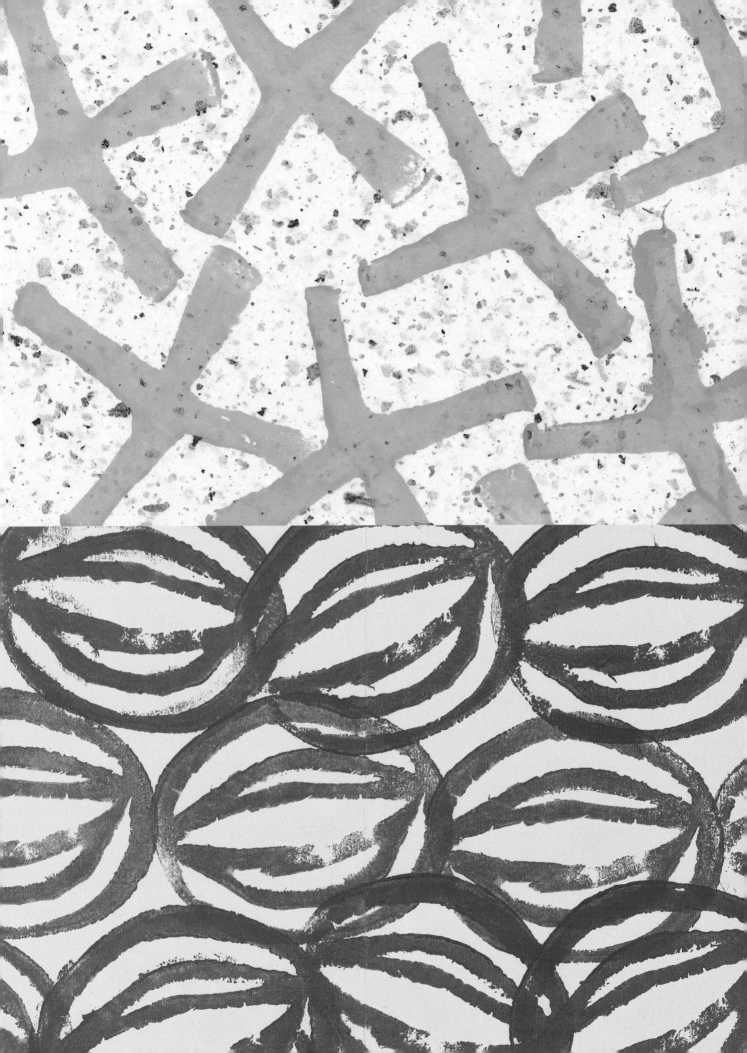

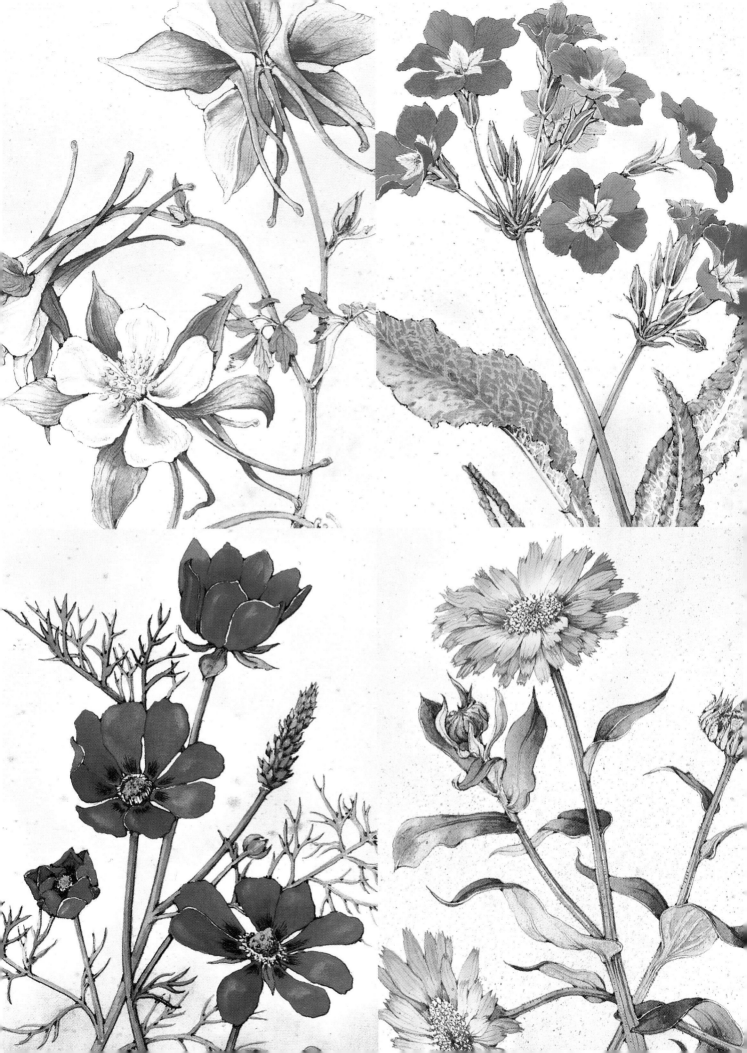

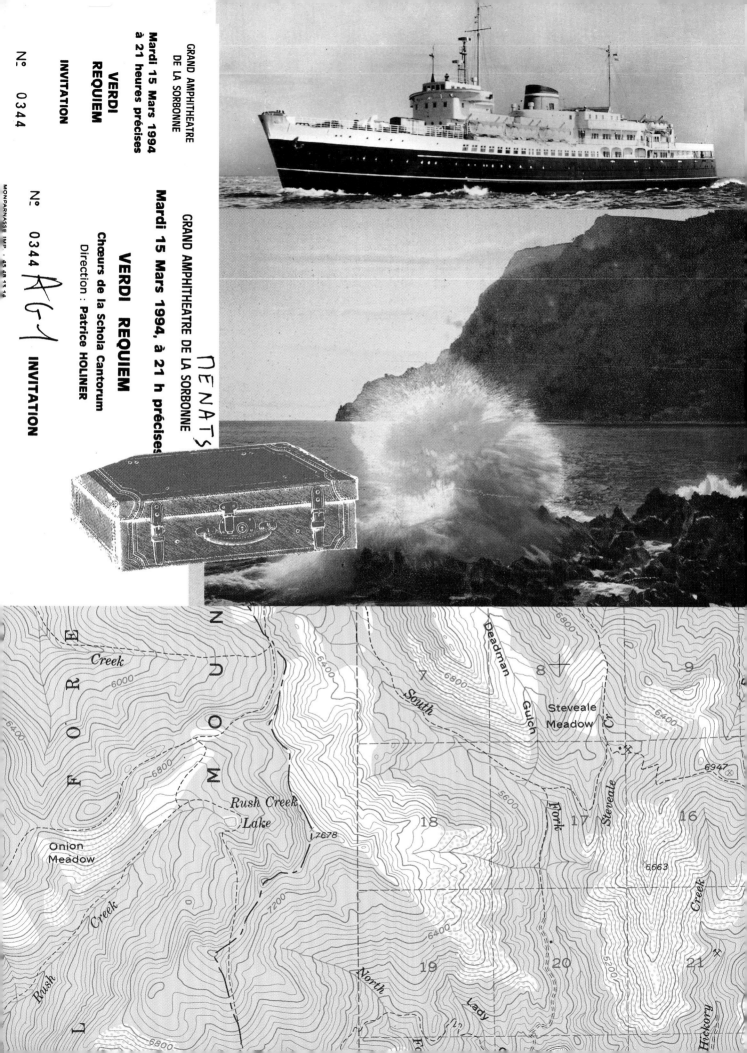

NENATS

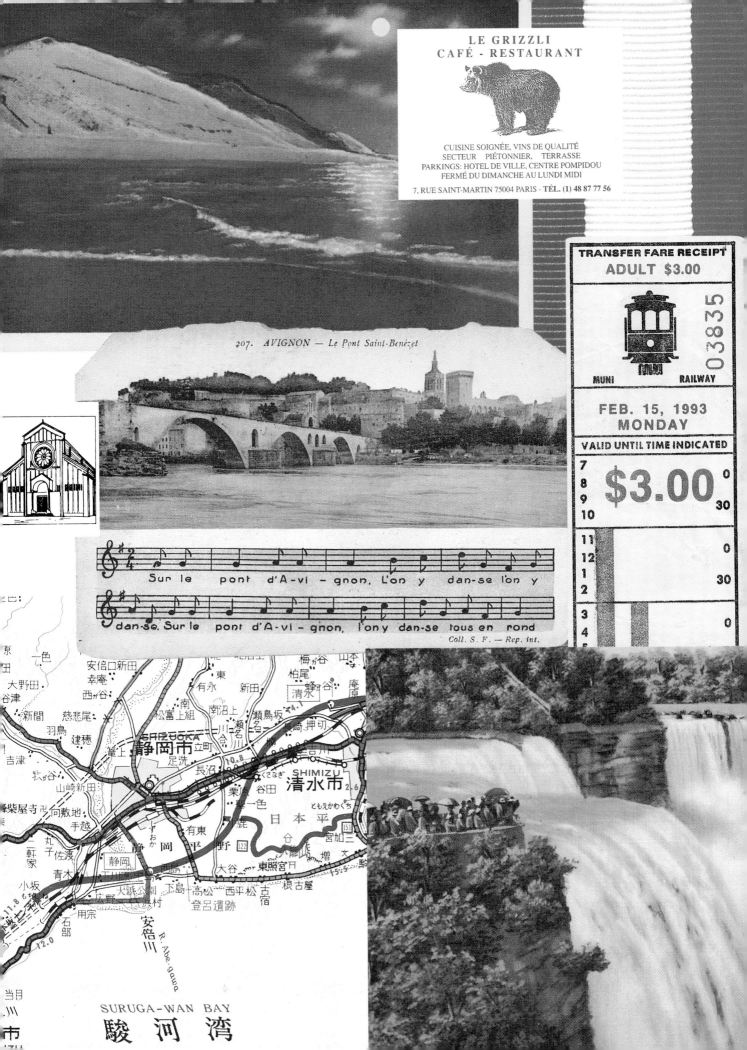

207. AVIGNON — Le Pont Saint-Benézet

TRANSFER FARE RECEIPT
ADULT $3.00

MUNI   RAILWAY   03835

FEB. 15, 1993
MONDAY

VALID UNTIL TIME INDICATED

7
8
9      $3.00
10

11
12
1
2

3
4

0

30

0

30

0

Sur le pont d'A-vi-gnon, L'on y dan-se l'on y
dan-se. Sur le pont d'A-vi-gnon, l'on y dan-se tous en rond

Coll. S. F. — Rep. int.

SHIZUOKA
静岡市

SHIMIZU
清水市

SURUGA-WAN BAY
駿河湾

R. Abe-gawa

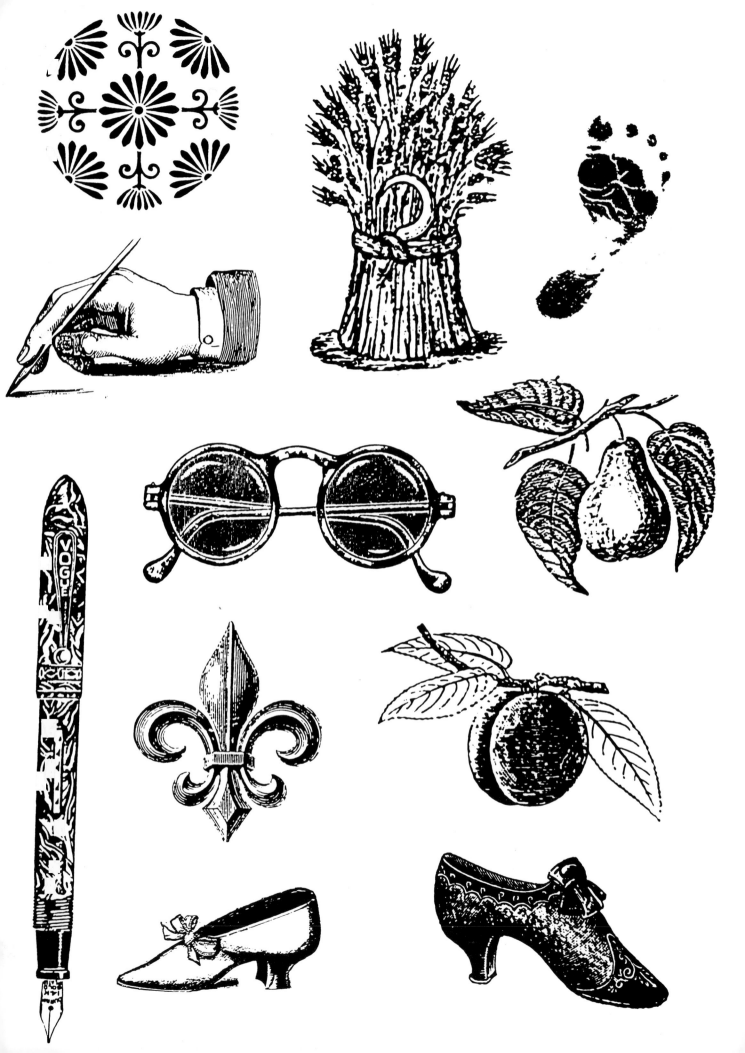

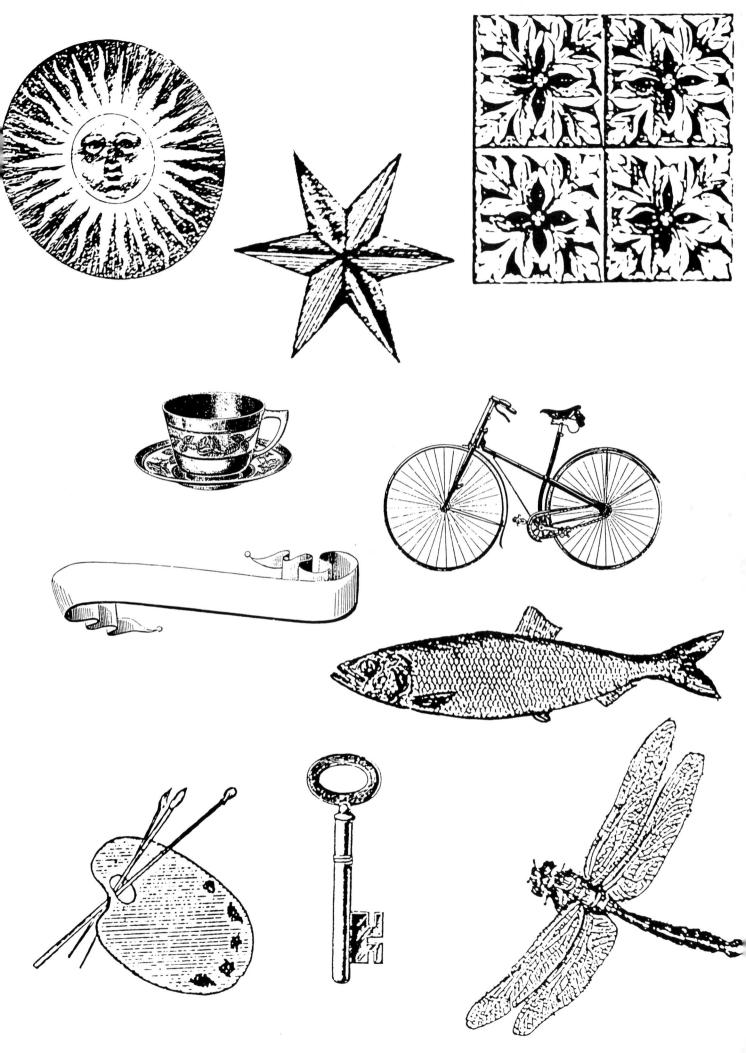

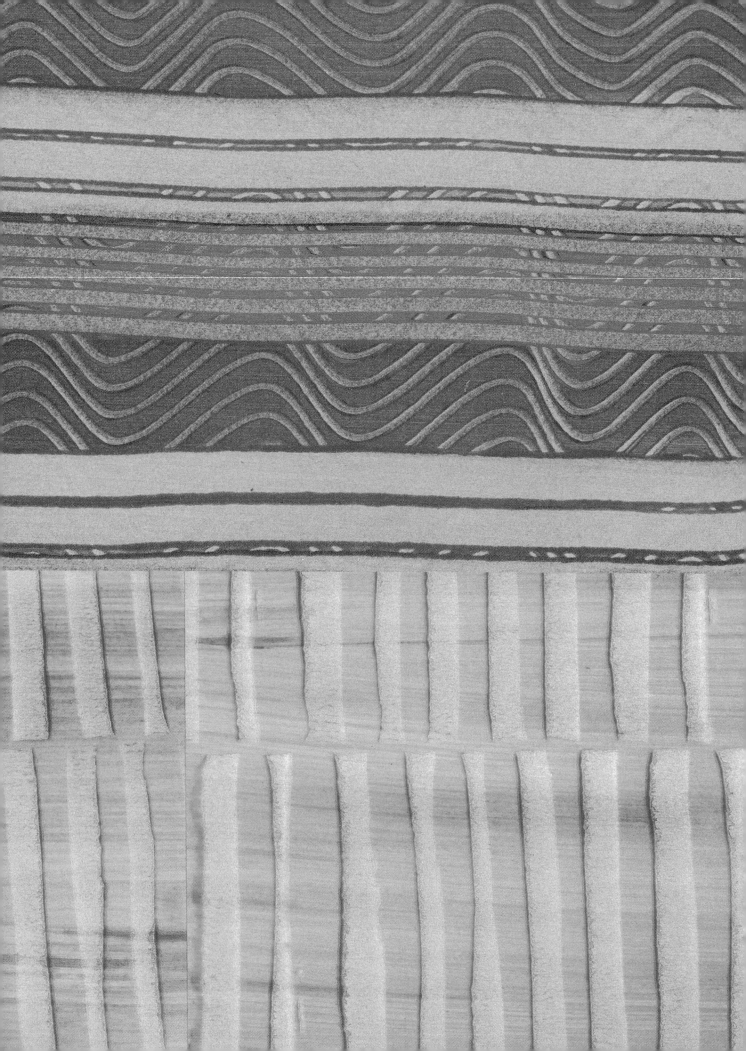

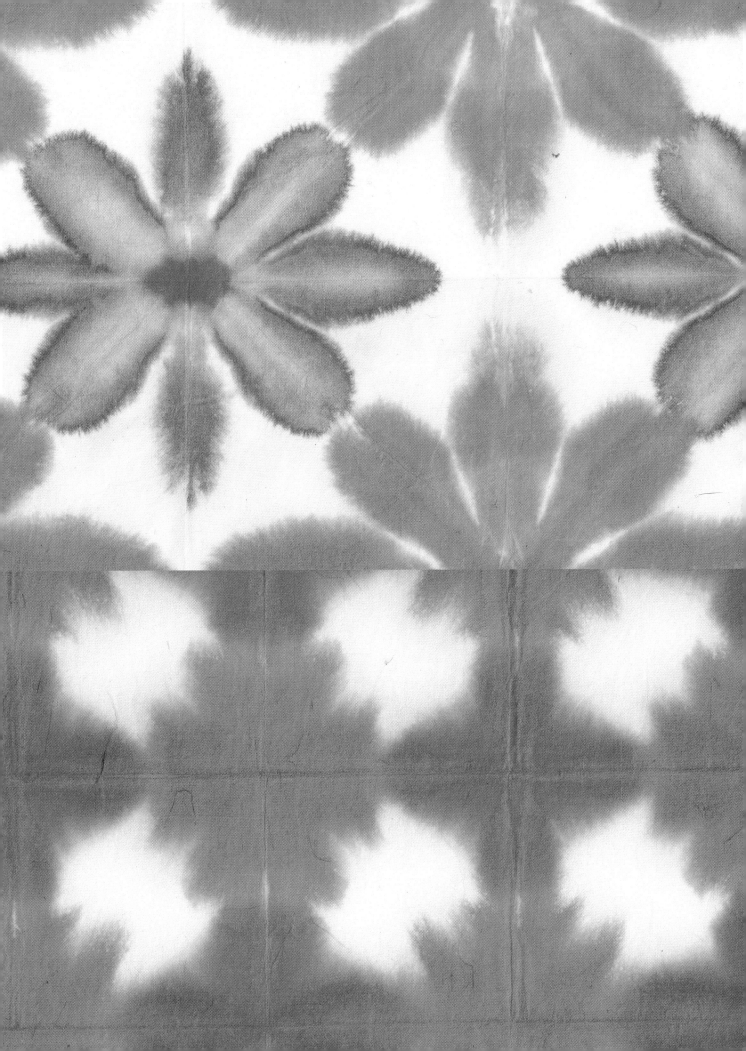

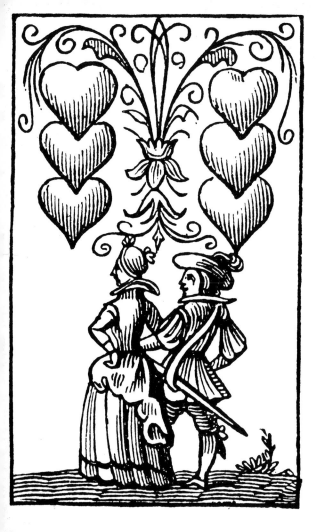

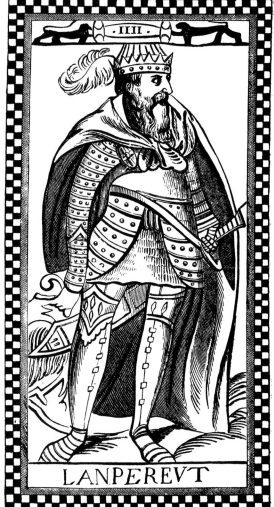

LANPEREVT

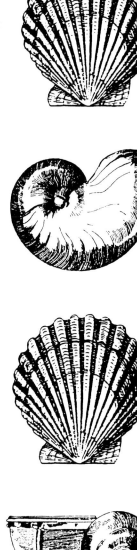

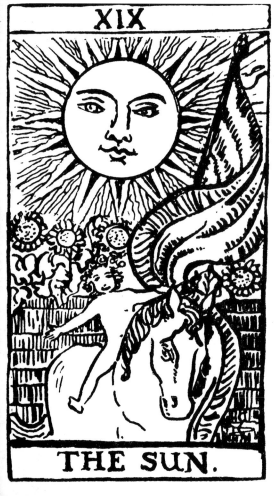

XIX

THE SUN.

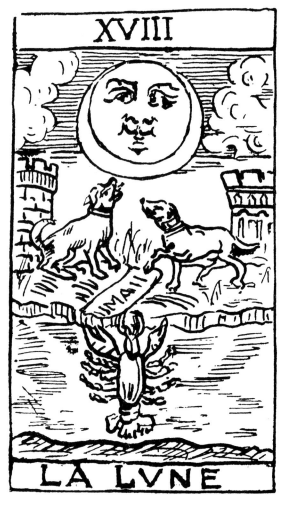

XVIIII

LA LVNE

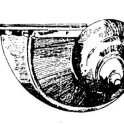

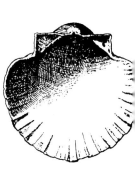

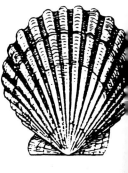

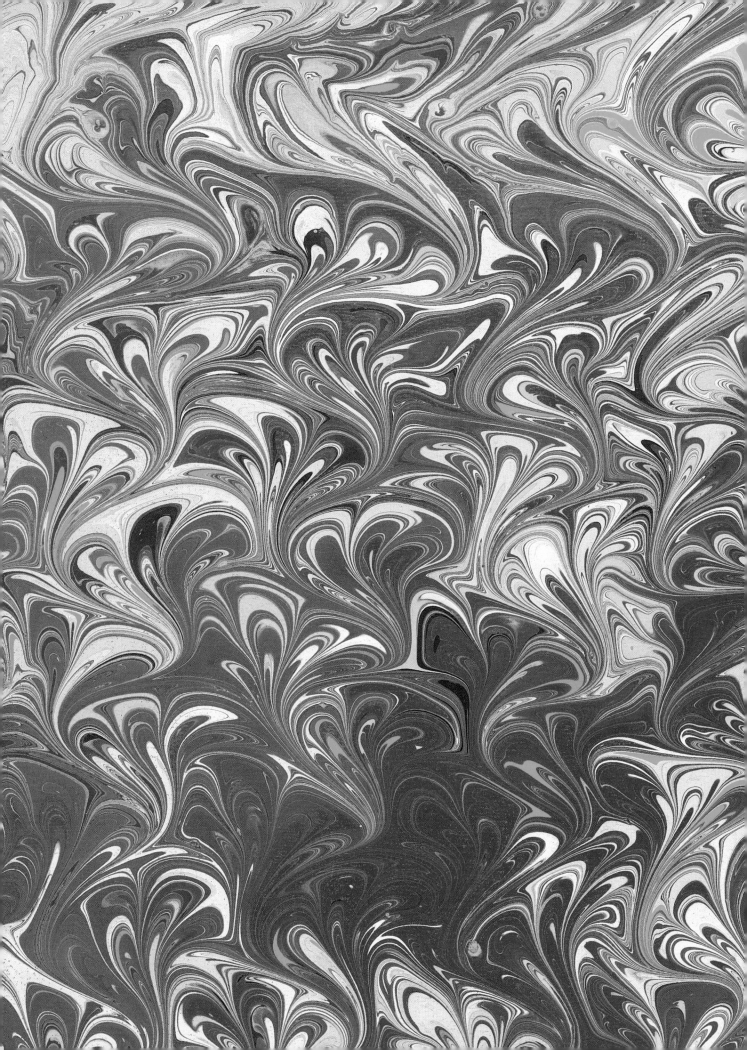